ACSM's
Sports Medicine
A Comprehensive Review

ACSM's
Sports Medicine
A Comprehensive Review

Senior Editor

Francis G. O'Connor, MD, MPH, FACSM
Uniformed Services University of the Health Sciences
Bethesda, Maryland

Editors

Douglas J. Casa, PhD, ATC, FACSM, FNATA
Korey Stringer Institute, University of Connecticut
Storrs, Connecticut

Brian A. Davis, MD, FACSM, FABPMR
University of California, Davis Medical Center
Sacramento, California

Patrick St. Pierre, MD, FAAOS
Eisenhower Desert Orthopedic Center
Rancho Mirage, California

Robert E. Sallis, MD, FACSM, FAAFP
Kaiser Permanente Medical Center
Fontana, California

Robert P. Wilder, MD, FACSM
University of Virginia
Charlottesville, Virginia

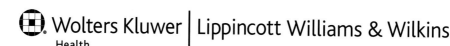

Wolters Kluwer | Lippincott Williams & Wilkins
Health

Philadelphia • Baltimore • New York • London
Buenos Aires • Hong Kong • Sydney • Tokyo

Senior Acquisitions Editor: Sonya Seigafuse
Senior Product Manager: Kerry Barrett
Vendor Manager: Alicia Jackson
Senior Manufacturing Manager: Benjamin Rivera
Senior Marketing Manager: Kim Schonberger
Design Coordinator: Terry Mallon
Production Service: Absolute Service, Inc.
ACSM's Publications Committee Chair: Walter R. Thompson, PhD, FACSM
ACSM's Group Publisher: Kerry O'Rourke

The views expressed by the author(s) do not necessarily reflect those of the Uniformed Services University of the Health Sciences, the U.S. Army, U.S. Air Force, U.S. Navy, or the Department of Defense.

Printed in China

Library of Congress Cataloging-in-Publication Data

ACSM's sports medicine : a comprehensive review / senior editor, Francis G. O'Connor ; editors, Douglas J. Casa ... [et al.].
   p. ; cm.
Sports medicine
Includes bibliographical references.
ISBN 978-1-4511-0425-7 — ISBN 1-4511-0425-1
I. O'Connor, Francis G. II. Title: Sports medicine.
[DNLM: 1. Sports Medicine—Outlines. 2. Athletic Injuries—Outlines. 3. Exercise—Outlines. QT 18.2]

617.1'027—dc23

2012018122

Care has been taken to confirm the accuracy of the information presented and to describe generally accepted practices. However, the authors, editors, and publisher are not responsible for errors or omissions or for any consequences from application of the information in this book and make no warranty, expressed or implied, with respect to the currency, completeness, or accuracy of the contents of the publication. Application of the information in a particular situation remains the professional responsibility of the practitioner.

The authors, editors, and publisher have exerted every effort to ensure that drug selection and dosage set forth in this text are in accordance with current recommendations and practice at the time of publication. However, in view of ongoing research, changes in government regulations, and the constant flow of information relating to drug therapy and drug reactions, the reader is urged to check the package insert for each drug for any change in indications and dosage and for added warnings and precautions. This is particularly important when the recommended agent is a new or infrequently employed drug.

Some drugs and medical devices presented in the publication have Food and Drug Administration (FDA) clearance for limited use in restricted research settings. It is the responsibility of the health care provider to ascertain the FDA status of each drug or device planned for use in their clinical practice.

To purchase additional copies of this book, call our customer service department at (800) 638-3030 or fax orders to (301) 223-2320. International customers should call (301) 223-2300.

Visit Lippincott Williams & Wilkins on the Internet: at LWW.com. Lippincott Williams & Wilkins customer service representatives are available from 8:30 am to 6 pm, EST.

10 9 8 7 6 5 4

CCS0420

Dedication
This textbook is dedicated to the success of all
students of sports medicine who are working hard
to keep athletes, recreational and elite, young
and old, in the game!

Contents

SECTION ii
Evaluation of the Injured Athlete

SECTION iii
Medical Problems in the Athlete

SECTION VII
Special Populations

Preface

The field of sports medicine is continually evolving, as new technologies and rapidly changing health care policies push the discipline forward at a dizzying pace. In 2005, my colleagues, Robert Wilder, Patrick St. Pierre, and Robert Sallis, and I sought to address a gap in the sports medicine world by publishing *Sports Medicine: Just the Facts* in an attempt to provide primary care physicians with a then-missing resource to prepare for Certificate of Added Qualification (CAQ) examinations (1). Since that short time, sports medicine has changed dramatically, as have the participants in the subspecialty certification examination process. Neuropsychological testing is now routinely performed in high schools across the country and conducted by certified athletic trainers. Ultrasound training and advanced treatments for the treatment of tendinopathy are common in most fellowship training programs (2). The physical medicine and rehabilitation (PMR) community is now eligible to sit for the CAQ, and the American Academy of Orthopedic Surgeons, starting in 2007, now offers a subspecialty certificate. Sports medicine practices are flourishing, and combinations of multidisciplinary groups, including orthopedic surgeons, primary care sports medicine physicians, PMR sports medicine physicians, and certified athletic trainers, are becoming more common in both private practice and in the world of academia.

As these changes have occurred, there has been a proliferation of sports medicine textbooks, as the literature has marched forward. As these texts continue to grow in number, however, there has continued to be a paucity of publications that have sought to directly address the single task of assisting the sports medicine student with succeeding on a subspecialty board examination.

In 2010, we approached the American College of Sports Medicine (ACSM) with the concept of creating a comprehensive review text that could address the needs of the clinical membership, including primary care physicians, specialists, and certified athletic trainers. Our intent was to model a text after the Just the Facts concepts to assist clinicians confronted with a test or to guide them with a direction during their sports medicine fellowship. The text was not intended to replace many of the fine sports medicine resources emerging on the market but to be comprehensive yet focused, well-referenced, and evidence-based. The idea was well received by the ACSM leadership, and we began to move forward.

Our first order of business was to address two gaps by identifying additional coeditors: an editor for the task of compiling and coordinating the questions that would support the review text and a member of the certified athletic trainer community. We were very fortunate that, at the time we were beginning to brainstorm, the ACSM leadership pointed Dr. Brian Davis, a PMR physician, in our direction as he was beginning to formulate a question text for PMR doctors looking to prepare for the CAQ. After a quick phone call, Brian became a member of our team, and we moved forward with our second challenge. For me personally, Douglas Casa was an easy choice. A leader in the National Athletic Trainers' Association (NATA), Doug has a history of high energy as he has tackled the world of exertional heat illness and hydration through research, clinical care, and advocacy. He was happy to join our team; we were happier to have him.

ACSM's Sports Medicine: A Comprehensive Review has one principal goal — to assist the reader with preparing for a subspecialty sports medicine certification examination. We have studied content identified by the medical specialties to identify what we believe to be the most important material to assist the reader with successfully passing the examination. The text is conveniently divided into seven sections to assist with your review: general considerations; evaluation of the injured athlete; medical problems in the athlete; musculoskeletal problems in the athlete; principles of rehabilitation; sports-specific populations; and special populations. The text is bulleted and well referenced. Where appropriate, tables, figures, and algorithms are provided to assist with important concepts. A quick review of the list of authors not only highlights the fact that we have compiled a "who's who" of sports medicine talent, but that we have members from nearly all medical specialties as well as leaders in athletic training and physical therapy.

To augment the text, we have nearly 1,000 board-type questions available online as a resource for the reader. Each question provides an explanation on why the right answer is correct and the other items are incorrect. In addition, references are provided. The online capability also provides for the reader a consolidated site for all key sports medicine reference documents produced by the ACSM, including Team Physician Statements and ACSM Position Stands.

We sincerely hope you enjoy the text and that this reference assists you in passing your particular examination.

1. Harmon KG, O'Connor FG. Musculoskeletal ultrasound: taking sports medicine to the next level. *Br J Sports Med*. 2010;44(16):1135–6.
2. O'Connor FG, Wilder RP, Sallis R, St Pierre P. *Sports Medicine: Just the Facts in Sports Medicine*. New York (NY): McGraw-Hill; 2005.

Acknowledgments

The editors would like to collectively acknowledge the support of our families and teachers, who daily have both supported and inspired us through this effort. In addition, we would like to thank Kerry Barrett from Lippincott Williams & Wilkins and Kerry O'Rourke from the American College of Sports Medicine who collaboratively teamed to see this project through to its completion. And finally, we want to thank our project manager, Jennifer Kowalak, who did the heavy lifting, kept us on task, and made this textbook a reality.

Contributor's List

Brian E. Abell, DO
Dwight David Eisenhower Army Medical Center
Fort Gordon, Georgia

Geoff Abrams, MD
Stanford University
Stanford, California

Jeffrey S. Abrams, MD
University Medical Center at Princeton
Princeton, New Jersey

William B. Adams, MD
Family Medicine/Sports Medicine
Quantico, Virginia

Terry Adirim, MD
Children's National Medical Center
Washington, District of Columbia

Venu Akuthota, MD
University of Colorado
Aurora, Colorado

Anthony S. Albert, MD
New England Baptist Hospital
Boston, Massachusetts

Anthony G. Alessi, MD
The William W. Backus Hospital
Norwich, Connecticut

Alan P. Alfano, MD
University of Virginia Health System
Charlottesville, Virginia

Carlos M. Alvarado, MD
NYU Hospital for Joint Diseases
New York, New York

Jeffrey M. Anderson, MD, FACSM
University of Connecticut
Storrs, Connecticut

Robert A. Arciero, MD
University of Connecticut Health Center
Farmington, Connecticut

Julia Arroyo
Universidad Complutense de Madrid
Madrid, Spain

Edward S. Ashman, MD
Nevada Orthopedic and Spine Center
Las Vegas, Nevada

Chad A. Asplund, MD, FACSM
Dwight David Eisenhower Army Medical Center
Fort Gordon, Georgia

Selasi Attipoe, MA
Uniformed Services University of the Health Sciences
Bethesda, Maryland

Wes Bailey, MD
Moses Cone Sports Medicine Fellowship
Greensboro, North Carolina

Thad J. Barkdull, MD, FAAFP, CAQSM
TriCity Medical, Inc.
Pleasant Grove, Utah

Kenneth P. Barnes, MD, MSc, CAQSM
Elon University
Elon, North Carolina

Kenneth B. Batts, DO, FAAFP
Womack Army Medical Center
Fort Bragg, North Carolina

Christopher C. Bell, MD
Intermountain Healthcare
Bountiful, Utah

Matthew C. Bessette, MD
University of Rochester
Rochester, New York

Anthony I. Beutler, MD
Uniformed Services University of the Health Sciences
Bethesda, Maryland

Richard M. Blyn, MS, ATC
Extreme Sports Medicine, Inc.
Milford, Massachusetts

Barry P. Boden, MD
The Orthopaedic Center
Rockville, Maryland

Nicholas A. Bontempo, MD
University of Connecticut Health Center
Farmington, Connecticut

Jay E. Bowen, DO
New Jersey Sports Medicine
Summit, New Jersey

Michael G. Bowers, DO
Town Center Family Medicine
Reston, Virginia

Fred H. Brennan, Jr, DO, FAOASM, FAAFP, FACSM
Seacoast Orthopedics and Sports Medicine
Somersworth, New Hampshire

Dean M. Brewer, DO
Reynolds Army Community Hospital
Fort Sill, Oklahoma

David L. Brown, MD, PhD
Madigan Healthcare System
Tacoma, Washington

Linda L. Brown, MD
Madigan Healthcare System
Tacoma, Washington

Eric J. Buchner, MD
University of Virginia
Charlottesville, Virginia

Jennifer Burke, MD
Scottsdale Healthcare - Thompson Peak Family Care
Scottsdale, Arizona

Dan Burnett, MD, MPH, FAAFP
Uniformed Services University of the Health Sciences
Bethesda, Maryland

Janus D. Butcher, MD, FACSM
Aerospace Medicine
Duluth, Minnesota

Dennis J. Caine, PhD
University of North Dakota
Grand Forks, North Dakota

Dennis A. Cardone, DO
New York University Hospital for Joint Diseases
New York, New York

Luis P. Carrilero, MD
Private Practice
Buenos Aires, Argentina

Eric W. Carson, MD
University of Virginia School of Medicine
Charlottesville, Virginia

A. Bobby Chhabra, MD
University of Virginia Health System
Charlottesville, Virginia

Marc Childress, MD
Fort Belvoir Community Hospital
Fort Belvoir, Virginia

Brian J. Cole, MD
Rush Oak Park Hospital
Chicago, Illinois

Loren A. Crown, MD
University of Tennessee College of Health Sciences
Covington, Tennessee

Gregory G. Dammann, MD
Tripler Army Medical Center
Honolulu, Hawaii

Emily A. Darr, MD
Medical University of South Carolina
Charleston, South Carolina

Courtney A. Dawley, DO
David Grant Medical Center – Family Medicine Residency
Travis AFB, California

Arthur Jason De Luigi, DO
MedStar Georgetown University Hospital
Washington, District of Columbia

D. Nicole Deal, MD
University of Virginia Health System
Charlottesville, Virginia

Thomas M. DeBerardino, MD
University of Connecticut Health Center
Farmington, Connecticut

Craig R. Denegar, PhD, PT, ATC, FNATA
University of Connecticut
Storrs, Connecticut

Patricia A. Deuster, MPH, PhD
Uniformed Services University of the Health Sciences
Bethesda, Maryland

Kevin deWeber, MD, FAAFP, FACSM
Uniformed Services University of the Health Sciences
Bethesda, Maryland

William W. Dexter, MD, FACSM
Maine Medical Center
Portland, Maine

Aman Dhawan, MD
UMDNJ-Robert Wood Johnson Medical School
New Brunswick, New Jersey

Paul T. Diamond, MD
University of Virginia Health System
Charlottesville, Virginia

Margarete DiBenedetto, MD
University of Virginia
Charlottesville, Virginia

Jay Dicharry, MPT, SCS
University of Virginia
Charlottesville, Virginia

John P. DiFiori, MD, FACSM
University of California, Los Angeles
Los Angeles, California

Matthew Diltz, MD
Eisenhower Desert Orthopedic Center
Rancho Mirage, California

Robert J. Dimeff, MD
University of Texas Southwestern Medical Center
Dallas, Texas

Lindsay J. DiStefano, PhD, ATC
University of Connecticut
Storrs, Connecticut

Jonathan A. Drezner, MD
University of Washington
Seattle, Washington

Sarah A. Eby, MD
University of Virginia
Charlottesville, Virginia

Richard P. Eide, III, MD
Dwight David Eisenhower Army Medical Center
Fort Gordon, Georgia

Robert W. Engelen, DO
Naval Health Clinic Charleston
Goose Creek, South Carolina

J. Richard Lee Evanson, DO
Dwight David Eisenhower Army Medical Center
Forth Gordon, Georgia

Nathan P. Falk, MD
Air Force Base/University of Nebraska Medical Center
Offutt AFB, Nebraska

Reginald S. Fayssoux, MD
Eisenhower Desert Orthopedic Center
Rancho Mirage, California

John F. Feller, MD
Desert Medical Imaging
Indian Wells, California

Karl B. Fields, MD
University of North Carolina
Chapel Hill, North Carolina

Kevin F. Fitzpatrick, MD
INOVA Fairfax Hospital
Falls Church, Virginia

Scott Flinn, MD
Arch Health Partners
Poway, California

Nicole L. Frazer, PhD
Defense Health Headquarters (DHHQ)
Falls Church, Virginia

Michael Fredericson, MD, FACSM
Stanford University School of Medicine
Stanford, California

Jason Friedrich, MD
Kaiser Permanente Colorado
Denver, Colorado

Michael C. Gaertner, DO
Parkland Health Center
Farmington, Missouri

Elizabeth Gannon, DO
South Riding Family Medicine
Chantilly, Virginia

Jennifer M. Garrison, DO
Blanchfield Army Community Hospital
Fort Campbell, Kentucky

Robert Giering, MD
Taconic Spine
Manchester, Vermont

John E. Glorioso, MD
Tripler Army Medical Center
Honolulu, Hawaii

John P. Goldblatt, MD
University of Rochester
Rochester, New York

Jeffrey L. Goodie, PhD, ABPP
Uniformed Services University of the Health Sciences
Bethesda, Maryland

David K. Gordon, MD
Pentagon Flight Medicine Clinic
Washington, District of Columbia

Carlos A. Guanche, MD
Southern California Orthopedic Institute
Van Nuys, California

Frank Winston Gwathmey, Jr, MD
University of Virginia
Charlottesville, Virginia

Mark Hamming, MD
Duke University
Durham, North Carolina

Kimberly G. Harmon, MD
University of Washington
Seattle, Washington

George D. Harris, MD, MS
Truman Medical Center-Lakewood
Kansas City, Missouri

Mark D. Harris, MD, MPH, MBA
Joint Task Force National Capital Medicine
Bethesda, Maryland

Joseph M. Hart, PhD, ATC
University of Virginia
Charlottesville, Virginia

C. Joel Hess, MD
University of Virginia Health System
Charlottesville, Virginia

R. Todd Hockenbury, MD
South Louisville Orthopedics
Louisville, Kentucky

Brian R. Hoke, DPT, SCS
Atlantic Physical Therapy, PC
Virginia Beach, Virginia

Thomas M. Howard, MD, FACSM
Fairfax Family Practice
Fairfax, Virginia

Shane Hudnall, MD
Cone Health Sports Medicine
Greensboro, North Carolina

Casey Hulsey, ATC
North Georgia College & State University
Dahlonega, Georgia

Garrett S. Hyman, MD, MPH
Lake Washington Sports & Spine
Bellevue, Washington

Christopher D. Ingersoll, PhD, ATC, FACSM, FNATA
Central Michigan University
Mount Pleasant, Michigan

Benjamin J. Ingram, MD
Womack Army Medical Center
Fort Bragg, North Carolina

Keith Lynn Jackson, II, MD
Dwight David Eisenhower Army Medical Center
Fort Gordon, Georgia

Carrie A. Jaworski, MD, FAAFP, FACSM
NorthShore University Health System
Glenview, Illinois

Mark D. Jeffords, MD
Tripler Army Medical Center
Honolulu, Hawaii

Jeffrey G. Jenkins, MD
University of Virginia School of Medicine
Charlottesville, Virginia

Michael W. Johnson, MD
Franciscan Medical Group
University Place, Washington

Christopher E. Jonas, DO, FAAFP
Uniformed Services University of Health Sciences
Bethesda, Maryland

Wayne B. Jonas, MD
Uniformed Services University of the Health Sciences
Bethesda, Maryland

Shawn F. Kane, MD, FAAFP, FACSM
Womack Army Medical Center
Fort Bragg, North Carolina

Vasili Karas, BS
Rush University Medical Center
Chicago, Illinois

Amanda Weiss Kelly, MD
Pediatric Sports Medicine, UH Case Medical Center
Cleveland, Ohio

John J. Klimkiewicz, MD
Georgetown University Hospital
Washington, District of Columbia

Roger J. Kruse, MD, FAAFP, FACSM
University of Toledo
Toledo, Ohio

Christopher M. Kuenze, MA, ATC
The University of Virginia
Charlottesville, Virginia

Catherine N. Laible, MD
Hospital for Joint Diseases
New York, New York

Vanessa Lalley, DO
St. Joseph's Hospital Health Center
Syracuse, New York

Connor R. LaRose, MD
Southern California Orthopedic Institute
Van Nuys, California

Christopher J. Lutrzykowski, MD
Maine-Dartmouth Family Medicine Residency
Augusta, Maine

James H. Lynch, MD, MS
Womack Army Medical Center
Fort Bragg, North Carolina

John M. MacKnight, MD, FACSM
University of Virginia Health System
Charlottesville, Virginia

Scott A. Magnes, MD, ATC, FAAOS, FACSM, FAAFP
Captain James A. Lovell Federal Health Care Center
North Chicago, Illinois

Eric M. Magrum, DPT, OCS, FAAOMPT
University of Virginia/Healthsouth
Charlottesville, Virginia

Gerard A. Malanga, MD
Morristown Medical Center
Morristown, New Jersey

Sean N. Martin, DO
Eglin Air Force Base
Eglin AFB, Florida

Ronica Martinez, MD
University of New Mexico
Albuquerque, New Mexico

Jason M. Matuszak, MD, FAAFP
Excelsior Orthopaedics
Amherst, New York

Jeffery A. May, BA, MA, BS, MD
May Medical Group, PC
Munford, Tennessee

Augustus D. Mazzocca, MS, MD
University of Connecticut Health Center
Farmington, Connecticut

Devin P. McFadden, MD
Bayne Jones Army Community Hospital
Fort Polk, Louisiana

J. Andrew McMahon, DO
Maine Medical Center
Portland, Maine

Andrew J. McMarlin, DO, CAQSM
Trident Medical Center
North Charleston, South Carolina

Mark Miller, MD
University of Virginia
Charlottesville, Virginia

Kambiz Motamedi, MD
Ronald Reagan Medical Center
Los Angeles, California

Sean W. Mulvaney, MD
Uniformed Services University of the Health Sciences
Bethesda, Maryland

Robert J. Nascimento, MD
Boston University Medical Center
Boston, Massachusetts

Michael Needham, MD
Dwight David Eisenhower Army Medical Center
Fort Gordon, Georgia

Bradley J. Nelson, MD
University of Minnesota
Minneapolis, Minnesota

Robert P. Nirschl, MD, MS
Nirschl Orthopedic Center
Arlington, Virginia

Rochelle M. Nolte, MD
NTC Clinic
San Diego, California

Elizabeth M. O'Connor, DDS
Advanced Family Dental Care
North Syracuse, New York

Francis G. O'Connor, MD, MPH, FACSM
Uniformed Services University of the Health Sciences
Bethesda, Maryland

Tracey O'Connor, MD
Roswell Park Cancer Institute
Buffalo, New York

Ralph G. Oriscello, MD, FACC, FACP
Veterans Administration Medical Center
East Orange, New Jersey

Andrea Pana, MD
University of Texas
Austin, Texas

Chris G. Pappas, MD, FAAFP
Womack Army Medical Center
Fort Bragg, North Carolina

Paul F. Pasquina, MD

Uniformed Services University of the Health Sciences
Bethesda, Maryland

Evan Peck, MD

Cleveland Clinic Florida
West Palm Beach, Florida

Andrew D. Perron, MD, FACEP

Maine Medical Center
Portland, Maine

Nicholas A. Piantanida, MD

Evans Army Community Hospital
Fort Carson, Colorado

Jessica M. Poole, M.ED, ATC

North Georgia College & State University
Dahlonega, Georgia

RM Barney Poole, PT, DPT, ATC

Performance Physical Therapy
Stockbridge, Georgia

Joel Press, MD

Rehabilitation Institute of Chicago
Chicago, Illinois

Scott W. Pyne, MD, FACSM, FAAFP

Uniformed Services University of the Health Sciences
Bethesda, Maryland

Catherine R. Rainbow, MD

Carolinas Healthcare System
Charlotte, North Carolina

Meghan F. Raleigh, MD

Evans Army Community Hospital
Fort Carson, Colorado

Dipak B. Ramkumar, BS

Dartmouth Medical School
Hanover, New Hampshire

Brian V. Reamy, MD

F. Edward Hebert School of Medicine, Uniformed Services University
Besthesda, Maryland

Jennifer L. Reed, MD

Naval Medical Center Portsmouth
Portsmouth, Virginia

John C. Richmond, MD, FAAOS

New England Baptist Hospital
Boston, Massachusetts

Nancy E. Rolnik, MD

California Sports and Orthopaedic Institute
Berkeley, California

Aaron Rubin, MD, FAAFP, FACSM

Kaiser Permanente
Fontana, California

Marc R. Safran, MD

Stanford University
Redwood City, California

Robert E. Sallis, MD, FACSM, FAAFP

Kaiser Permanente Medical Center
Fontana, California

Anthony A. Schepsis, MD

Boston University Medical Center
Boston, Massachusetts

Michael B. Schwartz, DO

Soundview Medical Associates
Darien, Connecticut

Keith A. Scorza, MD, MBA

Fort Belvoir Community Hospital
Fort Belvoir, Virginia

Leanne L. Seeger, MD, FACR

Ronald Reagan Medical Center
Los Angeles, California

Peter H. Seidenberg, MD

Penn State Hershey Bone and Joint Institute - State College
State College, Pennsylvania

Craig K. Seto, MD, FAAFP

University of Virginia
Charlottesville, Virginia

Joel Shaw, MD

Max Sports Medicine Institute
Columbus, Ohio

Manik Singh, MD

North Jersey Orthopaedic & Sports Medicine Institute
Clifton, North Jersey

Jay Smith, MD

Mayo Clinic
Rochester, Minnesota

James P. Sostak, II, MD

Southern California Orthopedic Institute
Van Nuys, California

Patrick St. Pierre, MD, FAAOS

Eisenhower Desert Orthopedic Center
Rancho Mirage, California

Scott P. Steinmann, MD

Mayo Clinic
Rochester, Minnesota

Mark B. Stephens, MD, MS, FAAFP

Uniformed Services University of the Health Sciences
Bethesda, Maryland

Eric J. Strauss, MD

New York University Hospital For Joint Diseases
New York, New York

Timothy L. Switaj, MD

Keller Army Community Hospital
West Point, New York

Michelle E. Szczepanik, MD

Dwight David Eisenhower Army Medical Center
Fort Gordon, Georgia

Dean C. Taylor, MD

Duke University Medical Center
Durham, North Carolina

Courtney T. Tripp, DO, LTC, USA, MC

Evans Army Community Hospital
Fort Carson, Colorado

Brian K. Unwin, MD

Uniformed Services University of the Health Sciences
Bethesda, Maryland

Ricardo J. Vasquez-Duarte, MD

University of Miami Miller School of Medicine
Miami, Florida

Heather K. Vincent, PhD
University of Florida
Gainesville, Florida

Kevin R. Vincent, MD, PhD
University of Florida
Gainesville, Florida

Katrina D. Warme
Bellevue, Washington

Winston J. Warme, MD
University of Washington
Seattle, Washington

Charles W. Webb, DO
Oregon Health & Science University
Portland, Oregon

C. Thayer White, MD
Oregon Health & Science University
Portland, Oregon

Russell D. White, MD
Truman Medical Center-Lakewood
Kansas City, Missouri

Bryan J. Whitfield, MD
Georgetown University Hospital
Washington, District of Columbia

John H. Wilckens, MD
Johns Hopkins Bayview Medical Center
Baltimore, Maryland

Robert P. Wilder, MD, FACSM
University of Virginia
Charlottesville, Virginia

Stacey A. Zeno, MS
Uniformed Services University of the Health Sciences
Bethesda, Maryland

Reviewer's List

Jeffrey M. Anderson, MD, FACSM
University of Connecticut
Storrs, Connecticut

Chad A. Asplund, MD, FACSM
Dwight David Eisenhower Army Medical Center
Evans, Georgia

Robert J. Baker, MD, FACSM
Michigan State University, Kalamazoo Center for Medical Studies
Kalamazoo, Michigan

Sherrie Lynn Ballantine-Talmadge, DO
Northwestern University
Evanston, Illinois

Steve J. Blivin, MD, FACSM
U. S. Navy
Cedar Point, North Carolina

Delmas J. Bolin, MD, FACSM
Radford University
Roanoke, Virginia

Kyle J. Cassas, MD, FACSM
Steadman Hawkins Clinic of the Carolinas, Greenville Hospital System
Greer, South Carolina

George T. Chiampas, DO
Northwestern University
Chicago, Illinois

Stephanie Chu, DO
University of Colorado
Denver, Colorado

Nailah Coleman, MD
Children's National Medical Center
Alexandria, Virginia

Kevin deWeber, MD, FAAFP, FACSM
Uniformed Services University of the Health Sciences
Bethesda, Maryland

Pierre A. D'Hemecourt, MD, FACSM
Children's Hospital Boston
Newton Highlands, Massachusetts

John P. DiFiori, MD, FACSM
University of California, Los Angeles
Los Angeles, California

Sameer Dixit, MD
Johns Hopkins University
Baltimore, Maryland

Jeffrey D. Fields, MD
Capital City Family Medicine
Boise, Idaho

Peter G. Gerbino, II, MD, FACSM
Monterey Joint Replacement and Sports Medicine
Monterey, California

Heather M. Gillespie, MD
University of California, Los Angeles
Santa Monica, California

Andrew Gregory, MD, FACSM
Vanderbilt University
Nashville, Tennessee

John Hatzenbuehler, MD
Maine Medical Center
Portland, Maine

Diana Lee Heiman, MD
ETSU Family Physicians of Johnson City
Johnson City, Tennessee

Duane R. Hennion, MD
U. S. Army
Honolulu, Hawaii

John C. Hill, DO, FACSM
University of Colorado-Denver
Aurora, Colorado

Allyson Howe, MD
Maine Medical Center
Portland, Maine

Mark R. Hutchinson, MD, FACSM
University of Illinois at Chicago
Chicago, Illinois

Shawn F. Kane, MD, FAAFP, FACSM
Womack Army Medical Center
Fort Bragg, North Carolina

Cynthia R. Labella, MD
Children's Memorial Hospital
Chicago, Illinois

Beverly C. Land, DO, FACSM
U. S. Army
West Point, New York

Timothy Stephen Lishnak, MD
Milton Family Practice
Shelburne, Vermont

David Knight Lisle, MD
University of Vermont
Charlotte, Vermont

Christopher D. Meyering, DO
U. S. Army
Evans, Georgia

Dilipkumar R. Patel, MD, FACSM

Michigan State University, Kalamazoo Center for Medical Studies
Kalamazoo, Michigan

Scott W. Pyne, MD, FACSM

U. S. Navy
Edgewater, Maryland

Rodney Riedel, MD

Mid Hudson Family Practice
Kingston, New York

Katherine Riggert, DO

University of Massachusetts
Boston, Massachusetts

William O. Roberts, MD, FACSM

University of Minnesota
Saint Paul, Minnesota

Elizabeth Rothe, MD

Central Maine Medical Center
Turner, Maine

Pierre A. Rouzier, MD, FACSM

University of Massachusetts
Amherst, Massachusetts

Mark Snowise, MD

Berkshire Medical Center
Pittsfield, Massachusetts

John Herbert Stevenson, MD

University of Massachusetts
Fitchburg, Massachusetts

Thomas H. Trojian, MD, FACSM

University of Connecticut
Hartford, Connecticut

L. Tyler Wadsworth, MD

St. Louis University
Saint Louis, Missouri

Jon Woo, MD

University of Washington
Newcastle, Washington

Question Writer's List

David C. Agerter, MD
College of Medicine, Mayo Clinic
Rochester, Minnesota

Marwa A. Ahmed, MD, MSc
New York Presbyterian Hospital - Columbia and Cornell
New York, New York

Joanne B. "Anne" Allen, MD, FAAPMR, FACSM
Allen Spine and Sports Medicine
Wilmington, North Carolina

Jessica Au, MD
New York Presbyterian Hospital - Columbia and Cornell
New York, New York

Darryl E. Barnes, MD
Mayo Clinic Health System
Austin, Minnesota

Kevin J. Burnham, MD
University of California, Davis Health System
Sacramento, California

Robert C. Cantu, MA, MD, FACS, FAANS, FACSM
Emerson Hospital
Concord, Massachusetts

Gretchen Casazza, PhD
University of California, Davis
Sacramento, California

John Cianca, MD
Baylor College of Medicine
Houston, Texas

Micky Collins, PhD
UPMC Sports Medicine Concussion Program
Pittsburgh, Pennsylvania

Brian A. Davis, MD, FACSM, FABPMR
University of California, Davis Medical Center
Sacramento, California

Russell Dunning, MSPT
Results Physical Therapy
Sacramento, California

Joseph H. Feinberg, MD, MS
Hospital for Special Surgery
New York, New York

Walter R. Frontera, MD, PhD
Vanderbilt University School of Medicine
Nashville, Tennessee

Brian W. Fullem, DPM
Bayshore Podiatry Center
Tampa, Florida

Libi Z. Galmer, DO
New York Presbyterian Hospital - Columbia and Cornell
New York, New York

Ellen T. Geminiani, MD
Boston Children's Hospital
Boston, Massachusetts

Eric Giza, MD
University of California, Davis
Sacramento, California

William M. Green, MD, FACEP
University of California, Davis Medical Center
Sacramento, California

Mederic M. Hall, MD
University of Iowa
Iowa City, Iowa

Marni G. Hillinger, MD
New York Presbyterian Hospital - Columbia and Cornell
New York, New York

Alan M. Hirahara, MD, FRCS(C)
Private Practice
Sacramento, California

Shawn Hsieh, MD
University of California, Davis Medical Center
Sacramento, California

Julie Ingwerson, BS Exercise Science, MD
University of California, Davis Medical Center
Sacramento, California

Brian J. Krabak, MD, MBA
University of Washington and Seattle Children's Sports Medicine
Seattle, Washington

Paul Krause, MD
Truckee Tahoe Medical Group
Tahoe, California

Jeffrey S. Kutcher, MD
University of Michigan
Ann Arbor, Michigan

Mously Le Blanc, MD
New York Presbyterian Hospital - Columbia and Cornell
New York, New York

Cassandra A. Lee, MD
Sports Medicine and Arthroscopy
Sacramento, California

Grant S. Lipman, MD
Stanford University School of Medicine
Stanford, California

Samuel Louie, MD

University of California, Davis Health System
Sacramento, California

Quang Luu, MD

University of California, Davis
Sacramento, California

Gerard A. Malanga, MD

UMDNJ-New Jersey Medical School
Newark, New Jersey

John P. Meehan, MD

University California, Davis
Sacramento, California

Melita N. Moore, MD

University of California, Davis Medical Center
Sacramento, California

Kyle Morgan, DO

Baylor College of Medicine/ University of Texas Medical School at Houston
Houston, Texas

Hien H. Nguyen, MD, MAS

University of California, Davis Health System
Sacramento, California

Ray Padilla, DDS, FASD

UCLA School of Dentistry, AEGD
Los Angeles, California

Luga Podesta, MD

Podesta Orthopedic & Sports Medicine Institute
Thousand Oaks, California

Hollis G. Potter, MD

Hospital for Special Surgery
New York, New York

Pamela T. Prescott, MD

University of California, Davis
Sacramento, California

Ashwin Rao, MD, CAQSM

University of Washington
Seattle, Washington

Amol Saxena, DPM

Palo Alto Foundation Medical Group
Palo Alto, California

Michael Schivo, MD, MAS

University of California, Davis School of Medicine
Sacramento, California

Jay Smith, MD

Mayo Clinic
Rochester, Minnesota

Nathan Swain, DO

University of California, Davis Medical Center
Sacramento, California

Jeffrey L. Tanji, MD

University California, Davis
Sacramento, California

Douglas Taylor, MD

University of California, Davis Medical Center
Sacramento, California

Joseph E. Tonna, MD

Stanford/Kaiser Emergency Medicine Residency
Stanford, California

James Van den Bogaerde, MD

University of California, Davis School of Medicine
Sacramento, California

Alan Vernec, MD, Dip. Sport Med

World Anti-Doping Agency
Montreal, Quebec, Canada

Brandee L. Waite, MD

University California Davis School of Medicine
Sacramento, California

Kenten Wang, DO

University of California, Davis Medical Center
Sacramento, California

Kyle M. Yamashiro, PT, CSCS

Results Physical Therapy, Sacramento State University
Sacramento, California

Michael Kenji Yamazaki, MD

Assistant Question Editor
Straub Bone & Joint Center, An Affiliate of Hawaii Pacific Health
Honolulu, Hawaii

The Team Physician

Anthony I. Beutler and John H. Wilckens

WHAT IS A TEAM PHYSICIAN?

- Very little has been published about the duties and responsibilities of a team physician, and few formal studies exist as to the qualifications and skills necessary to be effective in these duties.

- In 2000, the American College of Sports Medicine® (ACSM), American Medical Society for Sports Medicine (ASSM), American Orthopaedic Society for Sports Medicine, American Osteopathic Academy of Sports Medicine, and American Academy of Pediatrics issued a consensus statement on the duties and qualifications of a team physician (5). Since that time, the same conglomerate has published statements on sideline preparedness (6), concussion (4), and issues of the adolescent (3) and master athlete (9) for the team physician.

- The following consensus statement from the ACSM defines the unique role of a team physician:

  The Team Physician must have unrestricted medical license and be an M.D. or D.O. who is responsible for treating and coordinating the medical care of the athletic team members. The principal responsibility of the team physician is to provide for the well-being of individual athletes — enabling each to realize his or her full potential. The team physician should possess special proficiency in the care of musculoskeletal injuries and medical conditions encountered in sports. The team physician also must actively integrate medical expertise with other healthcare providers, including medical specialists, athletic trainers, and allied health professionals. The team physician must ultimately assume responsibility within the team structure for making medical decisions that affect the athlete's safe participation (5).

- Practitioners from many specialties serve in the role of team physician, with primary care physicians comprising the majority. The most common fields of medicine (percentage of the total in parentheses) are family practice (25.5%), orthopedic surgery (16.2%), osteopathic medicine (10.9%), internal medicine (10.1%), general practice (6.3%), pediatrics (5.4%), emergency medicine (4.9%), general surgery (4.5%), obstetrics/gynecology (2.8%), cardiology (2.0%), and all others (11.5%) (10).

- The team physician is part of a team of professionals that cares for the athletes and contributes to the athlete's success by maximizing training and competition preparation. He or she also assists by accurately diagnosing ailments and promptly, yet completely, rehabilitating injuries to return athletes to competition as quickly and safely as possible. In addition to expertise in the common medical conditions encountered in athletes, other necessary qualities include: flexibility and availability, good communication skills, a desire to educate, and an understanding of injury prevention principles (5).

TIME REQUIREMENTS OF A TEAM PHYSICIAN

- A team physician must have an office schedule that can accommodate athletes with urgent and time-sensitive medical needs.

- Most team physicians have designated training room time each week, at least one to two evenings, where they can evaluate new and follow-up existing injuries of team members. Training room time is an especially important setting in which to communicate with the athletic trainer on the rehabilitation progress of athletes' injuries (7). An athlete's behavior and responses can vary widely, depending on the familiarity of the environment; therefore, training rooms should ideally be held in the athlete's "native environment," at a location convenient to the athletes and close to practice or training facilities.

- Although knowledge and ability are certainly important, the most valuable asset to the team physician is trust. Trust is earned by connecting to the athletes, coaches, and school officials.

- Team physicians often neglect team practices. Although it is not necessary that all practices be attended, occasional, brief appearances during practice will allow the physician to gain insight into the environment and conditions in which the athletes train, the team's training regimen, and interactions between coaches and players. A better appreciation of all these factors can prove invaluable in the physician's medical decision making. Additionally, brief appearances at practice help the physician build collegial relationships with coaches

The views expressed herein are those of the authors and should not be construed as official policy of the Department of the Navy, the Department of the Air Force, or the Department of Defense.

and players, establishing his or her role as a part of the team and distinguishing the physician from other officials, support staff, and media representatives who participate only in game-day activities.

- The amount of time spent at the actual competition depends on the team physician's role and availability, as well as on state laws and the regulations of the governing athletic association. Some laws mandate that a physician be in attendance for every game. Other laws allow nonphysician medical personnel, such as an athletic trainer, to cover an event with on-call physician backup (6).

- The clinician who is the team physician for an entire institution must decide whether to attend all the games for a few teams, or to attend a few games for every team. We recommend that team physicians attend at least part of one practice and at least one game for each team they supervise. Providing good "team medicine" is very difficult without observing the interactions and conditions of play and practice.

CORE KNOWLEDGE OF A TEAM PHYSICIAN

- To perform his or her duties effectively, a team physician needs an understanding of the medical conditions common to the athlete. This knowledge should encompass many areas of medicine, including but not limited to, orthopedics, cardiopulmonary medicine, neurology, dermatology, and rehabilitation (5).

- The team physician also needs expertise in pharmacology. Practical pharmacology for the team physician includes knowing how to treat illnesses, but also an understanding of performance-enhancing drugs and herbal medicines. Team physicians must be familiar with which substances are banned by the governing athletic association so that an athlete does not inadvertently lose eligibility to compete (10).

- A team physician must have a general knowledge of behavioral medicine and psychology. Mood disturbances and mental illnesses such as depression affect athletes and can be very common in injured athletes.

- A team physician's knowledge of exercise science and nutrition can help prevent injuries as well as maximize an athlete's performance (3). Disordered eating and overtraining can prove devastating if not recognized early and treated effectively (5).

MEDICAL RESPONSIBILITIES OF THE TEAM PHYSICIAN

- The first responsibility of a team physician is to determine whether an athlete is fit to participate. This evaluation most commonly occurs during the preparticipation physical. This

examination may or may not be performed by the team physician, but the team physician should review its documentation so that he or she will be aware of any condition that may limit competition or predispose the athlete or other participants to injury. This preparticipation physical must be done before athletic training or participation — preferably 6–8 weeks before — so that all potentially disqualifying conditions can be fully evaluated without jeopardizing scheduled participation (6).

- Sideline and event coverage is the most obvious responsibility of the team physician. A physician should cover all collision and high-risk sports. Other athletic events can be covered by any allied health professional who is trained in recognition and initial treatment of athletic injuries (6). Team physicians must continually remind themselves that they are more than spectators. Each should be a "dispassionate observer," that is, the emotions of the competition must not affect medical decision making. Attention should be directed to the safety of the participants, not the immediate passions of the game.

- The team physician should focus attention on the aspects of play and the individuals who are prone to injury. In other words, the seasoned team physician will carefully follow the game, but not always follow the ball. For instance, in gridiron football, relatively little injury information can be gained by watching the flight of the ball on punts, kickoffs, and passes. Rather, injuries occur in — and attention should be focused on — lineman and quarterbacks after releasing the ball and wide receivers after catching the ball.

- The team physician must be prepared to handle nonparticipant emergencies because it is not uncommon for the team physician to be called on to treat an inadvertently involved coach, injured or sick referee, or emergently ill spectator. The team physician should verify that proper protocols and policies exist for medical emergencies involving spectators. The team physician may be the most qualified first responder, but he cannot assume final treatment responsibility for spectators because his first duty is to the athletes on the field of play.

- The team physician maintains a sense of sideline awareness and encourages others to do the same. The team physician recognizes that the energy to play carries well beyond the field's sideline. The more advanced the athletic level, the greater the area of potential injury beyond the field of play. Many sideline personnel are distracted: Cheerleaders, mascots, and photographers may be completely unaware of the action coming toward them. Even experienced coaches can be surprised and injured when the game suddenly "comes to them" (1,2). The individual who has a pass to the sidelines for the first time is often the most endangered person because he or she has very little concept of the speed of the game and the closeness of potential injury.

- The team physician ensures accurate diagnosis through use of additional studies and specialty consults, communicates information regarding the player's condition clearly and confidentially to those who "need to know," coordinates the rehabilitation process, and determines when the athlete is again able to compete. This essential process involves *active* communication with athletes, parents, athletic trainers, physical therapists, coaches, administrators, and other medical specialists as necessary (12).

- Pursuing active follow-up with medical specialists is a critical duty. Team physicians may refer athletes to subspecialty providers to assist in treatment or with clearance for athletic participation; however, information from these visits does not naturally flow back to the team physician. Assuming that the specialty provider will call with any important information or that all pertinent information will flow back through the health care system will result in confusion for the team physician and danger for the athletes. Shadow files, "tickler lists," and other reminder systems can help team physicians actively and personally follow up on referrals, preventing the always embarrassing and often dangerous situations that result from incomplete medical communication between subspecialists and the team physician.

- Documentation of medical care is often mistakenly neglected in the team setting. The team physician needs to keep formal and confidential medical records that detail communication with consultants, give home treatment and follow-up instructions, and provide details for insurance and reimbursement purposes (12).

- The team physician should have final say of when an athlete is initially cleared to begin competition and when a previously injured athlete may return to play (6). Although a detailed discussion of return-to-play criteria is beyond the scope of this chapter, several fundamental principles guide return-to-play decisions:

  - Injured athletes must have the muscular strength to perform adequately. Typically the injured body part should have approximately 90% strength compared with the uninjured side or the player's normative strength. Athletes returned without adequate muscular strength rapidly revisit to the training room, often with a subsequent injury that is more severe than the first.

  - Before an athlete can return to play, he or she must demonstrate adequate agility. Contact athletes require full agility to protect themselves on the fields of friendly strife. Agility in noncontact athletes indicates the return of normal motor patterns that help protect against overuse injury. Strength and agility requirements vary widely between sports. An injured toe may be catastrophic to a basketball or football athlete and completely inconsequential to a rifle marksman.

  - The returning athlete should pose no increased risk of injury to other players. Casts, splints, braces, and other protective equipment should be of a material suitable for safe competition.

  - Finally, it should be recognized that clear thinking and intact cognition are required before any return to play or practice is considered.

ADMINISTRATIVE RESPONSIBILITIES OF THE TEAM PHYSICIAN

- The team physician's primary concern is the coordination of medical supervision. This organization includes making sure qualified medical personnel are attending practices and competitions as needed, designing a plan for sideline evaluation, and having necessary medical equipment readily available. The team physician encourages defined roles and responsibilities for all involved in the medical care of the team, along with establishing a medical chain of command. The team physician may not make all the daily decisions but should have full authority concerning medical policy making.

- The team physician needs to lead the planning for and practicing of medical emergencies and urgencies. In addition to having an emergency treatment and transport plan, the team physician also must know the medical capabilities of surrounding hospitals — particularly around away competition sites — so that injured athletes are brought to medical facilities that are best equipped to handle their specific medical problem (6).

- Team physicians should become familiar and maintain familiarity with the rules and position statements established by the ACSM, the AMSSM, and other organizations. They should also maintain familiarity with regulations established by governing bodies of sport (state high school athletic boards, the National Collegiate Athletic Association, Major League Baseball, and National Football League).

- The team physician should implement protocols that facilitate timely and quality medical care for situations when he or she is not immediately available. Preestablished guidelines for return to play are very helpful, especially when injuries to impact athletes result in high pressure for returning to competition before appropriate healing has occurred (5). The ACSM consensus statement on return-to-play issues more fully details the responsibilities of the team physician when returning athletes to competition (8).

- The team physician oversees the playing environment. He or she should evaluate both practice and game facilities for safety. A safe playing environment also involves appropriate and properly fitting protective equipment, available hydration, and an activity level appropriate for the climate.

COMMUNICATION RESPONSIBILITIES OF A TEAM PHYSICIAN

- For a team to receive optimal medical care, the team physician and athletic trainer must communicate openly and clearly. Even before the season, they need to discuss medical treatment protocols, which preferably are documented in writing (12). When an injury occurs, there can be no confusion over who will go on the field for initial evaluation and who will communicate to the coach the extent of an athlete's injury and playing status.

■ A potentially contentious area between team physicians, athletes, coaches, and school officials is the ordering of a magnetic resonance imaging (MRI) study. For physicians in nonsport settings, MRI scans are typically used as a diagnostic tool, to confirm a suspected diagnosis. In sports medicine, however, the MRI scan is more of a management tool. Although the team physician may not need an MRI study to make the diagnosis, an early MRI scan can allow team officials, coaches, and the athlete to get on the same page with the team physician. This shared unity results in management decisions that are more timely, better coordinated, and ultimately more appropriate for the athlete. Total player management includes not only medical management, but also administrative management. Administrative management may involve placing the player on injured reserves or the disabled list or beginning an application for a redshirt year. In addition to building unity among the management team, MRI often has mystical healing powers! For worried athletes, an MRI scan has not only diagnostic, but also mentally therapeutic effects. Early and timely MRI scans often require a strong working relationship with musculoskeletal radiologists and local radiology departments. Making them part of the medical team by providing them access to games or sideline passes can assist in developing this rapport.

■ A team physician needs to develop good rapport with the coach. Offering injury prevention suggestions and player health education may demonstrate to the coach a shared desire to assist the team attaining their goals. Most importantly, a team physician must keep the coach informed of an injured player's ability to continue to compete safely. Without breaching player confidentially, the team physician should provide the coach with a time frame for further evaluation or the player's return. In general, this information should be communicated in terms of a sport-specific timeline, such as the player is out for a play, the player is out for a series, reassessment will be done at half-time or game's end, or the player is likely out for the rest of the season.

■ A team physician may also be required to discuss a player's medical condition with school officials. Administrators often need to know specifics regarding physician recommendations, for example, how long the player will miss class or be in the hospital. They seldom need to know medical or personal details of the athlete's situation. Remember that the athlete's confidentiality is the first concern.

■ Members of the media rarely, if ever, need information from the team physician. Well-defined criteria for dealing with the media should be established. If a team physician is encouraged to participate in an interview, insist that written questions be submitted beforehand so that appropriate remarks can be constructed for the record. These planned responses can be reviewed with team coaches, athletic trainers, and administrators to ensure consistency, accuracy, and regard for the athlete's privacy.

■ A team physician may need to discuss an athlete's medical condition with his or her parents, especially if the athlete is a minor. It may be beneficial to send a letter to all parents of athletes less than 18 years old before the season, describing the role of the team physician and the continued importance of the personal primary care physician to the athlete's overall heath.

■ As mentioned earlier, the team physician coordinates specialty care as medically indicated. In doing so, he or she should provide the pertinent information necessary to the respective medical consultant's care and receive written documentation of recommendations from medical specialists.

OTHER CONSIDERATIONS FOR THE TEAM PHYSICIAN

■ Sports medicine abounds with opportunities for research. Simply keeping accurate epidemiologic and injury data has the potential to impact training regimens, competition rules, or mandates for protective equipment (11). Injury surveillance is very important to preventative sports medicine and actually advances the safety of sport much better than does any surgical technique or new prescription drug.

■ The dedicated team physician uses his or her observations and recorded injury data to prevent future injuries on his or her teams. Observing a rise in concussions will prompt a review of the team's helmets or the tackling technique. An increase in acromioclavicular separations may trigger an inspection of shoulder pads. An outbreak of rashes, abscesses, or other skin conditions should prompt a review of sanitation, equipment, and laundry procedures.

■ The astute team physician ensures that injury and outcome data are gathered, stored, and shared using methods that are Health Insurance Portability and Accountability Act (HIPAA) compliant. Sharing data across team, league, and state boundaries is essential to future efforts to prevent injury, but the privacy of the individual athlete must be protected.

■ Judgment and good sense are required when evaluating new injury prevention programs. Team physicians must be open and responsive to proven changes that will benefit and protect their athletes, but they cannot afford to simply follow the latest fad. Judgment is also required when treating injuries to ensure that treatment decisions made for professional athletes are not automatically translated into other echelons of sport. Ulnar collateral surgery may be absolutely indicated in a 34-year-old major league pitcher. Does that make it right for a 16-year-old high school pitcher?

■ Every would-be team physician must research the medical liability risk and coverage associated with the position.

A written contract or memorandum of understanding with the institution or team that defines responsibilities and expected level of coverage is essential — even if no compensation is to be received (12). "Good Samaritan" laws exist in many states, but the exact law varies widely between different jurisdictions. Most such laws apply only if the physician is receiving no compensation for his or her services. Compensation may be defined by a specific dollar amount or be as little as receiving a team shirt to wear at games!

■ Compensation as a team physician is variable. Almost all work with teams competing at lower than the collegiate level is voluntary. Deferring offers for nominal remuneration in favor of paying an athletic trainer's salary will likely benefit the athletes and the team physician (12). Almost all team physicians work with athletic teams solely for professional and personal satisfaction because of their interest in sports and athletes.

REFERENCES

1. Associated Press. Paterno fractured leg bone during sideline collision [Internet]. 2011 [cited 2011 July 11]. Available from: http://sports.espn.go.com/ncf/news/story?id=2650560.

2. Associated Press. Weis tears ACL and MCL on sideline [Internet]. 2011 [cited 2011 July 2011]. Available from: http://nbcsports.msnbc.com/id/26690497.

3. Herring SA, Bergfeld JA, Bernhardt DT, et al. Selected issues for the adolescent athlete and the team physician: a consensus statement. *Med Sci Sports Exerc.* 2008;40(11):1997–2012.

4. Herring SA, Bergfeld JA, Boland A, et al. Concussion (mild traumatic brain injury) and the team physician: a consensus statement. *Med Sci Sports Exerc.* 2006;38(2):395–9.

5. Herring SA, Bergfeld JA, Boyd J, et al. Team physician consensus statement. *Med Sci Sports Exerc.* 2000;32(4):877–8.

6. Herring SA, Bergfeld J, Boyd J, et al. Sideline preparedness for the team physician: a consensus statement. *Med Sci Sports Exerc.* 2001;33(5):846–9.

7. Herring SA, Bergfeld J, Boyd J, et al. The team physician and conditioning of athletes for sports: a consensus statement. *Med Sci Sports Exerc.* 2001;33(10):1789–93.

8. Herring SA, Bergfeld J, Boyd J, et al. The team physician and return-to-play issues: a consensus statement. *Med Sci Sports Exerc.* 2002;34(7):1212–4.

9. Kibler WB, Putukian M. Selected issues for the master athlete and the team physician: a consensus statement. *Med Sci Sports Exerc.* 2010;42(4):820–33.

10. Mellion MB, Walsh WM. The team physician. In: Mellion MB, Walsh WM, Shelton GL, editors. *The Team Physician's Handbook.* Philadelphia: Hanley & Belfus; 1997. p. 1–8.

11. Rice SG. Development of an injury surveillance system: results from a longitudinal study of high school athletes. In: Ashare AB, editor. *Safety in Ice Hockey.* West Conshohocken (PA): ASTM; 2000. p. 3–18.

12. Rice SG. The high school athlete: setting up a high school sports medicine program. In: Mellion MB, Walsh WM, Madden C, Putukian M, Shelton GL, editors. *Team Physician's Handbook.* 3rd ed. Philadelphia: Hanley & Belfus; 2002. p. 67–77.

2 Ethical Considerations in Sports Medicine

Ralph G. Oriscello and Christopher E. Jonas

INTRODUCTION

- Ethics in general terms is the conforming to accepted standards or principles of conduct. No one achieves ethical perfection, but most sports physicians are good by nature and guided by high ethical standards. Sports themselves are considered to reflect values generally considered to be important to society: character building, health promotion, and the pursuit of competitive excellence and enjoyment (3).

- Ethical considerations in the area of sports medicine are similar to those in medicine in general, including basic principles and rules (10).

- Beneficence, the principle of performing acts or making recommendations only potentially beneficial to an athlete, is the overriding principle.

- Nonmaleficence ("first do no harm"), the principle of prohibiting recommendations or actions detrimental to an athlete's short-term and long-term health, is considered with every action taken in the training room or medical setting when tending to an injured athlete.

- Confidentiality, shared decision making, informed consent, and truthfulness are absolutely essential for the ethical management of any sports-related medical decision.

THE SPORTS PHYSICIAN'S RESPONSIBILITIES

- An athlete's autonomy, his or her interests and desires and the third principle of medical ethics, must always be taken into consideration in any decision made by a sports physician. Such decisions should always be made in the athlete's best interest (17).

- Whether the decision involves a diagnostic test or the athlete's eligibility, its end result is the maintenance of good health with the least risk to the athlete.

- Conflict between physician and athlete should always be minimal or absent. The physician should use all reasonable means possible to resolve a dispute with an athlete–patient (4).

- Although autonomy is respected, most athletes can and should rely on their sports physician to lead them in the shared decision-making process.

- Sports physicians recognize that one solution rarely applies to every athlete who presents the same problem, and the same set of circumstances can also lead to a different suggested solution by the same sports physician (3,5).

- Exactness and infallibility, while desirable, are not traits of even the finest sports physicians (11,13).

- The sports physician's primary duty is to make the best effort to maintain or restore health and functional ability (9). Despite the athlete's wishes, the sports physician cannot do less than seek the best possible outcome (1). The athlete's welfare must guide all efforts.

- A good sports physician must have a genuine appreciation for the importance of athletics in an athlete's life. Donald O'Donoghue, MD, suggests the following timeless precepts for sports physicians: accept athletics, avoid expediency, adopt the best methods, act promptly, and try to achieve perfection (14).

- The injured athlete must understand the diagnosis, comprehend its implications, and participate in all therapeutic decisions.

- All sports medicine physicians gain knowledge, wisdom, and better judgment with experience, soon recognizing that many recommendations or forms of therapy have risks as well as benefits.

- Harm can come to the athlete–patient from unnecessary or excessive restriction as well as from failure to restrict activity when appropriate.

- The sports physician does not operate in a vacuum. To make sports-oriented medical decisions, one must be well versed in current recommendations for eligibility and continued participation and not depend on his or her own limited personal experience or unscientific reasoning (4,7).

- Recognizing the wide range of opinions and individual fallibility, athlete–patients can assert their right to another opinion.

- Continuing education of the sports physician aids in the development of a suitable level of skill and knowledge and their maintenance (12).

- Although sports physicians will be able to treat most referrals, they must be aware of their own level of competence. They must know when and where to refer for specialized consultation or therapy. It is essential to know their colleagues' ability, personality, and empathy for athletes in order to make competent referrals (15).

- The referred patient should not be abandoned. The consultant may gain insight from the referring physician. This affords the athlete continuing support from his or her primary sports physician.
- There is no obligation to accept without question the recommendations of consultants, especially if incongruent with the referring physician's knowledge of the patient.
- All of the above lead to trust established between athlete and physician, allowing for more comfortable resolution of the decision-making process.

POTENTIAL FOR DIVIDED LOYALTIES

- Although rare in high school and uncommon in college sports, there is major distrust between professional athletes and team physicians (6).
- Athletes may feel there are too many instances when the quality of their treatment is secondary to the physician's obligation to team owners and coaches (2).
- A salaried position may interfere with the traditional doctor–patient relationship.
- A salaried physician has a potential conflict of interest. Objective professional duties are compromised by personal interests (e.g., the financial reward of the professional team association, as well as the publicity and high visibility one gets from such a position).
- The ultimate welfare of the athlete may seem in conflict with the wishes of parents, spouse, coaches, or team management, but the loyalty of the sports physician is to the continued well-being of the athlete and a healthy physician–patient relationship.
- Decisions must be made solely based on sound medical judgment; however, a third party (e.g., a university or professional team) that does not follow reasonable medical advice may be cause for the physician to cease providing services for that party (2).
- When the wishes of the athlete–patient conflict with what the physician believes to be in the athlete's best interest and the conflict cannot be resolved, the athlete should be reassigned to another physician (4).
- For the professional athlete, the unfavorable mix of high salaries and short careers can precipitate risky decision making by both the athlete and the physician. Coaches often encourage physicians to return players, and players themselves often desire to return to the field of play too quickly (17).
- An untimely death or worsening injury sets the stage for a potential lack of trust in the team physician.
- The physician must take great care to avoid becoming overly concerned with the team's record or athlete's statistics and remain most concerned with the athlete's health.

- The team physician's actions should demonstrate a primary responsibility to the players' safety and well-being, and the physician should not allow players to be on the field who are not truly medically qualified (16).

DRUG USE

- It is common knowledge that there is illicit drug use by athletes at all levels of play, including recreational drugs, anabolic steroids, pain-controlling agents, ergogenics, and alcohol (17).
- Therapeutic medications are an integral part of sports medicine. Used appropriately, they control pain and inflammation, speed recovery, and hasten return to function.
- It is the obligation of the sports physician to know each drug thoroughly, especially its potential effect(s) on the safety or effectiveness of the athlete's performance.
- The sports physician must not expose the athlete to potential disqualification (e.g., as in the prevention of exercise-induced asthma) when an effective legal medication can be found.
- Appropriate reference to World Anti-Doping Agency (WADA), United States Anti-Doping Agency (USADA), and other applicable banned substance listings is of utmost importance for the sports medicine physician.
- The available drug testing cannot detect all participants who use banned substances, but the testing capabilities are rapidly changing.

CONFIDENTIALITY

- All athletes have a right to full confidentiality, despite the fact that some athletes are very public persons (2).
- All inquiries made of sports physicians by the press or other interested parties should go unanswered unless specifically permitted by the athlete or should be referred to the athlete or representative.
- The permission to discuss medical information should be in writing and explicitly outline the information that can be revealed.
- Despite claims regarding the public's "right to know," the right to privacy remains with the athlete–patient (2).
- On occasion, the sports physician will advise the athlete–patient about the amount of information to release to coaches. This is important when restriction from practice or competition is necessary. Here we refer to the athlete's private sports physician, not one employed by a school or professional team.
- When a sports physician is employed by a school, team, or similar entity, the sports physician must always advocate for the athlete–patient's welfare, while fulfilling the role of protecting the team or school.
- An employed sports physician must still respect the athlete–patient's autonomy in medical decision making, while advising against any decision that could compromise the patient's future health and athletic career.

RELATIONSHIP WITH COLLEAGUES

- Conflict can arise between a team physician and other physicians participating in the care of the athlete–patient; there must be sensitivity demonstrated to the relationship of all medical professionals involved.

- The sports physician must never criticize the actions of another physician to the athlete–patient. Private discussions with the other physicians regarding recommended therapy should be undertaken.

- The sports physician is in a position to positively influence the knowledge of other physicians by providing positive, collegial input.

- If inappropriate playing restrictions or early return have been recommended by another physician, the sports physician should perform an individual assessment of the athlete's return-to-play status.

- Sports medicine is a team effort involving physicians and other medical professionals who can be helpful with the athlete's care; the sports physician must insist that all adhere to the same high ethical standards.

- The sports medicine physician has an obligation to expose quackery and unproven practices employed in the guise of improving performance, thus protecting athletes and their careers.

FEAR OF LEGAL ENTANGLEMENT

- There is always a question as to what the sports medicine physician should do in the presence of a life-threatening situation or a potentially disabling condition, and the physician must consider the athlete's safety while allowing the athlete–patient to share in the decisions.

- When operating at the highest ethical level with support from the medical literature and the medical community, such an event should never alter a physician's role in the future evaluation of other athletes.

- A sports physician who is not afraid to make the correct recommendation in a difficult medical situation should be sought out by other physicians and athletes.

SUMMARY

- Sports medicine requires ethical treatment of athletes in all situations (5).

- Familiarity with many disease states that can affect an athlete's ability to participate is required (1).

- Athletes can only participate if they do not endanger themselves or others (1).

- The physician must be familiar with unethical means of enhancing performance (8,17).

- The physician must be aware of resources available to aid him or her in rendering an authoritative opinion (1,3).

- The physician must be devoted to the rules of confidentiality, informed consent, and truthfulness. The physician must be aware that there is uncertainty in some decisions that have no right or wrong answer; the decisions should be made based on the literature and experience.

REFERENCES

1. American College of Sports Medicine. Code of ethics [Internet]. Available from: http://www.acsm.org/join-acsm/membership-resources/code-of-ethics.
2. Anderson L. Contractual obligations and the sharing of confidential information in sport. *J Med Ethics*. 2008;34(9):e6.
3. Anderson L. Writing a new code of ethics for sports physicians: principles and challenges. *Br J Sports Med*. 2009;43(13):1079–82.
4. Capozzi JD, Rhodes R, Gantsoudes G. Ethics in practice: terminating the physician-patient relationship. *J Bone Joint Surg Am*. 2008;90(1):208–10.
5. Dunn WR, George MS, Churchill L, Spindler KP. Ethics in sports medicine. *Am J Sports Med*. 2007;35(5):840–4.
6. George T. Care by team doctors raises conflict issue. *The New York Times*. July 28, 2002, section 8, column 5. Available at: http://www.nytimes.com/2002/07/28/sports/pro-football-care-by-team-doctors-raises-conflict-issue.html
7. Giordano S. A new professional code in sports medicine. *BMJ*. 2010; 341:c4931.
8. Holm S, McNamee M. Ethics in sports medicine. *BMJ*. 2009;339: b3898.
9. Howe WB. Primary care sports medicine: a part-timer's perspective. *Phys Sports Med*. 1988;16:103.
10. Johnson R. The unique ethics of sports medicine. *Clin Sports Med*. 2004; 23(2):175–82.
11. Maron B, Klues HG. Surviving competitive athletics with hypertrophic cardiomyopathy. *Am J Cardiol*. 1994;73(15):1098–104.
12. Maron BJ, Mitchell JH. 26th Bethesda Conference: recommendations for determining eligibility for competition in athletes with cardiovascular abnormalities. *J Am Coll Cardiol*. 1994;24(4):845–99.
13. Mitten MJ. *The Athlete and Heart Disease: Diagnosis, Evaluation & Management*. Philadelphia (PA): Lippincott Williams & Wilkins; 1999. 307 p.
14. O'Donoghue DH. *Treatment of Injuries to Athletes*. 4th ed. Philadelphia (PA): W.B. Saunders; 1984. 714 p.
15. Rizve AA, Thompson PD. Hypertrophic cardiomyopathy: who plays and who sits. *Curr Sports Med Rep*. 2002;1(2):93–9.
16. Salkeld LR. Ethics and the pitchside physician. *J Med Ethics*. 2008;34(6): 456–7.
17. Tucker AM. Ethics and the professional team physician. *Clin Sports Med*. 2004;23(2):227–41.

Legal Issues in Sports Medicine

Aaron Rubin

3

INTRODUCTION

- The advice of an attorney should be considered before making any legal decisions.
- Sports is a microcosm of society.
- There are rules of sports and society that must be created, interpreted, and, at times, debated.
- Medical practice in sports holds no exemption from any other medical practice.
- Legal issues present in the area include, but are not limited to, malpractice, contracts, licensure, insurance, "Good Samaritan" laws, and confidentiality issues (Health Insurance Portability and Accountability Act [HIPAA] and Family Educational Rights and Privacy Act [FERPA]).
- These issues may be complicated by the practice of sports medicine in the public arena and the traditions of team and game coverage.
- This chapter is by no means meant to substitute for the advice of an attorney, but is presented to draw attention to potential legal issues that may arise in the practice of sports medicine.

DEFINITIONS

- **Law:** A body of rules or standards of conduct promulgated or established by some authority.
  - That which is laid down, ordained, or established. A body of rules of action or conduct prescribed by controlling authority and having binding legal force. The law of a state is found in statutory and constitutional enactments as interpreted by its courts. The word "law" contemplates both statutory and case law (7).
- **Lawful:** That which is permitted or authorized by the law.
  - Legal, warranted, or authorized by the law. Not contrary to nor forbidden by the law; not illegal (7).
- **Contract:** An agreement between two or more parties that creates legally binding obligations. A valid contract must involve competent parties, proper subject matter, consideration, and mutuality of agreement and of obligation. Contracts are classified in many ways.

- An agreement between two or more persons that creates an obligation to do or not to do a particular thing. A legal relationship consisting of the rights and duties of the contracting parties; a promise or set of promises constituting an agreement between the parties that gives each a legal duty to the other and also the right to seek a remedy for the breach of those duties. Its essentials are competent parties, subject matter, and mutuality of agreement (7).
- **Expressed:** An Expressed contract is an actual agreement in terms that are openly declared at the time of making it, being stated in distinct and explicit language either orally or in writing (7).
- **Implied:** An implied contract is one inferred by law to exist because the parties' conduct or surrounding circumstances indicate a contractual relationship exists.
- **Bilateral:** A bilateral contract is one involving mutual promises between parties.
  - Bilateral or reciprocal contracts are those by which the parties expressly enter into mutual engagements such as sale or hire (7).
- **Unilateral:** A unilateral contract is a one-sided promise where one party undertakes an obligation without a reciprocal promise or obligation being made or undertaken.
- **Civil law:** Body of law that a nation or state has established for itself as distinguished from natural law. Law determining private rights and liabilities as distinguished from criminal law.
  - That body of law that every particular nation, commonwealth, or city has established peculiarly for itself; more properly called "municipal" law to distinguish it from the "law of nature," and from international law. Laws concerned with civil or private rights and remedies as contrasted with criminal laws (7).
- **Criminal law:** The branch of law that defines what public wrongs are considered crimes and assigns punishment for those wrongs.
  - The substantive criminal law is that law which, for the purpose of preventing harm to society, (a) declares what conduct is criminal, and (b) prescribes the punishment to be imposed for such conduct (7).

- **Natural law:** The moral or ethical law, formulated in accordance with reason, natural justice, and the original state of nature (7).
- **Case law:** Law based on judicial precedent rather than legislative enactment. The body of law founded in adjudicated cases as distinguished from statute, common law.
  - The aggregate of reported cases as forming a body of jurisprudence, or the law of a particular subject as evidenced or formed by the adjudged cases, in distinction to statutes and other sources of law. It includes the aggregate of reported cases that interpret statutes, regulations, and constitutional provisions (7).
- **Tort:** A wrongful injury; a private or civil wrong. A tort is some action or conduct by the defendant that results from a breach of a legal duty owed by the defendant to the plaintiff, which proximately causes injury or damage to the plaintiff. Torts may be "intentional" (when the defendant intends to violate a legal duty) or "negligent" (when the defendant fails to exercise the proper degree of care established by law).
  - A private or civil wrong or injury, including action for bad faith breach of contract, for which the court will provide a remedy in the form of an action for damages (7).
  - A legal wrong committed upon the person or property independent of contract. It may be (a) a direct invasion of some legal right of the individual; (b) the infraction of some public duty by which special damage accrues to the individual; or (c) the violation of some private obligation by which like damage accrues to the individual (7).
- **Negligence:** The inadvertent or unintentional failure to exercise that care that a reasonable, prudent, and careful person would exercise; conduct that violates certain legal standards of due care. Negligence constitutes grounds for recovery in a tort action if it is the proximate cause of injury to the plaintiff.
  - The omission to do something that a reasonable man, guided by those ordinary considerations that ordinarily regulate human affair, would do, or the doing of something that a reasonable and prudent man would not do (9).
- **Liability:** Any type of obligation or debt, fixed or contingent; an indebtedness owed to another party; a duty to pay money on funds owed. An obligation or mandate to do or refrain from doing something.
  - Broad legal term. It has been referred to as of the most comprehensive significance, including almost every character of hazard or responsibility, absolute, contingent, or likely. An obligation one is bound in law or justice to perform (7).
- **Plaintiff:** Person who brings a lawsuit; the complainant; the prosecution in a criminal case.

- A person who brings an action. The party who complains or sues in a civil action and is so named on the record. A person who seeks remedial relief for an injury to rights; it designates a complainant (7).
- **Defendant:** The person accused in a criminal case or sued in a civil action.
  - The person defending or denying; the party against whom relief or recovery is sought in an action or suit or the accused in a criminal case (7).
- **Captain of the ship doctrine:** This doctrine imposes liability on the surgeon in charge of the operation for negligence of his assistants during the period when those assistants are under the surgeon's control, even though the assistants are also employees of the hospital (7).

DUTIES, ROLES, AND RESPONSIBILITIES OF THE TEAM PHYSICIAN (2,5)

- The duties of the team physician to a team may be outlined in a letter of agreement or contract between the organization and physician.
- The duties to the individual athlete should be considered as with any other patient–physician relationship.
- Balancing this duty to team and athlete must be considered in every situation.
- A consensus statement on the duties of the team physician has been created by several organizations and is available in its entirety from the following groups:
  - American College of Sports Medicine (ACSM)
  - American Academy of Family Physicians (AAFP)
  - American Academy of Orthopedic Surgeons (AAOS)
  - American Medical Society for Sports Medicine (AMSSM)
  - American Orthopaedic Society for Sports Medicine (AOSSM)
  - American Osteopathic Academy of Sports Medicine (AOASM)
- Qualifications from this consensus statement include:
  - Medical or osteopathic degree with unrestricted license to practice medicine
  - Fundamental knowledge of emergency care regarding sporting events
  - Trained in cardiopulmonary resuscitation (CPR)
  - Working knowledge of trauma, musculoskeletal injuries, and medical conditions affecting the athlete
- Medical duties from this statement stated that the team physician has ultimate responsibility to include: coordination of the preparticipation screening; management of on-field injuries; medical management of injury and illness;

coordination of rehabilitation and return to participation; coordination of medical care; education; and documentation and record keeping.

- Administrative duties include: establishing relationships; education; development of a chain of command; plan and train for emergencies; address equipment and supply issues (as needed to provide adequate medical coverage); provide for event coverage; and assess environment concerns and playing conditions.

- Standard definitions of negligence generally apply. The physician is held to what the reasonable, prudent man would do.

- As guidelines become more established, these may become the basis for duties and responsibilities of the team physician

DUTIES, ROLES, AND RESPONSIBILITIES OF THE TEAM AND ATHLETES (2,5)

- The responsibilities of the team (organization, ownership, administration) should also be outlined in a contract.

- The team should provide a safe venue (including adequate security), appropriate safety equipment, supplies needed to treat injured or ill athletes (unless otherwise specified in the agreement), and appropriate response for emergency situations.

- The team (including coaching staff) should not interfere with the care of the athlete, including return-to-play issues.

- The athlete should be prepared for participation and participate safely and according to the rules of the sport. If not, the athlete may share in responsibility for the injury.

- The athlete or team has a duty to report conditions to the team physician and not conceal illnesses, injury, or symptoms that may occur.

CONTRACTS

- Traditionally, many team physicians work with as little as a handshake or loose agreement; one should consider "putting it in writing."

- This contract should outline duties, responsibilities for providing supplies, compensation, travel expectations, provision of coverage in the team physician's absence, length of contract, responsibilities for providing preparticipation examinations, liability coverage, and game decision processes (such as who has the final word on return-to-play issues).

- An attorney can be extremely helpful in creating such a document.

LIABILITY

Malpractice Coverage

- Malpractice is defined as unreasonable lack of skill or professional misconduct (7).
  - Failure to render professional services under circumstances in the community by the "average, prudent reputable member of the profession" with resultant injury or damage to the recipient of those services.

- Negligence is the predominant theory of liability in medical malpractice suits. It requires all of the following elements to occur:
  - Physician's **duty** to the plaintiff
  - **Violation** of applicable standard of care
  - **Injury** that can be compensated
  - **Connection** between the violation of care and harm

- A physician should have adequate coverage to defend any case brought against the physician and to compensate any judgments decided against the physician.

- Coverage may not be in effect if one is practicing outside of his or her scope of practice or in an area where not licensed.

- Physicians traveling out of state (or country) with teams should be aware of this possibility and check with their malpractice carrier.

- Malpractice insurance should include an adequate "tail" to cover the physician in the event the physician changes jobs or malpractice insurance before a case is brought.

Fallacy of the Good Samaritan

- Good Samaritan doctrine: One who sees a person in imminent and serious peril through negligence of another cannot be charged with contributory negligence as a matter of law, in risking his own life or serious injury in attempting to effect a rescue, provided the attempt is not recklessly or rashly made. Under this doctrine, negligence of a volunteer must worsen position of person in distress before liability will be imposed. This protection from liability is provided by statute in most states.

- These laws and protection vary from state to state.

- These are a defense in a lawsuit and must be presented by your attorney as such.

- A person expected to act, such as a team physician at a game, may not be covered by Good Samaritan doctrine, whether compensated or not.

- Good Samaritan doctrine should not be a substitute for adequate malpractice coverage.

- The doctrine should be adequate in most states to cover a physician who renders aid when an unexpected medical situation arises, such as at an auto accident or if, when a spectator at an event, another spectator has a cardiac arrest.

■ Some jurisdictions may **require** a physician to provide care under these circumstances.

PATIENT (ATHLETE)–PHYSICIAN RELATIONSHIP

■ The patient (athlete)–physician relationship should be one of mutual trust and teamwork.

■ The athlete (or parents or guardian if a minor) has rights to autonomy, self-determination, privacy, and appropriate medical care.

■ Even if a minor, the athlete has certain rights to seek medical care in most jurisdictions for treatment related to pregnancy, drugs, and sexually transmitted disease. Check with local laws.

■ HIPAA, FERPA, and Protected Health Information (PHI)

  ■ HIPAA

    ❏ Health Insurance Portability and Accountability Act of 1996

    ❏ Defines PHI

    ❏ *Individually identifiable health information* is information, including demographic data, that relates to the individual's past, present, or future physical or mental health or condition; the provision of health care to the individual; or the past, present, or future payment for the provision of health care to the individual, and that identifies the individual or for which there is a reasonable basis to believe it can be used to identify the individual.

      ▪ Individually identifiable health information includes many common identifiers (*e.g.*, name, address, birth date, social security number) (9).

  ■ FERPA

    ❏ Family Educational Rights and Privacy Act

    ❏ Relates primarily to protected educational information; could raise issues if acting as a team physician at an educational facility.

  ■ Effects of both laws have been to legislate protection of information that was once a moral and ethical issue for health care providers.

■ Privacy is a difficult issue due to the public nature of athletic events and evaluation done on the field or courtside. All attempts to maintain privacy must be attempted. Reporters, scouts, and others may be with the physician on the sidelines.

■ Professional and college organizations may consider waivers to allow certain information regarding athletic injuries or illnesses to be discussed with press representatives.

■ It is probably best to have an administrative person deal with press, such as a sports information director or public information officer, to keep the physician from accidentally releasing private issues.

DRUGS AND THE ATHLETE (2)

Medications: Prescribing and Dispensing

■ Legal medications are generally divided into two groups, prescription and over-the-counter (OTC). Prescription medications are further divided into controlled substances (*e.g.*, narcotics, sedatives), which have a higher potential for abuse and misuse, and standard prescription drugs (*e.g.*, antibiotics, anti-inflammatory, blood pressure, diabetes medications).

■ In some states, a special prescription is needed for dispensing of the highest level of controlled substances.

■ Medication prescribing and dispensing falls under many laws including state medical laws, pharmacy laws, and consumer safety laws.

■ The National Collegiate Athletic Association (NCAA) has well-referenced specific guidelines regarding dispensing in the training room that provides good direction if considering dispensing medication (6).

■ In general, a physician may prescribe medication or provide medications under the state laws, which usually include examination of the patient.

■ A licensed pharmacist may provide medication as prescribed by a licensed physician.

■ There are generally strict labeling requirements often including the name of the patient, name and strength of the medication, directions for use, date dispensed, quantity dispensed, and warnings of common side effects. In addition, many states require the pharmacist to counsel the patient on the medication.

■ Dispensing medications by individuals not licensed to do so, even if OTC, may not be allowed and could open those doing so to prosecution under appropriate laws. This may also open the individuals to liability for negligence if an untoward effect occurs.

Drug Testing (See Chapter 25)

■ The team physician may be asked to participate in drug testing program for teams.

■ Careful consideration regarding the physician's role as an "enforcer" of rules versus a counselor for medical care must be undertaken.

■ Proper protection of rights and "due process" of the athlete must be maintained.

- Testing may include recreational as well as performance-enhancing drugs.
- Testing may be voluntary or mandated by certain organizations such as the NCAA or International Olympic Committee (IOC).

"CAPTAIN OF THE SHIP"

- Although this doctrine relates to surgeons and assistants, the philosophy could be expanded to team physicians and those they work with.
- Choose your partners in sports medical care wisely to avoid being drawn into bad situations (1).

RISK MANAGEMENT (1)

- Manage risk by being prepared, documenting care, working with likeminded professionals, anticipating problems, and communicating with athletes and, where appropriate, their families.
- Advice of legal counsel should be sought in planning team coverage, in writing contracts, and if any events occur.
- Bad outcomes often lead to legal actions (lawsuits).

CASE LAW OF INTEREST TO THE TEAM PHYSICIAN

- Knapp versus Northwestern 1996 (4)
  - A competent, intelligent adult with Division I basketball skills signs a letter of intent to play with a Division I school.
  - Athlete suffers sudden cardiac arrest, is resuscitated, and has implantable cardioverter-defibrillator implanted.
  - School's team physician declares him ineligible quoting Bethesda Guidelines.
  - School does provide scholarship, but will not allow him to play or practice.
  - Player sues under Rehabilitation Act.
  - District court states school violated Act and must allow him to participate.
  - U.S. Seventh Circuit Court of Appeals reversed, stating school does have ability to refuse his participation.
  - ". . . medical determinations of this sort are best left to team doctors."
- Kleinknecht versus Gettysburg College, April 27, 1993 (3)
  - Athlete collapses, and coach runs to his side (not trained in CPR).

- Sends for trainer and to call for help.
  - Pre–cell phone era, pre–automated external defibrillator era.
- Student trainer arrives (2 minutes after collapse) but did not start CPR because student was breathing.
- Athletic Trainer, Certified arrives, notes athlete stopped breathing, and begins CPR with bystander emergency medical technician.
- Athlete dies, and parents filed wrongful death suit.
- College filed motion against, which was initially denied and then allowed.
- District court found for the college:
  - *College had no duty to anticipate and guard against the chance of a fatal arrhythmia in a young and healthy athlete.*
  - *Actions taken by school employees were reasonable. . . . College did not negligently breach any duty that might exist.*
- U.S. Court of Appeals overturned finding:
  - There is a duty of care.
  - There is a special relationship between athletes and the school.
  - Negligence should be determined by the jury.
  - Immunity (Good Samaritan law)
  - College did not assert defense, but the court found that would not have been allowed.
- Commonwealth of Kentucky versus David Jason Stinson, September 17, 2009 (8)
  - A 15-year-old high school football player dies of heat stroke days after coach had team run wind sprints on hot August day.
  - Parents file wrongful death lawsuit against head coach and five assistants.
  - Reckless homicide charges are filed against coach.
  - Coach also indicted by Grand Jury for wanton endangerment.
  - Coach found not guilty after 2-week trial.
  - Jury deliberated 90 minutes.
  - Civil case settled out of court.

REFERENCES

1. Birnie B. Legal issues for the team physician. In: Rubin AL, editor. *Sports Injuries and Emergencies, a Quick-Response Manual.* New York: McGraw-Hill; 2003.
2. Herring SA, Bergfeld J, Boyd J, et al. Team physicians consensus statement [Internet]. 2001. Available from: http://www.acsm.org/pdf/teamphys.pdf
3. Kleinknecht versus Gettysburg College. *United States Court of Appeals for the Third Circuit*; 1993 Apr 27: 25 Fed.R.Serv.3d 65; 61 USLW 2606; 989 F.2d 1360.

4. Knapp versus Northwestern. *United States Court of Appeals for the Seventh Circuit*; No. 96–3450.

5. Mitten MJ. Emerging legal issues in sports medicine: a synthesis, summary, and analysis. *St John's L Rev*. 2002;76(1):5–8.

6. NCAA Sports Medicine Handbook, 2011–2012 [Internet]. 2011 [cited 2011 Sep 10]. Available from: http://www.ncaapublications.com/product downloads/MD11.pdf.

7. Nolan JR, Nolan-Haley JM. *Black's Law Dictionary with Pronunciations*. 6th ed. St Paul (MN): West Publishing; 1990. 1657 p.

8. Riley J. Stinson found not guilty in PRP player's death [Internet]. 2011 [cited 2011 Sep 10]. Available from: http://www.courier-journal.com/article/20090917/SPORTS05/909170320/Stinson-found-not-guilty-PRP-player-s-death.

9. United States Department of Health and Human Services. Summary of the HIPAA Privacy Rule [Internet]. 2011 [cited 2011 Sep 10]. Available from: http://www.hhs.gov/ocr/privacy/hipaa/understanding/summary/privacysummary.pdf.

Orthopedic Sports Medicine Terminology

4

Scott A. Magnes, Vanessa Lalley, and Francis G. O'Connor

- One of the challenges facing sports medicine providers is the communication barrier that exists when interacting with others outside the specialty. Sports medicine has a vocabulary that is unique, and few health care providers outside of the field speak this language fluently.

- The purpose of this chapter is to attempt to make readers more fluent in this "language" in order to enhance meaningful communication.

- General terminology has been derived from authoritative textbooks in the field of sports medicine and related disciplines; specific terminology is referenced from current peer reviewed literature (1,3–5,8,10,11,14).

GENERAL TERMINOLOGY

- **Accessory or supernumerary bone:** Develops from separate center of ossification from parent bone; may or may not obtain bony union with parent bone.

- **Active-assisted motion:** Range of motion (ROM) of a joint that a patient is able to achieve with the assistance of the examiner.

- **Active motion:** ROM of a joint that a patient is able to achieve on his or her own.

- **Allograft:** Cadaver graft.

- **Anatomic axis (of lower extremity):** Angle formed by intersection of lines through the femoral and tibial shafts with patient standing. The difference between the mechanical and anatomic axis is usually $5+/-2$ degrees.

- **Apophysis:** Secondary growth center forming bony outgrowth or contour that remains a part of the native bone (*e.g.*, process, tubercle, tuberosity).

- **Apophysitis:** Inflammation of an apophysis.

- **Arthritis:** Deviation from normal structure and physiology of joint tissues; a form of joint disorder that involves inflammation of one or more joints.

- **Arthropathy:** Joint disease; does not specify the type of joint disease.

- **Arthrosis:** An arthrosis is a joint; an area where two bones are attached for the purpose of motion of body parts.

- **Atrophy:** Muscle "wasting"; loss of muscle mass.

- **Autograft:** Graft from one's own body.

- **Avascular necrosis (AVN), aseptic necrosis, osteonecrosis:** Blood supply to affected bone is insufficient, resulting in bony necrosis; etiologies include idiopathic, traumatic, steroids, heavy alcohol use, dysbaric illness (Caisson disease), blood dyscrasias (*e.g.*, sickle cell disease), high doses of radiation therapy, and Gaucher disease. Untreated, the natural disease progression is to degenerative joint disease.

- **Avulsion fracture:** Injury to tendinous insertion site where a small piece of bone is fractured in continuity with the tendon, rather than rupture at the tendon–bone interface.

- **Bone bruise:** Microfractures seen on magnetic resonance imaging. This is common with anterior cruciate ligament (ACL) injuries; with this injury, the lesions are located on the posterior portion of the lateral tibial plateau and the lateral femoral condyle.

- **Bursitis:** Inflammation of a bursa.

- **Chondromalacia:** Softening or damage to the articular cartilage of the patella; diagnosis is made under direct visualization at the time of surgery. This term is often used to describe similar lesions in other bones.

- **Chondrosis:** Chondral degeneration.

- **Diaphysis:** Midshaft, tubular portion of long bone.

- **Dislocation:** Complete loss of apposition of articulating bones that normally comprise a joint.

- **Effusion:** Excessive fluid within a joint.

- **Epiphysis:** Center of ossification; longitudinal growth center.

- **Extension lag:** Lack of normal active extension of a joint with normal passive extension; usually measured in degrees.

- **Flexion contracture:** Lack of normal active and passive extension of a joint usually measured in degrees.

- **Instability:** Functional term referring to symptomatic joint laxity; may be unidirectional or multidirectional, with the etiology being posttraumatic or congenital.

- **Laxity:** Degree of looseness; usually referring to a ligament. Symptomatic laxity is termed "instability."

- **Long bone:** Length > width; found in limbs.

- **Mechanical axis (of lower extremity):** Angle formed by intersection of lines drawn from center of femoral head to center of knee joint, and center of knee joint to center of ankle with patient standing.
- **Metaphysis:** The growing portion of a long bone that lies between the epiphyses (the ends) and the diaphysis (the shaft); consists of cancellous bone.
- **Osteochondritis dissecans (OCD):** A fragment of subchondral bone and its overlying chondral cartilage are separated from the underlying bone. The etiology is unclear, but most likely traumatic. Most often, it occurs in the knee, and the most common location is the lateral aspect of the medial femoral condyle.
- **Osteotomy:** Transection of a bone; often refers to the tibia or femur to correct for varus or valgus deformities. The surgeon alters the mechanical axis of the limb in an attempt to alleviate malalignment, arthrosis, and pain.
- **Passive motion:** ROM of a joint performed by the examiner.
- **Physis:** Growth plate; the segment of a bone that is responsible for lengthening. There are four zones within the physis: the resting cartilage zone, the proliferating cartilage zone, the zone of hypertrophy, and the zone of calcification.
- **Platelet-rich plasma (PRP):** PRP is blood plasma that has been enriched with platelets. As a concentrated source of autologous platelets, PRP contains (and releases through degranulation) several different growth factors and other cytokines that stimulate healing of bone and soft tissue. Localized injections of autologous blood with a supraphysiologic concentration of platelets are thought to enhance the healing process via a variety of potential mechanisms (13).
- **Proprioception:** Reflex mechanism whereby position sense receptors are able to detect the position of a joint in space and therefore provide a coordinated muscular response to aid in stabilization of a joint.
- **Recurvatum:** Hyperextension of a joint.
- **Sesamoid bone:** Bone located within tendons.
- **Short bone:** More cuboidal in shape; found in carpus and tarsals.
- **Sprain:** Injury to a ligament(s) around a joint; due to excessive stress
- **Strain:** Injury to a muscle or tendon due to excessive stress.
- **Stress views:** Radiographs used to assess ligamentous integrity by stressing the involved ligaments and assessing for increased laxity; often compared to the normal contralateral side.
- **Subluxation:** Partial dislocation of a joint.
- **Tendonitis (tendinitis):** Inflammation of a tendon.
- **Tendonopathy (tendinopathy):** Refers to injury or disease of a tendon.
- **Tendonosis (tendinosis):** Tendon degeneration (usually focal); suffix "osis" implies a pathology of chronic degeneration without inflammation (16).
- **Tenosynovitis:** Tendon sheath inflammation.
- **Tensile strength:** Maximum stress that a structure can sustain before failure.

EVIDENCE-BASED MEDICINE TERMINOLOGY

- **Bias:** Deviation of results or inferences from truth; systematic error in the design, conduct, or analysis of a study that results in a mistaken estimate of an exposure's effect on the risk of disease. Common forms of bias include selection and information bias.
- **Confidence interval (CI):** Accuracy of the study; the CI is the range of high to low values of the data with the true mean likely to be in the specified range (usually 90% to 95% CI acceptable). A narrow CI is good. If, when evaluating relative risk, the CI crosses 1, there is no real difference between groups.
- **Confounding:** A confounding variable (confounder) is an extraneous variable that correlates (positively or negatively) with both the dependent variable and the independent variable. Scientific studies therefore need to account for these variables either through controls or through statistical means; otherwise, an erroneous conclusion can be made that the dependent variables are in a causal relationship with the independent variable.
- **Incidence:** The number of new cases of a disease or injury that occurs during a specified period of time in a population at risk.
- **Number needed to harm (NNH):** Number of people needed to receive treatment to produce an adverse event. NNH = 1/Absolute risk increase.
- **Number needed to treat (NNT):** Number of people to be treated to prevent one more event or adverse outcome. NNT = 1/Absolute risk reduction.
- **P value:** The P value gives the interpreter the probability that the study results occurred by chance alone; acceptable P values are generally ≤ 0.05 and considered to be statistically significant.
- **Positive and negative predictive values (Table 4.1):** Percentage of patients with a positive or negative test for a disease who do or do not have the disease in question.
- **Power:** The ability of a study to demonstrate an association. Power = 1 − Probability of making a type II error; acceptable study power is 0.80.

Table 4.1	Statistics	
	Population at Risk	
Test Results	**Disease Present**	**No Disease**
Positive	A (true positives)	B (false positives)
Negative	C (false negatives)	D (true negatives)

Sensitivity = a/(a + c)
Specificity = d/(b + d)
Positive Predictive Value = a(a + b)
Negative Predictive Value = d(c + d)

- **Prevalence:** The amount of a disease or injury at a given time in a population.
- **Sensitivity (see Table 4.1):** Percentage of patients with disease who have a positive test for the disease in question.
- **Specificity (see Table 4.1):** Percentage of patients without disease who have a negative test for the disease in question.
- **Strength of recommendation grades (6):**
  - A: Consistent, good-quality, patient-oriented evidence
  - B: Inconsistent or limited-quality, patient-oriented evidence
  - C: Consensus, disease-oriented evidence, usual practice, expert opinion, or case series for studies of diagnosis, treatment, prevention, or screening
- **Study (evidence) quality:**
  - Level 1: Good-quality, patient-oriented evidence (systematic review, randomized controlled trial)
  - Level 2: Limited-quality, patient-oriented evidence with inconsistent results/findings (case-control or cohort studies)
  - Level 3: Other evidence (*i.e.*, consensus guidelines, disease-oriented evidence, and case series)
- **Type I error:** A type I error occurs in statistics when an association is demonstrated, but one does not actually exist. Probability of type I error is α. Studies generally need an α of 0.05 to minimize risk for a type I error.
- **Type II error:** A type II error occurs when no association is demonstrated, but one actually exists. This generally occurs because of too few subjects or because a study has inadequate power to detect a difference. Probability of type II error is β. Studies generally need to be powered to at least 0.80 $(1 - \beta)$ to avoid a type II error.
- **Types of studies**
  - Cohort: Observation of a population subset to determine incidence/mortality rates.
  - Case-control: Observation of population with disease versus those without disease.
  - Cross-section: Relationship between disease and other variables as they exist in a population at a particular time.
  - Double-blind trial: Where both the subjects and the observers in contact with the subjects are kept ignorant of study interventions.
  - Randomized controlled trial: Subjects in a population are randomly allocated into groups.
  - Randomized controlled, double-blind trial: Gold standard for research.
- **Validity:** The validity of a test is defined as its ability to distinguish between who has a disease and who does not.
- **Variable:** Variables are used in experiments to observe relationships and effects. The **dependent** variable is the event studied and expected to change whenever the **independent** variable is altered.

TERMINOLOGY REFERRING TO FRACTURES

- **Alignment:** Relationship of the longitudinal axis of one fracture fragment to another.
- **Angulation:** Position of distal fracture fragment in relation to the proximal fragment or direction of the apex of the angle formed by the fracture fragments (*e.g.*, apex dorsal).
- **Apposition:** Contact of the ends of the fracture fragments.
- **Avulsion:** Bony fragment is pulled away from its native bone by muscle contraction (*e.g.*, mallet finger) or a passive opposing force to a ligament (*e.g.*, tibial avulsion fracture of ACL).
- **Butterfly fragment:** Wedge-shaped fracture fragment that is separated from the main fracture fragment in a comminuted fracture.
- **Closed:** Intact skin.
- **Comminuted:** More than two fracture fragments.
- **Compression:** Usually refers to vertebral fracture where impaction occurs.
- **Delayed union:** Failure of union in the duration of time that healing usually takes place for that bone.
- **Depression:** An impaction-type fracture where the hard surface of one bone is driven into a second softer surface of bone (*e.g.*, tibial plateau fracture).
- **Diastasis:** Abnormal separation of two bones (*e.g.*, symphysis pubis diastasis secondary to ruptured ligaments, widened ankle mortise secondary to syndesmosis disruption).
- **Displacement:** Degree of loss of anatomic position.
- **Distraction:** Opposing ends of fracture fragments are not in contact (*e.g.*, secondary to musculotendinous forces, interposed soft tissue); suboptimal for fracture healing.
- **Extra-articular:** Does not penetrate the joint.
- **Fibrous union:** Healing with fibrous tissue rather than bony callus to stabilize fracture.
- **Fracture (fx or #):** Complete or incomplete discontinuity ("break") of bone or cartilage.
- **Impaction:** One fracture fragment is forcibly driven (telescoped) into another adjacent fragment (*e.g.*, Colles' fracture).
- **Incomplete fracture:** Only one cortex of the bone has been broken and the other remains intact.
- **Intra-articular:** Involves articular surface of a joint.
- **Malunion:** Healing of the fracture in an unacceptable position.
- **Nonunion:** Failure of bony union with cessation of healing process.
- **Oblique:** Fracture line is oblique to the long axis of the bone.
- **Open:** Fracture site communicates with ambient environment (old term was "compound").

- **Pathologic:** Fractures occurring in bones that have been weakened by disease (*e.g.,* osteoporosis leading to hip fractures).
- **Pseudoarthrosis:** Nonunion of a fracture resulting in a "false joint," where cartilaginous tissue forms over fracture and fills with fluid.
- **Remodeling:** Reshaping and reorganizing repair tissue to complete successful healing; occurs in skeletally immature patients with healed fractures such that future bony growth will serve to correct bony deformity if it is not rotational in nature. Potential for remodeling is greatest in younger children, with fractures occurring in close proximity to the physis, and if the bony displacement is in the plane of motion of the affected joint.
- **Rotation:** Degree of revolution about the central axis of one fracture fragment relative to another.
- **Segmental:** Comminuted fracture where a long bone is separated into at least three segments.
- **Spiral:** Caused by a torsional force and is akin to an oblique fracture that encircles the long bone.
- **Transverse:** Fracture is perpendicular to the long axis of the bone.
- **Union:** Healing of fracture.

FRACTURE EPONYMS

- **Aviator's astragalus:** General term referring to fracture or fracture-dislocation involving the talus.
- **Barton's fracture:** Dorsal articular margin fracture of the distal radius.
- **Bennett's fracture:** Triangular-shaped intra-articular fracture involving the radial portion of the base of the thumb metacarpal with proximal dislocation of the metacarpal shaft.
- **Boxer's fracture:** Fracture of the neck of the small metacarpal. This term is often incorrectly used to describe a similar fracture in other metacarpal bones.
- **Chance fracture:** Usually caused by a flexion injury to the spine resulting in a sagittally oriented fracture through the posterior spinous process and neural arch exiting the superior articular surface of the involved vertebral body just anterior to the neural foramina (spinal canal).
- **Chauffeur's fracture:** Triangular-shaped oblique articular fracture involving the radial portion of the distal radius.
- **Chopart's fracture and dislocation:** Injury involving the mid-tarsal joints (talonavicular and calcaneocuboid) of the foot.
- **Clay-shoveler's fracture:** Fracture of the posterior spinous process(es) of the lower cervical and/or upper thoracic vertebrae.
- **Colles' fracture:** Comminuted fracture of the distal radius occurring in osteopenic bone as a result of a fall on an outstretched hand, resulting in dorsal angulation of the fracture fragments.
- **Dashboard fracture:** Posterior wall acetabular fracture.

- **Essex-Lopresti fracture:** Comminuted radial head fracture with associated dislocation of the distal radioulnar joint.
- **Galeazzi fracture:** Radius fracture at the junction of the middle and distal thirds with concomitant subluxation of the distal ulna.
- **Greenstick fracture:** Incomplete, angulated fracture that occurs in skeletally immature patients that results in "bowing" of the affected bone, with the affected cortex always occurring on the convex surface.
- **Jones fracture:** Fracture of the base of the small metatarsal occurring at the metaphyseal-diaphyseal junction. The significance is that this is a vascular "watershed" area resulting in an increased propensity to nonunion requiring a short leg cast and non–weight bearing.
- **Lisfranc fracture/dislocation:** Occurring at the tarsometatarsal joint of the foot. There are two types: homolateral (all rays dislocate laterally) and divergent (lesser rays are dislocated laterally).
- **Maisonneuve fracture:** Fracture of the proximal one-third of the fibula associated with rupture of the tibiofibular syndesmosis and fracture of the medial malleolus or rupture of the deltoid ligament.
- **Mallet finger (baseball finger):** Flexion deformity of the distal phalanx resulting from a separation of the common extensor tendon at its insertion at the dorsal base of the distal phalanx with or without an avulsion fracture.
- **March fracture:** Stress or fatigue fracture usually referring to the metatarsals.
- **Monteggia fracture:** Fracture of the proximal third of the ulna with anterior dislocation of the radial head.
- **Nightstick fracture:** Fracture of the ulnar shaft.
- **Piedmont fracture:** Isolated, closed fracture of the radius at the junction of the middle/distal thirds.
- **Rolando fracture:** Y-shaped intra-articular fracture at the base of the thumb metacarpal.
- **Segond fracture (lateral capsular sign):** Avulsion fracture of the lateral capsule off the lateral tibial plateau associated with an ACL injury.
- **Torus fracture ("buckle" fracture):** Incomplete fracture with "buckling" of one cortex predominantly in skeletally immature patients. It usually occurs with a fall on an outstretched hand and is a stable fracture.

CLASSIFICATION SYSTEMS

- **Acromioclavicular joint injuries**
  - Type I: Acromioclavicular (AC) ligament sprain
  - Type II: Partial tear of the AC ligament; sprain of coracoclavicular (CC) ligaments
  - Type III: AC and CC ligaments disrupted with superior displacement of the clavicle < 100% of the width of the clavicle

- Type IV: AC and CC ligaments disrupted with clavicle displaced into or through trapezius
- Type V: As in type III, except that clavicle is displaced superiorly 100%–300%
- Type VI: AC and CC ligaments disrupted with clavicle displaced inferiorly

- **Acromion morphology:** Bigliani et al. (2) described the morphology of the acromion. It is felt that increasing curvature is associated with higher risk for rotator cuff pathology and "impingement." The classification system is based on morphology of the acromion as seen on the supraspinatus outlet (SSO) view radiograph. The increased curvature is most often associated with arthrosis of the acromion.
  - Type 1: Flat acromion
  - Type 2: Curved acromion
  - Type 3: "Hooked" acromion

- **Articular cartilage lesions:** Outerbridge (12) published his classification system for chondromalacia patellae. Today, it is used to classify chondrosis throughout the knee and other joints, as well.
  - **Modified Outerbridge Classification**
    - Grade 1: Cartilage softening and swelling
    - Grade 2: Fragmentation and fissuring < 1 cm in diameter
    - Grade 3: Fragmentation and fissuring > 1 cm in diameter
    - Grade 4: Erosion of cartilage to bone (*i.e.*, full-thickness damage)

- **American Medical Association Ligament Injury Classification**
  - Grade 1: Minor tearing without increase in translation of affected joint (with laxity testing on physical examination)
  - Grade 2: Partial tear with mild-moderate increased translation
  - Grade 3: Complete tear with marked increase in translation

- **Degenerative knee changes:** Fairbank (7) described changes commonly used to grade osteoarthritis of the knee.
  - Grade 0: normal
  - Grade 1: osteoarthritic changes from margin of femoral condyles
  - Grade 2: joint space narrowing
  - Grade 3: flattering of the femoral condyle.

- **Laxity:** Looseness, usually referring to a ligament compared with the normal contralateral side.
  - Grade 1 (1+): up to 5 mm
  - Grade 2 (2+): 6–10 mm
  - Grade 3 (3+): > 10 mm

- **Nerve injuries (Seddon Classification) (15)**
  - Neurapraxia: No structural damage to nerve with complete recovery expected. Although the integrity of the axon is preserved, there is disruption of conduction due to derangement of axonal transport and selective demyelination.

- Axonotmesis: Disruption of the axon and myelin sheath with resulting degeneration of the axon distal to the site of injury; intact endoneurium provides a guide for axonal regeneration with recovery expected.
- Neurotmesis: Partial or complete tear of nerve with disruption of axon, myelin sheath, and connective tissue elements; recovery not expected.

- **Nerve injuries (Sunderland Classification) (17)**
  - Type 1: Neuropraxia: same as Seddon Classification
  - Type 2: Axonotmesis: same as Seddon Classification
  - Type 3: Neurotmesis: loss of nerve fiber continuity with perineurium and epineurium intact
  - Type 4: Neurotmesis: loss of nerve fiber continuity with only epineurium intact
  - Type 5: Neurotmesis: complete transection of nerve

- **Strain (classification)**
  - First degree: Minimal damage to the muscle, tendon, or musculotendinous unit
  - Second degree: Partial tear to the muscle, tendon, or musculotendinous unit
  - Third degree: Complete disruption to the muscle, tendon, or musculotendinous unit

FITNESS TERMS (9)

- **Active commuting:** Traveling to or from work or school by means involving physical activity.
- **Biomarkers:** Specific biochemical indicator of a biologic process, event, or condition (*e.g.*, disease, aging).
- **Cardiometabolic:** Factors that are associated with increased risk of cardiovascular disease and metabolic abnormalities (*i.e.*, obesity, insulin resistance, glucose intolerance, and type 2 diabetes).
- **Energy expenditure:** The total amount of gross energy expended during exercise, including the resting energy expenditure (resting energy expenditure + exercise energy expenditure). Energy expenditure may be calculated in metabolic equivalents (METs), kilocalories, or kilojoules.
- **Exercise:** Physical activity that is planned, structured, and repetitive and that has final or intermediate objective to improve or maintain physical fitness.
- **MET:** An index of energy expenditure. MET is the ratio of the rate of energy expended during an activity to the rate of energy expended at rest (1 MET = the rate of energy expenditure while sitting at rest, which is equal to oxygen uptake of 3.5 mL $\cdot$ kg^{-1} $\cdot$ min^{-1}).
- **MET-minutes:** Index of energy expenditure that quantifies the total amount of physical activity performed in a standardized manner across individuals and types of activities (METs × minutes). Usually standardized per week or per day.

- **Physical activity:** Any bodily movement produced by skeletal muscles that results in energy expenditure above resting (basal) levels; encompasses exercise, sports, and activities as part of daily living, occupation, leisure, and active transportation.

- **Physical fitness:** The ability to carry out daily tasks with vigor and alertness, without undue fatigue, and with ample energy to enjoy leisure pursuits and to meet unforeseen emergencies. Physical fitness is a set of measurable health and skill-related attributes that include cardiorespiratory fitness, muscular strength and endurance, body composition and flexibility, balance, agility, reaction time, and power.

- **Physical function:** The capacity of an individual to carry out the physical activities of daily living. Reflects motor function and control, physical fitness, and habitual physical activity. Is an independent predictor of functional independence, disability, morbidity, and mortality.

- **Sedentary behavior:** Activity that involves little or no movement or physical activity. Energy expenditure of 1–1.5 METs (*e.g.*, sitting, watching television, playing video games, computer use).

REFERENCES

1. Beaty JH, Kasser JR, editors. *Rockwood & Green's Fractures in Children*. 7th ed. Baltimore (MD): Lippincott Williams & Wilkins; 2009. 1096 p.

2. Bigliani LU, Morrison D, April EW. The morphology of the acromion and its relationship to rotator cuff tears. *Orthop Trans*. 1986;10:228.

3. Bucholz R, Heckman J, Court-Brown C, Tornetta P. *Rockwood & Green's Fractures in Adults*. 7th ed. Baltimore (MD): Lippincott Williams & Wilkins; 2009. 2296 p.

4. DeLee JC, Drez D, editors. *Orthopaedic Sports Medicine: Principles and Practices*. 3rd ed. Philadelphia (PA): Elsevier Science; 2009. 2392 p.

5. Dorland WA, editor. *Dorland's Illustrated Medical Dictionary*. 31st ed. New York (NY): W. B. Saunders; 2007. 1724 p.

6. Ebell MH, Siwek J, Weiss BD, et al. Strength of Recommendation Taxonomy (SORT): a patient-centered approach to grading evidence in the medical literature. *Am Fam Physician*. 2004;69(3):548–56.

7. Fairbank TJ. Knee joint changes after meniscectomy. *J Bone Joint Surg Br*. 1948;30B(4):664–70.

8. Firestein G, Budd R, Harris E, McInnes I, Ruddy S, Sergent J. *Kelley's Textbook of Rheumatology*. 8th ed. Philadelphia (PA): Saunders Elsevier; 2009. 2064 p.

9. Garber C, Blissmer B, Deschenes M, et al. quantity and quality of exercise for developing and maintaining cardiorespiratory, musculoskeletal, and neuromotor fitness in apparently healthy adults: guidance for prescribing exercise. *Med Sci Sports Exerc*. 2011;43(10):1334–59.

10. Gordis L. *Epidemiology*. 3rd ed. Philadelphia (PA): Saunders Elsevier; 2004. 335 p.

11. Helms CL. *Fundamentals of Skeletal Radiology*. 2nd ed. New York (NY): W. B. Saunders; 1995.

12. Outerbridge RE. The etiology of chondromalacia of the patellae. *J Bone Joint Surg Br*. 1961;43(B):752–7.

13. Peerbooms J, Sluimer J, Bruijn D, Gosens T. Positive effect of an autologous platelet concentrate in lateral epicondylitis in a double-blind randomized controlled trial, platelet-rich plasma versus corticosteroid injection with a 1-year follow-up. *Am J Sports Med*. 2010;38(2):255–62.

14. Porta M, editor. *A Dictionary of Epidemiology*. 5th ed. New York (NY): Oxford University Press; 2008. 316 p.

15. Seddon JH. Three types of nerve injury. *Brain*. 1943;66(4):237–88.

16. Sharma P, Maffulli N. Tendon injury and tendinopathy: healing and repair. *J Bone Joint Surg Am*. 2005;87(1):187–202.

17. Sunderland S. A classification of peripheral nerve injuries producing loss of function. *Brain*. 1951;74(4):491–516.

Basics in Exercise Physiology

Patricia A. Deuster and Selasi Attipoe

5

SKELETAL MUSCLE PHYSIOLOGY

Skeletal Muscle Fibers

Basic Units

- The basic units of skeletal muscle include sarcomeres, myofilaments, myofibrils (basic units of contraction), muscle fibers (cells), fascicles (bundles of about 150 muscle fibers each), and a muscle (Fig. 5.1). Sarcomeres, areas from Z line to Z line and functional contraction units of myofibrils, contain two types of myofilaments: thick (myosin) and thin (actin) myofilaments, which are repeated throughout muscle myofibrils.

- Other structures within sarcomeres are I bands, A bands, H zones (absence of actin), and M bands (sarcomere's center). Transverse tubules (T tubules; see Excitation-Contraction Coupling), found at the A-I junction of sarcomeres, and the sarcoplasmic reticulum (SR) are the primary regulators of calcium influx into muscle units. The sarcolemma is the muscle cell membrane.

- Satellite cells are muscle "stem" cells. They are activated to a full cell cycle from the quiescent state in response to heavy resistance training and cell damage. Activation of satellite cells is necessary for normal growth and regeneration of tissue damage. Insulin growth factor-1 (IGF-1) is a primary regulator of satellite cells (27,28).

Muscle Proteins

- Key muscle proteins include actin, myosin, troponin, and tropomyosin. Actin and myosin constitute myofilaments within myofibrils; myosin is the site of adenosine triphosphate (ATP) binding. Troponin complexes on actin molecules are the calcium binding sites for initiating contraction. Tropomyosin, found in thin filaments of muscle fibers, inhibits contraction until modified by troponin.

Muscular Contraction

Motor Neurons

- Alpha and gamma motor neurons initiate and regulate muscle contraction. Alpha motor neurons initiate contractions in contractile (extrafusal) fibers, whereas gamma neurons innervate muscle spindle (intrafusal) fibers of muscle.

Motor Unit

- Motor units (basic functional unit of movement) consist of alpha motor neurons, synaptic junctions (motor endplate), and the muscle fibers they innervate.

- One motor neuron can innervate 10 to several thousand muscle fibers. Release of acetylcholine by neurons initiates contraction, and degradation of acetylcholine by cholinesterase terminates action potentials.

Excitation-Contraction Coupling

- Muscle contraction is triggered by an electrical impulse involving acetylcholine release, arrival of the impulse at the sarcolemma (after crossing the synaptic junction), and subsequent entry of calcium into myofibrils. Electrical impulses travel quickly into the interior of muscle cells, down the T tubules with release of calcium from the SR to myofibrils.

- Once calcium stores are released from the SR, a nonstoppable contraction is initiated: Calcium entry activates crossbridge linkages and contraction of sarcomeres.

- *Sliding-Filament Theory:* This theory states that muscle contraction occurs when two major myofilaments (actin and myosin) slide past one another through a series of crossbridge linkages. Myosin crossbridge linkages combine, detach, and recombine in an oscillatory pattern such that at any point in time about 50% of myosin heads are attached to actin binding sites. No myofilament actually changes length.

- *All or None Law:* A motor neuron initiating an action potential will contract all muscle fibers innervated by that motor neuron simultaneously. Muscle fibers achieve gradation of contraction strength by recruiting fewer or more motor neurons to initiate contraction and/or by changing the frequency of action potentials to sustain contractions.

Sensory Receptors

- *Muscle Spindles:* These specialized intrafusal muscle fibers are located between and among extrafusal fibers deep within the interior of muscles. These proprioceptors sense and relay the length or velocity of muscle movement (*e.g.,* patellar reflex).

- *Golgi Tendon Organs:* These sensory organs detect differences in tension and muscle length. Although quiescent during

The opinions and assertions expressed herein are those of the authors and should not be construed as reflecting those of the Uniformed Services University of the Health Sciences or the Department of Defense.

Figure 5.1: Basic anatomy and structure of skeletal muscle. Reprinted with permission from http://www.medicdirect.com and http://www.medicdirect.co.uk.

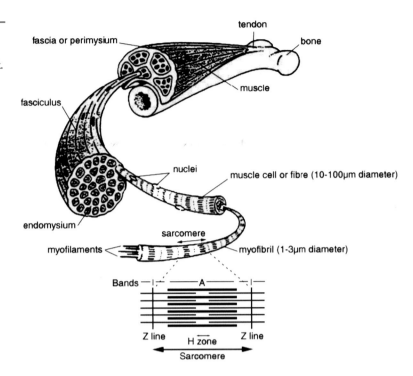

periods of slow to moderate muscle activity, they increase discharge when muscle load is excessive; they protect against injury due to overloading.

Skeletal Muscle Fiber Types

■ Skeletal muscle fiber types are characterized by differences in morphology, histochemistry, enzyme activity, surface characteristics, and functional capacity (17–19,23,24,27) (Table 5.1).

■ Human muscle fiber types include Type I, IIa, and IIx, due to the expression of different myosin heavy chain (MHC) forms (18,21,22,24).

■ Distribution of Type I (slow twitch) and Type II (fast twitch) fibers within normal populations depends on many factors

Table 5.1	Characteristics of Major Skeletal Muscle Fiber Types*		
Fiber Characteristics	**Slow Twitch**	**Fast Twitch**	
	Type I	Type IIa	Type IIx
Other Terminology	Slow Oxidative (SO)	Fast Oxidative Glycolytic (FOG)	Fast Glycolytic (FG)
Aerobic Capacity	High	Med/High	Low
Glycolytic Capacity	Low	High	High
Myoglobin Content	High	Med	Low
Color	Red	Red	Pink/White
Fatigue Resistance	High	Med	Low
Glycogen Content	Low	Med	High
Triglyceride Content	High	Med	Low
Time to Peak Tension	Slow	Med	High
Myosin ATPase Activity	Low	Med	Med
Myosin Heavy Chain (MHC)	MHCIβ	MHCIIa	MHCIIx
Tension Cost*	Low	Med	Med
ATP/ADP	Low	Med	Med

ADP, adenosine diphosphate; ATP, adenosine triphosphate; Med, medium.
This chart represents current nomenclature for human skeletal muscle fiber types. Type IIb human muscle fibers are currently referred to as Type IIx because of the MHCIIx isoform found in human muscle. Type IIb muscle fibers are found in rodents and other species, with MHCIIb (19,21–23).
*Tension cost = ATPase activity to isometric tension ratio.

and shows extraordinary adaptive potential in response to innervation/neuronal activity, hormones, neural signaling, training, functional demands, and aging (19).

- Muscle fiber types appear to change in response to these effectors in a sequential manner from either slow to fast or fast to slow (6,8,19).

BASIC DEFINITIONS IN EXERCISE PHYSIOLOGY

Pulmonary Ventilation

- Minute ventilation ($\dot{V}E$) is the total volume of air moved into and out of the lungs each minute; it is a function of *tidal volume* (V_T) and *respiratory rate* (f_B).
- At rest, $\dot{V}E$ is between 5 and 7 L · min^{-1}, whereas during exercise it increases to between 60 and 180 L · min^{-1}, depending on the health of the person (Fig. 5.2). V_T increases by expanding both inspiratory and expiratory volumes; these "extra" volumes are called inspiratory and expiratory reserve volumes (IRV and ERV), respectively. The increase in V_T allows $\dot{V}E$ to increase 5- to 10-fold during exercise. An increase in f_B further augments $\dot{V}E$ (1,2,26).

Maximal Voluntary Ventilation (MVV)

- MVV is the volume of air exchanged during repeated maximal respirations in a specified time (10–15 seconds). It is expressed as L · min^{-1} and represents a measure of maximum breathing capacity for comparing to maximal $\dot{V}E$ during exercise ($\dot{V}E_{max}$).

Breathing Reserve (BR)

- BR is the difference between MVV and $\dot{V}E_{max}$ and is sometimes expressed as $\dot{V}E_{max}$/MVV; it is the additional ventilation available during maximal exercise. If a person achieves maximal

work capacity prior to attaining MVV, the person has a normal BR, whereas if MVV = $\dot{V}E$, the person may have compromised pulmonary function. A typical BR is 11 L · min^{-1}, with normal $\dot{V}E_{max}$/MVV ranging between 60% and 75%.

Oxygen Uptake ($\dot{V}O_2$)

- Oxygen uptake ($\dot{V}O_2$), based on the Fick equation, can be expressed as: $\dot{V}O_2 = CO \times (a - vO_2) = HR \times SV \times (a - vO_2)$, where CO is cardiac output, $a - vO_2$ is arteriovenous O_2 content difference, SV is stroke volume, and HR is heart rate. For an average 70-kg adult, CO is about 5 L · min^{-1} at rest and can increase to 20 to 30 L · min^{-1} during strenuous exercise.
- $\dot{V}O_2$, determined during exercise by measuring respiratory gases, is related to the fractional percent of O_2 in inspired and expired air and $\dot{V}E$. Inspired air contains 20.93% O_2 and expired air around 17.0%.
- $\dot{V}O_2$ is usually expressed in absolute units (L · min^{-1}) or relative to body weight (mL · kg^{-1} · min^{-1}). Resting $\dot{V}O_2$ ranges from 0.25 to 0.4 L · min^{-1}, and maximal exercise $\dot{V}O_2$ values can exceed 5.0 L · min^{-1} (15–70 mL · kg^{-1} · min^{-1}) (Fig. 5.2). Higher relative values indicate higher aerobic fitness.

Carbon Dioxide Production ($\dot{V}CO_2$)

- Carbon dioxide (CO_2) is produced metabolically in tissues, transported in blood by venous return to the lung, and eliminated from the lung by breathing ($\dot{V}E$). Inspired air contains 0.03% CO_2 and expired air about 5% CO_2.
- Like $\dot{V}O_2$, $\dot{V}CO_2$ is usually expressed as L · min^{-1} or mL · kg^{-1} · min^{-1}. Resting and strenuous exercise values depend on metabolism and pulmonary function, but resting values are less than $\dot{V}O_2$.

Lactate

- Lactate, a product of glycolysis, is formed from pyruvate in the recycling of nicotinamide adenine dinucleotide (NAD+),

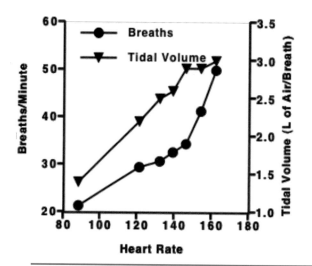
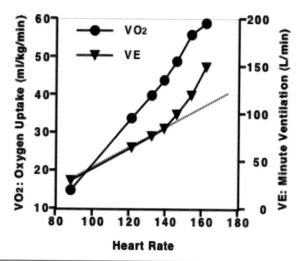

Figure 5.2: Tidal volume and breathing rate (left panel) and oxygen uptake and minute ventilation (right panel) in response to progressive maximal treadmill exercise. Dotted line through $\dot{V}E$ in right panel indicates departure from linearity.

or when the rate of pyruvate formation in the cytosol exceeds its rate of use by mitochondria. Lactate formation depends on the availability of pyruvate and NADH.

- Blood lactate at rest is 0.8 to 1.5 mM, but can exceed 18 mM during intense exercise.
- Muscle cells release lactate into the circulation during exercise, where it becomes a fuel for the heart and nonexercising muscles. Lactate released from the muscle can be converted to glucose in the liver by the Cori cycle.

Oxygen Pulse (O_2 pulse)

- O_2 pulse ($mL \cdot beat^{-1}$), or the ratio of $\dot{V}O_2$ ($mL \cdot min^{-1}$) to heart rate (bpm) when both measures are obtained simultaneously, is the product of stroke volume and a $- vO_2$ difference [see equation under Oxygen Uptake ($\dot{V}O_2$)].
- O_2 pulse increases with increasing work effort (range 4–30 $mL \cdot beat^{-1}$) and is affected by various factors, including anemia and heart disease. A low value during exercise indicates heart rate is too high for $\dot{V}O_2$ and may suggest heart disease (26).

Respiratory Quotient (RQ)/Respiratory Exchange Ratio (RER)

- RQ, the ratio of CO_2 produced by cellular metabolism to O_2 used by tissues, is used to quantify the relative amounts of carbohydrate and fatty acids being oxidized for energy. The RQ cannot exceed 1.0; an RQ of 0.7 implies dependence on free fatty acids, and a value of 1.0 indicates dependence on carbohydrate.
- RER represents pulmonary exchange of CO_2 and O_2 at rest and during exercise; it ranges between 0.7 and 1.0 during steady state exercise. RER often exceeds 1.0 during strenuous exercise because of increasing metabolic activity not matched by $\dot{V}O_2$ and additional CO_2 derived from bicarbonate buffering of lactate.
- The terms RQ and RER are often used interchangeably, but their distinction is important.

Ventilatory Equivalents ($\dot{V}E/\dot{V}O_2$ and $\dot{V}E/\dot{V}CO_2$)

- Ventilatory equivalents are unitless numbers derived from the ratio of $\dot{V}E$ to $\dot{V}O_2$ and $\dot{V}CO_2$. $\dot{V}E/\dot{V}O_2$ indicates the volume (L) of air required to use 1 L of O_2, and $\dot{V}E/\dot{V}CO_2$ indicates the appropriateness of ventilation (L of air required to remove 1 L of CO_2).
- During maximal exercise testing, $\dot{V}E$ is linearly related to $\dot{V}O_2$ and $\dot{V}CO_2$, but at high exercise intensities, $\dot{V}E$ increases more rapidly than $\dot{V}O_2$, and thus $\dot{V}E/\dot{V}O_2$ begins to increase, which is followed by an increase in $\dot{V}E/\dot{V}CO_2$. These increases reflect respiratory compensation for the corresponding rise in blood lactate (26).

Maximal Heart Rate

- The highest heart rate achieved during a standardized maximal exercise test is the maximal heart rate. If an exercise test

is not possible, then age-predicted heart rate formulas can be used. Two formulas for maximal heart rate are $208 - 0.7 \times$ age and $220 -$ age.
- The first formula, $208 - 0.7 \times$ age, is being recommended by the American College of Sports Medicine® (1) because it is more accurate for persons up to 80 years and independent of gender and habitual physical activity (25).
- An estimated maximal heart rate may be 5%–10% (10–20 bpm) higher or lower than the actual value.

Heart Rate Reserve (HRR)

- The difference between maximal heart rate during maximal exercise and resting heart rate is the HRR. If maximal heart rate is 205 bpm and resting heart rate is 55 bpm, then HRR would be $205 - 55 = 150$ bpm. The smaller the difference, the lower is the reserve and the narrower is the range for exercise.

Target Training Heart Rate

- A training program requires calculating a target heart range. To calculate the lower and upper target heart rates of the range, 60%–90% of maximal heart rate or 50%–85% of HRR can be used. For the first approach, the lower 60% and the upper 90% of the target heart rate range are determined as:

  $0.60 \times$ maximal heart rate (bpm) and $0.90 \times$ maximal heart rate (bpm)

- For the HRR or Karvonen formula, which may be a more valid approach, 50% and 85% of HRR are used for the lower and upper range:

  $0.50 \times$ HRR + resting heart rate and $0.85 \times$ HRR + resting heart rate

Muscular Contractions

Isometric/Static Contractions

- Isometric contractions refer to muscle fiber recruitment: No change in fiber length takes place, and no joint or limb motion occurs. Examples of isometric contractions are a person holding a weight in a particular position and postural stability.

Isotonic/Dynamic Contractions

- Isotonic contractions are when muscle fibers change length and movement at joints occurs. Specific types of dynamic contractions include *concentric*, *eccentric*, and *isokinetic*.
- *Concentric* contractions are movements where muscle fibers shorten as the muscle contracts, such as when a weight is being lifted. This is also known as positive work.
- When the direction is reversed and the weight is lowered, the contraction becomes an *eccentric* contraction (negative work), where muscle fibers lengthen as the muscle contracts. More fast twitch motor units are activated during eccentric contractions.

Isokinetic Contractions

- Isokinetic machines make these contractions possible: The muscular movement is performed at constant speed against a variable resistance. The applied resistance during the contraction is increased or lowered at various points across the full range of motion so a constant speed of movement can be maintained. Diagnostic strength equipment uses isokinetic tension to make more accurate measurements of strength at varying joint angles.

Borg Scale or Rating of Perceived Exertion (RPE)

- An RPE scale is used by an individual to rate his or her own "degree of physical strain." The original Borg scale ranges from 6 to 20, with each number anchored by a simple verbal expression (no exertion at all to maximum exertion). Also, a person exercising at 130 bpm is expected to report an RPE of 13, whereas a person exercising very strenuously and reporting an RPE of 19 is expected to have a heart rate around 190 bpm.

MEASUREMENTS OF ENERGY, WORK, AND POWER

Definitions of Energy, Work, and Power

- Physical exercise involves both mechanical and chemical work by the muscles; the degree of muscular effort depends on duration, frequency, and intensity. Together, these define energy, work, and power.
- *Energy:* The capacity to do work, with energy measured in joules (J): 4.186 J $= 1 \times 10^{-4}$ kcal and 1 J $= 2.3889 \times 10^{-4}$ kcal.
- *Work:* When a force acts against resistance to produce motion: Force $\times$ Distance. Work is often expressed in kilogram-meters or kgm, where 1 kcal $= 426.85$ kgm $= 4.186$ kJ.
- *Power:* Rate at which work is performed or the rate of energy transfer: Work/Time. Power is usually expressed as watts (W), where 1 W $= 1$ J $\cdot$ s^{-1}; 6.12 kpm $\cdot$ min^{-1}; and 0.01433 kcal $\cdot$ min^{-1}.

Energy Expenditure (EE)

- EE is usually determined by direct or indirect calorimetry. For direct calorimetry, both external work and heat output are measured, and heat production is used as an estimate of metabolic rate. For indirect calorimetry, either open or closed circuit spirometry can be used. With open circuit spirometry, $\dot{V}O_2$ and $\dot{V}CO_2$ are measured and the RER is calculated.
- To derive EE, add 4 to RER and then multiply by liters of $O_2 \cdot$ min^{-1} or $(4 + RER) \times O_2 \cdot$ min^{-1}. For example, if $\dot{V}O_2$ and RER determined from gas analysis were 0.3 L of $O_2 \cdot$ min^{-1} and 0.75 at rest and 2.5 L $\cdot$ min^{-1} and 0.95 during exercise, then EE at rest would be $(4.0 + 0.75) \times 0.3 =$ 1.4 kcal $\cdot$ min^{-1} and EE during exercise would be $(4.0 + 0.95) \times 2.5 = 12.4$ kcal $\cdot$ min^{-1}. Net EE would be $12.4 - 1.4$, or 11.0 kcal $\cdot$ min^{-1}.
- EE can also be estimated from $\dot{V}O_2$ by assuming 1 L of O_2 is approximately 5 kcal. If resting $\dot{V}O_2$ was 0.3 L $\cdot$ min^{-1}, energy costs would be (0.3×5) 1.5 kcal $\cdot$ min^{-1}.

Work Efficiency

- Gross work efficiency is the ratio of mechanical work output to energy expended; it typically ranges between 15% and 30%.
- Net work efficiency is the ratio of mechanical work output to total energy expended minus resting EE.
- Example: A woman with a resting $\dot{V}O_2$ of 0.3 L $\cdot$ min^{-1} rides a cycle ergometer for 30 minutes at 150 W (1 W $= 0.01433$ kcal $\cdot$ min^{-1}) and uses 2 L $O_2 \cdot$ min^{-1}.
  - *Mechanical work output:* 150 W $\times 0.01433 = 2.1$ kcal $\cdot$ min^{-1} or 63 kcal.
  - *Total energy expended:* 2 L $\cdot$ min$^{-1} \sim 10$ kcal $\cdot$ min$^{-1} \times 30 = 300$ kcal.
  - *Gross efficiency:* $63/300 = 21\%$.
  - *Resting EE:* 1.5 kcal $\cdot$ min^{-1}, or total of 45 kcal.
  - *Net efficiency:* $63/(300 - 45) = 24.7\%$.
- Factors influencing exercise efficiency include work rate, speed of movement, muscle fiber composition, and various biomechanical factors, such as equipment and clothing.

Exercise Economy

- Economy of movement is the efficiency of converting metabolic power into mechanical power/velocity. It is defined in terms of $\dot{V}O_2$ (energy required) for a specific power output or velocity (mL $\cdot$ min$^{-1} \cdot$ W^{-1} or mL $\cdot$ kg$^{-1} \cdot$ min^{-1} to km $\cdot$ min^{-1} or mile $\cdot$ min^{-1}). The more efficient a person is, the more power/velocity he or she can generate for the same $\dot{V}O_2$ cost.
- Selected factors affecting economy include age; body mass; heart rate; ventilatory rate; basal metabolic differences; leg length, stride frequency, and other biomechanical variations; shoes for running; aerodynamic positioning for cycling; and velocity. Values may range from 200 to 350 mL $\cdot$ kg$^{-1} \cdot$ km^{-1} for running and 10–15 mL $\cdot$ W^{-1} for cycling (10).

Metabolic Energy Equivalents (MET)

- MET is the energy cost of activities in multiples of resting metabolic rate. If 1 MET (resting metabolic rate) is taken as 3.5 mL of $O_2 \cdot$ kg$^{-1} \cdot$ min^{-1}, then 3 MET would be 10.5 mL $\cdot$ kg$^{-1} \cdot$ min^{-1}. These units are used by the Centers for Disease Control and Prevention to recommend exercise intensity.
- Energy expenditure for activities such as eating, dressing, and walking around the house range from 1 to 4 MET, whereas the cost of climbing a flight of stairs, walking on level ground, scrubbing floors, or playing a game of golf ranges from 4 to 10 MET. Strenuous sports, such as swimming, singles tennis, and football, often exceed 10 MET.

BASIC CONCEPTS IN AEROBIC AND ANAEROBIC EXERCISE

Maximal Aerobic Power

- Maximal aerobic power, or $\dot{V}O_{2max}$, is the greatest amount of O_2 a person can consume during physical exercise. It characterizes the functional capacity of the cardiovascular, pulmonary, and O_2 transport systems, and is considered "power" because it is a rate: L of $O_2 \cdot min^{-1}$.

- If two individuals had absolute $\dot{V}O_{2max}$ values of 4.2 and 3.2 $L \cdot min^{-1}$ and both weighed 70 kg, then normalizing for body weight would yield values of 60 and 45.7 $mL \cdot kg^{-1} \cdot min^{-1}$, respectively. If person 1 weighed 70 kg and person 2 weighed 53 kg, then normalized $\dot{V}O_{2max}$ values would be 60 $mL \cdot kg^{-1} \cdot min^{-1}$ for both persons. $\dot{V}O_{2max}$ values above 50 $mL \cdot kg^{-1} \cdot min^{-1}$ are considered high.

Testing for Maximal Aerobic Power

- The best tests for measuring $\dot{V}O_{2max}$ are incremental and progressive tests.

- $\dot{V}O_{2max}$ is measured by treadmill walking/running, cycle or arm ergometry, and step tests.

- Requirements for a valid maximal exercise test are as follows: standardized test conditions, involvement of large muscle groups, measurable and reproducible rates of work, little or no skill required, and tolerated by most people. Also, motivation should not be a major factor.

- Concept of plateau: During a progressive exercise test, when a step increase in work results in either no or a minimal increase in $\dot{V}O_2$, then $\dot{V}O_2$ has begun to level off. The leveling off or plateauing effect is considered the single best criterion for attaining a true $\dot{V}O_{2max}$.

- Criteria for achieving $\dot{V}O_{2max}$: If a leveling off or plateauing of $\dot{V}O_2$ is not seen, then at least two of the following criteria should be met for a true $\dot{V}O_{2max}$ test: blood lactate levels above 7 or 8 mM; heart rate equal to or within 15 beats of the age-estimated maximal heart rate; RER $\geq$ 1.15; and/or RPE $\geq$ 17.

- $\dot{V}O_{2peak}$: When an exercise test is terminated and the criteria described are not met, the highest $\dot{V}O_2$ achieved is referred to as $\dot{V}O_2$ peak ($\dot{V}O_{2peak}$).

- Ventilatory threshold: The point where $\dot{V}E$ begins to increase disproportionately to $\dot{V}O_2$ during incremental exercise testing.

- $\dot{V}O_{2max}$ can be estimated by using the linear relation between heart rate and $\dot{V}O_2$. Heart rates at submaximal work rates can be plotted against $\dot{V}O_2$, and then estimated maximal heart rate can be used to extrapolate to $\dot{V}O_{2max}$. Cycle tests are most appropriate because $\dot{V}O_2$ values can be defined as a function of watts (Table 5.2). Walking tests, step tests, endurance runs, and nonexercise data can also be used to estimate $\dot{V}O_{2max}$. Potential errors exist for all of these estimates, and care must be taken when interpreting these data.

Table 5.2	Expected $\dot{V}O_2$ Values at Designated Power Between 1 and 3 Minutes with Cycle Ergometry	
Power (Watts)	**Approximate Oxygen Uptake (L $\cdot$ min^{-1})**
50	0.9
100	1.5
150	2.1
200	2.8
250	3.5
300	4.2
350	5.0
400	5.7

Determinants of and Factors Affecting $\dot{V}O_{2max}$

- *Intrinsic and extrinsic factors:* Intrinsic factors affecting $\dot{V}O_{2max}$ include genetics, gender, body composition/muscle mass, age, and existing pathologies. Extrinsic factors include training/activity levels, dietary intake (alcohol, caffeine), nutritional and hydration status, and environmental conditions.

- *Determinants:* All systems serving a role in delivering O_2 can affect $\dot{V}O_{2max}$. Central factors include cardiac output, pulmonary ventilation, arterial pressure, hemoglobin (Hb) content, O_2 diffusion into and through the lungs, alveolar ventilation: perfusion ratio, and Hb-O_2 affinity. Peripheral determinants include muscle blood flow, capillary density, O_2 diffusion to and extraction by muscle cells, Hb-O_2 affinity, and skeletal muscle fiber profiles.

Aerobic and Anaerobic Exercise

Exercise Domains

- Three specific exercise domains have been suggested by Gaesser and Poole (7): moderate, heavy, and severe. Figure 5.3 depicts the domains for an incremental exercise test and constant load tests at three workloads. In panel 1, lactate threshold (T_{Lac}) represents the boundary between the moderate and heavy domain, and critical power (W_a) represents the boundary for the severe domain. These concepts are described below.

- Lactate threshold: T_{Lac} represents the lowest exercise intensity that can be maintained where blood lactate appearance exceeds removal and is sustained at about 1 mM above preexercise levels. Also known as aerobic T_{Lac}.

- Maximal lactate at steady state (MLSS): MLSS is the highest blood lactate concentration that can be sustained without progressive accumulation: A new steady state is achieved (between 3 and 8 mM). The upper boundary of the heavy domain likely demarcates MLSS. Also known as anaerobic T_{Lac}.

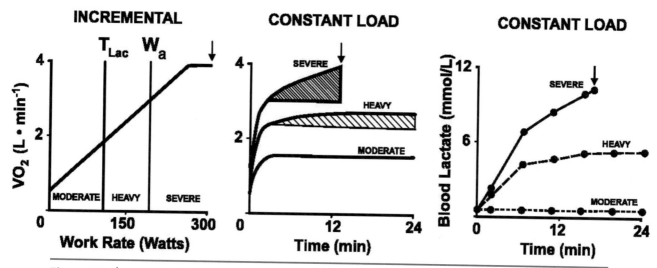

Figure 5.3: $\dot{V}O_2$ responses to incremental exercise (left panel), and $\dot{V}O_2$ (middle panel) and blood lactate (right panel) responses to constant load exercise as a function of exercise intensity domains. T_{Lac} represents the lactate threshold, and W_a represents critical power or work rate where maximal lactate at steady state occurs. Reprinted with permission from D.C. Poole (7,20).

- Critical power (W_a): W_a is the maximum power output that can be sustained without a continued and progressive anaerobic contribution. Exercise above W_a will elicit $\dot{V}O_{2max}$.

- Onset of blood lactate accumulation (OBLA): At a specific exercise intensity, muscle lactate production exceeds utilization and blood lactate begins to accumulate. W_a, MLSS, and OBLA may all demarcate transition between heavy and severe exercise domains.

- Steady state exercise: When lactate production is balanced by the rate of oxidative removal and $\dot{V}O_2$ is stabilized within 3–6 minutes. Cardiac output, heart rate, and pulmonary gas exchange are in a steady state and exercise can continue for an extended period of time.

- Maximal accumulated oxygen deficit (MAOD): The difference between the accumulated oxygen demand and the accumulated oxygen uptake of the exercise bout.

- Slow component of oxygen uptake: A continued rise in $\dot{V}O_2$ beyond the third minute when exercise is above the T_{Lac}. The rise in $\dot{V}O_2$ (see Fig. 5.3) usually stabilizes within 20 minutes when exercise is within the heavy domain or gradually increases to $\dot{V}O_{2max}$ when exercise is within the severe domain. The slow component may indicate additional recruitment of muscle fibers (3,7,11–13).

- Velocity at $\dot{V}O_{2max}$ ($v\dot{V}O_{2max}$) is the minimal running velocity that elicits $\dot{V}O_{2max}$. It is considered the best indicator of endurance performance (9,14–16).

Oxygen Kinetics

- Oxygen deficit or MAOD: When an individual begins to exercise, a certain $\dot{V}O_2$ is required that cannot immediately be met aerobically. $\dot{V}O_2$ gradually increases until it reaches a steady state. The MAOD is calculated by subtracting the accumulated $\dot{V}O_2$ (measured during the exercise bout) from the estimated accumulated $\dot{V}O_2$ demand (11).

- Oxygen debt: Upon termination of exercise, $\dot{V}O_2$ remains elevated to restore energy systems to their preexercise states, after having "borrowed" ATP at the beginning of exercise. The term, O_2 debt, was coined by A.V. Hill in the early 1900s, but is transitioning to EPOC (see below).

- Excess postexercise oxygen consumption (EPOC): EPOC is the integral of $\dot{V}O_2$ during recovery after terminating exercise. It consists of a fast and slow component and is highly correlated with exercise intensity. The fast portion may indicate resynthesis of stored phosphocreatine and restoration of muscle and blood O_2 stores. The slow component may represent elevated body temperature, catecholamines, accelerated metabolism (conversion of lactic acid to glucose/gluconeogenesis), and other hormonal/metabolic processes.

Resistance Exercise

- Resistance exercise is used to improve muscular strength, endurance, and power. Strength is the greatest force a muscle can exert in one effort; endurance is the muscle's ability to make repeated efforts; and power is a measure of how quickly muscular strength can be applied.

Weight Training Parameters

- When training with weights, the magnitudes of increase in muscle strength and endurance depend on specific training parameters: repetitions, sets, volume, and intensity.

- *Repetition maximum (RM)* is the amount of force a person can lift a given number of times (repetitions). For example, 5-RM is the maximal force the person could lift five times.

- *Repetitions* are the number of consecutive times a particular weight is lifted without a rest period. For examples, repetitions could be 5, 10, 12, 25, or 50.

- *Sets:* The number of sets delineates how many repetitions are repeated after a rest period. For example, a training session could consist of three sets of 12 repetitions.

- *Volume* equates to the total number of times a weight was lifted (Sets × Repetitions). For example, for three sets of 12 repetitions with 50 lb, the volume would be 3 × 12 × 50, or 1,800 lb. Volume indicates how much work was done: The greater the volume, the greater is the total work.

- *Intensity* depends on the actual resistance lifted and is expressed as a percent of maximum weight (1-RM). If 1-RM for an exercise is 80 kg, then weights of 40 and 60 kg would approximate 50% and 75% intensities, respectively.

Resistance Training Concepts

- *SAID (specific adaptation to imposed demand):* The specificity principle states that physiological, neurological, and psychological adaptations to training are specific to the "imposed demand." For example, to develop speed or power, the imposed demand must target those areas.

- *Strength-endurance continuum:* A weight training concept based on the premise that muscle strength and muscle endurance exist on a continuum, with muscle strength being 1-RM and muscle endurance representing the ability to exert a lower force repeatedly over time. Low numbers of repetitions (6- to 10-RM) are associated with increases in strength, and high numbers (20- to 100-RM) are associated with increases in endurance. As repetitions increase, we transition from strength to endurance.

- *Muscle hypertrophy:* Compensatory growth in skeletal muscle in response to an imposed load. The initial adaptation to an increased load is a neural response followed by an increase in muscle size.

- Muscle hypertrophy may take 2 months to begin. New contractile proteins appear to be incorporated into existing myofibrils, and there may be a limit to how large a myofibril can become: They may split at some point. Hypertrophy results primarily from growth of each muscle cell, rather than an increase in the number of cells.

- Muscle hypertrophy is observed in all three major fiber types (Types I, IIa, and IIx or Type IIb) when low, but not high, numbers of repetitions are performed. Physiological adaptations and performance are linked to both the volume and intensity of resistance training.

Biomechanical Factors in Muscle Strength

- Neural control, muscle cross-sectional area, arrangement of muscle fibers, muscle length, joint angle, velocity of muscle contraction, joint angular velocity, strength-to-mass ratio, body size, joint motion (joint mobility, dexterity, flexibility, limberness, range of motion), point of tendon insertion, and the interactions of these factors influence muscle strength.

Delayed Onset Muscle Soreness (DOMS)

- DOMS is a term used to describe temporary soreness that results primarily from eccentric exercise and resistance training. It is usually noted the day after the exercise and may last 3–4 days (4,5).

- Factors that may elicit DOMS include inflammation, osmotic changes within muscle tissue, microtrauma to the tissue, and/ or alterations in calcium metabolism.

Plyometrics

- Plyometrics is a specific method of training for power or explosiveness. Most plyometric exercises involve jumping, bounding, and hopping. The force generated by a lengthening contraction (eccentric) can be markedly increased if it is followed by a shortening contraction (concentric).

EXERCISE TRAINING

Principles of Training

- *FITT:* This is an acronym to describe physical training variables that can be altered to achieve various fitness goals. FITT stands for Frequency, Intensity, Time (duration), and Type of exercise.

- *Overload:* The overload principle states that gains in strength/ endurance come about only when progressively greater demands are placed on cardiopulmonary and musculoskeletal systems.

- *Periodization:* The altering of training variables (repetitions/ set, exercises performed, volume, rest interval between sets) to achieve well-defined training goals and performance gains.

- *Quantifying exercise intensity:* Exercise intensity can be estimated from METs, percent of maximal heart rate, percent of $\dot{V}O_{2max}$, or RPE.

- *Absolute and relative intensity:* If two individuals (Tom and Mark) have $\dot{V}O_{2max}$ values of 4.2 and 3.2 L $\cdot$ min^{-1}, respectively, and both work at 2.5 L $\cdot$ min^{-1}, they would be working at the same absolute power output, but at different relative intensities because of different $\dot{V}O_{2max}$ values. Tom would be working at 2.5/4.2 or 60% and Mark at 2.5/3.2 or 78% of $\dot{V}O_{2max}$.

Adaptations to Training

Endurance Training

- Adaptations to endurance exercise include improvements in neuromuscular and cardiovascular function, respiratory muscle efficiency and cost of breathing, decreases in body mass/body fat, improvements in heat tolerance, increases in self-esteem, lower blood lactate accumulation at higher power outputs, and increased insulin sensitivity.

Resistance Training

- Resistance training induces a variety of adaptations, with clear increases in strength.

- Neural adaptations include increases in strength with or without hypertrophy, greater synchronicity in activating motor units, and increased density of presynaptic and postsynaptic neurotransmitter receptors.

- Contractile adaptations include muscle hypertrophy through increased synthesis and accretion of intracellular myofibrillar proteins and activation of local satellite cells to add new nuclei to existing myofibers.

- Fiber type–specific adaptations depend on volume and intensity, but a common change is an increase in the percentage of Type IIa fibers, at the expense of Type IIx fibers.

- Resistance training is not usually associated with increases in $\dot{V}O_{2max}$, but may enhance cardiovascular function by improving strength and lessening the daily load.

ESTIMATING STRENGTH AND ENDURANCE

Aerobic and Anaerobic Power

- Simple in-office and field tests can be used to estimate $\dot{V}O_{2max}$. These include the 1-, 1.5-, or 2-mile run, 12-minute run, 3-minute step test, shuttle runs, and submaximal cycle ergometry. The vertical jump, Wingate anaerobic cycle, running-based anaerobic sprint (400 m), and 300-yd shuttle run tests are used for anaerobic power.

Muscular Strength and Endurance

- Tests to assess muscular strength include free weights (1-RM: back squats/bench presses), hand grip dynamometry (maximal strength), and isokinetic equipment $(60–120° \times s^{-1})$.

- Muscular endurance can be measured by maximal number of push-ups, pull-ups, and/or sit-ups, as well as hand grip dynamometry (sustained submaximal endurance) and isokinetic equipment $(180–300° \times s^{-1})$.

REFERENCES

1. American College of Sports Medicine. *ACSM's Guidelines for Exercise Testing and Prescription*. 8th ed. Philadelphia (PA): Lippincott Williams & Wilkins; 2009. 400 p.

2. Astrand PO, Rodahl K. *Textbook of Work Physiology: Physiological Bases of Exercise*. 4th ed. Vol. 4. Windsor, Canada: Human Kinetics; 2003. 656 p.

3. Billat VL, Richard R, Binsse VM, Koralsztein JP, Haouzi P. The V(O₂) slow component for severe exercise depends on type of exercise and is not correlated with time to fatigue. *J Appl Physiol*. 1998;85(6):2118–24.

4. Close GL, Ashton T, McArdle A, Maclaren DP. The emerging role of free radicals in delayed onset muscle soreness and contraction-induced muscle injury. *Comp Biochem Physiol A Mol Integr Physiol*. 2005;142(3):257–66.

5. Dannecker EA, Hausenblas HA, Kaminski TW, Robinson ME. Sex differences in delayed onset muscle pain. *Clin J Pain*. 2005;21(2):120–6.

6. Demirel HA, Powers SK, Naito H, Hughes M, Coombes JS. Exercise-induced alterations in skeletal muscle myosin heavy chain phenotype: dose-response relationship. *J Appl Physiol*. 1999;86(3):1002–8.

7. Gaesser GA, Poole DC. The slow component of oxygen uptake kinetics in humans. *Exerc Sport Sci Rev*. 1996;24:35–71.

8. He ZH, Bottinelli R, Pellegrino MA, Ferenczi MA, Reggiani C. ATP consumption and efficiency of human single muscle fibers with different myosin isoform composition. *Biophys J*. 2000;79(2):945–61.

9. Hill DW, Rowell AL. Running velocity at $\dot{V}O_{2max}$. *Med Sci Sports Exerc*. 1996;28(1):114–9.

10. Hunter GR, Bamman MM, Larson-Meyer DE, et al. Inverse relationship between exercise economy and oxidative capacity in muscle. *Eur J Appl Physiol*. 2005;94(5–6):558–68.

11. Jones AM, Burnley M. Oxygen uptake kinetics: an underappreciated determinant of exercise performance. *Int J Sports Physiol Perform*. 2009;4(4):524–32.

12. Jones AM, Carter H, Doust JH. A disproportionate increase in $\dot{V}O_2$ coincident with lactate threshold during treadmill exercise. *Med Sci Sports Exerc*. 1999;31(9):1299–306.

13. Krustrup P, Söderlund K, Mohr M, Bangsbo J. The slow component of oxygen uptake during intense, sub-maximal exercise in man is associated with additional fibre recruitment. *Pflugers Arch*. 2004;447(6):855–66.

14. Lacour JR, Padilla-Magunacelaya S, Chatard JC, Arsac L, Barthélémy JC. Assessment of running velocity at maximal oxygen uptake. *Eur J Appl Physiol Occup Physiol*. 1991;62(2):77–82.

15. McLaughlin JE, Howley ET, Bassett DR Jr, Thompson DL, Fitzhugh EC. Test of the classic model for predicting endurance running performance. *Med Sci Sports Exerc*. 2010;42(5):991–7.

16. Midgley AW, McNaughton LR, Wilkinson M. The relationship between the lactate turnpoint and the time at $\dot{V}O_{2max}$ during a constant velocity run to exhaustion. *Int J Sports Med*. 2006;27(4):278–82.

17. Pette D, Staron RS. Mammalian skeletal muscle fiber type transitions. *Int Rev Cytol*. 1997;170:143–223.

18. Pette D, Staron RS. Myosin isoforms, muscle fiber types, and transitions. *Microsc Res Tech*. 2000;50(6):500–9.

19. Pette D, Staron RS. Transitions of muscle fiber phenotypic profiles. *Histochem Cell Biol*. 2001;115(5):359–72.

20. Poole DC, Richardson RS. Determinants of oxygen uptake. Implications for exercise testing. *Sports Med*. 1997;24(5):308–20.

21. Schiaffino S. Fibre types in skeletal muscle: a personal account. *Acta Physiol (Oxf)*. 2010;199(4):451–63.

22. Schiaffino S, Reggiani C. Myosin isoforms in mammalian skeletal muscle. *J Appl Physiol*. 1994;77(2):493–501.

23. Staron RS. Human skeletal muscle fiber types: delineation, development, and distribution. *Can J Appl Physiol*. 1997;22(4):307–27.

24. Staron RS, Hagerman FC, Hikida RS, et al. Fiber type composition of the vastus lateralis muscle of young men and women. *J Histochem Cytochem*. 2000;48(5):623–9.

25. Tanaka H, Monahan KD, Seals DR. Age-predicted maximal heart rate revisited. *J Am Coll Cardiol*. 2001;37(1):153–6.

26. Wasserman K, Hansen JE, Sue DY, Stringer WW, Whipp BJ. *Principles of Exercise Testing and Interpretation: Including Pathophysiology and Clinical Applications*. 4th ed. Philadelphia (PA): Lippincott Williams & Wilkins; 2005. 568 p.

27. Wilborn CD, Taylor LW, Greenwood M, Kreider RB, Willoughby DS. Effects of different intensities of resistance exercise on regulators of myogenesis. *J Strength Cond Res*. 2009;23(8):2179–87.

28. Zammit PS. All muscle satellite cells are equal, but are some more equal than others? *J Cell Sci*. 2008;121(Pt 18):2975–82.

6 Articular Cartilage Injury

Aman Dhawan, Vasili Karas, and Brian J. Cole

- Articular cartilage is a complex structure lining the articulating surfaces of diarthrodial joints. It provides a smooth, low-friction surface, while minimizing peak stress on the underlying subchondral bone.

- Injuries to the chondral surfaces occur in all joints of the human body. Articular injury of the knee has received the most attention in the literature. This chapter will focus primarily on articular injury as it pertains to the knee joint; however, many of the principles of evaluation, grading, and management hold true for chondral injury in any anatomic joint.

- Injury to articular cartilage is very common; in one retrospective review of 31,516 knee arthroscopies, 63% of patients were found to have chondral injury (21). Cartilage injury of the knee affects approximately 900,000 Americans annually, resulting in over 200,000 surgical procedures (20). Notably, the literature analyzing the prevalence of articular cartilage pathology does not provide significant guidance or insight into the prevalence of lesions that are or become symptomatic and require treatment.

- Although nonsurgical management of articular cartilage injury has remained largely the same over the past decade, surgical treatment of chondral injuries continues to evolve. Reparative, restorative, and reconstructive techniques continue to be refined, giving surgeons more tools and options for biologic reconstruction of articular surfaces.

BASIC SCIENCE

- Articular cartilage is composed of water (65%–80% of wet weight), collagen (10%–20% of wet weight), proteoglycans (10%–15% of wet weight), and chondrocytes (5% of wet weight). The collagen in native cartilage is primarily type II, with smaller quantities of types V, VI, IX, X, and XI. Chondrocytes are the cells responsible for the production of the extracellular matrix. These cells differentiate from mesenchymal stem cells during skeletal morphogenesis and are subsequently a low turnover cell type. Chondrocytes receive their nutrition and oxygen from the surrounding synovial fluid via diffusion (16). In the intact, uninjured knee, the articular cartilage shares load-bearing responsibility with the menisci (up to 70% from the lateral meniscus), making the chondral surfaces significantly vulnerable to injury and degeneration with partial or complete injury or removal of the menisci.

- Because of the limited vascular, neural, and lymphatic access, in addition to the limited capacity of chondrocyte division and migration, the healing response of articular cartilage is poor. Partial-thickness injury that does not penetrate the tidemark, the demarcation between the deep layer and calcified layer of cartilage, will result in cellular insult with decreased matrix production by the underlying and surrounding chondrocytes and ultimately little healing. In artilage matrix and cell injuries, decreased proteoglycan concentration, increased hydration, and disorganization of the collagen network occur (16,21).

- Injury that penetrates the tidemark into the calcified cartilage layer and the subchondral bone (an osteochondral lesion) will illicit an inflammatory response that includes an influx of marrow contents (undifferentiated mesenchymal stem cells, cytokines, and growth factors including transforming growth factor-β [TGF-β] and platelet-derived growth factor [PDGF]) triggered by hemorrhage and fibrin clot. The osteochondral injury has potential for a more robust healing response including a resultant repair that more closely resembles fibrocartilage (vs. native hyaline cartilage) composed of primarily type I collagen. This fibrocartilage-like repair is less stiff and more permeable than normal articular cartilage (16,21). Fibrocartilaginous repair tissue is far less durable than native hyaline cartilage and often begins to show evidence of depletion of proteoglycans, increased hydration, fragmentation and fibrillation, increased collagen content, and loss of chondrocytes within 1 year (15).

- Although the natural history of chondral injuries is not completely understood, it is postulated that defects, particularly larger, full-thickness injuries, can progress via edge loading and elevated contact pressures on the adjacent articular surfaces. This progression may lead to degradation of the surrounding chondral surfaces and ultimately osteoarthrosis.

Patient Evaluation

- Articular cartilage injury can be caused by an acute injury that results in a focal chondral or osteochondral injury or chronic/subacute injuries or conditions that result in degenerative lesions. Damage to the chondral surfaces can occur in isolation or, as is often the case, in association with other intra-articular injury. The evaluating physician should maintain a high index of suspicion for chondral injury when evaluating the knee for any causes of pain, effusion, instability, or mechanical symptoms.

- A thorough history should include details related to the onset of symptoms (traumatic or insidious), mechanism of injury, previous injuries and surgery, and symptom-provoking activities.

- A thorough physical examination should evaluate formal alignment, abnormal gait, swelling, effusions, instability, meniscal symptoms, range of motion, strength, and neurovascular abnormalities. Crepitus, catching, locking, or grinding can occur with focal irregularities of the articular surfaces. Diagnosis of all concomitant pathology is critical to formulate a successful, global treatment plan.

- Radiographic workup should include posterior-anterior, weight-bearing, 45-degree plain films and patellofemoral, and non–weight-bearing lateral projections. Evaluation on plain films for joint space narrowing, subchondral sclerosis, osteophytes, and cysts should be performed. History and physical examination, along with these radiographs, are often all that is needed to make the appropriate diagnosis. Magnetic resonance imaging (MRI) can be valuable to assess the status of the knee ligaments and menisci but can underestimate the degree of cartilage abnormalities seen during arthroscopy (36). Use of 3.0-tesla magnets, cartilage imaging sequence techniques including fat-suppressed or fat-suppressed spoiled gradient-echo imaging, and balanced free precession steady-state sequences have improved detection and characterization of chondral injuries using MRI (6). Routine MRI sequences are typically sufficient to evaluate for subchondral abnormalities that may become useful findings during definitive decision making.

GRADING OF ARTICULAR CARTILAGE INJURY

- Although MRI is being used with more frequency to evaluate chondral injuries, arthroscopic evaluation remains the most accurate way to assess the location, depth, size, shape, and stability of a chondral or osteochondral defect of the articular surface. The Outerbridge classification is most widely used to grade these injuries (Table 6.1) (48). More recently, the International Cartilage Repair Society has modified this to a more comprehensive description and grading system (see Table 6.1) (13). The International Cartilage Repair Society grading system can be used to describe lesions both arthroscopically and using advanced radiologic imaging techniques.

NONSURGICAL TREATMENT

- As with most joint pathology, initial treatment of articular cartilage injuries is typically conservative with recommendations that include activity modification, judicious use of nonsteroidal anti-inflammatory drugs (NSAIDs), glucosamine and chondroitin sulfate, corticosteroid injections, and consideration for

Table 6.1	Modified International Cartilage Repair Society (ICRS) Classification System for Chondral Injury (40)
Grade of Injury	**Modified ICRS System**
Grade 0	Normal cartilage
Grade I	Superficial fissuring
Grade II	< 1/2 cartilage depth
Grade III	> 1/2 cartilage depth up to subchondral plate
Grade IV	Through subchondral plate, exposing subchondral bone

viscosupplementation (22). Patients with mechanical symptoms (including catching, locking, sensation of loose body, or giving way), acute motion loss, or failed nonsurgical management with pain and loss of function should be considered for surgical intervention.

SURGICAL TREATMENT

Arthroscopic Debridement and Lavage

- Arthroscopic debridement and lavage is a consideration for a first-line surgical intervention in a patient with a symptomatic articular cartilage injury. This treatment modality allows the surgeon to perform diagnostic arthroscopy to assess the chondral injury and the remainder of the joint. Patient expectations must be managed in that the results of this procedure can range from diagnostic to therapeutic due to the removal of degenerative debris, loose nonviable chondral fragments, and lavage of the associated inflammatory cytokines such as interleukin-1 and tumor necrosis factor-α (1). Care is taken to preserve intact, healthy articular cartilage. Arthroscopic lavage alone has been proven to provide at least short-term benefits in 50%–70% of patients (1,24). In a select group of highly active individuals, especially in season when return-to-sport time lines are critical, arthroscopic debridement may prove to be beneficial in the short term. In general, however, the results of arthroscopic debridement and lavage are often not durable and deteriorate over time, and the primary benefit that remains is the diagnostic information obtained to help guide future treatment decisions (Table 6.2) (10,32,33,54,58).

Fragment Fixation

- Fixation of a chondral lesion is predicated on the condition, size, shape, defect location, and adequacy of subchondral bone attached to the osteochondral fragment. Radiographic and MRI evaluation can help with the determination of many of these factors and appropriateness of this surgical option. Prior to fixation of the osteochondral fragment, both the fragment and defect must be prepared to create an adequate

Table 6.2 | **Results of Arthroscopic Debridement and Lavage**

Study	No. of Patients	Mean Follow-Up	Results
Kirkley et al., 2008 (37)	163	2 years	Randomized controlled trial: Arthroscopy and PT vs. PT alone showed no difference in WOMAC, or SF-36 between groups ($P = 0.22$).
Jackson and Dieterichs, 2003 (34)	121	4–6 years	Retrospective case series: Stage I: 100% excellent/good Stage II: 90.6% excellent/good Stage III: 48.7% excellent/good Stage IV: 11.9% excellent/good
Moseley et al., 2002 (47)	180	2 years	Randomized controlled trial: Debridement, lavage, and placebo showed no difference in KSPS, AIMS2-P, and SF-36 scores.
Steadman et al., 2001 (55)	75	11.3 years	Retrospective case series: Lysholm 58.8→89 Tegner 3.1→5.8 Work 4.9→7.6 Sports 4.2→7.1
Timoney et al., 1990 (58)	109	48 months	Retrospective case series: 63% good 37% fair/poor
Jackson, 1989 (33)	137	3.5 years (2–9 years)	Retrospective case series: 68% remained improved
Sprague, 1981 (54)	78	14 months	Retrospective case series: 74% good 26% fair/poor

AIMS2-P, Arthritis Impact Measurement Scales; KSPS, Knee-Specific Pain Scale; PT, physical therapy; WOMAC, Western Ontario and McMaster Universities Arthritis Index; SF-36, Short Form-36.

healing milieu. The fragment must be reduced anatomically into its bed, and fixation may then be completed using either absorbable or nonabsorbable implants. Occasionally, bone graft augmentation is required for deeper cavitating lesions. Treating osteochondral lesions with the same considerations as a fracture nonunion will lead to more predictable healing. These factors include debriding fibrocartilage at the base of the lesion, microfracture augmentation of the base to promote bleeding, and rigid fixation with compression. Resorbable fixation placed without the intention to remove the implant should be buried to or beneath the level of the subchondral bone because these lesions can subside over time. Metallic implants removed at 6 to 8 weeks allow the opportunity to verify fragment healing and prevent the untoward effects of prominent hardware that can develop over time. Successful healing of the osteochondral fragment with the use of headless metallic cannulated screws has been reported in up to 90% of patients (1).

Marrow-Stimulating Techniques

■ The goal of marrow stimulation techniques is the delivery of mesenchymal stem cell progenitors to the defect bed and the subsequent formation of a fibrocartilage-like repair tissue from these cells. This technique can be performed in a number of ways to include drilling, abrasion, and microfracture and always involves penetration of the calcified cartilage layer into the subchondral bone to allow the migration of progenitor cells to the articular surface. Because of the limited fill that may occur in some lesions, particularly larger ones greater than 2 cm^2, and the different structural and biomechanical properties of this fibrocartilage-like repair tissue (see earlier Basic Science section), the best results are typically achieved with relatively small defects in a low-demand patient population (1). Results of microfracture technique are summarized in Table 6.3.

Osteochondral Autograft

■ This procedure uses plugs of cartilage and bone obtained from load-sparing areas of the knee with transplantation into the area of a symptomatic chondral defect. This technique offers several advantages including transplantation of viable hyaline cartilage, a relatively brief rehabilitation period, and the ability to perform the procedure in a single operation. Limitations include the availability of low-contact harvest areas, donor site morbidity, and the potential for surface plug incongruity (23,38). Short- and mid-term results of this technique have been promising, showing greater than 90% good to excellent results (30,31). Treating defects larger than 1 to 2 cm^2, however, is associated with inferior outcomes.

| Table 6.3 | Results of Microfracture |

Study	No.	Mean Follow-Up*	Results
Solheim et al., 2010 (53)	110 patients	5 years (2–9 years)	Retrospective cohort: Lysholm 51→71 VAS function 41→74 VAS pain 52→30†
Mithoefer et al., 2009 (45)	Systematic review (3,122 patients)	3.4 ± 0.4 years (1–3 years)	Systematic review: Short-term clinical improvement rate (≤ 24 months): 75%–100% Long-term clinical improvement rate (≥ 24 months): 67%–80%
Asik et al., 2008 (2)	90 patients	5.2 years (2–9 years)	Retrospective case series: Lysholm 52.4→84.6 Tegner 2.6→5.2
Bae et al., 2006 (4)	47 knees	1 year	Second look arthroscopy: Extent of cartilage healing > 90% in 55% of cases; 80%–89% in 10% Radiographic evaluation: average joint space increase of 1.06 mm on anterior-posterior and 1.37 mm on lateral
Gobbi et al., 2005 (27)	25 competitive athletes	6 years (3–10 years)	Prospective cohort study: 30% improved Lysholm 56.8→87.2 Tegner 3.2→5
Steadman et al., 2002 (57)	71 knees Age ≤ 45 years	11 years (7–17 years)	Retrospective case series: 80% improved Lysholm 59→89 Tegner 6→9 Majority of improvement in first year Maximal improvement in 2 to 3 years Younger patients did better
Steadman et al., 2001 (55)	75 patients	11.3 years	Retrospective case series: Lysholm 58.8→89 Tegner 3.1→5.8 Work 4.9→7.6 Sports 4.2→7.1
Gill and Macgillivray, 2001 (25)	103 patients	6 years (2–12 years)	Retrospective case series: 86% rated knee as normal/nearly normal Acute (treated within 12 weeks) did better
Blevins et al., 1998 (12)	140 recreational athletes Mean age, 38 years Mean defect size, 2.8 cm² 38 high-level athletes Mean age, 26 years Mean defect size, 2.2 cm²	3.7 years	Prospective cohort study: 77% returned to sports
Steadman et al., 1997 (56)	203 patients	3 years (2–12 years)	Retrospective case series: 75% improved, 19% unchanged, 6% worse, 60% improved sports Poor prognosis: joint space narrowing, age > 30 years, no postoperative CPM

CPM, continuous passive motion; VAS, visual analog scale.

* Represents median number of years as reported by study.

† Lower values denote improvement.

Osteochondral Allograft

- Osteochondral allograft transplantation involves transplantation of a prolonged, freshly preserved (at 4°C) cadaveric graft consisting of intact, viable articular cartilage and its underlying subchondral bone into the articular cartilage defect. Potential advantages of this technique include the ability to achieve more precise surface architecture, immediate transplantation of viable hyaline cartilage as a single-stage procedure, the potential to replace large defects or even hemicondyles, and no donor site morbidity. Limitations of osteochondral allografting include limited graft availability, relatively high cost, a low but possible risk of immunologic rejection, incomplete graft incorporation, potential for disease transmission, and the technically demanding aspects of graft matching and sizing (5,7,18). Because freezing and cryopreservation have both been shown to decrease chondrocyte viability, fresh osteochondral allografts are typically used.

- Long-term chondrocyte viability after osteochondral allograft transplantation has been well demonstrated by a number of studies. Williams et al. (59) reported on 26 retrieved osteochondral allograft specimens after an average survival time of 42 months. The rate of chondrocyte viability was 82%, and there was evidence of allograft bone incorporation in most specimens. The allograft bone is replaced by creeping substitution, but it provides a structural scaffold to support the articular surface during this gradual incorporation. Outcome studies on osteochondral allograft transplantation for symptomatic chondral defects demonstrate 91% success at 5 years and 84% success at 10 years (3,17). McCulloch et al. (42) demonstrated improvements in Lysholm scores (39–67), International Knee Documentation Committee scores (29–58), all five components of the Knee Injury and Osteoarthritis Outcome Score (Pain, 43–73; Other Disease-Specific Symptoms, 46–64; Activities of Daily Living Function, 56–83; Sport and Recreation Function, 18–46; Knee-Related Quality of Life, 22–50), and Short Form-12 physical component scores (36–40). Overall, patients from this study reported 84% (range, 25%–100%) satisfaction with their results and believed that the knee functioned at 79% (range, 35%–100%) of their unaffected knee (42). Literature outcomes on osteochondral allografts are included in Table 6.4.

Autologous Chondrocyte Implantation

- Autologous chondrocyte implantation requires a two-stage procedure including the biopsy of chondrocytes from the knee, culturing and expansion of the chondrocyte cell line, and reoperation for transplantation into the cartilage defect beneath a periosteal or collagen matrix patch. The potential advantages of this procedure include the ability to fill defects as large as 10 cm^2, the development of hyaline-like cartilage rather than fibrocartilage in the grafted defect, and possibly better long-term outcomes and longevity of the healing tis-

Table 6.4	**Results of Osteochondral Allograft**			
Study	**No.**	**Location**	**Mean Follow-Up**	**Results**
LaPrade et al., 2009 (39)	23	F	3 years	Prospective cohort study: IKDC score 52→69 Good incorporation: 22/23
McCulloch et al., 2007 (42)	25	F	35 months	Prospective cohort study: 84% success rate
Gross et al., 2005 (29)	123	F, T, P	7.5 years	Prospective cohort study: 85% success rate
Aubin et al., 2001 (3)	60	F	10 years	Prospective cohort study: 84% good/excellent 20% failure
Shasha et al., 2003 (52)	65	T	> 5 years	Prospective cohort study: 95% success rate at 5 years 80% success rate at 10 years 65% success rate at 15 years
Bugbee, 2000 (17)	122	F	5 years	Prospective cohort study: 91% success rate at 5 years 75% success rate at 10 years 5% failure
Chu et al., 1999 (19)	55	F, T, P	75 months	Prospective cohort study: 76% good/excellent 16% failure

F, femur; IKDC, International Knee Documentation Committee; P, patella; T, tibia.

Table 6.5	Results of Autologous Chondrocyte Transplantation			
Study	**No.**	**Location**	**Mean Follow-Up**	**Results**
Moseley et al., 2010 (46)	72	F	> 5 years Mean, 9.2 years	Case series: 69% of patients improved from baseline 12.5% had no change 17% failed
Peterson et al., 2010 (51)	224	F, P, multiple	> 10 years Mean, 12.8 years	Case series: 92% patient satisfaction
Bhosale et al., 2009 (11)	80	F, P, Tr, multiple	> 2.7 years Mean, 5 years	Prospective cohort study: 81% clinical improvement 19% clinical decline
Peterson et al., 2002 (49)	18 14 17 11	F OCD P F/ACL	> 5 years > 5 years > 5 years > 5 years	Case series: 89% good/excellent 86% good/excellent 65% good/excellent 91% good/excellent
Micheli et al., 2001 (44)	50	F/Tr/P	> 3 years	Prospective cohort study: 84% significant improvement 2% unchanged 13% declined
Peterson et al., 2000 (50)	25 19 16 16	F P F/ACL Multiple	> 2 years > 2 years > 2 years > 2 years	Case series: 92% good/excellent 62% good/excellent 75% good/excellent 67% good/excellent
Gillogly et al., 1998 (26)	25	F, P, T	> 1 year	Case series: 88% good/excellent
Brittberg et al., 1994 (14)	16 7	F P	39 months 36 months	Prospective cohort study: 88% good/excellent 12% poor 29% good/excellent 71% fair/poor

ACL, anterior cruciate ligament; F, femur; OCD, osteochondritis dissecans; P, patella; T, tibia; Tr, trochlea.

sue. This procedure can be technically demanding, requiring the patient to undergo a relatively long rehabilitation in addition to a requirement for two surgical procedures. Additionally, although the overall complication rate appears to be relatively low, the adverse events that do occur following autologous chondrocyte implantation can result in subsequent operative intervention.

- Peterson et al. (51) demonstrated that 92% of patients were satisfied and would have the autologous chondrocyte implantation (ACI) surgery again at 10–20 years after transplantation. In their cohort of 50 patients, Micheli et al. (44) demonstrated that 84% of patients had significant improvement in their symptoms at 3 years postoperatively. A recent multicenter cohort study evaluated outcomes of autologous chondrocyte transplantation after failed previous articular cartilage surgery (60). After 48 months of follow-up, 76% of the 154 patients had a successful outcome, whereas 24% were deemed as having treatment failure. Interestingly, 49% of the patients (n = 76) had a subsequent surgical procedure

performed after the autologous chondrocyte implantation. These additional procedures, predominantly arthroscopic, were not predictive of failure. The use of type I/III bilayer collagen instead of a periosteal patch to cover the cells during the implantation procedure has been shown to decrease the reoperation rate significantly (28). A recent study evaluating 2- to 9-year outcomes of autologous chondrocyte implantation in a diverse patient population demonstrated that 75% of patients were completely or mostly satisfied with their outcomes and 83% would have the procedure done again (43,50). Outcomes of autologous chondrocyte implantation are summarized in Table 6.5.

TREATMENT DECISION MAKING

- Management of articular cartilage injuries can be challenging, and multiple options are described that can be used to treat similar lesions. Although there is not necessarily a

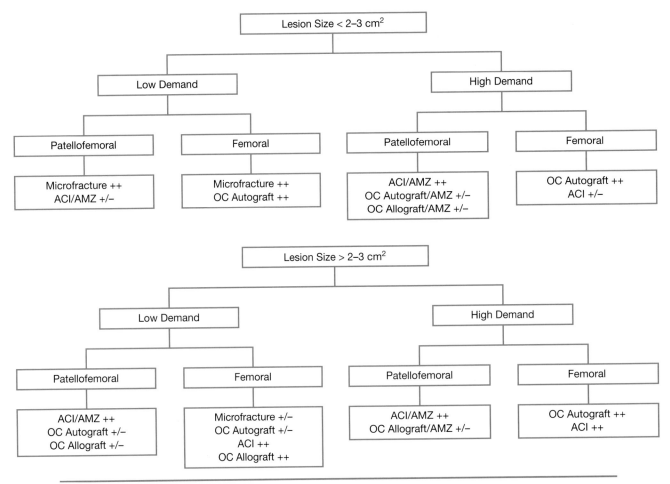

Figure 6.1: Surgical treatment algorithm of articular cartilage injuries. ACI, autologous chondrocyte implantation; AMZ, antero-medialization tibial tubercle osteotomy; OC, osteochondral.

consensus on optimal treatment, certain guidelines can be followed. Decision making must consider patient goals, physical demands, expectations, and perceptions, as well as defect size, depth, location, chronicity, previous treatments and response, and concomitant pathology. Ligament insufficiency, meniscal pathology, and/or mechanical malalignment must be addressed, particularly in treatment of articular cartilage injury of the femoral condyles. Not infrequently, concomitant procedures are performed that include meniscal allograft transplantation, distal femoral or high tibial osteotomy, and tibial tuberosity elevation. Our recommended primary treatment guideline is included in Figure 6.1.

■ Articular cartilage surgical restoration allows for a high rate of return to high-impact sports often at the preinjury competitive level. The time of return and durability can be variable and depend on repair technique and athlete-specific factors. Player age, competitive level, defect size, time to treatment, and repair tissue morphology all affect the ability and time to return-to-play. Sports participation after cartilage repair generally promotes joint restoration and functional recovery. Time to return to impact sports generally varies between 7 and 17 months, with the longest time after autologous chondrocyte transplantation.

FUTURE DIRECTIONS

■ Ongoing research in the area of articular cartilage continues. Indeed, it is one of the most studied topics in contemporary orthopedics. Additional treatments being evaluated include cell-based and scaffold-associated chondrocyte treatments. These techniques involve delivery of harvested autologous chondrocytes on a biologic scaffold that may avoid many of the limitations associated with our current techniques (49). In addition, the use of a scaffold with chondrocytes may make many of these procedures amenable to arthroscopic implantation, at least for many accessible lesions. Animal and basic science models have demonstrated early promise using these techniques; however, rigorous, well-conducted human trials need be conducted to elucidate the scope of additional benefits associated with these procedures (8,9,35,41,61).

REFERENCES

1. Alford JW, Cole B. Cartilage restoration, part 2: techniques, outcomes, and future directions. *Am J Sports Med.* 2005;33(3):443–60.

2. Asik M, Ciftci F, Sen C, Erdil M, Atalar A. The microfracture technique for the treatment of full-thickness articular cartilage lesions of the knee: midterm results. *Arthroscopy.* 2008;24(11):1214–20.

3. Aubin PP, Cheah HK, Davis AM, Gross AE. Long-term follow up of fresh femoral osteochondral allografts for posttraumatic knee defects. *Clin Orthop Relat Res.* 2001;(391 Suppl):S318–27.

4. Bae DK, Yoon KH, Song SJ. Cartilage healing after microfracture in osteoarthritic knees. *Arthroscopy.* 2006;22(4):367–74.

5. Bakay A, Csönge L, Papp G, Fekete L. Osteochondral resurfacing of the knee joint with allograft. Clinical analysis of 33 cases. *Int Orthop.* 1998;22(5):277–81.

6. Bauer JS, Barr C, Henning TD, et al. Magnetic resonance imaging of the ankle at 3.0 tesla and 1.5 tesla in human cadaver specimens with artificially created lesions of cartilage and ligaments. *Invest Radiol.* 2008;43(9):604–11.

7. Beaver RJ, Mahomed M, Backstein D, Davis A, Zukor DJ, Gross AE. Fresh osteochondral allografts for post-traumatic defects in the knee. A survivorship analysis. *J Bone Joint Surg Br.* 1992;74(1):105–10.

8. Bedi A, Feeley B, Williams RJ. Management of articular cartilage defects of the knee. *J Bone Joint Surg Am.* 2010;92(4):994–1009.

9. Behrens P, Bitter T, Kurz B, Russlies M. Matrix-associated autologous chondrocyte transplantation/implantation (MACT/MACI)—5-year follow-up. *Knee.* 2006;13(3):194–202.

10. Bernard J, Lemon M, Patterson MH. Arthroscopic washout of the knee—a 5-year survival analysis. *Knee.* 2004;11(3):233–5.

11. Bhosale AM, Kuiper JH, Johnson WE, Harrison PE, Richardson JB. Midterm to long-term longitudinal outcome of autologous chondrocyte implantation in the knee joint. *Am J Sports Med.* 2009;37(1 Suppl):131S–8S.

12. Blevins FT, Steadman JR, Rodrigo JJ, Silliman J. Treatment of articular cartilage defects in athletes: an analysis of functional outcome and lesion appearance. *Orthopedics.* 1998;21(7):761–8.

13. Brittberg M. Evaluation of cartilage injuries and cartilage repair. *Osteologie.* 2000;9:17–25.

14. Brittberg M, Lindahl A, Nilsson A, Ohlsson C, Isaksson O, Peterson L. Treatment of deep cartilage defects in the knee with autologous chondrocyte transplantation. *N Engl J Med.* 1994;331(14):889–95.

15. Buckwalter JA. Articular cartilage injuries. *Clin Orthop Relat Res.* 2002;(402):21–37.

16. Buckwalter JA, Rosenberg LA, Hunziker EB. Articular cartilage: composition and structure. In: Woo SL, Buckwalter JA, editors. *Injury and Repair of the Musculoskeletal Soft Tissues.* Park Ridge: American Academy of Orthopaedic Surgeons; 1988. p. 405–25.

17. Bugbee WD. Fresh osteochondral allografting. *Oper Techn Sport Med.* 2000;8(2):158–62.

18. Bugbee WD. Fresh osteochondral allografts. *J Knee Surg.* 2002;15(3):191–5.

19. Chu CR, Convery FR, Akeson WH, Meyers M, Amiel D. Articular cartilage transplantation: clinical results in the knee. *Clin Orthop Relat Res.* 1999;(360):159–68.

20. Cole BJ, Frederick R, Levy A, et al. Management of a 37 year old man with recurrent knee pain. *J Clin Outcomes Manag.* 1999;6(6):46–57.

21. Curl WW, Krome J, Gordon ES, Rushing J, Smith BP, Poehling GG. Cartilage injuries: a review of 31,516 knee arthroscopies. *Arthroscopy.* 1997;13(4):456–60.

22. Daher R, Chahine NO, Greenberg AS, Sgaglione NA, Grande DA. New methods to diagnose and treat cartilage degeneration. *Nat Rev Rheumatol.* 2009;5(11):599–607.

23. Feczkó P, Hangody L, Varga J, et al. Experimental results of donor site filling for autologous osteochondral mosaicplasty. *Arthroscopy.* 2003;19(7):755–61.

24. Friedman MJ, Berasi CC, Fox JM, Del Pizzo W, Snyder SJ, Ferkel RD. Preliminary results with abrasion arthroplasty in the osteoarthritic knee. *Clin Orthop Relat Res.* 1984;(182):200–5.

25. Gill TJ, Macgillivray JD. The technique of microfracture for the treatment of articular cartilage defects in the knee. *Oper Tech Orthop.* 2001;11(2):105–7.

26. Gillogly SD, Voight M, Blackburn T. Treatment of articular cartilage defects of the knee with autologous chondrocyte implantation. *J Orthop Sports Phys Ther.* 1998;28(4):241–51.

27. Gobbi A, Nunag P, Malinowski K. Treatment of full thickness chondral lesions of the knee with microfracture in a group of athletes. *Knee Surg Sports Traumatol Arthrosc.* 2005;13(3):213–21.

28. Gomoll AH, Probst C, Farr J, Cole BJ, Minas T. Use of a type I/III bilayer collagen membrane decreases reoperation rates for symptomatic hypertrophy after autologous chondrocyte implantation. *Am J Sports Med.* 2009;37(1 Suppl):20S–3S.

29. Gross AE, Shasha N, Aubin P. Long-term follow-up of the use of fresh osteochondral allografts for posttraumatic knee defects. *Clin Orthop Relat Res.* 2005;(435):79–87.

30. Hangody L, Feczkó P, Bartha L, Bodó G, Kish G. Mosaicplasty for the treatment of articular defects of the knee and ankle. *Clin Orthop Relat Res.* 2001;391(Suppl):S328–36.

31. Hangody L, Kish G, Kárpáti Z, Udvarhelyi I, Szigeti I, Bely M. Mosaicplasty for the treatment of articular cartilage defects: application in clinical practice. *Orthopedics.* 1998;21(7):751–6.

32. Hubbard MJ. Arthroscopic surgery for chondral flaps in the knee. *J Bone Joint Surg Br.* 1987;69(5):794–6.

33. Jackson RW. Meniscal and articular cartilage injury in sport. *J R Coll Surg Edinb.* 1989;34(6 Suppl):S15–7.

34. Jackson RW, Dieterichs C. The results of arthroscopic lavage and debridement of osteoarthritic knees based on the severity of degeneration: a 4- to 6-year symptomatic follow-up. *Arthroscopy.* 2003;19(1):13–20.

35. Kang JY, Chung CW, Sung JH, et al. Novel porous matrix of hyaluronic acid for the three-dimensional culture of chondrocytes. *Int J Pharm.* 2009;369(1–2):114–20.

36. Khanna AJ, Cosgarea AJ, Mont MA, et al. Magnetic resonance imaging of the knee. Current techniques and spectrum of disease. *J Bone Joint Surg Am.* 2001;83(A Suppl 2, Pt 2):128–41.

37. Kirkley A, Birmingham TB, Litchfield RB, et al. A randomized trial of arthroscopic surgery for osteoarthritis of the knee. *N Engl J Med.* 2008;359(11):1097–107.

38. LaPrade RF, Botker JC. Donor-site morbidity after osteochondral autograft transfer procedures. *Arthroscopy.* 2004;20(7):e69–73.

39. LaPrade RF, Botker J, Herzog M, Agel J. Refrigerated osteoarticular allografts to treat articular cartilage defects of the femoral condyles: a prospective outcomes study. *J Bone Joint Surg Am.* 2009;91(4):805–11.

40. Mainil-Varlet P, Aigner T, Brittberg M, et al. Histological assessment of cartilage repair: a report by the Histology Endpoint Committee of the International Cartilage Repair Society (ICRS). *J Bone Joint Surg Am.* 2003;85(Suppl 2):45–7.

41. Marcacci M, Berruto M, Brocchetta D, et al. Articular cartilage engineering with Hyalograft C: 3-year clinical results. *Clin Orthop Relat Res.* 2005;435:96–105.

42. McCulloch PC, Kang RW, Sobhy MH, Hayden JK, Cole BJ. Prospective evaluation of prolonged fresh osteochondral allograft transplantation of the femoral condyle. *Am J Sports Med.* 2007;35(3):411–20.

43. McNickle AG, L'Heureux DR, Yanke AB, Cole BJ. Outcomes of autologous chondrocyte implantation in a diverse patient population. *Am J Sports Med.* 2009;37(7):1344–50.

44. Micheli LJ, Browne JE, Erggelet C, et al. Autologous chondrocyte implantation of the knee: multicenter experience and minimum 3-year follow-up. *Clin J Sport Med*. 2001;11(4):223–8.

45. Mithoefer K, McAdams T, Williams RJ, Kreuz PC, Mandelbaum BR. Clinical efficacy of the microfracture technique for articular cartilage repair in the knee: an evidence-based systematic analysis. *Am J Sports Med*. 2009;37(10):2053–63.

46. Moseley JB, Anderson AF, Browne JE, et al. Long-term durability of autologous chondrocyte implantation: a multicenter, observational study in US patients. *Am J Sports Med*. 2010;38(2):238–46.

47. Moseley JB, O'Malley K, Petersen NJ, et al. A controlled trial of arthroscopic surgery for osteoarthritis of the knee. *N Engl J Med*. 2002;347(2):81–8.

48. Outerbridge RE. The etiology of chondromalacia patellae. 1961. *Clin Orthop Relat Res*. 2001;(389):5–8.

49. Peterson L, Brittberg M, Kiviranta I, Akerlund EL, Lindahl A. Autologous chondrocyte transplantation. *Am J Sports Med*. 2002;30(1):2–12.

50. Peterson L, Minas T, Brittberg M, Nilsson A, Sjögren-Jansson E, Lindahl A. Two to 9-year outcome after autologous chondrocyte transplantation of the knee. *Clin Orthop Relat Res*. 2000;(374):212–34.

51. Peterson L, Vasiliadis HS, Brittberg M, Lindahl A. Autologous chondrocyte implantation: a long-term follow-up. *Am J Sports Med*. 2010; 38(6):1117–24.

52. Shasha N, Krywulak S, Backstein D, Pressman A, Gross AE. Long-term follow-up of fresh tibial osteochondral allografts for failed tibial plateau fractures. *J Bone Joint Surg Am*. 2003;85(A Suppl 2):33–9.

53. Solheim E, Øyen J, Hegna J, Austgulen OK, Harlem T, Strand T. Microfracture treatment of single or multiple articular cartilage defects of the knee: a 5-year median follow-up of 110 patients. *Knee Surg Sports Traumatol Arthrosc*. 2010;18(4):504–8.

54. Sprague NF 3rd. Arthroscopic debridement for degenerative knee joint disease. *Clin Orthop Relat Res*. 1981;(160):118–23.

55. Steadman JR, Rodkey WG, Rodrigo JJ. Microfracture: surgical technique and rehabilitation to treat chondral defects. *Clin Orthop Relat Res*. 2001;391(Suppl):S362–9.

56. Steadman JR, Rodkey WG, Singleton SB, Briggs KK. Microfracture technique for full-thickness chondral defects: technique and clinical results. *Oper Tech Orthop*. 1997;7(4):300–4.

57. Steadman JR, Rodkey WG, Briggs K. Microfracture to treat full-thickness chondral defects: surgical technique, rehabilitation, and outcomes. *J Knee Sur*. 2002;15(3):170–6.

58. Timoney JM, Kneisl JS, Barrack RL, Alexander AH. Arthroscopy update #6. Arthroscopy in the osteoarthritic knee. Long-term follow-up. *Orthop Rev*. 1990;19(4):371–3, 376–9.

59. Williams SK, Amiel D, Ball ST, et al. Analysis of cartilage tissue on a cellular level in fresh osteochondral allograft retrievals. *Am J Sports Med*. 2007;35(12):2022–32.

60. Zaslav K, Cole B, Brewster R, et al. A prospective study of autologous chondrocyte implantation in patients with failed prior treatment for articular cartilage defect of the knee: results of the Study of the Treatment of Articular Repair (STAR) clinical trial. *Am J Sports Med*. 2009; 37(1):42–55.

61. Zheng MH, Willers C, Kirilak L, et al. Matrix-induced autologous chondrocyte implantation (MACI): biological and histological assessment. *Tissue Eng*. 2007;13(4):737–46.

Bone Injury and Fracture Healing

7

Connor R. LaRose and Carlos A. Guanche

- Fracture healing involves multiple orchestrated events that are intimately linked to each other (25). The goal of fracture healing is to restore the bone injury to the preinjury biologic and biomechanical state. To accomplish this task, the cellular content of bone and the ability of such cells to produce extracellular matrix and structure are altered.

BONE ANATOMY (5,6,9)

Bone Cells

Osteoprogenitor Cells

- Present on all bone surfaces, make up the deep layer of the periosteum and the endosteum, and can migrate from surrounding tissue.
- Osteoprogenitor cells are marrow stromal cells that differentiate into osteoblasts (9).
- The periosteum contains two layers: an outer layer of fibrous tissue and an inner layer (cambium) that contains cells capable of becoming osteoblasts.
- The endosteum is a single layer of osteogenic cells lacking a fibrous component.

Osteoblasts

- Mature, metabolically active bone-forming cells.
  - Secrete osteoid, the unmineralized matrix that subsequently undergoes mineralization.
  - Some osteoblasts are converted into osteocytes, whereas others remain on the surfaces of bone as lining cells.
  - Play a role in the activation of bone resorption by osteoclasts.

Osteocytes

- Mature osteoblasts trapped within the bone matrix.
- Form a network of cytoplasmic processes extending through cylindrical canaliculi to blood vessels and other osteocytes.
- Involved in extracellular calcium and phosphorus homeostasis.
- Act as in a paracrine function on active osteoblasts.

Osteoclasts

- Multinucleated bone-resorbing cells controlled by hormonal and cellular mechanisms.
- Differentiate from hematopoietic cells from the monocyte/macrophage cell lines (9).

- Function in groups termed *cutting cones* that attach to bare bone surfaces and dissolve inorganic and organic matrices of bone and calcified cartilage through the use of hydrolytic enzymes.
- Formation of ruffled border at bone–osteoclast interface leads to breakdown of organic and inorganic components (9).
- Process results in the formation of shallow pits on the bone surface called Howship's lacunae (5).

Types of Bone (6)

Woven Bone (Primary Bone)

- Primary bone formed during embryonic development, during fracture healing, and in some pathologic states such as hyperparathyroidism and Paget's disease (5,6).
- Composed of randomly arranged collagen bundles and irregularly shaped vascular spaces.
- Higher cellularity than lamellar bone and is not organized according to mechanical stress.
- Weaker and more easily deformed compared to lamellar bone secondary to irregular collagen orientation.

Lamellar Bone (Secondary Bone)

- Highly organized with densely packed collagen fibrils that are organized according to stress lines.
- Behaves anisotropically; the mechanical properties of the bone change depending on the direction of the applied force.
- Woven bone present at a fracture site must be eventually replaced by lamellar bone to restore the normal mechanical properties of bone.

Cortical Bone

- Dense compact bone that is primarily responsible for load bearing in the diaphysis of long bones.
- Remodeled from woven bone by means of vascular channels that invade the embryonic bone from its periosteal and endosteal surfaces.
- The primary structural unit of cortical bone is an osteon, also known as a Haversian system.
  - Consists of cylindrical-shaped lamellar bone that surrounds longitudinally oriented vascular channels called Haversian canals.
  - Horizontally oriented canals (Volkmann) connect adjacent osteons.

39

■ Mechanical strength of cortical bone is dependent on the concentration of the osteons.

Cancellous Bone (Trabecular)

■ Lies between cortical bone surfaces and consists of a network of honeycombed interstices containing hematopoietic elements and bony trabeculae.

■ Structurally important at epiphyseal–metaphyseal ends of long bone. Allows for absorption of loads across synovial joints.

■ Trabeculae are oriented perpendicular to external forces to provide structural support (48).

BONE BIOCHEMISTRY (9)

■ Bone is composed of organic matrix and mineral matrix.

■ Mineral matrix: Dry bone is made up of hydroxyapatite and tricalcium phosphate (65%–70% of the weight). Responsible for the compressive strength of bone.

■ Organic matrix: 90% type 1 collagen, 5% other collagen types, noncollagenous material, and growth factors (30%–35% of the weight).

■ Osteoid: Unmineralized organic matrix secreted by osteoblasts; composed of 90% type I collagen and 10% ground substance (noncollagenous proteins, glycoproteins proteoglycans, peptides, carbohydrates, and lipids). Mineralization of this substance by inorganic mineral salts provides bone with its strength and rigidity.

■ Inorganic bone contents: Primarily calcium phosphate and calcium carbonate with small quantities of magnesium, chloride, and sodium. Mineral crystals form hydroxyapatite, an orderly precipitate around the collagen fibers of the osteoid.

Regulators of Bone Metabolism (1,4,44)

■ Three of the calcitropic hormones that have the most effect on metabolism are parathyroid hormone, vitamin D, and calcitonin.

■ Parathyroid hormone is an amino acid made and secreted from the chief cells of the parathyroid gland. It is secreted in response to low plasma calcium. It directly activates osteoblasts to secrete receptor activator of nuclear factor κ-B ligand (RANKL), which stimulates osteoclastic development.

■ Vitamin D stimulates intestinal and renal calcium-binding proteins and facilitates active calcium transport.

■ Calcitonin is secreted by the parafollicular cells of the thyroid gland in response to rising plasma calcium level. Calcitonin serves to inhibit calcium-dependent cellular metabolic activity.

■ Miscellaneous proteins: Released from platelets, macrophages, and fibroblasts. Cause healing bone to vascularize, solidify, incorporate, and function mechanically. Induce mesenchymal-derived cells such as monocytes and fibroblasts to migrate, proliferate, and differentiate into bone cells (23,37).

■ Proteins that enhance bone healing include the *bone morphogenic proteins* (BMPs), insulin-like growth factors, transforming growth factors (TGFs), platelet-derived growth factor, and fibroblast growth factor, among others (10,14,50).

Bone Morphogenic Proteins (15,17)

■ Unique group of biologically active proteins that belong to the TGF-β superfamily.

■ Over 20 different BMPs have been discovered, but only BMP-2, -4, -6, -7, and -9 have been shown to have osteogenic properties.

■ In vivo, different BMPs act at different times and at differing concentrations during bone formation.

■ Currently BMP-2 and BMP-7 have been approved for use in treatment of tibial fractures and anterior spinal fusion (2,15,16,17).

BONE-HEALING PROCESS

■ Fracture healing restores the tissue to its original physical and mechanical properties and is influenced by a variety of systemic and local factors (26,39). Healing occurs in three distinct but overlapping stages (36,40).

Inflammatory Stage

■ A hematoma develops within the fracture site during the first few hours and days. Inflammatory cells and fibroblasts infiltrate the bone under prostaglandin mediation. This results in the formation of granulation tissue, ingrowth of vascular tissue, and migration of mesenchymal cells (4).

■ Osteoblast proliferation occurs at the fracture site from the surrounding osteoprogenitor cells.

■ Anti-inflammatory or cytotoxic medications during this first week are particularly detrimental to the initial inflammatory response to healing (41).

Repair Stage

■ Fibroblasts begin to lay down a stroma that helps support vascular ingrowth.

■ At this stage, nicotine can inhibit capillary ingrowth (11,45).

■ As vascular ingrowth progresses, a collagen matrix is laid down, while osteoid is secreted and subsequently mineralized. This leads to the formation of a soft callus around the repair site.

■ Soft callus is very weak in the first 4–6 weeks and requires adequate protection (29).

■ Eventually, ossified callus (hard callus) forms a bridge of woven bone between the fracture fragments. If proper immobilization is not employed, failure of ossification results in a fibrous union (7).

Remodeling Stage

- Healing bone is restored to its original shape, structure, and mechanical strength.
- Remodeling is a long-term process facilitated by mechanical stresses placed on the bone.
  - Axial loading across the fracture site leads to bone being deposited where it is needed and reabsorbed where it is not (26). Adequate strength is typically achieved in 3–6 months.

BIOMECHANICS OF FRACTURES

Stress Fractures (13,49,51)

- Cyclic loading repeated over a long period of time may cause disruption of the bony architecture.
- The susceptibility of bone to fracture under stresses of low magnitude is related to its crystal structure and collagen orientation.
- Under each cycle of loading, a small amount of strained energy may be lost through microscopic cracks along the cement lines of bone.
- Fatigue load under certain strain rates can cause progressive accumulation of microdamage in cortical bone.
  - Prolonged loading may eventually lead to failure through propagation of these cracks.
  - Bone may be created near the microscopic cracks through periosteal callus formation, thus arresting propagation.
- Fractures can be classified into low-risk and high-risk fracture types (13).
  - Low-risk fractures are typically treated without surgery with relatively quick healing.
    - Includes femoral shaft, medial tibia, ribs, ulna shaft, and first through fourth metatarsals.
  - High-risk fractures (those with osteoporosis) can be very difficult to treat and may require surgical intervention because they are at high risk for progression to displaced fractures as a result of relative avascularity at the fracture site.
    - Includes tension-sided femoral neck, patella, anterior tibial diaphysis, medial malleolus, talus, tarsal navicular, proximal fifth metatarsal, and first metatarsal phalangeal sesamoids.

Acute Fractures (3,14)

- Classified according to the magnitude and area of distribution of the force applied and the rate at which the force acts.
  - Soft tissue injury and fracture comminution directly proportional to the loading rate (27).
  - Modifies normal healing response by changing concentration of normal reparative mediators.

- Typically, force is applied to bone in many directions and generates compressive, tensile, or sheer stress (or some combination).
- The combination of the bone's material strength and anisometric properties dictates when, how, and along which path a fracture will occur.
  - Cortical bone is generally weak in tension and shear.
  - Area where tensile stresses arise fails first.
- Transverse fractures are the result of pure tensile forces or bending.
- Fractures from pure tensile force occur progressively across the bone, creating a transverse break without comminution.
- The pattern of fracture arising from pure bending is a simple transverse line.
- Bone undergoing rapid loading must absorb more energy than bone loaded at a slower rate.
  - At low speed, bending with tensile stress will cause a fracture with a single butterfly fragment.
  - High-speed bending will cause several butterfly fragments.
- The pattern of bone injury also impacts healing capacity (8).
  - Time to union is greatly prolonged in fractures with more soft tissue stripping.
  - Larger load under bending failure may cause the surrounding soft tissues and periosteum to sustain more damage and thus may affect the fracture healing potential.

FACTORS INFLUENCING FRACTURE REPAIR

- Systemic factors can inhibit bone healing, including the following:
  - Cigarette smoking (19)
  - Malnutrition (34)
  - Diabetes (33)
  - Rheumatoid arthritis
  - Osteoporosis (28)
  - Steroid medications (24)
  - Cytotoxic agents
  - Nonsteroidal anti-inflammatory medications (20)

Nutrition

- A typical diet including all food groups in proper amounts is enough to effect healing in a healthy individual.
  - Calcium usage is limited by absorption.
    - Preinjury calcium levels are predictive.
    - Intake of about $1 \text{ g} \cdot \text{d}^{-1}$ is optimal, along with supplemental vitamin D up to $1,000 \text{ IU} \cdot \text{d}^{-1}$.
  - True vegans with no alternative proteins are at risk for nonunion.

AUGMENTATION OF FRACTURE HEALING (14,18)

- In augmenting fracture healing, three basic components are required to enhance skeletal repair: osteogenesis, osteoconduction, and osteoinduction. Every bone graft used to enhance healing should incorporate one or more of these components (25).

Osteogenesis (3,43)

- The ability of the graft to produce new bone. This process is dependent on the presence of live bone cells in a graft material.
- Contains viable cells with the ability to form bone (osteoprogenitor cells) or the potential to differentiate into bone-forming cells.
- Osteogenesis is a property found only in fresh autogenous bone and in bone marrow cells.

Osteoconduction (22,45)

- The physical property of the graft to serve as a scaffold for viable bone healing.
- Allows for the ingrowth of neovasculature and the infiltration of osteogenic precursor cells into a graft site.
- Osteoconductive properties are found in cancellous autografts and allografts, demineralized bone matrix, hydroxyapatite, collagen, and calcium phosphate.

Osteoinduction (20,37)

- The ability of graft material to induce pluripotent mesenchymal stem cells from the surrounding tissues to develop into osteoprogenitor cells (25).
- Typically associated with the presence of bone growth factors within the graft material
- Growth-promoting proteins. Several factors are known to be associated with healing:
  - TGF-β
  - IGFs
  - BMPs
    - Glycoproteins known to induce bone.
    - Several BMPs are known to exist. BMP-3 (osteogenin) induces rapid differentiation of mesenchymal tissue to bone. BMPs induce endochondral bone formation in segmental defects (50).
- Systemic factors: Injury to bone marrow enhances osteogenesis at distant skeletal sites.
  - Factors thought to be responsible: (a) IGF-1 and IGF-2, (b) parathyroid hormone, and (c) prostaglandins.
  - Isolation and clinical development of these factors may lead to systemic treatment of fractures.

TYPES OF BONE GRAFT

Autologous Bone Graft (25,48)

- Graft is harvested from the patient, typically from a different site in the body, and used to augment fracture healing.
- Remains the gold standard of bone graft. Contains all of the properties required to help form bone.
- Donor site morbidity remains the biggest problem with autologous bone graft.

Types of Autologous Bone Graft

Autologous Cancellous Bone Graft (25).
- Cancellous grafts effect vascular ingrowth and progenitor mesenchymal cell invasion, osteoblastic appositional new bone formation, and ultimately, remodeling of the trabecular structure.
- Does not provide any initial structural support.
- Typical harvest sites: iliac crest, distal radius, and greater trochanter.

Autologous Cortical Bone Graft.
- Slow to revascularize when compared to cancellous bone graft.
- Primarily functions in osteoconductive manner with a lesser osteoinductive contribution.
- Must undergo osteoclastic resorption prior to osteoblastic new bone formation in a process called creeping substitution—an integrated process in which old necrotic bone is slowly reabsorbed and simultaneously replaced with new viable bone, thus incorporating bone grafts.
- Healing process begins at host–graft cortical junction.
- Provides initial structural support.

Autogenous Bone Marrow (30).
- Independent of cancellous or cortical bone.
- Undifferentiated progenitor cells form cells to aid in fracture healing.
- Typically can be harvested from iliac crest bone marrow.

Allograft Bone Grafting (18,30)

- Cadaveric tissue bank bone is used to augment fracture healing.
- Comes in several different preparations: cancellous graft, cortical grafts, osteochondral grafts, and demineralized bone matrix (DBM).
- Readily available in the United States.
- No harvest site morbidity.
- Risk of disease transmission is small but varies based on tissue preparation.
- Depending on the allograft used, can aid bone healing through osteoinductive and/or osteoconductive properties.

Bone Void Fillers (31,32)

- Synthetic calcium phosphate bone fillers are being more frequently used to help augment fracture fixation.
- Act as synthetic osteoconductive scaffold.
- Three subgroups: hydroxyapatites, solid tricalcium phosphates, and calcium phosphate cements (CPCs).
- The body resorbs the CPCs through an osteoclastic mediated process, which is then followed by new bone formation.
- Most commonly used to fill bone defects in subchondral bone to add mechanical strength to the fracture fixation as well as an osteoconductive scaffold.
- Most common areas of use: tibial plateau, distal radius, calcaneus, and spine.

PHYSICAL STIMULATION THERAPIES (35)

- Although the majority of fracture healing therapies are applied during surgical interventions, there are several non-invasive technologies that are being used to help fractures unite.

Electromagnetic Fields (21)

- Bone has a piezoelectric potential that is load induced due to two factors.
  - Current is induced by deformation of collagen.
  - Electrokinetic current is produced by the strain-induced flow of charged extracellular fluids.
- *Pulsed electromagnetic fields* (PEMFs) are intended to non-invasively induce electrical currents to replace endogenous currents in the absence of loading.
- Mollon et al. (38) published a recent meta-analysis that concluded a trend toward improved healing in delayed unions.

Low-Intensity Pulsed Ultrasound (LIPUS) (12,42)

- LIPUS has been shown to be effective in treatment of acute, delayed, and nonunion of bone (42).
- LIPUS has been shown in animal models to improve all phases of fracture healing.
- There is evidence that it can modulate gene expression, influence second messenger activity of chondroblasts and osteoblasts, enhance blood flow, and accelerate and augment fracture healing.
- In a study of distal radius fractures, the LIPUS-treated group had a 34%–38% decrease in time to union compared to controls (47).

Extracorporeal Shock Wave Therapy (ESWT) (52)

- Single high-amplitude sound waves propagate through tissue to create a change in tissue pressure.
- In vivo animal models have shown increased callus formation, decreased healing time, and improved mechanical properties (52).
- Wang et al. (46) demonstrated higher union rates in femur and/or tibia fractures treated with surgery and ESWT than surgery alone.
- The clinical efficacy of ESWT is still not fully understood secondary to limited randomized clinical trials available to evaluate efficacy.

REFERENCES

1. Boden SD, Kaplan FS. Calcium homeostasis. *Orthop Clin North Am.* 1990; 21(1):31–42.
2. Boden SD, Zdeblick TA, Sandhu HS, Heim SE. The use of rhBMP-2 in interbody fusion cages. Definitive evidence of osteoinduction in humans: a preliminary report. *Spine* (Phila Pa 1976). 2000;25(3):376–81.
3. Brighton CT. The biology of fracture repair. *Instr Course Lect.* 1984;33:60–82.
4. Brinker MR, O'Connor DP. Bone. In: Miller MD, Hart JA, editors. *Review of Orthopaedics.* Philadelphia: Saunders Elsevier; 2008. p. 1–43.
5. Buckwalter JA, Glimcher MJ, Cooper RR, Recker R. Bone biology. I: structure, blood supply, cells, matrix, and mineralization. *Instr Course Lect.* 1996;45:371–86.
6. Buckwalter JA, Glimcher MJ, Cooper RR, Recker R. Bone biology. II: formation, form, modeling, remodeling, and regulation of cell function. *Instr Course Lect.* 1996;45:387–99.
7. Burchardt H, Enneking WF. Transplantation of bone. *Surg Clin North Am.* 1978;58(2):403–27.
8. Carter DR, Blenman PR, Beaupré GS. Correlations between mechanical stress history and tissue differentiation in initial fracture healing. *J Orthop Res.* 1988;6(5):736–48.
9. Clohisy JC, Lindskog D, Abu-Amer Y. Bone and joint biology. In: Lieberman JR, editor. *AAOS Comprehensive Orthopaedic Review.* Rosemont: American Academy of Orthopaedic Surgeons; 2009. Chapter 5.
10. Connolly JF. Clinical use of marrow osteoprogenitor cells to stimulate osteogenesis. *Clin Orthop Relat Res.* 1998;355(Suppl):S257–66.
11. Daftari TK, Whitesides TE Jr, Heller JG, Goodrich AC, McCarey BE, Hutton WC. Nicotine on the revascularization of bone graft. An experimental study in rabbits. *Spine.* 1994;19(8):904–11.
12. Day SM, Ostrum RF, Chao EY. Bone injury, regeneration and repair. In: Buckwalter JA, Einhorn TA, Simon SR, editors. *Orthopaedic Basic Science.* Rosemont: American Academy of Orthopaedic Surgeons Press; 1999. p. 392–8.
13. Diehl JJ, Best TM, Kaeding CC. Classification and return-to-play considerations for stress fractures. *Clin Sports Med.* 2006;25(1):17–28.
14. Einhorn TA. Enhancement of fracture-healing. *J Bone Joint Surg Am.* 1995;77(6):940–56.
15. Garrison KR, Shemilt I, Donell S, et al. Bone morphogenetic protein (BMP) for fracture healing in adults. *Cochrane Database Syst Rev.* 2010; (6):CD006950.

16. Geesink RG, Hoefnagels NH, Bulstra SK. Osteogenic activity of OP-1 bone morphogenetic protein (BMP-7) in a human fibular defect. *J Bone Joint Surg Br.* 1999;81(4):710–8.

17. Giannoudis PV, Dinopoulos HT. BMPs: options, indications, and effectiveness. *J Orthop Trauma.* 2010;24(Suppl 1):S9–16.

18. Giannoudis P, Psarakis S, Kontakis G. Can we accelerate fracture healing? A critical analysis of the literature. *Injury.* 2007;38(Suppl 1):S81–9.

19. Glassman SD, Anagnost SC, Parker A, Burke D, Johnson JR, Dimar JR. The effect of cigarette smoking and smoking cessation on spinal fusion. *Spine.* 2000;25(20):2608–15.

20. Glassman SD, Rose SM, Dimar JR, Puno RM, Campbell MJ, Johnson JR. The effect of postoperative nonsteroidal anti-inflammatory drug administration on spinal fusion. *Spine.* 1998;23(7):834–8.

21. Goldstein C, Sprague S, Petrisor BA. Electrical stimulation for fracture healing: current evidence. *J Orthop Trauma.* 2010;24(Suppl 1):S62–5.

22. Hollinger JO, Brekke J, Gruskin E, Lee D. Role of bone substitutes. *Clin Orthop Relat Res.* 1996;(324):55–65.

23. Hynes RO. Integrins: versatility, modulation, and signaling in cell adhesion. *Cell.* 1992;69(1):11–25.

24. Jones JP Jr. Concepts of etiology and early pathogenesis of osteonecrosis. *Instr Course Lect.* 1994;43:499–512.

25. Kakar S, Einhorn AE. Biology and enhancement of skeletal repair. In: Jupiter J, Browner BD, Levine AM, Trafton PG, Krettek C, editors. *Skeletal Trauma: Basic Science, Management, and Reconstruction.* 4th ed. Philadelphia: Expert Consult: Online and Print; 2008.

26. Kalfas IH. Principles of bone healing. *Neurosurg Focus.* 2001;104(4):E1.

27. Karladani AH, Granhed H, Kärrholm J, Styf J. The influence of fracture etiology and type on fracture healing: a review of 104 consecutive tibial shaft fractures. *Arch Orthop Trauma Surg.* 2001;121(6):325–8.

28. Kelsey JL, Hoffman S. Risk factors for hip fracture. *N Engl J Med.* 1987;316(7):404–6.

29. Kenwright J, Gardner T. Mechanical influences on tibial fracture healing. *Clin Orthop Relat Res.* 1998;355(Suppl):S179–90.

30. Khan SN, Cammisa FP Jr, Sandhu HS, Diwan AD, Girardi FP, Lane JM. The biology of bone grafting. *J Am Acad Orthop Surg.* 2005;13(1):77–86.

31. Kirkpatrick JS, Cornell CN, Hoang BH, et al. Bone void fillers. *J Am Acad Orthop Surg.* 2010;18(9):576–9.

32. Larsson S. Calcium phosphates: what is the evidence? *J Orthop Trauma.* 2010;24(Suppl 1):S41–5.

33. Macey LR, Kana SM, Jingushi S, Terek RM, Borretos J, Bolander ME. Defects of early fracture-healing in experimental diabetes. *J Bone Joint Surg Am.* 1989;71(5):722–33.

34. Mankin HJ. Rickets, osteomalacia, and renal osteodystrophy. An update. *Orthop Clin North Am.* 1990;21(1):81–96.

35. Marsell R, Einhorn TA. Emerging bone healing therapies. *J Orthop Trauma.* 2010;24(Suppl 1):S4–8.

36. McKibbin B. The biology of fracture healing in long bones. *J Bone Joint Surg Br.* 1978;60-B(2):150–62.

37. Mohan S, Baylink DJ. Bone growth factors. *Clin Orthop Relat Res.* 1991;(263):30–48.

38. Mollon B, da Silva V, Busse JW, Einhorn TA, Bhandari M. Electrical stimulation for long-bone fracture-healing: a meta-analysis of randomized controlled trials. *J Bone Joint Surg Am.* 2008;90(11):2322–30.

39. Perlman MH, Thordarson DB. Ankle fusion in a high risk population: an assessment of non-union risk factors. *Foot Ankle Int.* 1999;20(8):491–6.

40. Perren SM. Physical and biological aspects of fracture healing with special reference to internal fixation. *Clin Orthop Relat Res.* 1979;(138):175–96.

41. Phillips AM. Overview of the fracture healing cascade. *Injury.* 2005;36(Suppl 3):S5–7.

42. Pounder NM, Harrison AJ. Low intensity pulsed ultrasound for fracture healing: a review of the clinical evidence and the associated biological mechanism of action. *Ultrasonics.* 2008;48(4):330–8.

43. Prolo DJ. Biology of bone fusion. *Clin Neurosurg.* 1990;36:135–46.

44. Reichel H, Koeffler HP, Norman AW. The role of the vitamin D endocrine system in health and disease. *N Engl J Med.* 1989;320(15):980–91.

45. Riebel GD, Boden SD, Whitesides TE, Hutton WC. The effect of nicotine on incorporation of cancellous bone graft in an animal model. *Spine.* 1995;20(20):2198–202.

46. Wang CJ, Liu HC, Fu TH. The effects of extracorporeal shockwave on acute high-energy long bone fractures of the lower extremity. *Arch Orthop Trauma Surg.* 2007;127(2):137–42.

47. Watanabe Y, Matsushita T, Bhandari M, Zdero R, Schemitsch EH. Ultrasound for fracture healing: current evidence. *J Orthop Trauma.* 2010;24(Suppl 1):S56–61.

48. White AA 3rd, Hirsch C. An experimental study of the immediate load bearing capacity of some commonly used iliac bone grafts. *Acta Orthop Scand.* 1971;42(6):482–90.

49. White AA 3rd, Panjabi MM, Southwick WO. The four biomechanical stages of fracture repair. *J Bone Joint Surg Am.* 1977;59(2):188–92.

50. Yasko AW, Lane JM, Fellinger EJ, Rosen V, Wozney JM, Wang EA. The healing of segmental bone defects, induced by recombinant human bone morphogenetic protein (rhBMP-2). A radiographic, histological, and biomechanical study in rats. *J Bone Joint Surg Am.* 1992;74(5):659–70.

51. Young AJ, McAllister DR. Evaluation and treatment of tibial stress fractures. *Clin Sports Med.* 2006;25:117–28.

52. Zelle BA, Gollwitzer H, Zlowodzki M, Bühren V. Extracorporeal shock wave therapy: current evidence. *J Orthop Trauma.* 2010;24(Suppl 1):S66–70.

Nerve Injury

Sarah A. Eby, Jeffrey G. Jenkins, and Eric J. Buchner

8

INTRODUCTION

- Trauma to peripheral nerves is a rare but important cause of sport-related injuries in the athlete (27).
- The type of peripheral nervous system (PNS) injury that occurs can vary based on numerous factors including type of sport, level of competition, and age of athlete (53).
- The segment of the PNS affected by injury, including nerve root, plexus, and peripheral nerve, also varies.
- It is important for the physician to be aware of the presentation, diagnosis, prognosis, and treatment of common peripheral nerve injuries associated with certain sports and athletic participation in general.
- This chapter will provide an overview of peripheral nerve anatomy and nerve injury diagnosis, classification, and prognosis, and identify common peripheral nerve injuries that will likely be encountered in the athletic population.

PERIPHERAL NERVE ANATOMY

- Cell body: Located in the anterior horn of the spinal cord for motor neurons or in the dorsal root ganglion for sensory neurons
- Axon: Projection from the cell body involved in propagation of an action potential and transport of cell nutrients. Axons may be myelinated or unmyelinated.
- Myelin: Substance produced by Schwann cells, layered to form a myelin sheath around axons, that acts as insulation for the conduction of current.
- Epineurium: Loose connective tissue that surrounds the entire nerve and protects it from compression.
- Perineurium: Strong layer of connective tissue surrounding fascicles or bundles of nerve fibers.
- Endoneurium: Connective tissue that surrounds an individual axon.

NERVE INJURY

- Etiology of peripheral nerve injury includes stretch or traction, compression, vibration, laceration, and ischemia (11).

- Most traumatic peripheral nerve injuries occur in the upper extremity, with the ulnar nerve most frequently injured (11).

Seddon Classification of Nerve Injury

- Neurapraxia denotes injury to myelin alone, with electrodiagnostic findings of conduction block and, later, conduction velocity slowing along the involved segment of nerve.
- Axonotmesis describes injury to axons resulting in wallerian degeneration. Early electrodiagnostic findings include loss of nerve conduction across the site of the injury (indistinguishable from neurapraxia). Later findings of decreased or absent evoked potential amplitudes distal to the site of injury are seen as wallerian degeneration occurs.
- Neurotmesis is complete disruption of the nerve, with injury to axons and wallerian degeneration as well as disruption of the supporting connective tissue. This type of injury carries a poor prognosis for recovery and usually requires urgent surgical intervention.
- Electrodiagnostic testing cannot differentiate between complete axonotmetic lesions and neurotmesis because the difference between these types of lesions is in the integrity of the supporting structures, which have no electrophysiologic function.

Sunderland Classification of Nerve Injury

- Organizes injury type based on the nerve anatomy involved.
- Class 1: Injury to myelin alone (*i.e.*, neurapraxia). Prognosis for recovery is excellent.
- Class 2: Axonotmesis with injury to axons with intact endoneurium, perineurium, and epineurium. Prognosis is good in general but varies depending on percentage of axons injured and distance of lesion from muscle.
- Class 3: Axonotmesis with injury to the endoneurium and sparing of the perineurium and epineurium. Prognosis is poor. Surgery may be required.
- Class 4: Axonotmesis with injury to the endoneurium and perineurium and sparing of the epineurium. Prognosis is poor. Surgery is required to restore nerve continuity.
- Class 5: Neurotmesis. Complete transection of the peripheral nerve. Surgery is required to restore nerve continuity. Prognosis for recovery is particularly poor (38).

DIAGNOSIS OF PERIPHERAL NERVE INJURY

■ Electrodiagnostic testing with nerve conduction studies (NCSs) and electromyography (EMG) is necessary to determine location, severity, and prognosis of nerve injury.

Timing of Electrodiagnostic Testing

■ Timing of testing depends on the question being asked.

■ Immediate to 7 days: Localization of injury with NCS, identifying conduction block versus axonotmesis (2,38).

■ 1–2 weeks: Distinguishes complete lesions from incomplete lesions. May also distinguish axonal from demyelinating lesions (axonotmesis and neurotmesis from neurapraxia) (2).

■ 3–4 weeks: Able to characterize lesion as EMG becomes useful. A single study at this point will yield the most information (2). Although EMG cannot accurately quantify axonal damage, it is the most sensitive indicator that axonal damage has occurred.

■ 3–4 months: Detects reinnervation of previously denervated muscles (2,38).

Prognosis

■ Prognosis is based on severity and type of damage to the nerve. Although purely neurapraxic (demyelinating) lesions have an excellent prognosis for fast and complete recovery, axonotmetic and neurotmetic lesions have variable outcomes based on the number of axons injured.

■ Axonal loss results in decreased evoked potential amplitudes. The best determination for degree of axonal loss is comparison to asymptomatic contralateral amplitude. A side-to-side amplitude difference of 50% is generally indicative of significant axonal loss.

■ EMG can determine complete versus partial functional denervation based on the absence or presence of motor unit action potentials. EMG can also demonstrate evidence of reinnervation based on the amplitude, phases, and duration of motor unit action potentials.

■ Most prognostication for motor recovery after peripheral nerve injury is extrapolated from a study of injured facial nerve compound motor action potential amplitudes in comparison with the asymptomatic contralateral side (45). Results indicated:

   ■ 0%–10% amplitude of contralateral side: poor prognosis

   ■ 10%–30% amplitude of contralateral side: good prognosis

   ■ > 30% amplitude of contralateral side: excellent prognosis

■ Mechanism of injury also contributes to prognosis, with avulsion-type injuries having the worst prognosis and compression injuries having the best prognosis (38).

Treatment of Nerve Injury

Pain Management

■ Early treatment is focused on pain control to allow for passive range of motion of the affected joint and limb.

■ Neuropathic pain is best managed with anticonvulsants, such as gabapentin, tricyclic antidepressants, and selective norepinephrine and serotonin reuptake inhibitors. Topical anesthetics and transcutaneous electrical nerve stimulation are good adjunct therapies (11,16,25).

■ Pain refractory to these medications and modalities can be managed with opioids, nonsteroidal anti-inflammatory medications, or in severe cases, a peripheral nerve or spinal block (11,25).

■ Desensitization techniques are important to reduce hypersensitivity and allodynia.

■ Function and range of motion are also preserved with static or dynamic splinting.

Surgical Management

■ Surgical management of nerve injury is dependent on the nerve injured, the type of injury, and the timing of injury (11,44,48).

■ Acute surgery (within 72 hours of injury) is indicated when there is a sharp nerve transection or laceration, or a hematoma or pseudoaneurysm is compressing the nerve (38).

■ Early surgery (within several weeks of injury) is indicated when there was blunt transection or avulsion of the nerve or when complete nerve lesions are noted during initial vascular repair surgery or on imaging (38).

■ Delayed surgery (3–6 months from injury) is indicated in most cases when degree of nerve damage is uncertain. Because patients with incomplete nerve lesions have better outcomes without surgery, appropriate management involves watching and waiting for clinical or electrodiagnostic evidence of recovery (11).

■ Surgical techniques for nerve repair include external neurolysis, which involves removal of the damaged epineurium, end-to-end nerve anastomosis, and nerve transfer or grafting (11,48).

■ Repair to reinnervate the muscle must be performed before 12–18 months after injury, when irreversible damage to the denervated muscle occurs (11).

■ Procedures such as tendon and muscle transfer can restore function when the primary muscle is irreversibly damaged.

PERIPHERAL NERVE INJURY IN NONCONTACT SPORTS

■ PNS injuries make up a small percentage of all sport-related traumas. However, there are certain relatively safe sports in which peripheral nerve injuries comprise a large proportion of all injuries incurred. These are volleyball, cycling, and racquet sports.

Volleyball

- Peripheral nerve injuries are unfortunately common in volleyball, with the most common being suprascapular nerve entrapment at the spinoglenoid notch.
- This presents as painless weakness and atrophy of the infraspinatus in the dominant serving arm of the player.
- Prevalence has been documented to range from 33% to 45% of symptomatic international-level players and to be 12% in asymptomatic players at the same level (17,19,53).
- EMG reveals isolated infraspinatus denervation and motor unit loss (32,53). Possible etiologies of this specific nerve entrapment related to volleyball serving include increased shoulder range of motion and impingement of the infraspinatus branch of the suprascapular nerve between the edge of the spine of the scapula and the medial tendinous margin between the infraspinatus and supraspinatus muscles (40,53).

Cycling

- Cycling is commonly associated with two peripheral nerve injuries: ulnar neuropathy at the wrist, or "cyclist's palsy," and pudendal neuropathy.
- Cyclist's palsy presents as numbness and paresthesias in the ulnar distribution of the hand (small finger and ulnar half of the ring finger) and weakness of hand intrinsic muscles (24).
- Ulnar neuropathy at the wrist is highly prevalent in long-distance cyclists and is independent of handlebar design (24,34)
- Injury is due to compression of the ulnar nerve at the wrist. NCSs have demonstrated significantly increased distal motor latencies in the deep branch of the ulnar nerve after a long-distance cycling event, suggesting the possibility of acute trauma (1,24).
- Treatment is usually conservative, including temporary rest from cycling, use of gloves and padded handlebars, and hand position changes during long rides (24,33,37). Conservative management leads to resolution of symptoms in the majority of cases, and surgical decompression of Guyon's canal is rarely indicated (24).
- Pudendal neuropathy presents as genital numbness affecting the penis, scrotum, and/or perianal area and erectile dysfunction. The area of sensory loss is dependent on the location of nerve compression, with more distal compression being associated with penile anesthesia alone.
- The pudendal nerve can be compressed proximally as the nerve crosses between the sacrospinal and sacrotuberous ligaments, within Alcock's canal, or distally between perineum and pubic symphysis (2,29).
- Pudendal neuropathy is highly prevalent in both competitive and recreational long-distance cyclists, with sensory symptoms present in 61% and impotency symptoms present in 24% of male cyclists riding more than 400 km per week (4,24,41,42,47).

- Treatment is usually conservative, including temporary rest from cycling; change of saddle design to shift weight from the perineum to the buttocks; switching to a wider, padded saddle with a flexible nose; positioning the saddle nose downward; decreasing height difference between seat and handlebar; and implementing riding breaks and position changes during longer rides (24,41). These modifications can prevent the need for surgical pudendal nerve decompression.

Racquet Sports

- Injuries in racquet sports are almost exclusively peripheral nerve injuries to the dominant arm (53).
- The posterior interosseous nerve can become entrapped with the arcade of Frohse. This presents as wrist and finger extensor weakness (22,31,53).
- Suprascapular neuropathy can also occur due to repetitive overhand serving. The pathology of nerve compression is similar to that in volleyball players, as discussed earlier (39,53).
- The use of constrictive wrist bands can cause superficial radial neuropathy (36,53).
- Neurogenic thoracic outlet syndrome has been diagnosed in the serving arm of tennis players (23,50,53).

SPORTS AND PERIPHERAL NERVE INJURY

- Sports in general can put peripheral nerves at risk for injury, due to the susceptibility of anatomy used to play the sport or the contact nature required for play.
- The nerves of the upper extremity are involved the majority of the time, with the most common injury being the "stinger" or "burner" (27).
- Case series describing peripheral nerve injuries in athletes have findings that are culture and country specific; thus, numbers reflect different levels of participation in various sports. However, studies done in the United States and Canada indicate that most peripheral nerve injuries are sustained playing football (27,52,53). Wrestling and throwing sports are also more highly associated with peripheral nerve injuries.

CONTACT SPORTS AND NERVE INJURY

Stingers and Burners

- Stingers, also referred to as "burners," are thought to be the result of compression, distraction, or direct blow injuries of the C5 and C6 cervical nerve roots or the upper trunk of the brachial plexus. This causes acute, temporary pain and paresthesias in the upper extremity (2,3,27,30).

- Studies that have employed electrodiagnostic testing of athletes with stingers have demonstrated lesions to the cervical nerve roots and brachial plexus (2,8,27,43).
- This is the most common nerve injury encountered in football players, particularly defensive players, and in wrestlers (15,26,52,53).
- The current recommendation for diagnostic evaluation and return to play is based on number of stingers, whether or not stinger recurrence occurred in the same season, and degree of clinical sequelae (49). Players with one stinger and no lasting sequelae are able to return to play the same day. Those with two or more stingers need a diagnostic evaluation, including magnetic resonance imaging and electrodiagnostic testing, before returning to play. Those with three stingers in the same season or three stingers in different seasons with persistent symptoms are out for the season (49).

Peroneal Nerve Injury

- The peroneal nerve is the most frequently injured lower extremity nerve in athletes (21,27).
- Injury at the fibular head is most common, followed by at the ankle. Mechanism of injury is direct blow to the knee or ankle sprain (27).
- Concomitant peroneal nerve injury with ligamentous trauma (involving the anterior cruciate, posterior cruciate, or lateral collateral ligament) and knee dislocation has also been described in athletes (27).
- Compartment syndrome in the lower leg can also put the peroneal nerve at risk for damage (27).

Axillary Nerve Injury

- Axillary nerve injury in athletes has been associated with anterior shoulder dislocation or direct shoulder trauma (27).

THROWING SPORTS AND NERVE INJURY

- Several upper extremity nerves, including the suprascapular, axillary, and ulnar nerves, are frequently injured in baseball and softball players due to the torque force that occurs during overhead throwing (5,7,13,53).

Ulnar Nerve Injury

- Ulnar neuropathy is most common in baseball pitchers, whereas radial neuropathy is common in softball pitchers due to the biomechanics of underhand or "windmill" pitching (5,14,46).
- The etiology of ulnar neuropathy is attributed to the valgus force placed on the medial elbow when the elbow is flexed and the wrist is extended during the acceleration phase of throwing with elbow flexion and wrist extension.

- With ulnar neuropathy at the elbow, electrodiagnostic studies will show slowed conduction velocity across the elbow and, in more severe cases, will demonstrate denervation in ulnar-innervated muscles
- Management of ulnar neuropathy at the elbow can include conservative treatment, but surgical decompression is usually most successful. Anterior subcutaneous transposition and submuscular transposition have demonstrated favorable outcomes when compared to simple decompression or medial epicondylectomy in the overhead-throwing athlete (5,6,11,13,14,20,36,54).

Suprascapular Nerve Injury

- The suprascapular nerve can be compressed in two different anatomic locations, producing different symptoms in the thrower:
  - In the suprascapular notch underneath the superior transverse scapular ligament (13,35). Injury at this location results in denervation of both the supraspinatus and infraspinatus muscles. Patients complain of posterior shoulder weakness and pain.
  - At the spinoglenoid notch. Patients will present with shoulder weakness; however, the infraspinatus muscle alone is involved because the branch to the supraspinatus has been spared. Posterior shoulder pain is not usually present due to the nerve injury being distal to the suprascapular sensory nerve fibers (13,19). A ganglion cyst can also compress the suprascapular nerve, with the most common location for a cyst to develop at the spinoglenoid notch (12,13,18).
- Electrodiagnostic studies can localize the suprascapular nerve injury, as well as rule out cervical radiculopathy and brachial plexopathy. NCSs can demonstrate an increased compound motor action potential latency, whereas EMG will determine if there is denervation of the supraspinatus, infraspinatus, or both.

Axillary Nerve Injury

- The axillary nerve is rarely injured in throwers, but when affected is usually due to the quadrilateral space syndrome. The syndrome involves compression of the axillary nerve in the quadrilateral space, due to a fibrous band or ganglion cyst within the space or decreased space between teres major and minor during the late cocking phase of pitch (10,13).
- Treatment of nerve injury in the throwing arm is usually conservative, consisting of throwing rest, physical therapy focusing on shoulder and trunk flexibility and strength, and correction of altered throwing mechanics (13).
- Surgery is indicated if there is no improvement with nonoperative management, if there is a mass lesion causing the symptoms, or if the neuropathy is severe (13).

CARPAL TUNNEL SYNDROME IN ATHLETES

- Cases of carpal tunnel syndrome (CTS) are usually found incidentally in asymptomatic athletes who undergo electrodiagnostic testing for other nerve injuries (27).
- Symptomatic CTS is most common in sports that require repetitive wrist maneuvers, such as weight lifting, cycling, and racquet sports (2,9,27,28,36,43,51).

CONCLUSION

- Peripheral nerve trauma is a rare but potentially debilitating occurrence in sports.
- Nerves of the upper extremity are more often affected than those in the lower extremity.
- Sports in general put nerves at risk, but certain sports are more highly associated with peripheral nerve injury than others.
- Diagnosis of nerve injury is achieved by combining clinical findings, appropriate imaging, and electrodiagnostic studies.
- Treatment can be conservative or surgical, depending on the type and severity of nerve injury.
- Prognosis of nerve injury is dependent on injury severity, mechanism of injury, and location of injury.

REFERENCES

1. Akuthota V, Plastaras C, Lindberg K, Tobey J, Press J, Garvan C. The effect of long-distance bicycling on ulnar and median nerves: an electrophysiologic evaluation of cyclist palsy. *Am J Sports Med.* 2005;33(8):1224–30.
2. Aldridge JW, Bruno RJ, Strauch RJ, Rosenwasser MP. Nerve entrapment in athletes. *Clin Sports Med.* 2001;20(1):95–122.
3. American College of Sports Medicine. Selected issues in injury and illness prevention and the team physician: a consensus statement. *Med Sci Sports Exerc.* 2007;39(11):2012–6.
4. Andersen KV, Bovim G. Impotence and nerve entrapment in long distance amateur cyclists. *Acta Neurol Scand.* 1997;95(4):233–40.
5. Andrews JR, Timmerman LA. Outcome of elbow surgery in professional baseball players. *Am J Sports Med.* 1995;23(4):407–13.
6. Aoki M, Kanaya K, Aiki H, Wada T, Yamashita T, Ogiwara N. Cubital tunnel syndrome in adolescent baseball players: a report of six cases with 3- to 5-year follow-up. *Arthroscopy.* 2005;21(6):758.
7. Bennett G. Elbow and shoulder lesions of the professional baseball pitcher. *Am J Surg.* 1959;98:484–92.
8. Bergfeld JA, Herschman EB, Wilbourn AJ. Brachial plexus injury in sports: a five-year follow-up. *Orthop Trans.* 1988;12:743–4.
9. Cabrera JM, McCue FC 3rd. Nonosseous athletic injuries of the elbow, forearm, and hand. *Clin Sports Med.* 1986;5(4):681–700.
10. Cahill BR, Palmer RE. Quadrilateral space syndrome. *J Hand Surg Am.* 1983;8(1):65–9.
11. Campbell WW. Evaluation and management of peripheral nerve injury. *Clin Neurophysiol.* 2008;199(9):1951–65.
12. Chochole M, Senker W, Meznik C, Breitenseher MJ. Glenoid-labral cyst entrapping the suprascapular nerve: dissolution after arthroscopic debridement of an extended SLAP lesion. *Arthroscopy.* 1997;13(6):753–5.
13. Cummins CA, Schneider DS. Peripheral nerve injuries in baseball players. *Neurol Clin.* 2008;26(1):195–215.
14. Del Pizzo W, Jobe FW, Norwood L. Ulnar nerve entrapment syndrome in baseball players. *Am J Sports Med.* 1997;5(5):182–5.
15. Diamond PT, Gale SD. Head injuries in men's and women's lacrosse: a 10 year analysis of the National Electronic Injury Surveillance System database. *Brain Inj.* 2001;15(6):537–44.
16. Dworkin RH, Backonja M, Rowbotham MC, et al. Advances in neuropathic pain: diagnosis mechanisms and treatment recommendations. *Arch Neurol.* 2003;60(11):1524–34.
17. Eggert S, Holzgraefe M. [Compression neuropathy of the suprascapular nerve in high performance volleyball players]. *Sportverletz Sportschaden.* 1993;7(3):136–42 [in German].
18. Fehrman D, Orwin J, Jennings R. Suprascapular nerve entrapment by a ganglion cyst: a report of six cases with arthroscopic finding and review of the literature. *Arthroscopy.* 1995;11(6):727–34.
19. Ferretti A, Cerullo G, Russo G. Suprascapular neuropathy in volleyball players. *J Bone Joint Surg Am.* 1987;69(2):260–3.
20. Glousman RE. Ulnar nerve problems in the athlete's elbow. *Clin Sports Med.* 1990;9(2):365–77.
21. Hirasawa Y, Sakakida K. Sports and peripheral nerve injury. *Am J Sports Med.* 1983;9(4):244–6.
22. Kaplan PE. Posterior interosseous neuropathies: natural history. *Arch Phys Med Rehabil.* 1984;65(7):399–400.
23. Karas SE. Thoracic outlet syndrome. *Clin Sports Med.* 1990;9(2):297–310.
24. Kennedy J. Neurologic injuries in cycling and bike riding. *Neurol Clin.* 2008;26(1):271–9.
25. Kingery WS. A critical review of controlled clinical trials for peripheral neuropathic pain and complex regional pain syndromes. *Pain.* 1997;73(2):123–39.
26. Kline DG, Judice DJ. Operative management of selected brachial plexus lesions. *J Neurosurg.* 1993;58(5):631–49.
27. Krivickas LS, Wilbourn AJ. Peripheral nerve injuries in athletes: a case series of over 200 injuries. *Semin Neurol.* 2000;20(2):225–32.
28. Kulund DN, McCue FC, Rockwell DA, Gieck JH. Tennis injuries, prevention and treatment. *Am J Sports Med.* 1979;7(4):249–53.
29. Leibovitch I, Mor Y. The vicious cycling: bicycling related urogenital disorders. *Eur Urol.* 2005;47(3):277–86.
30. Levitz CL, Reilly PJ, Torg JS. The pathomechanics of chronic, recurrent cervical nerve root neurapraxia. *Am J Sports Med.* 1997;25(1):73–6.
31. Lorei MP, Hershman EB. Peripheral nerve injuries in athletes. Treatment and prevention. *Sports Med.* 1993;16(2):130–47.
32. Montagna P, Colonna S. Suprascapular neuropathy restricted to the infraspinatus muscle in volleyball players. *Acta Neurol Scand.* 1993;87(3):174–80.
33. Munnings F. Cyclist's palsy making changes brings relief. *Phys Sportsmed.* 1991;19(9):113–9.
34. Patterson JM, Jaggars MM, Boyer MI. Ulnar and median nerve palsy in long-distance cyclists. A prospective study. *Am J Sports Med.* 2003;31:585–9.
35. Rengachary SS, Neff JP, Singer PA, Brackett CE. Suprascapular entrapment neuropathy: a clinical, anatomical and comparative study. Part 1: clinical study. *Neurosurgery.* 1979;5(4):441–6.
36. Rettig AC. Neurovascular injuries in the wrists and hands of athletes. *Clin Sports Med.* 1990;9(2):389–417.
37. Richmond DR. Handlebar problems in bicycling. *Clin Sports Med.* 1994;13(1):165–73.

38. Robinson LR. AAEM Minimonograph 28: traumatic injury to peripheral nerves. *Muscle Nerve*. 2000;23:863–73.

39. Romeo AA, Rotenberg DD, Bach BR Jr. Suprascapular neuropathy. *J Am Acad Orthop Surg*. 1999;7(6):358–67.

40. Sandow MJ, Ilic J. Suprascapular nerve rotator cuff compression syndrome in volleyball players. *J Shoulder Elbow Surg*. 1998;7(5):516–21.

41. Schrader SM, Breitenstein MJ, Clark JC, Lowe BD, Turner TW. Nocturnal penile tumescence and rigidity testing in bicycling patrol officers. *J Androl*. 2002;23(6):927–34.

42. Schwarzer U, Wiegand W, Bin-Saleh A, et al. Genital numbness and impotence rates in long distance cyclists. *J Urol*. 1999;161(4 Suppl):178.

43. Sicuranza MJ, McCue FC 3rd. Compressive neuropathies in the upper extremity of athletes. *Hand Clin*. 1992;8(2):263–73.

44. Siemionow M, Sari A. A contemporary overview of peripheral nerve research from the Cleveland Clinic microsurgery laboratory. *Neurol Res*. 2004;26(2):218–25.

45. Sillman JS, Niparko JK, Lee SS, Kileny PR. Prognostic value of evoked and standard electromyography in acute facial paralysis. *Otolaryngol Head Neck Surg*. 1992;107(3):377–81.

46. Sinson G, Zager EL, Kline DG. Windmill pitcher's radial neuropathy. *Neurosurgery*. 1994;34(6):1087–9.

47. Sommer F, König D, Graft C, et al. Impotence and genital numbness in cyclists. *Int J Sports Med*. 2001;22(6):410–3.

48. Spinner RJ, Kline DG. Surgery for peripheral nerve and brachial plexus injuries or other nerve lesions. *Muscle Nerve*. 2000;23(5):680–95.

49. Standaert CJ, Herring SA. Expert opinion and controversies in musculoskeletal and sports medicine: stingers. *Arch Phys Med Rehabil*. 2009;90(3):402–6.

50. Strukel RJ, Garrick JG. Thoracic outlet compression in athletes: a report of four cases. *Am J Sports Med*. 1978;6(2):35–9.

51. Szabo RM, Madison M. Carpal tunnel syndrome. *Orthop Clin North Am*. 1992;23(1):103–9.

52. Toth C. The epidemiology of injuries to the nervous system resulting from sport and recreation. *Neurol Clin*. 2008;26(1):1–31.

53. Toth C. Peripheral nerve injuries attributable to sport and recreation. *Neurol Clin*. 2008;26(1):89–113.

54. Treihaft MM. Neurologic injuries in baseball players. *Semin Neurol*. 2000;20(2):187–93.

Muscle and Tendon Injury and Repair

9

Luis P. Carrilero, Mark Hamming, Bradley J. Nelson, and Dean C. Taylor

SKELETAL MUSCLE INJURY AND REPAIR

■ Muscle injury is the most common musculoskeletal complaint in the athlete. Common muscle injuries include muscle strains, delayed muscle soreness, contusions, and cramps. Muscle injury results in 15%–50% of all injuries sustained in sports. More than 90% of these frequent injuries are contusions and strains, whereas laceration is considered the least frequent (20,27).

Anatomy and Physiology

■ Skeletal muscle is composed primarily of contractile proteins (myosin and actin), regulatory proteins (tropomyosin and troponin), and a connective tissue matrix (13).

■ The muscle fiber is the basic structural element of skeletal muscle. Muscle is a syncytium of multinucleated fibers (17). The functional unit of muscle is the sarcomere. Within each sarcomere are light and dark bands. The dark bands are made up of both the thick myosin and thin actin filaments, whereas the light bands are made up of just the thin actin filaments that connect to the Z lines.

■ A muscle fiber originates via a tendon from bone, traverses one or more joints, and joins with a tendon that inserts to bone. Fiber arrangement can be parallel or oblique (unipennate, bipennate, multipennate) in orientation. Fibers can be classified as Type I (slow-twitch oxidative) and Type II (fast-twitch). Type II fibers are further classified into Type IIa (fast-twitch oxidative glycolytic) and Type IIb (fast-twitch glycolytic).

■ Satellite cells are separate cells along the periphery of the muscle fiber that are important in cellular regeneration in response to injury. Satellite cells proliferate and transform into myotubes in response to growth factors and cytokines that mediate the repair process (62).

■ The musculotendinous junction is a specialized region of highly folded membranes that increase the surface area for force transmission (13). Most muscle strain injuries occur in this region.

■ The sarcoplasmic reticulum is a specialized cellular organelle that is responsible for calcium movement across the cell membrane and electrical transmission within the cell.

■ A motor unit is a motor neuron and all the muscle fibers it innervates. The motor neuron innervates each of its muscle fibers at a motor end plate. The number of myofibers in a motor unit and the number of motor units in a skeletal muscle are determined by the function of the muscle (20). The fewer the fibers in a motor unit, the finer is the control (e.g., ocular muscles), whereas many fibers in a motor unit lead to gross movements (e.g., quadriceps).

■ A muscle contraction begins when an electrical impulse travels down a motor neuron's axon to its motor end plates. This electrical impulse triggers the release of acetylcholine that migrates to receptors on the myofiber and causes a depolarization of the sarcolemma. The depolarization travels deep into the muscle by the transverse tubule, triggering the release of calcium from the sarcoplasmic reticulum. Calcium binds to troponin, which results in a conformational change in the tropomyosin, opening actin's active site and allowing the crossbridges of the myosin head to interact. The crossbridges then undergo their own conformational change that pulls the thin actin filament to slide past the myosin toward the center of the sarcomere. The process of sarcolemmal depolarization and the resulting sliding of the filaments is referred to as excitation–contraction coupling. The physical process of muscle contraction is the sliding of the actin filament past the myosin filament toward the center of the sarcomere pulling the ends of the sarcomere (the Z lines) toward each other. The whole muscle shortens when the process is multiplied over thousands of sarcomeres, thousands of conformational changes at the myosin crossbridge heads, and all of the activated fibers. This process is powered by the hydrolysis of adenosine triphosphate (ATP) to both bind and break the connection of the crossbridge with the actin filament (17,20).

■ Muscle contraction can be isometric, concentric, or eccentric. Isometric contraction is when the force by the muscle is equal to the load, and although there is no visible joint movement, the muscle does shorten. By recruiting more muscle fibers to overcome the external load, a concentric (or shortening) contraction can occur, and there is visible joint movement. Eccentric contraction is when the external load is greater than the force generated by the muscle and the muscle lengthens (20). For example, raising the weight in an arm curl is a concentric contraction of the elbow flexors, and lowering the weight is an eccentric contraction of the same flexors. Isometric strength measurements are strongly predictive of functional capacity and are sensitive in detecting changes in muscle strength (36).

Reparative Process

- The pathophysiology of the healing muscle is similar regardless of the type of injury. Healing occurs in three distinct phases: (a) degeneration and inflammation; (b) muscle regeneration; (c) development of fibrosis (20). The reparative process involves both inflammatory cells (neutrophils, macrophages) and myogenic (satellite) cells.

- Acute hemorrhage and inflammatory cell infiltration of the damaged muscle tissue occurs shortly after injury (40).

  - Initially, neutrophils infiltrate the injury site via cellular chemotaxis. Mediators such as *basic fibroblast growth factor* (BFGF), *platelet-derived growth factor* (PDGF), and *interleukin-1* (IL-1) regulate myoblast proliferation and differentiation to foster regeneration and repair of the muscle, as well as stimulation of macrophages and fibroblasts within the muscle tissue (17,20).

  - Macrophages are the most prevalent inflammatory cells present in injured muscle. Distinct subclasses of macrophages have been identified and play specific roles in the healing process. One subclass of macrophages is involved in the phagocytosis of damaged tissue and further stimulation of the inflammatory response. A second subclass of macrophages helps modulate the reparative process (61).

- Satellite cells are myogenic mononuclear cells responsible for muscle fiber repair and regeneration processes. They are located beneath the basal lamina of skeletal muscle fibers. Mechanical or chemical insults stimulate quiescent satellite cells through hepatocyte growth factor (HGF)/nitric oxide radical–dependent pathways (3,53). The activated satellite cells enter the cycle cell and differentiate into myoblasts, which fuse together and develop into multinucleated muscle fibers. Typically, these repaired myofibers attach to the extracellular matrix of the newly formed scar (32).

- Fibroblast proliferation and collagen matrix synthesis occur along with the inflammatory response and muscle regeneration. This connective tissue scar formation may inhibit the complete repair of injured muscle (32). Muscle degeneration and inflammation occur during the first days after injury. Regeneration then starts after 1 week, peaks at 2 weeks, and is typically complete by 3–4 weeks. Scar tissue starts to form 2–3 weeks after injury and increases (18).

- There has been considerable muscle-derived stem cell (MDSC) research recently, and the literature provides evidence that stem cells participate in myofiber regeneration. In addition, these pluripotent stem cells can differentiate into endothelial and neural lineages, which may be beneficial in vascular and neural supply to the regenerating muscle.

MDSCs have also been used to produce proregenerative and antifibrotic agents (18). However, the medical evidence in humans is limited, and further studies are needed.

Muscle Strain Injury

- Muscle strain is the most common injury sustained in sports. Muscle can be functionally limited from delayed muscle soreness (discussed later), partial muscle strain, or complete muscle disruption.

- A common feature in muscle tissue injury is muscle stretch in combination with a strong contraction in two-joint muscles (*e.g.*, rectus femoris, biceps femoris, gastrocnemius) or muscles with a complex architecture (*e.g.*, adductor longus). The injury occurs when selected muscles restrict range of motion of the joint they cross and a significant amount of tension is placed on that muscle (40).

- Clinically, muscle injury (strain/contusion) is classified depending on the level of damage generated: *mild* when the loss of strength and movement is minimal or nonexistent, *moderate* with inability to contract, and *severe* for absolute loss of function (22).

Mechanism of Injury

- Although a concentric muscle contraction alone is insufficient to create muscle strain injury, the force per fiber is higher in the relatively few muscle fibers needed during eccentric muscular contraction. The combination of passive stretch of the muscle past its resting length, eccentric loads, and the subsequent concentric contraction is required to injure the muscle (16). This overextension and tension development can then disrupt the myofibers near the myotendinous junction (26).

- Cellular disruption results in the hydrolysis of structural proteins and inflammation that further damages the muscle tissue (39).

- Animal studies reveal that muscle tissue sustaining a nondisruptive strain injury demonstrates decreased load to failure when subjected to stress (41,60). In addition, these partially injured muscles generate significantly less contractile force, which contributes to the clinical observation that significant muscle strain injuries are frequently preceded by a minor injury. These studies also underscore the importance of rest and complete recovery prior to the resumption of athletic activities.

Diagnosis and Imaging

- Although reviewing the athlete's history is essential, tenderness to palpation at the myotendinous junction is hallmark. When a complete rupture is present, a defect may be palpated, and weakness should be expected.

- Ultrasound, due to its lower costs and portability, is sometimes the first diagnostic modality. Evaluation of superficial structures such as the patellar tendon is easier with ultrasound; however, in athletes with a voluminous musculature, the evaluation of deep structures may be difficult due to dissipation of the sound waves and the lack of reflection over long distances (4).

- Magnetic resonance imaging is typically unnecessary for diagnosis of muscle strain, but it may help determine the severity of the strain, continuity of the myotendinous junction, and possible convalescent time, which is crucial for elite athletes. T1-weighted images show excellent anatomic detail such as the myotendinous junction disruption, whereas T2-weighted images are fluid-sensitive and reveal pathologic processes involved in edema, making muscle strains easy to visualize (4,40).

Reparative Response

- Similar to general reparative response of muscle described earlier.
- The presence of inelastic fibrotic tissue (scar) may make the muscle more susceptible to additional injury.

Treatment and Prevention

- Reduced activity is key in the treatment of muscle strain injuries. This helps control inflammation and prevents further tissue damage.
- The RICE principle (rest, ice, compression, and elevation) should be implemented immediately after skeletal muscle injury. Immobilization can diminish pain, reduce inflammation, and allow torn muscle ends to reapproximate. Prolonged muscle immobilization (> 7–14 days) results in lower loads to failure and should be avoided. Early motion also limits adhesions and provides quicker proprioceptive recovery (40).
- Therapeutic ultrasound is thought to relieve pain and promote muscle regeneration during the initial phase of muscle injuries. Its recommendation and use is promoted even though the results from animal studies have not been encouraging. In addition, its effectiveness in the complete healing process is questionable (47,64).
- Clinical trials have failed to demonstrate the benefits of hyperbaric oxygen therapy in the treatment of mild muscle injuries in athletes (12).
- **Nonsteroidal anti-inflammatory drugs**
  - Animal studies demonstrate that nonsteroidal anti-inflammatory drugs (NSAIDs) reduce the inflammatory response associated with muscle strain injury, providing more complete functional recovery by 1 week. A certain level of inflammation is necessary, however, to remove necrotic tissue and permit healing; thus, NSAIDs may delay complete healing of the damaged muscle tissue (39,41). The indication for the use of these drugs in muscle strain injury is unclear, and many physicians recommend only a short course of NSAIDs immediately after the acute strain (40).
  - Cryotherapy provides an analgesic effect, but its effect on inflammation is also unclear (40). Some authors state that icing injured skeletal muscle should be applied for 6 hours to limit the hemorrhage and tissue necrosis formation (51).
- **Muscle strengthening**
  - Muscle strengthening is an important factor in the recovery of injured muscle and the prevention of reinjury. Eccentric muscle strengthening exercises have been shown to decrease the rate of hamstring injuries in studies that compare conventional and eccentric strengthening exercises (6,7,14,15).
  - The gradual return to training activity should be considered when the athlete is able to stretch the injured muscle as far as the contralateral muscle and denies pain with basic movements (44). One prospective randomized study on hamstring strains highlighted that exercises of progressive agility and trunk stabilization resulted in fewer reinjuries and accelerated the return to practice of the athlete when compared to a stretch and strength protocol (54).
- **Muscle stretching and warm-up**
  - Muscle is viscoelastic material, and passive stretching can reduce stress for a given muscle length (59). In addition, preconditioned muscle and warm muscle fail at higher loads than control muscle (49). A recent review stated that a warm-up and stretching protocol implemented within the 15 minutes prior to starting physical activity results in better performance scores and fewer muscle injuries (67).
  - A systematic review of clinical and basic science literature, however, questioned this conclusion, stating that an intense period of stretching prior to exercise did not improve the athlete's performance, failed to prevent muscle injuries, and may make the muscle more susceptible to injury (55). It also points out that the study of stretching should not be limited to muscle injuries and the analysis should include other types of injuries (56–58). Additional studies are needed before definitive conclusions can be made.
  - A clinical study at the U.S. Military Academy examined the effects of dynamic warm-up versus a static stretching warm-up in running performance, underhand medicine ball throw for distance, and the five-step jump. The study concluded that dynamic warm-up enhanced the athlete's performance, whereas static stretching warm-up showed almost no effect and should be reassessed (37).

Delayed Muscle Soreness

- Delayed muscle soreness is defined as skeletal muscle pain 24–72 hours after unaccustomed physical activity. The pain lasts approximately 5–7 days and can range from mild soreness to severe discomfort (5). Loss of both muscle strength and joint range of motion, tenderness, and elevated muscle enzymes are also present.
- Strength loss can be explained by both the presence of pain and a decrease in the inherent force-producing capacity of the muscle fibers (5).
- Reduced range of motion and elevated levels of creatine kinase are common 1–2 days after the strenuous exercise; however, peak creatine kinase levels have not been shown to be correlated with the temporal aspects of pain or degree of tissue injury (34).

- No permanent muscle injury occurs, and complete muscle recovery is seen within 14 days. The adaptation to the unaccustomed exercise (*i.e.*, less soreness with successive bouts of the exercise) is rapid (9).
- Delayed muscle soreness occurs most commonly in fast-type muscle fibers when performing eccentric activity and is related to both the intensity and duration of activity.

Pathophysiology

- High tension over a small cross-sectional area (seen in eccentric muscular contraction) results in cytoskeletal disruption.
- Sarcolemma (cell membrane) and other myofibrillar disruption results in an influx of intracellular Ca^{2+} that induces proteolytic enzyme-mediated myoprotein degradation (5,34,45).
- Cellular damage results in the activation of the inflammatory process. This stimulates nociceptors within the muscle, resulting in the production of pain (5,34).

Treatment and Prevention

- Further exercise appears to be the most effective method of diminishing the symptoms of delayed muscle soreness (9). This is most likely due to exercise-induced production of endorphins, a stronger cytoskeleton, or alterations in neural pathways (5).
- Delayed muscle soreness diminishes with repetition of exercise; light activity and stretching preserve range of motion (40) for reasons that remain unclear. There is still continued muscle tissue damage with repetitive exercise, but to a progressively lesser extent. Perceptual discomfort associated with this tissue damage, however, is greatly diminished.
- NSAIDs demonstrate similar effects in an exercise-induced muscle injury model as they do in other muscle injury models. There is early benefit to the muscle by limiting inflammation, but the later negative effects on maximum muscle function discussed earlier persist (38).

Muscle Contusion Injury

- Muscle contusions are common injuries in collision and contact sports. These soft tissue injuries are frequently caused by impact with a blunt, nonpenetrating object. In most cases, contusions involve the lower extremity muscle groups such as the quadriceps, gastrocnemius, or anterior muscles of the leg (13).
- The initial clinical presentation includes pain, swelling, loss of joint range of motion, and the possibility of a palpable muscle defect. This can be followed by persistent swelling and warmth, a firm mass, and continued loss of motion.
- Animal studies of muscle contusion injury demonstrate muscle fiber rupture, resulting in hematoma formation, edema, and inflammation (63).

Reparative Response

- The process of muscle contusion healing is similar to the general process of muscle healing, involving a combination of the formation of scar tissue by fibroblasts and the regeneration of normal muscle by migrating myoblasts (10). There appears to be less scar formation from a contusion than with a muscle strain injury.

Diagnosis and Treatment

- RICE principle is usually the first treatment option for the athlete immediately after the injury.
- **Immobilization versus mobilization of contused muscle**
  - Brief immobilization (< 5 days) leads to faster healing without further tissue damage, whereas prolonged immobilization results in muscle atrophy and delayed muscle activity (in a rat model) (23,31). In addition, early mobilization results in increased tensile stiffness of contused muscle and more rapid resolution of the contusion injury (24).
  - Clinical studies from the U.S. Military Academy demonstrate that a brief period of immobilization (24–48 hours), with the involved muscle in a lengthened position, followed by mobilization results in earlier recovery than prolonged muscle immobilization (22,48).
  - Ultrasound has been useful in distinguishing swelling and edema from hematoma formation. This helps when considering surgical evacuation of the hematoma and when electing a less aggressive approach using compression and early mobilization (10).

Pharmacologic Treatment

- Animal studies have demonstrated that both corticosteroids and NSAIDs cause a decrease in the early inflammatory response (11); however, there is delayed muscle regeneration and a decrease in the later tensile properties of the healed muscle. Although the clinical use of anabolic steroids and growth factors has not been approved, recent animal studies show these can produce beneficial effects in the healing of contused muscle (10).
- Myositis ossificans is a complication of concern from muscle contusion injury. In the West Point study, 9% of the contusion injuries developed myositis ossificans as a complication (22,48). The etiology of this abnormal bone formation is unclear, but this diagnosis is related to the degree of muscle injury, the region injured (quadriceps and brachialis), and the number of times the muscle is subjected to trauma (10). Clinically, there is tenderness, swelling, loss of motion, persistent warmth, and a firm mass in the area of the bone formation. By 4 weeks, abnormal bone is evident on radiographs that resembles mature bone by 6 months (13). There are three forms of myositis ossificans: (a) a thin stalk of bone that connects the ossified muscle to the bone; (b) a broad-based ossification that has contact with the bone lying beneath; and (c) an ossification that originates entirely in the muscle and does not have connection with the underlying bone (10). Frequently, the calcium deposits are spontaneously reabsorbed after several months. Surgical resection, if necessary, should be delayed until the osteoblast activity has ceased (6 months to 1 year) and there is no evidence of increased tracer uptake on a bone scan.

Muscle Cramps

- Muscle cramps affect both athletes and nonathletes. The gastrocnemius, hamstrings, and quadriceps muscles are most commonly involved, but cramping can involve nearly any muscle group. Cramps begin with the muscle in a shortened position.

- The development of muscle cramps usually starts with a twitching of the muscle due to skeletal muscle fatigue ("cramp-prone state"), followed by spasmodic spontaneous contractions and pain. Electrical evidence suggests that the source of the abnormal activity is coming from the nerve within the muscle (13). Relief from cramping and pain is achieved with complete cessation of the activity.

- The etiology of muscle cramping is unclear. Historically, muscle cramps were thought to be associated with systemic electrolyte abnormalities (hyponatremia, hypokalemia, hypocalcemia, and hypomagnesemia), hydration status, metabolic abnormalities, and environmental factors. Recent research suggests that a primary factor is fatigue-induced alterations in neuromuscular control (52).

- Passive stretching is the most reliable immediate treatment to alleviate the cramped muscle group. Fluids and sodium replacement are still considered, but their use is controversial, and the effect is equivocal (52).

- A comprehensive and detailed assessment, including endocrine disorders, is needed for athletes who suffer from frequent cramps.

Muscle Laceration

- Muscle laceration is seen more often in trauma than sports. When a muscle is completely lacerated, 50% of its strength and 80% of its ability to shorten can be expected to be lost (40).

- In a murine model, immediate suturing of the fascia of the lacerated muscle has been shown to favor healing and to suppress the formation of deep scars, whereas with immobilization, the regeneration time of the injured muscle was longer and the scar was considerably larger (20).

TENDON INJURY REPAIR

- Tendon injuries are secondary to direct trauma (lacerations) or tensile overload.

- Tensile overload injuries are very common athletic injuries and can occur acutely or as a result of chronic overload.

- Acute tendon overload usually results in injury to the musculotendinous junction or a bony avulsion since tendons can withstand high tensile loads. A normal tendon does not rupture midsubstance.

- Chronic tendon overload is a common overuse injury and will be the focus of this section.

Anatomy and Physiology

- Tendons consist primarily of type I collagen fibrils, a proteoglycan matrix, and relatively few fibroblasts. A fibroblast is a contractile cell that produces procollagen that is secreted to the extracellular compartment as a soluble tropocollagen molecule, which after noncovalent cross-links results in insoluble collagen. The aggregation of this molecule forms collagen fibrils.

  - Type I collagen consists of two α-1 polypeptide chains and one α-2 chain that are organized into a triple helix stabilized by hydrogen and covalent bonds (65).

  - The collagen triple-helix molecules are aligned in quarter-staggered arrangement to make up the collagen microfibril. This alignment of oppositely charged amino acids contributes to tendon's strength.

  - The microfibrils are then arranged in a parallel, well-ordered, and densely packed fashion. This organization also contributes to the tendon's tensile strength. The microfibrils are combined with a proteoglycan and water matrix to form collagen fascicles. The tendon consists of groupings of these fascicles surrounded by connective tissue that contains blood vessels, nerves, and lymphatics (65). Tendons receive blood through the surrounding tissues, which reaches the cells through the paratenon, mesotenon, or vincula. The nervous supply is picked up through mechanoreceptors located near the musculotendinous junction.

- The insertion of tendons onto bone is usually via four zones: tendon, fibrocartilage, mineralized fibrocartilage, and bone.

- Tendons that bend at acute angles (*e.g.*, flexor tendons in the hands) are enclosed in a distinct sheath that acts as a pulley (65). Synovial fluid within the sheath assists in tendon gliding. Tendons that are not enclosed in a sheath (*e.g.*, Achilles tendon) are covered by a paratenon.

- Mechanical forces affect the characteristics of tendon. Tendons subjected to tensile loads have smaller densely packed collagen fibrils, increased collagen synthesis, smaller proteoglycan (decorin), and a higher collagen-to-proteoglycan ratio. Tendons sustaining compressive loads exhibit increased proteoglycan molecules and larger less dense collagen fibrils (21).

- Aging also affects the material characteristics of tendon. The decreased collagen synthesis, increased collagen fibril diameter, decreased proteoglycan content, decreased water content, and decreased vascularity of the aging tendon leads to a stiffer and weaker tendon (21).

Chronic Tensile Overload Injuries

Terminology

- There is significant confusion regarding the terminology of chronic tendon injuries. Tendinitis (or tendonitis) and tendinosis are frequently used terms to describe the clinical picture of pain, swelling, and stiffness in a tendon.

- Terminology based on pathology has been proposed (25).
  - Paratenonitis: Inflammation of the paratenon or tendon sheath. Peritendinitis and tenosynovitis are included in this category.
  - Paratenonitis with tendinosis: Tendon degeneration with concomitant paratenon inflammation.
  - Tendinosis: Tendon degeneration without inflammation.
  - Tendinitis: Inflammation within the tendon.
- *Tendinopathy* has been proposed as a generic term describing the clinical picture of pain, swelling, and impaired performance (35).

Etiology

- The etiology of chronic tendon injuries is multifactorial and involves a combination of intrinsic and extrinsic factors.
- Important intrinsic factors include *anatomic abnormalities* (*e.g.*, malalignment, muscle weakness/imbalance, decreased flexibility, and joint laxity), age, gender, weight, and predisposing diseases (1,2,29).
- Important extrinsic factors include excessive mechanical load (frequency, duration, and intensity), training, errors (overtraining, rapid progression, fatigue, running surface, and poor technique), and equipment problems (footwear, racquets, and seat height) (1,2,29).
- There are very few well-controlled studies that examine the etiologic factors involved in chronic tendon injuries.

Pathophysiology

- Repetitive load on a tendon that results in 4%–8% strain causes microscopic tendon fiber damage. Continued load on the tendon at this level overwhelms the tendon's ability for repair. Damage occurs to the collagen fibrils, the noncollagenous matrix, and microvasculature (21).
- Cellular damage results in inflammation of the surrounding paratenon (paratenonitis). Tissue edema, fibrin exudate, and capillary occlusion result in local tissue hypoxia. Audible crepitation may be noted in examination (29).
- The paratenon becomes thickened as fibroblast proliferation and fibrotic adhesions develop. This results in decreased tendon gliding and snapping.
- Intrinsic tendon damage (tendinosis) may occur with continued tendon overload. Tendon degeneration may appear as a number of histologic entities (*e.g.*, hypoxic degeneration, mucoid degeneration, fiber calcification) (29).
- The casual link between initial inflammation (paratenonitis) and tendon degeneration (tendinosis) is unclear. Chronic paratenonitis can result in tendon degeneration in an animal model (8); however, a large clinical study showed no previous evidence of paratenonitis in over 60% of patients who sustained an Achilles tendon rupture (30). The initial paratenonitis may be a causative factor for tendon degeneration or it may coexist independently.
- The exact cellular mechanism of tendon degeneration has not been fully defined. Important factors include tissue hypoxia, free radical–induced tendon damage, and tissue hyperthermia (29). Recent evidence shows that tendon overuse results in matrix metalloproteinase production, tendon cell apoptosis, chondroid metaplasia of the tendon, and release of protective factors like insulin-like growth factor 1 and nitric oxide synthetase (28,33). The disproportion between protective/regenerative changes and pathologic responses from tendon overuse results in *tendinopathy*.

Diagnosis

- The history often reveals repetitive mechanical overload. The athlete will usually be involved in either an endurance sport (*e.g.*, running, cycling, or swimming) or a sport that requires repetition of a specialized skill (*e.g.*, tennis, basketball, or baseball) (19). The athlete frequently will describe an increase in the duration, frequency, or intensity of the training regimen. The pain may be worse after a period of rest following the training period. Changes in footwear, equipment, or training surface may be present.
- The physical examination may reveal swelling or crepitation along the tendon sheath. The degenerative tendon may be tender to palpation or painful with compression (impingement signs). Range of motion may be restricted (2).
- Diagnostic tests include radiographs to exclude stress fractures or osteoarthritis. Ultrasound or magnetic resonance imaging can be useful in tendons that are not easily palpated (*e.g.*, the rotator cuff).

Treatment

- Removing or modifying the mechanical overload (relative rest) is the most important component in the treatment of chronic tendon injuries. Training errors and equipment problems should also be corrected.
- Prolonged immobilization should be avoided. Immobilization results in deceased tendon strength and stiffness due to proteolytic degradation of collagen (21).
- Physical therapy is often prescribed for chronic tendon disorders. Stretching and strengthening (particularly eccentric exercises) are thought to be beneficial. Modalities such as heat, ice, ultrasound, iontophoresis, deep transverse friction massage, and low-level laser therapy may also improve the patient's symptoms, but there is little evidence that these techniques accelerate tendon healing.
- NSAIDs are frequently taken for chronic tendon disorders. A recent review stated that five of nine placebo-controlled studies demonstrated the efficacy of NSAIDs in treatment of tendinopathy (2). There is no evidence that NSAIDs improve healing processes in tendon degeneration, and there is evidence in muscle injury that NSAIDs may actually be harmful to tissue healing (38). Short-term use of NSAIDs may be indicated to provide analgesia for the athlete.
- The use of corticosteroid injections in the treatment of tendinopathy is controversial. The rationale of using a local anti-inflammatory medication for a disease process that involves tissue degeneration is questionable. Corticosteroids may

decrease inflammation in the paratenon, reduce adhesions between the tendon and the peritendinous tissue, or block nociceptors in the damaged tendon (42); however, only three of eight placebo-controlled studies demonstrate the efficacy of corticosteroid injections (2). Direct injections into the tendon substance should be avoided because they result in elevated tissue pressure and tissue damage. The use of corticosteroid injections around weight-bearing tendons, such as the Achilles tendon and patellar tendon, remains controversial. There have been case reports of tendon rupture, but there are no controlled studies, and the tendon rupture may have occurred without injection. It is difficult to make recommendations on the use of corticosteroid injections because of the paucity of scientific evidence regarding their use.

- Platelet-rich plasma (PRP) is the plasma portion of autologous blood with a concentration of platelets above baseline. PRP contains a high concentration of growth factors that upregulate numerous modulators involved in muscle and tendon regeneration. It is thought that PRP interrupts macrophage proliferation and IL-1 production, which would prevent fibrous scar (66). Favorable outcomes have been reported for the use of PRP in lateral epicondylitis (43), Achilles ruptures (50), and rotator cuff tears (46). Although PRP is an encouraging treatment option, more controlled studies are needed to fully support the benefits of its use in muscle and tendon injuries.

- The surgical treatment of chronic tendon injury is usually reserved for those cases that do not resolve within 4–6 months of nonsurgical treatment. The surgical procedures usually involve debridement of the degenerative tendon tissue. Occasionally, grafting or complete resection and repair is required (1). Occasionally, removal of the involved paratenon or release of the tendon sheath is necessary. Bony prominences, osteophytes, or deformities may require removal (*e.g.*, Haglund tuberosity, around the acromion). There are case series reported in the literature that demonstrate the success of surgical management, but there are very few controlled studies.

ACKNOWLEDGEMENT

The authors acknowledge Donald T. Kirkendall for his assistance in preparing the revision of this chapter.

REFERENCES

1. Almekinders LC. Tendinitis and other chronic tendinopathies. *J Am Acad Orthop Surg.* 1998;6(3):157–64.
2. Almekinders LC, Temple JD. Etiology, diagnosis, and treatment of tendonitis: an analysis of the literature. *Med Sci Sports Exerc.* 1998; 30(8):1183–90.
3. Anderson JE. The satellite cell as a companion in skeletal muscle plasticity: currency, conveyance, clue, connector and colander. *J Exp Biol.* 2006;209(Pt 12):2276–92.
4. Armfield DR, Kim DH, Towers JD, Bradley JP, Robertson DD. Sports-related muscle injury in the lower extremity. *Clin Sports Med.* 2006;25(4):803–42.
5. Armstrong RB. Mechanisms of exercise-induced delayed onset muscular soreness: a brief review. *Med Sci Sports Exerc.* 1984;16(6):529–38.
6. Arnason A, Andersen TE, Holme I, Engebretsen L, Bahr R. Prevention of hamstring strains in elite soccer: an intervention study. *Scand J Med Sci Sports.* 2008;18(1):40–8.
7. Askling C, Karlsson J, Thorstensson A. Hamstring injury occurrence in elite soccer players after preseason strength training with eccentric overload. *Scand J Med Sci Sports.* 2003;13(4):244–50.
8. Backman C, Boquist L, Friden J, Lorentzon R, Toolanen G. Chronic Achilles paratenonitis with tendinosis: an experimental model in the rabbit. *J Orthop Res.* 1990;8(4):541–7.
9. Balnave CD, Thompson MW. Effect of training on eccentric exercise-induced muscle damage. *J Appl Physiol.* 1993;75(4):1545–51.
10. Beiner JM, Jokl P. Muscle contusion injuries: current treatment options. *J Am Acad Orthop Surg.* 2001;9(4):227–37.
11. Beiner JM, Jokl P, Cholewicki J, Panjabi MM. The effect of anabolic steroids and corticosteroids on healing of muscle contusion injury. *Am J Sports Med.* 1999;27(1):2–9.
12. Bennett M, Best TM, Babul-Wellar S, Taunton JE. Hyperbaric oxygen therapy for delayed onset muscle soreness and closed soft tissue injury. *Cochrane Database Syst Rev.* 2005;4:CD004713.
13. Best TM. Soft-tissue injuries and muscle tears. *Clin Sports Med.* 1997; 16(3):419–34.
14. Brooks JHM, Fuller CW, Kemp SPT, Reddin DB. Incidence, risk and prevention of hamstring muscle injuries in professional rugby union. *Am J Sports Med.* 2006;34(8):1297–306.
15. Crosier JL, Ganteaume S, Binet J, Genty M, Ferret JF. Strength imbalances and prevention of hamstring injury in professional soccer players: a prospective study. *Am J Sports Med.* 2008;36(8):1469–75.
16. Garrett WE Jr, Nilcolaou PK, Ribbeck BM, Glisson RR, Seaber AV. The effect of muscle architecture on the biomechanical failure properties of skeletal muscle under passive extension. *Am J Sports Med.* 1988;16(1):7–12.
17. Garrett WEJ, Best TM. Anatomy, physiology, and mechanics of skeletal muscle. In: Buckwalter JA, Einhorn TA, Sheldon S, editors. *Orthopaedic Basic Science.* Chicago: American Academy of Orthopaedic Surgeons; 2000.
18. Gates CB, Karthikeyan T, Fu FH, Huard J. Regenerative medicine for the musculoskeletal system based on muscle-derived stem cells. *J Am Acad Orthop Surg.* 2008;16(2):68–76.
19. Hess GP, Cappiello WL, Poole RM, Hunter SC. Prevention and treatment of overuse tendon injuries. *Sports Med.* 1989;8(6):371–84.
20. Huard J, Li Y, Fu FH. Muscle injuries and repair: current trends in research. *J Bone Joint Surg Am.* 2002;84-A(5):822–32.
21. Hyman J, Rodeo SA. Injury and repair of tendons and ligaments. *Phys Med Rehabil Clin N Am.* 2000;11(2):267–88.
22. Jackson DW, Feagin JA. Quadriceps contusions in young athletes. Relation of severity of injury to treatment and prognosis. *J Bone Joint Surg Am.* 1973;55(1):95–105.
23. Järvinen M. Healing of a crush injury in rat striated muscle. Part 2. A histological study of the effect of early mobilization and immobilization on the repair processes. *Acta Pathol Microbiol Scand (A).* 1975;83(3): 269–82.
24. Järvinen M. Healing of a crush injury in rat striated muscle. Part 4. Effect of early mobilization and immobilization on the tensile properties of gastrocnemius muscle. *Acta Chir Scand.* 1976;142(1):47–56.
25. Järvinen M, Józsa L, Kannus P, Järvinen TL, Kvist M, Leadbetter W. Histopathological findings in chronic tendon disorders. *Scand J Med Sci Sports.* 1997;7(2):78–85.

26. Järvinen TA, Järvinen TL, Kääriäinen M, et al. Muscle injuries: optimising recovery. *Best Pract Res Clin Rheumatol.* 2007;21(2):317–31.

27. Järvinen TA, Järvinen TL, Kääriäinen M, Kalimo H, Järvinen M. Muscle injuries: biology and treatment. *Am J Sports Med.* 2005;33(5):745–64.

28. Jones GC, Corps AN, Pennington CJ, et al. Expression profiling of metalloproteinases and tissue inhibitors of metalloproteinases in normal and degenerate human Achilles tendon. *Arthritis Rheum.* 2006;54(3):832–42.

29. Kannus P. Etiology and pathophysiology of chronic tendon disorders in sports. *Scand J Med Sci Sports.* 1997;7(2):78–85.

30. Kannus P, Józsa L. Histopathological changes preceding spontaneous rupture of a tendon. A controlled study of 891 patients. *J Bone Joint Surg Am.* 1991;73(10):1507–25.

31. Lehto M, Duance VC, Restall D. Collagen and fibronectin in a healing skeletal muscle injury. An immunohistological study of the effects of physical activity on the repair of injured gastrocnemius muscle in the rat. *J Bone Joint Surg Br.* 1985;67(5):820–8.

32. Lehto MU, Järvinen MJ. Muscle injuries, their healing process and treatment. *Ann Chir Gynaecol.* 1991;80(2):102–8.

33. Lian Ø, Scott A, Engebretsen L, Bahr R, Duronio V, Khan K. Excessive apoptosis in patellar tendinopathy in athletes. *Am J Sports Med.* 2007;35(4):605–11.

34. Lieber RL, Friden J. Morphologic and mechanical basis of delayed onset muscle soreness. *J Am Acad Orthop Surg.* 2002;10(1):67–73.

35. Maffulli N, Kahn KM, Puddu G. Overuse tendon conditions: time to change a confusing terminology. *Arthroscopy.* 1998;14(8):840–3.

36. Mafiuletti NA. Assessment of hip and knee muscle function in orthopedic practice and research. *J Bone Joint Surg Am.* 2010;92(1):220–9.

37. McMillian DJ, Moore JH, Hatler BS, Taylor DC. Dynamic vs. static-stretching warm up: the effect on power and agility performance. *J Strength Cond Res.* 2006;20(3):492–9.

38. Mishra DK, Fridén J, Schmitz MC, Lieber RL. Anti-inflammatory medication after muscle injury. A treatment resulting in short-term improvement but subsequent loss of muscle function. *J Bone Joint Surg Am.* 1995;77(10):1510–9.

39. Nikolaou PK, Macdonald BL, Glisson RR, Seaber AV, Garrett WE Jr. Biological and histological evaluation of muscle after controlled strain injury. *Am J Sports Med.* 1987;15(1):9–14.

40. Noonan TJ, Garrett WE Jr. Muscle strain injury: diagnosis and treatment. *J Am Acad Orthop Surg.* 1999;7(4):262–9.

41. Obremsky WT, Seaber AV, Ribbeck BM, Garrett WE Jr. Biomechanical and histologic assessment of a controlled muscle strain injury treated with piroxicam. *Am J Sports Med.* 1994;22(4):558–61.

42. Paavola M, Kannus P, Järvinen TA, Järvinen TL, Józsa SL, Järvinen M. Treatment of tendon disorders. Is there a role for corticosteroids injection? *Foot Ankle Clin.* 2002;7(3):501–13.

43. Peerbooms JC, Sluimer J, Bruijn DJ, Gosens T. Positive effect of an autologous platelet concentrate in lateral epicondylitis in a double-blind randomized controlled trial: platelet-rich plasma versus corticosteroid injection with a 1-year follow-up. *Am J Sports Med.* 2010;38(2):255–62.

44. Petersen J, Hölmich P. Evidence based prevention of hamstring injuries in sports. *Br J Sports Med.* 2005;39(6):319–323.

45. Proske U, Morgan DL. Muscle damage from eccentric exercise: mechanism, mechanical signs, adaptation and clinical applications. *J Physiol.* 2001;537(Pt 2):333–45.

46. Randelli PS, Arrigoni P, Cabitza P, Volpi P, Maffulli N. Autologous platelet rich plasma for arthroscopic rotator cuff repair. A pilot study. *Disabil Rehabil.* 2008;30(20–22):1584–9.

47. Rantajen J, Thorsson O, Wollmer P, Hurme T, Kalimo H. Effects of therapeutic ultrasound on the regeneration of skeletal muscle myofibers after experimental muscle injury. *Am J Sports Med.* 1999;27(1):54–9.

48. Ryan JB, Wheeler JH, Hopkinson WJ, Arciero RA, Kolakowski KR. Quadriceps contusions. West Point update. *Am J Sports Med.* 1991;19(3):299–304.

49. Safran MR, Garrett WE Jr, Seaber AV, Glisson RR, Ribbeck BM. The role of warmup in muscular injury prevention. *Am J Sports Med.* 1988;16(2):123–9.

50. Sánchez M, Anitua E, Azofra J, Andía I, Padilla S, Mujika I. Comparison of surgically repaired Achilles tendon tears using platelet–rich fibrin matrices. *Am J Sports Med.* 2007;35(2):245–51.

51. Schaser KD, Disch AC, Stover JF, Lauffer A, Bail HJ, Mittlmeier T. Prolonged superficial local cryotherapy attenuates microcirculatory impairment, regional inflammation, and muscle necrosis following closed soft tissue injury in rats. *Am J Sports Med.* 2007;35(1):93–102.

52. Schwellnus MP, Drew N, Collins M. Muscle cramping in athletes—risk factors, clinical assessment, and management. *Clin Sports Med.* 2008;27(1):183–94.

53. Sheehan SM, Tatsumi R, Temm-Grove CJ, Allen RE. HGF is an autocrine growth factor for skeletal muscle cells in vitro. *Muscle Nerve.* 2000;23(2):239–45.

54. Sherry MA, Best TM. A comparision of 2 rehabilitation programs in the treatment of acute hamstring strains. *J Orthop Sports Phys Ther.* 2004;34(3):116–25.

55. Shrier I. Stretching before exercise does not reduce the risk of local muscle injury: a critical review of the clinical and basic science literature. *Clin J Sport Med.* 1999;9(4):221–7.

56. Shrier I. Does stretching improve performance? A systematic and critical review of the literature. *Clin J Sports Med.* 2004;14(5):267–73.

57. Shrier I. Warm-up and stretching in the prevention of muscular injury. Letter to Editor. *Sports Med.* 2008;38(10):879–80.

58. Shrier I, Macdonald D, Uchacz G. A pilot study on the effects of preevent manipulation on jump height and running velocity. *Br J Sports Med.* 2006;40(11):947–9.

59. Taylor DC, Dalton JD Jr, Seaber AV, Garrett WE Jr. Viscoelastic properties of muscle-tendon units. The biomechanical effects of stretching. *Am J Sports Med.* 1990;18(3):300–9.

60. Taylor DC, Dalton JD Jr, Seaber AV, Garrett WE Jr. Experimental muscle strain injury. Early functional and structural deficits and the increased risk for reinjury. *Am J Sports Med.* 1993;21(2):190–4.

61. Tidball JG. Inflammatory cell response to acute muscle injury. *Med Sci Sports Exerc.* 1995;27(7):1022–32.

62. Ulibarri JA, Mozdziak PE, Schultz E, Cook C, Best TM. Nitric oxide donors, sodium nitroprusside and S-nitroso-N-acetylpencillamine, stimulate myoblast proliferation in vitro. *In Vitro Cell Dev Biol Anim.* 1999;35(4):215–8.

63. Walton M, Rothwell AG. Reactions of thigh tissues of sheep to blunt trauma. *Clin Orthop Relat Res.* 1983;176:273–81.

64. Wilkin LD, Merrick MA, Kirby TE, Devor ST. Influence of therapeutic ultrasound on skeletal muscle regeneration following blunt contusion. *Int J Sports Med.* 2004;25(1):73–7.

65. Wood SL, An KN, Frank CB, et al. Anatomy, biology, and biomechanics of tendon and ligament. In: Buckwalter JA, Einhorn TA, Sheldon S, editors. *Orthopaedic Basic Science.* Chicago: American Academy of Orthopaedic Surgeons; 2000.

66. Woodall J Jr, Tucci M, Mishra A, Asfour A, Benghuzzi H. Cellular effects of platelet rich plasmainterleukin1 release from prp treated macrophages. *Biomed Sci Instrum.* 2008;44:489–94.

67. Woods K, Bishop P, Jones E. Warm-up and stretching in the prevention of muscular injury. *Sports Med.* 2007;37(12):1089–99.

Basic Principles of Exercise Training and Conditioning

10

Kevin R. Vincent, Heather K. Vincent, and Craig K. Seto

INTRODUCTION

- Participation in exercise is a critical component of healthful living and reduced all-cause mortality. Moderate-intensity physical activity is related to numerous health benefits, including musculoskeletal adaptation, increased circulatory capacity, and improvements in metabolism and body composition. Regular exercise induces central nervous system benefits (1), improves mood, and reduces stress.

- The Centers for Disease Control and Prevention (CDC) and the American College of Sports Medicine® (ACSM) now recommend that every U.S. adult accumulate 30 minutes or more of moderate-intensity physical activity on most — and preferably all — days of the week. Those who follow these recommendations will experience many of the health-related benefits of physical activity, and if they are interested in achieving higher levels of fitness, they will be ready to do so (2,3,7).

- This chapter integrates and complements Chapters 5 (Basics in Exercise Physiology), 11 (Basics in Sports Nutrition), and 12 (Exercise Prescription), by specifically identifying appropriate principles for effective training to achieve the aforementioned fitness goals.

THE EXERCISE PRESCRIPTION AND TRAINING PROGRAM

Recommendations for Cardiorespiratory Endurance Training

- Chapter 12 details current guidelines from ACSM; this chapter elaborates upon those recommendations and outlines the integration of these guidelines into a sequenced exercise program.

Mode

- The best improvements in cardiorespiratory endurance occur when large muscle groups are engaged in rhythmic aerobic activity.

- Variety facilitates enjoyment and enhances compliance.

- Examples of activities include walking, jogging, cycling, rowing, stair climbing, aerobic dance (aerobics), water exercise, and cross-country skiing (2,3).

Intensity

- The ACSM recommends that exercise intensity be prescribed within a range of 70%–85% of maximal heart rate (HR_{max}), 50%–85% of maximal volume of oxygen consumed per unit time ($\dot{V}O_{2max}$), or 60%–80% of maximum metabolic equivalents (METs), or *heart rate reserve* (HRR).

  - Because there is variability with the HR_{max} from age, the use of an actual heart rate (HR) from a graded exercise test is optimal.

  - Lower intensities (40%–50% of $\dot{V}O_{2max}$) elicit a favorable response in low-fit individuals, inpatient populations, and those with musculoskeletal pain.

- **Calculating intensity:** The most common methods of setting the intensity of exercise to improve or maintain cardiorespiratory fitness use HR and rating of perceived exertion (RPE).

- **HR methods:** HR is used as a guide to set exercise intensity because of the relatively linear relationship between HR and *percentage of $\dot{V}O_{2max}$* (%$\dot{V}O_{2max}$). It is best to measure HR_{max} during a progressive exercise test whenever possible because HR_{max} declines with age. HR_{max} can be estimated by using the following equation: ($HR_{max} = 220 - age$).

- **HR_{max} method:** Using 70%–85% of an individual's HR_{max} approximates 55%–75% $\dot{V}O_{2max}$. Example: If $HR_{max} = 180$ bpm, then target HR (70%–85% HR_{max}) would range from 126 to 152 bpm. Given that there is variance around the HR of ± 15 bpm, the target HR should be calculated 10%–15% higher (7).

- **HRR method:** The HRR method is also known as the Karvonen method. Target HR range = [($HR_{max} - HR_{rest}$) × 0.60 and 0.85] + HR_{rest}. Using the HRR method allows a more direct correlation between HR and %$\dot{V}O_{2max}$ and accounts for the resting HR (7).

- **RPE:** The use of the RPE scale to guide exercise intensity is increasingly used in research and in the clinical setting. RPE may be used with HR for regulating intensity or alone if HR monitoring is not available. The RPE scales can be used to track exercise intensity and muscle fatigue during the session. One of two scales can be used: a 6- to 20-point scale (6 = no exertion, 20 = maximal exertion) and a 0- to 10-point scale (0 = no exertion, 10 = maximal exertion).

- For aerobic exercise, the onset of blood lactate generally occurs between 12 and 16 on the 6- to 20-point category scale and between 4 and 5 on the 0- to 10-point category-ratio scale (7).

- RPE is considered a reliable indicator of exercise intensity and is particularly useful when a participant is unable to monitor his or her pulse or when HR response to exercise has been altered by medications such as β-blockers (2,3).

- The average RPE range associated with physiologic adaptation to exercise is 12–16 ("somewhat hard" to "hard") on the Borg category scale. One should suit the RPE to the individual on a specific mode of exercise and not expect an exact matching of the RPE to a %HR$_{max}$ or %HRR. It should be used only as a guideline in setting the exercise intensity.

Duration

- The ACSM recommends 30–60 minutes of continuous activity per session for fitness and an accumulation of > 30 minutes of activity per day for general health (7)

- However, deconditioned individuals, older adults, or pregnant women with musculoskeletal discomfort may benefit from multiple, short-duration exercise sessions of < 10 minutes with frequent interspersed rest periods.

Frequency

- The ACSM recommends that aerobic exercise be performed 3–5 days per week for fitness and physical activity be performed on most if not all days per week for general health (7).

Recommendations for Muscular Strength and Resistance Training

- Overload and specificity are precepts of resistance training.

- **Overload** occurs when a greater than normal physical demand is placed on muscles or muscle groups. Muscular strength and endurance are developed by increasing the resistance to movement or the frequency or duration of activity to levels above those normally experienced.

- A training intensity of approximately 40%–60% of one-repetition maximum appears to be sufficient for the development of muscular strength in most normally active individuals (2,3). Lift intensity can be increased to near maximal if the goal is to increase muscle strength (7).

- **Specificity** relates to the nature of changes (structural and functional, systemic and local) that occur in an individual as a result of training. These adaptations are specific and occur only in the overloaded muscle groups or muscles (3).

- **Unilateral and bilateral strengthening:** Bilateral contractions induce less muscle activation per limb than unilateral contractions. Unilateral resistance exercise performed by one limb will induce training effects in the unexer-

cised contralateral limb, termed "cross-transfer" or "cross-education" (6).

- **Combined endurance and resistance exercise:** When endurance exercise is incorporated into a resistance exercise program, strength gains are not compromised when compared with resistance exercise alone (14).

ACSM Guidelines for Resistance Training

- A 5- to 10-minute warm-up period consisting of aerobic activity (walking on a treadmill or stationary cycling) or a light set (50%–75% of training weight) of the specific resistance exercise should precede the resistance exercise program (2,3).

- **Mode:** A minimum of 8–10 separate exercises that target major muscle groups (arms, shoulder, chest, abdomen, back, hips, and legs) is important for general strengthening. Free weights and weight machines are commonly used; however, springs, surgical or rubber tubing, and electronic devices are also used for resistance training. Choose different exercises for each body part every 2–3 training days where possible.

- **Intensity/duration:** For general health, perform a minimum of one set of 8–12 repetitions of each of the exercises to the point of volitional fatigue. Volitional fatigue refers to the inability to move a resistance through the appropriate range of motion with proper mechanical form. A set of 10–15 repetitions is recommended for developing muscular endurance and for those who are older or frailer. Using the target RPE values of 15–16 in persons with high cardiovascular risk or chronic comorbidities is appropriate (2,3).

- Progressive overload can be accomplished by increasing the load, increasing the repetitions for the current load, decreasing the rest period, or increasing the rest period with high loads (for strength and power development) (3).

- **Frequency:** Perform these exercises 2–3 days per week, usually with a day of rest in between. Another option is to alternate resistance exercises for upper and lower body on every other day, if time is a constraint.

- **Progression:** Resistance may be increased when the target repetition number can be completed with good technique and moderate effort (RPE rating of < 15).

- **Safety considerations:**
  - Perform every exercise in a controlled fashion through a full range of motion using proper technique during both concentric and eccentric phases.
  - Maintain a normal breathing pattern and avoid breath holding (*Valsalva maneuver*).
  - Exercise with a partner when possible for assistance and motivation; individuals achieve greater success with a successful exercise partner.

- Children may safely participate in resistance exercise using sets of 8–15 repetitions, for one to three sets, using both open- and closed-chain exercises no more than twice a week (3). Heavy weights and maximal strength testing are discouraged in children because of adverse effects on the growth plate development. Form is more important than weight in this population.

Recommendations for Flexibility Training

■ Static stretching involves slowly stretching a muscle to the point of mild discomfort and then holding that position for an extended period of time (usually 10–30 seconds). It is effective and requires little time, and the risk of injury is low. It is the most commonly recommended method.

■ Proprioceptive neuromuscular facilitation (PNF) involves a combination of alternating contraction and relaxation of both agonist and antagonist muscles through a designated series of motions. It is effective, but it is time consuming, requires a partner, may cause residual muscle soreness, and has potential for injury if applied to vigorously (3)

■ New evidence suggests that stretching is more effective after a light warm-up or after an exercise session, and stretching before resistance exercise may actually decrease the force-producing ability of muscle (2,3,7).

ACSM Recommendations for Flexibility Training

■ Flexibility exercises should be performed in a slow, controlled manner with a gradual progression to greater ranges of motion. A general stretching routine that exercises the major muscle and/or tendon groups can be done using static or PNF techniques — 10–30 seconds for static stretches and a 6-second contraction followed by a 10- to 30-second assisted stretch for PNF. Repeat the stretch three to four times. Stretching should be performed at a minimum of 2–3 days per week (7).

■ Progression should target a goal of performing stretches up to 5–7 days a week and hold for 30–90 seconds for each stretch. The intensity should be at the point of mild discomfort or tightness (7).

GENERAL COMPONENTS OF AN EXERCISE PROGRAM

■ Once the exercise prescription has been formulated, it is integrated into a comprehensive physical conditioning program that consists of the following components:

■ **Warm-up phase** (10 minutes): Warm-up phase facilitates the transition from rest to exercise, stretches postural muscles, augments blood flow, and increases the metabolic rate from the resting level (1 MET) to the aerobic requirements for endurance training.

■ **Endurance phase** (20–60 minutes): Endurance phase develops cardiorespiratory fitness and includes 20 to 60 minutes of continuous or intermittent (minimum of 10-minute bouts accumulated throughout the day) aerobic activity.

■ **Cool-down** (5–10 minutes): This phase provides a period of gradual recovery from the endurance phase and includes exercises of diminishing intensities. It permits appropriate circulatory adjustments and return of the HR and blood pressure to near resting values (2,18).

■ Although endurance training activities should be performed 3–5 days a week, complementary flexibility and resistance training may be undertaken at a slightly reduced frequency of 2–3 days a week. Flexibility training can be included as part of the warm-up or cool-down or undertaken at a separate time. Resistance training is often performed on alternate days when endurance training is not; however, both activities can be combined into the same workout.

■ This is "multimodal" exercise and is becoming commonly used in exercise research for a variety of healthy and diseased populations.

Rate of Progression

■ The recommended rate of progression in an exercise conditioning program depends on functional capacity, medical and health status, age, individual activity preferences and goals, and an individual's tolerance to the current level of training. For generally healthy adults, the endurance aspect of the exercise prescription has three stages of progression: initiation, improvement, and maintenance (2,3).

Initiation Stage

■ The initial stage should include light muscular endurance exercises and moderate-level aerobic activity exercises that are compatible with minimal muscle soreness, discomfort, and injury. If applicable, disease symptoms should be monitored during the exercise.

■ The duration of the exercise session during the initial stage depends on the starting point of the individual (healthy adults, 15–20 minutes; fit adults, 20–30 minutes; older, obese, very sedentary adults, 15–20 minutes). The content of the sessions can be modified to account for symptoms experienced by the individual; for example, increased stretching time or warm-up time can occur to minimize soreness or discomfort.

■ Proper form, technique, and education about the perceptual responses of the individual are important during this stage. It is recommended that individuals who are starting a moderate-intensity conditioning program should exercise three to four times per week (2,3).

Improvement Stage

■ This stage of training slowly increases the exercise stimulus to allow physiologic improvements in cardiorespiratory fitness to occur (termed **progressive overload**). Weekly increases in intensity and volume occur at a rate that stimulates adaptation. This stage typically lasts 2–5 months.

■ 10%–30% increases in aerobic capacity typically occur following these guidelines.

■ If the progression occurs too quickly, injury, aches and pains, lack of interest in training, and inability to complete a session may occur.

Maintenance Stage

■ This stage of training aims to maintain cardiorespiratory fitness over the long term. This stage begins when the participant has reached preestablished fitness goals; for most individuals, this occurs at approximately 6 months. The participant may no longer be interested in further increasing the conditioning stimulus. Further improvement may be minimal, but continuing the same workout routine enables individuals to maintain their fitness (3).

■ For general health, it is recommended that the weekly caloric expenditure should exceed 1,000 kcal.

■ **Cross-training** may be used to provide variety in the program. Adaptations achieved by one mode may be maintained with the substitution of other modes; for example, replacing a session of running with cycling or swimming at similar relative intensities can maintain the cardiorespiratory status and reduce the risk of fatigue and overuse of body parts used in the typical exercise plan (3).

The Concept of Periodization

■ **Periodization:** Planned sequencing of increased training loads and recovery periods within a training program. A periodized training program facilitates appropriate cycling of training volumes to facilitate peak performance (3).

■ A periodized training program consists of a series of microcycles, mesocycles, and macrocycles designed to emphasize unique aspects of training and adaptation (3).

    ■ Microcyle: several sessions separated by recovery days, lasting 1–2 weeks.

    ■ Mesocycle: two or more microcycles last 3–6 weeks. A mesocycle emphasizes one aspect of training such as endurance or speed. A number of mesocycles, arranged to produce physiologic adaptation, are known as a phase.

    ■ Macrocycle: three to four mesocycles comprise a macrocycle. Each macrocycle contains a preparatory phase, a competition phase, and a transition phase.

    ■ The final phase of a macrocycle is the transition phase, which allows for restoration/recovery. This phase should allow for complete recovery from the physiologic and psychological elements of training and competition.

Relaxation and Exercise

■ Additional exercise forms that involve balance, muscle strengthening, stretch, mental focus, and relaxation include yoga and t'ai chi. The popularity of these exercises has substantially increased over the last 10 years. Yoga and t'ai chi can be performed daily and are low impact.

■ In healthy and diseased populations, weeks to months of yoga may be just as effective or more effective as aerobic exercise in improving numerous health parameters (blood pressure, balance, baroreflex sensitivity, HR, HR variability, bodily pain, quality of life, stress, strength, and predisease biomarkers of oxidative stress and inflammation) (12).

■ T'ai chi is the most widely studied martial art, and established health benefits include stress reduction, improved agility and balance, posture control, and lower extremity

strength. T'ai chi can attenuate the decline of the muscularskeletal system that occurs with aging and counteract the risk of falls and hip fractures in older adults (5).

■ These techniques may improve physical and mental health through downregulation of the hypothalamic–pituitary–adrenal (HPA) axis and the sympathetic nervous system (SNS).

The Importance of Rest Periods During Training

■ As the volume of exercise training increases, the likelihood of injury increases, and performance may decline with excessive volume. This may be partly due to inadequate rest periods between exercise sessions. Irrespective of age, rest is a necessary part of exercise programming. By varying the intensity of exercise sessions during the week and including 1 or 2 days of rest among the sessions, performance can improve, and risk for injury can be reduced.

Detraining

■ The changes induced by regular exercise training generally are lost after 4–8 weeks of detraining. If training is reestablished, the rate at which the training effects occur do not appear to be faster (13).

Overtraining

■ Overtraining refers to a condition usually induced after prolonged heavy exercise over an extended period of time. Hallmark symptoms of overtraining include: decline in exercise performance, extreme fatigue, elevated resting HR, early onset of blood lactate accumulation, altered mood states, unexplained weight loss, insomnia, and injuries related to overuse.

■ HR variability and baroreceptor reflex sensitivity are reduced with overtraining, but recover to a large degree after 3–4 days of rest (4).

■ Overtraining may require weeks to months of complete rest in order to recover (13).

■ Treatment of overtraining includes 1 week of complete rest, followed by limited weekly training of one to three sessions (10–20 minutes of easy pace), progressing to longer sessions over a 6- to 12-week period.

■ Daily monitoring of exercise training volume, mood state, and well-being will assist the individual with moderating the return to full performance.

MEDICAL CLEARANCE

■ Exercise training may not be appropriate for everyone. Patients with severe disease may not be appropriate candidates for the recommended exercise guidelines (*e.g.*, osteoarthritis, heart disease, morbid obesity, movement disorders, chronic obstructive pulmonary disease) but may benefit from functional or disease-specific exercise instead. To determine the functional and cardiopulmonary capacity of the individual, disease history, current limitations, and presence of any contraindications to exercise should be documented. Based on the individual, a tailored physical activity program can be designed.

- The ACSM provides the guidelines for patients at high risk for adverse events during a high-intensity exercise testing session and exercise training. These **absolute contraindications** include unstable conditions such as recent acute myocardial infarction, unstable angina, ventricular tachycardia or other dangerous arrhythmias, severe aortic stenosis, acute infection and/or fever, recent systemic or pulmonary embolus, thrombophlebitis or intracardiac thrombi, active or suspected myocarditis or pericarditis, acute congestive heart failure, and dissecting aortic aneurysm (7).

- Once the condition has been stabilized and the physician has cleared the individual for testing, it is appropriate to proceed with exercise testing and programming as long as monitoring of blood pressure, HR, and symptoms occurs.

- There are cases in which individuals present with relative contraindications; if these patients have stable conditions and are managed and cleared by their physician, it is appropriate to proceed with testing and exercise prescription as long as monitoring of blood pressure, HR, and symptoms occurs.

- These **relative contraindications** include severe hypertension (uncontrolled or untreated), complicated pregnancy, moderate aortic stenosis, severe subaortic stenosis, supraventricular dysrhythmias, ventricular aneurysm, frequent or complex ventricular ectopy, cardiomyopathy, uncontrolled metabolic disease (thyroid or diabetes) or electrolyte abnormality, chronic or recurrent infectious disease (*e.g.*, malaria, hepatitis), and neuromuscular, musculoskeletal, or rheumatoid diseases exacerbated by exercise (7).

Identify Those Who Need an Exercise Stress Test

- Indications for an *exercise stress test* according to the American College of Cardiology (ACC), American Heart Association (AHA), and ACSM are as follows (2,3,8):
  - To evaluate patients for suspected coronary artery disease (typical and atypical angina pectoris)
  - To evaluate patients with known coronary artery disease (previous imaging tests, blood chemistries, electrocardiogram results)
  - To evaluate healthy asymptomatic individuals in the following categories:
    - ❏ High-risk occupations, such as pilots, firefighters, law enforcement officers, and mass transit operators
    - ❏ Men over age 40 and women over age 50 who are sedentary and plan to start vigorous exercise
    - ❏ Individuals with multiple cardiac risk factors or concurrent chronic diseases

  - To evaluate exercise capacity in patients with valvular heart disease, except severe aortic stenosis
  - Individuals with cardiac rhythm disorders for the following reasons:
    - ❏ Evaluate response to treatment of exercise-induced arrhythmia.
    - ❏ Evaluate response of rate-adaptive pacemaker setting.

- The ACSM and ACC/AHA guidelines discourage using exercise testing to screen asymptomatic adults unless they are at increased risk (2,3,8).

TRAINING EFFECTS OF AEROBIC EXERCISE

Cardiovascular System

Changes at Rest

- HR decreases likely secondary to decreased sympathetic tone, increased parasympathetic tone, and a decreased intrinsic firing rate of the sinoatrial node.
- Stroke volume (SV) increases secondary to increased myocardial contractility.
- Cardiac output is unchanged at rest.
- Oxygen consumption does not change at rest (13).
- Total blood volume increases due to an increased number of red blood cells and expansion of the plasma volume (10).

Changes During Submaximal Work

- Submaximal work is defined as a workload during which a steady state of oxygen use is achieved.
  - HR decreases at any given workload due to the increased SV and decreased sympathetic drive and improved metabolic and aerobic capacity of skeletal muscle.
  - SV increases due to increased myocardial contractility.
  - Cardiac output does not change significantly for a fixed workload; however, the same cardiac output is generated with a lower HR and higher SV.
  - Submaximal oxygen consumption does not change significantly because oxygen requirement is similar for a fixed workload.
  - Arteriovenous oxygen (AVO_2) difference increases during submaximal work.
  - Lactate levels are decreased due to metabolic efficiency and increased lactate clearance rates (13).

Changes at Maximal Work

- HR_{max} does not change with exercise training.
- SV increases due to increased contractility and/or increased heart size.
- Maximal cardiac output increases due to increased SV.
- Maximal oxygen consumption ($\dot{V}O_{2max}$) increases due to increased SV and AVO_2 difference.

■ AVO$_2$ difference increases due to improved ability of the mitochondria to use oxygen (13).

Blood Pressure

■ In normotensive individuals, regular exercise does not appear to have a significant impact on resting or exercising blood pressure.

■ In hypertensive individuals, there may be a modest reduction in resting blood pressure as a result of regular exercise (13).

Blood Lipids

■ Total cholesterol may be decreased in individuals with hypercholesterolemia.

■ *High-density lipoprotein* (HDL) *cholesterol* increases with exercise training.

■ *Low-density lipoprotein* (LDL) *cholesterol* may remain the same or decrease with regular exercise.

■ Triglycerides may decrease in those with elevated triglycerides initially. This change is facilitated by weight loss (13).

Body Composition

■ Total body weight usually decreases with regular exercise, the magnitude of which is directly dependent on the weekly exercise volume and caloric expenditure

■ Fat-free weight does not normally change and may decrease slightly, depending on the exercise volume over time.

■ Percent body fat declines (13).

■ Long-term participation in land-based exercise (walking, running, aerobic dancing, cycling) can attenuate age-related increases in body weight and fat content, whereas swimming does not appear to exert such effects (15).

Skeletal Muscle Adaptations

■ The levels of muscle glycogen and triglycerides stored within skeletal muscle fibers increase.

■ High-intensity aerobic exercise training increases the number of Type I fibers and decreases the number of Type II fibers, while the cross-sectional area remains unchanged.

■ The level of Type I myosin heavy chain content increases, while the content of Type IIa and IId/x decreases after aerobic training (11).

Nervous System Adaptations

■ Exercise training may induce brain mitochondrial biogenesis and increase central vasoreactivity (9).

■ Mood improves, and cognitive function is better maintained during aging.

Anti-Inflammatory Adaptations

■ Regular aerobic exercise can increase the production and release of anti-inflammatory cytokines and decrease the production of inflammatory cytokines and proteins such as C-reactive protein.

■ Exercise can reduce the number of circulating proinflammatory monocytes and can inhibit monocyte and macrophage infiltration into adipose tissue.

Adaptations to Resistance Exercise

■ Irrespective of age and presence of comorbid illness, dramatic improvements in muscle strength can occur after regular resistance exercise; bone density may increase, especially in locations such as the hip, lumbar spine, and lower extremities.

■ Functional ability (*e.g.*, stair climb, walking endurance, chair rise, sit to stand) and balance are improved after resistance training (17).

■ Blood pressure responses are lower for the same physical workload; HR and blood pressure recover more quickly after cessation of exercise; at rest, evidence is equivocal for improvement in these parameters (16).

■ Coordination of muscle activation patterns is improved, and antagonist muscle co-activation is reduced.

■ Economy during aerobic exercise (decreased oxygen consumption at an absolute workload) is improved.

■ Ability to recruit high-threshold motor units is increased.

■ Resistance exercise reduces the circulating levels of inflammatory cytokines and proteins such as C-reactive protein and biomarkers of disease such as homocysteine (17).

■ The myosin heavy chain IIa content and fiber number increase, whereas Type IId/x decreases (11).

■ Insulin resistivity and glucose disposal can improve by up to 48% from pretraining level. Mood, depressive symptoms, and self-efficacy improve.

SUMMARY

■ Numerous health and fitness benefits occur with exercise. Irrespective of age, gender, and physical condition, significant health benefits can be obtained by including a moderate amount of physical activity on most, if not all, days of the week. With a modest increase in daily activity, most patients will improve their health and quality of life.

■ Incorporation of aerobic, resistance, and flexibility components provides an overall exercise stimulus for health improvement and maintenance.

■ The musculoskeletal, cardiopulmonary, circulatory, and central nervous systems are plastic and able to adapt to exercise stimuli throughout the lifespan.

REFERENCES

1. Amann M. Central and peripheral fatigue: interaction during cycling exercise in humans. *Med Sci Sports Exerc.* 2011;43(11):2039–49.

2. American College of Sports Medicine. *ACSM's Resource Manual for Guidelines for Exercise Testing and Prescription.* 5th ed. Philadelphia (PA): Lippincott Williams & Wilkins; 2006. 848 p.

3. Baumert M, Bretchtel L, Lock J, et al. Heart rate variability, blood pressure variability, and baroreflex sensitivity in overtrained athletes. *Clin J Sports Med.* 2006;16(5):412–7.

4. Bu B, Haijun H, Yong L, Chaohui Z, Xiaoyuan Y, Singh MF. Effects of martial arts on health status: a systematic review. *J Evid Based Med.* 2010;3(4):205–19.

5. Gabriel DA, Kamen G, Frost G. Neural adaptations to resistive exercise: mechanisms and recommendations for training practices. *Sports Med.* 2006;36(2):133–49.

6. Garber CE, Blissmer B, Deschenes MR, et al. Quantity and quality of exercise for developing and maintaining cardiorespiratory, musculoskeletal, and neuromotor fitness in apparently healthy adults: Guidance for prescribing exercise. American College of Sports Medicine Position Stand. *Med Sci Sports Exerc.* 2011;43(7):1334–59.

7. Gibbons RJ, Balady GJ, Bricker JT, et al. ACC/AHA 2002 guidelines updates for exercise testing: summary article. A report of the American College of Cardiology/American Heart Association Task Force on Practice Guidelines (Committee to Update the 1997 Exercise Testing Guidelines). *J Am Coll Cardiol.* 2002;40(8):1531–40.

8. Martins-Pinge MC. Cardiovascular and autonomic modulation by the central nervous system after aerobic exercise training. *Braz J Med Biol Res.* 2011;44(9):848–54.

9. McArdle WD, Katch FI, Katch VL. *Exercise Physiology, Energy, Nutrition and Human Performance.* 5th ed. Philadelphia (PA): Lippincott Williams & Wilkins; 2001. 1158 p.

10. Putnam CT, Xu X, Gilles E, McLean IM, Bell GJ. Effects of strength, endurance and combined training on myosin heavy chain content and fiber-type distribution in humans. *Eur J Appl Physiol.* 2004; 92(4–5):376–84.

11. Ross A, Thomas S. The health benefits of yoga and exercise: a review of comparison studies. *J Altern Complement Med.* 2010;16(1):3–12.

12. Rupp J. Exercise physiology. In: Roitman J, Bibi K, Thompson W, editors. *ACSM's Health Fitness Certification Review.* Philadelphia: Lippincott Williams & Wilkins; 2001.

13. Shaw BS, Shaw I, Brown GA. Comparison of resistance and concurrent resistance and endurance training regimes in the development of strength. *J Strength Cond Res.* 2009;23(9):2507–14.

14. Stephens M, O'Connor F, Deuster P. *Exercise and Nutrition: AAFP Home Study—A Self-Assessment Program.* Leawood (KS): American Academy of Family Physicians; 2002. 73 p.

15. Tanaka H. Swimming exercise: impact of aquatic exercise on cardiovascular health. *Sports Med.* 2009;39(5):377–87.

16. Vincent KR, Vincent HK. Resistance training for individuals with cardiovascular disease. *J Cardiopulm Rehabil.* 2006;26(4):207–16.

17. Whaley MH, Brubaker PH, Otto RM. *American College of Sports Medicine: ACSM's Guidelines for Exercise Testing and Prescription.* 7th ed. Philadelphia (PA): Lippincott Williams & Wilkins; 2006. 400 p.

18. Wygand J. Exercise programming. In: Roitman J, Bibi K, Thompson W, editors. *ACSM's Health Fitness Certification Review.* Philadelphia: Lippincott Williams & Wilkins; 2001.

11

Basics in Sports Nutrition

Patricia A. Deuster, Stacey A. Zeno, and Selasi Attipoe

INTRODUCTION

■ This chapter focuses on the basic concepts of nutrition and sports. Topics include basics in energy metabolism, nutritional needs of athletes, hydration and fluid replacement, nutrient timing, selected nutritional issues, and information on ergogenic agents and nutritional supplements, to include sports drinks, bars, and energy drinks.

BASICS IN ENERGY METABOLISM

General Energy Needs

■ Energy balance is critical for all athletes and demands matching energy intake to total energy expenditure (TEE).

■ TEE is the sum of resting energy expenditure (REE), physical activity, and the energy used to digest foods (thermic effect of foods).

■ REE can easily be estimated for men and women as follows (26):

Men: $9.99 \times$ Weight (kg) $+ 6.25 \times$ Height (cm) $- 4.92 \times$ Age (yrs) $+ 5$, or $4.54 \times$ Weight (lbs) $+ 15.875 \times$ Height (inches) $- 4.92 \times$ Age (yrs) $+ 5$

Women: 9.99 Weight (kg) $+ 6.25 \times$ Height (cm) $- 4.92 \times$ Age (yrs) $- 161$, or $4.54 \times$ Weight (lbs) $+ 15.875 \times$ Height (inches) $- 4.92 \times$ Age (yrs) $- 161$

■ Physical activity levels (PAL) vary, but a factor can be applied to REE to estimate TEE. Table 11.1 presents suggested ranges for PAL factors. However, TEE may be overestimated in the low range of activity.

■ The Institute of Medicine (IOM) (41) also proposes formulas for TEE as follows:

Men: $662 - 9.53 \times$ Age (yrs) $+$ PAL $\times$ [$15.91 \times$ Weight (kg) $+ 539.6 \times$ Height (m)]

$662 - 9.53 \times$ Age (yrs) $+$ PAL $\times$ [$7.232 \times$ Weight (lbs) $+ 13.71 \times$ Height (inches)]

The opinions and assertions expressed herein are those of the authors and should not be construed as reflecting those of the Uniformed Services University of the Health Sciences or the Department of Defense.

Women: $354 - 6.9 \times$ Age (yrs) $+$ PAL $\times$ [$9.36 \times$ Weight (kg) $+ 726 \times$ Height (m)]

$354 - 6.9 \times$ Age (yrs) $+$ PAL $\times$ [$4.255 \times$ Weight (lbs) $+ 18.44 \times$ Height (inches)]

■ Comparison of the two formulas at the same PAL values reveals that the TEE estimated by the IOM formula is higher by $600–1,200$ kcal $\cdot$ d^{-1} for both men and women.

■ Failure to maintain energy balance can result in loss of muscle mass; menstrual disturbances; compromised bone density; increased risk of fatigue, injury, and illness; and overtraining (63).

Energy Sources and Stores

■ The universal source of metabolic fuel for energy is adenosine triphosphate (ATP) and the fuel sources to produce ATP are carbohydrates (CHO), fats (fatty acids), protein (amino acids), and alcohol. One gram of CHO (glucose, glycogen, etc.) yields 4 kcal; 1 g of protein yields 4 kcal; 1 g of fat provides 9 kcal; and 1 g of alcohol yields 7.4 kcal. These fuel sources are converted into energy.

■ ATP, glucose, and free fatty acids are stored in various amounts: ATP storage is sufficient for only 5–7 seconds of activity.

■ Glycogen, the storage form of CHO and a polymer of glucose, is found in both liver and muscle tissue.

■ Triglycerides, the storage form of lipids, consist of three fatty acids and a glycerol backbone.

■ Energy yields for glycogen (4 kcal $\cdot$ g^{-1}) in liver and skeletal muscle and triglycerides (9 kcal $\cdot$ g^{-1}) in skeletal muscle and adipose tissues are shown in Table 11.2.

■ Storing 1 g of glycogen requires at 2.7–4 g of water; thus, the energy yield is less than half of what would be expected: If 120 g of glycogen were stored, at least 80 g would be water, and the energy yield would be 160 rather than 480 kcal (69).

■ The breakdown of glycogen to form glucose for energy is called *glycogenolysis*.

■ The process of converting amino acids or lactate into glucose is called *gluconeogenesis*.

Energy Systems

■ Figure 11.1 presents the three different energy systems used in muscular activity, and Table 11.3 presents the length of time exercise can be maintained for these energy systems.

Table 11.1 | **Suggested Ranges for Physical Activity Factors Based on Activity**

Level of Physical Activity	PAL
Sedentary	1.2
Minimal regular physical activity	1.4–1.5
Some regular activity	1.6–1.7
Moderate physical activity	1.8–1.9
Strenuous physical activity	2.0–2.4

PAL, physical activity level.

Table 11.2 | **Energy Stores for a 60-kg Person with 15% Body Fat**

Energy Source	Energy (g)	Energy (kcal)
Liver and muscle glycogen	400–750	500–1,000
Glucose in body fluids	15–20	60–80
Total Carbohydrate Stores	**415–770**	**560–1,080**
Subcutaneous adipose triglycerides	9,000	81,000
Intramuscular triglycerides	150	1,350
Total Triglyceride Stores	**9,150**	**82,350**
Total Energy Stores	**9,565–9,920**	**82,910–83,430**

Skeletal Muscle

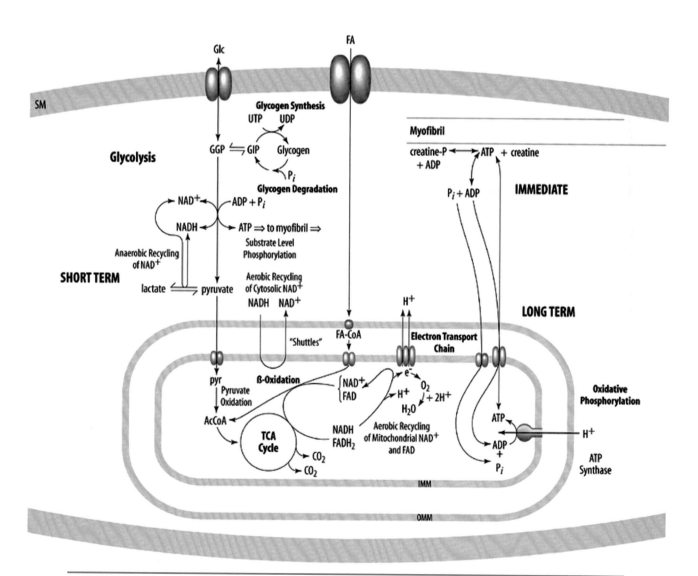

Figure 11.1: A schematic of the energy systems in skeletal muscle: immediate, short term, and long term. Glc, glucose; FFA, free fatty acid; IMM, inner mitochondrial membrane; OMM, outer mitochondrial membrane; SM, sarcolemma. Designed by Mark Roseman, PhD.

Table 11.3	Comparison of the Maximal Rates of Power and Length of Time Exercise Can be Maintained for the Immediate, Short-Term, and Long-term Energy Systems		

Energy Systems	Mole of ATP/min	Time to Fatigue
Immediate: phosphagen (phosphocreatine and ATP)	4	5–10 seconds
Short term: glycolytic (glycogen-lactic acid)	2.5	1.0–1.6 minutes
Long term: aerobic (glucose, fatty acids)	1	Unlimited time

ATP, adenosine triphosphate.

- The *immediate, or phosphagen, system* consists of ATP and creatine phosphate (PC or phosphocreatine) and allows for very short bursts of maximal power. It does not rely on oxygen.

- The *short-term, or glycogen-lactic acid, system* consists of glucose entering the glycolytic pathway and subsequent oxidation of pyruvate to lactate. The energy formed allows for only 1–1.6 minutes of maximal muscle activity at a reduced power output as compared to the phosphagen system. This often can happen in the absence of oxygen, but lactate can be both formed and used under fully aerobic conditions (10).

- The *aerobic, or long-term, system* involves glucose entering the glycolytic pathway through to pyruvate and its subsequent oxidation to acetyl-coenzyme A (acetyl-CoA) for entry into the tricarboxylic acid (TCA) cycle. Free fatty acids (FFAs) from triglycerides can be broken down into two-carbon acetyl fragments to form acetyl-CoA. This process, known as β-oxidation, can only occur under aerobic conditions (34).

- Amino acids can enter the TCA cycle after deamination/transamination and conversion into acetyl-CoA and/or acetoacetate. NADH and $FADH_2$, the reduced coenzymes formed during glycolysis and the TCA cycle, are shuttled to the electron transport chain within the mitochondria to be oxidized to NAD and FAD, respectively. ATP is regenerated from adenosine diphosphate (ADP) with 2.5 ATP per NADH and 1.5 ATP per $FADH_2$. The O_2 used for oxidation is tightly linked to aerobic ATP production.

- One molecule of glucose going through the glycolytic pathway to lactate yields 2 ATP, whereas one molecule of glucose going through the aerobic pathway yields 30 ATP.

Determinants of Fuel Utilization

- The primary determinant of substrate preference is exercise intensity. The higher the intensity, the greater is the demand on the immediate and short-term glycolytic energy system. Low-intensity exercise uses the aerobic system almost exclusively.

- The crossover point for metabolism is the power output (hard to maximal) at which an individual switches from a predominant reliance on FFA to a primary reliance on CHO utilization (glycogen; blood glucose; and blood, muscle, and liver lactate). Moreover, further increases in power elicit relative increments in CHO utilization and relative decrements in lipid oxidation (11).

- Use of FFA increases in proportion to the energy demand until the exercise intensity approaches 60% of $\dot{V}O_{2max}$, after which glucose becomes the dominant fuel source (35,65,66). Figure 11.2 shows the contributions of fat and CHO as substrate for various exercise intensities.

- Trained athletes are able to oxidize fatty acids as fuels at higher exercise intensities than untrained persons.

- During exercise and recovery from the exercise at altitude, CHO utilization is increased compared with conditions at sea level (45).

NUTRITIONAL REQUIREMENTS OF ATHLETES

- Most athletes can meet their nutritional needs by consuming a well-balanced diet. Athletes have increased energy needs, and if these needs are met by consuming a balanced diet, the nutritional requirement should be met as well.

Carbohydrates

- CHO intake is necessary to maintain blood glucose levels during exercise and restore muscle glycogen after exercise. Although the total intake will depend on TEE, intakes of 6–10 $g \cdot kg^{-1}$ body wt $\cdot d^{-1}$ (~2.7–4.5 $g \cdot lb^{-1}$ body wt $\cdot d^{-1}$), depending on energy needs, are currently recommended. This equates to 420–700 $g \cdot d^{-1}$ for a 70-kg (154-lb) person (63).

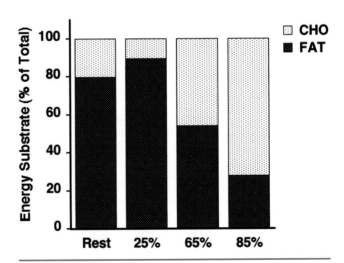

Figure 11.2: The relative contributions of fat and carbohydrate (CHO) to energy at rest and during exercise at 25%, 65%, and 85% of maximal aerobic capacity.

- The percentage of kilocalories in the diet from CHO should range between 55% and 70% of total energy intake. For a 70-kg person who requires 3,750 kcal · d^{-1}, 2,000–2700 kcal should come from CHO, which would equate to 500–675 g of CHO · d^{-1}.

Protein

- Approximately 10%–35% of the total energy should come from protein, depending on the actual energy intake.
- Protein needs of athletes are somewhat higher than for sedentary populations. The recommended range of intake for strength athletes is 1.2–1.7 g · kg^{-1} body wt · d^{-1} (0.5–0.8 g · lb^{-1} body wt · d^{-1}). This equates to a protein intake of 84–120 g · d^{-1} for a 70-kg (154-lb) person, which would be 9%–13% of the total kilocalories, if 3,750 kcal · d^{-1} were being consumed.
- The recommended protein intake for endurance athletes is 1.2–1.4 g · kg^{-1} body wt · d^{-1} (0.55–0.64 g · lb^{-1} body wt · d^{-1}) (63). This equates to a protein intake of 84–98 g · d^{-1} for a 70-kg (154-lb) person, which would be 336–392 kcal or 9%–10.5% of the energy, if total energy were 3,750 kcal.
- Essential amino acids (EAA) are not synthesized by the body and must be provided in the diet; they include leucine, isoleucine, valine, histidine, lysine, methionine, phenylalanine, threonine, and tryptophan (9,27).
- The requirement for protein can be met through diet alone, without using protein powders or amino acid supplements (63).
- When energy intake is low, it is important to consume the recommended amount of protein: Protein may contribute up to 35% of the total energy.

Fat

- Dietary fat intake should usually provide no more than 30% of the total energy. For example, a 70-kg (154-lb) person who consumes 3,750 kcal · d^{-1} would ingest ~125 g of fat (or 1,125 kcal from fat).
- Endurance athletes in training may decrease their intake of fat to only 20%–25% of total energy so they can consume adequate amounts of CHO.
- Ingestion of a high-fat, low-CHO diet is associated with lower resting muscle glycogen content and higher rates of fat oxidation during exercise as compared to a CHO-rich diet (18,32–34).

Vitamins and Minerals

- Active individuals should consume adequate vitamins and minerals to achieve the most recent Dietary Reference Intakes (DRIs) based on their life stage, gender, and activity level.
- Athletes who perspire heavily or engage in physical activity in hot conditions may be prone to increased losses of minerals in their sweat.

HYDRATION AND FLUID REPLACEMENT

- Water is the most important nutrient for regulating hydration status in individuals.
- Water losses during exercise occur primarily through sweat and can be considerable during prolonged exercise, particularly in warm or hot weather. Electrolyte losses in sweat can also be substantial.
- Sweat rate is influenced by ambient temperature, humidity, exercise intensity, training status, and rate of fluid intake.
- Fluid replacement is important for sustaining exercise performance and the current American College of Sports Medicine® (ACSM) guidelines note that the goal of fluid replacement is to prevent dehydration in excess of 2% weight loss and extreme changes in electrolyte balance to avoid performance decrements (67).
- ACSM recommends that people take personal responsibility for sustaining their hydration and develop fluid replacement programs to suit their individual needs (67).

Effects of Dehydration

- Dehydration (loss of body fluids) in excess of > 2% of body mass (> 1.4 L of water for a 70-kg person) can impair aerobic exercise performance, especially when the ambient temperature is warm.
- Dehydration between 3% and 5% of body mass (2.1–3.5 L of water for a 70-kg person) does not appear to compromise either strength or anaerobic performance (67).
- The greater the level of dehydration, the greater is the physiologic strain and degradation of aerobic exercise performance.
- Dehydration can increase the perceived effort of the task, degrade the ability to perform optimally, impair balance control, and is a risk factor for exertional heat illness, including heat stroke.

Monitoring Hydration

- The most effective way to evaluate the adequacy of a hydration program is to measure body mass before and after to quantify weight loss.
- Nude body mass should be measured before and after exercise. If body mass loss is greater than 2%, the individual is drinking too little; if body mass is greater than preexercise, the individual is drinking too much.
- Drinking in excess of sweat rate should be avoided.

Hydration Recommendations

- Fluid intake prior to exercise is necessary to increase the likelihood of starting the activity well hydrated. Consuming 400–600 mL (14–22 oz) of fluid 2 hours prior to exercise is recommended (63,67).

- Fluid intake during exercise is necessary to replace the fluid lost through sweat; fluid intake should approximate fluid losses. The practical recommendation is to consume 150–350 mL (5–12 oz) of water every 15–20 minutes of exercise if the activity lasts less than 1 hour (13).

- When exercise lasts more than 1 hour, a beverage containing 6%–8% CHO (glucose, sucrose, fructose, glucose polymers, and the like) and/or electrolytes can be beneficial (63,67,72). This amount of CHO with the addition of electrolytes ensures maximal stimulation of fluid absorption because of increased palatability and promotes gastric emptying.

- Restoration of hydration status can be accomplished by consuming regular foods and beverages.

- With excessive dehydration, persons should ingest approximately 1.5 L of fluid for each kilogram of body weight lost, and the fluid should contain more sodium than usual: A concentration of approximately 50 mmol $\cdot$ L^{-1} or 1 g of sodium per 1 L of fluid will stimulate thirst and fluid retention to enhance a more rapid and complete recovery (13,54,56,67,68).

ELECTROLYTES

- Electrolyte (sodium, potassium, chloride) and mineral (calcium, zinc, iron) losses from sweating can be substantial, depending on training status, sodium and potassium intake, genetics, sweat rate, prior heat exposure, and may lead to severe medical problems (67).

- Sodium losses, which have been associated with muscle cramps, can range from 60 to 5,000 mg $\cdot$ L^{-1} $\cdot$ d^{-1}, with higher values noted in heavy sweaters and those unaccustomed to working in the heat. Potassium losses may range from 25 to 2,000 mg (67).

- Electrolytes lost through sweating can be replaced by fluid replacement beverages and foods. Dried fruits are good food choices for potassium, and pretzels and pickles are good sources of sodium. A small box of raisins provides 322 mg of potassium, and a snack of 10 small, plain, hard salted pretzels (60 g) provides about 814 g of sodium. In addition, one small dill or kosher cucumber pickle provides about 569 g of sodium.

- Adding ½ teaspoon of table salt to food provides 1,200 mg of sodium. However, dietary intake of sodium may adversely affect blood pressure and cardiovascular disease risk, and the current published adequate intake is only 1,500 mg for young adults, slightly more than a half teaspoon of table salt (41).

NUTRIENT TIMING

- Nutrient timing is a concept developed by Drs. John Ivy and Robert Portman (42) to indicate that when food is eaten is as important as what is eaten. However, work on nutrient timing, particularly immediately after exercise to promote glycogen repletion, has been ongoing for many years (75).

- The proposed three phases of nutrient timing are during exercise, immediately after exercise (recovery), and throughout the rest of the day (maintenance) (Fig. 11.3).

Exercise

- Fluid and CHO ingestion during exercise depends on the duration and intensity.

- During exercise (training or competition), energy-providing beverages and foods are usually consumed only when the exercise is of sufficient duration to demand additional fuel (*e.g.*, marathons, triathlons, ultra-endurance events). The individual should consume what is familiar; no new fluids or foods should be consumed during competition.

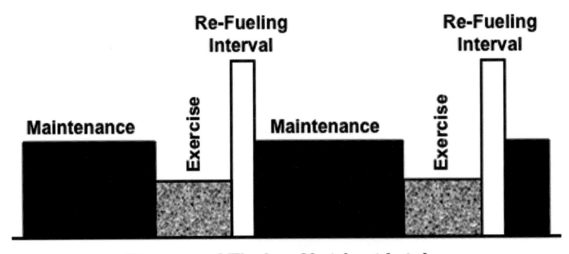

Figure 11.3: The three major phases for nutrient timing: maintenance and growth, exercise, and the refueling interval for recovery.

- For endurance activities longer than 1 hour, fluids should be consumed at regular intervals to replace fluid losses, and CHO (approximately 30–60 g · h^{-1}) should be ingested to maintain blood glucose levels.

- The above recommendations are particularly important when the exercise is under extreme environmental (heat, cold, or high altitude) conditions, in particular at high altitude.

Recovery

- During recovery, the goals are to provide adequate fluids, electrolytes, energy, and CHO to replace muscle glycogen and ensure rapid recovery.

- Ingesting CHO as a liquid, gel, or solid food (approximately 1.0–1.5 g · kg^{-1} or 0.5–0.7 g · lb^{-1} body wt) over several hours after endurance exercise, with a snack of approximately 50 g within 30 minutes, will enhance muscle glycogen synthesis (13,46,47,63).

- Protein consumed after exercise will provide amino acids for building and repair of muscle tissue but is unlikely to increase muscle glycogen repletion. The addition of protein to CHO may promote faster recovery and performance during multiple training sessions or competition.

- Ingestion of a small amount of protein (10–15 g) with the CHO during recovery can increase muscle protein synthesis and improve nitrogen balance compared with consuming only CHO (36–38,47).

Maintenance

- During the maintenance and growth phase of nutrient timing, a high daily intake of CHO, in combination with adequate protein and fat, should be consumed.

- CHO intake should match energy intensity and expenditure. As exercise intensity and/or workload increases, CHO intake should increase to ensure glycogen stores (63).

- The recommended amounts of vitamins and minerals should be consumed through proper choice of foods to meet nutritional demands of strenuous training (64).

- During the maintenance phase, it is important to develop nutritional strategies that consider nutrient timing as a

function of training schedule and competitive events. In particular, the time it takes to digest certain foods, what types of foods best meet the needs of the athlete, and ensuring snacks are available to provide CHO at regular intervals should be considered.

NUTRITIONAL ISSUES

Preexercise Meals

- The intensity of the exercise may dictate the preexercise meal. Foods consumed before low-intensity exercise may have adverse gastrointestinal effects at a higher intensity level. Try different foods to see what works best based on exercise intensity levels (53).

- Eating prior to exercise, as compared to exercising after an overnight fast, may improve performance (44,55,64).

- Consume a meal or snack 3–4 hours before heavy training or competition to minimize hunger, ensure food digestion and gastric emptying, and maximize endogenous glycogen stores. Table 11.4 presents several light preexercise meals.

- Ingesting a small meal 1 hour or less before heavy training or competition does not appear to benefit performance (63).

Glycemic Index

- The glycemic index (GI), a concept proposed by Jenkins et al. (43), describes how rapidly a particular food raises blood glucose levels after eating.

- CHOs come in different forms. Some contain dietary fiber, and the time required for digestion and absorption differs.

- High GI foods are usually digested and absorbed rapidly and release glucose into the circulation, whereas low GI foods take longer to digest and absorb (43). Figure 11.4 presents a comparison of blood glucose changes after the ingestion of a high and low GI food.

- On a scale of 0–100, foods with a GI > 70 are classified as high, whereas foods with a GI < 55 are considered low GI foods (43).

Table 11.4	Suggested Foods for Preexercise Meal or Snack			
Type of Food	**kcal**	**Carbohydrate (g)**	**Fat (g)**	**Protein (g)**
2 slices whole-wheat bread, 2 oz turkey, lettuce, and 1 medium orange	289	40	4	23
1 baked potato w/ yogurt	201	41	1	7
8 oz low-fat yogurt w/ fruit	255	47	3	11
½ cup low-fat granola w/ ½ cup skim milk	241	46	3	8
Bagel w/ 2 tbsp low-fat cream cheese	330	55	6	13
8 oz low-fat chocolate milk and 1 medium apple	264	51	3	9

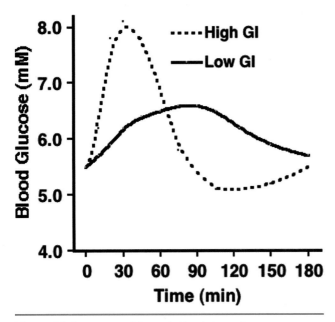

Figure 11.4: Patterns of change in blood glucose in response to high and low glycemic index (GI) foods.

■ High GI foods may be most effective in restoring glycogen after exercise because they produce a rapid rise in blood glucose (43,73).

■ Preexercise meals should consist of low GI foods to minimize a rapid rise in blood glucose (73).

Carbohydrate Manipulations

■ Individuals training for any sport must consume adequate amounts of CHO on a regular basis to maintain glycogen stores.

■ One effect of consuming a high-CHO diet is a greater reliance on CHO as the fuel of choice: CHO loading decreases oxidation of fatty acids (1,52).

■ A CHO manipulation termed "train low, compete high" has emerged. Train low means training with glycogen stores low (14,16,31,39). This is accomplished by ingesting a high-fat, low-CHO diet; having two training sessions daily and consuming no CHO between training sessions; and training after an overnight fast.

■ Training with low glycogen induces a variety of metabolic and training adaptations, but they do not benefit athletic performance (13,14,39,74).

High-Fat Diets

■ Consuming a high-fat diet ($> 65\%$ of energy as fat) for at least 5 days enhances fatty acid oxidation and spares glycogen (18,32,34,74) (Fig. 11.5). Such a practice will reduce muscle and liver glycogen stores, which can compromise exercise performance, particularly high-intensity exercise.

■ High-fat diets may be useful for ultra-endurance events where the intensity is typically low.

■ The type of running event would dictate whether a high-fat diet would confer any benefit.

ERGOGENIC AGENTS AND NUTRITIONAL SUPPLEMENTS

■ Dietary supplements can be found in various forms: pills, powders, beverages, and bars.

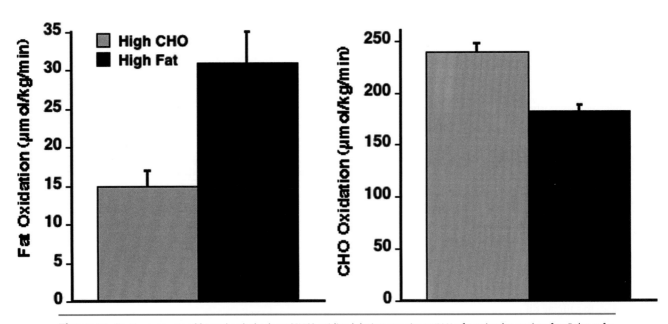

Figure 11.5: The amounts of fat and carbohydrate (CHO) oxidized during exercise at 70% of maximal capacity after 5 days of a high-fat diet (~68% of energy), followed by 1 day of rest with a high-CHO diet (~70% of energy).

- Manufacturers of dietary supplements often make claims that sound appealing, but many are not legal. No claims of preventing disease or improving health are allowed unless the Food and Drug Administration approves the claim. Claims related to structure and function can be made. For example, the statement "calcium promotes bone health" is legal because it relates to a structure — bone — but does not claim to improve health or disease.

- Multiple vitamin–mineral supplements may be necessary for athletes who restrict energy intake, engage in severe weight-loss practices, or eliminate food group(s) from their diet.

- When choosing supplements, look for a seal that demonstrates participation in a third-party verification program, such as U.S. Pharmacopeia (USP), NSF International, or Informed-Choice, which ensures quality and purity.

- Athletes should consider the tolerable upper intake levels (ULs) for nutrients when selecting dietary supplements. The UL is "the highest average daily nutrient intake level that is likely to pose no risk of adverse health effects to most individuals." Risk to the individual is minimal when intakes are below the UL.

- ULs for nutrients can be found at: http://www.wadsworth.com/nutrition_d/special_features/0-534-558986-7_C.pdf

- No supplements should provide more than 150% of the DRI of the nutrient.

Protein Powders

- The bioavailability of amino acids from various sources of protein is influenced by the source/type of protein and purification methods (19).

- Casein and whey are high-quality proteins but differ markedly in their digestion and absorption. Ingestion of whey protein produces a rapid, but transient (1–2 hours) peak in serum amino acids, whereas casein produces a more prolonged, modest increase (over 7 hours), which results in casein having a greater anabolic effect compared to whey (48).

- Protein hydrolysates are produced from purified proteins by hydrolysis with acid or by adding proteolytic enzymes (51).

- Hydrolysates are absorbed more rapidly than free-form amino acids and intact proteins, and whey hydrolysates are absorbed more rapidly than those of soy; both are absorbed more rapidly than casein hydrolysates (70).

Caffeine

- Caffeine is one of the substances most commonly used by athletes to enhance their performance.

- The optimal dose of caffeine for performance improvements is between 1 and 6 mg · kg^{-1} (28); higher doses may impair performance (15).

- Responses to caffeine differ among individuals due to varying abilities to metabolize caffeine: A single substitution in the CYP1A2 gene that codes for the protein, cytochrome

P450 1A2, causes those persons to be slow caffeine metabolizers (3).

- Trained athletes may experience greater performance benefits than recreational athletes when taking caffeine for exercise at high intensities (3).

- Caffeine can be ingested in capsule or powder form or as a constituent in energy drinks or in gum, but coffee may not be a good source of caffeine.

- Whereas normal caffeine intake poses no significant health risk, caffeine can cause multiple side effects, including insomnia, headaches, restlessness, nervousness, agitation, muscle twitching, tremors, gastric irritation, nausea, vomiting, and tachycardia.

- The Food and Drug Administration approved the addition of caffeine to soft drinks and limited the maximum caffeine content of cola-type soft drinks to 0.02% caffeine, or 71 mg per 12 oz of fluid (62).

Creatine

- Creatine is one of the supplements most widely used by athletes to increase muscle mass and enhance energy and athletic performance.

- Creatine exists in one of two forms in the body: free creatine (~40%), and a phosphorylated form, creatine phosphate (~60%) (12,21). Creatine phosphate (CP) is the energy reservoir that provides rapid phosphate-bond energy to resynthesize ATP from ADP and phosphate.

- Approximately 95% of the body's total creatine content (120–140 g for an average 154-lb/70-kg person) is located in skeletal muscles; a greater concentration is found in fast-twitch compared to slow-twitch muscle fibers (6,12,20–22).

- Most data suggest 2.0–3.0 g · d^{-1} of creatine is a safe and effective dose to maximize muscle creatine levels, regardless of weight (61).

- The typical washout period for creatine is 28–36 days (40).

Carnosine and β-Alanine

- Carnosine is one of the most abundant dipeptides found in skeletal muscle; it is synthesized from the amino acids L-histidine and β-alanine by carnosine synthase (23). β-Alanine is the rate-limiting factor, so increasing β-alanine increases the carnosine content of skeletal muscle (24).

- Increasing muscle carnosine content (via β-alanine supplementation) can improve high-intensity exercise performance probably by reducing contractile fatigue or enhancing muscle-buffering capacity (23).

- Consuming 3.2 or 6.4 g of β-alanine (regardless of weight) has been shown to elevate muscle carnosine content by 42% and 64%, respectively (30).

- Discontinuation of β-alanine supplementation causes carnosine to washout at a rate of 2.5%–3.5% per week; an increase of 55% would require a washout period of about 15 weeks (4).

Branched-Chain Amino Acids

- Branched-chain amino acids (BCAAs), which consist of the EAAs leucine, isoleucine, and valine, are metabolized in the muscle, rather than in the liver (60). They have received much attention with respect to exercise because they serve as precursors for the synthesis of other amino acids and proteins (60) and as an energy substrate during exercise and periods of stress.
- BCAAs, in particular leucine, have anabolic effects on human skeletal muscle under resting conditions and during recovery from endurance events (7,17,71).

Antioxidants

- Antioxidants are substances capable of inhibiting the oxidation of other molecules or delaying, preventing, or protecting cells from oxidative damage (29).
- Whether supplemental antioxidants decrease the damaging effects by scavenging reactive oxygen species (ROS) or preventing the transformation of ROS into more damaging compounds is not certain.

Sport Drinks

- Sport drinks are fluid replacement beverages containing electrolytes and CHO that help maintain hydration and provide fuel for working muscles during exercise. After exercise, they promote rehydration, replace electrolytes lost from sweating, and maximize muscle glycogen repletion (53,54).
- Sport drinks are not needed during exercise lasting less than 1 hour, but may be very important when exercising for extended periods of time, particularly in hot and humid conditions.
- The ideal commercial fluid replacement beverage provides sodium, potassium, and CHO; recommended ranges for sodium and potassium are 20–30 mEq $\cdot$ L^{-1} (460–700 mg $\cdot$ L^{-1}) and 5–10 mEq $\cdot$ L^{-1} (200–390 mg $\cdot$ L^{-1}), respectively, to offset sweat losses and promote fluid absorption; the anion, chloride, is recommended because it optimizes fluid absorption. The optimal CHO range is 5%–10%, or 50–100 g $\cdot$ L^{-1} of fluid (67).

Sport Bars

- Sport bars originated when it was shown that ultra-marathoners and other endurance athletes performed better when provided concentrated sources of easily absorbable CHO during long training and competitive events.
- Athletes use sport bars during training and competition to provide CHO and as recovery snacks to replete glycogen and restore protein balance.
- Sport bars should be ingested with fluids to enhance digestion and absorption of nutrients and should provide less than 100% of the Dietary Reference Intake (DRI) for vitamins and minerals.

- The CHO from sports bars is effectively oxidized during exercise and is a practical form of supplementation with other CHO forms (59).

Energy Drinks

- Energy drinks are beverages promoted as being able to increase alertness, improve cognitive tasks, enhance athletic performance, and promote weight loss; they are not fluid replacement beverages (25).
- Most energy drinks contain caffeine and a combination of other ingredients, including taurine, sucrose, guarana, ginseng, niacin, pyridoxine, glucuronolactone, and cyanocobalamin (5,25,57).
- Many energy drinks exceeded the caffeine limit of 0.02% in 2003: Doses of caffeine in energy drinks range from 50 to 505 mg per can or bottle as compared to only 100 mg in a 6-oz cup of coffee (62).
- Some energy drinks are also sold in combination with a 10%–12% alcohol content; thus, it is essential to read the nutrition label before purchasing and/or consuming such products.
- Weekly or daily energy drink use is strongly associated with alcohol dependence (2).

NUTRITION AND THE FEMALE ATHLETE

- Female athletes require special consideration because they typically consume diets too low in energy, which can place them at great risk of injury and limit exercise performance. A continual energy debt jeopardizes performance and health, as intake of essential nutrients is restricted (8,49).
- One of the most common nutrient deficiencies observed among female athletes is iron deficiency with low iron stores; iron deficiency, with or without anemia, will limit work capacity and can impair muscle function (50,58,63,64).

REFERENCES

1. Andrews JL, Sedlock DA, Flynn MG, Navalta JW, Ji H. Carbohydrate loading and supplementation in endurance-trained women runners. *J Appl Physiol.* 2003;95(2):584–90.
2. Arria AM, Caldeira KM, Kasperski SJ, Vincent KB, Griffiths RR, O'Grady KE. Energy drink consumption and increased risk for alcohol dependence. *Alcohol Clin Exp Res.* 2011;35(2):365–75.
3. Astorino TA, Roberson DW. Efficacy of acute caffeine ingestion for short-term high-intensity exercise performance: a systematic review. *J Strength Cond Res.* 2010;24(1):257–65.
4. Baguet A, Reyngoudt H, Pottier A, et al. Carnosine loading and washout in human skeletal muscles. *J Appl Physiol.* 2009;106(3):837–42.
5. Ballard SL, Wellborn-Kim JJ, Clauson KA. Effects of commercial energy drink consumption on athletic performance and body composition. *Phys Sportsmed.* 2010;38(1):107–17.

6. Bemben MG, Lamont HS. Creatine supplementation and exercise performance: recent findings. *Sports Med.* 2005;35(2):107–25.

7. Blomstrand E, Saltin B. BCAA intake affects protein metabolism in muscle after but not during exercise in humans. *Am J Physiol Endocrinol Metab.* 2001;281(2):E365–74.

8. Bonci CM, Bonci LJ, Granger LR, et al. National athletic trainers' association position statement: preventing, detecting, and managing disordered eating in athletes. *J Athl Train.* 2008;43(1):80–108.

9. Børsheim E, Tipton KD, Wolf SE, Wolfe RR. Essential amino acids and muscle protein recovery from resistance exercise. *Am J Physiol Endocrinol Metab.* 2002;283(4):E648–57.

10. Brooks GA. Cell-cell and intracellular lactate shuttles. *J Physiol.* 2009; 587(Pt 23):5591–600.

11. Brooks GA, Mercier J. Balance of carbohydrate and lipid utilization during exercise: the "crossover" concept. *J Appl Physiol.* 1994;76(6):2253–61.

12. Buford TW, Kreider RB, Stout JR, et al. International Society of Sports Nutrition position stand: creatine supplementation and exercise. *J Int Soc Sports Nutr.* 2007;4:6.

13. Burke L. Fasting and recovery from exercise. *Br J Sports Med.* 2010; 44(7):502–8.

14. Burke LM. New issues in training and nutrition: train low, compete high? *Curr Sports Med Rep.* 2007;6(3):137–8.

15. Burke LM. Caffeine and sports performance. *Appl Physiol Nutr Metab.* 2008;33(6):1319–34.

16. Burke LM. Fueling strategies to optimize performance: training high or training low? *Scand J Med Sci Sports.* 2010;20(Suppl 2):48–58.

17. Burke LM, Castell LM, Stear SJ, et al. BJSM reviews: A-Z of nutritional supplements: dietary supplements, sports nutrition foods and ergogenic aids for health and performance. Part 4. *Br J Sports Med.* 2009; 43(14):1088–90.

18. Burke LM, Hawley JA. Effects of short-term fat adaptation on metabolism and performance of prolonged exercise. *Med Sci Sports Exerc.* 2002; 34(9):1492–8.

19. Campbell B, Kreider RB, Ziegenfuss T, et al. International Society of Sports Nutrition position stand: protein and exercise. *J Int Soc Sports Nutr.* 2007;4:8.

20. Clarkson PM. Antioxidants and physical performance. *Crit Rev Food Sci Nutr.* 1995;35(1–2):131–41.

21. Dechent P, Pouwels PJ, Wilken B, Hanefeld F, Frahm J. Increase of total creatine in human brain after oral supplementation of creatine-monohydrate. *Am J Physiol.* 1999;277(3 Pt 2):R698–704.

22. Demant TW, Rhodes EC. Effects of creatine supplementation on exercise performance. *Sports Med.* 1999;28(1):49–60.

23. Derave W, Everaert I, Beeckman S, Baguet A. Muscle carnosine metabolism and beta-alanine supplementation in relation to exercise and training. *Sports Med.* 2010;40(3):247–63.

24. Derave W, Ozdemir MS, Harris RC, et al. beta-Alanine supplementation augments muscle carnosine content and attenuates fatigue during repeated isokinetic contraction bouts in trained sprinters. *J Appl Physiol.* 2007;103(5):1736–43.

25. Duchan E, Patel ND, Feucht C. Energy drinks: a review of use and safety for athletes. *Phys Sportsmed.* 2010;38(2):171–9.

26. Frankenfield D, Roth-Yousey L, Compher C. Comparison of predictive equations for resting metabolic rate in healthy nonobese and obese adults: a systematic review. *J Am Diet Assoc.* 2005;105(5):775–89.

27. Fujita S, Dreyer HC, Drummond MJ, et al. Nutrient signalling in the regulation of human muscle protein synthesis. *J Physiol.* 2007;582(Pt 2): 813–23.

28. Ganio MS, Klau JF, Casa DJ, Armstrong LE, Maresh CM. Effect of caffeine on sport-specific endurance performance: a systematic review. *J Strength Cond Res.* 2009;23(1):315–24.

29. Halliwell B. Biochemistry of oxidative stress. *Biochem Soc Trans.* 2007; 35(Pt 5):1147–50.

30. Harris RC, Tallon MJ, Dunnett M, et al. The absorption of orally supplied beta-alanine and its effect on muscle carnosine synthesis in human vastus lateralis. *Amino Acids.* 2006;30(3):279–89.

31. Havemann L, West SJ, Goedecke JH, et al. Fat adaptation followed by carbohydrate loading compromises high-intensity sprint performance. *J Appl Physiol.* 2006;100(1):194–202.

32. Helge JW. Adaptation to a fat-rich diet: effects on endurance performance in humans. *Sports Med.* 2000;30(5):347–57.

33. Helge JW. Long-term fat diet adaptation effects on performance, training capacity, and fat utilization. *Med Sci Sports Exerc.* 2002;34(9): 1499–504.

34. Helge JW, Watt PW, Richter EA, Rennie MJ, Kiens B. Fat utilization during exercise: adaptation to a fat-rich diet increases utilization of plasma fatty acids and very low density lipoprotein-triacylglycerol in humans. *J Physiol.* 2001;537(Pt 3):1009–20.

35. Horowitz JF, Mora-Rodriguez R, Byerley LO, Coyle EF. Substrate metabolism when subjects are fed carbohydrate during exercise. *Am J Physiol.* 1999;276(5 Pt 1):E828–35.

36. Howarth KR, Moreau NA, Phillips SM, Gibala MJ. Coingestion of protein with carbohydrate during recovery from endurance exercise stimulates skeletal muscle protein synthesis in humans. *J Appl Physiol.* 2009;106(4): 1394–402.

37. Howarth KR, Phillips SM, MacDonald MJ, Richards D, Moreau NA, Gibala MJ. Effect of glycogen availability on human skeletal muscle protein turnover during exercise and recovery. *J Appl Physiol.* 2010; 109(2):431–8.

38. Hulmi JJ, Lockwood CM, Stout JR. Effect of protein/essential amino acids and resistance training on skeletal muscle hypertrophy: a case for whey protein. *Nutr Metab (Lond).* 2010;7:51.

39. Hulston CJ, Venables MC, Mann CH, et al. Training with low muscle glycogen enhances fat metabolism in well-trained cyclists. *Med Sci Sports Exerc.* 2010;42(11):2046–55.

40. Hultman E, Söderlund K, Timmons JA, Cederblad G, Greenhaff PL. Muscle creatine loading in men. *J Appl Physiol.* 1996;81(1):232–7.

41. Institute of Medicine. *Dietary Reference Intakes: Water, Potassium, Sodium, Chloride, and Sulfate.* Washington, DC: The National Academies Press; 2005. 618 p.

42. Ivy J, Portman R. *Nutrient Timing: The Future of Sports Nutrition.* Laguna Beach, CA: Basic Health Publications, Inc; 2004. 224 p.

43. Jenkins DJ, Wolever TM, Taylor RH, et al. Glycemic index of foods: a physiological basis for carbohydrate exchange. *Am J Clin Nutr.* 1981; 34(3):362–6.

44. Jentjens RL, Cale C, Gutch C, Jeukendrup AE. Effects of pre-exercise ingestion of differing amounts of carbohydrate on subsequent metabolism and cycling performance. *Eur J Appl Physiol.* 2003; 88(4–5):444–52.

45. Katayama K, Goto K, Ishida K, Ogita F. Substrate utilization during exercise and recovery at moderate altitude. *Metabolism.* 2010;59(7): 959–66.

46. Kerksick C, Harvey T, Stout J, et al. International Society of Sports Nutrition position stand: nutrient timing. *J Int Soc Sports Nutr.* 2008;5:17.

47. Koopman R, Wagenmakers AJ, Manders RJ, et al. Combined ingestion of protein and free leucine with carbohydrate increases postexercise muscle protein synthesis in vivo in male subjects. *Am J Physiol Endocrinol Metab.* 2005;288(4):E645–53.

48. Lemon PW, Berardi JM, Noreen EE. The role of protein and amino acid supplements in the athlete's diet: does type or timing of ingestion matter? *Curr Sports Med Rep.* 2002;1(4):214–21.

49. Lynch SL, Hoch AZ. The female runner: gender specifics. *Clin Sports Med.* 2010;29(3):477–98.

50. Mann SK, Kaur S, Bains K. Iron and energy supplementation improves the physical work capacity of female college students. *Food Nutr Bull.* 2002;23(1):57–64.

51. Manninen AH. Protein hydrolysates in sports nutrition. *Nutr Metab (Lond).* 2009;6:38.

52. McLay RT, Thomson CD, Williams SM, Rehrer NJ. Carbohydrate loading and female endurance athletes: effect of menstrual-cycle phase. *Int J Sport Nutr Exerc Metab.* 2007;17(2):189–205.

53. Mondazzi L, Arcelli E. Glycemic index in sport nutrition. *J Am Coll Nutr.* 2009;28(Suppl):455S–463S.

54. Montain SJ. Hydration recommendations for sport 2008. *Curr Sports Med Rep.* 2008;7(4):187–92.

55. Moseley L, Lancaster GI, Jeukendrup AE. Effects of timing of pre-exercise ingestion of carbohydrate on subsequent metabolism and cycling performance. *Eur J Appl Physiol.* 2003;88(4–5):453–8.

56. Noakes TD. Hydration in the marathon: using thirst to gauge safe fluid replacement. *Sports Med.* 2007;37(4–5):463–6.

57. O'Brien MC, McCoy TP, Rhodes SD, Wagoner A, Wolfson M. Caffeinated cocktails: energy drink consumption, high-risk drinking, and alcohol-related consequences among college students. *Acad Emerg Med.* 2008;15(5):453–60.

58. Ostojic SM, Ahmetovic Z. Weekly training volume and hematological status in female top-level athletes of different sports. *J Sports Med Phys Fitness.* 2008;48(3):398–403.

59. Pfeiffer B, Stellingwerff T, Zaltas E, Jeukendrup AE. Oxidation of solid versus liquid CHO sources during exercise. *Med Sci Sports Exerc.* 2010;42(11):2030–7.

60. Platell C, Kong SE, McCauley R, Hall JC. Branched-chain amino acids. *J Gastroenterol Hepatol.* 2000;15(7):706–17.

61. Poortmans JR, Rawson ES, Burke LM, Stear SJ, Castell LM. A-Z of nutritional supplements: dietary supplements, sports nutrition foods and ergogenic aids for health and performance. Part 11. *Br J Sports Med.* 2010;44(10):765–6.

62. Reissig CJ, Strain EC, Griffiths RR. Caffeinated energy drinks—a growing problem. *Drug Alcohol Depend.* 2009;99(1–3):1–10.

63. Rodriguez NR, DiMarco NM, Langley S. American College of Sports Medicine position stand. Nutrition and athletic performance. *Med Sci Sports Exerc.* 2009;41(3):709–31.

64. Rodriguez NR, DiMarco NM, Langley S. Position of the American Dietetic Association, Dietitians of Canada, and the American College of Sports Medicine: nutrition and athletic performance. *J Am Diet Assoc.* 2009;109(3):509–27.

65. Romijn JA, Coyle EF, Sidossis LS, Rosenblatt J, Wolfe RR. Substrate metabolism during different exercise intensities in endurance-trained women. *J Appl Physiol.* 2000;88(5):1707–14.

66. Sahlin K, Harris RC. Control of lipid oxidation during exercise: role of energy state and mitochondrial factors. *Acta Physiol (Oxf).* 2008;194(4):283–91.

67. Sawka MN, Burke LM, Eichner ER, Maughan RJ, Montain SJ, Stachenfeld NS. American College of Sports Medicine position stand. Exercise and fluid replacement. *Med Sci Sports Exerc.* 2007;39(2):377–90.

68. Sharp RL. Role of sodium in fluid homeostasis with exercise. *J Am Coll Nutr.* 2006;25(3 Suppl):231S–9S.

69. Sherman WM, Plyley MJ, Sharp RL, et al. Muscle glycogen storage and its relationship with water. *Int J Sports Med.* 1982;3(1):22–4.

70. Tang JE, Moore DR, Kujbida GW, Tarnopolsky MA, Phillips SM. Ingestion of whey hydrolysate, casein, or soy protein isolate: effects on mixed muscle protein synthesis at rest and following resistance exercise in young men. *J Appl Physiol.* 2009;107(3):987–92.

71. Tipton KD, Wolfe RR. Protein and amino acids for athletes. *J Sports Sci.* 2004;22(1):65–79.

72. von Duvillard SP, Arciero PJ, Tietjen-Smith T, Alford K. Sports drinks, exercise training, and competition. *Curr Sports Med Rep.* 2008;7(4):202–8.

73. Wong SH, Chan OW, Chen YJ, Hu HL, Lam CW, Chung PK. Effect of preexercise glycemic-index meal on running when CHO-electrolyte solution is consumed during exercise. *Int J Sport Nutr Exerc Metab.* 2009;19(3):222–42.

74. Yeo WK, Lessard SJ, Chen ZP, et al. Fat adaptation followed by carbohydrate restoration increases AMPK activity in skeletal muscle from trained humans. *J Appl Physiol.* 2008;105(5):1519–26.

75. Zawadzki KM, Yaspelkis BB 3rd, Ivy JL. Carbohydrate-protein complex increases the rate of muscle glycogen storage after exercise. *J Appl Physiol.* 1992;72(5):1854–9.

Exercise Prescription

12

Dan Burnett and Mark B. Stephens

INTRODUCTION

- Over two-thirds (68%) of all Americans are either overweight or obese, a remarkable increase over the last 30 years (6). Physical inactivity and obesity are correlated with increases in coronary heart disease, diabetes, certain cancers, and all-cause mortality. Lack of physical activity is also associated with osteoporosis, falls, and mental health issues, including depression (12). Sufficient physical activity protects against these conditions.

- Guidelines from the Department of Health and Human Services (DHHS) and the American College of Sports Medicine® (ACSM) recommend a minimum of 150 minutes of moderate activity per week (2) or 75 minutes of vigorous activity per week to obtain substantial health benefits (14). The guidelines further advise that more extensive health benefits can be obtained with 300 minutes of moderate or 150 minutes of vigorous activity per week and explicitly recommend that adults also engage in muscle-strengthening activities on 2 or more days a week. The ACSM guidelines additionally further recommend flexibility exercises on 2 days per week to maintain joint range of motion, as well as neuromotor exercise training 2–3 days per week (exercises involving motor skills including balance, agility, and coordination) (2).

- Estimates from 2010 found that only 43.5% of U.S. adults met the minimum recommendations from the DHHS for aerobic activity, 21.9% met the muscle-strengthening guidelines, and only 18.2% met both the muscle-strengthening and minimum aerobic recommendations (4).

- From 1998 to 2008, improvements in these percentages improved minimally, ranging from 2.4% to 4.2% (4).

- Physical activity is one of the critically important Objective Topic Areas for Healthy People 2020 (8), the national effort to define public health priorities and goals for the United States. Multi-disciplinary targets include the DHHS guidelines for physical activity (14) and the ACSM Position Stand on the Quantity and Quality of Exercise for Developing and Maintaining Cardiorespiratory, Musculoskeletal, and Neuromotor Fitness in Apparently Healthy Adults: Guidance for Prescribing Exercise (2).

- Health care providers are poor at recognizing, addressing, and documenting the physical activity needs of patients. National data indicated that in 1995–1996 physicians provided exercise counseling for 18% of all visits by obese patients (13). A more recent study compared counseling trends across time and noted no improvement in counseling rates for exercise despite the highly documented increase in the prevalence of obesity from 1995 to 2004 (10).

- Current 2002 U.S. Preventive Services Task Force (USPSTF) recommendations (17) state that there is insufficient evidence to recommend for or against routine physical activity counseling ("I" recommendation). In a recent December 2010 draft statement the USPSTF recommended not routinely providing primary care dietary or physical activity counseling for adults without preexisting cardiovascular disease or its risk factors because the average benefit of counseling for such patients is small ("C" recommendation) (16).

- The USPSTF draft statement proposed that clinicians consider selectively providing or referring specific (higher risk) patients for more intensive counseling (16).

- The ACSM Position Stand strongly endorses interventions to increase physical activity for prevention of weight gain, for weight loss, and for weight maintenance after weight loss (1). A 2011 ACSM comprehensive review describes evidence-based summaries of the quantities and qualities of exercise appropriate for exercise prescriptions (2).

- The American Medical Association also recently published lifestyle medicine competencies that specifically call for primary care physicians to be able to assess lifestyle "vital signs" including physical activity and to be able to collaboratively develop appropriate prescriptions in response (9).

- The new Exercise Is Medicine initiative (http://www.exerciseismedicine.org), involving multiple commercial, medical, and academic entities and coordinated by ACSM, encourages physicians to include physical activity and exercise specifically in their prescribing practices for the treatment and prevention of chronic disease (5). Guidelines for preexercise graded exercise testing are discussed in Chapter 20 (Electrodiagnostic Testing).

BENEFITS OF PHYSICAL ACTIVITY (14)

- There is strong evidence that physical activity decreases adult risk for:
  - Early death
  - Coronary heart disease
  - Stroke

- ◼ Hyperlipidemia
- ◼ High blood pressure
- ◼ Type 2 diabetes
- ◼ Colon cancer
- ◼ Breast cancer
- ◼ Similar strong evidence suggests that physical activity helps with:
  - ◼ Prevention of weight gain
  - ◼ Weight loss (especially when combined with lower calorie intake)
  - ◼ Improved cardiorespiratory and muscular fitness (adults and children/adolescents)
  - ◼ Prevention of falls
  - ◼ Reduced depression
  - ◼ Better cognitive function in older adults
- ◼ Strong evidence linking physical activity with favorable body composition, improved bone health, and improved cardiovascular and metabolic health markers also exists specifically for children/adolescents.
- ◼ Other benefits of physical activity for which there is moderate evidence include improved sleep quality and reduced risk for cancer, hip fracture, and abdominal obesity.

THE EXERCISE PRESCRIPTION: WHAT TO INCLUDE

- ◼ An exercise prescription (also referred to as an activity prescription) should include clear descriptions of the frequency, intensity, type, and duration (time) of activities that individuals should engage in to achieve health benefits. Providing these recommendations as a written prescription (as with other medical treatments) may help patient adherence.
- ◼ The mnemonic "FITT" (frequency, intensity, type, time) is a useful aid for guiding clinicians when working with the patient on an exercise prescription.
- ◼ An individualized prescription should include specific recommendations for different physical activities (aerobic and muscle-strengthening) in the context of patient goals and preexisting health.

Frequency

- ◼ Patients should accumulate a minimum of 150 minutes of moderate or 75 minutes of vigorous exercise every week to positively influence health (14). For most patients, this can be accomplished by assuring at least 30 minutes of moderate-intensity walking most (preferably all) days of the week (7,15). Newer guidelines focus on total physical activity accumulated during a typical week. Activity sessions spread across at least 3 days per week may help reduce the risk of injury. The ACSM Position Stand (2) recommends 30 minutes of moderate-intensity cardiorespiratory exercise 5 days per week (totaling 150 minutes per week). An alternative is 20 or more minutes of vigorous-intensity exercise at least 3 days per week (totaling 75 minutes per week).
- ◼ Adults should perform muscle-strengthening activities of moderate or high intensity involving all major muscle groups at least 2 days per week for additional health benefits (2,14).

Intensity

- ◼ There are many ways to prescribe exercise intensity. The intensity of the exercise session should be tailored to the individual's preexisting state of health and individual goals.
- ◼ Individuals wishing to improve health and lower disease-specific risk should be advised that sufficient levels of physical activity can be accumulated through small bouts of activity throughout the day. A dedicated activity or training session is not necessary.
- ◼ The target heart rate is the most common method of prescribing exercise intensity. The training heart rate is based on an age-predicted maximal heart rate (based on the formula $HR_{max} = 220 -$ patient age). Patients are instructed to exercise at a range of 40%–80% of HR_{max} based on their specific goals.
- ◼ A modification of the target heart rate includes calculation of the heart rate reserve (HRR). This method takes into account the patient's resting heart rate (HR). Moderate activities typically are performed at 40%–60% of the HRR, whereas vigorous activities are performed at 60%–90% of HRR. To calculate the target HR based on this method:

  $HRR = \{(220 - \text{patient age}) - HR_{resting}\}$

  $HR_{target} = \{(HRR \times \text{training intensity}) + HR_{resting}\}$

- ◼ The *talk test* provides another safe and easy way to counsel individuals about exercise intensity. Patients should exercise at an intensity that allows them to carry out a conversation without undue shortness of breath.

Type

- ◼ The type of activity should be based on the individual's fitness level and interests.
- ◼ Activities involving repetitive movement of large muscle groups are recommended. Walking is the easiest activity on which to base an exercise prescription. Non–weight-bearing activities, such as swimming, rowing, and cycling, should be considered for individuals with orthopedic concerns.
- ◼ Helping an individual choose an activity that is fun and enjoyable for them increases the likelihood that an individual will keep doing it long term.
- ◼ Examples of vigorous-intensity activities include running, jogging, swimming, tennis (singles), aerobic dancing, bicycling (> 10 mph), jumping rope, and heavy gardening.
- ◼ Examples of typically moderate-intensity activities include walking briskly (> 3 mph), water aerobics, bicycling (< 10 mph), tennis (doubles), and ballroom dancing.

Duration (Time)

- Each individual bout of moderate- and vigorous-intensity exercise should be at least 10 minutes in duration. While shorter bouts may provide some health value, bouts of activity exceeding 10 minutes are known to have benefit (14).

- One approach to meet the activity guidelines would be to recommend 30–60 minutes of walking most if not all days of the week.

- An important point to help patients understand is that not all health benefits occur at minimum levels of physical activity. Additional benefits accrue as people increase levels of activity and move toward 300 minutes per week or more (colon and breast cancer risk reduction and prevention of unhealthy weight gain are two specific examples) (14).

THE EXERCISE PRESCRIPTION: BEYOND CARDIOVASCULAR ENDURANCE

- An exercise prescription should also include specific advice regarding muscular strength and endurance.

- The same FITT principle used to guide aerobic exercise prescriptions can be applied to muscular conditioning prescriptions as well.

- **Frequency:** Activities focused on improving muscular strength should be performed two to three times per week (2,14).

- **Intensity:** To develop muscular strength, individuals should perform exercises using 60%–70% of the one-repetition maximum (1-RM) level of resistance (1-RM is the maximum amount of weight that an individual can lift one time using proper technique). To develop muscular endurance, an individual should perform exercises using lower resistance, typically 50% of the 1-RM.

- **Sets/repetitions:** For strength, two to four sets of 8–12 repetitions are recommended. For muscular endurance, two sets of 15–20 repetitions are recommended.

- **Type:** Muscular strength and endurance can be developed using either free weights or dedicated resistance machines. Household items such as rubber tubing can also serve as creative forms of resistance.

- **Duration (time):** Typically, two sets are performed for each muscular group. Rest intervals consist of 2–3 minutes between sets; muscle groups require 48 hours of rest between exercise sessions.

THE EXERCISE PRESCRIPTION: OVERCOMING BARRIERS TO ACTIVITY

- **Time:** Patients commonly cite lack of time as a significant barrier to physical activity. Small bouts of physical activity scattered through the day can help overcome this barrier.

- **Convenience:** Patients also cite lack of convenience as a common obstacle. Efforts to incorporate physical activity and exercise into normal routines can help patients with this barrier. Walking or biking to work is a good example. Using public transportation in combination with walking or bicycling is another. Using available public facilities (parks, trails, courts, fields), particularly with an exercise partner, can be helpful.

- **Fatigue:** Physical activity actually improves energy levels.

- **Boredom:** Exercising with a friend or family member increases social support and accountability and reduces boredom. Choosing activities that are intrinsically fun can also help people overcome boredom.

- All of these common barriers may be addressed by both creating environments where it is physically and socially easier for people to exercise and by allowing them to come up with some of these ways to overcome the barriers themselves (see later information on motivational interviewing).

THE EXERCISE PRESCRIPTION: ASSESSING READINESS TO CHANGE

- Not all patients are immediately ready to engage in a program of increased physical activity. The likelihood of sustaining an active lifestyle can be quickly assessed using the stages-of-change model (18).

Precontemplation

- Individuals who are in the precontemplative stage have not seriously considered participating in regular physical activity. They are unlikely to significantly change their current pattern of behavior. Informing patients about risks associated with physical inactivity and encouraging them to be more active are useful counseling points for these individuals.

Contemplation

- Patients who are contemplating change are ready for an exercise prescription, but often describe barriers to an active lifestyle. Steady encouragement with suggestions for overcoming predictable barriers helps individuals in the contemplative stage.

Preparation/Action

- Patients in this stage particularly benefit from an individualized exercise prescription. Encouragement and support should be offered with specific follow-up to assess progress.

Maintenance

- Individuals in the maintenance stage have incorporated physical activity into their regular routine. The exercise prescription should be revised and updated periodically to ensure patients maintain physically active behaviors.

- Most individuals incorporating an exercise prescription into their routine lifestyle will progress through predictable phases of *acclimation*, *improvement*, and *maintenance*.

    - **Acclimation:** Acclimation typically lasts several weeks and is often the most psychologically challenging phase. Drop-out rates are highest during the acclimation phase. Patients should be encouraged to commit to the frequency of activity first, then to duration, and finally to intensity.

    - **Improvement:** Improvement occurs after patients have acclimated to regular activity. Patients experience predictable improvements in self-efficacy, physical fitness, and mood. The exercise prescription can be modified during the improvement phase as well to target patient goals.

    - **Maintenance:** In addition to the psychological characteristics described with the stages-of-change model, maintenance also has physical characteristics as well, including heart rate adaptations and exercise tolerance. The exercise prescription should be modified to account for changes in cardiovascular condition and enhanced muscular performance.

THE EXERCISE PRESCRIPTION: RESOLVING AMBIVALENCE ABOUT CHANGE

- Motivational interviewing is a helpful technique to use when helping people resolve ambivalence around health-related behaviors (11). Motivational interviewing is also helpful and effective for improving physical activity levels (3). The key questions in motivational interviewing are: (a) How important is the behavioral change to you? (b) How confident are you that you can make the necessary change? Patients who perceive behaviors as important and who are confident that they are able to make necessary changes are likely to succeed.

- Other helpful tips for motivational counseling include (11):

    - Providing an accurate and empathetic style

    - Being collaborative (rather than authoritarian)

    - Evoking the patient's own motivation (rather than trying to instill it)

    - Honoring patient autonomy

REFERENCES

1. American College of Sports Medicine. Position Stand: appropriate physical activity intervention strategies for weight loss and prevention of weight regain for adults. *Med Sci Sports Exerc.* 2009;41(2):459–71.

2. American College of Sports Medicine. Position Stand: quantity and quality of exercise for developing and maintaining cardiorespiratory, musculoskeletal, and neuromotor fitness in apparently healthy adults: guidance for prescribing exercise. *Med Sci Sports Exerc.* 2011; 43(7):1334–59.

3. Carels RA, Darby L, Cacciapaglia HM, et al. Using motivational interviewing as a supplement to obesity treatment: a stepped-care approach. *Health Psychol.* 2007;26(3):369–74.

4. Carlson SA, Fulton JE, Schoenborn CA, Loustalot F. Trend and prevalence estimates based on the 2008 Physical Activity Guidelines for Americans. *Am J Prev Med.* 2010;39(4):305–13.

5. Exercise Is Medicine Web site [Internet]. Indianapolis (IN): American College of Sports Medicine; [cited 2011 Sep 30]. Available from: http://www.exerciseismedicine.org.

6. Flegal KM, Carroll MD, Ogden CL, Curtin LR. Prevalence and trends in obesity among US adults, 1999–2008. *JAMA.* 2010;303(3):235–41.

7. Haskell WL, Lee IM, Pate RR, et al. Physical activity and public health: updated recommendation for adults from the American College of Sports Medicine and the American Heart Association. *Med Sci Sports Exerc.* 2007;39(8):1423–34.

8. Healthy People 2020 Web site [Internet]. Washington (DC): U.S. Department of Health and Human Services; [cited 2011 Mar 18]. Available from: http:www.healthypeople.gov.

9. Lianov L, Johnson M. Physician competencies for prescribing lifestyle medicine. *JAMA.* 2010;304(2):202–3.

10. McAlpine DD, Wilson AR. Trends in obesity-related counseling in primary care: 1995–2004. *Med Care.* 2007;45(4):322–9.

11. Miller WR, Rose GS. Toward a theory of motivational interviewing. *Am Psychol.* 2009;64(6):527–37.

12. Remington PL, Brownson RC, Wegner MV. *Chronic Disease Epidemiology and Control.* 3rd ed. Washington (DC): American Public Health Association; 2010. 659 p.

13. Stafford RS, Farhat JH, Misra B, Schoenfeld DA. National patterns of physician activities related to obesity management. *Arch Fam Med.* 2000; 9(7):631–8.

14. U.S. Department of Health and Human Services. 2008 physical activity guidelines for Americans [Internet]. Washington (DC): ODPHP Publication no. U0036. 2008 [cited 2011 Feb 21]. 61 p. Available from: http://www.health.gov/paguidelines/pdf/paguide.pdf.

15. U.S. Department of Health and Human Services. Physical activity and health: a report of the Surgeon General [Internet]. Atlanta (GA): U.S. Department of Health and Human Services, Centers for Disease Control and Prevention, National Center for Chronic Disease Prevention and Health Promotion. 1996 [cited 2011 Mar 18]. 300 p. Available from: http://www.cdc.gov/nccdphp/sgr/pdf/sgrfull.pdf.

16. U.S. Preventive Services Task Force Web site [Internet]. Rockville (MD): U.S. Preventive Services Task Force; [cited 2011 Mar 18]. Available from: http://www.uspreventiveservicestaskforce.org/draftrec.htm.

17. U.S. Preventive Services Task Force Web site [Internet]. Rockville (MD): U.S. Preventive Services Task Force; [cited 2011 Mar 18]. Available from: http://www.uspreventiveservicestaskforce.org/uspstf/uspsphys.htm#related.

18. Zimmerman GL, Olsen CG, Bosworth MF. A 'stages of change' approach to helping patients change behavior. *Am Fam Physician.* 2000; 61(5):1409–16.

Playing Surface and Protective Equipment

13

Jeffrey G. Jenkins and C. Joel Hess

PLAYING SURFACE

- In many sports, the athlete or event organizer has no choice with regard to playing surface — only one option exists. However, in some sports, different options offer their own advantages and disadvantages. These are addressed below.

Turf Sports

- Turf sports (*e.g.*, football, soccer, field hockey) may be played on either artificial turf or natural grass.
- First-generation artificial turf, AstroTurf, was introduced in the late 1960s and consisted of short pile carpet monofilament fibers on top of padding over concrete. Second-generation artificial turf incorporated longer fibers, sand filing, and a rubber base.
- Early studies comparing these surfaces with natural grass found a higher incidence of injuries when playing on these artificial surfaces (11,21).
- Third-generation artificial turf (*e.g.*, FieldTurf), which is composed of longer synthetic fibers and infill made of rubber pellets or sand, more closely mimics the physical properties of natural turf.
- Multiple studies have demonstrated no significant difference in overall injury incidence for soccer players when third-generation artificial turf is compared with natural grass (2,8–10,25).
- Evidence is sparse and less conclusive when comparing injury rates on third-generation artificial turf versus natural grass in American football. A 5-year study comparing injury rates in high school football players found a higher rate of injuries occurring during games played on third-generation turf (17). By contrast, Meyers' most recent study involving National Collegiate Athletic Association (NCAA) Division I-A football players found a significantly lower overall incidence of injury on artificial turf (16).
- Although overall injury incidence may be comparable between third-generation turf and natural grass, injury patterns differ.
- Ankle ligament injuries in soccer players tend to be more prevalent and have been shown to be the most common season-ending injury on artificial turf. By contrast, ligamentous knee injuries are the most common season-ending injury for soccer players on grass (8–10).
- Grass surfaces have been associated with a higher incidence of both ligamentous knee injuries and concussion in high school football players (17).
- Certain types of minor injuries are exclusive to artificial turf. These include *turf burns*, the common abrasions associated with the surface. In one study, college football players were seven times more likely to have a methicillin-resistant *Staphylococcus aureus* infection after acquiring *turf burn* (5).

Tennis

- Tennis is another sport with playing surface options, including hard court, clay, composition, grass, and carpet.
- Hard courts are associated with greater stress on the lower extremities as a result of the reduced shock-absorbing ability and increased traction between shoe and court.
- With its energy-absorbing properties, clay is more forgiving to the upper extremities due to reduced ball speed (20).
- During rehabilitation from injury, carpet, composition, and clay offer more cushion and are more forgiving to the lower extremities.

PROTECTIVE EQUIPMENT

- The purpose of protective equipment is to prevent injury and to protect injured areas from further injury. Sanctioning bodies (*e.g.*, the NCAA) of various sports have rendered certain protective equipment mandatory.

Football

- The NCAA mandates the use of a helmet, face mask, four-point or six-point chin strap, mouthguard, shoulder pads, and hip, coccyx, thigh, and knee pads during football competition.
- There are two types of helmets currently in use: (a) padded, and (b) air and fluid filled, with combinations of both types.

81

- All football helmets in use at the high school or college level must be certified by the National Operating Committee on Standards for Athletic Equipment (NOCSAE). This ensures that each helmet has been tested to withstand repeated blows of high mass and low velocity. A study by Cantu and Mueller (7) attributed in large part a dramatic reduction in brain injury–related fatalities from football to the adoption of NOCSAE helmet standards. These standards went into effect in 1978 for colleges and in 1980 for high schools.

- Proper fitting of a helmet is ensured by the following criteria: The frontal crown of the helmet should sit approximately one to two fingerbreadths above the eyebrows; the back edge of the helmet should not impinge on the neck as it extends; when the head is held straight forward, an attempt to turn the helmet on the head should result in only a slight movement; jaw pads should fit the jaw area snugly to prevent lateral rocking of the helmet; the chin strap should fit snugly with equal tension on both sides; the hair should be cut to normal length prior to fitting.

- Mouthguards include ready-to-wear, mouth-formed, and custom-fitted types. Ready-made guards are the least comfortable and least protective type (19). Mouthguards have been required equipment for high school football players since 1962 and for their collegiate counterparts since 1973. Mouth injuries, which at one time comprised 50% of all football injuries, have been reduced by more than half since the adoption of face masks and mouthguards for use in the sport (13).

- Two types of shoulder pads are in use: flat and cantilevered. Flat pads allow greater glenohumeral motion and are appropriate for limited contact positions, such as quarterback and receiver. Cantilevered pads are named for the cantilever bridge that extends over the shoulder, dispersing impact force over a wider area. These pads offer greater protection to the shoulder area and are appropriate for the majority of players.

- A proper shoulder pad fit is achieved when the tip of the inner pad extends just to the lateral edge of the shoulder. The sternum and clavicles should be covered, and the flaps or epaulets should cover the deltoid area.

- Hip and coccyx pads are mandatory equipment and should cover the greater trochanters, the iliac crests, and the coccyx. Snap-in, girdle, and wrap-around pads are available. Girdle pads are the most common type but also the most difficult to keep in place. Care should be taken to ensure coverage of the iliac crest.

- Controversy exists regarding the use of prophylactic knee braces in football. A study by Rovere et al. (22) in 1987 actually showed an increased rate of anterior cruciate ligament (ACL) injuries with brace use. Since then, however, a study carried out at West Point (23) and another from the Big Ten Conference (1) showed a consistent trend toward a reduction of medial collateral ligament (MCL) injuries with use of prophylactic braces. Due to these inconsistent findings and the lack of demonstrated proof of efficacy, both the American Academy of Pediatrics and the American Academy of Orthopedic Surgeons have recommended against the routine use of prophylactic knee bracing in football (15).

- ACL functional braces are available for players with ACL-deficient knees. Custom-fit braces have not been shown to perform better or offer more protection than off-the-shelf braces (28).

Baseball/Softball

- The NCAA mandates the use of a double earflap helmet for all batters and base runners as well as a mask and throat guard for catchers.

- Little League Baseball requires protective helmets for batters, catchers, base runners, first and third base coaches, and on-deck hitters.

- All helmets should be NOCSAE certified to ensure strength and safety and bear a "Meets NOCSAE Standard" seal on the outside.

- It is recommended that baseball batters age 4–14 wear helmets with face protectors to reduce the risk of eye and facial bone injury. This recommendation was originally made in 1984 by the Sports Eye Safety Committee of the National Society to Prevent Blindness.

- Breakaway bases are available, which can decrease sliding-associated injuries by approximately 98% (18).

Ice Hockey

- The NCAA mandates the use of helmets with fastened chin straps, face masks, and an internal mouthpiece.

- Shoulder pads, elbow pads, protective gloves, padded pants, and shin guards are also standard equipment.

- Athletic supporter and neck or throat guard are also recommended for goalies.

- The use of full face shields results in a significantly decreased risk of facial or dental injury (6). A systematic review found that face shields offer these protective benefits without increasing the incidence of head and neck injury (3).

- It has been shown that prophylactic knee braces do not significantly reduce the incidence of knee injury among hockey players (27).

Lacrosse

- The NCAA requires the use of a NOCSAE-certified helmet with face mask, chin strap, and chin pad, as well as protective gloves, shoulder and arm pads, and a mouthguard for all male lacrosse players. Goalies are additionally required to wear chest and throat protectors. Many players also wear rib protector vests.

Racquet Sports

- Some clubs require eye protection for badminton, squash, and racquetball players.

- Lenses should be composed of at least a 3-mm thick CR 39 plastic or polycarbonate plastic.

- Glass lenses are discouraged due to risk of breakage.

■ Lenses should be mounted in a nylon sports frame with a steep posterior lip and temples that rotate about 180 degrees. When a lens in a sports frame is struck, it projects forward rather than back and toward the eye (14).

Basketball

■ Mouthguards are recommended, but not mandatory, to reduce risk of dental trauma.

■ High top basketball shoes have been shown not to reduce the incidence of ankle sprains during play (4).

■ The use of a semirigid ankle stabilizing brace does seem to reduce the incidence of ankle injury, but not the severity of such injuries (24).

Wrestling

■ The NCAA requires use of ear protectors, which protect against the formation of auricular hematomas and the cosmetic deformity, *cauliflower ear*. It is recommended that all wrestlers use mouthguards.

Soccer

■ Shin guards should be worn to reduce incidence of tibia and fibula fractures, as well as compartment syndrome from anterior leg contusions. Shin guards should protect the entire length of the tibia (12). They are mandated by the NCAA and require NOCSAE certification.

■ Use of a semirigid ankle orthosis has been shown to decrease the incidence of recurrent ankle sprains in soccer players with previous history of sprains (26).

■ Mouthguards are recommended, especially for goalkeepers, to protect against not only dental injury but also concussion resulting from head-to-head collisions.

REFERENCES

1. Albright JP, Powell JW, Smith W, et al. Medial collateral ligament knee sprains in college football: effectiveness of preventive braces. *Am J Sports Med.* 1994;22(1):12–8.

2. Aoki H, Kohno T, Fujiya H, et al. Incidence of injury among adolescent soccer players: a comparative study of artificial and natural grass turfs. *Clin J Sports Med.* 2010;20(1):1–7.

3. Asplund C, Bettcher S, Borchers J. Facial protection and head injuries in ice hockey: a systematic review. *Br J Sports Med.* 2009;43(13):993–9.

4. Barret JR, Tanji JL, Drake C, et al. High- versus low-top shoes for the prevention of ankle sprains in basketball players. A prospective randomized study. *Am J Sports Med.* 1993;21(4):582–5.

5. Begier EM, Frenette K, Barrett NL, et al. A high-morbidity outbreak of methicillin-resistant *Staphylococcus aureus* among players on a college football team, facilitated by cosmetic body shaving and turf burns. *Clin Infect Dis.* 2004;39(10):1446–53.

6. Benson BW, Mohtadi NG, Rose MS, Meeuwisse WH. Head and neck injuries among ice hockey players wearing full face shields vs half face shields. *JAMA.* 1999;282(24):2328–32.

7. Cantu RC, Mueller FO. Brain injury related fatalities in American football, 1945–99. *Neurosurgery.* 2003;52(4):846–52.

8. Ekstrand J, Timpka T, Hägglund M. Risk of injury in elite football played on artificial turf versus natural grass: a prospective two-cohort study. *Br J Sports Med.* 2006;40:975–80.

9. Fuller CW, Dick RW, Corlette J, Schmalz R. Comparison of the incidence, nature and cause of injuries sustained on grass and new generation artificial turf by male and female football players. Part 1: match injuries. *Br J Sports Med.* 2007;41(Suppl 1);i20–6.

10. Fuller CW, Dick RW, Corlette J, Schmalz R. Comparison of the incidence, nature and cause of injuries sustained on grass and new generation artificial turf by male and female football players. Part 2: training injuries. *Br J Sports Med.* 2007;41(Suppl 1);i27–32.

11. Grippo A. *NFL Injury Study 1969–1972. Final Project Report (SRI-MSD 1961).* Menlo Park (CA): Stanford Research Institute; 1973.

12. Howe WB. Soccer. In: Morris MB, editor. *Sports Medicine Secrets.* 2nd ed. Philadelphia: Hanley & Belfus; 1999. p. 382–5.

13. Knapik JJ, Marshall SW, Lee RB, et al. Mouthguards in sport activities: history, physical properties and injury prevention effectiveness. *Sports Med.* 2007;37(2):117–44.

14. Kulund DN. Athletic injuries to the head, face, and neck. In: Kulund DN, editor. *The Injured Athlete.* 2nd ed. Philadelphia: J.B. Lippincott Company; 1988. p. 267–99.

15. Martin TJ. American Academy of Pediatrics Committee on Sports Medicine: knee brace use by athletes. *Pediatrics.* 1990;85(2):228.

16. Meyers MC. Incidence, mechanisms, and severity of game-related college football injuries on FieldTurf versus natural grass: a 3 year prospective study. *Am J Sports Med.* 2010;38(4):687–97.

17. Meyers MC, Barnhill BS. Incidence, causes, and severity of high school football injuries on FieldTurf versus natural grass: a 5-year prospective study. *Am J Sports Med.* 2004;32(7):1626–38.

18. Naftulin S, McKeag DB. Protective equipment: baseball, softball, hockey, wrestling, and lacrosse. In: Morris MB, editor. *Sports Medicine Secrets.* 2nd ed. Philadelphia: Hanley & Belfus; 1999. p. 110–6.

19. Newsome PR, Tran DC, Cooke MS. The role of the mouthguard in the prevention of sports-related dental injuries: a review. *Int J Paediatr Dent.* 2001;11(6):396–404.

20. Nicola TL. Tennis. In: Mellion MB, Walsh WM, Shelton GL, editors. *The Team Physician's Handbook.* 2nd ed. Philadelphia: Hanley & Belfus; 1997. p. 816–27.

21. Powell JW, Schootman M. A multivariate risk analysis of selected playing surfaces in the National Football League: 1980 to 1989. An epidemiologic study of knee injuries. *Am J Sports Med.* 1992;20(6):686–94.

22. Rovere GD, Haupt HA, Yates CS. Prophylactic knee bracing in college football. *Am J Sports Med.* 1987;15(2):111–6.

23. Sitler M, Ryan J, Hopkinson W, et al. The efficacy of a prophylactic knee brace to reduce knee injuries in football. A prospective, randomized study at West Point. *Am J Sports Med.* 1990;18(3):310–5.

24. Sitler M, Ryan J, Wheeler B, et al. The efficacy of a semirigid ankle stabilizer to reduce acute ankle injuries in basketball. A randomized clinical study at West Point. *Am J Sports Med.* 1994;22(4):454–61.

25. Steffen K, Andersen TE, Bahr R. Risk of injury on artificial turf and natural grass in young female football players. *Br J Sports Med.* 2007;41(Suppl 1):i33–7.

26. Surve I, Schwellnus MP, Noakes T, Lombard C. A fivefold reduction in the incidence of recurrent ankle sprains in soccer players using the Sport-Stirrup orthosis. *Am J Sports Med.* 1994;22(5):601–6.

27. Tegner Y, Lorentzon R. Evaluation of knee braces in Swedish ice hockey players. *Br J Sports Med.* 1991;25(3):159–61.

28. Wojtys EM, Huston LJ. "Custom fit" versus "off the shelf" ACL functional braces. *Am J Knee Surg.* 2001;14(3):157–62.

14 Field-Side Emergencies

Jeffery A. May, Loren A. Crown, and Michael C. Gaertner

INTRODUCTION

- Although most sports injuries are nonemergent and musculoskeletal in nature, there are certain life- and limb-threatening injuries that the field-side physician (FSP) must be prepared to handle immediately. The most important step in the management of on-field and field-side emergencies is preparation, and depending on the setting of the event and the level of competition, resources may be limited. The FSP must at a minimum have ready access to appropriate health care personnel to assist in an emergency, appropriate medical supplies and emergency equipment, immediate access to a telephone, and the ability to transport an athlete to a medical facility. It would also be advisable to be certified in basic life support (BLS) and have a working knowledge of advanced cardiac life support (ACLS), advanced trauma life support (ATLS), and the common and uncommon injuries specific to the event being covered.

GENERAL APPROACH TO THE FALLEN ATHLETE

- When approaching the collapsed athlete, the field-side evaluation should be both rapid and focused. The "primary survey" should follow the "ABCDE" approach taught by ATLS (7) and should occur where the athlete is found. The athlete should initially be left in that position unless the athlete is prone and unconscious or there is a problem performing the "ABCs" (3), in which case the athlete should be logrolled to a supine position.

- The logroll should ideally be a four-person technique in which the team leader is at the victim's head maintaining in-line immobilization of the head and neck, while the other three members of the team control the torso, hips, and legs. The athlete should be turned in the direction of the three assistants according to the count of the leader and then onto a spine board placed under the athlete.

- If an athlete is wearing an appropriately fitted helmet, neither the helmet nor its chin strap should be removed. Padding or sandbags should be placed around the helmet and the shoulders with the hips and legs immobilized. The face guard can easily be removed by prying or cutting it off for access to the airway. The helmet and shoulder pads should be considered a single unit — the removal of either one necessitates the removal of the other, as leaving only one of them in place forces the neck out of a neutral position (13). If the athlete is not wearing a helmet, a rigid cervical collar should be applied with in-line immobilization of the spine.

- After the primary survey is complete and the patient is stabilized, a more detailed secondary survey should be performed either on the field or on the sideline, depending on the status of the athlete and the environmental conditions.

- The factors to be considered while evaluating the fallen athlete include whether the injury was witnessed or traumatic. The age, general conditioning, and specific medical conditions of the athlete should be considered, as well as the general characteristics of the sport, such as the amount of contact (i.e., collision, limited contact, and noncontact), the degree of speed involved, and the duration of the event. Finally, the environmental conditions must be considered as both a potential causative and/or exacerbating factor in the injury.

- After the initial examination of the patient is completed, the FSP should identify any problem areas and categorize them as being of either an immediate or potential life-threatening/disabling nature and treat accordingly. Frequent reevaluation of the injured athlete is a must.

IMMEDIATE LIFE-THREATENING INJURIES

Respiratory Compromise

Upper Airway Obstruction

- Although rare in organized sports, respiratory arrest can result from upper airway obstruction (UAO). Signs include respiratory distress with little or no air movement, significant accessory muscle use, and stridorous, wheezing, or snoring breath sounds. If the athlete is unconscious, the airway should be opened with a jaw-thrust maneuver to keep the tongue from occluding the airway, and an oral or nasal airway should be inserted as necessary. In-line repositioning of the head and neck may be necessary to establish airway patency. The oropharynx should be inspected for foreign bodies, which should be removed if visualized; however, blind finger sweeps are not recommended in either children or adults. Significant facial or mandibular trauma with resultant loss of support of the tongue or with blood, secretions, and loose teeth in the pharynx can produce UAO, particularly in the unconscious athlete who has lost protective airway reflexes. Other causes of UAO, such as airway edema from anaphylaxis, inhalation burn injuries, or an expanding neck or retropharyngeal hematoma from neck trauma should be considered, with early intubation a priority. Surgical airway capability is a is a legitimate concern, and a cricothyrotomy kit might be prudent.

Laryngeal Fracture

■ This rare injury occurs after direct trauma to the anterior neck. Signs include stridor, hoarseness, subcutaneous emphysema, and perhaps bony crepitus and a palpable fracture. Although airway obstruction may not be immediate, it can rapidly progress to this stage because of resultant edema, and as with other causes of obstruction, early intubation is a priority; surgical airway capability is again a necessity.

Pneumothorax

■ A simple pneumothorax may be spontaneous (*i.e.*, rupture of a bleb) or traumatic, with spontaneous pneumothoraces occurring more often in sports that involve changes in intrathoracic pressure (*e.g.*, scuba diving and weightlifting) and traumatic pneumothoraces occurring secondary to rib fractures. Symptoms may include unilateral chest pain, dyspnea, and cough. Immediate treatment is rarely needed unless the patient is severely dyspneic or the pneumothorax is open or under tension. Those with a stable simple pneumothorax should be given oxygen and transported to a medical facility for further evaluation and management.

Open Pneumothorax

■ This is defined as a pneumothorax accompanied by an open wound to the chest (sucking chest wound). Treatment consists of placing an occlusive dressing over the open wound and taping it down on three sides to create a one-way valve that allows air to exit without reentering until a definitive thoracostomy tube can be placed.

Tension Pneumothorax

■ This occurs when a pneumothorax is accompanied by progressive accumulation of air in the pleural space with the resultant increase in intrathoracic pressure causing a shift of mediastinal structures away from the pneumothorax as well as a decrease in venous return and cardiac output. In addition to the previously listed symptoms, these athletes may have tracheal deviation away from the affected side with jugular venous distention and hypotension. This is a true medical emergency that requires immediate treatment by needle decompression of the chest with a large (14–16 gauge) needle or catheter inserted in the anterior chest wall in the second intercostal space at the midclavicular line, followed by placement of a thoracostomy tube.

Cardiac Arrest

■ Although devastating when it occurs in a young athlete, a cardiac sudden death is extremely rare, with incidence varying depending on the age of the athlete and the sporting event (17,23). The most common cause of sudden cardiac death in young athletes is congenital cardiovascular structural abnormalities, with hypertrophic cardiomyopathy leading the list, followed by coronary artery anomalies. The most common cause in middle-aged athletes is atherosclerotic heart disease causing acute ischemic events.

■ The field-side treatment of any cause of cardiac arrest should follow ACLS guidelines with attention to early cardiopulmonary resuscitation (CPR) and defibrillation as indicated. An equally important task for the FSP is to identify those athletes who have warning signs of cardiac disease and dysrhythmias, such as sudden unexplained syncope or collapse, exertional syncope, early fatigue, or anginal chest pain during or immediately following exertion, as well as a family history of early sudden cardiac demise. Strong consideration should be given to withholding these athletes from further competition until a thorough evaluation is performed (17,23).

■ Commotio cordis is a rare event caused by relatively low-energy chest trauma and results in a dysrhythmia very often unresponsive to treatment. With a huge proportion of cases being fatal, the most successful intervention has been immediate CPR and application of an automated external defibrillator (AED) to treat ventricular fibrillation, the predominant arrhythmia. Better protection from direct blows to the chest may be the best way to prevent this rare but often lethal injury.

Anaphylaxis

■ Anaphylactic reactions are acute systemic hypersensitivity reactions that can be idiopathic, exercise-induced, or allergen-induced, and although rare, they can progress very rapidly and prove fatal if unrecognized. Insect stings (especially Hymenoptera) may be a cause of sports-related anaphylaxis; inhalation of such insects is another possible cause in athletes.

■ The symptoms of anaphylaxis may include urticaria or angioedema, upper airway edema, dyspnea, wheezing, flushing of skin, dizziness, hypotension, syncope, gastrointestinal symptoms, rhinitis, and headache (2). Symptom onset is typically rapid (within 5–30 minutes of exposure), and in its most severe form, anaphylaxis can progress to severe bronchospasm, airway edema, and fatal cardiovascular collapse.

■ Treatment consists of prompt attention to the ABCs, followed by treatment with 100% oxygen, epinephrine (1:1,000) 0.3–0.5 mL in adults or 0.01 mg/kg in children (not to exceed 0.30 mg) given subcutaneously and repeated every 10–15 minutes as needed, intravenous (IV) fluids if hypotensive, β-agonists by nebulizer if bronchospasm is present, antihistamines (H$_1$ and H$_2$ blockers), and glucocorticoids if available. The athlete must be rapidly transported to a medical facility because continued observation will be required (15).

Severe Hemorrhage

- Hemorrhage in the athlete may be the result of lacerations, fractures, vascular disruptions, or visceral organ or muscle disruptions. It can manifest as either massive external bleeding or insidious and occult internal bleeding. Control of external bleeding should follow the basic principles of hemostasis, which include steady direct pressure over the bleeding site and over larger arteries proximal to the site of injury, as well as elevation of the affected body part. Blind clamping of bleeding vessels and tourniquet application (with the possible exception of a traumatic amputation) are not recommended.

- Scalp lacerations can cause significant hemorrhage and often go unnoticed if the athlete is lying on his back or is strapped to a spine board.

- Occult bleeding may produce delayed signs and symptoms, and what may at first appear to be an atraumatic incident may actually have been caused by recent unnoticed or unwitnessed trauma (3).

- Potential injuries that may be major sources of occult blood loss include hemorrhage into the thoracic and abdominal cavities, the soft tissues surrounding major long bone fractures, and the retroperitoneal space secondary to a pelvic fracture, and as a result of penetrating torso injury (7).

- Signs and symptoms of hypovolemic shock include altered sensorium; pale and cool extremities with a decreased capillary refill; weak, thready, and rapid pulses; hypotension; tachycardia; and tachypnea.

- Treatment should follow ATLS protocol, two large-bore peripheral IVs should be started and oxygen administered. Consideration should be given to starting crystalloid fluids, although there is some debate as to whether or not aggressive fluid resuscitation may actually be more detrimental to patients with certain types of injuries, and one should consider the concept of permissive hypotension when managing hypovolemic shock in the alert patient (11).

POTENTIAL LIFE-THREATENING/ DISABLING INJURIES: HEAD, NECK, AND SPINE

Head Injury

- Head injuries in sports are quite common and often provoke anxiety and uncertainty. The most common head injury in sports is a concussion, and 90% or more of concussions do not involve a loss of consciousness (LOC) (18,19). The FSP should know how to recognize concussions (which is not always easy) and manage the concussion on the sidelines

with a low threshold for transfer to an emergency facility if needed. A search for clues to more serious underlying injury should take place, and finally, a determination of if and when the athlete may return to play must occur (10). In most instances in nonprofessional sports, the player will be removed from play.

- When approaching the fallen athlete with a suspected head injury, the FSP should rapidly assess the ABCs and determine the level of consciousness as well as note any spontaneous movement and speech. Assessment for potential spine injury should be done, and once on the sidelines, a focused neurologic examination should be performed, including a more thorough sensory, motor, and cranial nerve examination as well as cognitive functioning and memory testing.

- Obvious signs of skull fracture or intracerebral bleeding, such as pupillary asymmetry, postauricular or periorbital ecchymosis, clear otorrhea, rhinorrhea, or hemotympanum, and any depression in the skull should be searched for (epidural hematoma is discussed in more detail later). It must be emphasized that even if the initial examination is completely normal, frequent reassessment is mandatory because victims of head injury may rapidly deteriorate, and many of the previously listed findings may be delayed.

- A concussion is generally agreed upon to be a trauma-induced alteration in mental status that may or may not involve loss of consciousness. Historically, the most commonly used systems assess severity based on the presence or absence of LOC and/or amnesia, as well as the duration of postconcussive symptoms; however, current guidelines refine decisions to a "yes" or "no" decision regarding concussion.

- Despite the multiple differences among the recognized guidelines, most authorities would agree with the following statements:
  - No athlete should return to play while any symptoms are still present either at rest or with exertion.
  - No athlete should return to play on the same day.
  - It must be emphasized that the safest maxim in the face of any uncertainty is "when in doubt, sit them out" (4).
  - Frequent reevaluation and serial examinations are *absolutely mandatory*.

Epidural Hematoma

- This most commonly results from a tear of the middle meningeal artery after high-velocity impact to the temporoparietal region and is associated with a skull fracture 80% of the time. Athletes will often experience a brief LOC followed by a lucid interval, which may last up to several hours, and then progress to rapid neurologic deterioration and eventually coma and brainstem herniation. Treatment is surgical, and immediate transfer to a medical facility is required.

Second Impact Syndrome

- This is defined as a second head injury occurring before the symptoms of a first head injury have resolved. A controversial topic, it is a catastrophic injury that may occur because of loss of cerebral autoregulation caused by the initial injury (8,12). When the second injury occurs, and it is often a very mild injury, cerebral edema may rapidly develop with subsequent brainstem herniation within a matter of seconds to minutes. Treatment consists of immediate intubation and hyperventilation, administration of an osmotic diuretic (*i.e.*, mannitol), and transport to a medical facility. Despite aggressive treatment, mortality and morbidity may range between 50% and 100%. Therefore, prevention may be the best management, which includes thoughtful consideration of return-to-play decisions (4,10).

Neck Injury

- Neck injuries, although relatively uncommon and usually self-limited (18), represent one of the most feared and potentially catastrophic injuries in sports. The FSP must promptly recognize the potential for spine injury, adhere strictly to spinal precautions (discussed previously in this chapter), and finally, determine whether an athlete requires immobilization and transfer to a medical facility, can return to play, or simply requires further sideline observation.

- Indications for spinal immobilization include posttraumatic LOC, subjective neck pain or bony tenderness on examination, significant neck/upper back trauma, significant head injury, mental status changes, peripheral neurologic abnormalities, or significant mechanism of injury (18,21).

- Usually minor, "burners" or "stingers" are nerve injuries resulting from trauma to the neck and/or shoulder that cause either a compressive or a traction injury to the fifth or sixth cervical nerve roots or the brachial plexus itself (13,18). The syndrome consists of immediate onset of burning pain radiating down the arm, is usually unilateral in distribution, and is often associated with other symptoms such as numbness, paresthesias, and muscle weakness or paresis. It is typically self-limiting, with most cases resolving in a matter of minutes, although some symptoms may persist for weeks to months.

- A "burner" should *not* be considered as an initial diagnosis if an athlete has any of the following:
  - Bilateral upper extremity involvement
  - Any lower extremity involvement
  - Neck pain or tenderness

- Although there are no definitive guidelines as to which athletes with neck injuries are safe to return to play, it is generally agreed on that only those players with no neck pain or neurologic symptoms and with completely normal examinations may return to play safely, with repeated evaluation being necessary (13,18,21).

Ophthalmologic (Globe) Injury

- Any injury to the eye warrants an immediate ocular examination, as seemingly minor injuries can be potentially vision threatening. Examination of the eyes should include an assessment of visual acuity, visual fields, the eyelids and periorbital bony structures, the surface of the globe (conjunctiva, sclera, cornea), the pupils (size, shape, reactivity), and extraocular movements, and funduscopic examination (9).

Eyelid Lacerations

- Any lacerations involving the lid margin or lacrimal system or those with significant tissue loss should be repaired by an ophthalmologist or plastic surgeon.

Corneal Abrasion

- An abrasion presents with pain, photophobia, tearing, and a foreign body sensation. Diagnosis is by fluorescein examination, and potential treatment consists of topical antibiotics, analgesia, and tetanus prophylaxis. The athletes may return to play if appropriate.

Corneal Foreign Body

- The presentation is similar to corneal abrasion, and corneal perforation must be ruled out if there is a history of high-velocity objects involved. Removal can be accomplished with a cotton tip applicator, eye spud, or 20- to 22-gauge needle under magnification and topical anesthesia.

Corneal Laceration

- Many of these are self-sealing and difficult to visualize, thereby requiring a high index of suspicion. Examination may show a teardrop pupil, hyphema, or flat anterior chamber. The eye should be covered with a hard shield and the athlete told not to move the eye. Intraocular pressures should *not* be measured, and immediate ophthalmology consult is required.

Hyphema

- A hyphema is blood within the anterior chamber, usually due to trauma, although atraumatic hyphemas may occur in the presence of coagulopathies. Presenting symptoms include decreased vision, pain, and a history of trauma. The size of the hyphema should be noted, the eye shielded, and immediate ophthalmology consult or emergency department evaluation obtained.

Subconjunctival Hemorrhage

- Although startling in appearance, subconjunctival hemorrhage is usually harmless and may be ignored unless accompanied by a significant mechanism of injury and/or medical history of bleeding disorders.

Intraocular Foreign Body

- Many sports involve objects that are propelled, thrown, or swung or are subject to fragmentation, possibly leading to an intraocular foreign body.

- Presenting symptoms include pain, irritation, and injection, and suspicion should be based on a history of any high-velocity projectile or metal striking metal. Fluorescein staining may reveal a positive Seidel sign (a washing away and streaking of fluorescein as aqueous humor leaks out of the globe). The eye should be shielded, intraocular pressure measurements avoided, and ophthalmology consultation obtained.

Globe Rupture

- This usually occurs from direct blunt trauma to the eye because of a sudden increase in intraocular pressure. Examination may reveal a total subconjunctival hemorrhage, enophthalmos, a teardrop pupil, or a flat anterior chamber. Treatment is the same as that of an intraocular foreign body or corneal laceration.

Retrobulbar Hemorrhage

- Retrobulbar hemorrhage usually occurs after trauma and presents with acute proptosis, pain, swelling, and limitation of extraocular muscle (EOM) movement. This is essentially an "orbital compartment syndrome." Irreversible vision loss can occur within 1 hour. Therefore, although only necessary in remote environments where perhaps logistics preclude rapid ophthalmologic or plastic surgery consultation, lateral orbital canthotomy may be necessitated; an excellent description of the technique is provided by Liu and Hackett (16).

Orbital Rim Fracture

- Blunt trauma may result in periorbital bony tenderness, crepitus, or paresthesias in the distribution of the infraorbital nerve, as well as limitation of EOM movement if there is entrapment. Athletes should be sent for radiographic evaluation, with treatment depending on the extent of injury.

Nasal Injury

- The field-side care of problematic nasal injuries generally involves identification of nasal fractures, control of epistaxis, or treatment of septal hematomas.

- Isolated nasal fractures are usually not corrected acutely unless associated with significant deformity or other soft tissue injury. Treatment includes ice, analgesics, nasal decongestants, and avoidance of further injury.

- Given that the vast majority of nosebleeds seen by the FSP are anterior in origin, most can be controlled with either direct pressure and, if necessary, cauterization of an identified bleeding site or packing with a nasal tampon.

- A potential complication of nasal injuries that must be carefully looked for is a septal hematoma, which is a red-blue, bulging mass on the nasal septum. These should be drained promptly by incision or aspiration followed by packing to prevent reaccumulation, because avascular necrosis and/or an abscess of the nasal septum may develop within a few days if left untreated. This procedure may be delayed if adequate equipment is unavailable field-side.

Ear Injury

- An auricular hematoma is a subperichondrial accumulation of blood following blunt trauma. If large enough and left untreated, it can cause avascular necrosis as well as asymmetrical regrowth of new cartilage with a resultant cosmetic deformity of the ear known as a *cauliflower ear*. Treatment involves drainage of the hematoma followed by a pressure dressing to prevent reaccumulation. This too is a nonemergent condition and may be referred.

- Tympanic membrane perforation, although not an acute emergency, must be recognized so that proper follow-up care is obtained to ensure proper healing and avoidance of hearing loss. Most will be caused by either blunt or noise-induced trauma, and greater than 90% will heal spontaneously. Antibiotics (either systemic or topical) are typically not necessary for uncomplicated perforations. Those that are caused by penetrating trauma should be promptly referred to an otolaryngologist (6).

Abdominal/Pelvic Injury

- Although potentially serious and even life threatening, most abdominal injuries can be managed nonoperatively with close observation. These injuries generally result from rapid deceleration, direct blunt trauma to the abdomen, or indirect trauma from a displaced lower rib fracture.

- Injuries to the abdominal wall include simple contusions and rectus sheath hematomas, both of which are benign and usually managed conservatively, although the latter can occasionally require surgical intervention. The importance of these injuries to the FSP lies in excluding associated intra-abdominal injuries, with mechanism of injury being perhaps the most important clue because a single field-side abdominal examination, even if benign, is often misleading and inadequate in excluding significant intra-abdominal injury.

- Exercise-related transient abdominal pain (ETAP) or "stitch" is an intense stabbing subcostal pain usually occurring early in the conditioning of the athlete and goes away as the athlete gets in shape. It may be due to diaphragmatic ischemia and is benign (1).

Splenic/Hepatic Injury

- The spleen and liver comprise two common organs injured in blunt abdominal trauma. There may be left or right upper quadrant and/or shoulder pain (Kehr sign), respectively, as well as signs of hypotension if bleeding is significant. All athletes with significant pain and/or appropriate mechanism of injury may require urgent ultrasound, computed tomography (CT) imaging, and/or observation.

Genitourinary Injury

- Injuries to the genitourinary system seldom require immediate intervention, and suspicion should be based on the mechanism of injury as well as the presence and degree of hematuria. One must keep in mind that injury to the kidney may be present without hematuria and that hematuria does not always signify significant renal injury. In terms of evaluating hematuria, usually only those athletes with gross hematuria accompanied by hypotension or associated nonrenal injuries require urgent radiographic evaluation of the genitourinary system.

- Gross blood may occur at the urethral meatus as a result of blunt trauma to the scrotal region. Displacement of the testicle into the perineum or inguinal canal may indicate rupture of the testicular capsule and require surgical intervention. Examination is often difficult because of pain and swelling; however, severe scrotal or testicular swelling or a nonpalpable testicle warrants further evaluation. In the absence of direct trauma, testicular torsion must be ruled out in the athlete presenting with acute onset of testicular pain. In either case, removal from the field of play and transfer to an emergency department for color flow Doppler ultrasound studies may define the nature or extent of the problem.

Musculoskeletal Injury

- Musculoskeletal injuries are the most commonly encountered injuries in sports. Most are minor and self-limited, and it is certainly beyond the scope of this chapter to discuss various specific fractures; however, a few general statements about fracture care can be made, and a handful of limb-threatening injuries can be discussed.

- In terms of fracture care, the FSP should ascertain the mechanism of injury and never assume that the obvious deformity is the only injury. Always check the neurovascular status of the affected body part distal to the fracture site. If there is vascular compromise, reduction of dislocations and/or fractures should be attempted in the field with gentle traction. Otherwise, fractures should be splinted in the position in which they are found, unless some degree of reduction is required because of neurovascular compromise. Finally, no athlete should return to play if there is a question of a fracture, no matter how minor the injury may seem, because this may transform a nondisplaced or a closed fracture into a displaced or open one.

- The following injuries represent a potential threat to a limb.

Open Fracture

- Previously known as a compound fracture, this is a fracture associated with overlying soft tissue injury with communication between the fracture site and the skin. These are at high risk for subsequent infection and osteomyelitis and require washout in the operating room. On the field, the open wound should be covered with moist sterile gauze and the extremity splinted with no attempts made to push extruding bone or soft tissue back into the wound or to reduce the fracture, unless neurovascular compromise is present.

Traumatic Amputations

- This is a very rare and dramatic injury that is easy to recognize. The proximal stump should be irrigated with a sterile solution and a sterile pressure dressing applied, with a tourniquet used only for severe, uncontrolled bleeding. The amputated portion should be irrigated, wrapped in a sterile fashion, placed in a bag, and put on ice with rapid transport to an appropriate medical facility.

Compartment Syndrome

- This is a state of increased pressure within a closed tissue compartment that compromises blood flow through nutrient capillaries supplying muscles and nerves within that compartment. The potential causes of compartment syndrome are numerous, although in terms of athletes, this is typically an injury with the most common site being the anterior compartment of the leg. Presentation typically occurs within a few hours after injury and will consist of severe and constant pain over the involved compartment and an increase in pain with both active contraction and passive stretching of the involved muscles. There may also be significant dysesthesias as well as an absent or diminished pulse, pallor, and/or paralysis of the affected neuromuscular group, although these are considered to be late findings that indicate that significant myoneural ischemia has already occurred. Treatment is an emergent fasciotomy and requires rapid transport of the athlete to a medical facility.

Knee Dislocation

- Extremely rare and usually associated with a high-velocity/high-energy mechanism of injury, this is a very serious injury that may require a high index of suspicion because many dislocations will have spontaneously reduced prior to evaluation. The knee will typically be very swollen and painful and will often demonstrate severe instability in multiple directions on examination. The seriousness of the injury lies in the high rate of associated complications, specifically popliteal artery injury and peroneal nerve injury (which may occur despite spontaneous reduction and normal pulses). Early reduction of a visible dislocation is important. Rapid transport of the patient with a known or suspected dislocation to a medical facility for orthopedic and/or vascular consultation is essential.

Hip Dislocation

- Like the knee, this dislocation is rare in sports and usually involves a high-velocity/high-energy mechanism of injury. Posterior dislocations are by far the most common type, and the seriousness of this injury lies in the risk for avascular necrosis (AVN) of the femoral head as circulation is disrupted. This occurs in a matter of hours, with 6 hours being the danger zone because approximately 60% of reductions beyond 6 hours develop AVN, whereas only 5% of reductions occurring within this time frame develop this complication (22).

Other Dislocations: Digits, Elbows, Shoulders, and Patellas

- Many FSPs are familiar with these entities and are quite capable of early reduction. However, there will be the occasional unreducible event that necessitates prompt referral. All dislocations need splinting, comfort care, and follow-up to ensure successful outcome.

Environmental Injury

Hypothermia

■ Defined as core body temperature < 95°F (< 35°C), this usually occurs as a result of prolonged exposure to cold environmental conditions. When approaching the hypothermic athlete, the FSP must keep the following points in mind.

   ■ Treatment should routinely start with passive external rewarming (*i.e.*, moving the athlete from a cold to a warm environment, removing all wet clothing, and covering with dry blankets). Active external rewarming and core rewarming should usually be deferred until the hospital environment because patients with moderate to severe hypothermia are at high risk of having significant electrolyte, acid-base, and cardiovascular changes associated with rewarming.

   ■ Significantly hypothermic patients are at very high risk of fatal cardiac arrhythmias.

   ■ Assessment for pulse/breathing may take a little longer than usual due to the difficulty of palpation in cold tissue as well as the bradycardia, but if none is detected in 30–60 seconds, CPR will be required. And if started, CPR should continue until the patient's temperature reaches 92°F (32°C); the phrase "they are not dead until they are warm and dead" still applies (14).

Hyperthermia

■ Heat-related illnesses are a spectrum of diseases ranging from heat cramps and edema to heat stroke and death. Dehydration may potentiate these processes but is not necessary as a causative factor. Heat stroke is a true medical emergency, with high mortality rates if unrecognized (5). It typically presents in warm, humid conditions with elements of overexertion on the part of the athlete, but has been documented in temperatures < 60°F. A temperature > 105°F (> 40.5°C) and prominent central nervous system (CNS) changes make the diagnosis in the field. Other signs include tachycardia autoregulatory changes and decompensation in the intrinsic ability of the vasculature to maintain blood pressure to end organs within a homeostatic range despite changes in perfusion pressure. Although end-organ perfusion failure only presents later on laboratory studies, blood pressure may be most indicative of changes in autoregulation when interpreted in the clinical setting of an insult to thermoregulation. The FSP must keep the following in mind when approaching the hyperthermic athlete.

   ■ Active and passive cooling measures (*e.g.*, removing from the heat, disrobing, placement of ice packs around the groin, neck, and axillae) should be instituted immediately with the goal being to lower the core temperature to < 102°F (< 39°C) as quickly as possible using immersion in a tub of ice water or rapidly rotating ice water–soaked towels around the entire body. A novel method of water ice therapy has been found safe and effective and is available for field-side use. Patients are placed on a stretcher

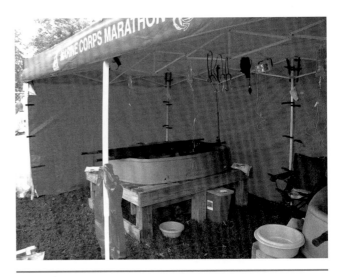

Figure 14.1: Heat deck used at Marine Corps Marathon for management of exertional heat stroke.

proximal to a cold water tub of about 50°F (10°C) and doused but not immersed, while being massaged with ice bags (20). (See Fig. 14.1.)

   ■ Oral fluid replacement is sufficient in most circumstances; however, IV fluids may be started if hypovolemia remains a problem. Caution must be exercised because overaggressive rehydration may put the victim at an increased risk of pulmonary edema and adult respiratory distress syndrome (ARDS). Victims who remain symptomatic despite simple measures of treatment should be transported to a medical facility for further care.

Lightning Injury

■ Although rare, lightning injury is one of the more frequent injuries by a natural phenomenon, with the largest number of injuries occurring in golf and water sports. Most injuries occur during the months of June through September. Although it is by definition an *electrical injury*, it differs significantly from high-voltage electrical injuries in the pattern and severity of injuries as well as the immediate treatment. While the voltage of lightning is extraordinarily high, it is usually an instantaneous contact that tends to flash over the outside of a victim's body, often creating superficial burns, but sparing extensive damage to internal organs and structures. Lightning may injure a person by striking either the person directly or something they are holding, or by splashing over from a nearby person or object that has been struck. It may also strike the ground and spread circumferentially, often creating multiple victims. Although it can potentially affect any organ system, injuries to the cardiovascular and neurologic systems tend to be the most serious, primarily due to asystole, with the immediate cause of death most commonly being cardiopulmonary arrest. Minor injuries include dysesthesias, minor burns, temporary LOC, confusion, amnesia, tympanic membrane perforation, and ocular injury. Long-term sequelae include peripheral neuropathies and mental impairment (24). The FSP should keep the following points in mind when approaching a victim of lightning injury:

- In lightning victims with cardiopulmonary arrest, cardiac automaticity and contractions will often resume spontaneously in a short period of time, whereas respiratory arrest from paralysis of the medullary respiratory center may be prolonged. Therefore, unless the victim is ventilated quickly, the victim will progress to a secondary hypoxic cardiac arrest despite normal cardiac activity. If promptly resuscitated and supported, full recovery may ensue.

  - Therefore, in a multicasualty situation from a lightning strike, the FSP should always resuscitate "the dead" first, a reversal of the standard rule of triage where the obvious moribund are left to the last.

- Standard ACLS protocols should be followed.

- Victims do not "retain charge" and are not dangerous to touch, so CPR should not be delayed for this reason.

- Contrary to popular belief, lightning can and often does strike the same place twice, so personal safety must be taken into consideration.

- Hypotension in a lightning victim should prompt a search for occult hemorrhage or fractures as a result of blunt trauma; spinal precautions are required.

- Pupils may become "fixed and dilated" because of the nature of lightning injuries, and this should not preclude resuscitation attempts as these changes do not necessarily indicate brain death in lightning victims.

- In lightning victims with cardiopulmonary arrest, cardiac automaticity and contractions will often resume spontaneously in a short period of time, whereas respiratory arrest from paralysis of the medullary respiratory center may be prolonged. Therefore, unless the victim is ventilated quickly, the victim will progress to a secondary hypoxic cardiac arrest despite normal cardiac activity. If promptly resuscitated and supported, full recovery may ensue.

- Long bone fractures, vertebral injuries, and dislocations may be found.

SUMMARY

- In conclusion, although most sports-related injuries are minor, for the few urgent/emergent events the FSP will encounter, planning is paramount. Medical equipment appropriate for the event and knowledge of life support techniques are essential. A study of the topics presented here should be helpful in preparing for field-side emergencies.

REFERENCES

1. Atkins JM, Taylor JC, Kane SE. Acute and overuse injuries of the abdomen and groin in athletes. *Curr Sports Med Rep.* 2010;9(2):115–20.

2. Barclay L, Vega C. New pediatric guidelines for self-injecting epinephrine for anaphylaxis treatment. *Medscape Medical News* [Internet]. 2007 [cited 2007 March 27]. Available from: http://www.medscape.org/viewarticle/554150.

3. Blue JG, Pecci MA. The collapsed athlete. *Orthop Clin North Am.* 2002;33(3):471–8.

4. Cantu R. When to disqualify an athlete after a concussion. *Curr Sports Med Rep.* 2009;8(1):6–7.

5. Centers for Disease Control and Prevention: Non-fatal sports and recreation heat illness treated in hospital emergency departments–United States, 2001–2009. *Morb Mortal Wkly Rep.* 2011;60(29):977–80.

6. Chao MT, Paletta C, Garza JR, et al. Facial trauma, sports-related injuries. *Medscape* [Internet]. 2010 [cited 2010 Sept 10]. Available from: http://emedicine.medscape.com/article/1284288-overview.

7. Committee on Trauma. *Advanced Trauma Life Support for Doctors: Student Course Manual.* 8th ed. Washington (DC): American College of Surgeons; 2008. 444 p.

8. Crump WJ. Managing adolescent sports head injuries: a case-based report. *Fam Prac Recert.* 2001;23(4):27–32.

9. Cuculino GP, DiMarco CJ. Common ophthalmologic emergencies: a systematic approach to evaluation and management. *Em Med Rep.* 2002;23(13):163–78.

10. Davis GA. Concussion in sport. *J Clin Neurosci.* 2009;16(6):731–2.

11. Fowler R, Pepe PE. Prehospital care of the patient with major trauma. *Emerg Med Clin North Am.* 2002;20(4):953–74.

12. Graber MA. Minor head trauma in children and athletes. *Emerg Med.* 2001;14,17,18,20.

13. Haight RR, Shiple BJ. Sideline evaluation of neck pain: when is it time for transport? *Phys Sportsmed.* 2001;29(3):45–62.

14. Hypothermia. 2005 American Heart Association guidelines for cardiopulmonary resuscitation and emergency cardiovascular care. *Circulation* [Internet]. 2005 [cited 2005 Dec 13];112(24, Suppl):IV-136–8. Available from: http://circ.ahajournals.org/content/112/24_suppl/IV-136.full.

15. Lieberman P, Nicklas RA, Oppenheimer J, et al. The diagnosis and management of anaphylaxis practice parameter: 2010 update. *J Allergy Clin Immunol.* 2010;126(3):477–80.

16. Liu LG, Hackett TS. Lateral orbital canthotomy. *Medscape* [Internet]. 2010 [cited 2010 May 19]. Available from: http://emedicine.medscape.com/article/82812-overview.

17. Maron BJ, Doerer JJ, Haas TS, et al. Sudden deaths in young competitive athletes: analysis of 1866 deaths in the United States, 1980–2006. *Circulation.* 2009;119(8):1085–92.

18. McAlindon RJ. On field evaluation and management of head and neck injured athletes. *Clin Sports Med.* 2002;21(1):1–14.

19. McCrory P, Meeuwisse W, Johnston K, et al. Consensus statement on concussion in sport—the 3rd International Conference in Sport, held in Zurich, November 2008. *J Clin Neurosci.* 2009;16(6):755–63.

20. McDermott BP, Casa DJ, O'Connor FG, et al. Cold-water dousing with ice massage to treat exertional heat stroke: a case series. *Aviat Space Environ Med.* 2009;80(8):720–2.

21. Sanchez AR 2nd, Sugalski MT, LaPrade RF. Field-side and pre-hospital management of the spine injured athlete. *Curr Sports Med Rep.* 2005;4(1):50–5.

22. Scopp JM, Moorman CT 3rd. Acute athletic trauma to the hip and pelvis. *Orthop Clin North Am.* 2002;33(3):555–63.

23. Thomas M, Haas TS, Doerer JJ, et al. Epidemiology of sudden death in young, competitive athletes due to blunt trauma. *Pediatrics* [Internet]. 2011 [cited 2011 July 1];128(1):e1–8. Available from: http://pediatrics.aappublications.org/content/128/1/e1.full. doi:10.1542/peds.2010-2743.

24. Whitcomb D, Martinez JA, Daberkow D. Lightning injuries. *South Med J.* 2002;95(11):1331–4.

15 Mass Participation Events

Scott W. Pyne

GOALS

- Mass participation events are those sporting events in which many people participate and are generally spread out over several miles and variable terrain.
- Advanced planning and preparation are critical to successfully accommodate the medical needs of the event participants.
- The medical director has numerous responsibilities of planner, communicator, and organizer in addition to the care of injured athletes.

Medical Coverage

- The needs of the athletes competing must be considered prior to the event.
- Specific considerations of the type of event, number of participants, course peculiarities, and environmental predictions are all very important in determining the medical coverage required.
- The formation and implementation of an emergency action plan have proven successful in numerous situations (5).

Safe Environment

- As a key advisor to the event director, the medical director must ensure that the event is conducted with the safety of the competitors being of utmost importance. Often, this is furthest from the minds of race organizers especially with competing priorities of sponsor, financial, and community concerns.
- In extreme conditions, the race may need to be cancelled or rescheduled (17). It is best that these possibilities and contingency plans be discussed and prepared prior to the race day.
- It is often necessary to review the course for any potential trouble spots and hazards that could cause injury. The start and finish are common sites of medical concern. The start area should be on a large level surface devoid of obstacles, thereby allowing the athletes to more easily accommodate the surge that invariably occurs. The finish area should also be large enough to prevent the athletes from bunching up and being forced to stand in one place. It should also have necessary facilities and resources to allow the athletes to properly cool down and recover after the event and easily access medical treatment areas as required.

- Biking, swimming, and skiing events carry additional risk elements (8,15,22), such as water safety and trauma potential associated with high speeds. Water temperature; sea conditions; road conditions; transition, acceleration, and deceleration zones; and protective equipment must be carefully scrutinized.

EPIDEMIOLOGY

Injury Rate

- Running (42 km), 1%–20%; running (< 21 km), 1%–5%; triathlon (225 km), 15%–30%; Nordic skiing (55 km), 5%; triathlon (51 km), 2%–5%; cycling (variable), 5% (20).
- Injury rate increases with increased distance and environmental temperature (9,10).

Predicting Injury Rate

- Previous years' experience is very helpful in planning for subsequent years. This also stresses the importance of a reliable injury data tracking system.
- Similar events in similar elements can be used in the initial planning and preparation stages.
- Fortunately, the risk for exertional death in marathons is quite small (13).

MEDICAL PHILOSOPHY

Level of Care

- The level of medical care that will be available on the course must be defined and agreed on between the medical director and the event director early in the planning stage.
- This may differ among the aid stations throughout the course with the most robust resources usually being provided at the finish area.
- It is essential to provide on-site basic first aid and cardiopulmonary resuscitation (CPR). It is desirable to provide on-site early defibrillation, advanced cardiac life support (ACLS), and advanced trauma life support (ATLS).

- The usage and type of intravenous fluids and availability of oxygen, medications, and advanced cardiac and trauma life support equipment are all areas requiring discussion.
- Coordination with the local emergency medical system (EMS) and emergency rooms and hospitals is absolutely required.
- Mobile medical assets in the form of bike or canoe/kayak teams or EMS units provide an excellent means to access injured competitors throughout the course (12,14).

Medication Plan

- A decision must be made as to the provision of medication on the race course and in the medical aid stations. It is recommended that these medications be tightly controlled and kept to a minimum if dispensed at all.
- In longer events, it is not uncommon for athletes to carry and take their own medication during the competition. This must be anticipated to best treat the competitor and prevent overprescribing.
- The availability of urgent or emergency medication, such as aspirin, epinephrine autoinjector, albuterol metered-dose inhaler, glucose, and ACLS medications, should be considered.

Laboratory Plan

- Medical aid stations may or may not have basic laboratory capability. The ability to assess an athletes' blood glucose and sodium levels will assist with their rapid evaluation and allow for the appropriate treatment of a collapsed athlete (6,11).
- Hand-held glucose and electrolyte monitors are readily available and have become part of the standard medical kit for many endurance events (21).

Communication Plan

- It is vital that medical support assets have the ability to communicate with each other, EMS assets, local hospitals, and the event director before, during, and after the competition.
- Various communication networks have been used to include cellular phones, computer networks, ham radio, and hand-held radios. These systems should be tested well before the event, and a backup plan should be established in the case of failure of the primary means of communication.
- A communication plan outlining how EMS will be requested and dispatched, where injured athletes will be taken, and when to contact the medical director will increase the efficiency of the medical care provided.

MEDICAL CHAIN OF COMMAND

- An individual must be identified to serve as the medical director. His or her responsibilities include advanced planning, event day medical decision making, and medical troubleshooting. The medical support staff, event director, and media all benefit from having one identified contact, rather than a committee, to answer all medical issues.
- It is also recommended that each aid station have an assigned medical leader well versed in the event medical philosophy. This medical leader can organize the support staff and coordinate medical care provided locally.

MEDICAL TRAINING

Medical Staff

- It is common that the medical support for mass participation events is gathered from diverse backgrounds and experience levels. Most are better versed in medical care within a clinical or hospital facility than in the field environment.
- The medical plan, chain of command, and level of care provided must be reviewed with the medical staff. It is helpful although not always practical to provide a didactic session prior to race day.
- Triage and treatment guidelines specific for the event provided in writing are useful, as well as administration information to include the course map; parking; proximity to water, food, and facility stations; communication; and transportation plans (16).

Competitors

- Preevent and on-site education may reduce injury risk and improve event safety (2). This is most easily provided with the race information and can be coordinated through the event director. Additions to event Web sites, handouts to accompany the race packet pick-up, and information posters displayed in common areas are several examples.
- Common medical conditions and their prevention, location of medical aid stations on the course, and available services at these areas assist the participants in their planning and preparation for a safe event.
- Medical presentations to the athletes and interest groups are often well received.
- Race-day information regarding weather conditions and health warnings has been used with success at numerous events (4).

STAFFING

Medical and Nonmedical Support

- The appropriate staffing of medical treatment areas with both medical and nonmedical staff is important in the safe conduct of the medical aid station. The composition and number of this staff will vary depending on the location and nature of the event.

- The number of staff can be best derived from previous experience or through comparison with similar events in similar conditions. A helpful guide from the American College of Sports Medicine® (3) is to provide the following medical personnel per 1,000 runners: 1 or 2 physicians, 4–6 podiatrists, 1–4 emergency medical technicians, 2–4 nurses, 3–6 physical therapists, 3–6 athletic trainers, and 1–3 assistants. Approximately 75% of these personnel should be stationed at the finish area.
- Nonmedical staff can assist with the transport of injured athletes, documentation, and medical tracking, and provide information within the medical aid station and to event staff.

Staff Feedback

- After the event, it is most important to elicit feedback from both medical and nonmedical staff. This often identifies areas that had not been considered in the initial planning and execution phases of the event.
- The follow-up of these comments in a written after-action report is highly recommended because it allows the documentation of areas of concern, develops solutions, and prepares for subsequent events.

TRIAGE AND TREATMENT GUIDELINES

- The majority of the medical conditions presenting at a given event can be predicted well in advance. Preparing, training, and practicing for these conditions are important in the evaluation, treatment, and disposition of injured participants.

Severe Versus Nonsevere

- The initial evaluation of an athlete in the medical aid station should focus on the severity of their injury (10). Fortunately, most complaints are nonsevere in nature and can be quickly treated and released.
- Severe medical conditions include cardiac events, hypothermia, hyperthermia, hyponatremia, near-drowning, and head and neck trauma. These can be quickly differentiated from nonsevere conditions by the evaluation of mental status, rectal temperature (19), blood pressure, and pulse. Serum glucose and sodium levels may also aid in the diagnosis.
- Depending on the medical care plan of the event, some of these severe conditions may be treated at the medical aid station or transported via EMS to the most appropriate medical treatment facility.

Medical Versus Musculoskeletal

- Medical conditions, such as exercise-associated collapse, heat stroke, chest pain, and hyponatremia, can be triaged from muscle cramps, blisters, and extremity pain in the treatment areas.
- This separation of care allows the assignment and preparation of support staff in the area of care for which they are most experienced. This also allows those with more severe conditions to be treated in the same area where they can be more closely monitored.
- The establishment of a medical holding area has proven successful (16). This area is reserved for athletes who are waiting for transportation for nonsevere conditions or who are not prepared to leave the medical area, but do not require further care. This group is continuously observed and encouraged to make their way back to the after-event areas.

Evaluation of Exercise-Associated Collapse

- The majority of cases of exercise-associated collapse are the result of predictable physiologic events associated with exertion and respond rapidly to positioning with the head down and legs and pelvis in an elevated position (10). These athletes generally have normal mental status.
- Individuals with altered mental status should be rapidly evaluated with a rectal temperature for hyperthermia or hypothermia (1). Persistent altered mental status with relatively normal rectal temperatures should be treated as suspected hyponatremia until proven otherwise (10).
- Hyperthermic individuals should be rapidly cooled on-site, preferably with ice water immersion (10,15).

FINANCE AND LOGISTICS

Financial Planning

- The conduct of mass participation events both requires and has the potential to generate money. Medical directors must ensure that the safety of the participants and the support staff is not compromised by decisions to increase revenue for the event. The medical director must be involved in any plans affecting the event that may have medical implications.
- Planning for the costs of medical supplies, transportation, and personnel compensation must be made and agreed on early in the event-planning process.

Medical Aid Station Location

- The spacing of medical aid stations throughout the course is determined by many variables. The course must be previewed and the location of medical aid stations established based on anticipated need, appropriate location, and course-specific considerations (4).
- Medical aid stations must be easily identifiable to competitors and EMS units.
- Medical evacuation routes must be established to avoid conflict with the event in progress and ensure the most efficient transport requirements.
- Adequate (unlimited) fluid must be available at all aid stations and at the finish. Runners should also be educated regarding the risk of hyponatremia associated with overhydration.

Transportation Plan

- It is not unusual for participants to decide that a medical treatment area is a good place to end their participation in the event. If this decision is realized in the middle of the course, a plan for the removal of these athletes must be used.

- Many races have a "sweep" vehicle that follows the last competitor and can transport these participants to the finish area. Other transport arrangements may be available depending on the nature of the event but must be anticipated prior to the event.

MEDICAL-LEGAL

- An additional responsibility of the medical director is the assurance of medical staff liability coverage (18).

- General event insurance packages usually exclude medical coverage (7).

- Options for medical liability coverage should be discussed with legal representation in advance of the event and include individual or group policies and Good Samaritan laws.

CONCLUDING COMMONSENSE PRINCIPLES

- Medical planning and preparation are absolute requirements for the successful conduct of mass participation events.

- Following established medical plans and treatment guidelines and remembering limitations with a focus on competitor and staff safety invariably result in a fulfilling experience for everyone involved.

REFERENCES

1. American College of Sports Medicine. Exertional heat illness during training and competition: a position stand. *Med Sci Sports Exerc.* 2007; 39(3):556–72.

2. American College of Sports Medicine. Mass participation event management for the team physician: a consensus statement. *Med Sci Sports Exerc.* 2004;36(11):2004–8.

3. Armstrong LE, Epstein Y, Greenleaf JE, et al. American College of Sports Medicine position stand. Heat and cold illnesses during distance running. *Med Sci Sports Exerc.* 1996;28(12):i–x.

4. Cianca JC, Roberts WO, Horn D. Distance running: organization of the medical team. In: O'Connor FG, Wilder RP, editors. *Textbook of Running Medicine.* New York: McGraw-Hill; 2001. p. 489–503.

5. Courson R. Preventing sudden death on the athletic field: the emergency action plan. *Curr Sports Med Rep.* 2007;6(2):93–100.

6. Davis DP, Videen JS, Marino A, et al. Exercise associated hyponatremia in marathon runners: a two-year experience. *J Emerg Med.* 2001; 21(1):47–57.

7. Dooley JW. Professional liability coverage (medical malpractice). *Road Race Manage.* 1999;Oct 3.

8. Greenland K. Medical support for adventure racing. *Emerg Med Australas.* 2004;16(5–6):465–8.

9. Hiller WD, O'Toole ML, Fortess EE, Laird RH, Imbert PC, Sisk TD. Medical and physiologic considerations in triathlons. *Am J Sports Med.* 1987;15(2):164–7.

10. Holtzhausen LM, Noakes TD. Collapsed ultraendurance athlete: proposed mechanisms and an approach to management. *Clin J Sport Med.* 1997;7(4):292–301.

11. Jaworski CA. Medical concerns of marathons. *Curr Sports Med Rep.* 2005;4(3):137–43.

12. Laird RH. Medical care at ultraendurance triathlons. *Med Sci Sports Exerc.* 1989;21(5 Suppl):S222–5.

13. Maron BJ, Poliac LC, Roberts WO. Risk for sudden cardiac death associated with marathon running. *J Am Coll Cardiol.* 1996;28(2):428–31.

14. Martinez JM. Medical coverage of cycling events. *Curr Sports Med Rep.* 2006;5(3):125–30.

15. Mayers LB, Noakes TD. A guideline to treating ironman triathletes at the finish line. *Phys Sportsmed.* 2000;28(8):33–50.

16. O'Connor FG, Pyne SW, Brennan FH, Adirim TA. Exercise-associated collapse: an algorithmic approach to race day management part I of II. *Am J Med Sports.* 2003;5:221–7, 229.

17. Roberts WO. Determining a "do not start" temperature for a marathon on the basis of adverse outcomes. *Med Sci Sports Exerc.* 2010;42(2): 226–32.

18. Roberts WO. Administration and medical management of mass participation endurance events. In: Mellion MB, Walsh WM, Madden C, Putukian M, Shelton GL, editors. *Team Physician's Handbook.* Philadelphia: Hanley & Belfus; 2002. p. 748–56.

19. Roberts WO. Assessing core temperature in collapsed athletes: what's the best method? *Phys Sportsmed.* 2000;28(9):71–6.

20. Roberts WO. Exercise-associated collapse in endurance events. A classification system. *Phys Sportsmed.* 1989;17:49–57.

21. Speedy DB, Noakes TD, Holtzhausen LM. Exercise-associated collapse. *Phys Sportsmed.* 2003;31(3):23–9.

22. Young CC. Extreme sports: injuries and medical coverage. *Curr Sports Med Rep.* 2002;1(5):306–11.

16 Catastrophic Sports Injuries

Barry P. Boden

INTRODUCTION

- In the United States, approximately 10% of all brain injuries and 7% of all new cases of paraplegia and quadriplegia are related to athletic activities (15).

- Information on catastrophic injuries in athletes is collected by the National Center for Catastrophic Sports Injury Research (NCCSIR), the U.S. Consumer Product Safety Commission (CPSC), and the professional league data registries.

- The NCCSIR defines catastrophic sports injury as "any severe spinal, spinal cord, or cerebral injury incurred during participation in a school- or college-sponsored sport." Concussions are not considered to be catastrophic injuries.

- The NCCSIR classifies injuries as direct, resulting from participating in the skills of a sport (*i.e.*, trauma from a collision), or indirect, resulting from systemic failure due to exertion while participating in a sport.

- The NCCSIR subdivides catastrophic injuries into three categories: fatal, nonfatal, and serious. A nonfatal injury is any injury where the athlete suffered a permanent, severe, functional disability. A serious injury is a severe injury with no permanent functional disability (*e.g.*, a fractured cervical vertebra without paralysis) (15).

- The CPSC operates a statistically valid injury and review system known as the National Electronic Injury Surveillance System (NEISS) (26). The NEISS estimates are calculated using data from a sample of hospitals that are representative of emergency departments in the United States. The CPSC does not provide data on injury specifics nor does it include information on injuries that initially presented to physician offices.

- The National Collegiate Athletic Association (NCAA) and the National Federation of State High School Associations (NFHS) review injury epidemiology annually and publish a rules book for each sport with the intent of promoting safe play (17,18).

EPIDEMIOLOGY

- For all sports followed by the NCCSIR, the total direct and indirect incidence of catastrophic injuries is approximately 1 per 100,000 high school athletes and 4 per 100,000 college athletes (16).

- The combined fatality rate for direct and indirect injuries in high school is 0.40 for every 100,000 high school athletes and 1.42 for every 100,000 college participants (16).

- Football is associated with the greatest number of catastrophic injuries for all major team sports.

- Pole vault, gymnastics, ice hockey, and football have the highest incidence of injury per 100,000 male participants (16).

- Cheerleading is associated with the highest number of direct catastrophic injuries for all female sports (16).

INDIRECT INJURIES

- Indirect or nontraumatic deaths in athletes have been identified to be predominantly caused by cardiovascular conditions such as hypertrophic cardiomyopathy (HCM), cardiac artery anomalies, myocarditis, aortic stenosis, and dysrhythmias. The most common etiology of sudden cardiac death is HCM for those under age 35 and coronary artery disease for those over age 35. Noncardiac conditions that cause fatalities are heat illness and miscellaneous diagnoses such as rhabdomyolysis, status asthmaticus, and electrocution caused by lightning.

Cardiac Conditions

- Most young athletes who die suddenly have HCM. These athletes typically have prodromal symptoms such as presyncope or syncope with or without exercise prior to the fatal event. A systolic murmur is often appreciated only in the standing position or with a Valsalva maneuver.

- Congenital coronary artery anomalies are a frequent cause of sudden cardiac death. These athletes may or may not have symptoms of syncope or chest pain with exercise, making diagnosis difficult.

- Athletes with aortic stenosis and mitral valve prolapse have abnormal auscultatory findings that should lead to the suspected diagnosis.

- The preparticipation physical is critical for detecting cardiac conditions that may be life threatening.

Heat Illness

Epidemiology

- Heat illness is the third most common cause of death in athletes.
- Risk factors for heat illness include obesity, fever, recent respiratory or gastrointestinal (GI) viral illness, sickle cell trait, stimulants, supplements such as ephedrine, illicit drugs, alcohol, sleep deprivation, sunburn, and underconditioned athletes (9).
- Heat illness usually occurs during unseasonable hot conditions at times of extreme exertion. A typical scenario is an obese football lineman wearing a football uniform and playing two-a-day practices during late summer tryouts in the Southeast United States.

Clinical Features

- Heat cramps is a misnomer and should be termed exercise cramps. Muscle cramping is triggered by fatigue and can occur at any temperature.
- Heat syncope is associated with an abrupt loss of consciousness in a heat-exposed athlete whose core temperature is normal or mildly elevated. The condition often occurs toward the completion of exercise due to reduced cardiac return and postural hypotension. Heat syncope usually occurs during the first few days of heat exposure before the body has been allowed to acclimatize.
- Heat exhaustion is defined as the inability to continue to exercise in the heat since the cardiovascular system fails to respond to workload. The condition occurs at core or rectal temperatures between 100.4°F and 104°F. Symptoms of heat exhaustion can include muscle cramping, mild confusion, headache, dizziness, chills, nausea, and often collapse.
- Heatstroke is exercise-associated collapse with thermoregulatory failure and central nervous system dysfunction. Heatstroke and mental status changes begin at temperatures in excess of 104°F. The athlete may or may not be sweating. The condition may result in a variety of life-threatening problems, such as rhabdomyolysis, renal failure, disseminated intravascular coagulopathy, liver failure, and brain injury.
- The athlete with repeated heat illness requires a workup for a muscle enzyme deficiency.

Diagnosis and Treatment

- A correct diagnosis is based on the history, physical examination, core body temperature, and differential including hyponatremia and cardiac conditions.
- Treatment involves rapid cooling, moving to a cooler environment, removing clothing, tepid water spray, fans, and ice to the neck, groin, and axilla. Hydration should include both oral intake and intravenous fluids. Rehydration with sports drinks containing electrolytes is preferred over water. Athletes with core temperatures greater than 104°F should be considered for cold water immersion. Emergency medical services (EMS) should be contacted for athletes with heat exhaustion and heat stroke.

Prevention

- The incidence of heat illness can be significantly reduced by frequent hydration, acclimatization, identifying at-risk athletes, and monitoring daily weights, medication use, and status of recent illnesses.

DIRECT INJURIES

Football

Epidemiology

- Football has the highest number of catastrophic head and neck injuries per year for all high school and college sports (16).
- From 1989 through 2002, the average number of quadriplegic events for high school and college football players was six per year (5).
- From 1989 through 2002, there was an average of seven catastrophic head injuries per year for high school and college football participants (6). The incidence is dramatically higher at the high school level than at the college level (6).

Mechanisms

- Spearing or tackling a player with the top of the head has been identified as a major cause of permanent cervical quadriplegia. When the neck is flexed 30 degrees, the cervical spine becomes straight, and the forces are transmitted directly to the spinal structures. In 1976, spearing was banned, and the rate of catastrophic cervical injuries dramatically dropped (24,25).
- Cervical cord neurapraxia (CCN) is an acute, transient neurologic episode associated with sensory changes with or without motor weakness or complete paralysis in the arms, legs, or both (25). Complete recovery usually occurs within 10–15 minutes but may take up to 2 days. The *pincer* mechanism involves cord compression either through hyperflexion or hyperextension of the neck. Axial compression may also cause CCN via shear forces on the cervical spine (5).
- An episode of CCN is not an absolute contraindication to return to football. It is unlikely that athletes who experience CCN are at risk for permanent neurologic sequelae with return to play. The overall risk of a recurrent CCN episode with return to football is approximately 50% and is correlated with the canal diameter size. The smaller the canal diameter, the greater is the risk of recurrence.
- The majority of catastrophic head injuries are subdural hematomas (6). Forty percent of players have been reported to be playing with residual neurologic symptoms from a prior head injury at the time of the catastrophic injury (6).

Prevention

- Banning spear tackling and teaching players to play "heads up" ball with no contact on the top of the helmet have dramatically reduced the incidence of permanent cervical quadriplegia. A recent change in the spear tackling rule to include intentional and unintentional spear tackling may further reduce the incidence of this injury.

- The development of a safety standard for the football helmet by the National Operating Committee on Standards for Athletic Equipment (NOCSAE) has also been a significant factor in reducing catastrophic head injuries.

- Careful surveillance for concussions and referral to medical personnel before return to play have reduced the incidence of catastrophic head injuries. Younger athletes often have a protracted recovery from concussion and may require delayed return to play compared to college and professional athletes.

- Training medical personnel to understand on-field management of athletic head and neck injuries and guidelines for return to contact or collision sport after an injury will also help to reduce injuries.

Pole Vaulting

Epidemiology

- Pole vaulting is a unique sport in that athletes often land from heights ranging from 10 to 20 ft. Prior to 2003, pole vaulting had one of the highest rates of direct, catastrophic injuries per 100,000 participants for all sports monitored by the NCCSIR (4).

- The vast majority of catastrophic pole vaulting injuries are head injuries in male athletes. The overall incidence of catastrophic pole vault injuries is two per year, whereas the incidence of fatalities is one per year. Most injuries occurred at the high school level (4).

Mechanisms

- Three common mechanisms of injury have been described (4). The most common mechanism occurs when a pole vaulter lands with his body on the edge of the landing pad and his head whips off the pad, striking the surrounding hard surface (in most cases, either concrete or asphalt). The second most common mechanism occurs when the vaulter releases the pole prematurely or does not have enough momentum and lands in the vault or planting box. The third most common mechanism occurs when the vaulter completely misses the pad and lands directly on the surrounding hard surface.

Prevention

- As of January 2003, both the NCAA and NFHS decided to increase the minimum pole vault landing pad size from 16′ × 12′ to 19′8″ × 16′5″.

- Any hard or unyielding surfaces such as concrete, metal, wood, or asphalt around the landing pad must be padded or cushioned.

- A new rule has been adopted placing the crossbar farther back over the landing pad. This should reduce the chance of an athlete landing in the vault or planting box.

- A coach's box or painted square in the middle of the landing pad is being promoted. This zone would help train athletes to instinctively land near the center of the landing pad. Other safety measures include marking the runway distances so athletes can better gauge their takeoff and prohibiting the practice of tapping or assisting the vaulter at takeoff.

- Pole vaulting is a complicated sport requiring extensive training. Certification by coaches is encouraged.

- The value of helmets in reducing head injuries in high school pole vaulters is controversial. Without conclusive data as to their protective effect, the use of helmets is optional for athletes at this time (22).

- Since the rule change in 2003, the number of catastrophic pole vaulting injuries reported from athletes missing the sides or back of the landing pad has dramatically dropped, but vault box injuries remain a problem.

Soccer

Epidemiology

- Injuries to the head, neck, and face in soccer account for between 5% and 15% of all injuries. Most head and neck injuries occur when two players collide, especially when jumping to head the ball.

- Direct fatalities in soccer are usually associated with either movable goalposts falling on a victim or player impact with the goalpost (11). The CPSC identified at least 21 deaths over a 16-year period associated with movable goalposts (26).

- The incidence of concussions in college soccer athletes is approximately one per team per season (2). There is a 50% chance for a professional athlete to sustain a concussion over a 10-year span. Most concussions occur as a result of contact with an opposing player, not with the soccer ball.

- There is no evidence that an isolated episode of heading a soccer ball can cause any head injury; however, there is controversy over whether repetitive soccer heading over a prolonged career can lead to neuropsychological deficits.

Prevention

- Children should never be allowed to climb on the net or goal framework. Soccer goalposts should be secured at all times. During the off-season, goals should be either disassembled or placed in a safe storage area. Goals should be moved only by trained personnel and should be used only on flat fields (26). The use of padded goalposts may also reduce the incidence of impact injuries with the goalposts (11).

- Children should use smaller soccer balls to reduce the risks of repetitive heading. Leather or water-soaked soccer balls should never be used. Proper heading techniques should be employed: contact on the forehead with the neck muscles contracted. Soccer players should be trained to hit the ball, not to be hit by the ball.

Wrestling

Epidemiology

- Indirect catastrophic wrestling injuries are often the result of rapid weight loss, which causes dehydration and potential cardiovascular compromise (13,19).

- There are approximately two direct catastrophic wrestling injuries per year at the high school and college levels (3). The direct catastrophic injury rate in high school and college wrestlers is approximately 1 per 100,000 participants. The majority of injuries occur in match competitions, where intense, competitive situations place wrestlers at a higher risk (3,12,20).

■ There is a trend toward more direct injuries in the low- and middle-weight classes.

■ Cervical fractures or major cervical ligament injuries constitute the majority of direct catastrophic wrestling injuries (3).

Mechanisms

■ The position most frequently associated with injury is the defensive posture during the takedown maneuver, followed by the down position (kneeling) and the lying position (3). There is no clear predominance of any one type of takedown hold that contributes to wrestling injuries.

■ The athlete is typically injured by one of three scenarios: (a) The wrestler's arms are in a hold such that he or she is unable to keep from landing on his or her head when thrown to the mat. (b) The wrestler attempts a roll but is landed on by the full weight of his opponent, causing a twisting, usually hyperflexion, neck injury. (c) The wrestler lands on the top of his head, sustaining an axial compression force to the cervical spine.

Prevention

■ A minimum body fat for high school and college wrestlers has been established to reduce weight loss injuries. The NFHS also instituted a rule that competitors cannot lose more than 1.5% body weight per week. Both the NCAA and NFHS have banned the use of laxatives, diuretics, and other rapid weight loss techniques such as rubber suits.

■ Referees should strictly enforce penalties for slams and gain more awareness of dangerous holds (3). There is particular vulnerability for the defensive wrestler who may be off balance, have one or both arms held, and then have his opponent land on top of him. Stringent penalties for intentional slams or throws are encouraged. The referee should have a low threshold of tolerance to stop the match during potentially dangerous situations.

■ Coaches can prevent serious injuries by emphasizing safe, legal wrestling techniques. Coaches should teach wrestlers to keep their head up during any takedown maneuver to prevent axial compression injuries to the cervical spine. Proper rolling techniques, with avoidance of landing on the head, need to be emphasized in practice sessions.

Cheerleading

Epidemiology

■ Over the past 20 years, cheerleading has evolved into an activity demanding high levels of skill, athleticism, and complex gymnastics maneuvers (1).

■ In 2002, cheerleading was one of the four most popular organized sports activities for women in high school.

■ Cheerleaders in college and high school account for more than half of the catastrophic injuries that occur in female athletes (16).

■ There are approximately two direct catastrophic cheerleading injuries per year. The catastrophic injury rate is 0.4 per 100,000 in high school cheerleaders, 2 per 100,000 college participants, or an overall rate of 0.6 per 100,000 cheerleaders (8).

■ In 2000, the CPSC estimated a total of 1,258 head injuries in cheerleaders, of which 604 were recorded as concussions and six as skull fractures. In the same year, there were 1,814 neck injuries with 76 fractures in cheerleaders that initially presented to an emergency department in the United States (26).

■ Compared with other sports, cheerleading has a low overall incidence of injuries but a high risk of catastrophic injuries.

■ The majority of injuries occur in female athletes because there are more female than male cheerleaders and the women are usually at the top of the pyramid or being thrown into the air during basket tosses. The majority of injuries occur during the winter months because cheerleaders perform on indoor hard surfaces.

■ College athletes are five times more likely to sustain a catastrophic injury than their high school counterparts due to the increased complexity of stunts at the college level (8). Catastrophic head injuries are twice as common as cervical injuries.

Mechanisms

■ The most common stunts resulting in catastrophic injury are the pyramid or the basket toss (8). The cheerleader at the top of the pyramid is most frequently injured. A basket toss is a stunt where a cheerleader is thrown into the air, often between 6 and 20 ft, by either three or four tossers. Poor judgment or inadequate training of the spotter is often the main problem leading to injury.

■ Less common mechanisms include advanced floor tumbling routines, participating on a wet surface, or performing a mount. The majority of injuries occur when an athlete lands on an indoor hard gym surface (8).

Prevention

■ Height restrictions on pyramids are limited to two levels in high school and 2.5 body lengths in college (17,18). The top cheerleaders are required to be supported by one or more individuals (base) who are in direct weight-bearing contact with the performing surface. The base cheerleaders must remain stationary and maintain constant contact with the suspended or top athlete. Spotters must be present for each person extended above shoulder level. The suspended person is not allowed to be inverted (head below horizontal) or to rotate on the dismount. Limiting the total number of cheerleaders in a pyramid as well as the quick transitions between pyramids and other complex stunts may also help reduce injuries.

■ Basket toss rules limit the stunt to four tossers, starting the toss from the ground level (no flips) and having one of the tossers behind the top person during the toss (17,18). The top person (flyer) is trained to be directed vertically and not allow the head to drop backward out of alignment with the torso or below a horizontal plane with the body. Other safety measures that may reduce the incidence of basket toss injuries include evaluating the height thrown, using mandatory landing mats for complex stunts, and improving the skills of the spotters.

- All stunts should be restricted when wet conditions are present.
- Injuries from floor tumbling routines can be prevented by proper supervision, progression to complex tumbling only when simple maneuvers are mastered, and using spotters as necessary.
- Mini trampolines, springboards, and any apparatus used to propel a participant have been prohibited since the late 1980s.
- A landing mat should be employed during all complex stunts.
- Cheerleading coaches need to place equal time and attention on the technique and attentiveness of spotters in practice compared with the athletes performing the stunts.
- Coaches are encouraged to complete a safety certification, especially for any teams that perform pyramids, basket tosses, and/or tumbling.
- Pyramids and basket tosses should be limited to experienced cheerleaders who have mastered all other skills and should not be performed without qualified spotters or landing mats.

Baseball

Epidemiology

- Baseball has a low rate of noncatastrophic injuries but a high incidence of catastrophic injuries.
- Head injuries constitute the majority of catastrophic injuries.
- There are approximately two direct catastrophic injuries reported to the NCCSIR per year or 0.6 injuries per 100,000 participants (16). The total incidence of catastrophic injuries and fatalities is 5 and 13 times higher, respectively, at the college level than at the high school level (7).

Mechanisms

- The most common mechanism is a pitcher hit by a batted ball, followed by a collision of two fielders and a collision of a runner and a fielder (7). An area of controversy in baseball is the safety of aluminum or enhanced bats. Nonwood bats are typically lighter than woods bats and can be swung faster with greater ball velocity off the bat.
- Commotio cordis is arrhythmia or sudden death from low-impact blunt trauma to the chest in subjects with no preexisting cardiac disease (10,14). The proposed mechanism is impact just prior to the peak of the T wave on an electrocardiogram, which induces ventricular fibrillation. The pediatric population may be more susceptible because of a thinner layer of soft tissue to the chest wall, increased compliance of the immature rib cage, and slower protective reflexes.

Prevention

- Protecting pitchers from a batted ball may be accomplished by requiring pitchers to wear helmets, using protective screens during batting practice, and regulating the bat and ball (7).
- In 2003, the NCAA and NFHS placed new regulations on bats. All bats must be certified as having a ball exit speed that cannot exceed 97 miles per hour as measured by the Baum hitting machine. In addition, certified bats may not weigh more than 3 oz less than the length of the bat (*e.g.*, a 34-in. long bat cannot weigh less than 31 oz) (18).
- Decreasing the ball's hardness and weight may significantly reduce injury severity. The coefficient of restitution or the measure of rebound that a ball has off a hard surface cannot exceed 0.555 at the high school and college levels.
- Preventive strategies for commotio cordis include teaching youth baseball players to turn their chest away from a batted ball. The use of chest protectors is controversial. Automatic external defibrillators hold promise for preventing fatalities but require further research (10,14).

Ice Hockey

Epidemiology

- Although the number of catastrophic injuries in ice hockey is low compared with other sports, the incidence per 100,000 participants is high (16).
- The majority of catastrophic injuries occur to the cervical spine.

Mechanisms

- Most injuries occur when an athlete is struck from behind by an opponent and contacts another object, especially the boards, with the crown of the head (21,23).
- Head and facial injuries are common from collisions or being hit by the puck or stick.
- Catastrophic accidents from collisions with goalposts were common before the advent of displaceable goalposts.

Prevention

- Enforce current rules against pushing or checking from behind.
- Encourage the use of helmets and face masks.
- Padding the boards and developing a potential space between the boards and the Plexiglass extension may reduce the frequency and severity of head and neck injuries.
- Ensure that the goals can slide out of position to protect athletes from colliding against an immovable object.
- Discourage aggression and fighting in hockey.

Swimming

Mechanisms

- Most catastrophic swimming injuries are related to the racing dive into the shallow end of pools (16).
- Hyperventilating just prior to swimming can rid the body of carbon dioxide. This fools the brain into thinking it doesn't need to breathe, even when its oxygen stores are dangerously low, which may lead to loss of consciousness and drowning.

Prevention

- At the high school level, swimmers must start the race in the water if the water depth at the starting end is less than 3.5 ft. If the water depth is 3.5 ft to less than 4 ft at the starting end, the swimmer may start from the deck or in the water. If the water depth at the starting end is 4 ft or more, the swimmer may start from a platform up to 30 in. above the water surface (18).

- The NFHS mandates that swimmers break the surface of water to breathe at or before 15 m to prevent shallow water blackout.

Rugby

Mechanisms

- Cervical spine injuries occur most frequently during a scrum, when the opposing sides of tightly bound players come forcibly together (engagement) (27).
- The hooker or central player on the front row of the scrum suffers the most injuries. If engagement does not occur properly or the hooker employs the top of the head as a weapon with the neck flexed during contact, an axial compression injury with quadriplegia may result (27).

Prevention

- Preventative methods include avoiding a mismatch in physical size of the hookers, not allowing unskilled players to participate on the front row, and restricting tackling with the top of the head.
- Sequential engagement or having the front rows engage separately from the pack is encouraged. A new international rugby rule in 2007 requires a "crouch, touch, pause, and engage" maneuver during the scrum. Front row players are not allowed to be more than an arm's length away from the opponent before engagement.

Gymnastics

- Most injuries are associated with a missed vault, a fall from the parallel bars or horizontal bar, or a faulty dismount (16).

GENERAL PREVENTION TIPS

- Preparticipation physicals
- Qualified coaches
- Proper strength and conditioning programs
- Supervision of athletes at all times
- EMS protocols in place at all times
- Continued research concerning catastrophic injuries and methods to prevent these injuries

REFERENCES

1. American Association of Cheerleading Coaches and Administrator Web site [Internet]. Available from: http://www.aacca.org.
2. Boden BP, Kirkendall DT, Garrett WE. Concussion incidence in elite college soccer players. *Am J Sports Med.* 1998;26(2):238–41.
3. Boden BP, Lin W, Young M, Mueller FO. Catastrophic injuries in wrestlers. *Am J Sports Med.* 2002;30(6):791–5.
4. Boden BP, Pasquine P, Johnson J, Mueller FO. Catastrophic injuries in pole-vaulters. *Am J Sports Med.* 2001;29(1):50–4.
5. Boden BP, Tacchetti RL, Cantu RC, Knowles SB, Mueller FO. Catastrophic cervical spine injuries in high school and college football players. *Am J Sports Med.* 2006;34(8):1223–32.
6. Boden BP, Tacchetti RL, Cantu RC, Knowles SB, Mueller FO. Catastrophic head injuries in high school and college foobaII players. *Am J Sports Med.* 2007;35(7):1075–81.
7. Boden BP, Tacchetti R, Mueller FO. Catastrophic injuries in high school and college baseball players. *Am J Sports Med.* 2004;32(5):1189–96.
8. Boden BP, Tacchetti R, Mueller FO. Catastrophic cheerleading injuries. *Am J Sports Med.* 2003;31(6):881–8.
9. Coyle JF. Thermoregulation. In: Sullivan JA, Anderson SJ, editors. *Care of the Young Athlete.* Elk Grove: American Academy of Pediatrics and American Academy of Orthopedic Surgeons; 2000. p. 65–80.
10. Janda DH, Bir CA, Viano DC, Cassatta SJ. Blunt chest impacts: assessing the relative risk of fatal cardiac injury from various baseballs. *J Trauma.* 1998;44(2):298–303.
11. Janda DH, Bir C, Wild B, Olson S, Hensinger RN. Goal post injuries in soccer. A laboratory and field testing analysis of a preventive intervention. *Am J Sports Med.* 1995;23(3):340–4.
12. Jarrett GJ, Orwin JF, Dick RW. Injuries in collegiate wrestling. *Am J Sports Med.* 1998;26(5):674–80.
13. Kiningham RB, Gorenflo DW. Weight loss methods of high school wrestlers. *Med Sci Sports Exerc.* 2001;33(5):810–13.
14. Maron BJ, Poliac LC, Kaplan JA, Mueller FO. Blunt impact to the chest leading to sudden death from cardiac arrest during sports activities. *N Engl J Med.* 1995;333(6):337–42.
15. Mueller FO. Introduction. In: Mueller FO, Cantu RC, VanCamp SP, editors. *Catastrophic Injuries in High School and College Sports.* Champaign: HK Sport Science Monograph Series; 1996.
16. Mueller FO, Cantu RC. NCCSIR nineteenth annual report. *National Center for Catastrophic Sports Injury Research: Fall 1982–Spring 2000.* Chapel Hill (NC): National Center for Sports Injury Research; 2000.
17. National Collegiate Athletic Association Web site [Internet]. Available from: http://www.ncaa.org.
18. National Federation of State High School Associations Web site [Internet]. Available from: http://www.nfhs.org.
19. Oppliger RA, Case HS, Horswill CA, Landry G, Shelter AC. American College of Sports Medicine position stand: weight-loss in wrestlers. *Med Sci Sports Exerc.* 1996;28(10):135–8.
20. Pasque CB, Hewett TE. A prospective study of high school wrestling injuries. *Am J Sports Med.* 2000;28(4):509–15.
21. Reid DC, Saboe L. Spine fractures in winter sports. *Sports Med.* 1989;7(6):393–9.
22. Sky Jumpers Vertical Sports Club Web site [Internet]. Available from: http://www.skyjumpers.com.
23. Tator CH, Edmonds VE, Lapczak L, Tator IB. Spinal injuries in ice hockey players, 1966–1987. *Can J Surg.* 1991;34(1):63–9.
24. Torg JS, Gennarelli TA. Head and cervical spine injuries. In: DeLee JC, Drez D Jr, editors. *Orthopaedic Sports Medicine: Principles and Practice.* Philadelphia: WB Saunders; 1994. p. 417–62.
25. Torg JS, Guille JT, Jaffe S. Current concepts review: injuries to the cervical spine in American football players. *J Bone Joint Surg.* 2002;84(1):112–22.
26. United States Consumer Product Safety Commission summary reports. *National Electronic Injury Surveillance System* [Internet]. Washington (DC): U.S. Consumer Product Safety Commission. Available from: http://www.cpsc.gov.
27. Wetzler MJ, Akpata T, Laughlin W, Levy AS. Occurrence of cervical spine injuries during the rugby scrum. *Am J Sports Med.* 1998;26(2):177–80.

17 The Preparticipation Physical Examination

Robert E. Sallis and Christopher C. Bell

INTRODUCTION

- It is estimated that approximately 10–15 million or more athletes from grade school to college require preparticipation examinations (PPEs) annually in the United States (20).
- No defined national standard exists for PPEs, and each state has different laws and statutes regarding them.

GOALS

- Ensure that athletes of all ages and skill levels are able to safely compete.
- Detect any condition, medical or musculoskeletal, that may limit an athlete's participation or require treatment, rehabilitation, or adequate control prior to participation.
- Detect any condition that may predispose an athlete to injury or lead to sudden death during competition.
- Meet legal or insurance requirements (49 of 50 states require yearly examinations).
- Determine general health of the athlete.
- Assess fitness level for specific sports.
- Counsel on lifestyle issues and high-risk behaviors.
- Answer health-related questions, and update vaccines.

QUALIFIED PROVIDERS

- It is recommended by the American Heart Association (AHA) that providers who perform screening PPEs have adequate medical training, particularly in cardiovascular auscultation (25).
- Currently, however, 18 states still allow chiropractors and naturopathic practitioners to screen athletes (25).

FORMAT

- Private office with primary care provider
  - Advantages: privacy, controlled environment, better continuity of care, and easier to perform counseling.
  - Disadvantages: higher cost, less communication with school athletic staff, and potential for providers who have insufficient knowledge and skills necessary for a complete and appropriate evaluation.
- Group examination (usually done as a station-based examination)
  - Advantages: more cost effective, more time efficient, usually done at school with athletic staff present.
  - Disadvantages: lack of privacy, loud and chaotic environment thereby impairing proper cardiac auscultation, and poor follow-up.

FREQUENCY AND TIMING OF EXAMINATION

- Most states require an examination to be done yearly for high school–aged and younger athletes. However, a comprehensive exam every 2 years with yearly updates as needed is recommended by the AHA.
- The National Collegiate Athletic Association (NCAA) requires an initial complete PPE prior to participation in intercollegiate athletics, with interim annual updates of the athlete's history. Further PPEs are not deemed necessary unless indicated by the updated history (28).
- Optimal timing for the examination is at least 6 weeks before the season starts to allow sufficient time for further evaluation, treatment, and/or rehabilitation of any problems that may be uncovered.

CONTENT

- Because the stress of sports and exercise falls primarily on the cardiovascular and musculoskeletal systems, these areas are essential for assessment as part of the PPE. This evaluation should begin with a thorough history, followed by a focused physical examination.
- Close attention should also be paid to the neurologic history to specifically address concussions, stingers, and other neurologic issues.

- In 1992, representatives from several national physician groups assembled to develop a comprehensive PPE tool for use among providers who perform athletic screening. Since then, there have been periodic updates.

  - *Preparticipation Physical Examination*, 4th Edition (PPE Monograph), is the most recent iteration of this work, which has been established through the collaboration of the American College of Sports Medicine®, American Academy of Family Physicians (AAFP), American Academy of Pediatrics (AAP), American Medical Society for Sports Medicine (AMSSM), American Orthopaedic Society for Sports Medicine (AOSSM), and American Osteopathic Academy of Sports (AOASM). It can be found at http://www.ppesportsevaluation.org (1).

  - It is recommended that all providers use this monograph as the primary template for the PPE.

MEDICAL HISTORY

- A thorough personal and family medical history has been shown to identify up to 75% of all medical problems affecting athletes (17).

- The easiest method for obtaining an athlete's history is to use a preprinted questionnaire (such as the one available in the PPE monograph) that the parent(s) of the athlete completes prior to the examination (Fig. 17.1). The history portion of these forms is best filled out by the parents and the athlete together, because the athlete may not be fully aware of his or her complete personal and/or family history.

- Key questions include asking about any major preexisting medical problems or injuries; if the athlete is taking any medicines or supplements; if the athlete has any significant environmental and/or medication allergies; and about the athlete's current state of health.

- Assess for cardiovascular risk:

  - Because most sudden death episodes in sports are due to cardiovascular causes, thorough cardiovascular screening is extremely important.

  - The relative risk for sudden cardiac death (SCD) has been found to be 2.5 times higher in athletes than in the general population (11).

  - The AHA has recommended eight history questions as the initial screening for cardiovascular risk.

  - The PPE Monograph uses those questions (see Fig. 17.1).

  - Positive answers to critical history questions such as "Have you ever passed out or nearly passed out DURING or AFTER exercise?" and "Have you ever had discomfort, pain, tightness, or pressure in your chest during exercise?" (Questions 5 and 6) may signal the presence of a structural heart problem.

  - It is also important to assess for family history of early unexplained death, cardiovascular abnormalities, or concerning signs and symptoms that may allude to possible undiagnosed cardiac abnormalities in family members.

- Assess for symptoms of exercise-induced bronchospasm (EIB):

  - Symptoms include coughing, wheezing, and/or chest tightness during or immediately after exercise, especially in those with a personal or family history of allergic rhinitis, eczema, or asthma.

  - Improvement of symptoms after using an inhaled bronchodilator is highly suggestive.

- Assess for concussion history:

  - It is important to ask about the symptoms of concussion because most who have had one may not have sought medical attention and been diagnosed.

  - Common symptoms include headache, nausea, dizziness, blurred vision, getting "dinged" or your "bell rung," fatigue, either hypersomnolence or insomnia, retrograde amnesia, emotional lability, inability to concentrate in school or with homework, irritability, confusion, "not feeling right," and "feeling like in a fog" (33,35).

    - If the patient can recall one or more of these symptoms in association with an impact to the head or body (possibly denoting a contrecoup injury), then he or she likely had a concussion.

- Assess for history of repeated "stingers" and/or "burners," which are symptoms of numbness and/or pain radiating down an arm after a blow to the head, neck, or ipsilateral shoulder; if present, they may indicate cervical stenosis or a similar condition.

- Screen females for signs and symptoms related to the "female athlete triad" (disordered eating, menstrual irregularities, history of stress fractures).

PHYSICAL EXAMINATION

Cardiovascular Assessment

- Cardiac auscultation should be done both standing and supine.

- Benign systolic murmurs are common in athletes. If a murmur is grade III or louder, or diastolic, further evaluation is recommended.

- The murmur associated with hypertrophic cardiomyopathy (HCM) is best heard while upright and may disappear with supine position as well as squatting.

- If there is a potentially concerning murmur, having the patient perform a Valsalva maneuver can provide additional information. Typically, Valsalva will accentuate murmurs due to outflow obstruction abnormalities such as HCM.

- Twenty-five percent of patients with HCM with left ventricular outflow obstruction have a murmur on physical exam (18).

■ PREPARTICIPATION PHYSICAL EVALUATION
HISTORY FORM

(Note: This form is to be filled out by the patient and parent prior to seeing the physician. The physician should keep this form in the chart.)

Date of Exam _____

Name _____ Date of birth _____

Sex _____ Age _____ Grade _____ School _____ Sport(s) _____

Medicines and Allergies: Please list all of the prescription and over-the-counter medicines and supplements (herbal and nutritional) that you are currently taking

Do you have any allergies? ☐ Yes ☐ No   If yes, please identify specific allergy below.
☐ Medicines   ☐ Pollens   ☐ Food   ☐ Stinging Insects

Explain "Yes" answers below. Circle questions you don't know the answers to.

GENERAL QUESTIONS	Yes	No
1. Has a doctor ever denied or restricted your participation in sports for any reason?		
2. Do you have any ongoing medical conditions? If so, please identify below: ☐ Asthma ☐ Anemia ☐ Diabetes ☐ Infections Other:		
3. Have you ever spent the night in the hospital?		
4. Have you ever had surgery?		

HEART HEALTH QUESTIONS ABOUT YOU	Yes	No
5. Have you ever passed out or nearly passed out DURING or AFTER exercise?		
6. Have you ever had discomfort, pain, tightness, or pressure in your chest during exercise?		
7. Does your heart ever race or skip beats (irregular beats) during exercise?		
8. Has a doctor ever told you that you have any heart problems? If so, check all that apply: ☐ High blood pressure ☐ A heart murmur ☐ High cholesterol ☐ A heart infection ☐ Kawasaki disease Other:		
9. Has a doctor ever ordered a test for your heart? (For example, ECG/EKG, echocardiogram)		
10. Do you get lightheaded or feel more short of breath than expected during exercise?		
11. Have you ever had an unexplained seizure?		
12. Do you get more tired or short of breath more quickly than your friends during exercise?		

HEART HEALTH QUESTIONS ABOUT YOUR FAMILY	Yes	No
13. Has any family member or relative died of heart problems or had an unexpected or unexplained sudden death before age 50 (including drowning, unexplained car accident, or sudden infant death syndrome)?		
14. Does anyone in your family have hypertrophic cardiomyopathy, Marfan syndrome, arrhythmogenic right ventricular cardiomyopathy, long QT syndrome, short QT syndrome, Brugada syndrome, or catecholaminergic polymorphic ventricular tachycardia?		
15. Does anyone in your family have a heart problem, pacemaker, or implanted defibrillator?		
16. Has anyone in your family had unexplained fainting, unexplained seizures, or near drowning?		

BONE AND JOINT QUESTIONS	Yes	No
17. Have you ever had an injury to a bone, muscle, ligament, or tendon that caused you to miss a practice or a game?		
18. Have you ever had any broken or fractured bones or dislocated joints?		
19. Have you ever had an injury that required x-rays, MRI, CT scan, injections, therapy, a brace, a cast, or crutches?		
20. Have you ever had a stress fracture?		
21. Have you ever been told that you have or have you had an x-ray for neck instability or atlantoaxial instability? (Down syndrome or dwarfism)		
22. Do you regularly use a brace, orthotics, or other assistive device?		
23. Do you have a bone, muscle, or joint injury that bothers you?		
24. Do any of your joints become painful, swollen, feel warm, or look red?		
25. Do you have any history of juvenile arthritis or connective tissue disease?		

MEDICAL QUESTIONS	Yes	No
26. Do you cough, wheeze, or have difficulty breathing during or after exercise?		
27. Have you ever used an inhaler or taken asthma medicine?		
28. Is there anyone in your family who has asthma?		
29. Were you born without or are you missing a kidney, an eye, a testicle (males), your spleen, or any other organ?		
30. Do you have groin pain or a painful bulge or hernia in the groin area?		
31. Have you had infectious mononucleosis (mono) within the last month?		
32. Do you have any rashes, pressure sores, or other skin problems?		
33. Have you had a herpes or MRSA skin infection?		
34. Have you ever had a head injury or concussion?		
35. Have you ever had a hit or blow to the head that caused confusion, prolonged headache, or memory problems?		
36. Do you have a history of seizure disorder?		
37. Do you have headaches with exercise?		
38. Have you ever had numbness, tingling, or weakness in your arms or legs after being hit or falling?		
39. Have you ever been unable to move your arms or legs after being hit or falling?		
40. Have you ever become ill while exercising in the heat?		
41. Do you get frequent muscle cramps when exercising?		
42. Do you or someone in your family have sickle cell trait or disease?		
43. Have you had any problems with your eyes or vision?		
44. Have you had any eye injuries?		
45. Do you wear glasses or contact lenses?		
46. Do you wear protective eyewear, such as goggles or a face shield?		
47. Do you worry about your weight?		
48. Are you trying to or has anyone recommended that you gain or lose weight?		
49. Are you on a special diet or do you avoid certain types of foods?		
50. Have you ever had an eating disorder?		
51. Do you have any concerns that you would like to discuss with a doctor?		

FEMALES ONLY		
52. Have you ever had a menstrual period?		
53. How old were you when you had your first menstrual period?		
54. How many periods have you had in the last 12 months?		

Explain "yes" answers here
_____
_____
_____
_____
_____
_____
_____

I hereby state that, to the best of my knowledge, my answers to the above questions are complete and correct.

Signature of athlete _____ Signature of parent/guardian _____ Date _____

Figure 17.1: Preparticipation physical examination form. *(continued)*

■ PREPARTICIPATION PHYSICAL EVALUATION

THE ATHLETE WITH SPECIAL NEEDS: SUPPLEMENTAL HISTORY FORM

Date of Exam _____

Name _____ Date of birth _____

Sex _____ Age _____ Grade _____ School _____ Sport(s) _____

	Yes	No
1. Type of disability		
2. Date of disability		
3. Classification (if available)		
4. Cause of disability (birth, disease, accident/trauma, other)		
5. List the sports you are interested in playing		
6. Do you regularly use a brace, assistive device, or prosthetic?		
7. Do you use any special brace or assistive device for sports?		
8. Do you have any rashes, pressure sores, or any other skin problems?		
9. Do you have a hearing loss? Do you use a hearing aid?		
10. Do you have a visual impairment?		
11. Do you use any special devices for bowel or bladder function?		
12. Do you have burning or discomfort when urinating?		
13. Have you had autonomic dysreflexia?		
14. Have you ever been diagnosed with a heat-related (hyperthermia) or cold-related (hypothermia) illness?		
15. Do you have muscle spasticity?		
16. Do you have frequent seizures that cannot be controlled by medication?		

Explain "yes" answers here

_____

_____

_____

_____

_____

Please indicate if you have ever had any of the following.

	Yes	No
Atlantoaxial instability		
X-ray evaluation for atlantoaxial instability		
Dislocated joints (more than one)		
Easy bleeding		
Enlarged spleen		
Hepatitis		
Osteopenia or osteoporosis		
Difficulty controlling bowel		
Difficulty controlling bladder		
Numbness or tingling in arms or hands		
Numbness or tingling in legs or feet		
Weakness in arms or hands		
Weakness in legs or feet		
Recent change in coordination		
Recent change in ability to walk		
Spina bifida		
Latex allergy		

Explain "yes" answers here

_____

_____

_____

_____

_____

I hereby state that, to the best of my knowledge, my answers to the above questions are complete and correct.

Signature of athlete _____ Signature of parent/guardian _____ Date _____

Figure 17.1:   *(continued)*

■ PREPARTICIPATION PHYSICAL EVALUATION
PHYSICAL EXAMINATION FORM

Name _____ Date of birth _____

PHYSICIAN REMINDERS

1. Consider additional questions on more sensitive issues
   - Do you feel stressed out or under a lot of pressure?
   - Do you ever feel sad, hopeless, depressed, or anxious?
   - Do you feel safe at your home or residence?
   - Have you ever tried cigarettes, chewing tobacco, snuff, or dip?
   - During the past 30 days, did you use chewing tobacco, snuff, or dip?
   - Do you drink alcohol or use any other drugs?
   - Have you ever taken anabolic steroids or used any other performance supplement?
   - Have you ever taken any supplements to help you gain or lose weight or improve your performance?
   - Do you wear a seat belt, use a helmet, and use condoms?
2. Consider reviewing questions on cardiovascular symptoms (questions 5–14).

EXAMINATION				
Height	Weight		☐ Male ☐ Female	
BP / (/) Pulse		Vision R 20/	L 20/	Corrected ☐ Y ☐ N

MEDICAL	NORMAL	ABNORMAL FINDINGS
Appearance • Marfan stigmata (kyphoscoliosis, high-arched palate, pectus excavatum, arachnodactyly, arm span > height, hyperlaxity, myopia, MVP, aortic insufficiency)		
Eyes/ears/nose/throat • Pupils equal • Hearing		
Lymph nodes		
Heart [a] • Murmurs (auscultation standing, supine, +/- Valsalva) • Location of point of maximal impulse (PMI)		
Pulses • Simultaneous femoral and radial pulses		
Lungs		
Abdomen		
Genitourinary (males only) [b]		
Skin • HSV, lesions suggestive of MRSA, tinea corporis		
Neurologic [c]		
MUSCULOSKELETAL		
Neck		
Back		
Shoulder/arm		
Elbow/forearm		
Wrist/hand/fingers		
Hip/thigh		
Knee		
Leg/ankle		
Foot/toes		
Functional • Duck-walk, single leg hop		

[a] Consider ECG, echocardiogram, and referral to cardiology for abnormal cardiac history or exam.
[b] Consider GU exam if in private setting. Having third party present is recommended.
[c] Consider cognitive evaluation or baseline neuropsychiatric testing if a history of significant concussion.

☐ Cleared for all sports without restriction

☐ Cleared for all sports without restriction with recommendations for further evaluation or treatment for _____
_____

☐ Not cleared

    ☐ Pending further evaluation

    ☐ For any sports

    ☐ For certain sports _____

      Reason _____

Recommendations _____
_____

I have examined the above-named student and completed the preparticipation physical evaluation. The athlete does not present apparent clinical contraindications to practice and participate in the sport(s) as outlined above. A copy of the physical exam is on record in my office and can be made available to the school at the request of the parents. If conditions arise after the athlete has been cleared for participation, the physician may rescind the clearance until the problem is resolved and the potential consequences are completely explained to the athlete (and parents/guardians).

Name of physician (print/type) _____ Date _____

Address _____ Phone _____

Signature of physician _____ , MD or DO

Figure 17.1: *(continucd)*

■ PREPARTICIPATION PHYSICAL EVALUATION
CLEARANCE FORM

Name _____ Sex ☐ M ☐ F Age _____ Date of birth _____

☐ Cleared for all sports without restriction

☐ Cleared for all sports without restriction with recommendations for further evaluation or treatment for _____
_____

☐ Not cleared

    ☐ Pending further evaluation

    ☐ For any sports

    ☐ For certain sports _____

    Reason _____

Recommendations _____
_____
_____
_____
_____
_____

I have examined the above-named student and completed the preparticipation physical evaluation. The athlete does not present apparent clinical contraindications to practice and participate in the sport(s) as outlined above. A copy of the physical exam is on record in my office and can be made available to the school at the request of the parents. If conditions arise after the athlete has been cleared for participation, the physician may rescind the clearance until the problem is resolved and the potential consequences are completely explained to the athlete (and parents/guardians).

Name of physician (print/type) _____ Date _____

Address _____ Phone _____

Signature of physician _____ , MD or DO

EMERGENCY INFORMATION

Allergies _____
_____
_____
_____
_____

Other information _____
_____
_____
_____
_____
_____
_____
_____
_____

Figure 17.1: *(continued)*

■ Ectopic beats are also common. Those that disappear with exercise are usually benign, while those brought on with exercise are more worrisome. Ventricular ectopy in young athletes should also raise suspicion for possible use of stimulants (*e.g.*, cocaine).

■ Simultaneous palpation of the radial and femoral pulses for asymmetry is a simple screen for coarctation of the aorta.

Blood Pressure

■ Readings that indicate hypertension vary for different age ranges and between genders (34). Three separate elevated blood pressure (BP) readings are needed to diagnose hypertension (8,34).

■ Hypertension in children and adolescents is based off of percentiles for each age according to gender and height; those with repeated measurements at or above the 95th percentile are considered hypertensive (34).

■ Those between the 90th and 95th percentiles are deemed "high normal," or the equivalent of the adult prehypertensive.

■ In people age 18 and over, the definitions of hypertension are as follows (8):

■ Prehypertension: systolic blood pressure (SBP) between 120 and 139 mm Hg or diastolic blood pressure (DBP) between 80 and 89 mm Hg.

■ Grade I hypertension: SBP between 140 and 159 mm Hg or DBP between 90 and 99 mm Hg.

■ Grade II hypertension: SBP ≥ 160 mm Hg or DBP ≥ 100 mm Hg.

■ Those who have prehypertension or grade I hypertension without evidence of end-organ damage need not be restricted from competitive sports.

■ Grade II hypertensives should be restricted from high static sports (*e.g.*, weightlifting) until their BP is controlled.

■ Systolic hypertension in young athletes is frequently related to anxiety or inappropriate cuff size in husky individuals.

■ If the initial measurement is high, it is recommended that another reading be taken after resting for 5 minutes.

Musculoskeletal Assessment

■ It is not necessary to perform a comprehensive joint-by-joint musculoskeletal exam on all PPEs.

■ The "2-minute musculoskeletal examination" can be a useful screen (Table 17.1).

■ Look for preexisting injuries, because they are likely to recur. The knees, shoulders, and ankles are most at risk.

■ Focus more of your examination on problem areas if they exist.

■ Keep in mind the demands of the particular sport the athlete will be playing, and focus more on areas of the body that will be under stress and prone to injury from that sport.

Table 17.1	The 2-Minute Musculoskeletal Examination for Screening Athletes During the Preparticipation Examination
Instructions	**Observation**
Stand facing examiner	Acromioclavicular joints, general habitus
Look at ceiling, floor, over both shoulders; touch ears to shoulders	Cervical spine motion
Shrug shoulders (examiner resists at 90 degrees)	Trapezius strength
Abduct shoulders 90 degrees (examiner resists at 90 degrees)	Deltoid strength
Full external rotation of arms	Shoulder motion
Flex and extend elbows	Elbow motion
Arms at sides, elbows 90 degrees flexed; pronate and supinate wrists	Elbow and wrist motion
Spread fingers; make fist	Hand or finger motion and deformities
Tighten (contract) quadriceps	Symmetry and knee effusion; ankle effusion
"Duck" walk four steps (away from examiner with buttocks on heels)	Ability to perform this rules out significant hip and knee abnormalities
Back to examiner	Shoulder symmetry, scoliosis
Knees straight, touch toes	Scoliosis, hip motion, hamstring tightness
Raise up on toes, raise heels	Calf symmetry, leg strength

SOURCE: Smith NJ. *Sports Medicine: Health Care for Young Athletes.* Evanston (IL): American Academy of Pediatrics; 1983. 1 p.

■ Musculoskeletal problems found during the PPE should be treated with appropriate rehabilitation and conditioning programs prior to returning to activity.

Other Areas for Assessment

■ Height/weight
■ Eating disorders, ideal body weight
■ General appearance
■ Stigmata of Marfan disease: kyphoscoliosis
■ Eyes
■ Vision
■ Pupils for the presence of anisocoria, which may be present in up to 10% of patients.
■ Ears/nose/throat
■ Lungs
■ Abdominal
■ Hepatosplenomegaly, masses
■ Skin
■ Infectious diseases, acne

- Neurologic
- Genitourinary
  - Single testicle, hernia, testicular mass
  - Tanner staging to assess physical maturity is no longer recommended.

DIAGNOSTIC TESTS

Laboratory Tests

- Consensus is that laboratory tests should not be done routinely during the PPE.
- Consider routine hematocrit in female athletes, especially those involved in endurance sports.
- Perform cholesterol testing if indicated by history.

Sickle Cell Trait

- Consider testing for sickle cell trait (SCT). The NCAA now requires testing for all Division I athletes in which the presence of SCT is unknown. However, individual athletes can opt out of testing if they prefer (28).

Concussion

- Consider formal neuropsychological testing if there is a history of multiple concussions, prolonged postconcussion symptoms, or inconsistent or significantly diminished school performance (see Chapter 26).

Exercise-Induced Bronchospasm

- EIB appears to be much more prevalent in endurance athletes (27).
- If there is concern for EIB, it is recommended to perform testing to confirm or rule out the condition, because it has been shown that the correlation between symptoms and actual disease is poor (7,16,32) (see Chapter 24).
- Although this testing may be difficult to accomplish and simply prescribing a trial of an inhaled β_2 agonist is much easier and more time efficient, one must be aware not only of misdiagnosis and subsequent unnecessary treatment but also of the potential for doping infractions for athletes competing at the collegiate or elite levels (27).
- There are NCAA restrictions regarding the use of inhaled β_2 agonists, and the International Olympic Committee (IOC) has them on the banned substances list except for the long-acting versions, which are restricted in use (38).

Cardiac Testing

- There has been considerable debate recently regarding the inclusion of routine screening electrocardiogram (ECG) as a part of the PPE in the United States.

- Routine ECG is being performed in Europe and is recommended by the European Society of Cardiology (ESC) and the IOC as part of their baseline screening programs. The recommendations are based on data that have come out of Italy that have shown that including ECG in regular screening has resulted in an 89% reduction in SCD (10).
- It has been shown that for HCM (the most common cause of SCD in the United States), ECG abnormalities are present in 75%–95% of those with the condition (22,23,29). However, most of the ECG findings are subtle and require added expertise to detect.
- In addition, the sensitivity and specificity of history and physical in detecting cardiac abnormalities responsible for SCD are quite low, and often SCD is the first manifestation of the underlying disorder (4,5,23,24,28,30,35,37).
- In a recent consensus statement (25), the AHA came to the conclusion that implementing a nationwide screening program that would include ECG for athletes in the United States is not viable for the following reasons:
  - Lack of medical resources and infrastructure to perform this testing on the large number of athletes in this country (estimated to be 10–15 million).
  - The need to enact federal statutes to establish mandatory compliance with the screening process and nationwide consensus regarding the disqualification standards in the face of more pressing public health care issues.
  - Lack of financial resources for this kind of endeavor within our current health care system.
  - The relatively large percentage of false-positives that result from these screening programs, mostly related to ECG interpretation. This leads to subsequent testing, further increasing the cost in addition to causing additional anxiety for the athlete and his or her family.
  - The detrimental effect of unnecessary disqualification from sport and activity of children and adolescents within the context of our current epidemic of inactivity and obesity.

SCREENING TO PREVENT EXERCISE-RELATED SUDDEN DEATH

- The cause of sudden death during exercise is usually cardiac: under 35 years, usually structural heart problem; over 35 years, usually coronary artery disease.
- The overall prevalence of cardiac abnormalities responsible for SCD is approximately 0.3% (18).
- Preparticipation screening is the primary preventive tool. Exercise-related SCD in the United States is rare, but its actual incidence is still in question. Estimates range from 0.3 to 3 per 100,000 athletes per year (2–4,6,8,9,11–14,19–21,31,34,36).
- The official recommendation of the AHA is to perform a thorough personal and family history, with questions specific for cardiac conditions (as noted earlier), and focused physical examination. Proceed with further testing only as indicated.

- Including routine screening ECG and/or echocardiogram would be the individual choice of certain communities and would be considered optional. However, it is warned that including these additional baseline tests brings with it added liability and increased (and likely unsustainable) financial and medical resource needs.
- If there are any concerning findings on history or physical exam, further evaluation is warranted. The subsequent workup will depend on the suspected abnormality.
- ECGs can usually be performed in most primary care offices but should also be interpreted by a cardiologist or someone well versed in ECG findings associated with young healthy athletes as well as those conditions known to cause SCD. As mentioned later, there are many ECG changes associated with normal adapted ("athletic") hearts, as well as very subtle findings that can alert one to concerning cardiac abnormalities.
- In the adult athlete, however, a resting ECG and/or exercise stress test may be indicated in males over the age of 40 and females over the age of 55 with two or more cardiac risk factors, prior to starting an exercise program (15).
- Causes of SCD in sports include the following.

Hypertrophic Cardiomyopathy

- Most common cause of SCD in the United States.
- Symptoms: may exhibit palpitations, syncope, chest pain, and dyspnea on exertion. Most are asymptomatic until an episode of sudden death.
- Examination: may have high-frequency systolic ejection murmur at the left lower sternal border while standing, increased with Valsalva, decreased with supine position and squatting.
- Diagnosis: echocardiogram (ventricular septum > 15-mm thick); cardiac magnetic resonance imaging (MRI) with enhancement. The presence of the "athletic heart syndrome" (see Chapter 27) may complicate screening.

Congenital Coronary Artery Anomalies

- Types:
  - Origin of left coronary artery from right sinus of Valsalva
  - Single coronary artery
  - Origin of coronary artery from the pulmonary artery
  - Coronary artery hypoplasia
  - Coronary bridging
- Symptoms: vast majority are asymptomatic; may have exertional chest pain or syncope.
- Diagnosis: angiogram; cardiac MRI.

Marfan Syndrome

- Quick screen for stigmata:
  - Tall stature, arachnodactyly (positive Walker and Steinberg signs), significant pectus carinatum or excavatum, arm span to height ratio greater than 1.05, reduced upper body to lower body ratio of 0.85 or lower, ectopic lens, significant pes planus, scoliosis > 20 degrees, systolic murmur, known family history of Marfan.
- If some characteristics are noted or there is a documented family history, patient should be referred for genetic and cardiovascular screening (including echocardiogram).

Coronary Artery Disease

- Consider exercise stress testing for the following:
  - Asymptomatic male over 45 or female over 55 (15).
  - Those with two or more risk factors: hyperlipidemia, hypertension, smoking, diabetes, personal history of stroke and/or peripheral vascular disease, and family history of heart attack or SCD in a first-degree relative younger than 60 years. An alternative approach might be to select patients with a Framingham risk score consistent with at least a moderate risk of serious cardiac events within 5 years (15).
  - Anyone with angina, syncope, or palpitations, exertional or otherwise.
- Those with a prior history of heart disease should be evaluated by their physician before initiating an exercise program (see Chapters 12 and 21).

Valvular Disorders

- Aortic stenosis:
  - Usually a result of congenital bicuspid valve.
  - This often results in sudden death, with or without exercise.
- Mitral valve prolapse: uncommon cause of SCD.

Cardiac Conduction System Abnormalities

- Idiopathic long QT syndrome
  - QT_c interval > 440 ms
- Wolff-Parkinson-White syndrome (accessory pathway disorder leading to tachyarrhythmias)
- Brugada syndrome (sodium channelopathy)
- Catecholaminergic polymorphic ventricular tachycardia
- All must be suspected in cases of sudden death in which no structural heart problems are found, and all may produce symptoms of palpitations, syncope, or near syncope.

Arrhythmogenic Right Ventricular Cardiomyopathy

- Condition in which normal myocardium is replaced by fibrofatty tissue, leading to arrhythmias that are potentially fatal.
- More common in Mediterranean populations than in the United States; most common cause of SCD in Italy.
- Cause of SCD in 4% of athletes in the United States in a recent study (18).

CLEARANCE

- If a problem is found, the following factors should be considered in deciding whether to clear an athlete to participate:

  - Does the problem place the athlete at increased risk of injury?

  - Is any other participant at risk of injury or illness because of the problem?

  - Can the athlete safely participate with treatment (medication, rehabilitation, bracing, or padding)?

  - Can limited participation be allowed while treatment is being initiated?

- If clearance is denied only for certain activities, in what activities can the athlete safely participate?

- "Medical Conditions Affecting Sports Participation," a policy statement released by the AAP, is a useful guide to help make decisions about clearance (Tables 17.2 and 17.3) (31).

- The article "36th Bethesda Conference: Eligibility Recommendations for Competitive Athletes with Cardiovascular Abnormalities" (26) is a great resource for clearance guidelines for athletes who have congenital heart disease and other cardiovascular abnormalities.

- A clearance form (see Fig. 17.1) is a useful tool to clearly express recommendations regarding clearance.

Table 17.2	The Classification of Sports by Contact	
Contact/Collision	**Limited Contact**	**Noncontact**
Basketball	Baseball	Archery
Boxing	Bicycling	Badminton
Diving	Cheerleading	Body building
Field hockey	Canoeing/kayaking (white water)	Bowling
Football (flag or tackle)	Fencing	Canoeing/kayaking (flat water)
Ice hockey	Field events	Crew/rowing
Lacrosse	High jump	Curling
Martial arts	Pole vault	Dancing
Rodeo	Floor hockey	Field events
Rugby	Gymnastics	Discus
Ski jumping	Handball	Javelin
Soccer	Horseback riding	Shot put
Team handball	Racquetball	Golf
Water polo	Skating	Orienteering
Wrestling	Ice	Power lifting
—	In-line	Race walking
—	Roller	Riflery
—	Skiing	Rope jumping
—	Cross country	Running
—	Downhill	Sailing
—	Water	Scuba diving
—	Softball	Strength training
—	Squash	Swimming
—	Ultimate Frisbee	Table tennis
—	Volleyball	Tennis
—	Windsurfing/surfing	Track
—	—	Weightlifting

SOURCE: American Academy of Pediatrics Committee on Sports Medicine. Recommendations for participation in competitive sports. *Pediatrics*. 1998;81(5):737–9.

Table 17.3	Recommendations Regarding Sports Participation with Common Medical Conditions

Condition	May Participate
Atlantoaxial instability (instability of the joint between cervical vertebrae 1 and 2)	Qualified yes
Explanation: Athlete needs evaluation to assess risk of spinal cord injury during sports participation.	
Bleeding disorder	Qualified yes
Explanation: Athlete needs evaluation.	
Cardiovascular disease	No
Carditis (inflammation of the heart)	
Explanation: Carditis may result in sudden death with exertion.	
Hypertension (high blood pressure)	Qualified yes
Explanation: Those with significant essential (unexplained) hypertension should avoid weight and power lifting, body building, and strength training. Those with secondary hypertension (hypertension caused by a previously identified disease) or severe essential hypertension need evaluation. The National High Blood Pressure Education Working Group (American College of Sports Medicine and American College of Cardiology, 1994) defined significant and severe hypertension.	
Congenital heart disease (structural heart defects present at birth)	Qualified yes
Explanation: Those with mild forms may participate fully; those with moderate or severe forms or who have undergone surgery need evaluation. The 26th Bethesda Conference (Franklin, 1997) defined mild, moderate, and severe disease for common cardiac lesions.	
Dysrhythmia (irregular heart rhythm)	Qualified yes
Explanation: Those with symptoms (chest pain, syncope, dizziness, shortness of breath, or other symptoms of possible dysrhythmia) or evidence of mitral regurgitation (leaking) on physical examination need evaluation. All others may participate fully (Koester and Amundson, 2003).	
Heart murmur	Qualified yes
Explanation: If the murmur is innocent (does not indicate heart disease), full participation is permitted. Otherwise, the athlete needs evaluation (see congenital heart disease and mitral valve prolapse) (Koester and Amundson, 2003).	
Cerebral palsy	Qualified yes
Explanation: Athlete needs evaluation.	
Diabetes mellitus	Yes
Explanation: All sports cart be played with proper attention to diet, blood glucose concentration, hydration, and insulin therapy. Blood glucose concentration should be monitored every 30 minutes during continuous exercise and 15 minutes after completion of exercise.	
Diarrhea	Qualified no
Explanation: Unless disease is mild, no participation is permitted, because diarrhea may increase the risk of dehydration and heat illness (see fever).	
Eating disorders	Qualified yes
Anorexia nervosa	
Bulimia nervosa	
Explanation: Patients with these disorders need medical and psychiatric assessment before participation.	
Eyes	Qualified yes
Functionally one-eyed athlete	
Loss of an eye	
Detached retina	
Previous eye surgery or serious eye injury	
Explanation: A functionally one-eyed athlete has a best-corrected visual acuity of less than 20/40 in the eye with worse acuity. These athletes would suffer significant disability if the better eye were seriously injured, as would those with loss of an eye. Some athletes who previously have undergone eye surgery or had a serious eye injury may have an increased risk of injury because of weakened eye tissue. Availability of eye guards approved by the American Society for Testing and Materials and other protective equipment may allow participation in most sports, but this must be judged on an individual basis (Kurowski and Chandran, 2000; Maron et al, 1996).	

Table 17.3	Recommendations Regarding Sports Participation with Common Medical Conditions (*continued*)
Condition	**May Participate**
Fever	No
Explanation: Fever can increase cardiopulmonary effort, reduce maximum exercise capacity, make heat illness more likely, and increase orthostatic hypertension during exercise. Fever may rarely accompany myocarditis or other infections that may make exercise dangerous.	
Heat illness, history of	Qualified yes
Explanation: Because of the increased likelihood of recurrence, the athlete needs individual assessment to determine the presence of predisposing conditions and to arrange a prevention strategy.	
Hepatitis	Yes
Explanation: Because of the apparent minimal risk to others, all sports may be played that the athlete's state of health allows. In all athletes, skin lesions should be covered properly, and athletic personnel should use universal precautions when handling blood or body fluids with visible blood (Risser et al, 1985).	
Human immunodeficiency virus infection	Yes
Explanation: Because of the apparent minimal risk to others, all sports may be played that the athlete's state of health allows. In all athletes, skin lesions should be covered properly, and athletic personnel should use universal precautions when handling blood or body fluids with visible blood (Risser et al, 1985).	
Kidney, absence of one	Qualified yes
Explanation: Athlete needs individual assessment for contact, collision, and limited contact sports.	
Liver, enlarged	Qualified yes
Explanation: If the liver is acutely enlarged, participation should be avoided because of risk of rupture. If the liver is chronically enlarged, individual assessment is needed before collision, contact, or limited contact sports are played.	
Malignant neoplasm	Qualified yes
Explanation: Athlete needs individual assessment.	
Musculoskeletal disorders	Qualified yes
Explanation: Athlete needs individual assessment.	
Neurologic disorders	
History of serious head or spine trauma, severe or repeated concussions, or craniotomy (Sallis, 1996; Smith and Laskowski, 1998).	Qualified yes
Explanation: Athlete needs individual assessment for collision, contact, or limited contact sports and also for noncontact sports if deficits in judgment or cognition are present. Research supports a conservative approach to management of concussion (Sallis, 1996; Smith and Laskowski, 1998).	
Seizure disorder, well-controlled	Yes
Explanation: Risk of seizure during participation is minimal.	
Seizure disorder, poorly controlled	Qualified yes
Explanation: Athlete needs individual assessment for collision, contact, or limited contact sports. The following noncontact sports should be avoided: archery, riflery, swimming, weight or power lifting, strength training, or sports involving heights. In these sports, occurrence of a seizure may pose a risk to self or others.	
Obesity	Qualified yes
Explanation: Because of the risk of heat illness, obese persons need careful acclimatization and hydration.	
Organ transplant recipient	Qualified yes
Explanation: Athlete needs individual assessment.	
Ovary, absence of one	Yes
Explanation: Risk of severe injury to the remaining ovary is minimal.	
Respiratory conditions	
Pulmonary compromise, including cystic fibrosis	Qualified yes
Explanation: Athlete needs individual assessment, but generally, all sports may be played if oxygenation remains satisfactory during a graded exercise test. Patients with cystic fibrosis need acclimatization and good hydration to reduce the risk of heat illness.	

(*Continued*)

Table 17.3	Recommendations Regarding Sports Participation with Common Medical Conditions (*continued*)
Condition	**May Participate**
Asthma	Yes
Explanation: With proper medication and education, only athletes with the most severe asthma will need to modify their participation.	
Acute upper respiratory infection	Qualified yes
Explanation: Upper respiratory obstruction may affect pulmonary function. Athlete needs individual assessment for all but mild disease (see fever).	
Sickle cell disease	Qualified yes
Explanation: Athlete needs individual assessment. In general, if status of the illness permits, all but high exertion, collision, and contact sports may be played. Overheating, dehydration, and chilling must be avoided.	
Sickle cell trait	Yes
Explanation: It is unlikely that persons with sickle cell trait have an increased risk of sudden death or other medical problems during athletic participation, except under the most extreme conditions of heat, humidity, and possibly increased altitude (Tanner, 1994). These persons, like all athletes, should be carefully conditioned, acclimatized, and hydrated to reduce any possible risk.	
Skin disorders (boils, herpes simplex, impetigo, scabies, molluscum contagiosum)	Qualified yes
Explanation: While the patient is contagious, participation in gymnastics with mats; martial arts; wrestling; or other collision, contact, or limited contact sports is not allowed.	
Spleen, enlarged	Qualified yes
Explanation: A patient with an acutely enlarged spleen should avoid all sports because of risk of rupture. A patient with a chronically enlarged spleen needs individual assessment before playing collision, contact, or limited contact sports.	
Testicle, undescended or absence of one	Yes
Explanation: Certain sports may require a protective cup.	

SOURCE: American Academy of Pediatrics Committee on Sports Medicine. Recommendations for participation in competitive sports. *Pediatrics*. 1998;81(5):737–9. Those listed with a "qualified" yes or no require individual assessment.

REFERENCES

1. American Academy of Family Physicians, American Academy of Pediatrics, American Medical Society for Sports Medicine, American Orthopedic Society for Sports Medicine, and American Osteopathic Academy of Sports Medicine. *Preparticipation Physical Evaluation*. 4th ed. Elk Grove Village (IL): American Academy of Pediatrics; 2010. 160 p.

2. American Academy of Pediatrics. Medical conditions affecting sports participation. Committee on Sports Medicine and Fitness. *Pediatrics*. 1994;94(5):757–60.

3. Asif I, Harmon K, Drezner J, Klossner D. Incidence and etiology of sudden death in NCAA athletes. *Clin J Sports Med*. 2010;20:136.

4. Atkins DL, Everson-Stewart S, Sears GK, et al. Epidemiology and outcomes from out-of-hospital cardiac arrest in children: the Resuscitation Outcomes Consortium Epistry-Cardiac Arrest. *Circulation*. 2009;119(11):1484–91.

5. Baggish AL, Hutter AM, Wang F, et al. Cardiovascular screening in college athletes with and without electrocardiography. *Ann Intern Med*. 2010;152(5):269–75.

6. Borjesson M, Pellicia A. Incidence and aetiology of sudden cardiac death in young athletes: an international perspective. *Br J Sports Med*. 2009;43(9):644–8.

7. Capão-Filipe M, Moreira A, Delgado L, Rodrigues J, Vaz M. Exercise-induced bronchoconstriction and respiratory symptoms in elite athletes. *Allergy*. 2003;58(11):1196.

8. Chobanian AV, Bakris GL, Black HR, et al. The Seventh Report of the Joint National Committee on Prevention, Detection, Evaluation, and Treatment of High Blood Pressure: the JNC 7 report. *JAMA*. 2003; 289(19):2560–72.

9. Chugh SS, Reiner K, Balaji S, et al. Population-based analysis of sudden death in children: the Oregon Sudden Unexpected Death Study. *Heart Rhythm*. 2009;6(11):1618–22.

10. Corrado D, Basso C, Pavei A, Michieli P, Schiavon M, Thiene G. Trends in sudden cardiovascular death in young competitive athletes after implementation of a preparticipation screening program. *JAMA*. 2006;296(13): 1593–1601.

11. Corrado D, Basso C, Rizzoli G, et al. Does sports activity enhance the risk of sudden death in adolescents and young Adults? *J Am Coll Cardiol*. 2003;42(11):1959–63.

12. Drezner JA, Rao AL, Heistand J, Bloomingdale MK, Harmon KG. Effectiveness of emergency response planning for sudden cardiac arrest in United States high schools with automated external defibrillators. *Circulation*. 2009;120(6):518–25.

13. Drezner JA, Rogers KJ, Zimmer RR, Sennett BJ. Use of automated external defibrillators at NCAA division I universities. *Med Sci Sports Exerc*. 2005;37(9):1487–92.

14. Eckart RE, Scoville SL, Campbell CL, et al. Sudden death in young adults: a 25-year review of autopsies in military recruits. *Ann Intern Med*. 2004;141(11):829–34.

15. Gibbons RJ, Balady GJ, Beasley JW, et al. ACC/AHA 2002 update for exercise testing: a report of the American College of Cardiology/American

Heart Association Task Force on Practice Guidelines (Committee on Exercise Testing) [Internet]. 2011 [cited 2011 Feb 3]. Available from: http://www.americanheart.org/downloadable/heart/1032279013658exercise.pdf.

16. Hammerman SI, Becker JM, Rogers J, Quedenfeld TC, D'Alonzo GE Jr. Asthma screening of high school athletes: identifying the undiagnosed and poorly controlled. *Ann Allergy Asthma Immunol.* 2002;88:380–4.

17. Kurowski K, Chandran S. The preparticipation athletic evaluation. *Am Fam Physician.* 2000;61(9):2683–90, 2696–8.

18. Maron BJ. Hypertrophic cardiomyopathy. *Lancet.* 1997;350(9071): 127–33.

19. Maron BJ. Sudden death in young athletes. *N Engl J Med.* 2003;349(11): 1064–75.

20. Maron BJ, Doerer JJ, Hass TS, Tierney DM, Mueller FO. Sudden deaths in young competitive athletes: analysis of 1866 deaths in the United States, 1980–2006. *Circulation.* 2009;119(8):1085–92.

21. Maron BJ, Gohman TE, Aeppli D. Prevalence of sudden cardiac death during competitive sports activities in Minnesota high school athletes. *J Am Coll Cardiol.* 1998;32(7):1881–4.

22. Maron BJ, Roberts WC, Epstein SC. Sudden death in hypertrophic cardiomyopathy: a profile of 78 patients. *Circulation.* 1982;65(7):1388–94.

23. Maron BJ, Seidman JG, Seidman CE. Proposal for comtemporary screening strategies in families with hypertrophic cardiomyopathy. *J Am Coll Cardiol.* 2004;44(11):2125–32.

24. Maron BJ, Shirani J, Poliac LC, Mathenge R, Roberts WC, Mueller FO. Sudden death in young competitive athletes. Clinical, demographic, and pathological profiles. *JAMA.* 1996;276(3):199–204.

25. Maron BJ, Thompson PD, Ackerman MJ, et al. American Heart Association Council on Nutrition, Physical Activity, and Metabolism. Recommendations and considerations related to preparticipation screening for cardiovascular abnormalities in competitive athletes: 2007 update: a scientific statement from the American Heart Association Council on Nutrition, Physical Activity, and Metabolism: endorsed by the American College of Cardiology Foundation. *Circulation.* 2007;115(12):1643–55.

26. Maron BJ, Zipes DP. 36th Bethesda Conference: eligibility recommendations for competitive athletes with cardiovascular abnormalities. *J Am Coll Cardiol.* 2005;45(8):1317–75.

27. McKenzie DC, Fitch KD. The asthmatic athlete: inhaled beta-2 agonists, sport performance, and doping. *Clin J Sport Med.* 2011;21(1): 46–50.

28. NCAA Sports Medicine Handbook 2010–2011 [Internet]. 21st ed. Indianapolis (IN): 2010 [cited 2011 Jan 30]. Available from: http://www.ncaapublications.com/productdownloads/MD11.pdf.

29. Pelliccia A, Di Paolo FM, Corrado D, et al. Evidence for efficacy of the Italian national pre-participation screening programme for identification of hypertrophic cardiomyopathy in competitive athletes. *Eur Heart J.* 2006;27(18):2196–200.

30. Pelliccia A, Maron B. Preparticipation cardiovascular evaluation of the competitive athlete: perspectives from the 30-year Italian experience. *Am J Cardiol.* 1995;75(12):827–9.

31. Rice SG, American Academy of Pediatrics Council on Sports Medicine and Fitness. Medical conditions affecting sports participation. *Pediatrics.* 2008;121(4):841–8.

32. Rundell KW, Im J, Mayers LB, Wilbur RL, Szmedra L, Schmitz HR. Self reported symptoms and exercise-induced asthma in an elite athlete population. *Med Sci Sports Exerc.* 2001;33(2):208–13.

33. Sport Concussion Assessment Tool 2, adapted from the 3rd International Consensus Meeting on Concussion in Sport held in Zurich, Switzerland in November 2008. *Br J Sports Med.* 2009;43(Suppl 1).

34. U.S. Department of Health and Human Services, National Institutes of Health, National Heart, Lung, and Blood Institute. The fourth report on the diagnosis, evaluation, and treatment of high blood pressure in children and adolescents [Internet]. Revised May 2005. 2011 [cited 2011 Feb 3]. Available from: http://www.nhlbi.nih.gov/health/prof/heart/hbp/hbp_ped.pdf.

35. Valovich McLeod TC, Bay RC, Heil J, McVeigh SD. Identification of sport and recreational activity concussion history through the preparticipation screening and a symptom survey in young athletes. *Clin J Sports Med.* 2008;18(3):235–40.

36. Van Camp SP, Bloor CM, Mueller FO, Cantu RC, Olson HG. Nontraumatic sports death in high school and college athletes. *Med Sci Sports Exerc.* 2005;27(5):641–7.

37. Wilson MG, Basavarajaiah S, Whyte GP, Cox S, Loosemore M, Sharma S. Efficacy of personal symptom and family history questionnaires when screening for inherited cardiac pathologies: the role of electrocardiography. *Br J Sports Med.* 2008;42(3):207–11.

38. World Anti-Doping Agency Web site [Internet]. Montreal, Canada. World Anti-Doping Agency; 2011 Prohibited List [cited 2011 Jan 30]. Available from: http://www.wada-ama.org.

18 Diagnostic Imaging

Leanne L. Seeger and Kambiz Motamedi

INTRODUCTION

- There are several modalities available for the imaging evaluation of sports injuries. The strengths and weaknesses of each modality, along with their specific indications are discussed in this chapter.
- The choice of the imaging modality depends on several factors, including the anatomic location of interest, chronicity of the symptoms, suspected pathology, and potential treatment alternatives. Guidelines for "what to use when" can be found on the American College of Radiology Web site "ACR Appropriateness Criteria" under Musculoskeletal Imaging at: http://www.acr.org/SecondaryMainMenuCategories/quality_safety/app_criteria.aspx.

IMAGING MODALITIES

- Imaging tools that are commonly available are plain radiography (with or without applied stress), conventional arthrography, magnetic resonance imaging (MRI), which may be combined with arthrography, computed tomography (CT), which may be combined with arthrography, ultrasonography (US), and radionuclide bone scans. Over the past several years, US has gained substantial popularity in sports medicine imaging. Radionuclide bone scans have diminished in popularity, having been largely replaced by MRI.

MODALITY STRENGTHS AND WEAKNESSES

- *Plain radiography* is widely available, relatively inexpensive, and provides excellent detail of bony structures and soft tissue calcifications. Although resolution has improved with digital radiography, the ability of radiography to depict soft tissue pathology remains far inferior to cross-sectional imaging (MRI, CT, and US).
- *Stress radiography* (*e.g.*, varus or valgus) reveals abnormal laxity of joints and can indirectly diagnose soft tissue injury. Stress must be applied by the referring physician.

Disadvantages include availability of the physician, radiation exposure, and subjectivity of the amount of stress needed. In some cases, it may exacerbate underlying pathology. For subtle cases, comparison with the contralateral side may be needed. Consequently, indirect evaluation of soft tissue injury with stress radiography has been replaced by MRI and US.

- *Arthrography* delineates the synovial space and intraarticular structures by joint distention. Although invasive, there are few inherent risks. Arthrography requires patient preparation and cooperation, informed consent, and the availability of a radiologist. Prior to the advent of cross-sectional imaging (MRI and CT), conventional arthrography was popular, consisting of a fluoroscopically guided injection of iodinated contrast and/or air, followed by spot imaging during provocative maneuvering. This procedure is now rarely done in isolation, having been supplanted with injection of dilute gadolinium for magnetic resonance arthrography or, less commonly, dilute iodinated contrast for CT arthrography when there is a contraindication to MRI (*e.g.*, cardiac pacemaker). For both of these procedures, coordination is needed for scheduling scanner time to immediately follow the procedure.
- *MRI* provides unparalleled soft tissue and bone marrow contrast. Soft tissue, marrow, and/or even periosteal edema is readily seen, even when subtle. MRI will demonstrate an early stress reaction of bone when plain radiographs and CT are normal. Structural abnormalities depicted with MRI include ligament and tendon tears, as well as the amount of retraction. There are several relative and absolute contraindications to MRI, including claustrophobia, cardiac pacemakers, certain kinds of neurosurgical aneurysmal clips, and inner ear implants. Although there is a plethora of pulse sequences that can be used with MRI, four are the mainstay of musculoskeletal imaging; T1, proton density (PD), T2, and inversion recovery (IR). T1, PD, and T2 sequences fall under the category of "spin echo" imaging. T1-weighted imaging displays anatomy. Fat (including fatty bone marrow) appears with high signal intensity, or bright; muscles appear with intermediate signal intensity; and cortex, tendons, and ligaments appear with low signal intensity, or dark. T2-weighted (usually undertaken with fat suppression) and IR imaging highlights tissues with increased water content, displaying them as bright. By suppressing fat signal (turning it dark),

T2 and IR imaging obscures normal anatomy but highlights edema and tears of muscles, tendons, and ligaments. Hematomas and most tumors also appear primarily bright, while surrounding normal tissue is dark. PD imaging takes advantage of both of these techniques by demonstrating anatomy but highlighting certain types of pathology. A primary role for PD scans in musculoskeletal imaging is for detection of meniscal pathology. Another technique called gradient recalled echo imaging is useful for demonstrating blood products and has been shown useful in imaging glenoid and acetabular labral pathology. Diffusion tensor imaging (DTI) is a newer technique that is commonly used in neuroimaging. In combination with the previously mentioned methods, DTI is proving to be an effective tool for assessing the severity of cerebral concussion, including minor head injury.

■ *CT* is superior to other modalities for fine bone detail and is an important tool for depicting the anatomy of complex fractures such as around the knee, hip, elbow, and shoulder. Newer generation multislice scanners have significantly diminished acquisition time and artifact and are capable of submillimeter slice thickness. CT is often used as a surrogate for MRI, in cases where MRI is contraindicated. Volumetric image acquisition enables rapid data reformation into not only standard axial, sagittal, and coronal planes, but also any obliquity desired to optimize depiction of anatomy. Reconstruction artifact commonly encountered with older scanners is far less of a problem with newer generation scanners. Disadvantages of CT are limited soft tissue contrast and radiation dose. To minimize radiation, scanning should be coned as tightly as possible to the area of interest.

■ Although popular in Europe and Asia for over three decades, musculoskeletal US was slow to be widely accepted in the United States. However, that has dramatically changed. Portable US equipment is now common at sporting events to provide a rapid assessment of injury severity and clearly competes with MRI in evaluation of muscle, tendon, and ligament injuries. One of the strengths of US lies in its ability to acquire dynamic images, depicting soft tissue structures while in motion. A normal control is readily available by acquiring images from the contralateral side. There is direct patient contact of the sonographer, facilitating immediate customization of the exam to the patient's symptoms. The major disadvantage is that US is strongly operator dependent, requiring intense training with extensive hands-on experience for competency. US does not provide adequate resolution of intraarticular structures.

■ *Radionuclide bone scanning* with technetium-99m methylene diphosphonate (Tc-99m MDP) is extremely sensitive for detecting areas of increased bone turnover. However, it is nonspecific, and traumatic lesions cannot be differentiated from inflammation or neoplasia. Correlation with plain films is usually needed. Bone scans also have poor spatial resolution, which may be improved by either obtaining oblique projections or using *single photon emission computed tomography* (SPECT). SPECT imaging produces multiplanar tomographic slices similar to CT and MRI, allowing precise localization of foci of abnormal tracer activity in complex structures such as the spine. The triple-phase (three-phase) bone scan includes an angiogram acquired at the time of tracer injection, a blood-pool phase within 5 minutes of injection, and 3-hour delayed (static) images. This technique assists in differentiating soft tissue from bone pathology. Soft tissue abnormalities generally show preferential uptake on the first two phases, whereas bone pathology should show increased activity on all three phases. For single- or triple-phase bone scans, pinhole collimation should be used for small parts such as feet and hands to provide magnification and increased spatial resolution. Over the past years, MRI has largely replaced radionuclide bone scans.

SPECIFIC USES OF DIFFERENT MODALITIES

■ *Radiography* should usually be used for the initial assessment of an acute traumatic event to assess for fracture and/or alignment abnormality. In the case of chronic disorders, radiographs can eliminate alternate diagnoses, such as arthritis or neoplasia. Radiography is also the standard method for following fracture healing and alignment abnormalities (subluxation or dislocation).

■ *Stress radiography* may find its niche in cases of chronic trauma with instability and suspected soft tissue injury. It has, however, been widely replaced by MRI and/or US.

■ *Arthrography* is used when joint distention is required for lesion detection. This may include cases of cartilage injury, labral or meniscal pathology, capsular tears, and intraarticular loose bodies.

■ *MRI* is used for suspected bone or soft tissue injury, especially when plain radiographs are normal. Indications for magnetic resonance arthrography include glenoid or acetabular labral tears, low-grade *superior labrum anterior-posterior* (SLAP) lesions, evaluating for retear of a repaired knee meniscus, and detection of noncalcified intraarticular loose bodies. MRI may also be useful in evaluation of pars defects of the spine, showing edema at sites of abnormal motion.

■ *CT* is indicated for demonstrating the extent and anatomy of fractures. It is especially useful with complex pelvic trauma, where plain radiography is limited and the pelvic three-dimensional architecture is complex. It is also useful for evaluation of complex elbow trauma, another joint that is difficult to depict three dimensionally with plain film. CT with multiplanar reformations provides an excellent road map for the surgeon in planning the appropriate operation. CT is also used for intra- versus extraarticular localization of periarticular mineralization seen on plain film and is well suited for demonstrating calcifications associated with ligaments and tendons. This latter finding is often associated with chronic injury. CT is useful for demonstrating pars defects but does not assist in determining if the defect may be the source of pain.

■ *US* is extremely useful when dynamic imaging is desired, as in cases with snapping ankle and hip tendons. It is sensitive in demonstrating minute calcium deposits and tiny abnormal fluid collections in and around tendons and ligaments. Mobile units allow immediate field-side evaluation of injured athletes for tendon tears, muscle strains, and hematomas. US is also gaining popularity as a device to guide diagnostic and therapeutic interventional procedures, including cyst aspiration and steroid and/or anesthetic injections around tendons.

■ *Radionuclide bone scans* are useful primarily for localizing the site of bone pathology in cases where symptoms are diffuse. In lesions such as pars defects, a bone scan done with SPECT will show if the lesion is associated with abnormal activity, implying an active and likely symptomatic lesion. It also provides information about the chronicity of an abnormality, because acute lesions show intense tracer accumulation and more chronic quiescent conditions appear more normal.

CONSIDERATIONS

■ Considering that different modalities have differing sensitivity to demonstrate certain pathology, it becomes evident that clinical information is paramount in not only deciding which method to use, but also in tailoring the imaging study to the patient's specific needs.

■ Clinical information also helps to choose the correct modality for acute versus overuse injury. In both cases, one should usually begin with plain radiography. In cases of normal radiographs and suspected acute bone injury, one may choose to obtain an MRI to evaluate edema and a possible nondisplaced fracture. MRI is also useful for more chronic injuries where a soft tissue abnormality is suspected. Complex acute fractures should be evaluated with CT if further imaging is needed.

■ The choice of imaging modality also depends on the level of the patient's activity. In the case of an elite athlete where the decision of return to play is important, one may choose to obtain MRI or US immediately after obtaining radiographs.

TISSUE OF INTEREST

■ *Bone* is the fundamental scaffolding of the musculoskeletal system and plays a central role in diagnostic imaging. With MRI, marrow edema in the context of an injury indicates at a minimum trabecular trauma and contusion. Specific patterns of marrow edema may prompt a closer search for injury to specific soft tissue structures. In the knee, for example, marrow edema in the posterior tibia and the lateral femoral condyle at the sulcus terminalis has a high association with an acute anterior cruciate ligament tear.

■ *Cartilage* outlines the bony surfaces of the joints. As a shock absorber, it is prone to wear and tear as well as acute injuries. Acute chondral fractures, often with an adjacent bone fragment (osteochondral fracture), are common in sports medicine. Cartilage is not directly visible with plain radiography; however, an initial evaluation of cartilage thickness may be performed with plain radiography to assess joint space narrowing. MRI, on the other hand, not only demonstrates acute injuries to the osteochondral unit, but also nicely shows intrinsic signal abnormalities of cartilage due to wear and tear (chondromalacia). MRI can also evaluate cartilage for focal areas of thinning, fissuring, and ulceration. One of the more common areas of interest for cartilage evaluation is the anterior knee for chondromalacia patellae. With newer high-field MRI scanners (3 T and greater), detailed evaluation of joint surfaces rarely requires arthrography.

■ Joint-stabilizing *ligaments* and *tendons* and the dynamic *muscle* and tendon units are prone to injuries. Certain sports are associated with specific injury patterns. The examples are innumerable, including jumper's knee (patellar tendon), tennis leg (plantaris tendon and/or gastrocnemius muscle), and tennis or golfer's elbow (collateral ligament). If plain films are normal or equivocal, MRI will provide the necessary soft tissue resolution for diagnosis. The spectrum of findings ranges from mild edema to hematoma, partial tear, and complete disruption. With experience, US is a viable alternative for evaluation of the more superficial tendons and muscles, especially around the elbow and ankle.

■ *Bursae* are fluid-filled structures with synovial linings that act as cushions at foci of increased motion or friction. They are classically found between bones and tendons or muscles and skin but can form anywhere protection is needed (adventitial bursa). Inherent to their function, bursae are prone to inflammation, especially in cases with overuse. MRI is excellent for demonstrating inflamed and fluid-filled bursal structures. US is suitable for detecting superficial fluid collections and possibly hyperemia in an inflamed superficial bursa. US may also provide guidance for therapeutic injections.

ACUTE INJURY VERSUS OVERUSE

■ Plain radiography is usually used to evaluate for acute fracture. With chronic complaints or overuse, plain films provide an effective screening tool for arthritis, inflammatory processes, and musculoskeletal tumors. Plain films may be helpful in demonstrating acute or chronic joint effusions (*e.g.,* knee and elbow) by demonstrating a soft tissue density displacing normal fat planes. In cases of chronic injuries, calcifications are easily seen with radiography. Plain films are also used to evaluate for periosteal new bone formation, abnormal bone sclerosis, and callus formation.

■ If plain films are deemed to be normal and symptoms warrant, MRI is usually the next modality undertaken. With chronic or overuse disorders, stress reaction or fracture will appear on MRI as edema in bone marrow, possibly with immature periosteal new bone formation. Focal abnormalities are also evident in muscles, tendons, and ligaments. When the suspicion of an acute fracture is high and plain films are normal, MRI will detect radiographically occult fractures. This is especially important in weight-bearing bones such as the tibial plateau and proximal femur. Early diagnosis can prevent fragment displacement with activity.

- If a patient's symptoms persist after adequate conservative treatment or seem out of proportion to the clinical setting, additional imaging is warranted. It is not uncommon for bone and soft tissue tumors to be initially diagnosed as a hematoma or muscle strain. Any palpable mass diagnosed as a hematoma should be followed clinically to maturation or resolution.

CHRONIC SEQUELAE TO TRAUMA

- Areas of prior hemorrhage, hematoma, or inflammation may undergo transformation into mature bone. This phenomenon is called heterotopic ossification. The term myositis ossificans has fallen out of favor, because this is not an inflammatory process of the muscles. Plain radiography and CT play a crucial role in recognizing this entity. The finding of peripheral calcification around a soft tissue mass is the hallmark of this entity. This is contrary to mineralized tumors such as osteosarcoma, where the osteoid is situated centrally. Unfortunately, these two entities may be confused histologically. With maturation, the mineralization of heterotopic ossification will often completely ossify with marrow induction centrally and cortex peripherally. An area of heterotopic ossification immediately adjacent to bone may result from an avulsion injury. This is termed periostitis ossificans.

- Calcific deposits may be seen not only in tendons and ligaments, but also in chronic inflammation of a bursa (calcific bursitis). These calcifications are usually hydroxyapatite bound and have a pasty appearance. They may be linear or globular. Depending on the location of the symptoms, radiographs, CT, or US may be used for diagnosis.

SITE-SPECIFIC PLAIN RADIOGRAPHY: STANDARD AND SPECIAL VIEWS

- Each institution has its own set of plain film series, and as such, it is useful to know what views are included in a given radiologic examination. The referring physician may then request a specific view that may be useful for the diagnosis of the suspected pathology, or the radiologist may add a study or vary the study according to the initial findings and the pathology suspected. In the setting of acute joint trauma, a three-view minimum is usually required. Two perpendicular views suffice for the long bone shafts, and two views are usually adequate for fracture follow-up.

Shoulder

- Internal and external rotation views in the anteroposterior (AP) projection are included in most shoulder series. Axillary and transscapular Y views are common third projections obtained and are needed for a perpendicular view of the glenoid. Grashey, outlet (caudally angulated transscapular), and West Point views may be obtained for evaluation of the glenohumeral joint space, anterior acromial shape and subacromial space, and anteroinferior glenoid rim, respectively.

Elbow

- AP and lateral views are standard. The lateral view should be obtained with the elbow in 90 degrees of flexion to allow detection of an elbow joint effusion. Displacement of the fat pads around the joint by intraarticular fluid or blood may be the only evidence of a nondisplaced fracture. Bilateral oblique views are helpful to depict soft tissue calcifications or acute fracture, and an angulated radial head view may show a nondisplaced fracture.

Hand/Wrist

- Posteroanterior (PA), lateral, and oblique views usually constitute a hand series. The basic wrist series consists of four projections, those above coned to the wrist, as well as a scaphoid view to lay the bone out on its long axis. The carpal tunnel view will show fractures of the hook of the hamate or the pisiform bone, and ulnar and radial deviation views may reveal widening of the scapholunate or lunotriquetral space, implying a ligament tear.

Cervical/Lumbar Spine

- AP and lateral views are the basic series, and oblique views are obtained to evaluate the neural foramina in the cervical spine and the facets in the lumbar spine. Lateral flexion and extension views may be added to evaluate for instability. When obtaining flexion/extension images, the patient should provide range of motion independently and never be forced into position. This is especially true in the setting of acute trauma. In the cervical spine, the open mouth view shows alignment of the first two vertebral segment lateral masses and the odontoid base. The Fuchs view shows the odontoid tip. The swimmer's view shows the lower cervical and upper thoracic segments that may be obscured by shoulder soft tissues on the conventional lateral projection. In the lumbar spine, a coned lateral view of the LS–S1 disc is often useful, and this level is subject to distortion from beam angulation on the standard lateral lumbar film.

Thoracic Spine

- AP and lateral views are standard. A swimmer's view is frequently obtained to evaluate the upper thoracic segments. Oblique views of the thoracic spine add no useful information. The thoracic facets are best assessed with CT.

Pelvis

- The most common view of the pelvis is the AP projection. Inlet/outlet and bilateral Judet (lateral oblique) views may also be obtained, but these are usually reserved for significant pelvic trauma. The PA view is preferred over an AP projection for imaging the sacroiliac (SI) joints because of their oblique orientation. This allows the x-ray beam to travel down the axis joint and minimizes overlap of the cortices of the lower synovial portion of the articulation. It should be coned to the SI joints and sacrum. The PA projection of both joints may be combined with oblique views of each side, oriented down the long axis of the joint.

Hip

- AP and frog-leg lateral views are standard. Although these provide two views of the proximal femur, they show the acetabulum in only one projection. A true acetabular lateral may be obtained with an axial lateral view.

Knee

- AP, lateral, and patellar views are standard for the plain radiographic series. Except in the setting of acute trauma where fracture is of clinical concern, these should be obtained in the upright position. In acute trauma, the lateral view should be positioned in a cross-table manner to allow demonstration of a lipohemarthrosis, a sign of an articular fracture. The patellar view (sunrise or Merchant) is obtained with the knee flexed, usually oriented superior-to-inferior. This shows the patellofemoral compartment to best advantage. Additional options for knee imaging include the flexed PA view. This gives insight into the intercondylar notch and may be more sensitive than the fully extended upright position for detecting early joint space narrowing. The flexed PA view can also be used to look for acute or chronic osteochondral lesions of the femoral condyles. Oblique views can be helpful to demonstrate a nondisplaced tibial plateau fracture.

Ankle/Foot

- AP, lateral, and oblique views are usually obtained. As with the knee, the images should be taken upright except when an acute fracture is suspected. Alignment abnormalities require weight bearing for proper evaluation. If a subtle Lisfranc injury is suspected, weight-bearing AP films of both feet may be needed to evaluate for mild widening through comparison with the uninjured side. The Harris view provides a perpendicular projection of the calcaneus. Coalitions are often only seen on an oblique view of the foot.

CONCLUSION

- When dealing with the athlete, plain radiography is usually the first imaging study that should be performed. This holds true whether dealing with an acute injury or overuse.
- MRI is preferred for the diagnosis of radiographically occult bone injury and soft tissue trauma, be it acute or chronic. This is not an urgent examination unless one is dealing with an elite athlete where return to play is an issue or there is concern for a radiographically occult fracture in a weight-bearing bone.
- US is a viable alternative to MRI for evaluation of superficial soft tissues, but it requires an experienced operator.
- CT is preferred for complex bone trauma.
- The clinical history will affect both image acquisition and interpretation. Open communication between clinician and radiologist is essential for optimal patient care.

SUGGESTED READING

1. Allen GM, Wilson DJ. Ultrasound in sports medicine — a critical evaluation. *Eur J Radiol.* 2007;62(1):79–85.
2. Brittenden J, Robinson P. Imaging of pelvic injuries in athletes. *Br J Radiol.* 2005;78(929):457–68.
3. Cubon VA, Putukian M, Boyer C, Dettwiler A. A diffusion tensor imaging study on the white matter skeleton in individuals with sports-related concussion. *J Neurotrauma.* 2011;28(2):189–201.
4. Healy JC, Lee JC. Sports injury of the lower extremity: role of imaging in diagnosis and management. *Semin Musculoskelet Radiol.* 2011; 15(1):1–2.
5. Khoury V, Guillin R, Dhanju J, Cardinal E. Ultrasound of ankle and foot: overuse and sports injuries. *Semin Musculoskelet Radiol.* 2007;11(2):149–61.
6. Parker BJ, Zlatkin MB, Newman JS, Rathur SK. Imaging of shoulder injuries in sports medicine: current protocols and concepts. *Clin Sports Med.* 2008;27(4):579–606.
7. Raissaki M, Apostolaki E, Karantanas AH. Imaging of sports injuries in children and adolescents. *Eur J Radiol.* 2007;62(1):86–96.
8. Robinson P. *Essential Radiology for Sports Medicine.* New York (NY): Springer; 2010. 268 p.
9. Sanchez TRS, Jadhav SP, Swischuk LE. MR imaging of pediatric trauma. *Radiol Clin N Am.* 2009;47(6):927–38.
10. Smits M, Houston GC, Dippel DW, et al. Microstructural brain injury in post-concussion syndrome after minor head injury. *Neuroradiology.* 2011;53(8):553–63.
11. Torriani M, Kattapuram SV. Musculoskeletal ultrasound: an alternative imaging modality for sports-related injuries. *Top Magn Reson Imaging.* 2003;14(1):103–11.

Musculoskeletal Ultrasound

Sean W. Mulvaney and Sean N. Martin

INTRODUCTION

- Musculoskeletal (MSK) ultrasound (US) is a rapidly emerging imaging modality in the field of sports medicine. It is a powerful tool in both the diagnosis and management of the injured athlete. MSK US is unique in that it provides previously unavailable point-of-care diagnostic imaging, completed by the clinician, and with the patient still in the examination room (3). This technology is the result of continued improvement of broadband high-frequency transducers and new developments in signal-processing software that have improved the image quality for evaluating MSK structures (10).
- Advantages of US imaging:
  - Portable, point-of-care imaging.
  - Direct, dynamic visualization of injured structure, aiding in a pathoanatomic diagnosis:
    - Many pathologic conditions are only apparent while a structure is in motion.
    - Magnetic resonance imaging (MRI) only allows the injured tissue to be viewed in one position.
  - Relatively inexpensive.
  - Focus: able to focus on the area of interest to a degree not possible with MRI.
  - Side-to-side comparison views are simple to obtain for anatomic variants/growth plate comparison.
  - Low-risk visualization of soft tissue and superficial bone:
    - No risk associated with iodinated contrast.
    - No risk associated with MRI contrast (*i.e.*, gadopentetate dimeglumine contrast resulting in gadolinium-associated nephrogenic systemic fibrosis).
    - No risks associated with ionizing radiation.
  - Ability to accurately image soft tissue structures despite metallic implants.
  - Immediate correlation of imaging with history and physical.
  - Superior imaging modality for peripheral nerve pathology (6,12).
  - Real-time visualization, allowing accurate percutaneous procedures.
    - Increases accuracy of medication placement.
    - Allows determination of the exact pain generator in cases when multiple pathologic structures are visualized.

- Disadvantages of US imaging:
  - Significant time, effort, and cost investment to become proficient.
    - Many providers initially rely upon attendance at dedicated MSK US courses to learn directly from industry leaders.
  - Although US can rule-in a fracture, it can neither rule-out nor characterize a fracture.
  - Due to reliance on direct visualization, US can be hindered by intervening bony structures. Intraarticular pathology is incompletely visible on US exam.
  - Labral pathology is incompletely visible on US.
  - Even if a surgical lesion is identifiable on US, many orthopedic surgeons are more comfortable with MRI imaging to justify surgery, for presurgery planning, and for use as a reference during surgery.
  - US is more limited with obese patients.

PHYSICS

- The US image is the product of sound waves that have been emitted by piezoelectric crystals on the US transducer, passed through tissues, some of which are reflected back to the transducer.
- Echo signature of bone, ligaments, tendons, muscles, and other soft tissues is based on the degree of absorption versus reflection of the sound waves.
- The US image is based on reflected sound or US waves. The processor translates the echo signatures of the US waves into a real-time two-dimensional image.
- Attenuation is the name for all interactions that decrease the intensity of the US beam except reflection. Attenuation includes the effects of scattering and absorption that reduce the US wave amplitude.
- Constant = frequency $\times$ wavelength:
  - The constant used is the velocity of sound in tissue (dermis, adipose, muscle, tendon, cartilage, and ligament), approximately 1,540 meters per second.
  - Because the position of any object measured with US can be determined only to an accuracy of about one wavelength, the limitation on image resolution is imposed by wavelength.

- The resolution required in diagnostic US is 1 mm or less.
  - ❏ Therefore: frequency = constant/wavelength
    - Frequency (MHz) = 1,540 meters per second · 0.001 m
    - 1.54×10^6 meters per second = 1.54 MHz = the minimum usable frequency for MSK US applications, which will yield a resolution of about 1 mm before significant attenuation degrades this.
- US technology allows for a degree of lateral resolution, which is defined as the ability to visualize and differentiate structures parallel to the transducer footprint and determined by:
  - Hardware: Chiefly the number of sound-emitting crystals on the transducer. This is a fixed number determined at the time the transducer is manufactured. The number of crystals determines the potential number of lines of sight (LOS) and is one of the primary quantitative indicators of the quality of a transducer.
  - Software: By sequencing of the sound emission by the crystals, the software is able to activate the sound-emitting crystals in different time sequences to generate multiple sound wave fronts. By having the computing power to process these multiple reflecting LOS, the software is able to generate a significantly more detailed two-dimensional image on the display screen than if all the crystals fired all only in one sequence. This sequence processing is referred to as "multibeam" or "crossbeam" imaging.
- Axial resolution allows for clearer visualization of structures at varying depths, in the same axis as the transducer. Axial resolution can be increased or decreased by adjusting the frequency.
  - Frequency refers to the time between emissions of sound waves.
  - Higher frequencies result in greater axial resolution, resulting in a more detailed US image; however, higher frequencies have less tissue penetration (the ability to see deeper structures clearly). High-frequency sound waves have less penetration because they are subject to more rapid *attenuation* of sound waves by refraction and absorption of sound waves by tissues (reflectors).
  - Lower frequencies result in less axial resolution, resulting in a less detailed US image; however, lower frequency sound waves have greater tissue penetration because they are less subject to attenuation by reflectors.
  - Higher frequency = higher resolution and less penetration (more attenuation). Use higher frequencies to view relatively shallow structures with greater detail.
  - Lower frequency = less resolution and higher penetration (less attenuation). Use lower frequencies to view deeper structures.
  - Contemporary transducer technology emits multiple (broadband) frequencies near simultaneously to generate the most useful real-time US image by maximizing potential resolution (using some higher frequencies) and penetration (using some lower frequencies). The particular mix of high and low frequencies may be manually or automatically selected depending on the particular US machine used. The mix of frequencies is based on the depth of the structure of interest, with the frequencies emitted for deeper structures viewed weighted toward lower frequencies and vice versa with superficial structures.
- There are two commonly used transducer styles that feature frequency ranges that are useful for MSK US, with the choice between the two dependent on the particular application.
- All transducers operate within a range of frequencies as determined by the manufacturer.
  - ❏ Broadband high-frequency linear transducer: Most universal in application. Appropriate for superficial and medium-depth applications such as hand, knee, and shoulder. These transducers have a higher degree of resolution compared to curvilinear transducers at more superficial depths.
  - ❏ Broadband low-frequency curvilinear transducer: Appropriate for viewing deeper structures such as hip, spine, and shoulders in large individuals.

TERMINOLOGY

- Anisotropy
  - US best interprets echo signatures when the transducer is positioned directly perpendicular to a structure.
  - The artificial lack of signal (artifact) caused by loss of perpendicular positioning is termed *anisotropy* and is a significant and omnipresent challenge in MSK US.
  - The physical explanation for this phenomenon remains largely undetermined; however, it is associated with viewing relatively fibrillar structures, and the effects of anisotropy are more pronounced as structures become more fibrillar.
  - Anisotropy is a commonly encountered artifact when visualizing bundles of fibers (ligaments, tendons, muscle) or fascicles (nerves) as they curve (with loss of perpendicular positioning of the transducer) and can be easily misinterpreted as a tear. It affects higher density (more fibrillar) structures before less fibrillar structures.
    - ❏ Ligament > tendon > muscle > nerve
  - Knowledge of the relative anisotropic nature of structures aids the scanner in identification of anatomy. For example, when viewing the carpal tunnel in a transverse axis, as the operator tilts the probe, the carpal ligament signal will drop out first, then the tendons, then the muscle, with the median nerve as the last fibrillar structure in view.
  - A tilt as small as 3–7 degrees away from a perpendicular plane can produce anisotropy and can be seen in both the longitudinal and transverse planes.

- This effect is particularly evident when scanning a curved structure, such as a tendon insertion, and can be corrected by positioning the probe to remain perpendicular to the curvature.
- Volume averaging
  - US transducers emit a shaft of sound about 1 mm thick. This 1-mm three-dimensional shaft of sound gradually spreads and becomes wider as it penetrates tissue. The reflected sound waves from this three-dimensional shaft of sound are then processed by the computer to render a two-dimensional image.
  - The resultant generated image is an *average* of the total volume of the reflected signal.
  - Disruption of normal echo signature of a structure is often not translated into the image until more than 50% of the 1-mm shaft is abnormal. Even if 75% of a tendon in a given image is disrupted, it may still appear to be grossly intact, although relatively hypoechoic compared to the other parts of the tendon.
    - ❑ This is a crucial concept when it comes to interpretation of partial-thickness tears.
  - If a defect is suspected, turn the transducer orthogonally to assess for relative hypoechoic areas consistent with partial tears.
  - Aside from traditional longitudinal and transverse scanning axis, oblique approaches should be undertaken when attempting to delineate a partial-thickness tear.
  - An understanding of volume averaging is crucial to successful visualization of US-guided needles in longitudinal axis.
    - ❑ Because needles are relatively narrow, if the needle is located within the outer 25% of the projected sound shaft, the signal from the needle will be "volume averaged out," and no needle will be seen on the screen.
    - ❑ The needle must be in the middle 50% of the projected shaft of sound to be visible; this requirement becomes more exacting with deeper injections.
    - ❑ A clinician's eye dominance needs to be accounted for when attempting to place a needle under a transducer. What looks to be the centerline of the probe may actually be slightly to the left or right of centerline.
- Through transmission enhancement
  - If a sound wave passes through relatively less echo-dense material, it will be less subject to attenuation and will result in a relatively stronger reflection back to the transducer. For example, if a sound wave passes through a fluid-filled cyst lying over a bone, the image of the bone beneath the fluid-filled cyst will appear brighter than the adjacent bone.
  - In the case of a defect in a tendon, the structure immediately deep to this defect exhibits a relatively hyperechoic echo signature. Through transmission enhancement is critical to help identify partial-thickness tears, fluid interfaces, and tenosynovitis.

- In the same case of a defect in a tendon overlying bone, through transmission enhancement produces an artifact of relatively more intense hyperechoic area beneath the defect, which is referred to as "crescent sign" or "cartilage interface sign."
- Shadowing
  - This phenomenon is seen as an anechoic area immediately deep to a structure that blocks or partially blocks sound wave transmission.
  - This can be seen at bony interfaces, under calcifications, and around foreign bodies (such as needles).
- Gain
  - Often described as the "volume button," gain adjusts the intensity of the acoustic pulse emitted by the piezoelectric crystals, with the result being a stronger echo return.
  - Increasing gain enhances the detection of weak reflectors.
- Artifacts are any visible structures in an image that do not correlate directly with the actual tissue.
- Sonopalpation: Visualization of the clinician's palpating finger directly over the area of maximum tenderness to assist in correlating a patient's area of maximum tenderness with a potential anatomic pain generator.
- Doppler imaging
  - Most US equipment allows adjustment of the mode to allow visualization of blood flow. This can assist in establishing anatomic landmarks, avoiding vascular structures during US-guided injections, and assessing blood vessels for normal flow.
    - ❑ Color Doppler: signals both the presence and the direction of flow within a structure using the indicator colors of blue (flowing away) and red (flowing toward).
    - ❑ Power Doppler: provides a very sensitive assessment of presence of flow by indicating the reflection of red blood cells using the indicator colors of red and yellow.

MUSCULOSKELETAL ULTRASOUND SIGNALS

- Echo signatures are based on density of tissue reflecting the US waves. These signatures can be thought of as representing a continuum of varying degrees of shading.
  - Anechoic (black): no or minimal reflection of sound waves: hyaline cartilage, fluid.
  - Hypoechoic (relatively darker): scant reflection of sound waves *or* relatively darker in appearance than other tissues within the viewed structure. A relatively reduced density (darker area) in a tendon.
  - Echoic: A structure of sufficient reflectiveness to be visible on US image.

- Mixed echogenicity: An image made up of both hypoechoic and hyperechoic structures: muscle tissue.
- Isoechoic: Similar reflectiveness relative to the compared tissue.
- Hyperechoic: Relatively brighter (whiter) in appearance than comparative structures on the screen (*e.g.*, cortical surfaces, fascial layers, foreign bodies).

- Classic US descriptions of tissues
  - Muscle: loosely compact fibrillar pattern.
    - ❑ Transverse axis: "Starry Night" appearance.
    - ❑ Longitudinal axis: pennate pattern.
  - Tendon: compact fibrillar pattern in longitudinal and transverse axis.
  - Ligaments
    - ❑ Transverse axis: very compact fibrillar pattern.
    - ❑ Longitudinal axis: trilaminar appearance.
      - ▪ Intrasubstance appears dark compared to whiter, adjacent surfaces (white-black-white appearance).
  - Nerves
    - ❑ Transverse axis: fascicular pattern.
      - ▪ "Bundle of grapes" appearance.
    - ❑ Longitudinal axis: striated fascicular appearance.

INDICATIONS FOR ULTRASOUND IN SPORTS MEDICINE (1)

- MSK US is a valuable tool in the evaluation and management of the injured athlete and has become invaluable to the practice of MSK medicine, as evidenced by its exponential increase in clinical usage within the past 10 years. New indications for this tool are constantly described, most of which fall under one of two primary categories:
  - Diagnostic scanning:
    - ❑ Static assessment
    - ❑ Dynamic assessment
  - Visualization of percutaneous procedures:
    - ❑ Injection
    - ❑ Aspiration
    - ❑ Fenestration
    - ❑ Neurolysis
- The remainder of this chapter is devoted to highlighting the value of real-time US imaging in several common MSK injuries (1).
- Anterior hip
  - Significant hip effusions are obvious on US imaging.
  - US-guided hip joint injections can safely and effectively replace the fluoroscopically guided injections.
  - The anterior labrum is visible, as is the bony contour of the femoral neck associated with femoral acetabular impingement.
  - A snapping iliopsoas tendon can be identified snapping over the pectineal eminence with hip extension. Holding

the transducer in position during this dynamic exam is challenging but possible.

- Posterior hip pain
  - US allows the astute clinician to differentiate what appears to be piriformis pain from an obturator internus tendinopathy as it sharply bends as it courses over the ileum. Sonopalpation or a US-guided diagnostic injection can quickly differentiate these two common sources of posterior hip pain, resulting in a more precise patho-anatomic diagnosis and appropriate treatment.
- Lateral hip pain
  - Often what clinically appears to be "greater trochanteric bursitis" (GTB) is a tendinopathy in one or both of the gluteus medius tendons as they insert onto the superior aspect of the greater trochanter.
  - Insertional tendinopathy of the piriformis as it inserts onto the superior/lateral aspect of the greater trochanter or an insertional tendinopathy of the obturator internus as it inserts on the posterior medial border of the greater trochanter can also clinically be misidentified as GTB.
  - With diagnostic US and a US-guided diagnostic injection of a small amount (1 mL) of local anesthetic, an astute clinician can formulate a precise diagnosis from a differential of overlapping or similar possibilities.
- Hamstring
  - Acute complete and partial hamstring tears and their associated hematomas are often obvious on US.
  - Hamstring origin tendinopathies at the conjoined tendon can be differentiated from adductor magnus origin tendinopathy, but a precise diagnosis may require a US-guided diagnostic injection.
  - Whenever considering an injection of the hamstring origin area, the sciatic nerve must be clearly identified because it runs immediately lateral to these structures.
- Quadriceps
  - Quadriceps tendon partial- and full-thickness tears are readily evident on US exam. Quadriceps hematomas are obvious and can be safely aspirated under US guidance.
- Knee
  - MSK US can quickly assess many common chronic and acute knee injuries.
  - Knee effusions are obvious on US exam of the suprapatellar pouch. Aspiration and injection of the knee joint at this location virtually negate the possibility of iatrogenic cartilage damage from the needle.
  - Baker cysts in the posterior knee can also be easily identified at the junction of the semimembranosus tendon and the medial gastrocnemius and safely aspirated under US guidance.
  - US can rule-in (but not rule-out) tears in the outer menisci. Meniscal tears are often visible on US, and US combined with positive sonopalpation and an effusion provide even stronger evidence of a tear.

- Meniscal cysts are an indication of a meniscal tear and are readily viewed.
- Full-thickness tears, partial tears, and tendinopathies of the patellar and quadriceps tendons are readily visible.
- Pathologic plical folds are visible.
- Injuries to the lateral and medial collateral ligaments are readily visible and gradable on a dynamic US exam.
- Cartilage thickness and some cartilage defects can be measured with US.
- The common peroneal nerve, an uncommon source of lateral knee pain, can be additionally identified as it branches off of the sciatic nerve and courses around the fibular head.
- Calf
  - Partial and complete tears of the gastrocnemius and soleus are readily visible, as are their associated hematomas.
  - Achilles tendon partial tears, complete tears, and tendinopathies are readily viewed and measured with US. The ability to definitively establish a diagnosis of a ruptured tendon may reduce the delay before surgical repair.
  - The os trigonum in the posterior heel can be viewed and injected under US guidance.
  - Nerve injuries and neuromas within the lower leg are also readily viewed with US.
- Ankle
  - Ligament sprains, including high ankle sprains, can be dynamically evaluated and accurately graded to establish appropriate treatment and prognosis.
  - Ankle joint effusions are readily viewed.
  - Tenosynovitis, such as a posterior tibial tenosynovitis, can be viewed in any of the tendons as they course over the ankle joint.
  - Split tears in the peroneal and tibial tendons are often difficult to image with other modalities and are often only viewed in the oblique axis.
- Foot
  - One of the more common running-related complaints is heel pain, with plantar fasciitis representing the "low back pain" of the runner.
  - MSK US allows the provider to assess a number of structures including the plantar fascia, tarsal tunnel, and plantar nerves.
  - The plantar fascia is readily measured; thickness > 4 mm is considered enlarged and consistent with a diagnosis of plantar fasciosis (5).
- Shoulder
  - Rotator cuff tears: The accuracy of US has been shown to be comparable to MRI in the detection of rotator cuff tears (11).
  - Dynamic US exam of the shoulder can impressively show anterior and posterior impingement, as well as acromioclavicular joint dysfunction and arthropathy.
- Diagnostic injections with as little as 1 mL of lidocaine can differentiate the pain generator in the presence of multiple pathologies.
- Glenohumeral joint injections can be performed while sparing the articular cartilage surfaces and the labrum from needle trauma.
- Elbow
  - Medial and lateral tendinopathies and partial tears can be assessed and accurately injected with US.
  - It is possible to assess less common sources of lateral elbow pain, such as anconeus tears, radial nerve entrapments, and annular ligament tears.
- Wrist
  - Scapholunate ligament injuries can be assessed by performing a dynamic exam by having the patient grip an object while observing for an instability and gapping between the scaphoid and lunate (Terry-Thomas sign).
  - It is possible to rule-in (but not rule-out) triangular fibrocartilage complex injuries.
  - Carpal dislocations and fractures can be ruled-in (but not ruled-out).
  - De Quervain tenosynovitis and intersection syndrome are readily assessed and accurately injected with US guidance.
- The median nerve is easily visualized and its cross-sectional area measured to assess for impingement (12).
- Hands
  - A potential gamekeeper's thumb can be assessed with a cautious dynamic exam.
  - Extensor and flexor tendons are readily assessed.
  - First carpometacarpal joints are easily assessed for arthropathies.

EVIDENCE FOR USE OF ULTRASOUND IN SPORTS MEDICINE

- Although there are hundreds of studies in the peer-reviewed medical literature demonstrating the benefit of US both in diagnosis and for procedure guidance, included in the remaining section of this chapter are several studies that address clinical questions that are pertinent to physicians seeking to adopt US into their practice.
- US improves clinical efficiency. A retrospective record review of 1,012 patients treated by MSK and sports physicians over a 10-month period by Sivan et al. (9) concluded that the use of clinic-based MSK US enables a one-stop approach, reduces repeated hospital appointments, and improves quality of care in an outpatient MSK clinic.
- The question of clinical outcomes from US-guided injections was addressed by Sibbitt et al. (8) in a randomized controlled study of 148 painful joints that were randomized

to intraarticular corticosteroid injection by conventional palpation-guided or sonographic image-guided injection. Relative to conventional palpation-guided methods, sonographic guidance resulted in 43% reduction in procedural pain ($P > 0.001$), 58% reduction in absolute pain scores at the 2-week outcome ($P > 0.001$), 75% reduction in significant pain ($P > 0.001$), and 62% reduction in nonresponder rate. Sonography also increased detection of effusion by 200% and volume of aspirated fluid by 337%. The authors concluded that sonographic guidance significantly improved clinical outcomes (8).

- Naredo et al. (7) concluded that US-guided subacromial injection resulted in improved pain (as assessed on a visual analog scale) and shoulder function assessment scores at 6 weeks versus clinically guided injections ($P < 0.001$) .

- The need for US guidance for standard injections such as knee injections has been questioned. In a prospective series of 240 consecutive injections in patients without clinical knee effusion, Jackson et al. (4) tested the accuracy of clinically guided intraarticular knee injections by an experienced orthopedic surgeon. Accuracy rates for needle placement were confirmed with fluoroscopic imaging to document the dispersion pattern of injected contrast material. Of 80 injections performed through an anterolateral portal, 57 were confirmed to have been placed in the intraarticular space on the first attempt (an accuracy rate of 71%). The authors demonstrated the difficulty of accurately placing a needle into the intraarticular space of the knee when an effusion is not present. They concluded that their study highlights the need for clinicians to refine injection techniques for delivering intraarticular therapeutic substances that are intended to coat the articular surfaces of the knee joint (4).

- Curtiss et al. (2), in their study of US-guided versus clinically guided injections into the suprapatellar pouch of the knee (an approach that does not risk injury to the cartilage surfaces by the needle), concluded that the US-guided knee injections that use a superolateral approach are very accurate in a cadaveric model, whereas the accuracy of palpation-guided knee injections that use the same approach is variable and appears to be significantly influenced by clinician experience. Their findings suggest that US guidance should be considered when one performs knee injections with a superolateral approach that require a high degree of accuracy (2).

- US is comparable to MRI in the detection of rotator cuff tears. In their prospective study of 124 patients, Teefey et al. (11) compared the accuracy of the two tests (MRI vs. US) for detection and measurement of the size of rotator cuff tears, with arthroscopic findings used as the standard. They concluded that US and MRI had comparable accuracy for identifying and measuring the size of full-thickness and partial-thickness rotator cuff tears (11).

- Ziswiler et al. (12), in their prospective study of 110 patients, determined the largest cross-sectional area of the median nerve at the carpal tunnel and compared this to nerve conduction studies (NCS) and clinical signs and symptoms. They concluded that measurement of the nerve cross-sectional area was diagnostically as accurate as NCS and can be used to rule-in or rule-out carpal tunnel syndrome (12).

RESOURCES

American Institute of Ultrasound in Medicine (free resource):
- Located at: http://www.aium.org
- Discussion forums, practice guidelines

European Society of Musculoskeletal Radiology (free resource):
- Located at: http://www.essr.org
- Technical guidelines

American Medical Society for Sports Medicine (membership restricted):
- Located at: http://www.amssm.org
- Business plan, protocols, practice cases, listing of training courses

University of Michigan Health System (free resource):
- Located at: http://www.med.umich.edu/rad/muscskel/mskus/index.html
- Tutorials

RadiologyInfo.Org (free resource):
- Located at: http://www.radiologyinfo.org/en/info.cfm?pg=musculous
- Patient information

Musculoskeletal Ultrasound (free resource)
- Located at: http://www.mskus.com
- Protocols, listing of training workshops

REFERENCES

1. Bianchi S, Martinoli C. *Ultrasound of the Musculoskeletal System*. Berlin Heidelberg (Germany): Springer-Verlag; 2007. 990 p.
2. Curtiss HM, Finnoff JT, Peck E, Hollman J, Muir J, Smith J. Accuracy of ultrasound-guided and palpation-guided knee injections by an experienced and less-experienced injector using a superolateral approach: a cadaveric study. *PM R*. 2011;3(6):507–15.
3. Harmon KG, O'Connor FG. Musculoskeletal ultrasound: taking sports medicine to the next level. *Br J Sports Med*. 2010;44(16):1135–6.
4. Jackson DW, Evans NA, Thomas BM. Accuracy of needle placement into the intraarticular space of the knee. *J Bone Joint Surg Am*. 2002;84-A(9):1522–7.
5. McMillan M, Landorf KB, Barrett JT, Menz HB, Bird AR. Diagnostic imaging for chronic plantar heel pain: a systematic review and meta-analysis. *J Foot Ankle Res*. 2009;2:32.
6. Mulvaney S. Ultrasound guided percutaneous neuroplasty of the lateral femoral cutaneous nerve for the treatment of meralgia paresthetica: a case

report and description of a new ultrasound guided technique. *Curr Sports Med Rep*. 2011;10(2):99–104.

7. Naredo E, Cabero F, Beneyto P, et al. A randomized comparative study of short term response to blind injection versus sonographic-guided injection of local corticosteroids in patients with painful shoulder. *J Rheumatol*. 2004;31(2):308–14.

8. Sibbitt WL Jr, Peisajovich A, Michael AA, et al. Does sonographic needle guidance affect the clinical outcome of intraarticular injections? *J Rheumatol*. 2009;36(9):1892–902.

9. Sivan M, Brown J, Brennan S, Bhakta B. A one-stop approach to the management of soft tissue and degenerative musculoskeletal conditions using clinic-based ultrasonography. *Musculoskeletal Care*. 2011;9(2):63–8.

10. Tagliafico AS, Michaud J, Marchetti A, Garello I, Padua L, Martinoli C. US imaging of the musculocutaneous nerve. *Skeleletal Radiol*. 2011;40(5):609–16.

11. Teefey SA, Rubin DA, Middleton WD, Hildebolt CF, Leibold RA, Yamaguchi K. Detection and quantification of rotator cuff tears. Comparison of ultrasonographic, magnetic resonance imaging, and arthroscopic findings in seventy-one consecutive cases. *J Bone Joint Surg Am*. 2004; 86-A(4):708–16.

12. Ziswiler HR, Reichenbach S, Vögelin E, Bachmann LM, Villiger PM, Jüni P. Diagnostic value of sonography in patients with suspected carpal tunnel syndrome: a prospective study. *Arthritis Rheum*. 2005; 52(1):304–11.

20 Electrodiagnostic Testing

Venu Akuthota and Jason Friedrich

INTRODUCTION

■ Electrodiagnostic (EDX) testing can be a useful tool in the evaluation of athletes with neurologic problems (1,26).

■ Although clinical recognition of patterns of pain and sensory or motor abnormalities is the first step toward the identification of a nerve problem, EDX testing can augment the clinical examination to better localize and characterize neuropathology (2).

■ A thorough EDX consultation integrates the history, physical examination, and selected nerve conduction and electromyographic studies into a meaningful diagnostic conclusion.

■ Whereas imaging studies identify structural abnormalities, EDX studies evaluate the physiology and function of the peripheral nervous system.

■ A negative EDX examination does not rule the possibility of pathology because electrophysiologic studies are time and severity dependent (1,2).

■ Clinical judgment is used in EDX; therefore, EDX studies are highly dependent on the quality of the electromyographer (7,11,12).

■ This chapter will describe the pathophysiology of nerve injury and associated chronology of electrophysiologic findings, as well as describe the components of an EDX evaluation.

■ EDX testing involves both nerve conduction studies (NCS) and needle examination (NE). The NE is also referred to as electromyography (EMG).

■ The purpose of this chapter is to provide the clinician a basis for ordering EDX consultations and understanding proper EDX reports.

ANATOMY

■ EDX studies evaluate the peripheral nervous system or lower motor neuron pathway (11,12).

■ Standard EDX studies typically give little information regarding central nervous system pathology (upper motor neuron pathway).

■ The components of the peripheral nervous system include afferent sensory nerves and efferent motor nerves.

Sensory (Afferent) Pathway

■ Cutaneous receptors → sensory axons → pure sensory or mixed nerves → nerve plexus (*e.g.*, brachial plexus, lumbosacral plexus) → cell bodies in the dorsal root ganglion (usually within intervertebral foramina) → dorsal roots synapse in the dorsolateral spinal cord.

■ This pathway is evaluated during NCS of pure sensory or mixed nerves.

Motor (Efferent) Pathway

■ Anterior horn cell (spinal cord) → spinal nerves, subsequently dividing into ventral and dorsal rami. Ventral rami → nerve plexus → peripheral motor nerve → neuromuscular junction → muscle fibers. Entire pathway is referred to as a motor unit.

■ This pathway is evaluated during NCS of motor or mixed nerves, from the point of stimulation to the recording site.

■ Individual motor units can be evaluated during NE with voluntary muscle activation.

PATHOPHYSIOLOGY OF NERVE INJURY

■ Peripheral nerves can either be myelinated or unmyelinated.

■ Myelinated fibers conduct much more rapidly by way of saltatory ("jumping") conduction, in which depolarization occurs only at interspersed nodes of Ranvier, allowing current to jump from node to node (2).

■ NCSs evaluate the fastest-conducting fibers within a given nerve; typically, these are the A alpha myelinated fibers.

Seddon Classification

■ Divides peripheral nerve injury into neurapraxia, axonotmesis, and neurotmesis (Table 20.1).

Neurapraxia

■ Neurapraxia is a comparatively mild injury that affects only the myelin sheath and causes focal conduction slowing or conduction block as a result of current leakage between nodes of Ranvier (32). Although the myelin is injured, the

Table 20.1	Classification of Nerve Pathophysiology (2)			
Type	**Pathology**	**EDX Correlation**		**Prognosis**
Neurapraxia	Myelin injury	CV slowing across segment DL prolonged across segment to months Loss of amplitude proximal but not distal NE normal		Recovery in weeks
Axonotmeses	Axonal injury with variable stromal disruption	Loss of amplitude distal and proximal NE shows spontaneous activity NE shows abnormal voluntary motor units		Longer recovery and more variable
Neurotmeses	Severance of entire nerve	No waveform with proximal or distal stimulation NE shows spontaneous activity NE shows no recruited motor units		Poor recovery, surgery required

CV, conduction velocity; DL, distal latency; NE, needle examination.

nerve fibers remain in axonal continuity. This results in motor or sensory loss from impaired conduction across the demyelinated segment. However, impulse conduction is normal in the segments proximal and distal to the injury, where the myelin remains intact.

- Demyelination is typically seen with focal nerve entrapments (*e.g.*, carpal tunnel syndrome). It may also occur in peripheral polyneuropathies either as a patchy process (*e.g.*, Guillain-Barré syndrome) or a diffuse process (*e.g.*, diabetic peripheral neuropathy).

- Runners often experience neurapraxic injury of the tibial nerve branches with putative tarsal tunnel syndrome due to repeated traction injury with the foot in pronation (2,21).

Axonotmesis and Neurotmesis

- Axonotmesis and neurotmesis refer to axonal injury with Wallerian degeneration of nerve fibers disconnected from their cell bodies. These types of injuries result in loss of nerve conduction at the site of injury and distally. Axonotmetic injuries involve damage to the axon, with some preservation of the surrounding stroma (endoneurium, perineurium, epineurium), whereas neurotmetic injuries imply complete disruption of the enveloping nerve sheath (2,32).

- EDX studies typically cannot distinguish axonotmesis from neurotmesis.

- Athletes can experience axonal injury with conditions such as radiculopathy.

SPECIFIC ELECTRODIAGNOSTIC STUDIES

- EDX studies typically consist of NCS and NE.

- Each part of the evaluation has its own strengths and shortcomings; therefore, it is imperative that a well-trained consultant performs EDX studies and can recognize sources of error during testing (1,2).

Nerve Conduction Studies

- NCSs may be performed on motor, sensory, or mixed nerves.

- There are numerous pitfalls associated with performing NCSs (Table 20.2). Both motor and sensory NCSs test only the fastest, myelinated axons of a nerve; thus, the lightly myelinated or unmyelinated fibers (*e.g.*, C pain fibers) are not examined (7,18,19).

- Motor nerves are stimulated at accessible sites, and the compound motor action potential (CMAP) is recorded over the motor points of their target muscles. Motor points represent regions of high concentration of neuromuscular junctions, typically in the central muscle belly.

- Deep motor nerves and deep proximal muscles are more difficult to study and interpret (15).

- Sensory nerves can be studied along the physiologic direction of the nerve impulse (orthodromic) or opposite the physiologic direction of the afferent input (antidromic).

- A stimulated sensory nerve produces the recorded sensory nerve action potential (SNAP).

- Frequently, sensory nerves are tested within mixed nerves, such as the plantar nerves, and produce a mixed nerve action potential (MNAP).

- CMAP, SNAP, and MNAP waveforms are analyzed and interpreted by the clinician.

Table 20.2	Sources of Error with Nerve Conduction Studies (1,2)

- Temperature
- Inadequate or excessive stimulation
- Improper placement of electrodes
- Tape measurement error
- Not adjusting values for age
- Anomalous innervation
- Volume conduction of impulse to nearby nerve
- Improper filter settings
- Improper electrode montage setup
- Involuntary muscle contractions

- Waveform parameters include amplitude, latency, and conduction velocity.
- Amplitude evaluates the number of functioning axons in a given nerve and, for motor nerves, the number of muscle fibers activated.
- Latency refers to the time (milliseconds) from the stimulus to the recorded action potential.
- With motor NCSs, latency accounts for peripheral nerve conduction (distal to the site of stimulation), neuromuscular junction transition time, and muscle fiber activation time (12).
- With sensory nerves, latency measures only the conduction time within the segment of nerve stimulated. Conduction velocity is calculated by dividing the distance travelled between a distal and proximal stimulation site by the impulse conduction time.

Late Responses

- Whereas routine NCSs typically evaluate distal nerve segments, late responses, such as the H reflex and F wave, travel the full length of a nerve.

H Reflex

- The H reflex is the electrophysiologic analog to the ankle stretch reflex. It measures afferent and efferent conduction along the S1 nerve root pathway (16).
- A latency difference of at least 1.5 milliseconds is significant in most laboratories.
- Amplitude of < 50% compared with the uninvolved side is also significant.
- Because the amplitude of this reflex is sensitive to contraction of the plantar flexor muscles, amplitude changes without associated latency abnormalities should be interpreted with caution (31).
- The H reflex evaluates the afferent and efferent pathway; thus, it gives information about the sensory pathway that is not tested on NE.
- The S1 nerve injury can be due to S1 radiculopathy from a herniated disc or lumbar stenosis, peripheral neuropathy (usually with bilaterally abnormal H reflexes), or sciatic/tibial nerve injuries (2).

F Wave

- The F wave is a late muscle potential that results from a motor nerve volley created by supramaximally stimulated anterior horn cells (16). Thus, the F wave represents conduction up and down a motor nerve, without any sensory afferent contribution.
- Unlike the H reflex, the F wave can be elicited at many spinal levels and from any muscle.
- Like the H reflex, F wave studies examine long nerve pathways, which consequently obscure small focal abnormalities.
- Abnormalities of F wave values may be due to injury anywhere along the pathway evaluated; thus, specificity may be limited.

Magnetic Stimulation

- Proposed by some as an alternative to electrical stimulation for peripheral NCS (5,33).
- Potential advantages over conventional electrical stimulation are less discomfort with stimulations and improved access to deeper nerve segments, including roots of the lumbosacral plexus and the proximal sciatic nerve (5).
- Utility remains extremely limited due to inability to reliably produce a controlled focal stimulus and reproduce maximum amplitude CMAPs, which hinders detection of focal conduction block (28,34).

Needle Examination

- Evaluates the entire motor unit (lower motor neuron pathway), but not the sensory pathway.
- Assesses muscles at rest (to detect potential axonal injury) and with volitional activity (to evaluate voluntary motor unit morphology and recruitment) (9).
- Needs to be timed such that abnormalities are optimally detected.
- If performed too early (i.e., < 2–3 weeks after the initial injury), spontaneous muscle fiber discharges (denervation potentials) may not have had time to develop (2).
- If performed too late (i.e., > 6 months after the initial injury), reinnervation from collateral sprouting may have stabilized the muscle membrane and halted spontaneous muscle fiber discharges (31).
- At rest, the electrical activity of selected muscles is studied for abnormal spontaneous waveforms. Of these, the most common are fibrillation potentials and positive sharp waves. They are found when the muscle tested has been denervated (12).
- Fibrillations and positive sharp waves are graded on a scale from 0 to 4+ (Table 20.3).
- Complex repetitive discharges (CRDs) are also common and represent ephaptic spread of a spontaneous discharge ("cross-talk") from a single muscle fiber to neighboring fibers. CRDs may be present in the setting of longstanding cycles of denervation and reinnervation.
- Fasciculation potentials represent spontaneous discharges of an entire motor unit; thus, they are much larger than

Table 20.3	Grading of Fibrillations and Positive Waves	
Grading	**Characteristics**
0	No activity
1+	Persistent (longer than 1 second) in 2 muscle regions
2+	Persistent in 3 or more muscle regions
3+	Persistent in all muscle regions
4+	Continuous in all muscle regions

fibrillations and positive waves and can sometimes be grossly observed as muscle twitches. They can be found in a variety of benign or malignant conditions. Benign fasciculations may be found in runners following heavy exercise, dehydration, anxiety, fatigue, coffee consumption, or smoking (1,2).

■ With muscle activation, motor unit action potentials (MUAPs) may be analyzed. Motor unit analysis provides opportunity to distinguish between neuropathic and myopathic processes based on MUAP morphology and recruitment pattern differences (1,2).

■ NE also may help differentiate acute from chronic neuropathic conditions.

■ The amplitude of fibrillation potentials can grade nerve injury as occurring for less than or more than 1 year (with smaller potentials for the latter) (23). This can be particularly helpful in identifying an athlete's acute on chronic nerve injury.

■ Chronic nerve injuries, without significant ongoing denervation, may additionally show large-amplitude, long-duration, polyphasic MUAPs (31).

Provocation Electrodiagnostics

■ Some authors advocate performing EDX testing after exercise or with the limbs in provocative positions. These techniques have still not been validated with sound research and are subject to measurement error (1,2).

■ Anecdotally, these techniques may have limited use in certain circumstances, such as peroneal nerve entrapments in runners detected only with EDX testing following exercise (24). Runners diagnosed with chronic exertional compartment syndrome and potential nerve entrapment (e.g., superficial peroneal nerve entrapment as it exits the fascia of the lateral compartment) have also been postulated to need EDX testing following exercise (3).

■ Some suggest that electrophysiologic evidence of piriformis syndrome is more apparent when an H reflex is performed with the sciatic nerve on stretch (hip flexed to 90 degrees, maximally adducted, and knee flexed to 90 degrees) (17).

■ Studies of other peripheral nerves have not supported the notion that EDX sensitivity is improved in dynamic positions (27). Spuriously slow and fast nerve conduction velocity can be recorded with the limb in various positions, most famously described with ulnar nerve studies around the elbow (6).

■ These techniques need to be interpreted with caution because many "abnormal" readings occur based on measurement error alone.

Dynamic or Quantitative Electromyography

■ Demonstrates the sequence of muscle recruitment and muscle force for a given activity; in this capacity, only available in specialized gait laboratories (1,2).

■ Employs surface or needle electrodes to record EMG signals through multiple channels. Fine wire electrodes may be used to record signal from deeper muscles.

■ Caution should be used in correlating EMG amplitude with muscle force generated because the relationship is not consistently linear (4).

■ In research, quantitative EMG has also been used to assess degree of muscle fatigue and biomechanics of sports activities or adaptations following injury (such as knee mechanics after anterior cruciate ligament tear) (15,20).

■ The kinesiology of the running gait has been elucidated with dynamic EMG. The gluteal muscles and hamstrings are more active in running than in walking, particularly at the termination of swing phase in preparation for foot strike. The quadriceps and posterior calf group also work during a greater proportion of the swing and stance phases of running compared to walking. The calf muscle in particular becomes much more active as the speed of gait increases (25).

■ Surface EMG can be used as a biofeedback technique in runners to improve their running biomechanics (i.e., the use of hip extensors may be trained with the use of surface EMG) (2).

INDICATIONS FOR ELECTRODIAGNOSTIC TESTING

■ The utility of EDX testing in a given athlete can be estimated following a thorough history and physical examination, by a review of supplemental information (e.g., imaging studies), and through an appreciation for the chronology of the electrophysiologic changes that occur following nerve injury (1,2).

■ Some useful generalizations about the indications for EDX testing are discussed below (7,31,32):

■ Establish and/or confirm a clinical diagnosis:
  ❏ EDX study can rule in a suspected diagnosis or rule out a competing diagnosis.
  ❏ EDX may alert the examiner to the possibility of an unsuspected concomitant pathologic process (e.g., an athlete with tarsal tunnel syndrome and superimposed radiculopathy).

■ Localize nerve lesions:
  ❏ Nerve injury location often needs to be objectively confirmed prior to contemplating invasive or surgical treatment.
  ❏ For example, an athlete presenting with plantar surface numbness and tingling may have a sciatic nerve lesion anywhere along the course of the sciatic nerve or its branches.
  ❏ EDX studies can be used to localize the injury within the nerve roots, plexus, or peripheral nerves.

■ Determine the extent and chronicity of nerve injury:
  ❏ Properly timed EDX studies can differentiate a neurapraxic injury from axonal degeneration. This may have a significant impact on the aggressiveness of treatment for the nerve injury.

Table 20.4 | **Timing of Wallerian Degeneration, Nerve Recovery and EDX Findings with Axonal Injury (1,2)**

Time	Nerve Degeneration	Nerve Recovery	NCS Correlate	NE
Day 0	None	None	Proximal-recorded segment abnormal; distal segment CMAP normal	Decreased recruitment
Day 3	NMJ impaired	Nodal and terminal sprouts		
Day 9	Motor axons lost		Decreased distal segment CMAP	Increased insertional activity
Day 11	Sensory axons lost			
Day 14	*See nerve recovery*		Decreased distal segment SNAP	Large denervation potentials in proximal muscles
Day 21		Increased fiber density		Denervation potentials in distal muscles
Week 6-8		Axonal sprouting	CMAP/SNAP increasing back towards normal	Nascent reinnervation potentials
Week 16		Axonal regrowth 1mm/day		Maturing reinnervation proximal muscles
Week 20				Maturing reinnervation distal muscles
Year 1				Smaller denervation potentials
Year 2		Muscle no longer viable		

NCS, nerve conduction study; NE, needle examination; NM, neuromuscular junction; CMAP, compound muscle action potential; SNAP, sensory nerve action potential.

- ❏ The acuteness and chronicity of a nerve lesion may also be assessed using fibrillation amplitude measurement and motor unit analysis, as well as clinical history (23).
- ■ Correlate findings of anatomic studies:
  - ❏ Because EDX studies examine nerve physiology, they can provide a correlate of nerve function within a region of structural pathology found on imaging studies.
  - ❏ This may be particularly useful in the spine where structural pathology, such as disc herniations effacing nerve roots, can be seen in asymptomatic individuals (22).
- ■ Assist in prognosis and return to play (see following section).

Nerve Recovery and Return to Play

- ■ By determining the degree of nerve injury, the clinician can predict nerve recovery (1,32).
- ■ In general, neurapraxic injuries recover sooner than axonal injuries.
- ■ NCSs can determine if neurapraxic injury is present.
- ■ Motor CMAP amplitudes of weak muscles can be compared to the asymptomatic side to estimate the extent of injury. A side-to-side difference of > 50% is probably significant.
- ■ NE of volitional motor units can also help predict prognosis.
- ■ If no motor units are detected during the early stages and NCSs do not reveal conduction block, a severe axonal injury is present and full recovery is unlikely.
- ■ After a couple of months, motor unit analysis can indicate reinnervation by means of terminal reorganization or sprouting from preserved axons (1,32).

- ■ EDX studies should not be the *sine qua non* for return to play because they may lag behind clinical recovery.
- ■ The best determination of return to play remains the athlete's functional performance in simulated sports activities (15).

Timing of Electrodiagnostic Testing

- ■ When ordering EDX studies, the timing of findings should be kept in mind (Table 20.4) (1,2).
- ■ With traumatic injuries, serial EDX studies, including an immediate study, may be helpful to thoroughly determine the extent of injury.
- ■ EDX studies performed before postinjury day 9 may show normal distal segment motor nerve conduction parameters (or before postinjury day 11 in the case of sensory nerve conduction).
- ■ EDX testing performed around the 1-month mark can help quantify the number of surviving axons.
- ■ NE findings can take from 2 to 6 weeks to manifest.

LIMITATIONS OF ELECTRODIAGNOSTIC TESTING

- ■ EDX testing has limitations and should not be performed in every athlete with neurologic signs and symptoms (1,2).
- ■ Some diagnoses are unequivocal, and treatment should be initiated without delay (*e.g.*, progressive neurologic deficits, such as after traumatic posterior knee dislocation, requiring emergent care. The results from EDX will not change management.).

- The clinician must also understand that the probability of a false-positive result increases with the number of tests performed (*e.g.*, the probability of obtaining one false-positive result out of five tests is 12%, and increases to 20% with nine tests) (11).

- EDX findings always need to be considered in the full clinical context, and EDX impressions should emphasize patterns of abnormalities, rather than isolated findings.

- Relative to other body regions, EDX evaluation of the foot more often yields less definitive results (2).

- Some authors report NE abnormalities in the intrinsic foot muscles of asymptomatic subjects (29), but recent analysis indicates this may only occur 0%–2% of the time (13). Therefore, NE of the foot intrinsics (*e.g.*, abductor hallucis and extensor digitorum brevis) could be considered in the EDX evaluation for suspected nerve entrapment in the foot and ankle region (29).

- Relative contraindications to EDX testing include pacemaker (no Erb's point stimulation), arteriovenous fistula, open wound, coagulopathy, lymphedema, anasarca, and pending muscle biopsy (1,2,12).

SPECIFIC CONDITIONS

- Many pain complaints in athletes present as neurologic signs and symptoms (*e.g.*, numbness or tingling and focal weakness in the foot).

- Although most runners do not complain of symptoms of neuropathy, they do appear to have subclinical changes in nerve physiology in the lower leg and foot: increased vibratory sensory thresholds and delayed nerve conduction velocities (8,14). Some runners do present with symptoms and sign of focal nerve entrapments (2) (Table 20.5).

- Athletes with nerve pain describe a burning, shooting, tingling, numb, and/or electric quality to their pain. Athletes commonly present with tibial or peroneal nerve problems that can be evaluated by EDX techniques.

Tibial Nerve

- Specific techniques exist to evaluate the tibial nerve and its terminal branches (29).

- The tibial nerve has four terminal branches: (a) medial plantar nerve, (b) lateral plantar nerve, (c) inferior calcaneal nerve, and (d) medial calcaneal nerve (29).

- The medial plantar nerve is easily tested as a motor NCS, stimulating at the tibial nerve proximal to the medial malleolus and recording over the abductor hallucis.

- The lateral plantar motor nerve study is performed by stimulating the tibial nerve proximal to the medial malleolus and recording over the flexor digiti minimi.

- The inferior calcaneal motor nerve study is performed to the abductor digiti minimi pedis.

- The medial calcaneal nerve can be studied as a sensory nerve antidromic study with the recording electrode placed over the skin of the medial calcaneus.

- The sensory components of the medial and lateral plantar nerves may be practically tested with a mixed nerve study.

Table 20.5	Focal Entrapment Neuropathies Seen in Runners (2)	
Syndrome/Nerve	**Symptoms**	**Entrapment Site**
■ Tarsal tunnel syndrome (tibial nerve proper)	Plantar pain/paresthesias Worse at night and with prolonged standing or walking	Under flexor retinaculum
■ Medial calcaneal neuritis	Medial heel pain	At medial heel
■ Inferior calcaneal nerve (first branch of lateral plantar nerve)	Chronic heel pain No numbness Weakness of ADM	Between AH and QP or calcaneal heel spur
■ Medial plantar nerve (Jogger's foot)	Medial arch pain (hypertrophy of AH)	At master knot of Henry
■ Morton's toe (interdigital nerve)	N/T in toes	At intermetatarsal ligament
■ Superficial peroneal nerve	Lateral ankle pain Fascial herniation	At deep crural fascia as exits lateral compartment
■ Deep peroneal nerve (anterior tarsal tunnel)	Dorsum of foot pain Tightly laced shoes	At inferior extensor retinaculum
■ Common peroneal nerve	N/T in lateral leg, dorsum of foot	Compression in fibular tunnel by fibrous edge of peroneus longus Traction from ankle sprains
■ Sural nerve	Posterolateral calf pain, worse with physical exertion	Superficial sural aponeurosis

ADM, abductor digiti minimi; AH, abductor hallucis; N/T, numbness/tingling; QP, quadratus plantae.

■ The medial and lateral plantar nerves are stimulated individually at the plantar aspect of the foot, and the SNAP is recorded posterior to the medial malleolus.

Peroneal Nerve

■ The peroneal nerve's motor and sensory components can be consistently studied with NCS.

■ The motor nerve study is performed by stimulating the peroneal nerve at the ankle, the fibular head, and the popliteal fossa. Recording is usually over the extensor digitorum brevis; however, the anterior tibialis can be used as an alternative and may have more functional significance (10).

■ The sensory nerve study is performed by stimulating the superficial peroneal branch as it exits the lateral compartment and recording over the ankle.

Tarsal Tunnel Syndrome

■ EDX evaluation is often used to confirm and localize suspected tarsal tunnel syndrome.

■ NCSs for tarsal tunnel syndrome include: (a) tibial motor study to abductor hallucis and abductor digiti minimi pedis, (b) medial and lateral plantar mixed nerve study, and (c) medial and lateral plantar sensory study (30).

■ Abnormal plantar nerve SNAP response is thought to be the most sensitive finding but is nonspecific (30).

■ Focal tibial motor abnormalities are thought to be specific when present.

■ Mixed nerve study of the medial and lateral plantar nerves may be the most sensitive and specific test for tarsal tunnel syndrome.

■ NE of the foot intrinsics may offer additional useful information (29).

ELECTRODIAGNOSTIC REPORT

■ The EDX report should include a number of important pieces of data for the referring physician.

■ The electrophysiologic findings should correlate with the physical findings, and any discrepancies should be identified. Inconsistencies may have as much importance in the clinical treatment of the patient as consistent results (1,2).

■ Also, the degree of definitiveness of the findings needs to be conveyed to the referring physician. A diagnosis of S1 radiculopathy by H reflex alone will carry different weight than abundant spontaneous activity in the S1 myotomal distribution.

■ One abnormal finding does not make the diagnosis if all other evidence is pointing to a different diagnosis (11).

■ When possible, the report should include (1,2):
  ■ Sufficient evidence to rule out alternative possibilities and to identify superimposed conditions

■ The degree of injury and chronicity
■ Prognostic information
■ Comparison with previous EDX data

SUMMARY

■ EDX studies (including NCS and NE) serve as an extension of the physical exam to better characterize and localize nerve injury.

■ EDX studies evaluate the physiology and function of the largest fibers of the peripheral nervous system (lower motor neuron pathway).

■ NCSs attempt to localize peripheral entrapment neuropathies by identification of conduction block (focally decreased amplitude or conduction slowing) and can often differentiate demyelination (prolonged latency/slow conduction velocity) from axonal injury (low amplitude).

■ Neurapraxic injuries are limited to the nerve myelin and tend to have more rapid recovery than axonal injuries.

■ NE can identify patterns of denervation from axonal injury, including information about chronicity. Acute denervation changes include abnormal spontaneous activity, such as fibrillations and positive sharp waves. Chronic changes may include long-duration, large-amplitude, or polyphasic MUAPs.

■ The timing of EDX study is important. Although immediate study after a trauma can provide useful information (such as presence of conduction block), some NE abnormalities may take 2–6 weeks to manifest.

■ Although EDX studies are considered reliable for detecting nerve pathology, they are dependent on the quality of the examiner.

REFERENCES

1. Akuthota V, Casey E. Diagnostic tests for nerve and vascular injuries. In: Akuthota V, Herring SA, editors. *Nerve and Vascular Injuries in Sports Medicine.* New York: Springer; 2009. p. 17–26.

2. Akuthota V, Friedrich JM. Electrodiagnosic testing in runners. In: Wilder RP, O'Connor FG, Magrum E, editors. *Textbook of Running Medicine.* 2nd ed. New York: McGraw-Hill; in press.

3. Bachner EJ, Friedman MJ. Injuries to the leg. In: Nicholas JA, Hershman EB, editors. *The Lower Extremity and Spine in Sports Medicine.* St. Louis: Mosby; 1995.

4. Basmajian JV, DeLuca CJ. *Muscles Alive: Their Functions Revealed by Electromyography.* 5th ed. Baltimore (MD): Williams & Wilkins; 1988. 561 p.

5. Chang CW, Shieh SF, Li CM, et al. Measurement of motor nerve conduction velocity of the sciatic nerve in patients with piriformis syndrome: a magnetic stimulation study. *Arch Phys Med Rehabil.* 2006;87(10):1371–5.

6. Checkles NS, Russakov AD, Piero DL. Ulnar nerve conduction velocity—effect of elbow positon on measurment. *Arch Phys Med Rehabil.* 1971;53(8):362–5.

7. Chémali KR, Tsao B. Electrodiagnostic testing of nerves and muscles: when, why, and how to order. *Cleve Clin J Med.* 2005;72(1):37–48.

8. Colak T, Bamaç B, Gönener A, et al. Comparison of nerve conduction velocities of lower extremities between runners and controls. *J Sci Med Sport.* 2005;8(4):403–10.

9. Daube JR, Rubin DI. Needle electromyography. *Muscle Nerve.* 2009; 39(2):244–70.

10. Derr JJ, Mickleson PJ, Robinson LR. Predicting recovery after fibular nerve injury: which electrodiagnostic features are most useful? *Am J Phys Med Rehabil.* 2009;88(7):547–53.

11. Dillingham, TR. Electrodiagnostic medicine II: clinical evaluation and findings. In: Braddom RL, editor. *Physical Medicine & Rehabilitation.* 3rd ed. Philadelphia (PA): Elsevier; 2007. 1532 p.

12. Dumitru D. *Electrodiagnostic Medicine.* Philadelphia (PA): Hanley and Belfus; 2001. 1524 p.

13. Dumitru D, Diaz CA, King JC. Prevalence of denveration in paraspinal and foot intrinsic musculature. *Am J Phys Med Rehabil.* 2001;80(7):482–90.

14. Dyck PJ, Classen SM, Stevens JC, O'Brien PC. Assessment of nerve damage in the feet of long-distance runners. *Mayo Clin Proc.* 1987;62(7): 568–72.

15. Feinberg JH. The role of electrodiagnostics in the study of muscle kinesiology, muscle fatigue and peripheral nerve injuries in sports medicine. *J Back Musculoskelet Med.* 1999;12(2):73–88.

16. Fisher MA. H reflexes and F waves: fundamentals, normal and abnormal patterns. *Neurol Clin.* 2002;20(2):339–60, vi.

17. Fishman LM, Dombi GW, Michaelson C, et al. Piriformis syndrome: diagnosis, treatment and outcome—a 10-year study. *Arch Phys Med Rehabil.* 2002;83(3):295–301.

18. Gooch CL, Weimer LH. The electrodiagnosis of neuropathy: basic principles and common pitfalls. *Neurol Clin.* 2007;25(1):1–28.

19. Horowitz SH. The diagnostic work-up of patients with neuropathic pain. *Med Clin North Am.* 2007;91(1):21–30.

20. Hurd WJ, Snyder-Mackler L. Knee instability after acute ACL rupture affects movement patterns during the mid-stance of gait. *J Orthop Res.* 2007;25(10):1369–77.

21. Jackson DL, Haglund BL. Tarsal tunnel syndrome in runners. *Sports Med.* 1992;13(2):146–9.

22. Jensen MC, Brant-Zawadzki MN, Obuchowski N, et al. Magnetic resonance imaging of the lumbar spine in people without back pain. *N Engl J Med.* 1994;331(2):69–73.

23. Kraft GH. Fibrillation potential amplitude and muscle atrophy following peripheral nerve injury. *Muscle Nerve.* 1990;13(9):814–21.

24. Leach RE, Purnell MB, Saito A. Peroneal nerve entrapment in runners. *Am J Sports Med.* 1989;17(2):287–91.

25. Mann RA. Biomechanics of running. In: Nicholas JA, Hershman EB, editors. *The Lower Extremity and Spine in Sports Medicine.* St. Louis: Mosby; 1995.

26. McKean KA. Neurologic running injuries. *Neurol Clin.* 2008;26(1): 281–96, xii.

27. Mysiew WJ, Colachis SC 3rd. The pronator syndrome: an evaluation of dynamic maneuvers for improving electrodiagnostic sensitivity. *Am J Phys Rehabil.* 1991;70(5):274–7.

28. Olney RK, So YT, Goodin DS, et al. A comparison of magnetic and electrical stimulation of peripheral nerves. *Muscle Nerve.* 1990;13(10): 957–63.

29. Park TA, Del Toro DR. Electrodiagnostic evaluation of the foot. *Phys Med Rehabil Clin North Am.* 1998;9(4):871–96, vii–viii.

30. Patel AT, Gaines K, Malamut R, et al. Usefulness of electrodiagnostic techniques in the evaluation of suspected tarsal tunnel syndrome: an evidence-based review. *Muscle Nerve.* 2005;32(2):236–40.

31. Press JM, Young JL. Electrodiagnostic evaluation of spine problems. In Gonzalez G, Materson RS, editors. *The Nonsurgical Management of Acute Low Back Pain.* New York (NY): Demos Vermande; 1997. p. 191–203.

32. Robinson LR. AAEM minimonograph 28: traumatic injury to peripheral nerves. *Muscle Nerve.* 2000;23(6):863–73.

33. Rossini PM, Barker AT, Berardelli A, et al. Non-invasive electrical and magnetic stimulation of the brain, spinal cord and roots: basic principles and procedures for routine clinical application. Report of an IFCN committee. *Electroencephalogr Clin Neurophysiol.* 1994;91(2):79–92.

34. Weber M, Eisen AA. AAEM minimonograph 35: magnetic stimulation of the central and peripheral nervous system. *Muscle Nerve.* 2002; 25(2):160–75.

21 Exercise Testing

Russell D. White and George D. Harris

INTRODUCTION

- Various anatomic, electric, and physiologic tests are used in evaluation of the heart. The exercise test (ET), formerly the exercise stress test (EST), endures as one of the few valuable and practical physiologic tools to evaluate cardiac perfusion and function under controlled conditions. With the advent of newer cardiovascular imaging techniques, many physicians have moved away from this traditional physiologic test, but numerous evidence-based guidelines as established by the American College of Cardiology (ACC)/American Heart Association (AHA), as well as the American College of Sports Medicine® (ACSM), have shown that many of the new technologies do not necessarily have better diagnostic characteristics than the standard ET (21).
- ET is useful for diagnosis of ischemia (sensitivity of 50%–70%, specificity of 80%–90%), prognosis of known cardiac disease, and exercise prescription (21,24).
- When performing an ET, one should understand its physiology, indications, contraindications, and interpretation, with special consideration given to athletes whose abnormal responses may, in fact, be normal variations.

EXERCISE TEST TERMINOLOGY

- It is essential to understand the basic ET terminology prior to performing the test:
  - **PR segment:** The isoelectric line from which the ST segment and the J point are measured at rest. With exercise, the PR segment slopes downward and shortens in duration, at which point the PQ junction becomes the point of reference for determining the ST segment.
  - **J point:** The point that distinguishes the QRS complex from the ST segment; the point at which the slope changes; the point against which the ST segment deviation (depression or elevation) is measured.
  - **ST segment:** ST segment level is measured relative to the PQ junction. If the baseline is depressed, the deviation from that level to the level during exercise or recovery is measured. The ST segment is measured at 60 or 80 milliseconds after the J point. (At ventricular rates > 145 bpm, it is measured at 60 milliseconds after the J point) (20,25).
- **$\dot{V}O_{2max}$:** The greatest amount of oxygen a person can use while performing dynamic exercise involving a large part of their muscle mass. This is a function of a person's functional aerobic capacity and defines the limits of the cardiopulmonary system. It is defined by the Fick equation, which incorporates both heart rate (HR) and stroke volume (SV):

$$\dot{V}O_{2max} = \text{Maximum cardiac output} \times \text{Maximum arteriovenous } O_2 \text{ difference}$$

$$\dot{V}O_{2max} = (HR_{max} \times SV_{max}) \times (CaO_{2max} - CvO_{2max})$$

- $\dot{V}O_{2max}$ is defined by a central component (cardiac output), which describes the capacity of the heart to function as a pump, and by peripheral factors (arteriovenous-oxygen difference), which describe the capacity of the lungs to oxygenate the blood delivered to it and the capacity of the working muscles to extract this oxygenated blood (39). Many factors affect each of these variables.
  - HR is affected most importantly by age and (220 − age) ± 12 beats (1 standard deviation [SD]) gives a good estimate of maximum HR (HR_{max}). However, in medicine, we use 2 SDs, which renders an extremely wide range. The scientific method for determining the individual HR_{max} is to perform an ET on the individual. HR is also affected by activity type, body position, fitness level, presence of heart disease, medications, blood volume, and environment (27).
  - SV is affected by factors such as genetics, conditioning (heart size), and cardiac disease. In normal subjects, an increase in both end-diastolic and end-systolic volume occurs in response to moving from an upright, at rest position to a moderate level of exercise. End-systolic volume decreases progressively as exercise intensifies in order to maintain SV. At peak exercise, end-diastolic volume may even decline.
  - Arterial oxygen content is related to the partial pressure of arterial oxygen, which is determined in the lung by alveolar ventilation and pulmonary diffusion capacity and in the blood by hemoglobin content. In the absence of pulmonary disease, arterial oxygen content and saturation generally remain similar to resting values throughout exercise, even at high levels (39).

❑ Venous oxygen content is determined by the amount of blood flow directed to the muscle and by capillary density. Muscle blood flow increases with exercise not only because of increased cardiac output, but also because of the preferential redistribution of the cardiac output (> 85% of total cardiac output) to the exercising muscle. A decrease in local and systemic vascular resistance also facilitates greater skeletal muscle flow. Finally, there is an increase in the overall number of capillaries with ongoing physical training (39).

■ **Metabolic equivalents (METs):** A convenient measure for expressing oxygen uptake. One MET is a unit of sitting, resting oxygen requirements (3.5 mL $O_2 \cdot$ kg body weight/min).

❑ 1 MET = Basal O_2 requirements (*e.g.*, sitting, lying)

❑ 5 METs = Energy cost for activities of daily living; poor prognosis for anginal patients; consider catheterization

❑ 10 METs = Similar prognosis with medical treatment versus interventional therapy in coronary artery disease (CAD)

❑ 13 METs = Excellent prognosis regardless of other exercise responses

❑ 18 METs = Elite athletes

■ **Myocardial oxygen consumption:** The "double product," an indirect measurement of myocardial oxygen consumption, measures the product of maximum or peak HR and systolic blood pressure (32). Angina normally occurs at the same double product rather than at same external workload. A normal value is considered greater than 25,000.

PERFORMING THE EXERCISE TEST

Indications

■ The three major cardiopulmonary reasons for ET relate to diagnosis, prognosis, and therapeutic prescription (25,28,45).

CLASS I

■ Conditions for which there is general consensus that ET is justified:

▪ To assist in the diagnosis of CAD in those adult patients with an intermediate (20%–80%) pretest probability of disease

▪ To assess functional capacity and to aid in the prognosis of patients with known CAD

▪ To evaluate the prognosis and functional capacity of patients with known CAD soon after an uncomplicated myocardial infarction (MI)

▪ To evaluate patients with symptoms consistent with recurrent, exercise-induced cardiac arrhythmias

CLASS II

■ Conditions for which ET is frequently used but in which there is a divergence of opinion regarding medical effectiveness of ET:

▪ To evaluate asymptomatic males > 45 years (females > 55 years) with special occupations

▪ To evaluate asymptomatic males > 45 years (females > 55 years) with two or more cardiac risk factors

▪ To evaluate asymptomatic males > 45 years (females > 55 years) who plan to enter a vigorous exercise program

▪ To assist in the diagnosis of CAD in adult patients with a high or low pretest probability of disease

▪ To evaluate patients with a class I indication who have baseline electrocardiogram (ECG) changes

CLASS III

■ Conditions for which there is general agreement that ET is of little or no value, inappropriate, or contraindicated:

▪ To assist in the diagnosis of CAD in patients with left bundle branch block (LBBB) or Wolff-Parkinson-White (W-P-W) syndrome on a resting ECG

▪ To evaluate patients with simple premature ventricular contractions (PVCs) on a resting ECG with no other evidence for CAD

▪ To evaluate men or women with chest discomfort not thought to be cardiac in origin

■ The above classes group the indications based on risk according to ACSM guidelines. Patients are categorized into low-, moderate-, and high-risk groups prior to beginning an exercise program. Risk stratification is based on age, sex, presence of CAD risk factors, major symptoms of disease, or known heart disease (1,19) (Tables 21.1 and 21.2).

■ **Low risk:** Asymptomatic younger individuals (men < age 45 years; women < age 55 years) and no more than one risk factor from Table 21.1.

■ Moderate risk: Older individuals (men age ≥ 45 years; women age ≥ 55 years) or those individuals with ≥ two risk factors from Table 21.1.

■ High risk: Individuals with one or more signs or symptoms from Table 21.2 or known cardiovascular, pulmonary, or metabolic disease.

■ In addition, level of activity is divided into low, moderate (3–6 METS or 40%–60% of $\dot{V}O_{2max}$), and vigorous (> 6 METS or > 60% of $\dot{V}O_{2max}$) exercise. Clinicians use these factors to recommend which patients need an ET (1):

▪ Low-risk individuals do not need an ET regardless of level of activity.

Table 21.1	**Atherosclerotic Cardiovascular Disease (CVD) Risk Factor Thresholds for Use with ACSM Risk Stratification**
Positive Risk Factors	**Defining Criteria**
Age	Men > 45 years; women > 55 years
Family history	Myocardial infarction, coronary revascularization, or sudden death before 55 years of age in father or other male first-degree relative, or before 65 years of age in mother or other female first-degree relative
Cigarette smoking	Current cigarette smoker or those who quit within the previous 6 months or exposure to environmental tobacco smoke
Sedentary lifestyle	Not participating in at least 30 minutes of moderate-intensity exercise (40%–60% $\dot{V}O_2R$) physical activity on at least 3 days of the week for at least 3 months
Obesity	Body mass index $\geq$ 30 kg · m^2 *or* waist girth > 102 cm (40 inches) for men and $\geq$ 88 cm (35 inches) for women
Hypertension	Systolic blood pressure > 140 mm Hg and/or diastolic blood pressure $\geq$ 90 mm Hg, confirmed by measurements on at least two separate occasions, *or* on hypertensive medication
Dyslipidemia	Low-density lipoprotein cholesterol $\geq$ 130 mL · kg^{-1} · min^{-1}) or high-density lipoprotein (HDL) cholesterol < 40 mL · kg^{-1} · min^{-1} or on lipid-lowering medication. If total serum cholesterol is all that is available, use $\geq$ 200 mL · kg^{-1} · min^{-1}.
Prediabetes	Impaired fasting glucose = fasting plasma glucose > 100 mL · kg^{-1} · min^{-1} but < 126 mL · kg^{-1} · min^{-1} *or* impaired glucose tolerance = 2-hour values in oral glucose tolerance test > 140 mL · kg^{-1} · min^{-1} but less than 200 mL · kg^{-1} · min^{-1} confirmed by measurements on at least two separate occasions
Negative Risk Factor	**Defining Criteria**
High-serum HDL cholesterol	$\geq$ 60 mL $\geq$ kg^{-1} · min^{-1}

SOURCE: American College of Sports Medicine. *ACSM's Guidelines for Exercise Testing and Prescription.* 8th ed. Baltimore (MD): Lippincott Williams & Wilkins; 2010. p. 28.

- Moderate-risk individuals should have an ET prior to beginning vigorous exercise only.
- High-risk individuals need an ET before any moderate or vigorous activity.
- Risk stratification of patients for diagnosis of CAD divides patients into those with typical angina, atypical angina, non-anginal chest pain, or no chest pain. There are also special disease groups (*e.g.*, diabetes mellitus) that have specific indications for testing (6,7,29,41). The Duke Treadmill Score has been validated in persons with diabetes (34).

Table 21.2	**Major Signs or Symptoms Suggestive of Cardiovascular, Pulmonary, or Metabolic Disease**

1. Pain or discomfort (or other anginal equivalent) in the chest, neck, jaw, arms, or other areas that may result from ischemia
2. Shortness of breath at rest or with mild exertion
3. Dizziness or syncope
4. Orthopnea or paroxysmal nocturnal dyspnea
5. Ankle edema
6. Palpitations or tachycardia
7. Intermittent claudication
8. Known heart murmur
9. Unusual fatigue or shortness of breath with usual activities

SOURCE: American College of Sports Medicine. *ACSM's Guidelines for Exercise Testing and Prescription.* 8th ed. Baltimore (MD): Lippincott Williams & Wilkins; 2010. p. 26–7.

Contraindications

- In some individuals, there may be contraindications to performing the procedure.

Absolute Contraindications

- Acute MI
- A recent significant change in ECG
- Unstable angina
- Rapid ventricular or atrial arrhythmias
- History suggesting medicine toxicity
- Severe aortic stenosis
- Uncontrolled congestive heart failure (CHF)
- Suspected dissecting aortic aneurysm
- Active myocarditis or pericarditis
- Active thrombophlebitis
- Recent embolism
- Active infection
- Uncooperative patient

Relative Contraindications

- Risks of performing procedure may outweigh benefits.
  - Uncontrolled tachyarrhythmias or bradyarrhythmias
  - Frequent ventricular ectopic activity
  - Untreated pulmonary hypertension
  - Resting systemic blood pressure (BP) > 200/110
  - Ventricular aneurysm
  - Moderate aortic stenosis/hypertrophic cardiomyopathy

- Marked cardiac enlargement
- Uncontrolled metabolic disease
- Chronic infectious disease
- Known left main artery disease
- Electrolyte abnormalities
- Neuromuscular, musculoskeletal disorders that prohibit exercise or are exacerbated by exercise

Special Considerations

- There are special situations in which the physician must evaluate the patient carefully before undertaking ET or should consider an alternative test. For example, a post–cerebrovascular accident patient may be unable to exercise and require a chemical test for evaluation. Other special situations fall into one of three groups: conduction disturbances (atrioventricular [AV] blocks, LBBB, W-P-W) (25), medication effects (β-blockers, calcium channel blockers, digoxin) (1), and special clinical situations (unstable hypertension, previous MI, known CAD) (4). With either chemical or exercise testing, one may couple imaging modalities (echocardiography or nuclear scanning) (28).

Physician Responsibilities

- During exercise testing, the physician's responsibilities include the following.

Pretest Patient Evaluation and Clearance

- Review of medical history including recent symptoms, cardiac risk factors, and previous exercise testing
- Pertinent clinical exam, including a cardiac exam to evaluate for murmurs or gallops
- Clarification of ET indications and exclusion of those patients with contraindications
- Obtaining a resting baseline ECG and evaluation for abnormalities
- Consent of patient and documentation of risks versus benefits

Protocol Selection

- The selected protocol must be customized to the individual patient to allow 8–12 minutes of exercise (22). The physician must decide whether the patient needs a maximal or submaximal test. Most information is obtained from performing a maximal test where a true peak, individual, maximal HR is achieved, rather than an age-predicted maximal HR. If one chooses a symptom-limited maximal test, the patient is in control, and ultimate information is obtained. If the ECG and BP are normal and the patient follows the Borg Scale of perceived exertion, minimal risk is posed for the patient. Examples of exercise protocols include the following:
  - Bruce (most common, extensive research database)
  - Modified Bruce (less rigorous)
  - Balke-Ware (smaller workloads, used in cardiac/older patients)

- Ramp (most accurate; excellent correlation with $\dot{V}O_{2max}$ determinations; slow, continuous increase in workload)
- Cycle or arm ergometry (if unable to use treadmill)

PERFORMING THE TEST

- A pretest checklist should be instituted that includes an equipment and safety check, consent and pretest assessment, supine and standing ECGs, BP measurements, and protocol selection (45). During the ET, the patient should be monitored continuously along with ECG and BP readings at each stage. The patient should be alerted to stage changes, and the test should be terminated when the patient reaches maximal effort or exhibits clinical signs requiring termination of the test:
  - Absolute indications for termination of ET:
    - Acute MI
    - Onset of progressive angina or angina equivalents
    - Exertional hypotension with increasing workload
    - Serious dysrhythmias (*e.g.*, ventricular tachycardia)
    - Signs of poor perfusion (pallor, cyanosis, nausea or cold, clammy skin)
    - Central nervous system symptoms (ataxia, vertigo, visual or gait problems)
    - Failure of increasing HR with increasing workload
    - Technical problems or equipment failure
    - Patient requests to stop
  - Relative indications for termination of ET
    - Pronounced ECG changes from baseline, including more than 2 mV of horizontal or downsloping ST segment depression or 2 mV of ST segment elevation
    - Progressive or increasing chest pain
    - Pronounced fatigue or dyspnea
    - Wheezing
    - Leg cramps or intermittent claudication
    - Hypertensive response (systolic BP > 250 mm Hg or diastolic BP > 115 mm Hg)
    - Less serious dysrhythmias such as supraventricular tachycardia
    - Exercise-induced bundle branch block that cannot be distinguished from ventricular tachycardia
    - Moderate chest pain, claudication, or dyspnea
- Recovery includes either immediately placing the patient in the supine position or allowing a "cool-down walk" for 5–6 minutes and then placing the patient in a chair. Maximal test sensitivity is achieved with the patient supine after exercise.
  - Auscultate for abnormal heart sounds such as a new-onset heart murmur or third heart sound.
  - Auscultate lungs for any evidence of exercise-induced bronchospasm that might cause chest pain
  - Obtain BP and ECG at 1 minute and then every 2 minutes thereafter (10,43,44).

- Carefully monitor patient for 8–10 minutes until clinically stable and ECG has returned to normal.
- Monitor carefully for any recovery-only ST segment depression (33).

INTERPRETATION OF THE TEST

- Interpreting the ET involves much more than describing whether the test was "positive" or "negative" for ischemia. The written report should include the HR and BP response, the presence or absence of symptoms, any dysrhythmias, the functional aerobic capacity, ECG changes, and the presence or absence of myocardial ischemia (3,14,17).

Heart Rate Response

- An increase in HR occurs with aerobic exercise secondary to a withdrawal of vagal tone and an increase in sympathetic tone. The increase is linear and correlates with workload and oxygen uptake. The maximum HR should be reported as a percentage of the predicted maximal HR (220 − age). The failure of the HR to elevate above 120 with maximum exercise is defined as chronotropic incompetence and suggests possible underlying CAD. Chronotropic incompetence is an independent predictor of mortality (13,35). Abnormal HR recovery (HRR), defined as the failure of the HR to decrease by 12 bpm during the first minute in recovery, portends an increased mortality for the patient (10).

Blood Pressure Response

- As work increases, there is a corresponding increase in the systolic BP that peaks at maximum exercise. A decrease in systolic BP during exercise is very suggestive of ischemic dysfunction of the myocardium (23). Diastolic BP remains the same or decreases. An increase in diastolic BP of > 10 mm Hg is abnormal and can be considered a hypertensive response to exercise. The postexercise systolic BP response has also been described. A 3-minute postexercise systolic BP/peak systolic BP ratio > 0.90 is considered abnormal with a diagnostic accuracy of 75% for CAD and comparable to that of ST segment depression (43,44).

Signs and Symptoms

- The presence or absence of symptoms such as chest pain, claudication, or exercise-induced wheezing should be mentioned in the report. Patients with exercise-induced angina have been shown to have a worse prognosis compared to patients with only ST depression (12). Therefore, these patients, even in the absence of ECG ischemic changes, should be regarded as having a test "suggestive of myocardial ischemia." The rating of perceived exertion (RPE) is valuable to measure during exercise testing because it correlates well with

HR and $\dot{V}O_{2max}$. The nonlinear Borg Scale (RPE) assigns a number of 0–10, with the higher number indicative of more difficult exertion (8).

Dysrhythmias/Conduction Disturbances

- Ectopy or dysrhythmias that occur during the ET should be mentioned on the report. Unifocal PVCs are seen frequently during testing and are not necessarily specific for myocardial ischemia, although, if frequent, they may increase the long-term risk of cardiovascular death in asymptomatic patients (15,16,31). High-grade ectopy (couplets, mutiform/multifocal PVCs, ventricular tachycardia) is more suggestive of severe ischemic heart disease and higher mortality than those without ectopy (9). Supraventricular dysrhythmias (atrial fibrillation/flutter) require termination of the test and further intervention. Intracardiac blocks can occur before, during, or after testing, and advanced forms of AV block (Mobitz II and higher) are abnormal. Bundle branch blocks occur very infrequently with exercise and require further evaluation, especially LBBB, which may portend an increased mortality if structural heart disease is present (15,16).

Aerobic Capacity

- The ET can either measure the maximal functional aerobic capacity ($\dot{V}O_{2max}$) by direct gas analysis or estimate it from workload performed in a maximal test. A nomogram is used to convert minutes (or METs) into $\dot{V}O_{2max}$. The results can then be compared with standard tables of fitness levels for age and sex (2).

Electrocardiographic Responses to Exercise Testing

- ST segment changes are the most common signs of ischemia. ST segment *depression* represents subendocardial ischemia, and one cannot anatomically localize the ischemia based on ECG location/changes of the ST depression. ST segment *elevation* represents transmural ischemia, and the location of the anatomic ischemia does correlate with associated ECG changes.

Normal Responses with Exercise

- The PR segment shortens and slopes downward in the inferior leads. The QRS complex may show increased Q wave negativity and a decrease in R wave amplitude with an increased S wave depth. The J point becomes depressed with exercise. If already elevated at rest, it will commonly normalize. The T wave decreases in amplitude, and the ST segment develops a positive upslope that returns to baseline within 60–80 milliseconds.

Abnormal Responses with Exercise

- ST segment depression: This is the hallmark of ischemia and a positive test (see next section).

- ST segment normalization: ST segments that are depressed and return to normal (pseudonormalization) are suggestive of ischemia.
- ST segment elevation: In patients without a prior history of MI, consider acute MI (if accompanied by chest pain) or serious transmural ischemia involving proximal high-grade stenosis of the left anterior descending artery or right coronary artery. This may also be seen with severe coronary artery spasm (Prinzmetal angina) (14). ST elevation over Q waves in patients with a previous history of an MI suggests areas of dyskinesis or ventricular aneurysm (18).
- U wave inversion: U wave inversion during exercise is suggestive of ischemia.

Final Determination for Myocardial Ischemia

- One of four descriptions should appear in the patient's written report to represent the final determination for myocardial ischemia (14,20,33,42).
  - Positive
    - Horizontal ST segment depression that is ≥ 1 mm at 60–80 milliseconds past the J point
    - Downsloping ST segment depression that is ≥ 1 mm at the J point or J + 20 milliseconds
    - Upsloping ST depression that is ≥ 1.5 mm depressed at 80 milliseconds past the J point
  - Suggestive
    - Horizontal ST segment depression between 0.5 and 1 mm at 60–80 milliseconds past the J point
    - Upsloping ST segment depression between 0.7 and 1.5 mm at 80 milliseconds past the J point ST elevation between 0.5 and 1.0 mm
    - Exercise-induced hypotension
    - Chest pain occurring with exercise typical of angina
    - Frequent, high-grade, ventricular ectopy
    - A new third heart sound or murmur at peak exercise
    - Abnormal 1-minute HRR or 3-minute systolic BP response in recovery
    - Recovery-only ST segment depression
    - Normalization of abnormal ST segments/T wave inversion
  - Negative
    - Above criteria are not met and the patient exercised to at least 85% of maximum predicted HR.
  - Inconclusive
    - The patient does not reach 85% of maximum predicted HR and there is no evidence of ischemia based on the above criteria. (Confirm the patient is not on β-blockers or does not have chronotropic incompetence.)

CLINICAL DECISION MAKING

- Physicians can use the results of the ET to guide them in the management of their patients. This approach should include

a probability statement of CAD and a prediction of severity of CAD, prognosis of the likelihood of future adverse events in a patient based on the exercise treadmill score or Duke Treadmill Score, the functional capacity of the patient, and an exercise prescription.

Probability of Coronary Artery Disease

- The ET has a role in the diagnosis of CAD, with an overall 75% sensitivity and 80% specificity. Froelicher and Myers (24) found that combining standard exercise testing with an evidence-based score strategy (*e.g.*, Duke Treadmill Score) yielded an 85% sensitivity, 92% specificity, and 88% predictive accuracy. These data confirm ET as an excellent screening test for CAD. The predictive value, however, depends on the prevalence of CAD in the population tested. It is, therefore, imperative to determine a pretest probability of CAD in a patient and then use the results of the ET to determine a new posttest likelihood. ET has the greatest value in individuals who have a pretest probability between 20% and 80% (11). Diamond and Forrester (12) have created tables to predict the pretest/posttest likelihood of disease based on age, sex, and clinical symptoms. Two examples serve to illustrate this point:
  - A 40-year-old male with atypical angina has a pretest probability of about 35%. If he has between 1 and 2 mm of ST depression on ET, his posttest probability of CAD becomes nearly 70%, a much more significant risk elucidated by ET.
  - A 40-year-old female with atypical angina has a pretest probability of less than 10%. If she has between 1 and 2 mm of ST depression, her posttest probability of CAD still is less than 20%, and little is gained from the ET.

Prediction of Severity of CAD

- A suggestive or positive written report may be used to further manage patients by predicting the severity of CAD. Upsloping, horizontal, and downsloping ST depression correlate respectively with a worsening extent of CAD. The following are important ET predictors of severe CAD (26):
  - ST depression > 2.5 mm
  - ST depression beginning at low workload, < 5 METS
  - Downsloping configuration (99% predictive of CAD) or ST elevation
  - Prolonged ST depression lasting > 8 minutes into rest
  - Global ST depression
  - Serious dysrhythmias at low HR (< 130 bpm)
  - U wave inversion
  - Low workload ability, < 5 METs
  - Exercise-induced hypotension
  - Chronotropic incompetence
  - Anginal symptoms

- ST depression only at high workloads (HR > 160 bpm or changes only after stage IV—Bruce protocol at 12 minutes) correlates with a low mortality and good prognosis in patients. In fact, the ability to exercise at > 13 METs has a good prognosis regardless of the ECG changes. Many cardiologists recommend repeating the ET in 6 months without further workup in these patients (26).

Exercise Treadmill Score

- This tool supports the above concepts by assigning a score to determine prognosis and applies to either inpatient or outpatient populations (36,37):

  Exercise treadmill score (Duke Treadmill Score) 5 Exercise duration (minutes) − 5 × ST deviation (mm) − 4 × treadmill angina index; (treadmill angina index = 0 if no exercise-associated angina, 1 for exercise-associated angina, and 2 for exercise-limiting angina)

- If the score is up to +5 or greater, the patient has a very good prognosis and can be followed safely with regular ET. The 5-year survival for this group is 97%.

- If the score is −10 to +4, the patient has an intermediate prognosis.

- A patient in the high-risk group (treadmill score of −11 or less) has a poor prognosis, with a 5-year survival rate of 72%. The ET score is thus valuable for prognosis and should be calculated in all patients undergoing CAD evaluation.

Exercise Prescription (4,5,25)

- The ET can assist in writing the exercise prescription. A maximum symptom-limited test establishes a baseline fitness level and establishes a parameter for improving fitness. The ACSM recommends exercise intensities between 55% and 90% of HR_{max}, or 50%–85% of $\dot{V}O_{2max}$. The conditioning range for most adults to improve cardiorespiratory fitness is between 70% and 85% of HR_{max} (65%–80% $\dot{V}O_{2max}$).

SPECIAL CONSIDERATIONS IN ATHLETES

- There are no specific indications for testing athletes, although they are tested for diagnosis of CAD, fitness evaluation, generating an exercise prescription, and guiding training. The Bruce protocol, with gas exchange, to establish a $\dot{V}O_{2max}$, is most often employed. The Astrand, Costill, or ramp protocols may also be used (38,40).

- Athletes manifest many differences compared with the general population both clinically and on ECG. They commonly have increased ventricular volume and mass along with sinus bradyarrhythmias. It is not uncommon to see certain ECG findings such as first-degree AV blocks, right axis deviation, ventricular hypertrophy with repolarization abnormalities, or incomplete right bundle branch block.

All these findings are normal variants known as the athletic heart syndrome (30).

- Interpretation of the ET in this population incorporates the same criteria as the general population; however, because of the variants stated above, there is a greater probability of a false-positive test.

SUMMARY

- The ET remains a valuable tool for diagnosing CAD, evaluating prognosis, and developing an exercise prescription. By implementing the test appropriately, the primary care physician can enhance its validity and usefulness in clinical decision making.

REFERENCES

1. American College of Sports Medicine. Preparticipation health screening and risk stratification. In: Thompson WR, editor. *ACSM's Guidelines for Exercise Testing and Prescription*. 8th ed. Baltimore: Lippincott Williams & Wilkins; 2010. p. 18–39.

2. American College of Sports Medicine. Health-related physical fitness testing and interpretation. In: Thompson WR, editor. *ACSM's Guidelines for Exercise Testing and Prescription*. 8th ed. Baltimore: Lippincott Williams & Wilkins; 2010. p. 60–104.

3. American College of Sports Medicine. Interpretation of clinical exercise test data. In: Thompson WR, editor. *ACSM's Guidelines for Exercise Testing and Prescription*. 8th ed. Baltimore: Lippincott Williams & Wilkins; 2010. p. 135–51.

4. American College of Sports Medicine. General principles of exercise prescription. In: Thompson WR, editor. *ACSM's Guidelines for Exercise Testing and Prescription*. 8th ed. Baltimore: Lippincott Williams & Wilkins; 2010. p. 152–82.

5. American College of Sports Medicine. Exercise prescription for healthy populations and special considerations. In: Thompson WR, editor. *ACSM's Guidelines for Exercise Testing and Prescription*. 8th ed. Baltimore: Lippincott Williams & Wilkins; 2010. p. 183–224.

6. American College of Sports Medicine. *ACSM's Guidelines for Exercise Testing and Prescription*. 8th ed. Baltimore: Lippincott Williams & Wilkins; 2010. p. 308–9.

7. American Diabetes Association. Clinical practice recommendations 2011: physical activity/exercise and diabetes mellitus. *Diabetes Care*. 2011;34(Suppl 1):S73–7.

8. Bax JJ, Young LH, Frye RL, et al. Screening for coronary artery disease in patients with diabetes. *Diabetes Care*. 2007;30(10):2729–36.

9. Borg G, Holmgren A, Lindblad I. Quantitative evaluation of chest pain. *Acta Med Scand Suppl*. 1981;644:43–5.

10. Califf RKM, McKinnis RA, McNeer M, et al. Prognostic value of ventricular arrhythmias associated with treadmill exercise testing in patients studied with cardiac catheterization for suspected ischemic heart disease. *J Am Coll Cardiol*. 1983;2(6):1060–7.

11. Cole CR, Blackstone EH, Pashkow EJ, et al. Heart rate recovery immediately after exercise as a predictor of mortality. *N Engl J Med*. 1999; 341(18):1351–7.

12. Diamond GA, Forrester JS. Analysis of probability as an aid in the clinical diagnosis of coronary artery disease. *N Engl J Med*. 1979; 300(24):1350–8.

13. Ellestad MH. Rhythm and conduction disturbances in stress testing. In: Ellestad MH, *Stress Testing: Principles and Practice*. 5th ed. Philadelphia: FA Davis; 2003. p. 241–70.

14. Ellestad MH. Predictive implications. In: Ellestad MH, *Stress Testing: Principles and Practice*. 5th ed. Philadelphia: FA Davis; 2003. p. 271–308.

15. Evans CH, Ellestad MH. Interpretation of the exercise test. In: Evans CH, White RD, editors. *Exercise Testing for Primary Care and Sports Medicine Physicians*. New York: Springer; 2009. p. 81–108.

16. Evans CH, Froelicher VF. Common abnormal responses seen with exercise testing and how to manage them. In: Evans CH, White RD, editors. *Exercise Testing for Primary Care and Sports Medicine Physicians*. New York: Springer; 2009. p. 109–20.

17. Evans CH, Froelicher VF. Some common abnormal responses to exercise testing: what to do when you see them. *Prim Care*. 2001;28(1): 219–32, ix.

18. Evans CH, Harris G, Mendold V, Ellestad MH. A basic approach to the interpretation of the exercise test. *Prim Care*. 2001;28(1):73–98, vi.

19. Evans CH, Pyhel HJ, White RD. Case studies: lessons learned from interesting cases. In: Evans CH, White RD, editors. *Exercise Testing for Primary Care and Sports Medicine Physicians*. New York: Springer; 2009. p. 375–99.

20. Expert Panel on Detection, Evaluation, and Treatment of High Blood Cholesterol in Adults. Executive summary of the third report of the National Cholesterol Education Program (NCEP) Expert Panel on Detection, Evaluation, and Treatment of High Blood Cholesterol in Adults (Adult Treatment Panel III). *JAMA*. 2001;285(19):2486–97.

21. Fletcher GF, Balady GJ, Amsterdam EA, et al. Exercise standards for testing and training: a statement for healthcare professionals from the American Heart Association Scientific Statement. *Circulation*. 2001;104(14):1694–740.

22. Froelicher VF, Fearon WF, Ferguson CM, et al. Lessons learned from studies of the standard exercise test? *Chest*. 1999;116(5):1442–51.

23. Froelicher VF, Myers J. *Exercise and the Heart*. 5th ed. Philadelphia (PA): Saunders-Elsevier; 2006. p. 11–39.

24. Froelicher VF, Myers J. *Exercise and the Heart*. 5th ed. Philadelphia (PA): Saunders-Elsevier; 2006. p. 113–7.

25. Froelicher VF, Myers J. *Exercise and the Heart*. 5th ed. Philadelphia (PA): Saunders-Elsevier; 2006. p. 228.

26. Gibbons RJ, Balady GJ, Beasley JW, et al. ACC/AHA Guidelines for Exercise Testing. A report of the American College of Cardiology/American Heart Association Task Force on Practice Guidelines (Committee on Exercise Testing). *J Am Coll Cardiol*. 1997;30(1):260–311.

27. Hammond HK, Froelicher VF. Normal and abnormal heart rate responses to exercise. *Prog Cardiovasc Dis*. 1985;27(4):271–96.

28. Harris GD, White RD. Performance of the exercise test. In: Evans CH, White RD, editors. *Exercise Testing for Primary Care and Sports Medicine Physicians*. New York: Springer; 2009. p. 23–44.

29. Hughes BC, White RD. Testing special populations. In: Evans CH, White RD, editors. *Exercise Testing for Primary Care and Sports Medicine*. New York: Springer; 2009. p. 55–77.

30. Hughston TP, Puffer JC, Rodney WM. The athletic heart syndrome. *N Engl J Med*. 1985;313(1):24–32.

31. Jouven X, Zuriek M, Desnos M, Courbon D, Ducimetière P. Long-term outcome in asymptomatic men with exercise-induced premature ventricular depolarizations. *N Engl J Med*. 2000;343(12):826–33.

32. Kitamura K, Jorgensen CR, Gobel FL, Taylor HL, Wang Y. Hemodynamic correlates of myocardial oxygen consumption during upright exercise. *J Appl Physiol*. 1972;32(4):516–22.

33. Lachterman B, Lehmann KG, Abrahamson D, Froelicher VF. "Recovery only" ST segment depression and the predictive accuracy of the exercise test. *Ann Intern Med*. 1990;112(1):11–6.

34. Lakkireddy DR, Bhakkad J, Korlakunta HL, et al. Prognostic value of the Duke Treadmill Score in diabetic patients. *Am Heart J*. 2005;150(3):516–21.

35. Lauer MS, Francis GS, Okim PM, Pashkow FJ, Snader CE, Marwick TH. Impaired chronotropic response to exercise stress testing as a predictor of mortality. *JAMA*. 1999;281(6):524–9.

36. Mark DB, Hlathy MA, Harrell FE Jr, Lee KL, Califf RM, Pryor DB. Exercise treadmill score for predicting prognosis in coronary artery disease. *Ann Intern Med*. 1987;106(6):793–800.

37. Mark DB, Shaw L, Harrell FE Jr, et al. Prognostic value of a treadmill exercise score in outpatients with suspected coronary artery disease. *N Engl J Med*. 1991;325(12):849–53.

38. Marolf GA, Kuhn A, White RD. Exercise testing in special populations: athletes, women, and the elderly. *Prim Care*. 2001;28(1):55–72, vi.

39. Myers JN. The physiology behind exercise testing. *Prim Care*. 2001;28(1): 5–28, v.

40. Price DE, Warren ET, White RD. Testing athletic populations. In: Evans CH, White RD, editors. *Exercise Testing for Primary Care and Sports Medicine*. New York: Springer; 2009. p. 341–51.

41. Sigal RJ, Kenny GP, Wasserman DH, Castaneda-Sceppa C, White RD. Physical activity/exercise and type 2 diabetes: a consensus statement of the American Diabetes Association. *Diabetes Care*. 2006;29(6):1433–8.

42. Stuart RJ, Ellestad MH. Upsloping S-T segments in exercise stress testing. Six year follow-up of 438 patients and correlation with 248 angiograms. *Am J Cardiol*. 1976;37(1):19–22.

43. Taylor AJ, Beller GA. Post-exercise systolic blood pressure response: association to presence and extent of perfusion abnormalities on thallium-201 scintigraphy. *Am Heart J*. 1995;129(2):227–34.

44. Taylor AJ, Beller GA. Postexercise systolic blood pressure response: clinical application to the assessment of ischemic heart disease. *Am Fam Physician*. 1998;58(5):1126–30.

45. White RD, Evans CH. Performing the exercise test. *Prim Care*. 2001; 28(1):29–53, vi.

22 Gait Analysis

Timothy L. Switaj, Brian R. Hoke, and Francis G. O'Connor

INTRODUCTION

- The ultimate goal of gait analysis is to understand the complex relationships between an individual's capabilities/impairments and the person's gait pattern, so as to enhance performance while preventing injury (2).
- Our gait cycle is unique to humans, forming the building block for all motion from walking to running.
- The complexity of gait physiology has been made more evident as technology advances, allowing providers to examine minute abnormalities in detail to fine-tune performance.
- Gait analysis is also used to understand the effects of both internal and external biomechanical factors. Modern gait analysis techniques can be used to evaluate for subtle muscle weaknesses and flexibility deficits while also evaluating the effects of shoes and orthoses on the gait pattern.
- Gait can be analyzed in multiple different ways, but with advancing technology, providers have become more and more reliant on the use of video and computer analysis software. Advances in technology have allowed for the identification of minute discrepancies, yielding an improved ability to help patients.
- Gait analysis techniques are actively used in rehabilitation protocols, most notably after stroke, in amputee care, in pediatric rehabilitation for children with cerebral palsy, and for the fine-tuning of elite athletes (4).

GAIT CYCLE

- The basic unit of walking and running is the *gait cycle,* or *stride.* Perry (9) described various temporal and functional variables within the gait cycle, which has become a standard reference to describe gait.
- Walking gait cycle timing is primarily divided into *double support* and *single support* phases.
- When focusing on each leg's activity, the cycle is divided into the *stance* and *swing* periods, which begin at initial and final contact of the foot, respectively.
- When focusing on functional aspects of gait, the walking gait cycle can be divided into three functional tasks: *weight acceptance, single limb support,* and *limb advancement,* with the first two occurring during stance and the third occurring primarily during swing. The tasks are further subdivided into eight phases: weight acceptance comprises *initial contact* and *loading response*; single-limb support comprises *midstance, terminal stance,* and *preswing*; and limb advancement comprises *initial swing, midswing,* and *terminal swing.*

- Temporal-spatial gait parameters consist of the following: *stride time* refers to the time from initial contact of one foot to initial contact of the same foot; *step time* refers to the time from initial contact of one foot to initial contact of the opposite foot; and *stride length* and *step length* refer to the distances traversed during the respective times. *Gait velocity* is the ratio between stride length and stride time. *Cadence* of gait refers to the stride (or step) frequency (*i.e.,* the number of strides [or steps] per unit of time).

- Temporal-spatial parameters can be effectively measured during either walking or running with pressure mats (cellular mats measuring foot pressure), force platforms (dynamometers sensing ground reaction forces in time), and motion analysis (system of stereophotogrammetric cameras for three-dimensional reconstruction of body motion, including foot contact timing). Temporal, but not spatial, parameters can be measured with foot switches (on/off devices detecting foot contact timing).

- Temporal-spatial features of walking and running differ substantially. During walking, at least one foot is always on the ground, whereas during the majority of running, neither foot is in contact with the ground. Although walking has two double-support phases, running has two phases of *double float* during the swing period. The percentages of time in stance and swing are reversed in walking and running: about 60% and 40%, respectively, for walking and about 40% and 60%, respectively, for running (7,9). During normal walking at an average walking speed, each double-limb support time comprises approximately 10% of the gait cycle, whereas single-limb support comprises about 40%. Typical values (5) of temporal gait parameters in healthy young adults, walking comfortably on a level surface, are summarized in Table 22.1. At slower walking speeds, double-limb support times are greater. Conversely, with increasing walking speeds, double-limb support time intervals decrease. Walking becomes running when there is no longer an interval of time in which both feet are in contact with the ground.

Table 22.1	Typical Values of Some Temporal and Spatial Walking Gait Variables	
Temporal/Spatial Variable		**Average Value**
Velocity (m · min^{-1})		~80
Cadence (steps · min^{-1})		113
Stride length (m)		1.41
Stance (percent of gait cycle)		~60
Swing (percent of gait cycle)		~40
Double support (percent per leg per gait cycle)		~10

KINEMATICS

- The kinematics (motion) of an individual while walking or running can be effectively assessed by modeling the individual's body as a multibody system. A multibody system is composed of links (body segments) and joints between the links. The kinematics of the system is completely known when orientation and position of each of its segments are known. Joint angles are obtained from the kinematics of both joint distal and proximal segments. Joint angular velocities are obtained from the joint angles and refer to the rapidity of variation of such angles. Joint accelerations are similarly obtained from joint velocities.

- Each segment possesses a center of mass (CoM). A whole-body CoM can also be defined as the point at the center of the body mass distribution. As segments move, the whole-body CoM moves. Its position in time is important for both balance and energy-related issues (2).

- With quantitative three-dimensional gait analysis, joint angles throughout the gait cycle are described with respect to flexion/extension, abduction/adduction, and internal/external rotation (6). CoM position in time is expressed in vertical, anterior-posterior, and mediolateral time histories.

- Both joint and CoM kinematics are obtained from the instantaneous three-dimensional position of markers attached on the individual's body segments.

- Joint kinematics patterns during running differ somewhat from the patterns during walking. Hip flexion/extension and abduction/adduction ranges are wider in running (about 60 and 15 degrees, respectively) than in walking (about 40 and 10 degrees, respectively) (7,9). Hip and knee full extension is reached only during walking. Maximum knee flexion is higher in running (about 90 degrees) than walking (about 60 degrees). Ankle joint angle ranges are greater in running (about 50 degrees) than in walking (about 30 degrees).

- During walking, the CoM trajectory reaches its highest point in stance when its speed is minimum. During running, the CoM trajectory reaches its maximum height during the double floating phase, at which time its velocity is maximum.

KINETICS

- *Kinetics* is defined as the study of forces and moments that cause movement.

- *Ground reaction forces* refer to the forces exerted on the foot during foot contact. They are measured with force platforms embedded in the ground, over which the individual walks or runs. The center of the distribution of these forces is called *center of pressure*. Knowing segment kinematics and ground reaction forces, in addition to some segment characteristics such as mass and CoM location, it is possible to estimate joint kinetics (*joint forces* and *moments*). Joint moments refer to forces applied at a distance from a joint and are expressed as either external (due to the ground reaction force, gravity, and inertia) or internal (due to internal structures including muscle, ligamentous, and bony structures). Joint *powers* indicate the rate of work operated by the joint muscles and are obtained by multiplying the joint moment by the joint angular velocity.

- To measure ground reaction forces and center of pressure trajectory, one force platform per foot contact is sufficient. To measure joint kinetics, a combination of measurements synchronously obtained from force platforms and a motion analysis system is necessary.

- The vertical ground reaction force typically demonstrates an initial peak at the very first contact of the heel and then a force absorption and a force generation phase. During walking, in addition to a peak at initial contact at the heel, the pattern of the vertical reaction force shows two maxima—one during the force absorption phase and another during the force generation phase. During running, a single maximum is present that divides absorption from generation. In running, maximum and minimum values are dependent on the speed of the runner. The amplitude of the pattern during running can be threefold the amplitude during walking (7).

- Sagittal ankle joint moment (flexion/extension moment) patterns in running and walking are similar. In running, the joint moment activity is faster (shorter stance phase) and more intense (greater maximum amplitude). Knee sagittal moment in running demonstrates higher amplitude after initial contact than during walking. Hip sagittal moment patterns are similar during walking and running, except for the amplitude, which is greater in running (7).

- Ankle, knee, and hip power patterns during walking are very similar to those obtained during running; however, the amplitudes of power absorption and generation are directly related to the individual speed (greater powers for higher speeds).

DYNAMIC ELECTROMYOGRAPHY

- Knowledge of the activation phases of the main lower limb muscles, in association with the joint moment patterns, can provide an effective description of overall gait function.

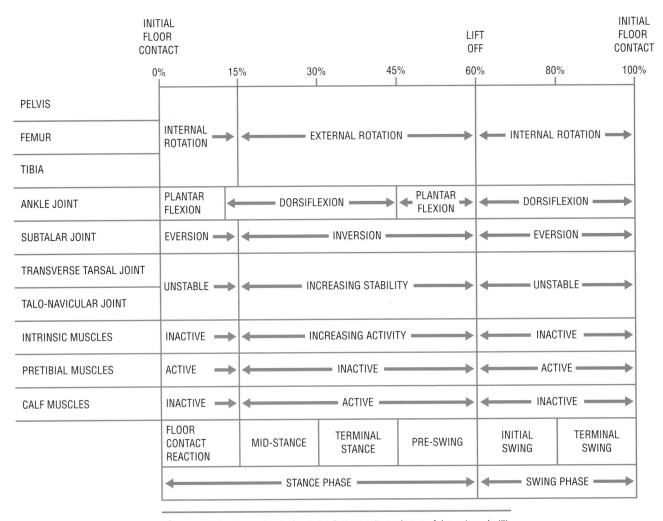

Figure 22.1: Biomechanical activity during various phases of the gait cycle (7).

Although joint moments provide information regarding the effect of action of all the muscles involved, the knowledge of the activation patterns allows us to discriminate in time the muscle groups that are responsible for the observed joint moment (9).

■ Surface electromyography (EMG) is the most common method for detecting muscle activity during gait. Current dynamic EMG systems allow one to detect EMG signals from up to 16 muscles at a time, which can be synchronized to both motion analysis systems and force platforms.

■ Activation patterns of lower limb muscles during a running gait cycle are different from those observed during a walking gait cycle with respect to both timing and duration of activity. Figure 22.1 illustrates the phases of muscle activity during running. In general, muscle activity during running begins earlier in the swing period and lasts for a relatively longer time during the stance period. During walking, the quadriceps are active at the end of swing through 25% of the stance period, while during running and sprinting, they continue to be active through 50%–100% of the stance period. Similarly, the hamstrings are active earlier in swing during

running and continue nearly to the end of the stance period, while in walking, they cease activity early in stance. The ankle dorsiflexors during walking are active from late stance until early stance, while during running, they continue to be active through midstance. During walking, the ankle plantar flexors are active only during stance from loading response or midstance to terminal stance, while in running, they are active in terminal swing through midstance to terminal stance (9).

OXYGEN CONSUMPTION

■ Measurement of oxygen consumption is typically obtained with pulmonary gas exchange devices, which are usually wearable and can be used outside a laboratory. Respiratory volumes of oxygen (O_2) and carbon dioxide (CO_2) can be monitored during the execution of the motor task.

■ The measurement of oxygen consumption provides information regarding the economy of gait. Walking energy expenditure per unit of distance is highly dependent on walking speeds. At natural walking speed, energy expenditure is lower than at both lower and higher speeds. In running, this dependency is not as evident. In both running and walking, the highest energy expenditure per distance unit occurs at slower speed.

GAIT EVALUATION

- Clinically meaningful information can be obtained from the wealth of data gathered from the measurement instruments and analysis techniques reported here. By relating EMG, kinetic, and kinematic patterns, it is possible to describe and evaluate the function of gait at a local level (*i.e.*, the joint). By combining CoM time histories and more complete segmental kinematic information with oxygen consumption measurements, an overall evaluation of the energetics of gait at a global level is possible.

- While during walking the total energy (kinetic plus potential) is almost constant throughout the cycle, in running the potential and the kinetic energies are in phase (*i.e.*, when one is minimum or maximum, so is the other), which means that energy is periodically stored and released. This action is performed mainly by the muscle tendons, which behave as springs activated by the relevant muscles.

- In analyzing gait (in particular, an atypical gait pattern or an effect of a shoe type, brace, musculoskeletal injury, or impairment), at least two distinct qualities need to be considered. The first is energetics (*i.e.*, how does the pattern, shoe, etc., affect energetics); this can be measured directly with oxygen consumption and indirectly with CoM calculations and by observing if EMG activities are consistent with kinetic needs. The second is risk for biomechanical injury (*i.e.*, how does the pattern affect risk over time, for ligamentous, muscle, tendon, cartilage, or bone injury); this is best estimated with joint kinetics, in particular joint moments, which may be higher than normal, indicating a greater risk for biomechanical injury.

Videotaped Observational Gait Analysis

- Videotaped observational gait analysis (VOGA) techniques can assist in the identification of minute discrepancies that are not visible in real-time analysis by clinical observation.

- VOGA starts with the placement of reflective tape, or other markers, on key landmarks of the human body. Commonly used landmarks are listed in Table 22.2 and depicted in Figure 22.2.

- VOGA is conducted through a scripted protocol with differing views across all phases of gait during both walking and running. Table 22.3 represents a sample taping protocol.

- Provider analysis of videotaped results is of variable reliability based on degree of training and experience of the provider. Advances in computer software make VOGA more reliable in the detection of fine abnormalities. (1)

Table 22.2	Retroflective Taping Landmarks	
Position	**Body Part**	**Landmark**
Lateral	Head	Zygomatic arch
	Shoulder	Acromion
	Elbow	Lateral epicondyle
	Wrist	Ulnar styloid
	Hip	Greater trochanter
	Knee	Central femoral condyle
	Ankle	Fibular malleolus
	Foot	Lateral border parallel to floor
Posterior	Lower back	Posterior sacroiliac spine
	Knee	Popliteal fossa
	Lower leg	Bisection of distal third of tib/fib
	Foot	Calcaneal bisection
Anterior	Hip	Anterior sacroiliac spine
	Patella	Midpoint
	Lower leg	Tibial tuberosity
	Foot	Midline of second metatarsal

- Dartfish Technologies has produced a gait analysis software package that is currently in use by multiple British sports teams, U.S. Colleges, and the U.S. Special Olympic and Paralympic Training Center (3). Initial results provided through case studies are promising, but there are no current peer-reviewed publications evaluating Dartfish Technologies software in the application of gait analysis at this time.

- VOGA presents a systematic approach toward identifying pathology in runners. After the systematic identification and taping of landmarks and the conduction of a taping session protocol, the trained provider must perform an analysis of the video footage. This is best performed by working through the footage from the feet to the head and in all phases of motion (static, walking, and running). Using Dartfish Technologies software, needed measurements will be provided; however, in the absence of the software, the provider must make measurements and comparisons by hand. Angles between retroflectively taped landmarks are the most common measurements needed and the most likely to yield fine abnormality findings.

- Subtle pathology can easily be detected using a strict VOGA protocol. For example, an abnormality in the symmetrical movement pattern of the shoulders is suggestive of a contralateral lower extremity injury; arm movements that cross the midline are suggestive of pelvic rotation; excessive vertical displacement of the head, more than 4 cm, during heel lift is

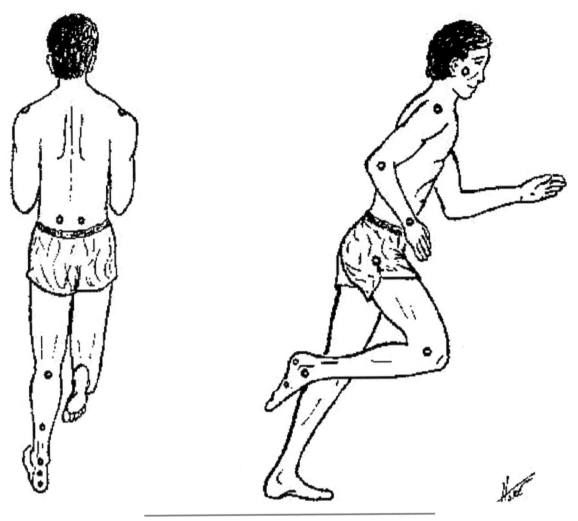

Figure 22.2: Placement of retroflective tape on bony landmarks.

Table 22.3	Taping Session Protocol

Static posture: head to feet	**Lateral view**
Anterior – 10 seconds	Head to feet – 30 seconds
Lateral – 10 seconds	Hips to feet – 30 seconds
Posterior – 10 seconds	**Anterior view (optional)**
Posterior view	Head to feet – 30 seconds
Head to feet – 30 seconds	Hips to feet – 30 seconds
Hips to feet – 30 seconds	Lower leg and feet – 30 seconds
Lower leg and rear foot	
Shoes on – 30 seconds	
Shoes off (walking) – 30 seconds	
Shoes off (running) – 30 seconds	

suggestive of a leg length discrepancy; forward leaning while running is indicative of weak back musculature or tight hip flexors; external rotation of the hip during the gait cycle is indicative of tight hip flexors, whereas excessive internal rotation is indicative of piriformis syndrome; close examination of knee flexion when cushioned can differentiate between quadriceps and hamstring weaknesses; and lastly, close examination of foot range of motion and flexibility through the gait cycle can help differentiate between gastrocsoleus problems, metatarsalgia, plantar fasciitis, and hallux limitus (8). Of course, these are just a few examples of the power of VOGA because it is impossible to describe every identifiable abnormality here.

■ In addition to traditional two-dimensional imaging and the newer Dartfish Technologies software, three-dimensional multiplanar imaging for gait analysis has hit the marketplace. As of today, there is no peer-reviewed literature on three-dimensional gait analysis, but preliminary work shows no significant difference in its ability to detect fine abnormalities compared with two-dimensional imaging or Dartfish Technologies software (6).

REFERENCES

1. Baker R. The history of gait analysis before the advent of modern computers. *Gait Posture.* 2007;26(3):331–42.
2. Birrer RB, Buzermanis S, DellaCorte MP, et al. Biomechanics of running. In: O'Connor F, Wilder R, editors. *The Textbook of Running Medicine.* New York: McGraw-Hill; 2001. p. 11–9.
3. Dartfish Technologies Case Studies [Internet]. Available from: http://www.dartfish.com/en/index.html.
4. Dicharry J. Kinematics and kinetics of gait: from lab to clinic. *Clin Sports Med.* 2010;29(3):347–64.
5. Kerrigan DC, Edelstein JE. Gait. In: Gonzalez EG, Myers SJ, Edelsteinet JE, et al., editors. *The Physiological Basis of Rehabilitation Medicine.* Boston: Butterworth-Heinemann; 2001. p. 397–416.
6. McGinley JL. The reliability of three-dimensional kinematic gait measurements: a systematic review. *Gait Posture.* 2009;29(3):360–9.
7. Novacheck TF. The biomechanics of running. *Gait Posture.* 1998;7:77–95.
8. O'Connor FG, Switaj TL. Gait analysis. In: Seidenberg PH, Beutler A, editors. *The Sports Medicine Resource Manual.* Philadelpha: Elsevier Health Sciences; 2008. p. 536–48.
9. Perry J. *Gait Analysis: Normal and Pathological Function.* Thorofare (NJ): Slack; 1992. 556 p.

Compartment Syndrome Testing

John E. Glorioso and John H. Wilckens

INTRODUCTION

- Exertional leg pain is a common complaint in the running athlete. The differential diagnosis includes stress fracture, tibial stress reaction such as periostitis or medial tibial stress syndrome (shin splints), tendonitis, nerve compression or entrapment, and chronic exertional compartment syndrome (CECS).

- Although a classic history may suggest the diagnosis of CECS, an exercise challenge and measurement of compartmental pressures are essential to confirm the diagnosis.

- Intracompartmental pressure measurement is the most clinically useful test to rule out or confirm CECS as the etiology of exertional leg pain.

COMPARTMENT SYNDROMES

- Compartment syndrome exists when tissue pressures are elevated in a restricted fascial space, resulting in decreased perfusion causing nerve and muscle ischemia.

- Compartment syndromes in the athlete can occur in two forms, acute and chronic. The distinction between the two is in the reversibility of the ischemic insult.

- In acute compartment syndrome, the ischemia is irreversible and rapidly leads to tissue necrosis unless emergently decompressed via fasciotomy.

  - Most commonly occurs with acute trauma (fracture) or soft tissue/muscle injury (crush injury, rhabdomyolysis).

  - A clinical diagnosis is made by historical and physical examination findings. Characteristic findings include pain out of proportion to injury, presence of paresthesias and sensory deficits, tense and swollen compartment on palpation, decreased or loss of active motion, and severe pain with passive stretch.

  - Treatment is emergent surgical decompression via fasciotomy.

  - If doubt exists as to the diagnosis in the acute presentation, intracompartmental pressure measurements may be indicated prior to emergent fasciotomy.

  - Resting intracompartmental pressure of > 30 mm Hg is the generally accepted level that can be associated with

decreased blood flow and resultant muscle and nerve ischemia (2).

- CECS involves reversible ischemia that is exercise induced and occurs at a predictable distance/intensity of exertion.

  - This form is much more common in athletes.

  - The reversible ischemia of exertional compartment syndrome occurs secondary to a noncompliant osseofascial compartment that is not responsive to the expansion of muscle volume that occurs with exercise.

  - CECS is characterized by recurrent episodes of a transient elevation in the intracompartmental pressure, which subsides with rest or cessation of activity.

  - Any athlete can develop CECS; however, runners are most commonly affected (6,15,20).

- Although compartment syndrome testing is useful in the diagnosis of acute compartment syndrome, the following discussion applies to the use of intracompartmental pressure measurements for the chronic exertional form of compartment syndrome.

The Leg Compartments

- The leg contains four anatomically distinct muscle compartments with structural support provided by the tibia and fibula. Each compartment is covered by a tight fascia and has a unique neurovascular supply that creates distinct pathology (Table 23.1).

- The anterior compartment contains muscles used for extension of the toes and dorsiflexion of the ankle: the tibialis anterior, the extensor hallucis longus, and the extensor digitorum longus. Blood supply to the anterior compartment is from the anterior tibial artery. The deep peroneal nerve provides innervation as it passes through the compartment.

- The lateral compartment contains the evertors of the foot: the peroneus longus and the peroneus brevis. Nerve supply is via the superficial peroneal nerve. Blood supply is from branches of the peroneal artery.

- The superficial posterior compartment contains the plantarflexors of the foot: the gastrocnemius, soleus, and plantaris. These muscles are supplied by branches of the tibial nerve.

- The deep posterior compartment contains the muscles of toe flexion, ankle plantar flexion and inversion, the flexor hallucis longus, the flexor digitorum longus, and the tibialis

Table 23.1	Muscle Compartments		
Compartment	**Nerve**	**Muscles**	**Vascular**
Anterior	Deep peroneal	Tibialis anterior Extensor hallucis longus Extensor digitorum longus Peroneus tertius	Anterior tibial artery and vein
Lateral	Superficial peroneal	Peroneus longus Peroneus brevis	
Superficial posterior	None	Gastrocnemius Soleus Plantaris	None
Deep posterior	Tibial nerve	Posterior tibialis Flexor hallucis longus Flexor digitorum longus Popliteus	Posterior tibial artery and vein Peroneal artery and vein

posterior. These muscles are supplied by the tibial nerve and posterior tibial artery.

- A fifth compartment has been described. The fascia surrounding the posterior tibialis has been described as a separate and distinct compartment (5).

PATHOPHYSIOLOGY

- Four factors have been identified that may contribute to an increase in the intracompartmental pressure seen during exercise (17):
  - Enclosure of compartmental contents in an inelastic fascial sheath
  - Increased volume of the skeletal muscle with exertion resulting from blood flow and edema
  - Muscle hypertrophy as response to exercise
  - Dynamic contraction factors due to the gait cycle
- The transient increase in pressure within the myofascial compartment compromises blood flow. When tissue perfusion is not adequate to meet the metabolic demands, the result is traversing neurologic and muscular ischemia, pain, and impairment of muscular function.

CLINICAL PRESENTATION

- In CECS, the characteristic complaint is recurrent exercise-induced leg discomfort that occurs at a well-defined and reproducible point of activity and increases if the training persists.
- The quality of pain is described as a tight, cramp-like, or squeezing ache over a specific compartment of the leg. Relief of symptoms occurs only with discontinuation of activity.

- Neurologic complaints such as paresthesias of the leg or foot with exertion may indicate involvement of the nerve traversing the compartment.
  - Nerve entrapment syndromes of the lower extremity often present with similar complaints and should be included in the differential diagnosis.
- At rest, the physical examination is commonly unremarkable with a normal gait and normal lower extremity examination. A muscle herniation through a fascial defect may be the only clinical abnormality noted.
- An exercise challenge followed by postexercise clinical examination is helpful in establishing the diagnosis (11).
  - After reproduction of discomfort, the athlete should be assessed for tenderness, tightness, and swelling over the involved compartment.
  - The tenderness noted should involve the muscle mass and not the bone or muscle–tendon junction.
  - Neurologic and vascular examination should be completed.
- Although history may be suggestive of CECS, no physical examination finding can firmly establish the diagnosis (14,25). Diagnosis based solely on clinical presentation can lead to misdiagnosis, inappropriate therapy, and/or delay of proper therapy (20).

INDICATIONS FOR INTRACOMPARTMENTAL PRESSURE MEASUREMENTS

- Any patient with clinical evidence of CECS should be considered for intracompartmental testing.
  - Significant historical features include a recurrent, exercise-induced leg discomfort that increases as the training persists and dissipates on cessation of activity.

- Pain quality described as a tight, cramp-like, or squeezing ache over a specific compartment of the leg.
- Paresthesias of the leg or foot with exertion.
- An exercise challenge with detailed physical examination immediately after reproduction of symptoms will lead to a more judicious use of invasive techniques (11).

TECHNIQUES TO MEASURE COMPARTMENT PRESSURES

- Multiple techniques have been described for measuring both static and dynamic intramuscular pressures. Techniques include the needle manometer (29), the wick catheter (18), slit catheter (22), continuous infusion (16), and a solid-state transducer intracompartmental catheter (17).
- The Stryker Intra-Compartmental Pressure Monitor (Stryker Corporation, Kalamazoo, MI) is a battery-operated, hand-held, digital, fluid pressure monitor. This device has been found to be more accurate, versatile, convenient, and much less time consuming in the clinical setting (3,13).
- Using an in vitro model to compare compartment pressure measuring techniques, both the arterial line manometer and Stryker have been found to be accurate (4).

PERFORMANCE OF THE PROCEDURE

- Because intracompartmental pressure measurement is an invasive procedure, proper technical performance and patient safety demand a thorough knowledge of the anatomy of the leg. Prior to attempting to measure compartment pressures, the physician should ensure an understanding of the anatomic structures in each compartment so as to avoid damage to neurovascular structures.
- The athlete must be made aware of the indications of the procedure, and consent should be obtained and the athlete counseled on the risk of infection, scarring, damage to nerve and vascular structures, and reaction to local anesthesia.
- Two types of measurements may be obtained during the procedure, *static* or *dynamic.*
  - Static, or intermittent, pressures are performed with a straight needle. Here, intracompartmental pressures are determined with a needle stick at rest and then again after exertion. The benefits of this procedure are that the athlete can perform activity causing symptoms without the measuring device attached to the leg and without an indwelling catheter in the compartment. Also, several compartments can be measured. A negative aspect of this technique is that it requires at least two needle sticks into each compartment being evaluated (one before and one after exertion). This procedure is most commonly used.

- Dynamic monitoring is performed with the use of a slit catheter inserted prior to exertion and taped/attached to the athlete's leg for continuous measurements. The benefits of this procedure are that the clinician can monitor the pressure changes during exertion without halting activity and that pressure monitoring during activity may be a more precise indicator of pathology (17). There are several negative aspects of this technique. Problems include maintaining the placement of catheter in the compartment during activity, attachment of the system to the athlete, and restrictions of the athlete's gait as he or she runs to reproduce symptoms. The procedure must be performed on a treadmill in order to continuously monitor pressure changes. Thus, the athlete cannot run outdoors on his or her usual training surface. In addition, only one compartment can be measured at a time. Some believe that with this technique, the results are inconsistent and difficult to obtain and interpret (21,23).
- Using an in vitro model to compare compartment pressure measuring techniques, side port needles, and slit catheters were found to be more accurate than straight needles, which had the tendency to overestimate pressure (4).
- With the static technique, measurements should be obtained at rest (prior to exertion), immediately after (1 minute) the reproduction of symptoms, and 5–10 minutes into rest.
- To properly reproduce symptoms, athletes should perform the specific activity that causes pain/discomfort.
- Three factors may alter the pressure measurements:
  - Proper calibration of the monitor is essential for reliable readings. The monitor must be zeroed at the same angle that will be used to penetrate the skin, and this angle must be maintained with repeated sticks.
  - Joint position at both the knee and ankle affect pressures (10).
  - Compression or squeezing the leg can alter pressures. Externally applied pressure is additive to any pressure already existing within the compartment (16).
- Each compartment should be approached with an understanding of the anatomic contents of each compartment so as to avoid injury to neurovascular structures.

APPROACH TO EACH LEG COMPARTMENT

- Measurement of intracompartmental pressures is an invasive procedure. To avoid damage to neurovascular structures, each compartment should be approached with an understanding of the anatomic contents (11).

Anterior Compartment

- Identify the muscle belly of the anterior tibialis just lateral to the anterior tibial border. Approach should have needle penetrate through fascia and into muscle belly of anterior tibialis at the level of the mid-third of the tibia.

- Anatomic structures to avoid include the neurovascular bundle containing the deep peroneal nerve, anterior tibial artery, and veins. This neurovascular bundle sits just above the interosseous membrane.

Lateral Compartment

- The muscle bellies of the peroneus longus and brevis are palpable on the lateral surface of the leg just superficial to the shaft of the fibula.
- Helpful technique to enter this compartment involves palpation of the head of the fibula and lateral malleolus and palpating the muscle bellies at the midpoint between these two bony landmarks.
- The superficial peroneal nerve resides within this compartment and provides innervation. The lateral compartment receives it blood supply from branches of the peroneal artery, but does not itself run through the lateral compartment.

Posterior Superficial Compartment

- The muscle bellies of the gastrocnemius and soleus muscles are easily identified and palpated.
- Approach to this compartment just medial to the midline will avoid the small saphenous vein and the medial and lateral sural cutaneous nerves.
- Branches of the tibial nerve innervate these muscles.

Posterior Deep Compartment

- The approach to the posterior deep compartment is technically more difficult because of the proximity of neurovascular structures.
- Two bundles are contained within this compartment that should be understood anatomically prior to needle insertion. A vascular bundle consisting of the peroneal artery and veins lies medial to the posterior aspect of the fibula. A neurovascular bundle consisting of the tibial nerve, posterior tibial artery, and veins lies in the posterior aspect of this compartment behind the mass of the tibialis posterior muscle.
- The posterior medial aspect of the mid-tibia must first be palpated. The needle should then be inserted just posterior to the tibia, closely approximating the posterior border of the bone. The needle will first enter the flexor digitorum longus muscle and if guided deeper will enter the posterior tibialis muscle. As long as it is not driven too deeply, this approach will keep the needle anterior and medial to the neurovascular structures.

Diagnostic Criteria

- Compartment pressure must be obtained both preexercise and postexercise. Postexercise pressures should be performed immediately after an exercise challenge that reproduces the patient's symptoms.

- Findings consistent with the diagnosis of CECS include an elevated resting pressure and increased postexertion pressure, and/or a delayed return to normal pressure after exertion.
- For CECS, the diagnostic criteria described by Pedowitz et al. (20) are commonly used. One or more of the following criteria must be met in addition to an appropriate history and physical examination:
  - Preexercise $\geq$ 15 mm Hg
  - 1 minute postexercise $\geq$ 30 mm Hg
  - 5 minutes postexercise $\geq$ 20 mm Hg

DIFFERENTIAL DIAGNOSIS

- Stress fractures, periostitis/medial tibial stress syndrome, and tendonitis can usually be differentiated from CECS by clinical presentation; however, several syndromes present very similar to CECS and must be suspected when intracompartmental pressures are found to be normal.
- Nerve entrapment and compression may cause exertional leg pain. This diagnosis should always be suspected when the patient presents with symptoms consistent with CECS but has normal pressures.
  - Common peroneal nerve entrapment presents as activity-related pain, paresthesias, and/or numbness in the anterolateral aspect of the leg.
  - Superficial peroneal nerve entrapment presents with a history very similar to that of CECS of the lateral compartment.
  - Saphenous nerve entrapment presents as medial knee and medial leg pain.
  - Sural nerve entrapment will present with posterior calf symptoms and can be almost indistinguishable from CECS of the superficial posterior compartment.
  - Proximal tibial nerve entrapment also presents similar to CECS of the posterior compartment.
- Lumbosacral radiculopathy should be suspected in athletes with the complaints of leg pain, especially if associated with back or buttock discomfort.
- Popliteal artery entrapment is often misdiagnosed as posterior CECS because of the ischemic etiology in the pathogenesis of symptoms in both syndromes (12).

OTHER DIAGNOSTIC OPTIONS

- Measurement of compartment pressure assesses only one aspect of CECS. Altered tissue perfusion, neurologic and muscular ischemia, and increased interstitial fluid all play a role in the pathophysiologic process.
- Recent attention has focused on noninvasive techniques that can detect these pathophysiologic alterations that are

associated with or a result of the pressure elevations. These emerging diagnostic options potentially offer an alternative to direct intracompartmental pressure measurements in those cases where the athlete is adverse to invasive procedures or where the results of pressure monitoring may be nondiagnostic.

■ **Triple-phase bone scan:** Scintigraphy has been investigated in the diagnosis of CECS (7,19,24). The utility of this study is based on the detection of abnormalities in tracer uptake in muscle compartments. As pressure increases in an anatomic compartment, blood flow through it declines. This is evident as the identification of decreased postexertional muscle perfusion and radionuclide concentration in the compartment with increased pressure when compared to resting images (7,19).

■ **Magnetic resonance imaging (MRI):** Considerable interest has focused on the use of MRI in the evaluation and diagnosis of CECS (9,28). MRI is sensitive to changes in water distribution in skeletal muscle. Soft tissue edema that occurs in muscle compartments can be visualized on postexercise MRI (8,9,14). Specifically, the T2-weighted signal intensity has been reported to show a statistically significant increase in signal intensity with exercise in affected compartments compared to unaffected compartments (28). Functional MRI techniques used to evaluate postexertion muscle perfusion and muscle oxygenation have not shown statistically significant differences between patients with exertional compartment syndrome and controls (1).

■ **Near infrared spectroscopy (NIRS):** Focusing on the induced ischemia as a result of impaired perfusion, NIRS has been used as a noninvasive method to measure tissue oxygen saturation and thereby support the diagnosis of CECS. When compared to controls, patients with CECS display significant differences in peak exercise and postexercise tissue oxygen saturation as measured by NIRS (27). Consistent with the induced ischemia theory, patients with CECS demonstrated greater deoxygenation with exercise compared to controls. The sensitivity of NIRS has been shown in one study to be clinically equivalent to intracompartmental pressure measurement (26).

■ **Neurosensory testing:** Transient neurologic ischemia due to increased compartment pressures can be assessed by sensory nerve function. Noninvasive neurosensory testing has been shown to detect reversible alterations in sensory nerve function when postexertion values are compared to preexertion/rest (30).

REFERENCES

1. Andreisek G, White LM, Sussman MS, et al. T2*-weighted and arterial spin labeling MRI of calf muscles in healthy volunteers and patients with chronic exertional compartment syndrome: preliminary experience. *Am J Roentgenol.* 2009;193(4):W327–33.
2. Andrish JT. The leg. In: DeLee JC, Drez DD, Miller MD, editors. *DeLee and Drez's Orthopaedic Sports Medicine: Principles and Practice.* 2nd ed. Philadelphia: Saunders; 2003. p. 2155–81.
3. Awbrey BJ, Sienkiewicz PS, Mankin HJ. Chronic exercise induced compartment pressure elevation measured with a miniaturized fluid pressure monitor. A laboratory and clinical study. *Am J Sports Med.* 1988;16(6):610–5.
4. Boody AR, Wongworawat MD. Accuracy in the measurement of compartment pressures: a comparison of three commonly used devices. *J Bone Joint Surg Am.* 2005;87(11):2415–22.
5. Davey JR, Rorabeck CH, Fowler PJ. The tibialis posterior muscle compartment. An unrecognized cause of exertional compartment syndrome. *Am J Sports Med.* 1984;12(5):391–7.
6. Detmer DE, Sharpe K, Sufit RL, Girdley FM. Chronic compartment syndrome: diagnosis, management, and outcomes. *Am J Sports Med.* 1985;13(3):162–70.
7. Edwards PD, Miles KA, Owens SJ, Kemp PM, Jenner JR. A new noninvasive test for the detection of compartment syndromes. *Nucl Med Commun.* 1999;20(3):215–8.
8. Elsayes KM, Lammle M, Shariff A, Totty WG, Habib IF, Rubin DA. Value of magnetic resonance imaging in muscle trauma. *Curr Probl Diagn Radiol.* 2006;35(5):206–12.
9. Eskelin MK, Lötjönen JM, Mäntysaari MJ. Chronic exertional compartment syndrome: MR imaging at 0.1 T compared with tissue pressure measurement. *Radiology.* 1998;206(2):333–7.
10. Gershuni DH, Yaru NC, Hargens AR, Lieber RL, O'Hara RC, Akeson WH. Ankle and knee position as a factor modifying intracompartmental pressure in the human leg. *J Bone Joint Surg Am.* 1984;66-A(9):1415–20.
11. Glorioso JE, Wilckens JH. Compartment syndrome testing. In: O'Connor FG, Wilder RP, editors. *Textbook of Running Medicine.* New York: McGraw-Hill; 2001. p. 95–9.
12. Glorioso JE, Wilckens JH. Exertional leg pain. In: O'Connor FG, Wilder RP, editors. *Textbook of Running Medicine.* New York: McGraw-Hill; 2001. p. 181–97.
13. Hutchinson MR, Ireland ML. Chronic exertional compartment syndrome: gauging pressure. *Phys Sportsmed.* 1999;27(5):101–2.
14. Kiuru MJ, Mantysaari MJ, Pihlajamaki HK, Ahovuo JA. Evaluation of stress related anterior lower leg pain with magnetic resonance imaging and intracompartmental pressure measurement. *Mil Med.* 2003;168(1):48–52.
15. Martens MA, Moeyersoons JP. Acute and recurrent effort-related compartment syndrome in sports. *Sports Med.* 1990;9(1):62–8.
16. Matsen FA 3rd, Mayo KA, Sheridan GW, Krugmire RB Jr. Monitoring of intramuscular pressure. *Surgery.* 1976;79(6):702–9.
17. McDermott AGP, Marble AE, Yabsley RH, Phillips MB. Monitoring dynamic anterior compartment pressures during exercise. A new technique using the STIC catheter. *Am J Sports Med.* 1982;10(2):83–9.
18. Mubarak SJ, Hargens AR, Owen CA, Garetto LP, Akeson WH. The wick catheter technique for measurement of intramuscular pressure. A new research and clinical tool. *J Bone Joint Surg Am.* 1976;58-A(7):1016–20.
19. Owens S, Edwards P, Miles K, Jenner J, Allen M. Chronic compartment syndrome affecting the lower limb: MIBI perfusion imaging as an alternative to pressure monitoring: two case reports. *Br J Sports Med.* 1999;33(1):49–51.
20. Pedowitz RA, Hargens AR, Mubarak SJ, Gershuni DH. Modified criteria for the objective diagnosis of chronic compartment syndrome of the leg. *Am J Sports Med.* 1990;18(1):35–40.
21. Rorabeck CH, Bourne RB, Fowler PJ, Finlay JB, Nott L. The role of tissue pressure measurement in diagnosing chronic anterior compartment syndrome. *Am J Sports Med.* 1988;16(2):143–6.
22. Rorabeck CH, Castle GS, Hardie R, Logan J. Compartmental pressure measurements: an experimental investigation using the slit catheter. *J Trauma.* 1981;21(6):446–9.

23. Rorabeck CH, Fowler PJ, Nott L. The results of fasciotomy in the management of chronic exertional compartment syndrome. *Am J Sports Med.* 1988;16(3):224–7.

24. Samuelson DR, Cram RL. The three phase bone scan and exercise induced lower leg pain: the tibial stress test. *Clin Nucl Med.* 1996;21(2):89–93.

25. Styf JR, Körner LM. Diagnosis of chronic anterior compartment syndrome in the lower leg. *Acta Orthop Scand.* 1987;58(2):139–44.

26. van den Brand JG, Nelson T, Verleisdonk EJ, van der Werken C. The diagnostic value of intracompartmental pressure measurement, magnetic resonance imaging, and near-infrared spectroscopy in chronic exertional compartment syndrome: a prospective study in 50 patients. *Am J Sports Med.* 2005;33(5):699–704.

27. van den Brand JG, Verleisdonk EJ, van der Werken C. Near infrared spectroscopy in the diagnosis of chronic exertional compartment syndrome. *Am J Sports Med.* 2004;32(2):452–6.

28. Verleisdonk EJ, van Gils A, van der Werken C. The diagnostic value of MRI scans for the diagnosis of chronic exertional compartment syndrome of the lower leg. *Skeletal Radiol.* 2001;30(6):321–5.

29. Whitesides TE Jr, Haney TC, Harada H, Holmes HE, Morimoto K. A simple method for tissue pressure determination. *Arch Surg.* 1975;110(11):1311–3.

30. Williams EH, Detmer DE, Guyton GP, Dellon AL. Non-invasive neurosensory testing used to diagnose and confirm successful surgical management of lower extremity deep distal posterior compartment syndrome. *J Brachial Plexus Peripher Nerve Inj.* 2009;4:4.

24 Exercise-Induced Bronchoconstriction Testing

Meghan F. Raleigh and Fred H. Brennan, Jr

EPIDEMIOLOGY

- Exercise-induced bronchoconstriction (EIB) is a common medical condition that affects at least 10%–15% of athletes (9).
- Exercise-induced asthma (EIA) is the presence of similar symptoms in a patient with a known diagnosis of asthma (18). The prevalence of EIB in asthmatic patients is 80%–90% (19).
- Respiratory symptoms alone are insensitive in predicting bronchospasm in athletes (11).
- Common respiratory symptoms suggestive of asthma (coughing, wheezing, etc.) have only a 60%–70% positive predictive value for EIB (15,16).

INDICATIONS FOR EIB TESTING

- An athlete with signs or symptoms suggestive of EIA.
- An athlete with known chronic asthma may be tested for an exercise-triggering event.
- An athlete with exertional dyspnea, once cardiac etiologies have been clinically and/or diagnostically eliminated.

CONTRAINDICATIONS FOR EIB TESTING

- Active or recent pulmonary infection within past 30 days.
- Ongoing or recent exacerbation of asthma.
- Known allergy to methacholine (methacholine challenge).
- An athlete using inhaled corticosteroids may still be tested; however, the provocation test may be falsely negative in up to 50% of patients (2,17).

EIB PROVOCATIVE TESTING

Exercise Challenge

- A baseline pulmonary function test (PFT) should be performed and results recorded prior to this provocative test.

- The sensitivity and specificity of this test for identifying EIB in athletes are approximately 65% (6,9).
- The challenge should be sport-specific and conducted in the environment in which athletes most commonly experience their symptoms (7).
- An exercise challenge may be used as a first-line diagnostic study.

Conducting an Exercise Challenge

- Allow athletes to stretch, but do not allow them to exercise or warm up prior to the challenge. A warm-up period may result in a false-negative result.
- Obtain a baseline PFT or peak expiratory flow rate (PEFR). Record FEV_1 (forced expiratory volume in 1 second) and FEF_{25-75} (force expiratory flow during the middle portion of expiration), or PEFR.
- The sport-specific exercise should be conducted for 8–10 minutes at 85%–90% of maximum calculated heart rate (220 − age in years = calculated maximum heart rate).
- After 10 minutes of exercise, allow a 1-minute rest. Check PFT or PEFR three times and record the best result.
- Repeat these measurements at 3, 5, 10, 15, and 20 minutes after termination of the exercise challenge.
- A decrease of > 10% in the FEV_1 or PEFR and/or a decrease in FEF_{25-75} of > 20% are diagnostic for EIB (10,13,14).

EUCAPNIC VOLUNTARY HYPERVENTILATION TEST

- Used by the International Olympic Committee–Medical Committee (IOC MC) to verify EIB and the need for pre-competition β-agonist (3,10).
- Sensitivity and specificity in athletes have been shown to be 50% and up to 100%, respectively (1,9).
- Eucapnic voluntary hyperventilation (EVH) is a well-known and accepted provocative test for EIB (11,13).
- This test is more sensitive than an exercise challenge in the field or in the lab (11,13).

- EVH is more sensitive than methacholine in response to dry air hyperpnea (11).
- Negative test is highly likely to exclude EIB (1).

Conducting the Test

- Obtain a baseline PFT. Record the best FEV_1.
- The Argyros and colleagues (5) protocol, which is based on single-level ventilation of 85% of the maximum voluntary ventilation (MVV), is used. MVV is calculated as 35 times the best recorded pretest FEV_1 and is used to calculate the volume of dry gas ventilated per minute.
- The athlete inhales dry gas consisting of 5% carbon dioxide, 21% oxygen, and the remainder nitrogen gas. The volume of ventilated gas is measured by a metered instrument. The athlete gauges and adjusts the rate of ventilation based on the volume of dry gas ventilated.
- The athlete breaths at a rate of 85% MVV for 6 minutes.
- At the completion of the 6 minutes, the FEV_1 is measured twice at 1, 3, 5, 7, and 8 minutes post challenge. The best FEV_1 value is used.
- A drop in FEV_1 of at least 20% is diagnostic for EIB (11).
- A bronchodilator may be administered at the conclusion of the study to decrease the patient's symptoms and document reversibility of airway hyperresponsiveness.

METHACHOLINE CHALLENGE

- Methacholine stimulates muscarinic receptors located in the airway smooth muscle (12).
- The sensitivity and specificity of this test are estimated to be 55% and up to 100%, respectively (9).
- The positive predictive value may be as high as 100%, with a negative predictive value of 61% (11).
- Negative test in symptomatic patients is useful to exclude asthma, but does not exclude EIB (1).

Conducting the Methacholine Challenge

- Obtain a baseline PFT. Record the best FEV_1.
- Solutions of methacholine are prepared in the following concentrations: 0.025, 0.25, 2.5, 0, and 25 mg · mL^{-1}.
- The athlete inhales five breaths of the lowest concentration solution via nebulizer. A PFT is performed 3 minutes after inhalation of the methacholine.
- The concentration of methacholine solution is increased to the next highest concentration, and a PFT is performed 3 minutes after inhalation.
- This provocative test is concluded and considered positive if there is a decline in the FEV_1 of at least 20%. The test is concluded but considered negative if the maximum solution concentration of 25 mg · mL^{-1} is administered without the diagnostic drop in FEV_1 (9).

- Albuterol may be given 3 minutes after a positive test to demonstrate airway bronchospasm reversibility that is consistent with asthma.

EVALUATING ATHLETES WITH SUSPECTED EIB

- The most appropriate provocative test for identifying EIB remains controversial (2,8,16).
- EVH may be the preferred method of laboratory provocative testing because of its relative ease and excellent sensitivity. It is also more sensitive than an exercise challenge in a lab or field environment (11,13). EVH provocative testing is the preferred diagnostic study of the IOC-MC.
- If EVH testing is unavailable, a sport- and climate-specific exercise challenge is an acceptable alternative. A methacholine challenge is also an acceptable option.
- Avoid empirically treating for EIB without formal provocative testing. Classic symptoms alone are unreliable and may lead to over- or underusage of the appropriate medical therapy.

REFERENCES

1. Anderson SD. Provocative challenges to help diagnose and monitor asthma: exercise, methacholine, adenosine, and mannitol. *Curr Opin Pulm Med.* 2008;14(1):39–45.
2. Anderson SD, Argyros GJ, Magnussen H, Holzer K. Provocation by eucapnic voluntary hyperpnea to identify exercise-induced bronchoconstriction. *Br J Sports Med.* 2001;35(5):344–7.
3. Anderson SD, Fitch K, Perry CP, et al. Response to bronchial challenge submitted for approval to use inhaled beta 2 agonists before an event at the 2002 winter Olympics. *J Allergy Clin Immunol.* 2003;111(1): 45–50.
4. Anderson SD, Lambert S, Brannan JD, et al. Laboratory protocol for exercise asthma to evaluate salbutamol given by two devices. *Med Sci Sports Exerc.* 2001;33(6):893–900.
5. Argyros GJ, Roach JM, Hurwitz KM, Eliasson AH, Phillips YY. The refractory period after eucapnic voluntary hyperventilation challenge and its effect on challenge technique. *Chest.* 1995;108(2):419–24.
6. Avital A. Exercise, methacholine, and adenosine 5' monophosphate challenges in children with asthma: relation to decreased severity of disease. *Pediatr Pulmonol.* 2000;30(3):207–14.
7. Brennan FH Jr. Exercise-induced asthma testing. In: O'Connor FG, Wilder R, editors. *Textbook of Running Medicine.* New York: McGraw-Hill; 2001. p. 101–7.
8. Eliasson AH. Blow dry your asthma. *Chest.* 1999;115(3):608–9.
9. Eliasson AH, Phillips YY, Rajagopal KR, Howard RS. Sensitivity and specificity of bronchial provocation testing. An evaluation of four techniques in exercise-induced bronchospasm. *Chest.* 1992;102(2):347–55.
10. Fitch KD, Sue-Chu M, Anderson SD, et al. Asthma and the elite athlete: summary of the International Olympic Committee's consensus conference, Lausanne, Switzerland, January 22–24, 2008. *J Allergy Clin Immunol.* 2008;122(2):254–60.
11. Holzer K, Anderson SD, Douglass J. Exercise in elite summer athletes: challenges for diagnosis. *J Allergy Clin Immunol.* 2002;110(3):374–80.

12. Lin CC, Wu JL, Huang WC, Lin CY. A bronchial response comparison of exercise and methacholine in asthmatic subjects. *J Asthma.* 1991;28(1):31–40.

13. Mannix ET, Manfredi F, Farber MO. A comparison of two challenge tests for identifying exercise-induced bronchospasm in figure skaters. *Chest.* 1999;115(3):649–53.

14. Provost-Craig MA, Arbour KS, Sestili DC, Chabalko JJ, Ekinci E. The incidence of exercise-induced bronchospasm in competitive figure skaters. *J Asthma.* 1996;33(1):67–71.

15. Rice SG, Bierman CW, Shapiro GG, Furukawa CT, Pierson WE. Identification of exercise-induced asthma among intercollegiate athletes. *Ann Allergy.* 1985;55(6):790–3.

16. Rundell KW, Im J, Mayers LB, Wilber RL, Szmedra L, Schmitz HR. Self-reported symptoms and exercise-induced asthma in elite athletes. *Med Sci Sports Exerc.* 2001;33(2):208–13.

17. Waalkans HJ, van Essen-Zandvliet EE, Gerritsen J, Duiverman EJ, Kerrebijn KF, Knol K. The effect of inhaled corticosteroid (budesonide) on exercise-induced asthma in children. Dutch CNSLD Study Group. *Eur Respir J.* 1993;6(5):652–6.

18. Weiller JM, Bonini S, Coiffman R, et al. American Academy of Allergy, Asthma & Immunology Work Group Report: exercise-induced asthma. *J Allergy Clin Immunol.* 2007;199(6):1349–58.

19. Weiss P, Rundell KW. Imitators of exercise-induced bronchoconstriction. *Allergy, Asthma Clin Immunol.* 2009;5(1):7.

Drug Testing

Aaron Rubin

INTRODUCTION

- Drug testing of the athlete is an ethical, moral, legal, regulatory, and possible medical issue.
- Team physicians, athletic trainers, team psychologists, coaches, administrators, and others dealing with the care of the athlete may become involved with drug testing.
- Care should be exercised to keep the punitive aspect of drug testing separate from the therapeutic care for athlete's problems.
- Drug testing is performed for many reasons:
  - To prevent "cheating" by use of drugs and chemicals
  - To "level the playing field" by keeping "clean" athletes from having to compete with anabolic using athletes
  - To prevent drug-induced illness and death
  - To prevent public relations problems for teams and organizations

SCOPE OF PROBLEM

- Olympic drug testing began in the 1968 Mexico City Olympics (2).
- Between the 1968 and 2008 Olympics, over 28,000 athletes were tested at competition, and 123 tested positive (including six horses at the Beijing Olympics) (2).
- Various studies suggest that 5%–11% of high school males and 0.5%–2.5% of high school females have tried anabolic steroids (1,3).
- This is not merely a problem of athletes; of the high school students, 33% using anabolic steroids were not athletes (1,3).

REGULATING AGENCIES

- United States Anti-Doping Agency (USADA)—http://www.usantidoping.org
  - Independent antidoping agency for Olympic sports in the United States (5).
- World Anti-Doping Agency (WADA)—http://www.wada-ama.org
  - The mission of WADA is to promote and coordinate at international level the fight against doping in sport in all forms (6).

- National Collegiate Athletic Association (NCAA)—http://www.ncaa.org/drugtesting
  - Regulate and provide safety guidelines for student athletes from member colleges in the United States (4).

DRUGS, MEDICATIONS, AND OTHER SUBSTANCES

- There are no inherently good, bad, dangerous, safe, legal, or illegal substances.
- In terms of athlete testing, it is best to consider **allowed** or **not allowed** substances.
- Illegal substances are determined by rule of law and may vary from jurisdiction to jurisdiction. Use of illegal substances can be punished by criminal law. (Marijuana and "crack" cocaine are illegal substances in most jurisdictions in the United States.)
- Components of these substances may be legal. (Dronabinol is a derivative of marijuana and legal under prescription of a licensed physician. Cocaine is a legal medicine for specific indications).
- Some legal substances can be used illegally (anabolic steroids are legal substances but can be obtained and used illegally).
- Over-the-counter medications are generally legal but may not be allowed for athletic competitions (such as high-dose caffeine in NCAA testing).
- Some substances are legal but not allowed under certain circumstance (alcohol and β-blockers may not be allowed for some events).
- The ultimate decision regarding allowed or not allowed substances falls to the regulating agencies responsible for establishing the rules for the various sports teams, leagues, and organizations.
- Therapeutic drugs:
  - Prescribed drugs are those given to the athlete under the direction (prescription) of a licensed physician or dentist. Just because a medication is prescribed does not exempt an athlete from sanctions.
  - Over-the-counter medications may be taken by the athlete on his or her own or by direction of a physician or other health care provider. Again, this does not exempt an athlete from sanctions if products are not allowed.

- "Natural" products are often a misnomer. Many drugs (legal and illegal, prescription and nonprescription) are based on natural products. To complicate matters even more, many of these products may not be fully labeled with all ingredients. The athletes are ultimately responsible for what they put in their body.

- Use of banned substances for therapy requires that a therapeutic use exemption (TUE) be applied. A TUE may be granted only if the following four criteria are fulfilled (7).
  - ❏ "The *Athlete* would experience a significant impairment to health if the *Prohibited Substance* or *Prohibited Method* were to be withheld in the course of treating an acute or chronic medical condition."
  - ❏ "The therapeutic *Use* of the *Prohibited Substance* or *Prohibited Method* would produce no additional enhancement of performance other than that which might be anticipated by a return to a state of normal health following the treatment of a legitimate medical condition. The *Use* of any *Prohibited Substance* or *Prohibited Method* to increase 'low-normal' levels of any endogenous hormone is not considered an acceptable therapeutic intervention."
  - ❏ "There is no reasonable therapeutic alternative to the *Use* of the otherwise *Prohibited Substance* or *Prohibited Method*."
  - ❏ "The necessity for the *Use* of the otherwise *Prohibited Substance* or *Prohibited Method* cannot be a consequence, wholly or in part, of prior nontherapeutic *Use* of any substance from the *Prohibited List*."

- Recreational drugs:
  - Alcohol is banned by the NCAA for rifle competition and by the Olympic Movement "where the rules of the governing body so provide." Use of alcohol by minors is illegal (4).
  - Tobacco is generally not tested, although use of tobacco is not allowed at NCAA practice or competitions (4).
  - Marijuana is not allowed and is tested by the NCAA and WADA.
  - Stimulants such as amphetamine, cocaine, ephedrine, caffeine (at set concentrations for the NCAA), methylenedioxymethamphetamine (MDMA or ecstasy), and related products are banned.
  - Hallucinogens such as LSD are listed as banned substances (as recreational drugs) and are illegal.
  - Many narcotics are generally banned as therapeutic or recreational substances (by WADA, but not NCAA) (6).

- Performance enhancements:
  - Stimulants as discussed earlier are prohibited.
  - Androgenic/anabolic agents such as anabolic steroids, testosterone, clenbuterol, and related compounds are banned by the NCAA and Olympic movement.
  - Recombinant erythropoietin and related compounds and blood doping are not allowed. Blood doping is the removal of one's own blood (or using donor blood) and later transfusing it to improve aerobic capacity.

- In addition, techniques to mask drug testing or fool drug testers are not allowed. These include diuretics, urine substitution, masking agents, and other techniques.

- NCAA publishes a list that bans classes of drugs and substances related chemically to the classes.

- In addition, NCAA has procedures subject to restrictions:
  - ❏ Blood doping
  - ❏ Local anesthetics (under some conditions)
  - ❏ Manipulation of urine Samples
  - ❏ β_2-Agonists permitted only by prescription and inhalation
  - ❏ Caffeine if concentrations in urine exceed 15 μg · mL^{-1} (4).

- WADA publishes a prohibited list that is also available for hand-held devices.

- WADA adds the following caveat:
  - ❏ "Any pharmacological substance which is not addressed by any of the subsequent sections of the List and with no current approval by any governmental regulatory health authority for human therapeutic use (i.e., drugs under preclinical or clinical development or discontinued) is prohibited at all times" (6).

- Warnings regarding use of nutritional supplements are prominent in NCAA materials, including the lack of regulation of the industry and inability for the athlete to know about contaminated or unlabeled ingredients (4).

- Although not as prominent, WADA gives similar precautions (6).

TESTING PROCEDURES (BASED ON THE NCAA DRUG TESTING PROGRAMS)

- Selection process must be fair and based on random testing, universal testing, or testing based on probable cause (evidence of drug use or previous positive test).

- Testing may be done out-of-competition (year round) or in-competition (postseason championship) (4).

POSTSEASON TESTING

- Facilities and procedures are fully outlined in the NCAA Drug-Testing Programs Site Coordinators Manual.

- WADA urine testing procedures are similar, and WADA has procedures for blood testing as well as developing the Athlete Biological Profile, which attempts to set "normal" standards for an individual athlete as opposed to a population (such as hemoglobin/hematocrit to try to prevent blood doping or use of recombinant erythropoietin).

- The athlete is notified of testing by a drug-testing courier and given a written notification form instructing the athlete to accompany the courier to the collection station. The athlete must report within 1 hour and remain in visual contact with the courier until the athlete signs in at the testing center. Only authorized agents for testing and the athletes are allowed in the testing center.

■ Sealed beverages without caffeine or other banned substances are allowed at the testing center.

■ The athlete selects a sealed beaker to provide their specimen. Sample will be given as an observed specimen.

■ Specimen must be at least 90 mL. If the specimen is not sufficient, it is discarded, and the athlete is asked to provide another specimen. The athlete is not allowed to leave the test center until adequate specimen is provided.

■ Specific gravity and pH are checked. If the specific gravity is less than 1.005 (1.010 if checked with a reagent strip), the specimen is discarded. If the pH is greater than 7.5 or less than 4.5, the specimen is discarded.

■ The specimen is processed if the specific gravity is above 1.005 (1.010 if using a reagent strip) and the pH is between 4.5 and 7.5.

■ Containers and unique bar-coded labels are selected by the athlete.

■ The specimen is divided into the "A vial" and the "B vial" by the crewmember. The vials are sealed, forms are filled out, and the specimens prepared for shipping. All is done in the presence of the athlete.

■ Chain of evidence must be maintained. The specimen must be controlled and signed at every step in the process.

■ The specimens are sent to an approved laboratory for testing. Specimen A is tested.

■ Results of positive tests are reported to the National Center for Drug Free Sport who breaks the number code and identifies the athlete. The athletics director or designate is notified by overnight mail marked confidential, who in turn must notify the athlete.

■ The athlete may be represented at the laboratory when testing specimen B. Different lab personnel will test specimen B.

■ The results of specimen B are considered final (4).

INSTITUTIONAL DRUG TESTING

■ Extreme care must be taken to protect the rights of the athlete.

■ Goals of testing, education program, punishment, selection process, procedures for testing, notification, confidentiality, appropriate follow-up, and legal issues must be carefully thought out and put into writing.

■ Multiple individuals may be involved in creating such a policy, including but not limited to administrators, legal counsel, medical advisors, psychologists, and representatives of the athletes.

■ Selection of athletes for testing may not be arbitrary.

■ After notification, the athlete must present to a testing center within a set amount of time.

■ Testing may be performed at an on-campus center or a designated industrial clinic for drug testing. If sent to an outside

facility, the school or organization must assure that proper conduct and procedures are followed.

■ Testing procedures should be similar to those discussed earlier under "Postseason Testing."

■ Lists of substances that are not allowed must be published and the athletes educated regarding the substances, health risks, treatment options, and sanctions for positive tests.

TESTING TECHNIQUES

■ Initial screening may be done by the relatively lower cost thin-layer chromatography or radioimmunoassay (RIA) methods.

■ Confirmation and definitive testing should be performed by gas chromatography and mass spectroscopy (6).

LEGAL ISSUES

■ Expect legal challenges to testing procedures and especially to positive tests.

■ Athletes should be afforded due process of law.

■ Institutions should define rights of appeal.

PUBLIC RELATIONS

■ Privacy of the athlete must be maintained.

■ The public and press often feel they have a "right to know" about the dealings of "their" teams, schools, and athletes.

■ The loss of an athlete from a team for "disciplinary" reasons is often assumed to be for positive drug tests.

REFERENCES

1. Greydanus DE, Patel DR. Sports doping in the adolescent athlete the hope, hype, and hyperbole. *Pediatr Clin North Am.* 2002;49(4):829–55.

2. International Olympic Committee. The fight against doping and promotion of athletes' health update-January 2010 [Internet]. [cited 2011 Feb 14]. Available from: http://www.olympic.org/Documents/Reference_documents_Factsheets/Fight_against_doping.pdf.

3. Knopp WD, Wang TW, Bach BR. Ergogenic drugs in sports. *Clin Sports Med.* 1997;16(3):375–93.

4. National Collegiate Athletic Association. Drug testing program [Internet]. [cited 2011 Sept 12]. Available from: http://www.ncaapublications.com/productdownloads/dt11.pdf.

5. United States Anti-Doping Agency (USADA) Web site [Internet]. [cited 2011 Feb 14]. Available from: http://www.usantidoping.org.

6. World Anti-Doping Agency (WADA) Web site [Internet]. [cited 2011 Sept 12]. Available from: http://www.wada-ama.org.

7. World Anti-Doping Agency. Therapeutic Use Exemption Guidelines Version 5, January 2011 [Internet]. [cited 2011 Sept 25]. Available from: http://www.wada-ama.org/Documents/World_Anti-Doping_Program/WADP-IS-TUE/2011/WADA_TUE_Guidelines_V5.0_EN_01JAN11.pdf.

26 Neuropsychological Testing in Concussion

Andrea Pana

INTRODUCTION

- It is estimated that 1.6–3.8 million sports concussions occur annually in the United States (1,9). This number may underestimate the total number of sports concussions because the athlete, coach, or parent may not report or may not recognize the symptoms of concussion.

- Animal studies have demonstrated a cascade of physiologic events that adversely affect cerebral functioning for a period of days to weeks after concussion (22).

- Diagnosis and management of concussion involve a careful assessment of the history of the injury and subsequent symptoms, a thorough clinical examination, as well as the consideration of advanced diagnostic testing. Neuropsychological (NP) testing is one of several tools currently used in the management of concussion.

- The Zurich Consensus statement on concussion states: "The application of neuropsychological (NP) testing in concussion has been shown to be of clinical value and continues to contribute significant information in concussion evaluation. It must be emphasized, however, that NP assessment should not be the sole basis of management decisions; rather, it should be seen as an aid to the clinical decision-making process in conjunction with a range of clinical domains and investigational results" (24).

- The Team Physician Consensus Statement on Concussion states that NP testing "is recommended as an aid to clinical decision-making but not a requirement for concussion management." The document also states that "the value of NP testing is enhanced when used as part of a multifaceted assessment and treatment program" and that it is "one component of the evaluation process and should not be used as a stand-alone tool to diagnose, manage or make RTP decisions in concussion" (12).

WHY IS NEUROPSYCHOLOGICAL TESTING USEFUL IN THE EVALUATION OF CONCUSSION?

- Returning an athlete to participation before complete recovery may increase the risk of a second concussive injury, a catastrophic injury, or chronic, long-term cognitive impairment (18). Postconcussive symptoms and clinical recovery patterns vary in individual athletes, and not all have a typical course. Up to 10%–20% of concussed athletes may have a postconcussion syndrome in which symptoms of concussion such as headache, fatigue, and memory impairment persist for a month or more after the injury (18).

- Self-reported symptoms are not reliable as a sole indicator of resolution of concussion. Several studies have shown that NP testing has a greater sensitivity than self-reported concussion symptoms in detecting resolution of concussion. Van Kampen et al. (33) found that 64% of their concussed athletes reported symptoms at 2 days, whereas 83% had deficits on NP testing compared to their baseline. Broglio et al. (2) showed that the sensitivity of symptoms in detecting concussion at 24 hours post injury was 68% compared to 78.6% and 79.2% for HeadMinder test and Immediate Post-Concussion Assessment and Cognitive Test, respectively.

- There are many reasons why athletes may underreport symptoms. Athletes may blatantly deny symptoms due to internal or external pressures to compete (fear of losing position, losing respect, seeming weak, letting team down). They may mislabel or fail to identify symptoms when they occur; attributing them to stress, dehydration, and tight-fitting helmet. Mild postconcussive symptoms may be viewed as their baseline level of functioning. Athletes may not be aware that symptoms of fatigue or sleep deprivation are postconcussive. Lastly, an athlete may truly be asymptomatic but still have neurocognitive deficits associated with concussion (11).

- Absence or resolution of symptoms is not indicative of complete recovery. Significant cognitive deficits remained in approximately 35% of concussive injuries when players were tested on computerized test battery after symptoms had resolved (20).

- NP testing is an objective measure of cognition that is more sensitive than sideline cognitive tests in identifying cognitive deficits and tracking recovery in concussed athletes.

TYPES OF NEUROPSYCHOLOGICAL TESTING

- Sideline assessment tools: These are basic NP tests designed for sideline assessment of players with concussion. Specifically, they involve tests of orientation, memory, concentration, and delayed recall.

- Clinician-administered NP tests: Consist of paper-and-pencil NP tests to assess cognitive function. Concussion assessment batteries typically focus on cognitive function, but additional tests assessing related psychological dysfunction can be added in cases where more extensive NP testing may be warranted in a given patient.

- Computerized NP tests: These are computer-based NP tests that measure various aspects of memory (new learning), cognitive processing speed, working memory, or executive functions. (The rationale for choosing tests from these domains is that these are functions typically affected by traumatic brain injury, as opposed to language or visuospatial skills, which are more resistant to the effects of brain injury) (9,28).

STATISTICAL FACTORS NECESSARY IN CHOOSING A NEUROPSYCHOLOGICAL TEST

- For NP testing to be valuable in the evaluation and treatment of concussion, certain statistical parameters should be met to demonstrate that as a clinical tool it has added value to the clinical armamentarium. Ultimately, one would like to be able to say that using this tool changes outcomes in the individuals one is treating with concussion.

- In the literature, statistical parameters applied in assessing NP test batteries include: reliability, validity, sensitivity, reliable change, and clinical utility.

Reliability

- This is a measure of the stability of a score or test over time.

- Test-retest reliability measures should ideally reflect clinically relevant intervals. For concussed athletes, that means scores need to be stable for months to more than a year in time.

- Test-retest reliability measures can be affected by practice effects. Some of these effects can be accounted for in the statistical measure used.

- Pearson coefficient and intraclass correlation coefficient (ICC) are two measures used in reliability. A minimally acceptable score for reliability is 0.60, with 0.90 being the ideal score to achieve (1,29).

- Pearson coefficient is a statistic that is a bivariate measurement of the relationship between two independent variables. It is limited by insensitivity to systematic changes in the score means due to learning or practice effects. It is known to overestimate the correlation when sample sizes are limited (1).

- The ICC is a univariate measure estimate of the agreement between two scores on the same test at two points in time. It accounts for some of the practice effects and is more commonly used in current studies as a measure of test-retest reliability.

Validity

- The basic concept behind validity is establishing that a test measures what it is supposed to measure.

- Concurrent validity: the degree to which a test under development correlates with established measures of the ability in question.

- Validity may also be established by demonstrating that a test is sensitive to the impairment in clinical populations with known defects. (For example, is a test of memory decreased in patients with known memory deficits?)

Sensitivity and Specificity

- One must establish that the test can differentiate between clinical patients (athletes with concussion) and controls (normal athletes). Is the test "positive in disease" (sensitivity) and "negative in health" (specificity)?

- One can measure sensitivity of a test with analysis of a group (comparing group means in those with and without concussion) or in analysis of individuals (requires a prospective age-matched study of controls to athletes with concussion).

- Specificity goes hand in hand with discussing sensitivity. In specificity, one looks at whether a test is negative in individuals without the disease in question. Is the test negative in an athlete who does not have a concussion? If not, then one has a false positive.

Change Scores

- This is a measure of the variability of a test over time.

- Variability is made up of a "real or normal fluctuation" of a test from one session to the next and an "error variance" or change in the test that is due to flaws in the measurement technique.

- The degree of change can be measured with the following measures: simple change scores, true change scores, standard deviations, standard error of measurement index, simple regression, multiple regression, reliable change index (RCI), and modified RCI. These techniques provide a degree of change measurement that accounts for one or more of the following: measurement error, regression to the mean, practice effects, and variables such as age, education, socioeconomic status, and history of concussion (only multiple regression).

- In the sports medicine/neuropsychology literature, the two most commonly applied techniques are RCIs and regression analyses (6).

- RCIs provide a value above which an observed change can be said to be meaningful. A standard RCI does not correct for the effects of measurement error caused by practice effects or other confounding variables. A modified RCI controls for measurement errors and practice effects.

- Simple and multiple regression techniques can be used to calculate or predict a subject's score after concussion. Multiple regression equations may include estimates of effects of variables such as age, education, socioeconomic status, and prior concussion history. A significant change is said to occur when the difference between the observed and predicted score is greater than a certain criterion (6).

Clinical Utility

- Is the test clinically useful? A test can have high reliability and high sensitivity but not necessarily be useful as a clinical decision-making tool.

- For concussion, an NP test would be clinically useful if it is sensitive in detecting neurocognitive impairments once concussion symptoms have resolved.

- It could also be added that a test would be clinically useful if the decision made from using it changes clinical outcomes. Does holding the athlete beyond the time during which they are asymptomatic until the time in which their NP tests return to baseline change their clinical outcome?

SIDELINE ASSESSMENT: BRIEF NEUROPSYCHOLOGICAL TESTS

How Are Neuropsychological Tests Used in Sideline Assessment of Concussion?

- Sideline NP assessment consists of brief tests of orientation, memory, concentration, and delayed recall used to assess an athlete's cognitive functioning to determine if the athlete sustained a concussion as well as to follow the concussion while on the field. It is used in conjunction with history, symptom assessment, and physical exam in the initial diagnosis and assessment of a concussed athlete.

- Serial cognitive sideline assessment of concussion was also used along with signs and symptoms to determine whether an athlete could return to the competition that day. However, recent changes in legislation (National Football League [NFL], National Collegiate Athletic Association [NCAA], state athletic associations) and medical practice have by in large restricted the return of an athlete into the competition in which he or she sustained a concussion.

- Serial NP assessment, along with serial symptom and exam evaluation, is used on the sideline to assess for worsening of cognitive status and necessity for further emergent evaluation such as imaging for a bleed.

Common Sideline Assessment Tools Used in the Evaluation of Concussion

- Maddocks questions, which are composed of questions of orientation and recent memory, were validated in a 1995 study. It was in this study that it was concluded that questions relating to orientation (person, date of birth, age, and month) were not sensitive in discriminating between a concussed and nonconcussed athlete. Questions relating to recall of recently acquired events (ground, quarter, how far into quarter, last team to score, team played last, who won last) were sensitive in detecting concussion (19).

- Standardized Assessment of Concussion (SAC) was developed in 1996 in response to the need for a standardized concussion assessment tool. It is a validated tool assessing orientation, immediate and delayed memory, and concentration. It is a scored tool that is optimally used when compared to a preseason baseline (26).

- Sport Concussion Assessment Tool (SCAT) is a validated tool developed from the Second International Consensus Conference on Concussion in Sport (Prague). It was created by combining several existing assessment tools used by medical and sports organizations into a new standardized tool. SCAT consists of evaluation of signs, memory assessment, symptoms, cognitive assessment, and neurologic screening (26).

- SCAT2 was a product of the Third International Consensus Conference on Concussion in Sport (Zurich). This tool consists of eight sections: symptoms, physical signs, Glasgow Coma Scale, sideline assessment-Maddocks score, cognitive assessment-SAC, balance examination, coordination examination, and cognitive assessment-delayed recall. Each section is scored with an overall total possible score of 100. This tool is not yet validated (24).

COMPREHENSIVE (CLINICAL) NEUROPSYCHOLOGICAL TESTING

Paper-and-Pencil (Clinician-Administered) Neuropsychological Testing

- A variety of paper-and-pencil test batteries have been used for neurocognitive assessment. In patients with concussion, tests that measure various aspects of memory (new learning), cognitive processing speed, working memory, attention, or executive functions have been most commonly used. The rationale for choosing tests from these domains is that these are functions typically affected by traumatic brain injury, as opposed to language or visuospatial skills, which are more resistant to the effects of brain injury (28).

- Examples of traditional paper-and-pencil neurocognitive tests (28):
  - Hopkin's Verbal Learning (memory/verbal learning)
  - Brief Visuospatial Memory Test (memory)

- Wechsler Adult Intelligence Scale, Third Edition (WAIS-III) Digit Symbol subtest (processing speed)
- Symbol Digit Modalities Test (SDMT) (processing speed)
- Trail Making Test (processing speed, executive)
- Controlled Oral Word Association (processing speed, executive)
- Stroop Color Word Test (executive)
- WAIS-III Digit Span Test (working memory)
- WAIS-III Letter-Number Sequencing Test (working memory)
- Paced Auditory Stimulation Test (working memory, speed of processing)

- Statistical support for use:
  - Paper-and-pencil tests have been used for years and have many studies looking at their validity. The validity of the tests has been well documented (28).
  - Reliability of individual tests have been documented through various studies. Reliability measures range from 0.39–0.93 for these individual tests, with most being in the 0.63–0.75 range; almost all are below the ideal of 0.90 but above the minimally acceptable 0.60 (9,13). There have been no attempts to combine several tests with similar cognitive domain measures into a composite score. This method is used with computer NP batteries and increases the reliability.
  - Randolph et al. (28) reviewed seven studies involving paper-and-pencil NP testing with respect to sensitivity. They concluded that the studies demonstrated "some evidence that standard paper-and-pencil tests are sensitive

to the effects of concussions, at least within the first five days of concussion" (28).

- Clinical utility has not been demonstrated; most studies have not demonstrated that paper-and-pencil NP tests can detect concussion once players are asymptomatic.

Computerized Neuropsychological Testing

- Computerized batteries measure domains of memory, attention, concentration, processing speed, and reaction time, as well as symptoms.
- Five computerized NP tests are currently available for the evaluation of sports-related concussions:
  - Automated Neuropsychological Assessment Metric (ANAM)
  - CogSport/Axon Sports Computerized Cognitive Assessment Tool (CCAT)
  - HeadMinder Concussion Resolution Index (CRI)
  - Immediate Post-Concussion Assessment and Cognitive Testing (ImPACT)
  - Concussion Vital Signs
    - ❏ This test will not be discussed; as of October 2011, there were no evidence-based studies in the literature on its use in sports-related concussions.
- Advantages and Disadvantages of Paper-and-Pencil, and Computerized NP Testing: see Table 26.1.

ANAM

- ANAM was the result of 30 years of test development. It was developed for serial testing and precision management of

Table 26.1	Advantages and Disadvantages of Neuropsychological (NP) Tests	
	Paper-and-Pencil NP Test	**Computerized NP Test**
Advantages	■ Extensive/thorough battery ■ Validity in diagnosis ■ Lower cost of equipment	■ Instant scoring; instant information to provider ■ More precise timing measures (reaction time measured to 1/100 of second) ■ Multiple equivalent forms, which decreases practice effects ■ Standardization of stimuli ■ Efficient in sports medicine setting ■ Practitioner need not be present; athletic training staff/medical assistants may administer ■ Large numbers of athletes can be tested at once ■ Short administration time (< 25 minutes) ■ Useful in serial testing ■ Centralized data storage, analysis, and reporting ■ Internet-based delivery possible ■ Do not need neuropsychologist to interpret
Disadvantages	■ Not ideal for serial use ■ Lack of equivalent alternative forms ■ Poor test-retest reliability ■ Susceptibility to interrater biases and practice effects ■ Time required by athlete and neuropsychologist ■ Must be interpreted by neuropsychologist ■ Cost of administration and interpretation	■ Practitioner need not be present ■ Tests specific domains, and at times, patient may need more global assessment of cognitive functioning ■ Baseline testing needed (to provide a better individual comparison) ■ Cost of computers, software

cognitive function in the U.S. Military. It was not specifically developed for concussion assessment, but a sport medicine battery evolved.

- ANAM Sports Medicine Battery (ASMB) (16,31):
  - Code Substitution (CDS): Concentration
  - Code Substitution-Delayed (CDD): Concentration, mental processing
  - Continuous Performance Test (CPT): Attention and concentration
  - Mathematical Processing (MTH): The test of mental processing speed and efficiency
  - Match to Sample (MSP): The test of visual memory
  - Simple Reaction Time (SRT): Test designed as a pure reaction time assessment
- Statistical support for use:
  - Cernich et al. (4) combined results of several studies on ANAM and concluded that there were significant practice effects (when individuals were tested 30 times in 4 days). Test-retest reliability measures in military cadets ranged from 0.38–0.87 on subsets tested (4,31).
  - A study by Segalowitz et al. (31) showed strong reliability (with a 1-week retest interval) in all subsets except reaction times, with Pearson coefficients of 0.67–0.81 and ICCs of 0.58–0.72. When aggregate scores were produced, the ICC increased to 0.86 (31).
  - A 2009 study by Kaminski et al. (16) examined test-retest reliability in the collegiate age group. Five trials 2 weeks apart showed an ICC of > 0.75. There was significant change from trial 1 to trial 2 before the score became stable, indicating support for double baseline testing (16). This study had participants tested at the same time of day to minimize effects of circadian rhythm, fatigue, and time since last meal; to have higher reliability, one should probably control these factors.
  - Several studies have shown that ANAM has consistent correlations with traditional NP tests, suggesting adequate concurrent validity (4,28,31).
  - Cernich et al. (4) compared ANAM's sensitivity to mild traumatic brain injury relative to a comprehensive battery of traditional NP measures; ANAM detected significant differences on four of five ANAM measures (4).
  - U.S. Military Academy surveillance data showed that SRT and CPT subtests were more sensitive in detecting cognitive changes after concussion; this was seen most prominently 1–2 days after concussion. Recovery in cognitive performance occurred in the 3- to 7-day time frame (4).

CogSport/Axon Sports CCAT

- Background: Computerized NP test that was developed in Australia and first available for use in sports concussion in 2002. Axon Sports CCAT is the online version of this test. This test is designed to be brief and keep the athlete

motivated. It is not intended to be a complete NP battery but focuses on speed and accuracy to detect change in cognitive measures over time.

- Test battery: The online version takes 12–15 minutes to complete and is composed of an initial response mapping, familiarizing the subject with the "yes" (K key) and "no" (D key) used in response during the following four tests below.
  - Processing speed task: This is a simple reaction time test.
  - Attention task: This is a choice reaction time task.
  - Learning task: This is a visual episodic recognition memory test.
  - Working memory task.
- A baseline report is marked as acceptable (check mark) or unacceptable. A baseline is unacceptable if it fails to meet integrity checks or is more than two standard deviations from the age group mean.
- A practice test is recommended prior to taking the test, and baselines are repeated if unacceptable.
- A postinjury report is given with the scores, along with a conclusion of acceptable (or a green check mark) or "not returned to baseline" (or a red "X"). A performance on any task that is worse than 1.65 standard deviations from baseline is flagged as impaired.
- The test developer recommends that baseline testing be done at least once a year or before each contact sport season; it should be done more often if the athlete sustained a concussion that season or is a young athlete going through cognitive maturation.
- Statistical support for use:
  - In a 2003 study by Collie et al. (5), test-retest reliability at 1 hour and 1 week were studied. ICCs at 1 hour ranged from 0.08–0.90, with those subsets for speed ranging from 0.69–0.90 and those for accuracy ranging from 0.08–0.45. At 1 week, ICCs were 0.31–0.82, with speed subsets ranging from 0.69–0.82 and accuracy subsets ranging from 0.31–0.51 (5).
  - Broglio (1) also looked at test-retest reliability for CogSport, testing at baseline, 45 days, and 50 days. ICCs were 0.23–0.65 from baseline to day 45 and 0.39–0.66 from day 45 to day 50. (Of note, three NP programs were tested back to back, which may have affected scores) (1).
  - Validity of CogSport compared to conventional NP tests was evaluated in 2003. ICCs between CogSport and Digit Symbol Substitution Test were 0.02–0.86, with speed ICCs of 0.42–0.86 and accuracy ICCs of 0.02–0.35. Comparing CogSport to Trail Making Tests, the ICCs were 0.04–0.44, with speed ICCs of 0.23–0.44 and accuracy ICCs of 0.04–0.38 (5).
  - Schatz and Putz (30) looked at cross-validation of CogSport SRT and Complex Reaction Time (CRT) with Trail Making Tests A and B and Digit Symbol test and found Pearson's coefficients for SRT to be 0.28, 0.17, and 0.08, respectively. Coefficients (r) with CRT were 0.54, 0.54, and 0.28, respectively (30).

- In a 2010 study, RCIs were used to assess concussed individuals' return to baseline. The value of 1.65 standard deviation from the mean was used (based on 2004 study); a clinically relevant change from baseline was considered to be 50 milliseconds (20).

- There is no evidence that composite scores are being produced for Axon Sports CCAT tests.

- Makdissi et al. (20) demonstrated both sensitivity and clinical utility; 70.8% of concussed patients in their cohort showed declines from baseline in one or more tests while symptomatic; 18% of patients showed deficits at 7 days. Computerized tests showed deficits 2–3 days longer on average than symptoms and paper-and-pencil tests (20).

- Reaction time measures have been shown to be the most sensitive index to cognitive changes following head injury (32).

HeadMinder CRI

- Background: The CRI is composed of six subtests measuring reaction time, visual recognition, and speed of information processing. Three factors are derived from the subtests: Simple Reaction Time (SRT), Complex Reaction Time (CRT), and Processing Speed (PS). The CRI primarily assesses cognitive change through online tests of attention and reaction time.

- Test battery (10):
  - The Reaction Time subtest
  - The Cued Reaction Time subtest
  - The Animal Decoding subtest
  - Visual Recognition 1
  - Visual Recognition 2
  - Symbol Scanning

- Statistical support for use:
  - Test-retest reliability over a 2-week interval demonstrated correlation coefficients of 0.82 for processing speed, 0.70 for simple reaction time, and 0.68 for complex reaction time (10).
  - In a study by Broglio (1), ICCs were 0.15–0.66 from baseline to day 45 and 0.03–0.66 between days 45 and 50 (three NP tests were tested back to back).
  - In a 2001 study, Erlanger et al. described the sensitivity of 88% when administered 1 to 2 days after injury (2).
  - In a 2003 paper, CRI was 77% sensitive (using 90% confidence interval) in detecting concussion; when combined with symptoms, sensitivity was 96% (10).
  - In a 2007 study, Broglio et al. (2) showed a sensitivity of 78.6% for detecting concussion at 24 hours, compared with 68% for self-reported symptoms, 62% for postural changes, and 43% for paper-and-pencil tests. A complete battery together had a sensitivity of 89.3% (2).
  - Validity was looked at in multiple studies. Erlanger showed that response speed scores correlated with Trail Making Test A (0.73) and Trail Making Test B (0.74) and that PS scores correlated with WAIS-III Digit Span (0.53) and SDMT (0.66). In a cross-validation study, less significant correlations were seen between HeadMinder SRT and CRT and Trail Making A, Trail Making B, and Digit Symbol tests, with correlations (r) of 0.43, 0.23, and 0.53 and 0.06, 0.32, and 0.30, respectively. However, PS correlated with Trail Making Test B ($r = 0.60$) and Digit Symbol Test ($r = 0.61$) (30). Finally, in a 2003 study, concurrent validity was looked at in comparing CRI PS, SRT, and CRT indices to a variety of paper-and-pencil tests. PS showed the best correlation (0.57–0.66) with the WAIS, SDMT, and Grooved Pegboard tests. SRT index correlated best with Grooved Pegboard (0.46–0.60), and correlation of CRT was 0.40 with Trail Making Test A and 0.59–0.70 with Grooved Pegboard (10).
  - Erlanger et al. (10) examined CRI, RCI, and REG (multiple regression) with 90% confidence intervals in a cohort of concussed patients.

ImPACT

- Background: The ImPACT test was developed in the United States in the 1990s. This 20-minute test assesses symptoms along with cognitive domains of attention span, working memory, sustained and selective attention, response variability, nonverbal problem solving, and reaction time.

- Test battery: Consists of six modules, which are individually scored and then used to calculate five composite scores.
  - Word Discrimination: This module evaluates attentional processes and verbal recognition memory.
  - Design Memory: This test evaluates attentional processes and visual recognition memory.
  - X's and O's: This measures visual working memory as well as visual processing speed.
  - Symbol Matching: This test evaluates visual processing speed, learning, and memory
  - Color Match: This module is a choice reaction time task and also measures impulse control and response inhibition.
  - Three Letter Memory: This measures working memory and visual-motor response speed.

- Composite scores: verbal memory, visual memory, processing speed composite, reaction time composite, and impulse control composite

- A total symptom score composite is also part of the test (22 symptoms rated from 1 to 6).

- Statistical support for use:
  - Broglio (1) looked at ImPACT scores at 45 and 50 days compared to baseline and found ICCs to be 0.23–0.39 from baseline to day 45 and 0.39–0.61 from baseline to day 50. These were lower than previous studies, but testing involved doing three NP tests back to back, which may have affected performance.

- Iverson et al. (14) reported 7-day test-retest reliabilities for ImPACT to be 0.65–0.86 for the five domain scores, with processing speed and reaction time being the highest.

- Schatz (29) looked at 2-year test-retest reliability in 2010. ICCs were as follows: verbal memory = 0.46, visual memory = 0.65, reaction time = 0.68, processing speed = 0.74, and symptoms scale = 0.43.

- In 2006, Schatz et al. (2) showed sensitivity of ImPACT to be 82% when administered 72 hours after injury.

- The Broglio et al. (2) study published in 2007 found the sensitivity of ImPACT to be 79.2%, compared with 68% for self-reported symptoms, 62% for postural changes, and 43% for paper-and-pencil tests. A complete battery together had a sensitivity of > 90%.

- Validity is demonstrated for performance on SDMT, which was shown to correlate significantly with ImPACT processing speed ($r = 0.70$) and reaction time ($r = 0.60$) (30).

- Postconcussive symptoms were significantly related to decreased performance on ImPACT reaction time, visual and verbal memory, and processing speed, indicating that ImPACT is sensitive to acute effects of concussion (11).

- A cross-validation study in 2006 showed correlations (Pearson's or r) between ImPACT reaction time and Trail Making Test A, Trail Making Test B, and Digit Symbol test to be 0.64, 0.44, and 0.46, respectively. Correlations between PS and Trail Making Test B and Digit Symbol test were found to be 0.51 and 0.54, respectively (30).

- An article on interpreting change in ImPACT delineates RCI and specific measures for each of the composite scores that are the reliable change variables set by 80% confidence intervals (based on changes in a group of nonconcussed athletes). Using these RCIs in evaluation, the study in concussed athletes at 72 hours showed that 64% had declines in two or more of the five composite scores and 76% had declines in one or more scores. They note that RCIs are used to supplement interpretation and not replace clinical judgment (14).

- McClincy et al. (21) showed that ImPACT scores demonstrated changes 4–7 days after clinical symptoms had resolved.

- Iverson et al. (15), in 2003, showed that symptoms in high school athletes resolved, on average, after 7 days, but ImPACT showed changes, on average, until 10 days.

- Lovell (15), in 2007, showed that average symptoms in high school students lasted 17 days compared with 26 days of NP test changes.

- In a study of high school and college students, Van Kampen et al. (33) noted that 2 days after injury, 64% reported symptoms, but 83% had neurocognitive changes seen on ImPACT (93% were identified as concussed with either symptoms or NP changes).

CONSIDERATIONS IN NEUROPSYCHOLOGICAL TESTING

Baseline Testing

- The principle behind baseline testing is to compare an athlete's neurocognitive functioning after concussion to his or her own neurocognitive function (as measured by an NP test) rather than to a group norm or age-matched control. Given that multiple issues can affect testing, comparing to one's own baseline will help control for some of these variables.

- "Post-injury neuropsychological test data are more useful if compared to the athlete's pre-injury baseline" (12).

- Baseline testing can be used to track recovery.

- Baseline testing is ideally performed in a quiet environment with no distractions, with the athlete well rested and a person who knows how to administer the test.

- Recommendations for frequency of baseline testing vary. The frequency could be every contact sport season, every year, or every 2 years.

- It has been observed that baseline NP tests change with cognitive maturity in the adolescent years. In a study with paper-and-pencil NP tests, average baselines were different among different grades in high school (13).

- Test-retest reliability studies on individual tests give some indication of the stability of the testing in different populations (high school vs. college vs. postcollege athletes).

- "Double baseline testing," or repeating the test twice in a 1- to 2-week span, has been suggested by some NP test developers to control for the learning effect seen in studies in the first two repetitions of the test.

- Practice effects can also be controlled for with statistical measures such as RCI and regression-based measures.

Factors Affecting Testing (23,26)

- Psychological: Test or general anxiety, fear, depression, stress, other emotional states

- Physiological: Sleep, alertness, pain, medication, nutrition, hormonal, severity of present concussion

- Cultural: education, language, previous exposure to testing or use of computers

- Premorbid conditions/past history: learning disorders (attention deficit hyperactivity disorder or others), developmental disorders, personality disorders, previous concussions or head injuries, drug use, alcohol use

- Genetic: age, intelligence, sex, race, handedness, visual acuity, auditory acuity

- Methodologic: test setting/atmosphere (temperature, quiet), time of day, size of computer display, practice/learning effects, administrator expertise

- Other: random variance/chance, motivation, effort, prior testing (affect of multiple tests in 1 week or a short period of time)

Interpretation of Testing

- Individual states may have laws that pertain to who may interpret and administer NP tests.

- Paper-and-pencil tests should be administered and interpreted by a neuropsychologist or other practitioner who is trained in the administration and interpretation of the tests.

- Computerized NP testing batteries have different reports that are generated from the testing. Some give composite scores that can be compared to baseline, and some give an overall assessment of acceptable or not returned to baseline. Depending on the type of report, there may be ability to interpret the scores with respect to an individual patient's situation. Ability to look at individual tests allows one to use clinical judgment and incorporate NP tests results with the rest of the clinician's armamentarium for concussion assessment.

- Test interpretation requires understanding patient symptoms, psychometric properties of the test, complex interactions of test data, sources of error, extra-test variables, and intraindividual variables (8).

- While some believe that only neuropsychologists should interpret the computerized NP tests, a more appropriate statement may be that NP tests should be interpreted by a medical provider trained in the use and interpretation of that particular NP test.

- Some of the computerized NP tests offer training in the use and interpretation of the tests Interpretation of testing should take into account the factors affecting testing described earlier.

Administration of Testing

- Testing should be administered by a qualified health professional appropriately instructed in the administration of that test. For computer NP testing in the collegiate, professional, and high school setting, this role has been largely delegated to the athletic trainer.

- There are no evidence-based guidelines on when and how often to administer a computerized NP test.

- Some providers use NP tests when symptomatic to document a postinjury starting point when there is no baseline, to prove there are neurocognitive changes to the athlete/coach/parent, to confirm diagnosis if it is in question, or to help guide academic considerations.

- Another common time to do the first post-injury NP test is when the player is asymptomatic to determine if the athlete can be started in an exercise progression.

- Lastly, some practitioners choose to start an exercise progression when asymptomatic and use the NP test at the end of exercise progression before clearance to full-contact sports.

- It is not uncommon for an athlete to take two or more NP tests before return to sport. One must be careful not to administer too many tests in a short time span because factors of learning, interference (of word groups, card numbers, etc.), and decreased motivation may affect test scores.

Factors Affecting Baseline Scores, Postinjury Scores, and Recovery Course

Age

- Younger brains may be more vulnerable to injury. This may be related to less myelination, greater head to body ratio, or thinner cranial bones. However, the primary factor is thought to be cognitive maturity (13) and possibly increased susceptibility to the neurometabolic changes associated with mild traumatic brain injury (15).

- Cognitive maturity increases through adulthood, with executive functioning the last to mature at age 24 (13).

- A study on baseline neurocognitive testing with paper-and-pencil test in high school students showed leveling off of the Trail Making A, Trail Making B, and SDMT at age 15, but reaction time continued to change (13).

- In one study, those high school students classified as having simple concussions recovered in an average of 5.7 days (43.5% of cases), while those classified as having complex concussions took an average of 29.3 days (56.5%) (17).

- In a study of high school and college Australian rules football players (age 16–35), the majority of players returned to play by 7 days (when using NP testing along with clinical assessment) with the mean return to play of 4.8 days. However, 17.9% still had cognitive changes at 1 week (20).

- In professional and college players, average time to return to play in studies is < 3 days and 5–7 days, respectively (15).

Sex

- Female athletes may be at greater risk for concussion due to differences in head-neck dynamics. They may also may experience different symptoms and recovery patterns (7).

- A study by Colvin et al. (7) showed decreased reaction times in female soccer players as compared to male counterparts. There was also a trend of decreased performance on memory and visual motor speed. These differences were found to be unrelated to body mass index. They also saw an increased number of symptoms and a different recovery pattern in the female soccer players (7).

- Brown et al. (3) found differences in several subset scores on ANAM in men and women, with women scoring higher than men on the Sternberg memory search (ST6) subtest and men scoring higher on SRTs 1 and 2, and Matching to sample pairs (MSP).

History of Prior Concussion

- A study on soccer players showed that those with no history of concussion performed better on ImPACT than those with more than one concussion (7). This is different than what has been shown in several other studies that found no association between athletes reporting two or more concussions and those reporting with none or one concussion (3). However, in a study examining multiple concussions in college football players, Collins and colleagues demonstrated long-term mild deficits in executive functioning and speed of information processing in athletes who sustained two or more concussions (15). A retrospective study surveying a sample of retired NFL athletes found that those who had experienced three or more concussions were more likely to report symptoms of cognitive impairment and depression (15).

Dehydration

- A study by Patel et al. (25) showed that dehydration led to greater symptom reporting and greater severity of symptoms at time of baseline testing but no NP test differences. This might indicate that symptoms alone may be misleading in a dehydrated athlete with a possible concussion.

Symptomatology and Recovery

- Headache is the most often reported symptom, documented in 40%–86% of concussions. Presence of headache, regardless of severity, is associated with higher levels of postconcussion symptoms, memory dysfunction, and decreased reaction time at 1 week after injury (11).

- Concussed athletes with headache were more likely to have had retrograde amnesia and five times more likely to have experienced mental status changes > 5 minutes after concussion (11).

- Concussed athletes with posttraumatic migraine have the most postinjury impairment, with significant decreases in visual memory, verbal memory, processing speed, and reaction time at 4 days post-injury (11). Athletes who experience headaches accompanied by typical migraine-type symptoms of nausea, vomiting, vision changes, and photophobia or phonophobia may experience a greater severity of symptoms and prolonged recovery (15).

- Iverson looked at fogginess and found that any fogginess after concussion was related to a higher number of concussion symptoms and a decreased performance in memory, reaction time, and processing speed at 5 and 10 days (11).

Arguments Against Baseline Neuropsychological Testing in Concussion

- If it is mandated, it could be costly to test all age groups and all college and professional athletes.

- True risks of returning an athlete to play before symptoms have resolved may be overstated (27). Incidence of second impact syndrome is low, and if ongoing research confirms a genetic predisposition, it may not be preventable. The rate of second concussion in a season was reported to be 6.5% in a study by Guskiewicz, which is not higher than the range of 3%–8% of primary concussions in a season reported in the literature. However, there may be a vulnerable postconcussion period; in one study, 90% of second concussions occurred in the within 10 days of the initial concussion (27).

- Utilization of testing may not modify risks or change outcome (27).

- There is currently no adequate research to show that baseline testing changes long-term outcomes with respect to multiple concussions and head trauma over a career and the individual's cognitive functioning or abilities in the future (27).

FUTURE DIRECTIONS

- NP testing has increasingly been used in the management of sport-related concussions. There are many studies on the various computer-based tests, each demonstrating some aspect of testing and evidence to support its use. Not all aspects of all of the computer-based (or even the paper-and-pencil) tools have been proven in terms of meeting statistical standards that we apply to clinical tests. The research will continue to grow as researchers and clinicians explore and validate these tests and their use in the realm of sports concussion.

- It is important to realize that NP testing is not meant to be and has not been proven to be the gold standard single test in the evaluation of concussion and should not replace clinical judgment. It is one of several tools along with history, physical exam, and balance testing that together can provide information that can assist the treating physician in decision making for the treatment and return-to-play decisions in athletes with concussion.

REFERENCES

1. Broglio SP, Ferrara MS, Macciocchi SN, Baumgartner TA, Elliott R. Test-retest reliability of computerized concussion assessment programs. *J Athl Train.* 2007;42(4):509–14.
2. Broglio SP, Macciocchi SN, Ferrara MS. Sensitivity of the concussion assessment battery. *Neurosurgery.* 2007;60(6):1050–8.
3. Brown CN, Guskiewicz KM, Bleiberg J. Athlete characteristics and outcome scores for computerized neuropsychological assessment: a preliminary analysis. *J Athl Train.* 2007;42(4):515–23.
4. Cernich A, Reeves D, Sun W, Bleiberg J. Automated neuropsychological assessment metrics sports medicine battery. *Arch Clin Neuropsychol.* 2007;22(Suppl 1):S101–14.
5. Collie A, Maruff P, Makdissi M, McCrory P, McStephen M, Darby D. CogSport: reliability and correlation with conventional cognitive tests used in postconcussion medical evaluations. *Clin J Sport Med.* 2003;13(1):28–32.
6. Collie A, Maruff P, Makdissi M, McStephen M, Darby DG, McCrory P. Statistical procedures for determining the extent of cognitive change following concussion. *Br J Sports Med.* 2004;38(3):273–8.
7. Colvin AC, Mullen J, Lovell MR, West RV, Collins MW, Groh M. The role of concussion history and gender in recovery from soccer-related concussion. *Am J Sports Med.* 2009;37(9):1699–704.
8. Echemendia RJ, Herring S, Bailes J. Who should conduct and interpret the neuropsychological assessment in sports-related concussion? *Br J Sports Med.* 2009;43(Suppl 1):i32–5.
9. Ellemberg D, Henry LC, Macciocchi SN, Guskiewicz KM, Broglio SP. Advances in sport concussion assessment: from behavioral to brain imaging measures. *J Neurotrauma.* 2009;6(12):2365–82.
10. Erlanger D, Feldman D, Kutner K, et al. Development and validation of a web-based neuropsychological test protocol for sports-related return-to-play decision-making. *Arch Clin Neuropsychol.* 2003;18(3):293–316.
11. Fazio VC, Lovell MR, Pardini JE, Collins MW. The relation between post concussion symptoms and neurocognitive performance in concussed athletes. *NeuroRehabilitation.* 2007;22(3):207–16.
12. Herring SA, Cantu RC, Guskiewicz KM, et al. Concussion (mild traumatic brain injury) and the team physician: a consensus statement. *Med Sci Sports Exerc.* 2011;43(12):2412–22.

13. Hunt TN, Ferrara MS. Age-related differences in neuropsychological testing among high school athletes. *J Athl Train.* 2009;44(4):405–9.

14. Iverson GL, Lovell MR, Collins MW. Interpreting change on ImPACT following sport concussion. *Clin Neuropsychol.* 2003;17(4):460–7.

15. Johnson EW, Kegel NE, Collins MW. Neurological assessment of sports related concussion. *Clin Sports Med.* 2011;30(1):73–88, viii–ix.

16. Kaminski TW, Groff RM, Glutting JJ. Examining the stability of Automated Neuropsychological Assessment Metric (ANAM) baseline test scores. *J Clin Exp Neuropsychol.* 2009;31(6):689–97.

17. Lau B, Lovell MR, Collins MW, Pardini J. Neurocognitive and symptom predictors of recovery in high school athletes. *Clin J Sport Med.* 2009;19(3):216–21.

18. Lovell M. The management of sports-related concussion: current status and future trends. *Clin Sports Med.* 2009;28(1):95–111.

19. Maddocks DL, Dicker GD, Saling MM. The assessment of orientation following concussion in athletes. *Clin J Sport Med.* 1995;5(1):32–5.

20. Makdissi M, Darby D, Maruff P, Ugoni A, Brukner P, McCrory PR. Natural history of concussion in sport: markers of severity and implications for management. *Am J Sports Med.* 2010;38(3):464–71.

21. McClincy MP, Lovell MR, Pardini J, Collins MW, Spore MK. Recovery from sports concussion in high school and collegiate athletes. *Brain Inj.* 2006;20(1):33–9.

22. McCrea M, Guskiewicz KM, Marshall SW, et al. Acute effects and recovery time following concussion in collegiate football players: the NCAA Concussion Study. *JAMA.* 2003;290(19):2556–63.

23. McCrory P, Makdissi M, Davis G, Collie A. Value of neuropsychological testing after head injuries in football. *Br J Sports Med.* 2005;39(Suppl 1):i58–63.

24. McCrory P, Meeuwisse W, Johnston K, et al. Consensus statement on concussion in sport: the 3rd International Conference on Concussion in Sport, held in Zurich. *Clin J Sports Med.* 2009;19(3):185–200.

25. Patel AV, Mihalik JP, Notebaert AJ, Guskiewicz KM, Prentice WE. Neuropsychological performance, postural stability, and symptoms after dehydration. *J Athl Train.* 2007;42(1):66–75.

26. Patel DR, Shivdasani V, Baker RJ. Management of sport-related concussion in young athletes. *Sports Med.* 2005;35(8):671–84.

27. Randolph C. Baseline neuropsychological testing in managing sports-related concussion: does it modify risk? *Curr Sports Med Rep.* 2011;10(1):21–6.

28. Randolph C, McCrea M, Barr WB. Is neuropsychological testing useful in the management of sport-related concussion? *J Athl Train.* 2005;40(3):139–54.

29. Schatz P. Long-term test-retest reliability of baseline cognitive assessments using ImPACT. *Am J Sports Med.* 2010;38(1):47–53.

30. Schatz P, Putz BO. Cross-validation of measures used for computer-based assessment of concussion. *Appl Neuropsychol.* 2006;13(3):151–9.

31. Segalowitz SJ, Mahaney P, Santessoa DL, MacGregor L, Dywan J, Willer B. Retest reliability in adolescents of a computerized neuropsychological battery used to assess recovery from concussion. *NeuroRehabilitation.* 2007;22(3):243–51.

32. Straume-Naesheim TM, Andersen TE, Bahr R. Reproducibility of computer based neuropsychological testing among Norwegian elite football players. *Br J Sports Med.* 2005;39:i64–9.

33. Van Kampen DA, Lovell MA, Pardini JE, Collins MW, Fu FH. The "value added" of neurocognitive testing after sports-related concussion. *Am J Sports Med.* 2006;34(10):1630–5.

27 Cardiovascular Considerations

Marc Childress, Jonathan A. Drezner, Ralph G. Oriscello, and Francis G. O'Connor

INTRODUCTION

- Exercise is clearly associated with improved cardiovascular health. In addition to a direct conditioning effect, physical activity is critical in the management and prevention of several chronic medical conditions that impact overall health (47).

- However, vigorous exercise also can be a trigger for sudden cardiac arrest in individuals with underlying cardiovascular disease (43).

- Sudden death in athletes is most often attributable to a cardiovascular disorder. Sudden cardiac death represents 75% of fatalities in National Collegiate Athletic Association (NCAA) athletes during training or competition, more than deaths related to blunt trauma, heat stroke, and sickle cell trait combined (1).

- A high index of suspicion must be maintained during screening to detect conditions associated with sudden death, including appropriate individual assessments as well as reasonable measures to evaluate large populations.

- When a serious cardiovascular condition is identified, appropriate treatment and activity modification may decrease the risk of sudden death.

CARDIOVASCULAR BENEFITS OF EXERCISE

- The lack of regular physical activity has clearly been associated with an increase in coronary heart disease and the incidence of adverse cardiac events (4,34,41,48,49). Multiple studies have confirmed the benefit of aerobic exercise with a reduction in the number of cardiac events and a reduction in mortality (3,18,34,36,50). Although there is an increased risk for adverse cardiac events during activity, there is overwhelming evidence that the net benefits of consistent and regular physical exercise outweigh these risks in the primary prevention of cardiovascular disease (22,45).

THE ATHLETIC HEART SYNDROME

- Vigorous athletic training is associated with specific physiologic and structural cardiovascular changes, so-called *athletic heart syndrome* (15,28). These changes represent normal adaptations to physical conditioning.

- Studies demonstrate a constellation of morphologic changes that vary depending on the type of training (39).

- In endurance-trained athletes, a chronic volume overload results in an increase in both left ventricular end-diastolic diameter and left ventricular wall thickness. This eccentric hypertrophy allows a larger stroke volume and thus a greater overall cardiac output at faster heart rates. Biatrial enlargement and right ventricular dilation also can be seen.

- Strength-trained athletes develop a concentric hypertrophy with an increase in absolute and relative wall thickness without significant changes in end-diastolic diameter. Right-sided and atrial dimensions typically remain unchanged.

- It is important to remember that the adaptive structural and physiologic response of the normal athletic heart does not rule out the presence of an underlying pathologic condition. In fact, it makes the task of diagnosing that condition more challenging for the primary care physician, sports medicine physician, and cardiologist (21). Criteria for distinguishing the characteristics of athletic heart syndrome from significant underlying pathology have been defined and, in some circumstances, may require detraining for 2–3 months (21). In benign cases, full resolution should be observed, whereas residual hypertrophic changes may suggest underlying concerns (38).

Physical Examination

- The heart rate of well-conditioned athletes is usually between 40 and 60 bpm, secondary to enhanced vagal tone, decreased sympathetic tone, and a larger stroke volume. Thus, sinus bradycardia is a common finding, and sinus arrhythmia may be more noticeable.

- The physiologic splitting of S2 may be slightly delayed during inspiration due to the larger stroke volume. An S3 may be noted in endurance-trained athletes secondary to the increased rate of left ventricular filling associated with the relative left ventricular dilatation (13,28).

- Although an S4 may be noted in strength-trained athletes secondary to concentric hypertrophy, its presence always warrants clinical evaluation. Functional (flow) murmurs characterized by a soft 1–2/6 ejection murmur often present when supine and diminished with standing or Valsalva may be noted in 30%–50% of athletes on careful examination (15).

Table 27.1	**Common ECG Findings in Athletic Heart Syndrome**
Sinus bradycardia	Sinus arrhythmia
First-degree AV block	Wenckebach AV block
Incomplete RBBB	Notched P waves
RVH by voltage criteria	LVH by voltage criteria
Early repolarization changes	QTc interval at upper limit
Tall, peaked T waves	

AV, atrioventricular; ECG, electrocardiogram; LVH, left ventricular hypertrophy; RBBB, right bundle branch block; RVH, right ventricular hypertrophy.
SOURCE: Adapted from Huston TP, Puffer JC, Rodney WM. The athletic heart syndrome. *N Engl J Med.* 1985;313:24–32.

Electrocardiographic Changes

■ Several electrocardiographic changes can be seen in well-conditioned athletes. In most cases, these changes are benign reflections of structural and functional changes. However, some findings are abnormal and may suggest underlying pathology. It can be challenging to distinguish adaptive versus pathologic changes in trained athletes, and modern electrocardiogram (ECG) criteria should be used to assist in interpretation (8,9,14,15) (Tables 27.1 and 27.2).

■ ECG is helpful in the initial evaluation of cardiac conditions in athletes who present with cardiovascular symptoms or have abnormal findings on physical examination.

■ The role of ECG in the preparticipation screening of athletes is controversial. Opponents of ECG screening are concerned about false-positive results, cost effectiveness, and unnecessary disqualifications in athletes (46). Proponents of ECG screening recognize that the sensitivity of a history and physical examination alone to detect potentially lethal cardiovascular disorders in athletes is very low, that the addition of an ECG greatly increases the sensitivity, and that it can be accomplished with a low and acceptable false-positive rate when performed by experienced physicians guided by modern ECG criteria (11,35).

SUDDEN CARDIAC DEATH IN EXERCISE

■ The overall risk of sudden death during exercise varies depending on age, gender, and sport. Estimates from studies in runners range from 1:15,000 joggers per year to 1:50,000 marathon participants per race (24,43). For high school and college-aged athletes, the range is 1:45,000 to 1:160,000 per year, and sudden deaths occur disproportionally more often in males, African Americans, and basketball and football players (1,23).

■ The specific etiologies contributing to sudden cardiac death are strongly related to age. For sudden death in persons over age 35, more than 75% are associated with coronary artery disease. This association increases with age, consistent with the rising prevalence of atherosclerosis (18).

Table 27.2	**Classification of Abnormalities of the Athlete's Electrocardiogram**
Group 1: Common and Training-Related ECG Changes	
Sinus bradycardia	
First-degree AV block	
Incomplete RBBB	
Early repolarization	
Isolated QRS voltage criteria for left ventricular hypertrophy	
Group 2: Uncommon and Training-Unrelated ECG Changes	
T-wave inversion	
ST-segment depression	
Pathologic Q waves	
Left atrial enlargement	
Left axis deviation/left anterior hemiblock	
Right axis deviation/left posterior hemiblock	
Right ventricular hypertrophy	
Ventricular pre-excitation	
Complete LBBB or RBBB	
Long- or short-QT interval	
Brugada-like early repolarization	

AV, atrioventricular; ECG, electrocardiogram; LBBB, left bundle branch block; RBBB, right bundle branch block.
SOURCE: Reproduced with permission from Corrado D, Pelliccia A, Heidbuchel H, et al. Recommendations for interpretation of 12-lead electrocardiogram in the athlete. *Eur Heart J.* 2010;31:243–59.

■ In younger athletes, sudden cardiac death is most often the result of intrinsic structural or electrical abnormalities. Hypertrophic cardiomyopathy (HCM) is the most common cause of sudden cardiac death, followed by coronary artery anomalies, myocarditis, and arrhythmogenic right ventricular cardiomyopathy (ARVC). Other etiologies include genetic conductive system abnormalities such as ion channel disorders (long QT syndrome), aortic rupture from Marfan syndrome, premature coronary artery disease, idiopathic left ventricular hypertrophy, substance abuse (cocaine or steroids), aortic stenosis, mitral valve prolapse, sickle cell trait, and blunt chest trauma (commotio cordis). This list reflects cases of sudden death in athletes over the past two decades in the United States (23). It is important to note that the relative prevalence of many of these conditions is variable, based on regional and ethnic differences. For example, ARVC is the leading cause of sudden cardiac death in the Veneto region of Italy (12).

Screening for Sudden Death

■ The American Heart Association (AHA) Science and Advisory Committee published consensus guidelines for preparticipation cardiovascular screening for high school and college athletes in 1996 and reaffirmed their recommendations in 2007 (25,26). A complete personal and family history and physical examination should be done for all athletes. It should focus on identifying those cardiovascular conditions known to cause sudden death. The recommended interval for evaluation begins in middle school and is repeated every 2 years with an interim history between examinations (Table 27.3).

■ Family history should include a specific inquiry for a family history of premature coronary artery disease, diabetes mellitus, hypertension, sudden death, syncope, death or significant disability from cardiovascular disease in relatives younger than age 50, or the presence of inherited cardiac disorders such as HCM, ARVC, Marfan syndrome, and long QT syndrome.

■ Personal past history should include specific inquiries on the detection of a heart murmur; risk factors for coronary artery disease such as diabetes mellitus, hypertension, hyperlipidemia, and smoking; and a history of syncope, near

Table 27.3	The 12-Element AHA Recommendations for Preparticipation Cardiovascular Screening of Competitive Athletes

Medical History*

Personal History

1. Exertional chest pain/discomfort

2. Unexplained syncope/near syncope**

3. Excessive exertional and unexplained dyspnea/fatigue, associated with exercise

4. Prior recognition of a heart murmur

5. Elevated systemic blood pressure

Family History

6. Premature death (sudden and unexpected, or otherwise) before age 50 years due to heart disease, in ≥ 1 relative

7. Disability from heart disease in a close relative < 50 years of age

8. Specific knowledge of certain cardiac conditions in family members: HCM, long QT syndrome, or other ion channelopathies, Marfan syndrome, or clinically important arrhythmias

Physical Examination

9. Heart murmur#

10. Femoral arterial pulses to exclude aortic coarctation

11. Physical stigmata of Marfan syndrome

12. Brachial blood pressure (sitting position)##

* Parental verification is recommended for high school and middle school athletes.
** Judged not to be neurocardiogenic (vasovagal); of particular concern when related to exertion.
# Auscultation should be performed in both supine and standing positions (or with Valsalva maneuver), specifically to identify murmurs of dynamic left ventricular outflow tract obstruction.
Preferably taken in both arms.
AHA, American Heart Association; HCM, hypertrophic cardiomyopathy.
SOURCE: Reproduced with permission from Maron BJ, Thompson PD, Ackerman MJ. Recommendations and considerations related to preparticipation screening for cardiovascular abnormalities in competitive athletes: 2007 update: a scientific statement from the American Heart Association Council on Nutrition, Physical Activity, and Metabolism: endorsed by the American College of Cardiology Foundation. *Circulation.* 2007;115(12):1643–55.

Table 27.4	Features of Marfan Syndrome on Physical Examination

Musculoskeletal

Tall stature

Thin body habitus (arm span to height ratio > 1.05)

Arachnodactyly (long thin fingers; able to wrap hand around opposite wrist and overlap thumb and small finger)

Pectus deformity

High arched palate

Kyphoscoliosis

Joint laxity

Cardiovascular

Systolic murmur (mitral valve prolapse)

Diastolic murmur (aortic regurgitation)

Ocular

Myopia

Retinal detachment

Lens subluxation

SOURCE: Adapted from De Paepe A, Devereux RB, Dietz HC, Hennekam RC, Pyeritz RE. Revised diagnostic criteria for the Marfan syndrome. *Am J Med Genet.* 1996;62(4):417–26.

syncope, exercise intolerance, exertional chest pain, dyspnea, or excessive fatigue.

■ Physical examination should specifically address blood pressure, heart rhythm, cardiac auscultation, and the physical stigmata associated with Marfan syndrome (10) (Table 27.4).

■ Cardiac auscultation should be performed in the supine and standing positions. The classic murmur of obstructive HCM increases with maneuvers that decrease venous return such as Valsalva or moving from squatting to standing. In contrast, the murmur of aortic stenosis intensifies with squatting and decreases with Valsalva (31).

■ Simultaneous radial and femoral artery pulses should be assessed to exclude coarctation of the aorta. Brachial blood pressure should be measured with the appropriately sized cuff in the sitting position, and in the pediatric population, normative values should be adjusted for age, gender, and height (29).

■ The use of ECG as a screening tool for conditions associated with sudden cardiac death continues to be the subject of much debate. An increasing number of governing bodies have endorsed the use of ECG screening for athletes, including the International Olympic Committee, European Society for Sports Medicine, Fédération Internationale de Football (FIFA), and all of the major U.S. professional sports leagues. However, concerns remain as to the feasibility of widespread ECG screening in younger or amateur populations (11). The normal adaptations of the "athletic heart" can make interpretation of ECG and echocardiogram problematic (37). False-positive rates, high relative costs, limited availability, and low prevalence of disease have all been cited as concerns for using ECG as a broad-based screening tool (25).

■ However, the prevalence of occult cardiac conditions at risk for sudden death in young athletes is higher than once thought, and consistently 0.2%–0.7% in studies using ECG (1). In addition, integrated programs using ECG offer the only screening model shown to reliably identify athletes at risk for sudden cardiac death and the only evidence that such a program can reduce the rate of sudden death in athletes. Concern about excessively high abnormal results does not reflect more contemporary standards of ECG interpretation. Advancements in physician education and improvements to our health system infrastructure are needed as ECG screening becomes more available.

■ Exercise testing may be advisable prior to beginning an exercise program in older athletes with risk factors for coronary artery disease. See Chapters 12 (Exercise Prescription) and 21 (Exercise Testing) for further discussion and recommendations.

■ Many conditions that cause sudden death in young athletes are familial (HCM—autosomal dominant defect in sarcomere formation; long QT syndrome—autosomal dominant sodium channel defect; Marfan syndrome—autosomal dominant mutation of *FBN1* fibrillin gene; Brugada syndrome—autosomal dominant SCN5A channelopathy; ARVC—autosomal dominant defect). Although genetic testing is not routinely recommended for screening, it may be helpful in the evaluation of

athletes or family members when a relative is identified with an inheritable cardiac disease.

SYNCOPE AND EXERCISE-ASSOCIATED COLLAPSE

■ Syncope is defined as a sudden loss of consciousness for a brief duration, in the absence of head trauma. Syncope occurs secondary to a sudden drop in cerebral blood flow or metabolic change (*e.g.*, hypoglycemia or hypoxemia). Athletes who present with a history of exercise-related syncope (ERS) require a careful history and physical to differentiate benign from life-threatening etiologies (17,32) (Table 27.5).

■ Exercise-associated collapse (EAC) refers to athletes who are unable to stand or walk unaided after exertion because of weakness, lightheadedness, faintness, or dizziness (42).

■ Although ERS and EAC are not mutually exclusive, they demonstrate the spectrum of adverse events that can occur in the context of exercise. The history in each case becomes critical in the appropriate evaluation and treatment. The occurrence of collapse or syncope *during* exertion is an ominous sign of potential underlying pathology, whereas events occurring immediately *after* stopping exertion are more often associated with benign etiology (7).

Table 27.5	**Clinical Clues to Common Etiologies Presenting with Exertional Syncope**		
Diagnosis	**Clinical Clues**	**ECG**	**Suggested Diagnostic Testing**
Neurocardiogenic syncope	Noxious stimulus, prolonged upright position	Normal	Exercise testing
Supraventricular tachyarrhythmias	Palpitations, response to carotid sinus pressure	Pre-excitation	Electrophysiologic study and definitive therapy
HCM	Grade III/VI systolic murmur, louder with Valsalva (when present)	Deep inverted T waves, Q waves, pseudoinfarction pattern, left ventricular hypertrophy with strain	Echocardiography with Doppler, consider cardiac MRI with gadolinium
Myocarditis	Prior upper respiratory tract infection, pneumonia, exertional fatigue, shortness of breath, recreational drug use	Simulating a myocardial infarction with ectopy	Viral studies, echocardiogram, drug screening
Aortic stenosis	Exertional syncope, grade III/VI harsh systolic crescendo-decrescendo murmur	Left ventricular hypertrophy	Echocardiography with Doppler
Mitral valve prolapse	"Thumping heart," Midsystolic click with or without a murmur	Normal	Echocardiography with Doppler
Prolonged QT syndrome	Recurrent syncope with family history of sudden death	Prolonged corrected QT interval (> 0.47 males, > 0.48 females)	Family history; exercise stress test with ECG after exercise
Coronary anomalies	Syncope, exertional chest pain	Normal resting ECG	Cardiac MRI or CT angiography
Acquired coronary artery diseases	Acute coronary syndrome (chest pain), family history	Ischemia, may be normal	Exercise testing with or without perfusion or contractile imaging
ARVC	Syncope, tachyarrhythmias	T wave inversion V1-V3 PVCs with LBBB configuration	Echocardiography with Doppler study, cardiac MRI

ARVC, arrhythmogenic right ventricular cardiomyopathy; CT, computed tomography; ECG, electrocardiogram; HCM, hypertrophic cardiomyopathy; LBBB, left bundle branch block; MRI, magnetic resonance imaging; PVC, premature ventricular contraction.
SOURCE: Adapted from Giese EA, O'Connor FG, Brennan FH, Depenbrock PJ, Oriscello RG. The athletic preparticipation evaluation: cardiovascular assessment. *Am Fam Physician.* 2007;75(7):1008–14.

- The presence of prodromal symptoms may help to identify specific conditions. Careful attention should be paid to any history of palpitations (arrhythmia), chest pain (ischemia or aortic dissection), nausea (ischemia or vagal activity), wheezing, or pruritus (anaphylaxis). Patients who suffer vasovagal reflex syncope often experience brief prodromal symptoms such as lightheadedness, tunnel vision, diaphoresis, and nausea. In contrast, abrupt syncope is concerning for a ventricular arrhythmia.

- A detailed physical examination should include a careful assessment of orthostatic vital signs, precordial auscultation attentive to the murmurs of HCM and aortic stenosis, and a careful search for any morphologic features of Marfan syndrome. An ECG should be obtained in all cases and should be evaluated closely for conditions that predispose to sudden death. This includes careful ECG assessment of rate, rhythm, QT interval,

repolarization abnormalities (T wave inversion, ST depression), left or right ventricular hypertrophy, preexcitation pattern, and complications of ischemic heart disease (Q waves) (5).

- Initial blood test and additional ancillary evaluation should be directed by clinical suspicion based on the history and physical. In cases where no clear noncardiac cause is identified, it is recommended that an echocardiogram and stress testing be completed.

- Advanced cardiac imaging, including cardiac MRI and coronary CT angiography, may be advisable in cases of suspected cardiac etiology when the preceding evaluation has been nondiagnostic (40). These advanced imaging modalities provide detailed morphologic assessments to further evaluate for cardiomyopathy or coronary artery anomalies.

- Figure 27.1 provides a suggested algorithm for the primary care evaluation of exertional syncope in the athlete (32).

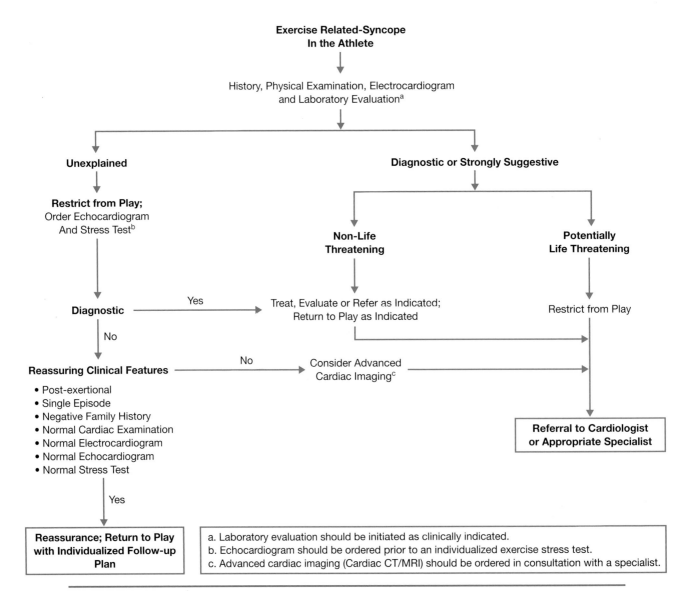

Figure 27.1: Algorithm for the evaluation of exercise-related syncope in the athlete. Reproduced with permission from O'Connor FG, Levine BD, Childress MA, Asplundh CA, Oriscello RG. Practical management: a systematic approach to the evaluation of exercise-related syncope in athletes. *Clin J Sport Med.* 2009;19(5):429–34.

HYPERTENSION IN ATHLETES

- Systemic hypertension remains one of the most common cardiovascular disorders in the United States and affects athletes of all ages and sports. The diagnosis, workup, and initial nonpharmacologic approach to treatment does not differ between athletes and nonathletes. This approach is consistent with current recommendations. (Joint National Committee on Prevention, Detection, Evaluation, and Treatment of High Blood Pressure, 2003) (6).

- Care must be taken not to overdiagnose the condition in young athletes and to use proper fitting cuffs with three different measures on 3 different days, adjusting for norms for age, gender, and height (20) (Table 27.6).

- Updated blood pressure tables are published by the National Heart, Lung, and Blood Institute (http://www.nhlbi.nih.gov/guidelines/hypertension/child_tbl.htm).

- An appropriate search for secondary etiologies and assessment for target end-organ damage should guide the history, physical, laboratory evaluation, and ancillary testing.

- History should inquire about substances that may affect blood pressure (*e.g.*, nonsteroidal anti-inflammatory drugs [NSAIDs], stimulants, anabolic steroids), and testing should include ECG, urinalysis, complete blood count (CBC), electrolytes, fasting glucose, lipid profile, blood urea nitrogen (BUN), and creatinine (19). All athletes with stage 1 or 2 hypertension should have an echocardiogram evaluating for target organ disease. An echocardiogram should also be considered in athletes with abnormal ECG findings (16).

- Nonpharmacologic treatment should be initiated, including engagement in moderate physical activity, maintenance of ideal body weight, limitation of alcohol, reduction in sodium intake, maintenance of adequate potassium intake, and consumption of a diet high in fruits and vegetables and low in total and saturated fat (16,30,33).

- When indicated, pharmacologic treatment should be initiated. Generally, angiotensin-converting enzyme (ACE) inhibitors, calcium channel blockers, and angiotensin-II receptor blockers are excellent choices for athletes with hypertension. Their low side effect profile and favorable physiologic hemodynamics make them generally safe and effective. It is preferable to avoid diuretics and β-blockers in young athletes. Volume and potassium balance issues limit diuretic use, and β-blockers adversely impact maximum cardiovascular performance (16,30,33). Additional care must be taken in prescribing antihypertensives in elite athletes because some may be prohibited by sport governing bodies, including the NCAA, International Olympic Committee, and the World Anti-Doping Agency (http://www.wada-ama.org).

- Restriction of activity for athletes with hypertension depends on the degree of target organ damage and on the overall control of the blood pressure (16).

- The presence of mild to moderate hypertension (stage 1) without target organ damage or concomitant heart disease should not limit eligibility for competitive sports (27). Athletes with severe hypertension (stage 2) should be restricted, particularly from static sports, until their hypertension is controlled. When hypertension coexists with other cardiovascular diseases, eligibility for competitive sports is

Table 27.6	**Classification of Hypertension in Children and Adolescents, With Measurement Frequency and Therapy Recommendations**			
	SBP or DBP Percentile*	**Frequency of BP Measurement**	**Therapeutic Lifestyle Changes**	**Pharmacologic Therapy**
Normal	< 90th	Recheck at next scheduled physical examination	Encourage healthy diet, sleep, and physical activity	—
Prehypertension	90th to < 95th or if BP exceeds 120/80 even if < 90th percentile up to < 95th percentile†	Recheck in 6 mo	Weight-management counseling if overweight; introduce physical activity and diet management‡	None unless compelling indications such as chronic kidney disease, diabetes mellitus, heart failure, or LVH exist
Stage 1 hypertension	95th–99th percentile plus 5 mm Hg	Recheck in 1–2 wk or sooner if the patient is symptomatic; if persistently elevated on 2 additional occasions, evaluate or refer to source of care within 1 mo	Weight-management counseling if overweight; introduce physical activity and diet management‡	Initiate therapy based on indications in Table 6 or if compelling indications (as shown above) exist
Stage 2 hypertension	> 99th percentile plus 5 mm Hg	Evaluate or refer to source of care within 1 wk or immediately if the patient is symptomatic	Weight-management counseling if overweight; introduce physical activity and diet management‡	Initiate therapy§

* For gender, age, and height measured on at least 3 separate occasions; if systolic and diastolic categories are different, categorize by the higher value.

† This occurs typically at 12 years old for SBP and at 16 years old for DBP.

‡ Parents and children trying to modify the eating plan to the Dietary Approaches to Stop Hypertension Study eating plan could benefit from consultation with a registered or licensed nutritionist to get them started.

§ More than 1 drug may be required

usually based on the severity of the other associated condition (16).

- In children and adolescents, the presence of severe hypertension (stage 2) or target organ disease warrants restriction until hypertension is under adequate control. The presence of mild to moderate hypertension (stage 1) should not limit a young athlete's eligibility for competitive athletics (29).

CORONARY ARTERY DISEASE IN ATHLETES

- Individuals diagnosed with coronary artery disease (CAD) require careful risk stratification prior to continuing or initiating exercise. Such an evaluation may require procedures for left ventricular assessment, maximal treadmill testing to determine functional capacity, and stress testing for inducible ischemia. Patients should be tested on their medications when possible.

- The 36th Bethesda Conference defines clear stratification criteria (Table 27.7) accompanied by activity recommenda-

---

Table 27.7 | Stratification Categories for Coronary Artery Disease Patients by the 36th Bethesda Conference

Mildly Increased Risk

- LVEF > 50%

- Normal exercise tolerance for age:
  - > 10 METS if age < 50
  - > 9 METS if age 50–59
  - > 8 METS if age 60–69
  - > 7 METS if age > 70

- Absence of exercise-induced ischemia and exercise-induced or postexercise complex ventricular arrhythmias

- Absence of hemodynamically significant stenosis (generally regarded as 50% or more luminal diameter narrowing) in any major coronary artery by coronary angiography

- Successful myocardial revascularization by surgical or percutaneous techniques if such revascularization was performed

Substantially Increased Risk

- Impaired LV systolic function at rest (EF < 50%)

- Evidence of exercise-induced myocardial ischemia or complex ventricular arrhythmias

- Hemodynamically significant stenosis (generally regarded as 50% or more luminal diameter narrowing) of a major coronary artery if coronary angiography was performed

EF, ejection fraction; LV, left ventricular; LVEF, left ventricular ejection fraction; MET, metabolic equivalent.
SOURCE: Adapted from Thompson PD, Balady GJ, Chaitman BR, Clark LT, Levine BD, Myerburg RJ. Task Force 6: coronary artery disease. *J Am Coll Cardiol*. 2005;45(8):1348–53.

Table 27.8 | Summary of 36th Bethesda Conference Recommendations for Patients With Coronary Artery Disease

- Athletes in the mildly increased risk group can participate in low dynamic and low/moderate static competitive sports, but should avoid intensely competitive situations. Selected athletes with mildly increased risk may be permitted to compete in sports of higher levels of intensity when their overall clinical profile suggests very low exercise risk.

- All athletes should understand that the risk of a cardiac event with exertion is probably increased once coronary atherosclerosis of any severity is present.

- Athletes with mildly increased risk engaging in competitive sports should undergo reevaluation of their risk stratification at least annually.

- Athletes in the substantially increased risk category should generally be restricted to low-intensity competitive sports.

- Athletes should be informed of the nature of prodromal symptoms (such as chest, arm, jaw, and shoulder discomfort, unusual dyspnea) and should be instructed to cease their sports activity promptly and to contact their physician if symptoms appear.

- Those with a recent MI or myocardial revascularization should cease their athletic training and competition until recovery is deemed complete.

- All athletes with atherosclerotic CAD should have their atherosclerotic risk factors aggressively treated as studies suggest that comprehensive risk reduction is likely to stabilize coronary lesions and may reduce the risk of exercise-related events.

CAD, coronary artery disease; MI, myocardial infarction.
SOURCE: Adapted from Thompson PD, Balady GJ, Chaitman BR, Clark LT, Levine BD, Myerburg RJ. Task Force 6: coronary artery disease. *J Am Coll Cardiol*. 2005;45(8):1348–53.

---

tions (Table 27.8) (44). This provides a general and conservative approach to the individual in regards to competitive sports.

ARRHYTHMIAS IN ATHLETES

- Lethal cardiac arrhythmias represent the most serious risk for sudden death in athletes. Symptoms of a potential ventricular arrhythmia may include syncope, near syncope, palpitations, exertional chest discomfort, severe dyspnea, or uncommon exertional fatigue.

- Structural heart disease must be ruled out before the athlete is allowed to return to sports (20,32,44,51).

- This will include a meticulous history, physical examination, and ECG, and in many circumstances, an echocardiogram, stress test, and possibly advanced cardiac imaging. These investigations should be pursued in conjunction with appropriate specialty consultation.

- Various supraventricular arrhythmias may be compatible with competitive sports once they are diagnosed and controlled. Task Force 7 of the 36th Bethesda Conference offers explicit details as to the recommended evaluations and allowed return-to-play recommendations for most encountered arrhythmias (51).

■ The Committee on Sports Medicine and Fitness for the American Academy of Pediatrics specifically recommends that the presence of a symptomatic dysrhythmia requires exclusion from physical activity until the athlete's problem can be adequately evaluated by a cardiologist and controlled (2).

REFERENCES

1. Asif I, Harmon K, Drezner J, Klossner D. Incidence and etiology of sudden death in NCAA athletes. *Clin J Sports Med*. 2010;20:136.
2. Berlin JA, Colditz GA. A meta-analysis of physical activity in the prevention of coronary heart disease. *Am J Epidemiol*. 1990;132(4):612–28.
3. Blair SN, Kohl HW 3rd, Barlow CE, Paffenbarger RS Jr, Gibbons LW, Macera CA. Changes in physical fitness and all-cause mortality. A prospective study of healthy and unhealthy men. *JAMA*. 1995;273(14):1093–8.
4. Cardiac dysrhythmias and sports. American Academy of Pediatrics Committee on Sports Medicine and Fitness. *Pediatrics*. 1995;95(5):786–8.
5. Childress MA, O'Connor FG, Levine BD. Exertional collapse in the runner: evaluation and management in fieldside and office-based settings. *Clin Sports Med*. 2010;29(3):459–76.
6. Chobanian AV, Bakris GL, Black HR, et al. The Seventh Report of the Joint National Committee on Prevention, Detection, Evaluation, and Treatment of High Blood Pressure: the JNC 7 report. *JAMA*. 2003;289(19):2560–72.
7. Colivicchi F, Ammirati F, Santini M. Epidemiology and prognostic implications of syncope in young competing athletes. *Eur Heart J*. 2004;25(19):1749–53.
8. Corrado D, Biffi A, Basso C, Pelliccia A, Thiene G. 12-Lead ECG in the athlete: physiological versus pathological abnormalities. *Br J Sports Med*. 2009;43(9):669–76.
9. Corrado D, Pelliccia A, Heidbuchel H, et al. Recommendations for interpretation of 12-lead electrocardiogram in the athlete. *Eur Heart J*. 2010; 31(2):243–59.
10. De Paepe A, Devereux RB, Dietz HC, Hennekam RC, Pyeritz RE. Revised diagnostic criteria for the Marfan syndrome. *Am J Med Genet*. 1996;62(4):417–26.
11. Drezner J, Berger S, Campbell R. Current controversies in the cardiovascular screening of athletes. *Curr Sports Med Rep*. 2010;9(2):86–92.
12. Firoozi S, Sharma S, Hamid MS, McKenna WJ. Sudden death in young athletes: HCM or ARVC? *Cardiovasc Drugs Ther*. 2002;16(1):11–7.
13. Giese EA, O'Connor FG, Brennan FH, Depenbrock PJ, Oriscello RG. The athletic preparticipation evaluation: cardiovascular assessment. *Am Fam Physician*. 2007;75(7):1008–14.
14. Holly RG, Shaffrath JD, Amsterdam EA. Electrocardiographic alterations associated with the hearts of athletes. *Sports Med*. 1998;25(3):139–48.
15. Huston TP, Puffer JC, Rodney WM. The athletic heart syndrome. *N Engl J Med*. 1985;313(1):24–32.
16. Kaplan NM, Gidding SS, Pickering TG, Wright JT Jr. Task Force 5: systemic hypertension. *J Am Coll Cardiol*. 2005;45(8):1346–8.
17. Kapoor WN. Syncope. *N Engl J Med*. 2000;343(25):1856–62.
18. Kohl HW 3rd, Powell KE, Gordon NF, Blair SN, Paffenbarger RS Jr. Physical activity, physical fitness, and sudden cardiac death. *Epidemiol Rev*. 1992;14(1):37–58.
19. Leddy JJ, Izzo J. Hypertension in athletes. *J Clin Hypertens (Greenwich)*. 2009;11(4):226–33.
20. Luckstead EF Sr. Cardiac risk factors and participation guidelines for youth sports. *Pediatr Clin North Am*. 2002;49(4):681–707, v.

21. Maron BJ. Distinguishing hypertrophic cardiomyopathy from athlete's heart physiological remodelling: clinical significance, diagnostic strategies and implications for preparticipation screening. *Br J Sports Med*. 2009;43(9):649–56.
22. Maron BJ. The paradox of exercise. *N Engl J Med*. 2000;343(19):1409–11.
23. Maron BJ, Doerer JJ, Haas TS, Tierney DM, Mueller FO. Sudden deaths in young competitive athletes: analysis of 1866 deaths in the United States, 1980–2006. *Circulation*. 2009;119(8):1085–92.
24. Maron BJ, Poliac LC, Roberts WO. Risk for sudden cardiac death associated with marathon running. *J Am Coll Cardiol*. 1996;28(2):428–31.
25. Maron BJ, Thompson PD, Ackerman MJ, et al. Recommendations and considerations related to preparticipation screening for cardiovascular abnormalities in competitive athletes: 2007 update: a scientific statement from the American Heart Association Council on Nutrition, Physical Activity, and Metabolism: endorsed by the American College of Cardiology Foundation. *Circulation*. 2007;115(12):1643–55.
26. Maron BJ, Thompson PD, Puffer JC, et al. Cardiovascular preparticipation screening of competitive athletes. A statement for health professionals from the Sudden Death Committee (clinical cardiology) and Congenital Cardiac Defects Committee (cardiovascular disease in the young), American Heart Association. *Circulation*. 1996;94(4):850–6.
27. Maron BJ, Zipes DP. Introduction: eligibility recommendations for competitive athletes with cardiovascular abnormalities-general considerations. *J Am Coll Cardiol*. 2005;45(8):1318–21.
28. Mukerji B, Alpert MA, Mukerji V. Cardiovascular changes in athletes. *Am Fam Physician*. 1989;40(3):169–75.
29. National High Blood Pressure Education Program Working Group on High Blood Pressure in Children and Adolescents. The fourth report on the diagnosis, evaluation, and treatment of high blood pressure in children and adolescents. *Pediatrics*. 2004;114(2 Suppl 4th Report):555–76.
30. Niedfeldt MW. Managing hypertension in athletes and physically active patients. *Am Fam Physician*. 2002;66(3):445–52.
31. O'Connor FG, Kugler JP, Oriscello RG. Sudden death in young athletes: screening for the needle in a haystack. *Am Fam Physician*. 1998;57(11): 2763–70.
32. O'Connor FG, Levine BD, Childress MA, Asplundh CA, Oriscello RG. Practical management: a systematic approach to the evaluation of exercise-related syncope in athletes. *Clin J Sport Med*. 2009;19(5):429–34.
33. O'Connor FG, Meyering CD, Patel R, Oriscello RP. Hypertension, athletes, and the sports physician: implications of JNC VII, the Fourth Report, and the 36th Bethesda Conference Guidelines. *Curr Sports Med Rep*. 2007;6(2):80–4.
34. Paffenbarger RS Jr, Hyde RT, Wing AL, Lee IM, Jung DL, Kampert JB. The association of changes in physical-activity level and other lifestyle characteristics with mortality among men. *N Engl J Med*. 1993;328(8): 538–45.
35. Papadakis M, Sharma S. Electrocardiographic screening in athletes: the time is now for universal screening. *Br J Sports Med*. 2009;43(9): 663–8.
36. Pate RR, Pratt M, Blair SN, et al. Physical activity and public health. A recommendation from the Centers for Disease Control and Prevention and the American College of Sports Medicine. *JAMA*. 1995;273(5):402–7.
37. Pelliccia A, Maron BJ, Culasso F, et al. Clinical significance of abnormal electrocardiographic patterns in trained athletes. *Circulation*. 2000; 102(3):278–84.
38. Pelliccia A, Maron BJ, De Luca R, Di Paolo FM, Spataro A, Culasso F. Remodeling of left ventricular hypertrophy in elite athletes after long-term deconditioning. *Circulation*. 2002;105(8):944–9.
39. Pluim BM, Zwinderman AH, van der Laarse A, van der Wall EE. The athlete's heart. A meta-analysis of cardiac structure and function. *Circulation*. 2000;101(3):336–44.

40. Prakken NH, Cramer MJ, Olimulder MA, Agostoni P, Mali WP, Velthuis BK. Screening for proximal coronary artery anomalies with 3-dimensional MR coronary angiography. *Int J Cardiovasc Imaging.* 2010;26(6):701–10.

41. Richardson CR, Kriska AM, Lantz PM, Hayward RA. Physical activity and mortality across cardiovascular disease risk groups. *Med Sci Sports Exerc.* 2004;36(11):1923–9.

42. Roberts WO. Exercise-associated collapse care matrix in the marathon. *Sports Med.* 2007;37(4–5):431–3.

43. Siscovick DS, Weiss NS, Fletcher RH, Lasky T. The incidence of primary cardiac arrest during vigorous exercise. *N Engl J Med.* 1984;311(14):874–7.

44. Thompson PD, Balady GJ, Chaitman BR, Clark LT, Levine BD, Myerburg RJ. Task Force 6: coronary artery disease. *J Am Coll Cardiol.* 2005;45(8): 1348–53.

45. Thompson PD, Franklin BA, Balady GJ, et al. Exercise and acute cardiovascular events placing the risks into perspective: a scientific statement from the American Heart Association Council on Nutrition, Physical Activity, and Metabolism and the Council on Clinical Cardiology. *Circulation.* 2007;115(17):2358–68.

46. Thompson PD, Levine BD. Protecting athletes from sudden cardiac death. *JAMA.* 2006;296(13):1648–50.

47. Villeneuve PJ, Morrison HI, Craig CL, Schaubel DE. Physical activity, physical fitness, and risk of dying. *Epidemiology.* 1998;9(6):626–31.

48. Warren TY, Barry V, Hooker SP, Sui X, Church TS, Blair SN. Sedentary behaviors increase risk of cardiovascular disease mortality in men. *Med Sci Sports Exerc.* 2010;42(5):879–85.

49. Wei M, Kampert JB, Barlow CE, et al. Relationship between low cardio-respiratory fitness and mortality in normal-weight, overweight, and obese men. *JAMA.* 1999;282(16):1547–53.

50. Williams PT. Relationships of heart disease risk factors to exercise quantity and intensity. *Arch Intern Med.* 1998;158(3):237–45.

51. Zipes DP, Ackerman MJ, Estes NA 3rd, Grant AO, Myerburg RJ, Van Hare G. Task Force 7: arrhythmias. *J Am Coll Cardiol.* 2005;45(8): 1354–63.

Dermatology

Mark D. Jeffords and Kenneth B. Batts

28

- Skin serves as a protective barrier against mechanical, environmental, and infective forces.
- Sport-specific dermatoses may incapacitate or disqualify an athlete or expose a teammate to a potential infection, placing him or her at risk for disqualification or impaired performance.

MECHANICAL INJURY

Abrasions

- Commonly known as *rug burn*, *strawberry*, or *road rash*, abrasion may occur on any surface, but primarily artificial turf, floor mats, synthetic courts, and asphalt roads.
- Treatment consists of cleaning and debriding the tissue with warm, soapy water and applying a topical antibacterial ointment.
- Topical anesthesia facilitates easier exploration and debridement and may be achieved with 2% lidocaine jelly or one of several commercially available anesthetics (lidocaine, epinephrine, tetracaine [LET]; eutectic mixture of local anesthetics [EMLA]; Ela-Max) (23).
- A thin covering of antibacterial ointment (mupirocin) or an adhesive hydrocolloid dressing (DuoDERM, OpSite) promotes healing (23).
- Because of the risk of bloodborne pathogens and subsequent disease transmission, all wounds should be covered with an occlusive dressing during participation.
- National Collegiate Athletic Association (NCAA) mandates that an athlete with active bleeding must be removed from competition, the bleeding stopped, and a dressing applied to withstand the rigors of competition prior to continued participation (8).

Acne Mechanica

- An occlusive obstruction of the follicular pilosebaceous units.
- The pustular eruption commonly occurs in a warm, moist environment occluded by protective equipment across the back and shoulders or on the chin (15).
- Wearing sweat-wicking underclothing, good personal hygiene, and regular cleaning of equipment help prevent outbreaks of lesions.

- Acne mechanica in dark-skinned athletes may evolve into acne keloidalis on the nape of the neck (36).
- The condition can be treated with various topical keratolytics with astringents (3% salicylic acid, 70% resorcinol) and antibiotics (tetracycline, clindamycin) (3).
- Athletes should be clearly informed of side effects including muscle soreness, joint pain, and lethargy prior to the use of isotretinoin for severe pustular acne (3).

Athletic Nodules

- Fibrotic connective tissue (collagenomas) formed as a result of repetitive pressure, friction, or trauma over bony prominences.
- Commonly located on knuckles (boxers, football players), tibial tuberosity (surfers), or dorsal feet (hockey "skate bites," runners, hikers) (36).
- Treatment includes intralesional steroids, protective taping and padding, and excision (36).
- Resolve after the discontinuation of causal activity.

Black Heel

- Black heel, or talon noir, refers to bluish-black petechiae within the stratum corneum on the posterior or posterolateral aspect of the heel caused by shearing forces between epidermis and dermis.
- Commonly occurs in basketball, tennis, track, and similar events requiring sudden changes in direction.
- A similar condition, black palm or tache noir, has been described in baseball players, golfers, gymnasts, mogul skiers, mountain climbers, and weightlifters (36).
- Self-limiting and will resolve spontaneously once the season ends.
- The use of heel cups, felt pads, cushioned athletic socks, and properly fitted footwear may help prevent black heel formation.

Black Toenail

- Rapid deceleration of the forefoot against the shoe toe box may produce painful subungual hemorrhages of the first and second toenail beds.
- The condition occurs with greater frequency in sports requiring quick stops, such as tennis, skiing, hiking, and rock climbing (36).

- The hematoma can be drained by carefully boring a hole through the nail with an 18-gauge needle or an electrocautery unit.
- Appropriate running shoes (2 cm from the longest toe to the end of the shoe), lacing shoes tightly enough to prevent the foot from sliding forward, and properly trimming the distal nail to its shortest length in a straight cut line will reduce the likelihood of developing this condition (31).
- Notable exceptions are the persistence of a linear black band or streak running the entire length of the nail representing a melanocytic nevus or the more serious involvement of the proximal nail fold as in malignant melanoma (2).

Blisters

- Vesicles or bullae filled with serosanguinous fluid or blood.
- Repeated pressure or friction over bony prominences associated with excessive perspiration and improperly fitted equipment leads to the formation of blisters.
- Treat early blisters with moleskin donuts and nylon foot stockings to decrease friction, talcum powder or antiperspirant to keep feet dry, and benzoin to harden the epidermis (15,30).
- Bullous blisters should be drained at the edge with a small needle leaving the roof of the blister as a protective layer.
- Ruptured and deroofed blisters may require the application of a hydrocolloidal dressing (DuoDERM) or an adhesive polyurethane dressing (OpSite) as a second-skin layer to reduce discomfort and enhance healing (5).
- Primary prevention includes wearing properly fitted and broken-in footwear, use of absorbent socks or two pairs of socks of different materials, and applying petrolatum jelly or commercial antichafing preparations (Bodyglide) over bony prominences (21).

Corns and Calluses

- Corns are small, soft or hard, deep painful conical lesions with a translucent central core in the web spaces of the toes and the plantar surface over the distal heads of the metatarsals (36).
- Calluses tend to be larger, hyperkeratotic, nonpainful lesions that serve as a protective skin layer and are considered an advantage in gymnastics, racquet sports, and rowing.
- The development of small black dots representing thrombosed capillaries implies the presence of plantar warts, compared to calluses that display a thickened epidermis with intact dermatoglyphics.
- The most important factor for successful recovery and prevention of the condition is redistributing pressure away from the lesion.
- The shaping of a metatarsal pad to the plantar surface, creating a wider shoe toe box, adding cotton or foam padding between the toes, and applying moleskin will all aid in decreasing the pressure over the existing lesion and prevent further injury.

- Keratolytic agents such as 5%–10% salicylic acid in colloid, 40% salicylic acid plaster, and 12% lactic acid will eliminate the lesions (26).

Follicular Keloiditis

- An inflammatory proliferation of fibrous tissue that is usually painless and is more prevalent in dark-skinned athletes.
- Multiple, small keloids commonly develop where the headgear comes in contact with the forehead, cheeks, and posterior neck or where the undergarment pads cover the thighs, knees, and shoulders.
- Treatment involves gradual reduction of the lesion with intralesional steroid injections or topical application of a steroid-impregnated adhesive tape (46).

Ingrown Toenail

- This condition is caused by nail bed pressure forcing the lateral edge of the nail plate into the lateral nail fold.
- The distal nail should be trimmed straight across, and at least one thumbnail in distance should exist from the longest distal toenail to the end of the shoe to prevent recurrence.
- Acute treatment options include soaks in an Epsom salt or soapy water bath followed by application of topical antibiotic or a mid- to high-potency topical steroid, gentle manual nail elevation, placing a small piece of cotton or dental floss under the corner of the nail to elevate the lateral margin, use of antibiotics, and excision of the lateral one-third of the nail with electrodesication or chemical matricectomy with 80%–88% phenol (10,20).

Jogger's Nipples

- Irritation and friction from coarse, cotton fabrics on an unprotected nipple and areola leading to pain and bleeding.
- The majority of jogger's nipples occur in male athletes, especially long-distance runners and triathletes (3).
- Preventive measures include wearing of soft, natural, silk fiber shirts or no shirt or application of breast padding, electrocardiographic lead pads, band-aids, or a double coat of fingernail polish over the nipples prior to running to prevent chafing.
- Treat by washing and gently drying and applying petroleum jelly, antibiotic ointment, or topical steroid cream to alleviate inflammation (31).

Piezogenic Papules

- Flesh-colored papules noticeable only on weight-bearing are found in up to 20% of the general population.
- Herniations of subdermal fat into the dermis visibly evident on either side of the heel.
- Typically asymptomatic, but may become painful, possibly due to herniation of nerve fibers with subdermal fat (38).

- More common in endurance athletes.
- Padding, compression stockings, taping for support, heel cups, and steroid injections may help reduce the pain (38).

Rower's Rump

- Rower's rump develops in the gluteal cleft of rowers training on small, unpadded scull seats and metal rowing machines (42).
- Repeated friction produces a lichen simplex chronicus of the buttocks.
- Treatment consists of padding the rowing seat and the use of potent, fluorinated topical steroids.

Runner's Rump

- A collection of ecchymotic lesions on the superior portion of the gluteal cleft of long-distance runners (3,31).
- Results from constant friction between the gluteal folds with each running stride.
- The hyperpigmentation will spontaneously resolve with rest.

ENVIRONMENTAL INJURY

Sun and Heat

Sunburn

- Prolonged exposure to ultraviolet B (UVB) (290–320 nm) may burn skin, producing symptoms ranging from mild erythema to intense blistering, edema, and pain.
- Ultraviolet A (UVA) (320–400 nm) is 1,000-fold less burning to the skin than UVB but is more penetrating and produces chronic damage.
- Ultraviolet exposure increases with altitude and with reflection off snow or water (23).
- Preventive measures include avoiding exercise between 10 a.m. and 2 p.m., applying sun protective factor (SPF) 15 or greater sunscreens with para-aminobenzoic acid (PABA) at least 20 minutes prior to sun exposure, and recoating after water exposure or sweating (23,40).

Miliaria

- Miliaria rubra, or prickly heat, occurs in hot, humid summer environments.
- Fine, pruritic, erythematous, vesiculopapular rash develops over eccrine sweat glands occluded by clothing (spares the palms and soles).
- Cooling and drying the skin to stop further sweating and application of hydrophilic ointments (Eucerin) and mild topical corticosteroids can open the occluded ducts (5,41).

Solar Urticaria

- Solar urticaria is an uncommon cause of urticaria in athletes.
- Manifested by itching and burning of the skin within minutes after exposure to UVA, UVB, or both wavelengths (17).

- Erythema and wheal formation will follow and clear within 2 hours after exposure (17,36).
- Normally unexposed skin areas of the trunk will be more prone to develop a urticarial reaction than the regularly exposed face or distal extremities.
- Phototesting is recommended to determine the type and treatment of solar urticaria.
- Desensitization by sunlight and a combination of oral psoralen and long-wave ultraviolet light (PUVA) has been shown to decrease symptoms (17).
- Treatment includes sunlight avoidance, sunscreen or zinc lotion, high-dose antihistamines, cyclosporine, chloroquine, and intravenous immunoglobulin (17).

Cholinergic Urticaria

- Pruritic dermatosis occurring during exercise, heat, emotional stress, or eating spicy foods believed to be mediated by increased sympathetic tone and acetylcholine activity (13).
- Most commonly affects trunk and extremities, sparing face and neck.
- The condition is characterized by the eruption of pinpoint papular wheals with a surrounding subcutaneous erythematous flare during and after heat exposure or exercise.
- Provocative testing with exercise under controlled circumstances is the safest and surest means to reproduce symptoms. Full resuscitative measures should be available because exercise-induced anaphylaxis may be included in the differential diagnosis (13).
- Treatment with H_1 antihistamines (hydroxyzine and cetirizine) and danazol has been found to be effective if taken 1 hour prior to exercise (13).
- Danazol should be avoided or used with caution in females because it is a strong androgenizing agent.
- Propranolol may be effective in refractory cases (13).
- A hot shower the night prior may deplete histamine and provide a refractory period for the athlete to compete (19).
- The condition can be exacerbated with the use of aspirin (19).

Cold

Chilblain

- Chilblain or pernio is the result of repeated or prolonged exposure to cold, but not freezing, temperatures in moist conditions (11).
- Athletes may initially be asymptomatic, but later complain of reddish-blue patches that are pruritic, painful, and tender and then lead to blisters or ulcerations (18).
- Injury is due to hypoxia from local vasoconstriction occurring primarily on the feet, hands, and face, particularly in young, white females (47).
- The area should be rewarmed and protected from further environmental exposure; rubbing or massaging is contraindicated as this may further damage the injured tissue (25).

- Topical corticosteroids or a short burst of oral corticosteroids may be used to minimize the painful, inflammatory skin lesions.
- Insulated and water-resistant outer clothing, moisture-wicking socks and gloves, frequent sock and glove changes, and protective covering over the face aid in preventing this injury.

Frostnip

- Frostnip is the most common of cold injuries and involves only the superficial skin.
- The skin and superficial subcutaneous tissue of the fingertips, toes, nose, cheeks, and ears become pallid and painful, develop paresthesias, and finally lose sensation.
- Penile frostnip has been reported in joggers wearing polyester trousers and cotton undershorts (11).
- Frostnip is completely reversed with rewarming of the affected area, but it is possible for paresthesia to persist for several weeks after the injury (11).
- Prevention includes insulation and skin protection from both wind and cold, not shaving prior to participation to preserve the natural skin oils, and application of a sunscreen or petrolatum-based emollient (11).

Frostbite

- Frostbite occurs when tissue temperature falls below 28°F (−2°C) and intra- and extracellular fluid sludges and then crystallizes, mechanically disrupting cell membranes (18).
- The tissue appears cold, white, and hard and will not exhibit pain or sensation to tactile stimulation until thawing occurs.
- Initial management is immobilization and evacuation. Rewarming should not be attempted until the risk of refreezing is eliminated because further freeze–thaw cycles greatly increase tissue damage.
- Once hypothermia has been ruled out or treated, affected areas should be rapidly warmed in a circulating water bath at 104–108°F (40–42°C) avoiding rubbing, which increases tissue damage and loss (25).
- Thawing is often intensely painful, and narcotic pain medication may be employed. Consideration should also be given to administration of tetanus toxoid and antibiotic therapy (18).
- Surgical therapy is often delayed up to 2–3 months until dry gangrene or mummification clearly demarcates nonviable tissue (25).

Cold Urticaria

- Cold urticaria is characterized by pruritic wheals or hives in response to exposure to cold weather or objects and flare after the area is rewarmed (11).
- Urticarial plaques are usually confined to the exposed area, but may be generalized.
- Provocative testing of the forearm with ice cubes for 5 minutes will produce wheals upon warming the skin and confirm the diagnosis (36).
- Symptoms will likely recur, so exposure avoidance is recommended.

- The prophylactic use of nonsedating antihistamines such as cyproheptadine (Periactin), 2 mg once or twice a day, or doxepin (Sinequan), 10 mg two or three times daily, has been useful in preventing recurrence (29).

INFECTIOUS INJURY

- Skin infections account for 1%–2% of time loss injuries in all sports and up to 20% of time loss injuries in wrestling.
- Prevention is important and is possible through athlete self-reporting, preparticipation examinations, personal and equipment hygiene, hand sanitization, avoidance of sharing toiletries or towels, and prompt treatment and isolation of infected individuals (48).

Bacterial

Impetigo

- Serosanguinous, honey-crusted pustules on an erythematous base.
- *β-Hemolytic streptococci* more commonly produce impetigo, but staphylococcal species have been isolated from cultured wounds.
- Very contagious and common among contact sports, although cases and outbreaks are documented among weightlifters, fencers, and cross-country runners (27).
- Recommended treatment includes both topical antibiotic (mupirocin twice daily) and a second-generation cephalosporin or penicillinase-resistant penicillin derivative for 10 days (1).
- The NCAA requires all wrestlers to be without new lesions for 48 hours before a meet, have completed 72 hours of antibiotic therapy, and have no moist or draining lesions prior to competition (8).

Furunculosis

- Erythematous, nodular abscesses found most commonly in the hairy areas of the axillae, buttocks, and groin.
- Highly contagious, so routine screening, prompt treatment, and event disqualification of infected players can prevent outbreaks (1).
- Staphylococci are the most frequent bacteria isolated, but all wounds should be cultured to guide therapy because methicillin-resistant *Staphylococcus aureus* (MRSA) is common (48).
- Acute treatment consists of warm compresses and a 10-day course of a cephalosporin, erythromycin, or penicillinase-resistant penicillin derivative (1).
- Topical mupirocin may be used to eradicate nasal carriage of *Staphylococcus* species among team members if an outbreak occurs (1).
- Incision and drainage are necessary because of the poor hematogenous antibiotic penetration.

- The NCAA guidelines for participation of wrestlers with bacterial infections are described in the previous section on impetigo (8).

Pitted Keratolysis

- A scalloped-bordered plaque with sculpted pits of variable depth forms on the weight-bearing plantar surfaces (heel and toes) and is often misdiagnosed as tinea pedis.
- Hyperhidrosis and gram-positive bacteria, most commonly *Corynebacterium* and *Micrococcus* species, found in the stratum corneum have been implicated in producing the pungent foot odor (1).
- Application of topical antibiotics 2–4 weeks (5% erythromycin or 1% clindamycin in 10% benzoyl peroxide) will reduce the bacterial inflammatory component and result in clearing (43).
- Prophylactic therapy includes washing with benzoyl peroxide soap and adding topical foot powders with 20% aluminum chloride (Drysol) to control hyperhidrosis (43).

Erythrasma

- Chronic, bacterial infection affecting the intertriginous areas.
- The causative organism is a gram-positive rod, *Corynebacterium minutissimum.*
- The sharply demarcated reddish-brown plaques are similar in appearance to tinea cruris, but diagnosis can be confirmed by examination with a Wood's lamp, which reveals coral-red fluorescence (32).
- Treatment options include a topical erythromycin cream or gel and oral erythromycin 250 mg four times a day for 14 days.
- The areas should be covered for athletes to participate in close-contact drills or events.

MRSA

- Community-acquired MRSA (CA-MRSA) is an increasingly common condition affecting athletes.
- MRSA typically presents similar to other bacterial infections as furuncles, carbuncles, and abscesses and is sometimes mistaken as spider bites, and any of these presentations should be evaluated for possible CA-MRSA (27).
- Any suspicious lesion should be cultured to isolate the infective organism and determine susceptibilities.
- Prevention measures are identical to those general principles listed earlier with the addition of showering using antibacterial soap after every practice and game, as well as eliminating cosmetic body shaving because shaving has been demonstrated to increase rates of CA-MRSA (48).
- Definitive treatment of cutaneous lesions is incision and drainage.
- Antibiotic therapy must be guided by culture and sensitivity as well as local susceptibility information.
- Antibiotic regimens most often include oral clindamycin 300–450 mg three times daily or trimethoprim-sulfamethoxazole two double-strength tablets daily.

- MRSA infections can be severe, leading to hospitalization and requiring intravenous antibiotic therapy including vancomycin, clindamycin, or linezolid.

Viral

Verrucae

- The human papilloma virus induces warts, or verrucae vulgaris.
- Plantar warts disrupt the normal dermatoglyphics of the pressure points of the feet and often coalesce to form a gyrate or mosaic pattern.
- Small black dots representing thrombosed capillaries within a hyperkeratotic plaque confirm the diagnosis (31).
- The NCAA requires wrestlers to be able to cover multiple digitate verrucae of the face with a mask, and verrucae plana or vulgaris must be adequately covered to compete (8).
- Salicylic acid preparations or topical imiquimod can be applied with an occlusion wrap during the season (31).
- Liquid nitrogen cryotherapy can be used concurrently or alone every 2 weeks, but may delay return to training due to pain.

Molluscum Contagiosum

- Characterized by flesh-colored, dome-shaped papules with a central umbilication.
- The pox virus is highly contagious and spreads by direct skin transmission from person to person, autoinoculation, water transmission, and gymnasium equipment (37).
- The papules are typically self-limiting and resolve over weeks to months.
- NCAA wrestling rules require that lesions be removed by sharp curettage or liquid nitrogen and any solitary lesions be covered with a gas-permeable dressing (OpSite, Bioclusive) and tape in a manner that can withstand the rigors of competition (8).
- Liquid nitrogen, 0.7% cantharidin, topical tretinoin (Retin-A), electrodesication, and the use of imiquimod 5% cream have been successful but may require several treatments (37).

Herpes Gladiatorum

- Herpes gladiatorum or rugbeiorum refers to a herpes simplex virus (HSV-1) outbreak on the face or body of wrestlers or rugby players during "lock-up" or in a scrum.
- Classic lesions appear as a cluster of painful vesicles on an erythematous base, and diagnosis is made on clinical appearance, but may be confirmed by Tzanck smear or viral culture (12).
- The virus is passed by direct face-to-face or body-to-body transmission between athletes, and headgear does not decrease the risk of transmission (37).
- Antiviral therapies for acute outbreaks include acyclovir 800 mg twice daily, valacyclovir 500 mg twice daily, or famciclovir 125 mg twice daily for 5 days (37).
- Athletes with recurrent outbreaks may use suppressive therapy during the season, most commonly with valacyclovir 500–1,000 mg daily (37).

- In the pediatric population ages 2 to 18 years, the standard of care is acyclovir 1200 mg/day divided 3–5 times per day for 7–10 days.
- The NCAA allows a wrestler to participate if free of systemic symptoms, has not developed new lesions during the last 72 hours, all lesions have a firm adherent crust, and the wrestler has been on antiviral therapy for 120 hours (8).

Fungal

Tinea Pedis

- A papulosquamous fungal infection producing a pruritic, red, scaly rash on the lateral soles of the feet and between the toes.
- The superficial dermatophytic fungal infection is caused by *Trichophyton rubrum*, *Trichophyton mentagrophytes*, or *Epidermophyton floccusum* (9).
- The majority of cases respond promptly to topical antifungal creams, such as ketoconazole, clotrimazole, itraconazole, or terbinafine (48).

Tinea Corporis

- A dermatophyte infection producing an annular lesion with a sharply demarcated, red scaly border, and central clearing.
- Tinea corporis gladiatorum has been frequently isolated and reported in wrestlers on their head, neck, and upper arms (1).
- In the majority of cases, *Trichophyton tonsurans* is the causative fungus (48).
- Recent studies reveal that oral fluconazole, 100 mg taken once daily for 3 days prior to the season and once again 6 weeks later, decreased the incidence of tinea among wrestlers from 67.4% to 3.5% (7).
- The NCAA requires a minimum of 72 hours of topical therapy for skin lesions, a minimum of 2 weeks of oral therapy for scalp lesions, and all lesions to be adequately covered after evaluation and disposition by a team physician or certified athletic trainer (8).

Tinea Cruris

- An erythematous, pruritic plaque with well-demarcated, scaly borders that extends to the groin, upper thighs, abdomen, and perineum, but typically spares the genitalia (34).
- The appearance of an inflammatory, red rash with satellite lesions involving the scrotum is candidiasis and requires treatment with imidazole creams.
- Diagnosis can be confirmed by the presence of fungal hyphae on a potassium hydroxide slide.
- Topical antifungals are effective, and clotrimazole is the recommended firstline therapy (34).
- Addition of topical corticosteroid with topical antifungal may speed resolution of symptoms (33).
- Oral antifungal agents may be required in recalcitrant cases, if the hair roots are involved.
- Tinea cruris must be differentiated from candida intertrigo (scrotal involvement and satellite lesions), erythrasma

(coral-red fluorescence under Wood's lamp), or a chronic irritant dermatitis from elasticized undergarments (34).

Tinea Versicolor

- Also called pityriasis versicolor, overgrowth of the active fungal form of *Malassezia furfur* (also known as *Pityrosporum orbicular*) causes a chronic, asymptomatic, hyper- or hypopigmented, scaling, macular dermatosis (24).
- Wood's lamp reveals a characteristic yellow-green fluorescence (6).
- Treatment consists of washing the affected area with zinc pyrithione or selenium sulfide shampoo or with topical imidazole treatments such as ketoconazole or clotrimazole (24).
- In extensive or recurrent disease, oral ketoconazole 200 mg daily for 7–15 days or fluconazole 400 mg for one dose may be effective (6).
- The athlete needs to continue exercise and perspire for at least 1 hour after taking ketoconazole to promote absorption into the hair root (5).

Onychomycosis

- Onychomycosis is the most common disease of the nails and represents a fungal infection, with *Trichophyton rubrum*, *Trichophyton mentagrophytes*, or *Epidermophyton floccosum* being the causative organism in 90% of cases (45).
- Risk factors include repeated nail trauma, moist environment, occlusive footwear, genetic predisposition, poor circulation, concurrent diabetes, and immunosuppression.
- Multiple treatment regimens of oral and topical antifungal medications are described, but combination therapy has been shown to be most effective (45).
- Oral itraconazole 200 mg daily for 12 weeks with topical amorolfine 5% lacquer applied weekly for 6 months has been shown to have a 94% cure rate (45).
- Prescriber should review medication interactions because these are common among systemic antifungals.
- Baseline liver function tests must be performed, and laboratory monitoring for hepatotoxicity and pancytopenia should be considered during therapy.

MISCELLANEOUS

Contact Dermatitis

- Primary irritant dermatitis is a nonallergic reaction that leads to symptoms within minutes of the exposure. The dermatitis is localized to the contact site and exhibits erythema and a burning sensation. Common irritants are detergents and soaps, adhesive pretape sprays, sunscreens, and fiberglass (1).
- Allergic contact dermatitis is an acquired immune response that develops hours to days after recurrent exposure to an allergen. The dermatitis exhibits patches of erythema, edema, vesicle formation, and extreme pruritus. Equipment

with protective rubber coverings (golf clubs), black rubber seals (swim gear), tanned leather straps, latex products, iodine preparations, topical antibiotic ointments, adhesive tape, shoe dyes, and poison ivy or oak have all produced allergic reactions (28).

- Initial treatment includes avoidance and washing with water in an attempt to physically remove the irritant and prevent further systemic progression.

- Alternative equipment has been manufactured using polyurethane, neoprene, and silicone to alleviate allergic reactions.

- Antihistamines, corticosteroids, analgesics, and H₂ antagonists are commonly used for moderate to severe systemic hypersensitivity reactions by either oral or intravenous routes.

- Patch testing can often help identify the allergen triggering the dermatitis.

Envenomation

- Most allergic reactions are from hornets and wasps.

- Hymenoptera venom can be neutralized with meat tenderizer or shaving cream at the site.

- Antihistamines and nonsteroidal anti-inflammatory agents are commonly prescribed for allergic reactions to stings.

- Participants with known allergic reactions to hymenoptera should be advised to use sunscreens with insect repellent formulas.

- Athletic trainers or physicians covering events should always carry an injectable subcutaneous 1:1,000 epinephrine syringe (EpiPen kit).

- In the United States, 4,000–6,000 venomous snake bites occur yearly, and about 70% require antivenom (44).

- Initial treatment of venomous snake bite includes splinting the limb below the level of the heart, removing restrictive clothing from the extremity, and evacuating to a medical facility immediately (44).

- Contraindicated first aid techniques include arterial tourniquet, incision and suction, ice or cryotherapy, venom extractors, electric shock, and application of papain or meat tenderizer (44).

- Antivenom is the primary treatment for envenomations, but should only be given based on the severity of envenomation because antivenom also has a significant risk of causing an allergic reaction.

Swimmer's Itch

- A parasitic dermatitis produced by the cercarial form of freshwater schistosomes commonly found in freshwater lakes of the United States (1).

- One- or 2-mm macules develop into papules on exposed areas, not under the bathing suit.

- Self-limiting, but symptoms may be reduced with cold packs, antihistamines, and topical steroids (4).

Seabather's Eruption

- Pruritic papules and wheals with onset 2–24 hours after saltwater swimming and occurring in areas covered by a swimming suit, especially under the waistband or shoulder straps (4).

- Free-swimming, larval forms of *Edwardsiella lineata* and *Linuche unguiculata* containing stinging nematocysts are trapped in the swimming suit (16).

- Symptoms typically resolve within 3–7 days, but resolution may take as long as 6 weeks in severe cases (16).

- Oral antihistamines and topical corticosteroid are effective (4).

Green Hair

- Regular swimmers with natural or tinted blonde, gray, or white hair may develop a green tint to their hair from the release of copper from pipes or algicides in swimming pools (22,35).

- Immediately washing the hair and maintaining the pool pH between 7.4 and 7.6 will prevent this condition (36).

- Copper chelating shampoo applied for 30 minutes, hydrogen peroxide soak for 2–3 hours, and ethylenediaminetetraacetic acid (EDTA) conditioner once or twice per season have been effective in returning hair to original color (2).

Exercise-Induced Anaphylaxis

- Exercise-induced anaphylaxis (EIA) is a rare and unpredictable condition that typically occurs with a short duration of submaximal exercise and may occur in sedentary individuals or elite athletes (39).

- Pruritus with large wheals may progress to systemic symptoms of wheezing, nausea, diarrhea, angioedema, hypotension, and shock.

- Running has been found to be the most common exercise predisposed to EIA (1).

- Food-dependent exercise-induced anaphylaxis (FDEIA) is a subtype in which symptoms result only when a particular food is ingested prior to exercise and no symptoms occur with the food or exercise alone.

- FDEIA has been associated with many food allergens, with wheat being the most common (39).

- EIA is a clinical diagnosis, and it is important to differentiate it from more common triggers including foods, ingredients in sports drinks, and latex.

- Plasma histamine levels are elevated in all forms of EIA.

- Preventive measures include not exercising in extremes of either hot or cold weather and the use of nonsedating antihistamines 1 hour prior to exercise (14).

- Athletes who want to continue vigorous exercise should be instructed to exercise with someone (jogging partner) who has knowledge of their condition and can administer an injectable subcutaneous 1:1,000 epinephrine syringe (EpiPen kit).

REFERENCES

1. Adams BB. Dermatologic disorders of the athlete. *Sports Med.* 2002;32(5):309–21.

2. Adams BB, Kindred C. Common and uncommon hair and nail problems in sports. *Cutis.* 2005;75(5):269–75.

3. Basler RS. Skin injuries in sports medicine. *J Am Acad Dermatol.* 1989;21(6):1257–62.

4. Basler RS, Basler GC, Palmer AH, Garcia MA. Special skin symptoms seen in swimmers. *J Am Acad Dermatol.* 2000;43(2 Pt 1):299–305.

5. Bergfeld WF, Elston DM. Diagnosis and treatment of dermatologic problems in athletes. In: Fu FH, Stone DA, editors. *Sports Injuries: Mechanisms, Prevention, Treatment.* Baltimore: Williams & Wilkins; 1994. p. 781.

6. Bonifaz A, Gómez–Daza F, Paredes V, Ponce RM. Tinea versicolor, tinea nigra, white piedra, and black piedra. *Clin Dermatol.* 2010;28(2):140–5.

7. Brickam K, Einstein E, Sinha S, Ryno J, Guiness M. Fluconazole as a prophylactic measure for tinea gladiatorum in high school wrestlers. *Clin J Sport Med.* 2009;19(5):412–4.

8. Bubb RG. *2010 and 2011 NCAA Wrestling Rules and Interpretations.* Indianapolis (IN): The National Collegiate Athletic Association; 2009.

9. Buescher SE. Infections associated with pediatric sport participation. In: Luckstead EF, editor. *Pediatric Clinics of North America.* Philadelphia: Saunders; 2002. p. 743.

10. Daniel CR 3rd, Iorizzo M, Tosti A, Piraccini BM. Ingrown toenails. *Cutis.* 2006;78(6):407–8.

11. Englund SL, Adams BB. Winter sports dermatology: a review. *Cutis.* 2009;83(1):42–8.

12. Fatahzadeh M, Schwartz RA. Human herpes simplex virus infections: epidemiology, pathogenesis, symptomatology, diagnosis, and management. *Am Acad Dermatol.* 2007;57(5):737–63.

13. Feinberg JH, Toner CB. Successful treatment of disabling cholinergic urticaria. *Mil Med.* 2008;173(2):217–20.

14. Fisher AA. Sports related allergic dermatology. *Cutis.* 1992;50(2):95–7.

15. Freiman A, Barankin B, Elpern DJ. Sports dermatology part 1: common dermatoses. *CMAJ.* 2004;171(8):851–3.

16. Freiman A, Barankin B, Elpern DJ. Sports dermatology part 2: swimming and other aquatic sports. *CMAJ.* 2004;171(11):1339–41.

17. Gambichler T, Al-Muhammadi R, Boms S. Immunologically mediated photodermatoses diagnosis and treatment. *Am J Clin Dermatol.* 2009;10(3):169–80.

18. Golant A, Nord RM, Paksima N, Postner MA. Cold exposure injuries to the extremities. *J Am Acad Orthop Surg.* 2008;16(12):704–15.

19. Habif TP. *Clinical Dermatology: A Color Guide to Diagnosis and Therapy.* 3rd ed. St. Louis (MO): Mosby; 1996. Chap. 7.

20. Heidelbaugh JJ, Lee H. Management of the ingrown toenail. *Am Fam Physician.* 2009;79(4):303–8.

21. Heymann WR. Dermatologic problems of the endurance athlete. *J Am Acad Dermatol.* 2005;52(2):345–6.

22. Hinz T, Klingmüller K, Bieber T, Schmid-Wendtner MH. The mystery of green hair. *Eur J Dermatol.* 2009;19(4):409–10.

23. Honsik KA, Romeo MW, Hawley CJ, Romeo SJ, Romeo JP. Sideline skin and wound care for acute injuries. *Curr Sports Med Rep.* 2007;6(3):147–54.

24. Hu SW, Bigby M. Pityriasis versicolor: a systematic review of interventions. *Arch Dermatol.* 2010;146(10):1132–40.

25. Jurkovich GJ. Environmental cold–induced injury. *Surg Clin North Am.* 2007;87(1):247–67.

26. Kantor GR, Bergfeld WF. Common and uncommon dermatologic diseases related to sports activities. In: Pandolf KB, editor. *Exercise and Sport Sciences Reviews.* New York: Macmillan; 1988. Chap. 7.

27. Kirkland EB, Adams BB. Methicillin-resistant *Staphylococcus aureus* and athletes. *J Am Acad Dermatol.* 2008;59(3):494–502.

28. Kockentiet B, Adams BB. Contact dermatitis in athletes. *J Am Acad Dermatol.* 2007;56(6):1048–55.

29. Krause K, Zuberbier T, Maurer M. Modern approaches to the diagnosis and treatment of cold contact urticaria. *Curr Allergy Asthma Rep.* 2010;10(4):243–9.

30. Levine N. Dermatologic aspects of sports medicine. *J Am Acad Dermatol.* 1980;3(4):415–24.

31. Mailler-Savage EA, Adams BB. Skin manifestations of running. *J Am Acad Dermatol.* 2006;55(2):290–301.

32. Miller SD, David-Bajar K. A brilliant case of erythrasma. *N Engl J Med.* 2004;351(16):1666.

33. Onsun N, Pirmit S, Ummetoglu O. Successful therapy of tinea cruris with topical isoconazole in combination with a corticosteroid. *Mycoses.* 2008;51(Suppl. 4):27–8.

34. Patel GA, Wiederkehr M, Schwartz RA. Tinea cruris in children. *Cutis.* 2009;84(3):133–7.

35. Peterson J, Shook BA, Wells MJ, Rodriguez M. Cupric keratosis: green seborrheic keratoses secondary to external copper exposure. *Cutis.* 2006;77(1):39–41.

36. Pharis DB, Teller C, Wolf JE Jr. Cutaneous manifestations of sports participation. *J Am Acad Dermatol.* 1997;36(3 Pt 1):448–59.

37. Pleacher MD, Dexter WD. Cutaneous fungal and viral infections and athletes. *Clin Sports Med.* 2007;26(3):397–411.

38. Redboard KP, Adams BB. Piezogenic pedal papules in a marathon runner. *Clin J Sport Med.* 2006;16(1):81–3.

39. Robson-Ansley P, Toit GD. Pathophysiology, diagnosis and management of exercise-induced anaphylaxis. *Curr Opin Allergy Clin Immunol.* 2010;10(4):312–7.

40. Seité S, Fourtanier A, Moyal D, Young AR. Photodamage to human skin by suberythemal exposure to solar ultraviolet radiation can be attenuated by sunscreens: a review. *Br J Dermatol.* 2010;163(5):903–14.

41. Seto CK, Way D, O'Connor N. Environmental illness in athletes. *Clin Sports Med.* 2005;24(3):695–718.

42. Tomecki KJ, Mikesell JF. Rower's rump (letter to editor). *J Am Acad Dermatol.* 1987;16(4):890–1.

43. Vlahovic TC, Dunn SP, Kemp KK. The use of a clindamycin 1%-benzoyl peroxide 5% topical gel in the treatment of pitted keratolysis: a novel therapy. *Adv Skin Wound Care.* 2007;22(12):564–6.

44. Weinstein SA, Dart RC, Staples A, White J. Envenomations: an overview of clinical toxicology for the primary care physician. *Am Fam Physician.* 2009;80(8):793–802.

45. Welsh O, Vera-Cabrera L, Welsh E. Onychomycosis. *Clin Dermatol.* 2010;28(2):151–9.

46. Wolfram D, Tzankov A, Pülzl P, Piza-Katzer H. Hypertrophic scars and keloids—a review of their pathophysiology, risk factors, and therapeutic management. *Dermatol Surg.* 2009;35(2):171–81.

47. Yang X, Perez OA, English JC 3rd. Adult perniosis and cryoglobulinemia: a retrospective study and review of the literature. *J Am Acad Dermatol.* 2010;62(6):e21–2.

48. Zinder SM, Basler RSW, Foley J, Scarlata C, Vasily DB. National Athletic Trainers Association position statement: skin diseases. *J Athl Train.* 2010;45(4):411–28.

Genitourinary

29

Sean N. Martin and Michael W. Johnson

EPIDEMIOLOGY

- Hematuria and proteinuria are the most common urinary findings in athletes. It is estimated that between 17% and 22% of marathon runners experience postrace gross or microscopic hematuria (5,14). Similarly, 55% of rowers and football players, 73% of boxers, and 80% of swimmers, lacrosse players, and track athletes experience postexertional hematuria (1,3). Further, 30%–69% of runners develop proteinuria following the completion of a marathon regardless of gender (5,15).

- Acute renal failure in athletes is a rare event and is usually associated with volume depletion, rhabdomyolysis, or the nephrotoxic effects of nonsteroidal anti-inflammatory drugs (NSAIDs).

- Although the incidence has not been directly studied, studies have demonstrated that sports are responsible for up to 30% of renal trauma in the pediatric population (2). Contusion is the most frequent kidney and bladder injury, whereas laceration and rupture may be life threatening. Athletes in gymnastics, horseback riding, football, ice hockey, rugby, boxing, and soccer have the highest incidence of renal trauma, whereas bicycle riding is the most common sports-related cause of renal injury (8). Overall, individual sports, rather than team sports, account for the majority renal injuries (13).

- The male genitalia are often subjected to trauma ranging from testicular contusions to penile frostbite. Bikers are at risk for overuse pudendal nerve injury and straddle injuries.

- The prevalence of sexually transmitted diseases (STDs) in athletes is similar to that of the general population, although a study of college athletes showed they tend to be at higher risk for certain lifestyle behaviors. These maladaptive behaviors include less safe sex, greater number of sexual partners, and less contraceptive use when compared with their nonathlete peers (14).

PATHOPHYSIOLOGY

Anatomy

- The genitourinary system is comprised of the kidneys, ureters, bladder, urethra, and genital organs and is located in the lower abdomen and pelvis.

- The kidneys can be found high in the retroperitoneum bilaterally and are well protected. A malpositioned kidney is prone to injury, while the presence of a solitary kidney places the athlete at especially higher risk. The urinary bladder is located in the anterior pelvis and is rarely acutely injured.

Physiology

- The kidneys receive more blood flow per unit weight than any other organ in the body. Renal blood travels to the glomerulus via the afferent arteriole and exits through the efferent arteriole. With afferent arteriole constriction, a pressure drop occurs within the glomerulus and filtration fraction decreases. With efferent arteriole vasoconstriction, pressure increases within the glomerulus thereby increasing the filtration fraction.

- Exercise causes acute changes in a variety of organ systems, as exercising muscle requires a significantly larger proportion of cardiac output. Blood flow is shunted away from the kidney to meet the demands of working muscle. Studies have noted a drop in renal blood flow from 1,000 mL/min to as little as 200 mL/min with exercise, a decrease that is proportional to the intensity of exercise (6,11). Interestingly, there are conflicting data correlating intensity and duration of exercise as independent variables causing hematuria (9,17).

- In an attempt to maintain glomerular filtration rate, the efferent arteriole constricts to a greater degree than the afferent arteriole, creating a "pressure head" at the glomerulus. Additionally, the nephron becomes partially hypoxic, causing increased glomerular permeability. These two mechanisms account for the increased urinary erythrocyte concentration.

- The increase in filtration fraction is attenuated by improving the runner's hydration status. Poorly hydrated individuals have a significantly larger decrease in renal blood flow compared with normally hydrated individuals.

- With moderate exercise (50% $\dot{V}O_{2max}$), renal plasma flow decreases by 30%, whereas with heavy exercise (65% $\dot{V}O_{2max}$), renal plasma flow decreases by 75%. These changes are temporary, and renal blood flow typically returns to preexercise levels within 60 minutes of exercise cessation (7).

HEMATURIA

Clinical Features

■ Exercise-induced hematuria is known by a variety of names, including *sports hematuria*, *stress hematuria*, *athletic pseudonephritis*, and *10,000-m hematuria*, and is defined as hematuria, gross or microscopic, that occurs following vigorous exercise and, except in the case of ultramarathoners, resolves promptly within 24–72 hours of decreased physical activity. Resolution within this time period is the hallmark for the diagnosis of exercise-induced hematuria.

■ Because exercise-induced hematuria is a diagnosis of exclusion, other causes of hematuria should be first ruled out. A thorough history should be obtained in athletes who present with gross hematuria, including the presence of urinary urgency, dysuria, frequency, or clots. Furthermore, a history of trauma, penile discharge, or nephrolithiasis should be ascertained. General historical questions include the presence of bleeding disorders, ongoing menses, recent streptococcal infection, generalized swelling, or risk factors for urologic cancer, such as tobacco use, age greater than 40, and pelvic irradiation. Other important questions include prescription and over-the-counter drug use, dietary supplement use, family history, and diet history.

■ A complete exercise history should be obtained when microscopic hematuria is discovered incidentally.

■ The timing of gross hematuria is an important historical feature. Presence of blood on initiating urination is likely urethral in origin. Hematuria on termination of urination originates from the bladder, prostate, or posterior urethra. Continuous hematuria likely originates from the upper urinary tract. The presence of clots suggests the pathology is distal to the nephron and the thickness of the clots increases with more distal pathology.

■ A thorough and meticulous physical examination should be completed. Vital signs — especially blood pressure — should always be obtained. The back, flank, abdomen, and genitalia are examined, paying particular attention to signs of trauma or infection.

Return to Play

■ Exercise-induced hematuria has not been shown to result in chronic sequelae. Athletes may return to sport once their symptoms have resolved and it can be concluded that their symptoms are purely related to exertion (10).

Differential Diagnosis and Treatment

■ Differential diagnosis includes exertional hematuria, urinary tract infection, nephrolithiasis, hydronephrosis, urethritis, prostatitis, glomerulonephritis, cancer of the urologic system, sickle cell disease, polycystic kidney disease, medication effect, kidney/bladder trauma, and myoglobinuria. Furthermore, ingestion of certain foods (beats, berries) is known to cause red-colored urine. Resolution of clinical signs after activity indicates exercises-induced pseudonephritis versus activity-independent nephritis.

■ Grossly bloody urine should always be dipstick tested for blood and red blood cells confirmed by microscopy. When myoglobin or hemoglobin is present, urine will test positive for blood, but red blood cells are absent on microscopic examination. Medications, dyes, and food coloring often discolor urine. In this case, dipstick testing and microscopy will be negative for blood.

■ See Figure 29.1 for evaluation and treatment.

PROTEINURIA

Clinical Features

■ Proteinuria is defined as more than 150 mg of protein excreted in a 24-hour period. Normal urine protein is composed of 30% albumin, 30% serum globulins, and 40% tissue proteins. Postexercise proteinuria is relatively common and has been described well for over 120 years. It occurs in a variety of sports, both contact and noncontact, and is associated with strenuous effort.

■ Important historical questions include exposure to nephrotoxic medications, intravenous (IV) drug use, and chronic conditions, such as diabetes, systemic lupus erythematosus, or chronic active hepatitis. A family history of hereditary nephritis or polycystic kidney disease is important.

■ Often, the proteinuria is an incidental finding and the patient should be questioned about prior exercise, its duration, and, more importantly, its intensity.

■ Vital signs, especially blood pressure, are essential, followed by a meticulous physical examination. The back, flank, abdomen, skin, and genitalia are examined in routine fashion. The extremities should be evaluated for any signs of edema.

Differential Diagnosis and Treatment

■ Differential diagnosis includes exercise-induced proteinuria, orthostatic proteinuria, glomerulonephritis, nephrotic syndrome, and multiple myeloma.

■ Proteinuria is usually identified through dipstick testing and, when exercise-induced, is usually 2+ to 3+.

■ False-positive results occur because of very concentrated urine, gross hematuria, alkaline urine, or phenazopyridine.

■ See Figure 29.2 for evaluation and treatment.

ACUTE RENAL FAILURE

Clinical Features

■ Acute renal failure in athletes is typically secondary to acute tubular necrosis caused by complications associated with strenuous exercise such as rhabdomyolysis, dehydration, or hyperpyrexia leading to hemolysis. Obstructive uropathy is rarely a cause.

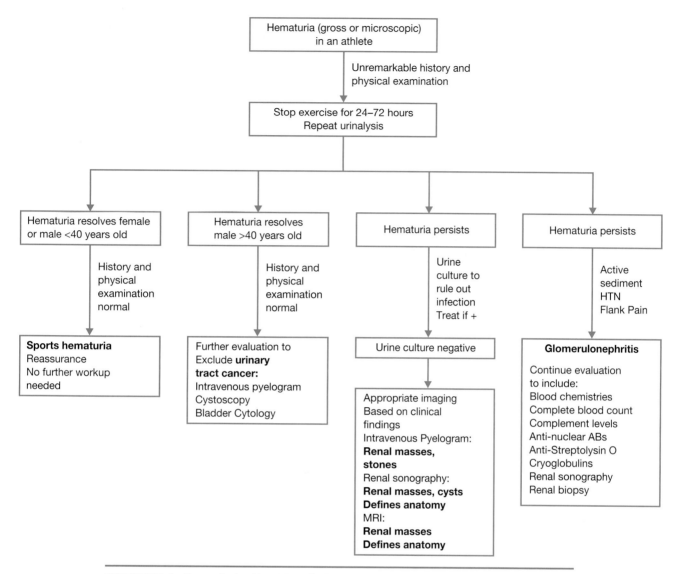

FIGURE 29.1: Hematuria algorithm. AB, antibody; HTN, hypertension; MRI, magnetic resonance imaging.

■ NSAIDs inhibit prostaglandins, thereby decreasing renal blood flow, and contribute to acute renal failure in athletes. Experienced athletes are at much lower risk of developing acute renal failure than untrained athletes.

■ The athlete in acute renal failure often presents with nonspecific complaints, such as malaise, weakness, loss of appetite, nausea, anuria or oliguria, and symptoms of dehydration.

Diagnosis and Treatment

■ Serum laboratory tests include a complete blood count, blood urea nitrogen (BUN), creatinine, and basic chemistry panel. Urine tests include osmolality, sodium, and creatinine. With these data, a fractional excretion of sodium (FE_{Na}) can be calculated to differentiate between prerenal azotemia and acute tubular necrosis as the cause of kidney failure.

■ Treatment of prerenal azotemia involves rapid and aggressive volume replacement.

■ Identification of the endogenous nephrotoxin such as myoglobin in rhabdomyolysis or the exogenous nephrotoxin as in NSAID-induced renal failure is crucial. All reversible causes must be sought and treated.

■ Treatment involves appropriate IV fluid hydration, electrolyte management, and cardiovascular monitoring. Diuretics are only indicated in fluid overload states. Indications for dialysis include the need for ultrafiltration of a volume-overloaded state or the need for solute clearance.

GENITOURINARY TRAUMA

Renal

■ The kidneys are normally well protected by surrounding muscles, ribs, and pericapsular fat in adults; these protective factors are not as pronounced in the pediatric population.

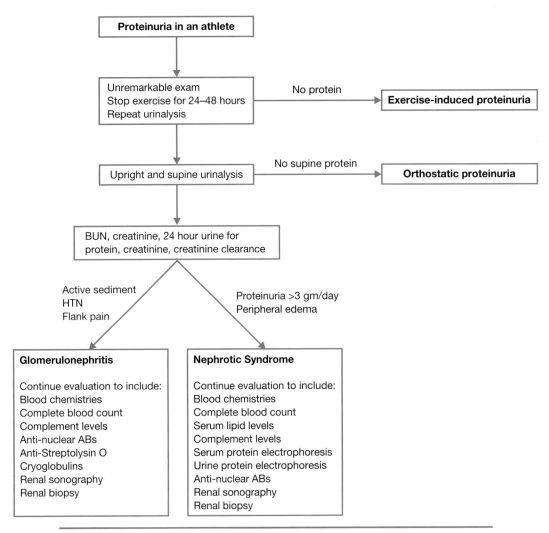

FIGURE 29.2: Proteinuria algorithm. AB, antibody; BUN, blood urea nitrogen; HTN, hypertension.

A blow to the flank or abdomen produces a coup or counter-coup mechanism of injury. Abnormally located or anomalous kidneys are more prone to injury.

- Flank pain and hematuria are the most common presenting complaint.
- Kidney injuries are divided into five classes based on severity and type of injury:
  - Class I: Contusion — most common renal sports injury
  - Class II: Superficial cortical laceration
  - Class III: Deep cortical laceration (> 1 cm)
  - Class IV: Laceration of cortex and collecting system
  - Class V: Complete avulsion of vascular pedicle/shattered kidney or multiple lacerations of class IV severity — again, rare in sports
- Flank pain or gross hematuria after blunt trauma in an athlete requires consideration of possible renal injury. Physical examination may reveal flank ecchymosis and tenderness.
- Athletes with severe renal injuries (class IV and V) often present in hypovolemic shock. Aggressive intravascular volume replacement, transfusion, and surgical exploration to control life-threatening bleeding are often required for these injuries.
- Computed tomography has become the imaging modality of choice for the evaluation of renal injuries in hemodynamically stable athletes. Laboratory examination of blunt trauma should include urinalysis, complete blood count, electrolyte panel, and a pregnancy test in females.
- Treatment of class I–III injuries involves observation, bed rest, and repeat urinalysis to assess for resolution of hematuria.

Ureters

- Ureteral injury is associated with severe trauma, such as pelvic fractures and lower lumbar vertebrae fractures.
- Trauma to flank or pelvis raises the possibility of ureteral injury. Hematuria is present in 90% of ureteral trauma. The diagnosis is best established using IV pyelogram and retrograde pyelogram.
- Treatment is accomplished with placement of a ureteral stent in a partially intact ureter or, as is often the case, open surgical repair.

Bladder

- Repetitive microtrauma is the most common cause of blunt abdominal trauma as demonstrated in a cohort of athletes who received cystoscopy following a run greater than 10,000 m (4). Being that proximity of the bladder walls increases this microtrauma, performing with residual urine in the bladder is thought to be protective.

- Patients with bladder contusion present with a history of trauma, suprapubic pain, guarding, hematuria, and possibly dysuria.

- *Biker's bladder is* a complication of aggressive bicycling and presents with abrupt onset of urinary frequency, diminished urinary stream, nocturia, and terminal dribbling.

- Bladder rupture may be intra- or extraperitoneal and is usually associated with pelvic fracture. Extraperitoneal rupture is often treated with catheter drainage and close observation. Intraperitoneal rupture, however, is often surgically repaired (16).

- Cystography is the definitive study for the diagnosis of bladder rupture. If bladder rupture is present, assessment for pelvic fracture is mandatory. Bladder contusions are treated with catheter drainage for a few days.

Genitalia

- Genital trauma may occur in any sport, although it's often seen in gymnastics, cycling, martial arts, and contact sports.

- Testicular injuries result from direct trauma and include contusion, torsion, or fracture.

- The extent of testicular trauma and testicular blood flow can be evaluated by ultrasound. Testicular rupture is a urologic emergency requiring surgical management if the testis is to be salvaged. Testicular contusions are treated symptomatically.

- Penile injuries are unusual in athletes. The penis may be injured in straddle-type injuries or by direct blow. Irritation of the pudendal nerve in bicycle racers can cause priapism or ischemic neuropathy of the penis. Symptoms usually resolve once the race is over.

- Penile frostbite occurs in runners who wear inadequate clothing in extremely cold conditions.

- Female genitalia may be injured by direct trauma and results in contusion, lacerations, or vulvar hematoma.

- Prostate and distal urethra trauma is most commonly observed in cyclists and is often mediated by reduction of seat height (12). This phenomenon is seen more often in triathletes compared to other types of cyclists as they adopt a forward leaning aerodynamic posture.

Return to Play

- In the case of contusion or minor laceration, athletes may return to sport following resolution of hematuria. They should be withheld from contact sports for a further 6 weeks (10). Extensive injury may necessitate withdrawal from contact sports for 6–12 months.

- Persistence or recurrent hematuria requires imaging evaluation.

REFERENCES

1. Alyea EP, Parish HH Jr. Renal response to exercise-urinary findings. *J Am Med Assoc.* 1958;167(7):807–13.
2. Amaral JF. Primary care of the injured athlete, part II: thoracoabdominal injuries in the athlete. *Clin Sports Med.* 1997;16(4):739–53.
3. Amelar RD, Solomon C. Acute renal trauma in boxers. *J Urol.* 1954;72(2):145–8.
4. Blacklock NJ. Bladder trauma in the long distance runner: "10,000 metres haematuria." *Br J Urol.* 1977;49(2):129–32.
5. Boileau M, Fuchs E, Barry JM, Hodges CV. Stress hematuria: athletic pseudonephritis in marathoners. *Urology.* 1980;15(5):471–4.
6. Castenfors J. Renal function during prolonged exercise. *Ann NY Acad Sci.* 1977;301:151–9.
7. Cianflocco AJ. Renal complications of exercise. *Clin Sports Med.* 1992;11(2):437–51.
8. Gerstenbluth RE, Spimak JP, Elder JS. Sports participation and high grade renal injuries in children. *J Urol.* 2002;168(6):2575–8.
9. Gerth J, Ott U, Fünfstück R, et al. The effects of prolonged physical exercise on renal function, electrolyte balance and muscle cell balance. *Clin Nephrol.* 2002;57(6):425–31.
10. Holmes FC, Hunt JJ, Sevier TL. Renal injury in sport. *Curr Sports Med Rep.* 2003;2(2):103–9.
11. Jones GR, Newhouse I. Sports-related hematuria: a review. *Clin J Sport Med.* 1997;7(2):119–25.
12. LeRoy JB. Banana-seat hematuria. *N Engl J Med.* 1972;287(6):311.
13. McAleer IM, Kaplan GW, Lo Sasso BE. Renal and testis injuries in team sports. *J Urol.* 2002;168(4 Pt 2):1805–7.
14. Nattiv A, Puffer JC, Green GA. Lifestyle and health risks of collegiate athletes: a multi-center study. *Clin J Sport Med.* 1997;7(4):262–72.
15. Reid RI, Hosking DH, Ramsey EW. Haematuria following a marathon run: source and significance. *Br J Urol.* 1987;59(2):133–6.
16. Sagalowsky AI, Peters PC. Genitourinary trauma. In: Walsh PC, Retik AB, Vaughan ED Jr, et al., editors. *Campbell's Urology.* 7th ed. Philadelphia (PA): Saunders; 1998. p. 3085–108.
17. Ubels FL, van Essen GG, de Jong PE, Stegeman CA. Exercise induced macroscopic haematuria: run for a diagnosis? *Nephrol Dial Transplant.* 1999;14(8):2030–1.

30 Ophthalmology

Ronica Martinez

BACKGROUND

- The emphasis in medicine is changing to preventive care, and more people are taking part in athletics and sport activities.
- Primary care providers are going to see a significant amount of injuries that occur during sports.
- Eye injuries account for a relatively small number of injuries when including all sport injuries, but an eye injury can have a significant impact especially if vision is lost.
- It is estimated that eye injuries from sports account for more than 100,000 visits to a physician each year, making the cost greater than $175 million (17).

EPIDEMIOLOGY

- There are over 40,000 sports-related eye injuries a year in the United States (5,7,9,14,16).
- Approximately 90% of sports-related eye injuries are preventable (1,5,12,14,16,17,20,24).
- Approximately 72% of sports-related eye injuries occur in people less than 25 years old, and approximately 43% occur in children younger than 15 years old (10).
- In the United States, baseball and basketball are associated with the most eye injuries in people between 5 and 24 years old (8,23,24).
- Another study showed that hockey, baseball, and racquet sports account for the majority of injuries (17).
- There are a significant number of ocular injuries in Europe and South America due to soccer, and the number is rising in the United States due to increased participation in soccer (2,3,4).
- A study over a 10-year span showed that 75% of severe eye injuries are due to squash, paintball, bungee jumping, and soccer (4).

CLASSIFICATIONS OF SPORTS FOR OCULAR INJURY RISK

- There are four different classifications: high risk, moderate risk, low risk, and eye safe (1,24).

- Generally, sports that involve a ball, racquet, or stick are considered high risk for eye injuries. Other sports that are high risk include boxing and full-contact martial arts (11).
- Moderate-risk sports include golf, fishing, football, tennis, badminton, soccer, water polo, and volleyball.
- Low-risk sports include diving, swimming, bicycling, non-contact martial arts, skiing, and wrestling.
- Eye-safe sports include gymnastics and track and field.

PREPARTICIPATION

- The eye exam is a very important part of the preparticipation exam. A thorough ocular history should be performed, paying close attention to prior injuries or surgeries and the presence of severe myopia, infection, and any retinal detachments. All these may predispose the athlete to a more severe or vision-threatening injury (16,20,25). Any athlete found to have a positive ocular history should be evaluated by an ophthalmologist or eye care professional prior to clearance for participation of a high-risk sport (16,20).

OCULAR EVALUATION OF THE INJURED ATHLETE

History

- A detailed description of the mechanism of injury should be obtained.
- The visual acuity needs to be measured on both the injured eye and noninjured eye immediately following the injury. Ideally, this should be compared to baseline.
- The history of the timing of any visual loss must also be obtained.
- Ask the athlete if there is any photophobia, diplopia, floaters, pain, flashing lights, tearing, nausea, or headache.

Physical Exam

- It is critical that a thorough eye exam be done and that it not just focus on the obvious area involved. Ideally, it should be done on site.

- Exam should be done in an orderly fashion, using the unaffected eye as baseline for comparison. If asymmetry is noted, further investigation is needed.

- Remove contact from the affected eye.

- **Visual acuity:** This is the most important part of any eye exam and should be done first using either a Snellen card or other text source. If an athlete is not able to read text, light perception or finger count should be documented.

- **Visual fields:** A defect could suggest an injury to the optic nerve, retina, or central nervous system.

- **Pupils:** Evaluate the pupils using a bright light. Pupils should be round, reactive, and symmetric. Normally, the pupils will constrict equally and quickly to accommodation and light directed to the affected eye and uninjured eye (consensual light reflex). If a diminished light reflex is found, a swinging flashlight test can be done to better determine if the problem is due to an efferent (pupillary muscle or third nerve) lesion or an afferent (optic nerve or retina) lesion. Pupillary irregularity is almost always pathologic.

- **Anterior chamber:** The anterior chamber can be examined with a penlight to check for any hyphema, foreign bodies, lacerations, or abrasions. Look closely for any blood in the anterior chamber, being sure to compare to the unaffected side.

- **Extraocular range of motion:** Both eyes should ensure full motility in all positions of gaze. An orbital floor fracture may exhibit limitation in gaze elevation. Double vision may suggest a serious problem in one or both eyes.

- **External examination:** Palpate and examine the bony orbits and eyelids. Closely examine the adnexal structures, periorbital skin, cornea, conjunctiva, and iris. Make note of any bony step-offs of the orbital rim, proptosis, edema, or periorbital ecchymosis. Pain with opening the mouth (trismus) often occurs with a fracture of the lateral orbital wall. A fracture of the inferior orbital floor can be suggested if there is paresthesia in the V2 distribution of the trigeminal nerve (20).

- **Sclera and conjunctiva:** Pay close attention to signs that suggest a ruptured globe. These include a 360-degree subconjunctival hemorrhage, lacerations, or extruding pigment (uveal tissue) or gel (vitreous humor).

- **Cornea:** The cornea needs to be examined for clarity. Apply fluorescein to identify any foreign bodies or epithelial defects. A pocket Wood's light or ophthalmoscope with blue light is an appropriate light source for this exam.

- **Funduscopic examination:** A funduscopic exam is required for all eye exams to evaluate the red reflex. Asymmetry of the red reflex may be the only subtle finding that is seen on exam if the athlete has a ruptured globe. Even a small amount of bleeding into the ocular media can obscure the red reflex. Any abnormality must be referred to an ophthalmologist immediately. Other ocular signs and symptoms that require an ophthalmology referral are found in Table 30.1.

Table 30.1	Ocular Signs and Symptoms Requiring Referral to an Ophthalmologist (16,20,21)
Diplopia	Photophobia
Hyphema	Sudden decrease in vision
Visual field loss	Pain with eye movement
Suspected globe perforation	Halos around lights
Irregularly shaped pupil	Foreign body sensation
Embedded foreign body	Laceration of lid margin
Laceration near medial canthus	Proptosis of the eye
Light flashes or floaters	Shattered eye glasses or broken contact
Red and inflamed eye	

COMMON EYE INJURIES

- Some of the more common eye injuries in sports will be reviewed. These include traumatic iritis, hyphema, corneal abrasions, eyelid lacerations, corneal and conjunctival lacerations, subconjunctival hemorrhages, retinal detachments, orbital wall fractures, ruptured globe and penetrating injuries, and foreign bodies. Each section will include the symptoms, examination, treatment, and return-to-play (RTP) recommendations, although RTP guidelines can vary depending on the extent of the injury and practitioner.

Traumatic Iritis

- Irritation in the anterior chamber usually occurring days to weeks after blunt trauma.

- Athletes will complain of a dull ache or throbbing pain, photophobia, and tearing.

- This requires a slit-lamp to diagnose, so if suspected, send athlete for an urgent referral to an ophthalmologist.

- Treatment is with a topical steroid drop.

- Athletes can RTP when asymptomatic and visual fields and acuity have normalized.

Hyphema

- The iris is torn either at the pupil margin or the iris root (15).

- A hyphema is defined as blood in the anterior chamber and can occur with any type of significant blunt trauma.

- Symptoms include blurred vision, photophobia, and pain and may be associated with traumatic iritis.

- A complete eye exam must be performed including intraocular pressure and a slit-lamp exam. Generally, the blood can layer, but clots or stranding can be seen by slit-lamp. Red blood cells floating can be identified, which would suggest a microhyphema.

- An ophthalmology referral is needed because often the athlete may be admitted for observation.
- Strict bed rest is emphasized, with elevation of head at 30 degrees.
- An eye shield should be used to help decrease the risk of re-bleed, which occurs in as many as 30% of cases.
- Ophthalmologist should treat with atropine 1% drops two or three times a day for a microhyphema.
- Athletes should not be on any anti-inflammatory medicine.
- Daily follow-up by an ophthalmologist is needed to assess intraocular pressure and evidence for rebleed.
- Restrict activity for 4 days because there is risk for rebleed, and monitor for resolution.
- RTP when resolved.

Corneal Abrasions

- Corneal abrasions are one of the most common eye injuries in sports (28).
- They account for 12% of eye injuries in the National Basketball Association (30) and 33% of eye injuries in the Major League Baseball (29).
- Symptoms include sharp pain, photophobia, tearing, and foreign body sensation.
- Exam should be done with a topical anesthetic drop, which will improve pain.
- Full examination of eye should be performed, including inversion of the upper lid to exclude foreign body.
- An epithelial defect is seen with fluorescein dye and a cobalt blue light confirming the diagnosis.
- Treat with a broad-spectrum topical antibiotic if there are signs of infection. If the athlete is a contact wearer, the topical antibiotic must have adequate *Pseudomonas* coverage.
- With patients with significant photophobia, cyclopentolate 1% three times a day is prescribed for 2–3 days.
- Close follow-up with daily slit-lamp exams are recommended.
- Patching could be used for comfort for large corneal abrasions but is not recommended for small corneal abrasion because it slows healing on the first day (22).
- Protect from the sunlight during healing by wearing sunglasses when outdoors.
- Patching is usually avoided especially if patient wears contacts (6).
- Keep athlete out of contact sports until completely healed, which usually takes about 3 days.

Eyelid Lacerations

- Eyelid lacerations are seen after blunt or sharp trauma to the eye. They may also occur indirectly from a broken pair of spectacles.
- Localized pain and bleeding around the eye are usually present.

- Check for involvement of the lid margin and assess the depth of laceration to see if orbital fat is exposed.
- If the laceration is medial to the pupil, the lacrimal drainage system needs to be thoroughly examined. A ruptured globe must be ruled out.
- **Need to refer:** Lid laceration repairs should be based on the team physician's level of comfort, but any laceration involving the lacrimal duct drainage system, full-thickness lacerations, exposure to orbital fat, and lacerations involving the lid margin require an immediate ophthalmology referral.
- **No referral needed:**
  - Clean the area with betadine and inject lidocaine locally for anesthesia.
  - Explore wound for a foreign body and irrigate with normal saline or lactated Ringer's.
  - Suturing is done using a 5–0 nylon.
  - Antibiotic ointment is then applied to the area, and a protective shield is placed.
  - Sutures can be removed within 7–10 days.
- Athletes can return to play with sutures but will need to wear proper eye protection until sutures are removed and wound is fully healed.

Corneal/Conjunctival Lacerations

- Often, a subconjunctival hemorrhage is seen with a conjunctival laceration.
- Corneal laceration: patient usually complains of severe eye pain, tearing, and blurred vision.
- Conjunctival laceration: patient presents with mild eye pain, a red eye, and a foreign body sensation.
- A thorough ocular exam should be done.
- The cornea is best viewed with a slit-lamp, but may be seen with a penlight. Any irregularities of the iris, a flattened anterior chamber, or a fold in the cornea are indicative of a corneal tear.
- Fluorescein exam may show a tear.
- The team physician should pay close attention for a scleral laceration or other evidence for a ruptured globe or subconjunctival foreign body.
- If suspected, a rigid eye shield should be placed, with immediate referral to an ophthalmologist.
- Treatment of conjunctival lacerations requires application of a topical broad-spectrum antibiotic and an overnight pressure patch if there is no evidence of a ruptured globe.
- Large lacerations (1–1.5 cm) can require suturing, but this should be reserved for the ophthalmologist.
- Athletes with corneal lacerations can RTP when released by an ophthalmologist and evidence of epithelium healing has occurred.
- Proper eye protection should be worn during sport until patient is fully released by eye specialist.

Subconjunctival Hemorrhage

- Subconjunctival hemorrhages are very common after blunt trauma.
- Usually the athlete does not complain of any discomfort or maybe just very mild irritation and a red eye.
- Assessment is mainly focused on ruling out a ruptured globe or foreign body.
- Treatment includes reassurance to the athlete, and most hemorrhages resolve in 2–3 weeks.
- Athletes can RTP immediately without restrictions.

Retinal Detachment

- Retinal detachment can occur after any direct trauma to the orbit or from significant head trauma.
- Athletes with myopia are at higher risk.
- Presentation includes the athlete complaining of floaters or flashing lights, and athlete may have a blind spot on the edge of a visual field. Timing may be remote to trauma, occurring even hours after trauma.
- The team physician must check confrontational visual field for defects.
- An afferent pupil defect may be present if there is a large area of detachment.
- A funduscopic exam should be performed, but a detachment can be hard to identify; they usually begin peripherally.
- If there is suspicion for a retinal detachment, an urgent referral to an ophthalmologist is warranted for a dilated exam.
- Treatment can include laser (tears or holes) or surgery (detachment).
- The athlete can RTP when released by an ophthalmologist, depending on extent of damage, but 2 weeks is the minimum out of activity (19).

Ruptured Globe/Penetrating Injuries

- These types of injuries occur from direct trauma to the orbit or significant head trauma.
- Like retinal detachments, athletes with myopia are at higher risk.
- The athlete may not have any symptoms or may present similarly to a retinal detachment (floaters, flashing lights, visual field loss).
- Athlete may complain of vision loss or eye pain.
- A thorough exam should be done, but **NO** pressure should be applied to the globe.
- Pay close attention to any dark pigmented tissue exposed (uveal tissue), leaking gel or fluid (vitreous or aqueous humor), or a flattened anterior chamber.
- The presence of a 360-degree subconjunctival hemorrhage strongly suggests a ruptured globe.
- Place an eye shield on the athlete and send the athlete for an immediate ophthalmology consultation.

- **DO NOT** attempt to remove the penetrating object.
- Athlete is to remain NPO (nothing by mouth) due to the high probability for surgical exploration and repair.
- RTP should be in conjunction with an ophthalmologist. If full vision returns, the athlete can RTP, but if partial vision returns, then the team physician must follow recommendations for the monocular athlete.

Orbital Wall Fracture

- Mostly seen after significant blunt eye trauma.
- Athletes present with localized pain and swelling or crepitus with nose blowing.
- The athlete may have diplopia, which can suggest extraocular muscle entrapment.
- Numbness on the cheek can be indicative of infraorbital nerve involvement.
- A complete eye exam should be done, with focus on extraocular motility, palpitation of the orbits, and facial numbness.
- A ruptured globe should be ruled out.
- A CT scan of the orbits should be ordered to further assess orbital wall fracture.
- Evaluation from ophthalmologist is warranted.
- Cephalexin 500 mg four times a day for 7 days and oxymetazoline nasal spray twice a day for 3 days should be given to prevent orbital cellulitis.
- Instruct athlete NOT to blow nose.
- Apply ice for the first 24–48 hours.
- Athlete needs clearance from eye specialist to return to contact play because timing depends on extent of injury. Some orbital wall fractures need immediate repair, while others may need repair 1–2 weeks after initial trauma.

Foreign Bodies

- Most common sports-related eye injury.
- More common with outdoor sports (dust, debris).
- Athletes will complain of eye irritation, tearing, pain, and possibly a "sandy/gravelly sensation" in affected eye.
- Conjunctival injection can occur due to the constant irritation.
- A thorough eye exam should be done including eversion of the upper eye using a cotton applicator. Fluorescence dye must be done to exclude a corneal abrasion, which occurs if the foreign body gets lodged under the lid.
- A topical anesthetic in the eye may be used to relieve pain and keep the athlete more comfortable, but the anesthetic should not be administered on a regular basis.
- Foreign body can be removed with a saline-moistened cotton applicator.
- If foreign body is unable to be removed or is embedded, removal must be done using a slit-lamp by an ophthalmologist.
- If the foreign body was metal, a rust ring may be seen after removal, thus warranting a referral to an ophthalmologist.

■ Athletes can usually RTP immediately once the foreign body has been removed and visual acuity restored. Protective eyewear may be needed for a short time.

PROTECTIVE EQUIPMENT

■ Should be made of polycarbonate or Trivex lenses (1,4,5, 13,16,20).

■ Proper fitting protective eyewear can reduce risk for serious eye injury by 90% (9).

■ Contact lenses offer no protection, and prescription glasses offer inadequate protection.

■ A protective shield may be integrated if helmet is required for particular sport.

■ Eye protectors should be replaced if they show damage or are yellowed with age (1).

■ Protective eyewear must meet American Society for Testing and Materials (ASTM) standards (1,13).

  ▪ ASTM F803 for selected sports (basketball, racket sports, women's lacrosse, baseball fielders, soccer, and field hockey [27])

  ▪ ASTM F910 for youth batter and base runner in youth baseball and softball.

  ▪ ASTM 513 facemask on helmet for street hockey and ice hockey.

  ▪ ASTM F1587 for ice hockey goaltenders.

  ▪ ASTM 659 for skiing (18).

  ▪ ASTM F1776 for paintball.

■ Additional certification on eye protection is needed from the Hockey Equipment Certification Council and the Canadian Standards Association for street and ice hockey.

■ Ultraviolet protection is needed for skiers, mountain climbers, and water sports.

Choosing Eye Protection

■ Use eye protection that is up to standard.

■ Get professional assistance to properly select eye protection. Professional can be an ophthalmologist, optometrist, athletic trainer, or optician.

■ Know the athlete's eye and vision history.

THE MONOCULAR ATHLETE

■ A child athlete is considered monocular when best-corrected visual acuity in the weaker eye is less than 20/40, and an adult is functionally monocular when he or she believes that if vision is lost in the better eye, quality of life would be affected having to rely on the weaker eye (14).

■ The monocular athlete must wear eye protection at all times regardless of sport (1,4,14,18).

■ The athlete must understand that there is still a chance for eye injury while participating in sport, despite proper wear of eye protection.

■ Full-contact martial arts, boxing, and wrestling are contraindicated for the monocular athlete (1,9).

CONCLUSION

■ Although eye injuries may be smaller in number compared to total injuries in sport, they can be more severe and detrimental when they occur.

■ Physicians, athletic trainers, and coaches should educate people who partake in sports to be more aware of potential hazards if proper eye protection is not worn.

■ Professionals need to identify people at high risk for eye injury including the monocular athlete, people with previous eye injury or surgery, or people who wear corrective lenses and participate in a potentially high-risk sport for eye injury (26).

■ Most eye injuries caused by sport can be prevented with proper eye protection that is certified by the Protective Eyewear Certification Council (4).

REFERENCES

1. American Academy of Pediatrics Committee on Sports Medicine and Fitness, Eye Health, and Public Information Task Force. Protective eyewear for young athletes. *Pediatrics.* 2004;113(3 Pt 1):619–22.

2. Capão Felipe JA. Soccer (football) ocular injuries; an important eye health problem. *Br J Ophthalmol.* 2004;88(2):159–60.

3. Capão Felipe JA, Fernandes VL, Barros H, Falcão-Reis F, Castro-Correia J. Soccer-related ocular injuries. *Arch Ophthalmol.* 2003;121(5):687–94.

4. Capão Felipe JA, Rocha-Sousa A, Falcão-Reis F, Castro-Correia J. Modern sports eye injuries. *Br J Ophthalmol.* 2003;87(11):1336–9.

5. Cassen JH. Ocular trauma. *Hawaii Med J.* 1997;56(10):292–4.

6. Ehlres JP, Shah CP, Fenton GL, Hoskins EN, Shelsta HN. *The Wills Eye Manuel: Office and Emergency Room Diagnosis and Treatment of Eye Disease.* 5th ed. Philadelphia (PA): Lippincott Williams & Wilkins; 2008. p. 97–8.

7. Heimmel MR, Murphy MA. Ocular injuries in basketball and baseball: what are the risks and how can we prevent them? *Curr Sports Med Rep.* 2008;7(5): 284–8.

8. Huffman EA, Yard EE, Fields SK, Collins CL, Comstock RD. Epidemiology of rare injuries and conditions among United States high school athletes during the 2005–2006 and 2006–2007 school years. *J Athl Train.* 2008;43(6):624–30.

9. Jeffers JV. An ongoing tragedy: pediatric sports-related eye injuries. *Semin Ophthal.* 1990;5:216–23.

10. Kent JS, Eidsness RB, Colleaux KM, Romanchuk KG. Indoor soccer-related eye injuries: should eye protection be mandatory? *Can J Ophthalmol.* 2007;42(4):605–8.

11. Larrison WI, Hersch PS, Kunzweiler T, Shingleton BJ. Sports-related ocular trauma. *Ophthalmology.* 1990;97(10):1265–9.

12. Leivo T, Puusaari I, Mäkitie T. Sports-related eye injuries: floorball endangers the eyes of young players. *Scand J Med Sci Sports.* 2007; 17(5):556–63.

13. Lexington Eye Associates Inc. Web site [Internet]. Massachusetts (MA): Vinger PF. The mechanism and prevention of sports eye injuries; [cited 2010 Dec 10]. Available from: http://www.lexeye.com/pdf/The-Mech-and-Prev-of-Sports-Eye-Injuries.pdf.

14. Lexington Eye Associates Inc. Web site [Internet]. Massachusetts (MA): The recommendations of the American Academy of Ophthalmology for sports eye wear; [cited 2010 Dec 10]. Available from: http://www.lexeye.com/pdf/AAO.pdf.

15. MacEwen CJ, McLatchie GR. Eye injuries in sport. *Scott Med J.* 2010; 55(2):22–4.

16. Martinez RA, Ellini KA. Ophthalmology. In: O'Conner FG, Sallis RE, Wilder RP, St. Pierre P, editors. *Just the Facts Sports Medicine.* New York: McGraw-Hill; 2005. p. 162–5.

17. Napier SM, Baker RS, Sanford DG. Easterbrook M. Eye injuries in athletics and recreation. *Surv Ophthalmol.* 1996;41(3):229–44.

18. National Collegiate Athletic Association. NCAA Guideline 4b. *Eye Safety Sports.* 2001;92–3.

19. Patel DR, Greydanus DE, Baker RJ. *Pediatric Practice Sports Medicine.* 1st ed. New York (NY): McGraw-Hill; 2009. 552 p.

20. Pieper P. Epidemiology and prevention of sports-related eye injuries. *J Emerg Nurs.* 2010;36(4):359–61.

21. Rodriguez JO, Lavina AM, Agarwal A. Prevention and treatment of common eye injuries in sports. *Am Fam Physician.* 2003;67(7):1481–8.

22. Shah A, Blackhall K, Ker K, Patel D. Educational interventions for the prevention of eye injuries. *Cochrane Database Syst Rev.* 2009;4:CD006527.

23. Turner A, Rabiu M. Patching for corneal abrasion. *Cochrane Database Syst Rev.* 2006;2:CD004764.

24. U.S. Consumer Product Safety Commission. *Sports and Recreational Eye Injuries.* Washington (DC): U.S. Consumer Product Safety Commission; 2000.

25. Vinger PF. A practical guide for sports eye protection. *Phys Sportsmed.* 2000;28(6):49–69.

26. Vinger PF. Sports medicine and the eye care professional. *J Am Optom Assoc.* 1998;69(6):395–413.

27. Vinger PF, Capão Filipe JA. The mechanism and prevention of soccer eye injuries. *Br J Ophthalmol.* 2004;88(2):167–8.

28. Youn J, Sallis RE, Smith G, Jones K. Ocular injury rates in college sports. *Med Sci Sports Exerc.* 2008;40(3):428–32.

29. Zagelbaum BM. Treating corneal abrasions and lacerations. *Phys Sportsmed.* 1997;25(3):38–44.

30. Zagelbaum BM, Hersh PS, Donnenfeld ED, Perry HD, Hochman MA. Ocular trauma in major league baseball players. *N Engl J Med.* 1994; 330(14):1021–3.

31 Otorhinolaryngology

Charles W. Webb and C. Thayer White

INTRODUCTION

- Facial injuries are among the most common injuries in athletics. They comprise 4%–19% of all sports-related injuries depending on age and gender. Of all facial injuries, 3%–29% are sports related, with the majority (60%–90%) occurring in males ages 10–29 (8,9). The gender difference increases with age from 1.5:1 male to females during the ages of 1–10 years to 12:1 during the ages of 16–18 (10,13). With the addition of facemasks and mouth guards in football and hockey (1950s and 1970s, respectively), the number of severe facial injuries has declined dramatically (3).

ASSESSMENT OF FACIAL INJURIES ON THE SIDELINE

- Sideline management of the athlete with a facial injury begins with the ABCs (airway, breathing, circulation). Blood, avulsed teeth, mouth guards, or other objects are airway hazards. Cervical spine precautions must be observed in all head injuries, especially when the player is unconscious.
- The history should include the mechanism of injury and assess for related injuries and the presence of any other injuries past or present (9).
  - Most facial injuries are the result of direct trauma. Assess the nature of the impact and the presence or absence of protective equipment.
  - Ask about alertness, orientation, headaches, vision symptoms, and neurologic deficits to assess for concussion or intracranial injury.
  - Ask about neck pain and take appropriate cervical spine precautions.
  - Other questions to ask include the following: Can you breathe through both sides of your nose? Are you having any trouble speaking? Is your hearing normal? Have you had any previous facial injuries or surgeries, including procedures to correct vision (*e.g.*, laser-assisted in situ keratomileusis [LASIK])?

- Physical examination includes observation, palpation, and imaging (if there is any question about the diagnosis).
  - Observation includes evaluation of facial symmetry, bruising, lacerations, and swelling. Asymmetry is especially important to assess on the sideline because it may be a clue to facial fracture and can become obscured by swelling and hematoma (9).
  - Bruising around the mastoid process is called Battle's sign and is suggestive of a basilar skull fracture.
  - Observation of the nares includes the septum, which can be seen with an otoscope. A bluish-tinted bulge represents a septal hematoma.
  - Palpation includes the orbital rim, nasal bones, maxillary bones, mandible, temporomandibular joint, mastoid process, and the upper and lower jaws
  - The nares should be inspected for any type of fluid drainage. This may be blood or cerebrospinal fluid (CSF). The "ring test" is a method of detecting CSF on the sideline. It is done by placing a drop of blood from the nares on a piece of paper or gauze; CSF will form a halo (clear fluid ring) around the drop of blood. This represents a severe facial fracture and requires immediate transport.
  - Imaging is usually of limited value. X-rays may be helpful in determining the presence of a facial fracture; however, computed tomography (CT) is the gold standard.
  - Return-to-play guidance is based on the history and physical examination. Suspected fractures (except some nasal fractures), airway obstruction or impending obstruction, uncontrolled bleeding, loss of consciousness, and changes in vision are contraindications for return to play.

EAR INJURIES

Ear Laceration

- The more common ear injuries encountered in sports include lacerations, hematomas, otitis externa and exostosis of the outer ear, and tympanic membrane (TM) rupture (traumatic and barometric) of the inner ear.
- The auricle consists of avascular cartilage, which derives its nutrition from the tightly adhered perichondrium. Overlying that is closely adhered skin with little subcutaneous tissue (1).

- **Signs and symptoms:** Pain and bleeding around the ear with history of trauma.
- **Examination:** Must evaluate for cartilage involvement and for radial extension to the scalp.
- **Treatment**
  - Cartilage tear must be repaired unless it is very small and can be readily approximated. Absorbable 5-0 suture is preferred.
  - Local anesthesia is best achieved with nerve blocks of the great auricular nerve (along the superficial body of the sternocleidomastoid muscle 6.5 cm inferior to the auditory canal) and V3 nerve (2.5 cm anterior to the tragus in the notch between the condyle and coronoid process of the mandible) to avoid local tissue swelling (15).
  - Laceration should be irrigated thoroughly prior to suturing, being careful to avoid removing the perichondrium.
  - Debridement of cartilage should be kept to a minimum to maintain cosmetic appearance and minimize risk of chondritis.
  - All exposed cartilage must be covered after the repair.
  - After the repair, apply a pressure dressing to prevent formation of auricular hematoma.
  - Prophylactic antibiotics may be used to prevent chondritis.

Auricular Hematoma

- "Wrestler's ear" or "cauliflower ear" is caused by bleeding between the skin (perichondrium) and the auricular cartilage. This occurs secondary to repetitive contusions to the auricle. This can evolve into a permanent cosmetic deformity with chronic hematomas, secondary to an increased pressure and eventual necrosis of the cartilage.
- **Signs and symptoms:** Acute throbbing pain, tenderness, and edema.
- **Examination:** Soft hematoma within the auricle.
- **Treatment**
  - Definitive treatment is incision and complete evacuation of hematoma as soon as possible, followed by compression (2).
  - Compression may be achieved by mattress sutures through the ear with or without cotton bolstering. A circumferential pressure dressing is also acceptable but less desirable.
  - The athlete should not return to play until after the removal of the compression device in 7–10 days and should always wear proper ear protection (head gear).
  - An alternative treatment method is repeated aspiration of the hematoma. This allows the athlete to return to play quickly (same day with head gear); however, this treatment method usually leads to a permanent cauliflower ear. Both the athlete and the parents should be informed of the risk and the permanence of this defect (11).

Otitis Externa (OE)

- Infection of the external auditory canal is most commonly caused by bacteria (90%), primarily *Pseudomonas aeruginosa*, *Staphylococcus aureus*, or occasionally other aerobic and anaerobic species. Fungal infections cause 10% of cases (7).
- Acute OE is unilateral in 90% of patients.
- OE is most common in children 7–12 years old and rare after age 50.
- Risk factors include high humidity, warm water, ear trauma, and compromised immune system. It is most common in water sports and has an increased incidence in poorly chlorinated pools and fresh water.
- **Evaluation**
  - Mild: erythema of the canal with mild discomfort and pruritus and a watery discharge.
  - Moderate: developing edema and mucopurulent discharge.
  - Severe: obstruction of the lumen with surrounding cellulitis, parotitis, or adenopathy.
  - Debris may be seen in the lumen, which should be removed to visualize the TM and facilitate effective treatment.
  - Always ensure TM integrity before irrigation or using ototoxic topical medications.
- **Differential diagnosis**
  - Other dermatologic conditions may manifest in the ear, such as contact dermatitis, eczema, or psoriasis.
  - Contact dermatitis from ototopicals is not uncommon, occurring in 5%–18% of patients using neomycin.
  - Consider fungal causes if not responding to antibacterial treatment.
- **Treatment**
  - Mild cases, including most fungal causes, may be treated with astringents, such as 2% acetic acid, 2.75% boric acid, or rubbing alcohol.
  - Moderate to severe cases should be treated with a topical antibiotic with or without topical corticosteroid. Commonly used medications include aminoglycosides, Cortisporin Otic (neomycin/polymyxin B/hydrocortisone), and fluoroquinolones.
  - Fluoroquinolones are the only topical antibiotic approved for ruptured TM.
  - Tolnaftate or clotrimazole can be used for fungal infections.
  - Pain control can be achieved with nonsteroidal anti-inflammatory drugs (NSAIDs) or mild opiates.
  - Consider oral antibiotics after getting a culture for severe cases or moderate disease in high-risk patients (elderly, immunocompromised, or diabetics).
  - If the canal is swollen, a cotton wick may be used to help deliver the antibiotic.
  - Swimmers may use alcohol or acidifying drops to prevent OE.

Tympanic Membrane Rupture

- This usually occurs secondary to a diving, water skiing, surfing, or slap injury.
- **Signs and symptoms:** Acute pain, sudden unilateral hearing loss, nausea, and vertigo.
- **Examination:** Visualization of the defect with an otoscope.
- **Treatment:** Observation and reassurance are the treatments of choice, as 90% will heal in 8 weeks.
  - Antibiotics are recommended only if an infection develops.
  - No water sports until perforation is completely healed.

Auditory Exostoses

- Exostoses are benign broad-based osseous lesions typically presenting after a history of cold water exposure.
- They are usually multiple and bilaterally symmetrical.
- More common in male teenagers or young adults.
- Present with conductive hearing loss, from external auditory canal obstruction.
- Pain with palpation or with cold water exposure.
- Bony outgrowths of the temporal bone into the auditory canal.
- Related to cold water exposure, primarily in surfers.
- Surgical referral for excision is advised for large growths or progressive hearing loss.
- Protective equipment, such as ear plugs, is used for treatment, as well as prevention for cold water athletes.
- Treatment involves ear plugs, avoidance of cold water, and surgery in severe cases (12).

NASAL INJURIES

Nasal Fractures

- Most common sports-related facial fracture, as well as the most common facial structure injured. Direct end-on blows usually result in comminuted fractures of both the bone and the cartilage. Side blows usually result in simple fractures with deviation to the opposite side.
- **Signs and symptoms:** Acute pain, tearing, epistaxis, facial swelling, and ecchymosis.
- **Examination:** Crepitus over the nasal bridge and observation of nasal deformity.
  - If bleeding is present, a ring test should be performed.
  - Careful evaluation for other injuries.
- **X-rays:** Seldom helpful for treatment decisions in the clinic or emergency room, but may be useful in documentation.
- **Treatment:** Reduction of the displaced nasal fracture may be done on the sideline and is semi-painless if done immediately.
  - If unable to reduce, an otorhinolaryngology referral is required in 5–7 days for reduction.

- Follow-up within 48 hours to ensure no septal hematoma.
- Athletes should not return to play the same day unless there are absolutely no other associated injuries and the nose can be protected. Return to play is typically not advised for at least the first week after reduction. External protective devices are recommended for the first 4 weeks after injury.

Septal Hematoma

- Accumulation of blood between the septal cartilage and the overlying perichondrium.
- Septal hematomas are prone to abscess formation and may lead to pressure necrosis of the underlying bone and cartilage (saddle nose deformity) if not treated (9).
- **Signs and symptoms:** Acute pain, facial swelling, and nasal obstruction.
- **Examination:** A bluish bulge is seen on the nasal septum.
- **Treatment:** Prompt aspiration is the key to successful treatment.
  - Aspiration is done using an 18- to 20-gauge needle or scalpel, and then packing the nose with bilateral nasal packing for 4–5 days to prevent recurrence.
  - The use of prophylactic broad-spectrum antibiotics for 10–14 days to prevent abscess formation, especially in children, is often recommended, although it is not proven to reduce complications.
  - **Complications:** Minor: minor aesthetic deformities and septal alterations with no airway compromise. Major: nasal deformation causing aesthetic impairment, deviation of the septum with nares obstruction, and swelling of the cartilage or complete erosion of the septal cartilage with saddle deformity of the nose.

Epistaxis

Anterior Epistaxis

- Of all nosebleeds, 90%–95% are anterior. The most common site for bleeding is from the Kiesselbach's plexus in Little's area on the anterior septum (6).
- Causes include blunt trauma, digital trauma, dry mucosa, chemical irritants, mucosal atrophy (topical steroids), and illicit drug use. NSAIDs are a common medication in athletes that may worsen bleeding. Other antiplatelet or anticoagulant medications are important to ask about.
- **Signs and symptoms:** Dripping blood from the nostrils.
- **Examination:** Every effort should be made to locate the bleeding when simple compression or nasal plugging does not stop the bleeding. Common equipment needed for complete nasal examination includes bayonet forceps; nasal speculum; Frazier suction tip; posterior double balloon system and syringe for balloon inflation; and packing materials, including nonadherent gauze impregnated with petroleum jelly and 3% bismuth tribromophenate (Xeroform), Merocel, and Gelfoam.

- **Treatment:** Ice and compression of the nasal ala are the mainstays of treatment.
  - Topical vasoconstrictors can be used, such as phenylephrine and oxymetazoline (Afrin).
  - Cautery may be considered if pressure fails and the bleeding site can be identified (silver nitrate or electrocautery pen).
  - Nasal packing may also be used for compression if bleeding site cannot be identified. Strenuous activity should be restricted if nasal packing is required, until the packing can be removed. The packing is often coated with antibiotic ointment. It should be removed in 1–5 days to prevent pressure necrosis of the nasal septum. Oral antibiotics may be given to prevent toxic shock syndrome.
  - Return to play should not be allowed with nasal packing in place because the potential for airway obstruction exists.
  - If no packing is required and the bleeding is controlled, the athlete may return to play.

Posterior Epistaxis

- Of all nosebleeds, 5%–10% are posterior.
- Bleeding occurs from branches of the sphenopalatine artery.
- **Signs and symptoms:** Bleeding that drains mainly through the posterior pharynx and does not stop with direct pressure.
- **Evaluation:** The bleeding cannot be directly visualized. Must evaluate for other facial trauma, including orbital fracture and nasal fracture. Most posterior bleeds require more than an on-the-field assessment. These athletes should be evacuated to a hospital for ear, nose, and throat (ENT) surgical consultation.
- **Treatment:** Emergent hemostasis can be achieved with a small Foley catheter inserted through the nares, inflated in the posterior pharynx, and then pulled snug against the posterior nares, tamponading the bleeding and protecting the airway (6).

FACIAL INJURIES

Lacerations

- Knowledge of facial anatomy is important for assessing damage to underlying structures, such as nerves, blood vessels, glands, ducts, and delicate facial musculature.
- Superficial facial lacerations should be thoroughly irrigated and all foreign bodies removed. Repair can be done with 6-0 or smaller sutures or skin adhesives such as Dermabond. Tissue adhesive works especially well on lacerations smaller than 4 cm, not under tension, and in children (8).
- Deeper lacerations may be repaired in the training room using absorbable sutures for subcutaneous approximation and skin closure, as above. Care must be taken to assess for damage to underlying structures and cosmetically sensitive areas.
- Lip lacerations should be referred if they cross the vermillion border or affect the orbicularis oris muscle

- With cheek lacerations, evaluate for damage of the parotid duct.
- Tongue lacerations may be repaired with absorbable suture or covered with saline-soaked gauze and referred.
- Eyelid lacerations should be closed within 12–36 hours. Packing with iced saline gauze can decrease swelling to allow for better repair. Some simple lacerations may be repaired on site, but referral to a qualified provider is strongly recommended for any involvement of the lid margins, tear ducts, lacrimal sac, or levator palpebrae muscle (1).
- Tetanus status should be assessed.

Fractures

- Assessment should be done immediately before swelling obscures bony deformity.
- The nose, zygoma, and mandible are involved in 75% of facial fractures (9).
- With all suspected facial fractures other than simple nasal fractures (discussed separately), the athlete should be removed from competition and referred for further evaluation.
- CT is the gold standard for imaging facial bones.
- Zygomatic fractures are caused by blunt trauma to the cheek. They can affect vision, jaw function, and the width of the face (8).
- Mandibular fractures may present with malocclusion or numbness of the inferior alveolar nerve in addition to pain and swelling. Fifty percent of fractures are multiple. Treatment consists of surgical reduction and fixation.
- Orbital fractures are caused by direct blunt trauma to the orbit. They most commonly affect the inferior wall and less commonly the medial wall. Vision and extraocular movement should be assessed. A deficit in either is an indication for emergent transfer due to risk of globe rupture or extraocular muscle entrapment.
- Maxillary fractures are classified according to the Le Fort system. These fractures may create an unstable midface that could complicate the airway. Surgical airway is sometimes needed.
- Return to play for noncombat athletes can begin with light activity at 21 days, noncontact training at 31 days, and full contact at 41 days. Protective masks may speed the return to contact. Combat athletes should wait 3 months before return to activity.

TRACHEAL INJURIES

- Blunt trauma to the anterior neck can have devastating effects on the larynx and the trachea, causing serious airway compromise. Hockey, football, softball, baseball, wrestling, soccer, lacrosse, and gymnastics are the sports more commonly associated with tracheal/laryngeal injury. Hockey, baseball, softball, lacrosse, and fencing all require the athlete to wear neck-protecting extensions or masks to protect the anterior neck. Blunt trauma to this region can produce both contusions and fractures of the larynx and the trachea.

Laryngeal Fracture

■ Typically a result of high-force trauma and associated with other maxillofacial injuries.

■ The signs and symptoms include airway compromise, voice changes, subcutaneous emphysema, and palpable fracture.

■ It is of the utmost importance to establish an airway, protect it, and then transport the athlete to the nearest health care facility. If there is an associated facial injury, it may be impossible to place an orotracheal tube or a nasotracheal tube. In these cases, the surgical airway of choice is the cricothyroidotomy (14).

Cricothyroidotomy

■ Cricothyroidotomy is placement of a catheter through the cricothyroid membrane to establish an airway. This surgical airway may be used as a temporizing airway when oral and nasal intubation is not possible.

　■ This is done by first identifying the anatomy. The cricothyroid membrane is located between the thyroid cartilage and the cricoid cartilage. The first landmark to find is the thyroid cartilage (Adam's apple), and then move inferiorly to the groove below the thyroid cartilage. The cricothyroid membrane is in the space between the thyroid cartilage and the cricoid cartilage located as the next hard ring of tissue inferior to the thyroid cartilage.

　■ If time permits, the neck should be prepped with alcohol or povidone-iodine and the skin anesthetized locally before the first incision is made.

　■ The initial incision is made **vertically** through the skin (3–4 cm) over the cricothyroid membrane.

　■ The next step is to identify the cricothyroid membrane immediately inferior to the thyroid cartilage. Once it is identified, a 1- to 2-cm **horizontal** incision is made.

　■ Insert a tracheostomy tube or a 5- to 6-mm endotracheal tube (3 mm for a child) and secure the tube with tape.

■ If there is not enough time to perform the surgical procedure, a needle cricothyroidotomy may be performed by locating the cricothyroid membrane as above and inserting a 12- to 16-gauge needle catheter that is attached to a syringe. This allows the syringe to be connected to a pressurized oxygen source or a 3.0 endotracheal tube for ventilation while transport is taking place.

Table 31.1	Sideline Cricothyroidotomy Kit
Alcohol pads	Povidone-iodine pads or swabs
#11 scalpel	3- or 5-cc syringe with needle
25-gauge needle	1% or 2% lidocaine with or without epinephrine
4-inch hemostat	5- to 6-mm endotracheal tube or tracheostomy tube
3-mm endotracheal tube	12–16 gauge catheter over needle

Table 31.2	Risks and Contraindications for Surgical Airway	
	Contraindications	
Risks	**Absolute**	**Relative**
Hemorrhage	Ability to place another type of airway	Coagulopathy
Esophageal perforation		Overlying tumor
Subcutaneous emphysema		Hematoma
Tracheal stenosis		Age less than 10 years
Vocal cord damage		Indistinct landmarks
Aspiration		Previous intubation
Infection		Longer than 3 days

■ There are prepackaged cricothyroidotomy kits available commercially. These kits will come prepackaged for either the blind percutaneous method or insertion through the skin incision. The contents for a sideline cricothyroidotomy kit are outlined in Table 31.1. The complications to this procedure should be weighed against the risk of death in the athlete prior to availability of definitive care. The complications and contraindications are listed in Table 31.2 (4,5).

CONCLUSION

■ Ear, nose, and throat injuries are common injuries seen on the sidelines and can be quite serious in nature. The team physician must have a thorough knowledge of the anatomy in order to provide adequate care to the injured athlete. These injuries can range from cosmetic (wrestler's ear) to severely life threatening (laryngeal fracture). Essential equipment and training for the team physician can mean the difference between life and death.

REFERENCES

1. Brown DJ, Jaffe JE, Henson JK. Advanced laceration management. *Emerg Med Clin North Am.* 2007;25(1):83–99.

2. Giles WC, Iverson KC, King JD, Hill FC, Woody EA, Bouknight AL. Incision and drainage followed by mattress suture repair of auricular hematoma. *Laryngoscope.* 2007;117(12):2097–9.

3. Hart LE. Full facial protection reduces injuries in elite young hockey players. *Clin J Sport Med.* 2002;12(6):406.

4. Hsiao J, Pacheco-Fowler V. Videos in clinical medicine. Cricothyroidotomy. *N Engl J Med.* 2008;358(22):e25.

5. Jaworski CA. Advances in emergent airway management. *Curr Sport Med Rep.* 2002;1(3):133–40.

6. Manes RP. Evaluating and managing the patient with nosebleeds. *Med Clin North Am.* 2010;94(5):903–12.

7. Osguthorpe JD, Nielsen DR. Otitis externa: review and clinical update. *Am Fam Physician.* 2006;74(9):1510–6.

8. Reehal P. Facial injury in sport. *Curr Sport Med Rep.* 2010;9(1):27–34.

9. Romeo SJ, Hawley CJ, Romeo MW, Romeo JP, Honsik KA. Sideline management of facial injuries. *Curr Sport Med Rep.* 2007;6(3):155–61.

10. Shaikh ZS, Worrall SF. Epidemiology of facial trauma in a sample of patients aged 1–18 years. *Injury.* 2002;33(8):669–71.

11. Swinson B, Lloyd T. Management of maxillofacial injuries. *Hosp Med.* 2003;64(2):72–8.

12. Taylor KS, Zoltan TB, Achar SA. Medical illnesses and injuries encountered during surfing. *Curr Sport Med Rep.* 2006;5(5):262–7.

13. Truman BI, Gooch BF, Sulemana I, et al. Reviews of evidence on interventions to prevent dental caries, oral and pharyngeal cancers, and sports-related craniofacial injuries. *Am J Prev Med.* 2002;23(1)(suppl):21–54.

14. Verschueren DS, Bell RB, Bagheri SC, Dierks EJ, Potter BE. Management of laryngo-tracheal injuries associated with craniomaxillofacial trauma. *J Oral Maxillofac Surg.* 2006;64(2):203–14.

15. Zide BM, Swift R. How to block and tackle the face. *Plast Reconstr Surg.* 1998;101(3):840–51.

INTRODUCTION

- There are many benefits to participating in athletic activities, such as enhanced physical fitness and the enjoyment from competition. Sport, however, also increases the risk of sustaining an injury, especially injuries to the teeth and mouth.
- Sports medicine physicians are in an ideal position to facilitate early intervention to preserve dental health and promote proper preventative strategies.

EPIDEMIOLOGY

- An oral injury can be defined as dental avulsions; dental fractures; dental luxations; lacerations or contusions to the gum, cheeks, tongue, and lips; and jaw injuries (fracture, locked open or closed, temporomandibular joint (TMJ) pain, and chewing difficulty). A concussion from a blow under the chin can also be included (9).
- Contact sports, such as basketball, hockey, and football, have a great risk of orofacial-related injuries. These injuries are the result of an increased risk of body-to-body or object/surface-to-oral cavity contact and are incrementally compounded by the speed of the sport. According to a study by Tesini and Soporowski (15), based on 159 injuries reported by pediatric dentists during a 1-year period, the sports receiving the most orofacial injuries were baseball and biking, followed by hockey and basketball.
- Noncontact sports, such as golf, billiards, and bowling, have a much lower incidence of orofacial injury. Although not a contact sport, biking, as previously noted, has a great risk of orofacial injury (15).
- Dental trauma data report that 25% of people ages 6–50 have sustained an injury to their anterior teeth (12).
- The literature suggests that more boys than girls (3:1) are involved in orofacial sports-related injuries. Parents additionally seem more inclined to have their sons wear mouthguards as opposed to their daughters (15).
- Studies have also shown that by the time a student graduates from secondary school, one out of three boys and one out of four girls will have suffered from a traumatic dental injury (15).

- Injury rates appear to be highest from about 7 to 14 years of age (6).

ANATOMY

- The tooth is composed of three layers: enamel, dentin, and the pulp chamber (Fig. 32.1).
- The enamel is the most external layer of the three. Enamel protects the crown of the tooth because of its hardness and structure.
- The next layer is called the dentin. The dentin is softer than the enamel and has dentinal tubules that contain neurovascular structures. When dentin is exposed, it is very prone to decay.
- The internal structure of a tooth is the pulp. The pulp contains the blood vessels and nerves that supply the tooth from the jaw.
- The *periodontal ligament* (PDL) connects the alveolar bone to the root and anchors the tooth in the socket.

FIELD-SIDE ASSESSMENT

- It is important not to overlook dental injuries as part of the sideline evaluation (4,14).
- Initial examination should be external, beginning with checking for lacerations of the head or injury to the neck. The TMJ can be externally palpated while the patient opens and closes the jaw. The opening pattern should be closely evaluated to check for deviation, which could indicate a unilateral mandibular fracture. Palpation of the zygomatic arch, angle, and lower border of the mandible should be checked for tenderness, swelling, and bruising to rule out bone fracture.
- Intraoral examination of the lips, tongue, cheek, palate, and floor of the mouth should be done to check for laceration. Tenderness, swelling, and bruising of the facial and lingual gingiva need to be checked. The anterior border of the ramus can be palpated intraorally.
- If there is a laceration to the lip or tongue, it must be palpated and, if need be, radiographed to rule out embedded foreign bodies.

Longitudinal Section of a Tooth

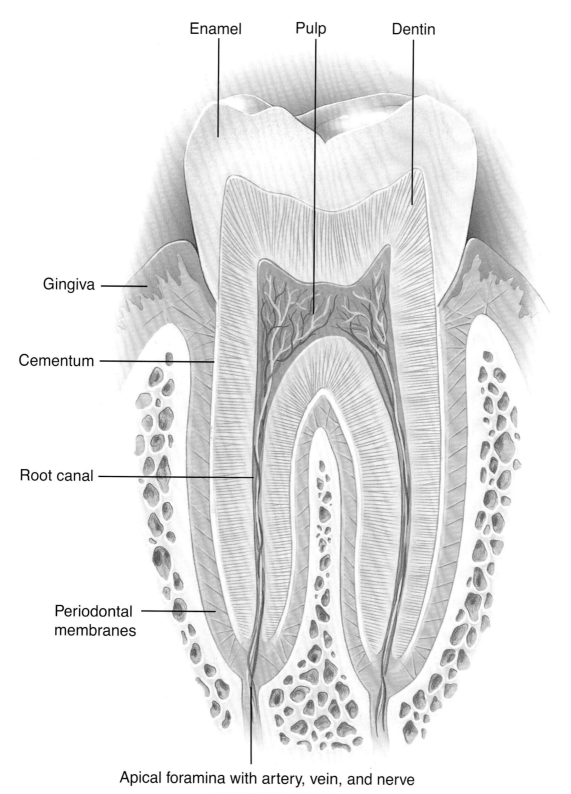

Enamel   Pulp   Dentin

Gingiva

Cementum

Root canal

Periodontal
membranes

Apical foramina with artery, vein, and nerve

Figure 32.1: Anatomy of the tooth.

SPECIFIC INJURIES

Trauma

- Maxillomandibular relationships can increase risk for oro-facial injury. Many studies have shown that the orthodontic status increases the rate of incisal trauma. A class 11 molar relationship (a malocclusion where the upper teeth protrude past the lower teeth, also called an *overbite* or *buck teeth*), having an overjet greater than 4 mm, having a short upper lip, having incompetent lips, and being a mouth breather will increase the chance of dental injury. A referral to an orthodontist to evaluate for orthodontic correction to reduce such risks is very important (14).

- A tooth fracture can be classified as a root fracture, crown fracture, or a chipped tooth. The most serious complication of the tooth fracture would involve injury to the pulp. Pulpal involvement can be seen by examining the fractured area and looking for a bleeding spot or a red dot. This type of involvement can be painful, so care should be taken not to expose the tooth to air, saliva, and temperature changes. A patient with such a tooth fracture involving injury to the pulp should see their dentist for an examination and treatment on an emergent basis. A patient with dentin involvement should also not return to play and seek immediate dental attention. A patient with enamel-only involvement does not need immediate referral and can return to normal play with a protective mouthguard but must see a dentist for follow-up within 24 hours.

- A tooth with a minor chip and without displacement does not need immediate dental attention but should be evaluated at a near future date, preferably within 24–48 hours (7). Any tooth fragments that can be saved should be given to the patient to bring to the dental examination.

- Intrusion is the most complicated and controversial type of luxation injury. If the intrusion is > 6 mm, then the prognosis is extremely poor. The eventual outcome of an intrusive injury depends on the severity of the injury, concurrent crown fracture, and treatment methods. The permanent tooth loss of severe intrusions is quite possible. This type of injury needs an immediate referral to a dentist. The tooth should not be attempted to be put back in correct position (14).

- A tooth that has had an extrusion injury will interfere with normal occlusion — the patient seems to contact prematurely on the injured tooth. The displaced tooth will be in front of or behind the normal tooth row. These teeth will be quite painful to return to normal position; therefore, these patients need immediate dental evaluation, treatment, and follow-up. An extruded tooth may be gently attempted to be repositioned in the field if not too painful (14,16).

- An avulsed tooth is a tooth that has completely come out of the socket. The tooth has been separated from the socket, and often, there are vital PDL cells on the root surface. The prognosis is much higher for successful reimplantation if the tooth is not given a chance to dry out. The tooth must first be located; it may be in the patient's mouth, on their clothing, or near the injury site. The avulsed tooth should be handled very carefully — only by the crown/enamel, therefore not causing further damage to the root surface. The tooth should be implanted within the first 20 minutes of injury to increase success of reimplantation. Immediate reimplantation onsite gives the best prognosis but requires onsite knowledge of emergency treatment (7). The tooth should be gently cleansed with saline and repositioned in the socket, if the patient is alert. The tooth will click into place, but make sure the tooth is properly positioned. After reimplantation onsite temporary splinting can be done with aluminum foil, silly putty, or chewing gum to the surrounding teeth (7). The athlete should then follow up with a dentist immediately for definitive diagnosis and management (10).

- If reimplantation is not able to be done onsite, then a proper medium for tooth transport is critical, and immediate referral to a dentist is necessary because speed of treatment affects prognosis. A tooth that has been out of the mouth for greater than 30 minutes decreases chance of survival. If the tooth is reimplanted within 15–30 minutes, there is a 90% chance the tooth will be retained for life (6).

- The most suitable transport medium is Hank's balanced salt solution (HBSS) because of its pH-preserving fluid and trauma-reducing suspension. Save-a-Tooth (Biologic Rescue Products, Conshohocken, PA) is one HBSS-type product. HBSS should be readily available at schools, in emergency rooms, in athletic coach trainer kits, and at private medical offices.

- If HBSS is not available, then milk, saliva, and physiologic saline are good alternatives. Tap water is not a good alternative because it can cause periodontal cell death within minutes (7). Cool milk has been shown to work as a better medium than warm milk. Also, getting the tooth into a medium within the first 15 minutes increases cell survival and reimplantation success (16).

- Primary avulsed teeth should not be reimplanted because this could injure the permanent tooth follicle (6).

Infection

- Pulpitis is when an inflamed pulp becomes necrotic, causing inflammation around the apex of the tooth. The tooth will then have localized pain and swelling and sensitivity to percussion. Referral to dentist for either a root canal or extraction is needed. Pain medication may be given, but antibiotics are not necessary (6).

- An apical abscess is localized, but if not treated, a cellulitis may follow. Cellulitis is a diffuse painful swelling. This infection may spread into the fascial spaces of the head and neck, possibly causing airway problems. The infection may spread to the periorbital area with complications, such as loss of vision, cavernous sinus thrombosis, and central nervous system (CNS) involvement. A patient with cellulitis should be placed on antibiotics, and incision and drainage should be performed whether cellulitis is indurated or fluctuant to allow for a pathway of drainage.

- Patients with severe swelling in the head/neck with possible airway compromise often need hospitalization. These patients will need surgical drainage and intravenous broad-spectrum antibiotics immediately.

- Periodontal disease is an inflammatory destructive process resulting in loss of attachment of tooth and bone. The PDL and alveolar bone are destroyed by bacterial plaque. Athletes with evidence of periodontal disease should be referred to the care of a periodontist.

- Dental decay or caries is caused by oral bacterial demineralizing tooth enamel and dentin. The acid production from the fermentation of dietary carbohydrates by oral bacteria demineralizes the tooth. Dental caries begins with no symptoms but can be seen as opaque areas on the enamel that progress to brownish cavities (11).

- Antibiotics should be prescribed for most sport-related and through-and-through oral lacerations. They are also recommended when there is an avulsed tooth, root fracture, or fracture of alveolar bone, mandible, or maxilla. Amoxicillin clavulanate or a cephalosporin is recommended (12).

Prevention

- A properly fitted mouthguard should be protective, comfortable, resilient, tear resistant, odorless, tasteless, not bulky, cause minimal interference to speaking and breathing, and have excellent retention, fit, and sufficient thickness in critical areas. Mouthguards are worn in football, and football has been reported to have 0.07% orofacial injuries. On the contrary, in basketball where mouthguards are not routinely worn, the orofacial injury rate is 34% (5). The American Dental Association (ADA) estimates mouthguards have prevented 200,000 injuries per year. A properly fitting mouthguard will protect the teeth and may reduce the incidence of concussion from a blow to the jaw (11).

- Overall injury reduction from a recent literature review was noted to be between 1.6- and 1.9-fold (8).

- The literature to this point does not support mouthguards preventing concussions (2).

- There are four types of mouthguards: stock, boil and bite, vacuum custom, and pressure laminated custom.

- Stock mouthguards are available at most sporting good stores and are the least expensive and least protective. They are ready to use out of the package but considered bulky and have little retention.

- Boil and bite mouthguards are the most common on the market. The mouthguard is immersed in boiling water and formed in the mouth by fingers, tongue, and biting pressure. This mouthguard does not cover all the posterior teeth, decreasing the protective qualities and possibly increasing concussion chance.

- Custom mouthguards are made by a dentist after a complete dental examination and proper questioning. An impression is taken of the athlete's mouth, allowing the dentist to make a stone cast of the mouth. A single-layer thermoplastic mouthguard material is adapted over the cast. A vacuum custom mouthguard can be made in the office.

- Increased evidence has shown that a multilayer guard or laboratory pressure laminated guard may be preferred to a single-layer guard. These either can be made by the dentist in the office if proper materials are available or need to be sent to a qualified laboratory.

- When properly worn, helmets and facemasks will increase safety and decrease morbidity. They protect the skin and bones of the head and face. Full face shields should be worn in hockey because wearing half shields is associated with a 2.31% increased risk of facial laceration and 9.90% increased risk of dental injury (3).

- The ADA recommends mouthguard use for 29 sports: acrobatics, basketball, bicycling, boxing, equestrian, extreme sports, field events, field hockey, football, gymnastics, handball, ice hockey, inline skating, lacrosse, martial arts, racquetball, rugby, shot putting, skateboarding, skiing, skydiving, soccer, softball, squash, surfing, volleyball, water polo, weightlifting, and wrestling (1).

- Injury rates in football have gone from 50% to less than 1% since the onset of mouthguard and face mask use (9).

- In athletes who are undergoing orthodontic treatment (braces are a greater risk for orofacial injuries), a custom mouthguard is indicated (9).

- Compliance can be a problem with mouthguard use — coaches, parents, and athletic trainers are encouraged to explain to the athletes the benefit of mouthguard use (13).

DENTAL MAINTENANCE

- It is important for athletes as well as the general public to have regular dental checkups. An initial comprehensive dental examination should be performed, including chief complaint, health history, intraoral and extraoral examination, and radiographs where applicable; then the dentist will recommend a recall schedule as needed dictated by the evaluation.

- Oral jewelry has become a recent fad with the youth of this country. Dental professionals are advised to give these patients information about the problems that can occur with the jewelry. Tongue piercing can cause teeth fractures and also gingival stripping. Dental professionals should also inform patients that the jewelry should be removed prior to any contact sports participation.

- Dentists can also screen patients who are using smokeless (spit) tobacco and inform them that it is not a safe substitute for smoking.

■ Anorexia and bulimia nervosa can also be picked up during routine dental checkup. The clinical signs are erosion of the lingual enamel of the teeth, bilateral swelling of the parotid gland, and floating amalgam because of quicker erosion of enamel versus metal.

■ It is important for patients to follow through with any recommended dental treatment, thereby preventing any future problems.

REFERENCES

1. American Dental Association. For the dental patient. The importance of using mouthguards. Tips for keeping your smile safe. *J Am Dent Assoc.* 2004;135(7):1061.

2. Benson BW, Hamilton GW, Meeuwisse WH, McCrory P, Dvorak J. Is protective equipment useful in preventing concussion? A systematic review of the literature. *Br J Sports Med.* 2009;43(supp 1):i56–67.

3. Benson BW, Mohtadi NG, Rose MS, Meeuwisse WH. Head and neck injury among ice hockey players wearing full face shields vs half face shields. *JAMA.* 1999;282(24):2328–32.

4. Cohen S, Burns RC. Traumatic injuries. In: Cohen S, Burns RC, editors. *Pathways of the Pulp.* 8th ed. St. Louis: Mosby; 2002. p. 605.

5. Dorn SO. Sports dentistry for endodontists. *J Endod.* 2002;28(9):669.

6. Douglas AB, Douglas JM. Common dental emergencies. *Am Fam Physician.* 2003;67(3):511–6.

7. Kenny DJ, Barrett EJ. Recent developments in dental traumatology. *Pediatr Dent.* 2001;23(6):464–8.

8. Knapik JJ, Marshall SW, Lee RB, et al. Mouth guards in sports activities: history, physical properties and injury prevention effectiveness. *Sports Med.* 2007;37(2):117–44.

9. Kvittem B, Hardie NA, Roettger M, Conry J. Incidence of orofacial injuries in high school sports. *J Public Health Dent.* 1998;58(4):288–93.

10. Lee JY, Vann WF Jr, Sigurdsson A. Management of avulsed permanent incisors: a decision analysis based on hanging concepts. *Pediatr Dent.* 2001;23(4):357–60.

11. Padilla RR. Sports Dentistry site [Internet]. Dental communications; [cited 2010 Nov 1]. Available from: http://www.sportsdentistry.com.

12. Ranalli DN. Dental injuries in sports. *Curr Sports Med Rep.* 2005;4(1):12–7.

13. Ranalli DN. Sports dentistry and dental traumatology. *Dent Traumatol.* 2002;18(5):231–6.

14. Roberts WO. Field care of the injured tooth. *Phys Sportsmed.* 2000;28(1):101–2.

15. Tesini D, Soporowski N. Epidemiology of orofacial sports-related injuries. In: Holland K, editor. *The Dental Clinic of North America Advances in Sports Dentistry.* Philadelphia: Saunders; 2000. p 8.

16. Trope M. Clinical management of the avulsed tooth: present strategies and future directions. *Dent Traumatol.* 2002;18(1):1–11.

Infectious Disease and the Athlete 33

Mark D. Harris and Thomas M. Howard

INTRODUCTION

- Sports participation has increased 7% in the United States since 1999 (44).
- Many athletes and providers associate sports medicine with orthopedic injuries, but up to 50% of visits to high school and college training rooms are for infectious diseases (41).
- Seventy-six percent of Masters athletes in one study perceived themselves to be less vulnerable than their sedentary peers to viral illnesses (55).
- Many studies suggest a drop in upper respiratory tract infection (URTI) incidence in moderate exercisers compared to sedentary people (11,33,34), some by as much as 20%–30% (40).
- Special needs athletes have fewer infections than nonathletes with similar needs (25).

IMMUNOLOGY AND EXERCISE

- The immune system includes the innate immune system, which provides nonspecific but immediate response to a wide variety of pathogens, and the acquired immune system, which provides delayed-onset but precisely targeted immunity (1).
- The innate immune system includes infection-fighting cells such as natural killer (NK) cells, phagocytes (neutrophils, monocytes, and macrophages), tumor necrosis factor, other cytokines, and complement factors (1). It includes barriers such as the skin, mucous membranes, and nasal hairs. Areas of turbulent airflow, temperature and pH, and pathogen and debris removal systems, such as the gastrointestinal tract and the mucociliary elevator, are also important parts of the innate immune system (7). Barriers can be breeched by environmental conditions, such as sun, wind, humidity, temperature, and trauma.
- The acquired immune system is composed of B and T lymphocytes, the immunoglobulins (Ig) that they produce, and cytokines that regulate the immune response (1). Secretory IgA in mucus is an especially important early defense (30).
- Nasal breathing allows moderate volumes of air to be warmed, hydrated, and filtered by the nasal mucosa, hairs, and turbulent air flow. This removes harmful particles for disposal via expectoration, sneezing, coughing, or gastrointestinal elimination (8).

- During strenuous exercise, the body's requirement for oxygen increases and the athlete transitions from nose breathing to mouth breathing. This brings in greater volumes of air but overloads or bypasses the warming and filtering mechanisms. Colder and drier air thickens the mucus and disrupts the mucociliary elevator while absence of filtering causes more foreign particles to be deposited in the lower airways (8). The ability of airways to remove them is also diminished, and airway inflammation is a common result (5).
- Moderate exercise, defined as exercise for 5–60 minutes within a range of 40%–60% of maximum heart rate (MHR), improves many aspects of immunity. Neutrophil and NK cell counts and salivary IgA increase with moderate exercise (7,8,30,45,46).
- Intense exercise, defined as 5–60 min of exercise at 70%–80% of MHR, and prolonged exercise, often defined as greater than 60 minutes, can have detrimental effects on the immune system (7). Cellular immunity is impaired because cortisol and adrenaline concentrations chronically increase (9). Immunomodulators prolactin and growth hormone also increase, but the result is less clear. The function of lymphocytes and B cells decreases, as do neutrophil counts. CD4–CD8 T-cell ratios are normally about 1.5:1 but decrease after intense or long-duration exercise, diminishing immune effectiveness (8). Prolonged, intense exercise causes NK cell number concentrations to fall (41). Salivary lactoferrin and lysozyme concentrations fall (62). Serum neutrophil levels decline (64), and nasal and salivary IgA concentrations fall (47), as do serum IgG and IgE concentrations (42).

INFECTIONS AND EXERCISE

- Infections can compromise athletes' ability to perform (8). Fever impairs coordination, concentration, muscle strength, and aerobic power (41). It also hinders fluid and temperature regulation and endurance. Viral illnesses contribute to tissue wasting, muscle catabolism, and negative nitrogen balance (41).
- Drugs commonly used to treat symptoms of infectious disease can also affect athletes. Acetaminophen is generally safe, but antibiotics can cause diarrhea, and quinolones may be associated with tendon rupture. Antihistamines can cause sedation, and usage of ephedrine-containing compounds, banned by many sports organizations, will lead to positive

drug tests and disqualification of an athlete during the competitive season (31,41).

- Fever can be treated with acetaminophen (up to 4 g per day divided into doses every 4–6 hrs) or nonsteroidal anti-inflammatory drugs (NSAIDs), such as ibuprofen or indomethacin. In dehydrated patients, NSAIDs may contribute to renal insufficiency.

RHINORRHEA AND NASAL CONGESTION

Upper Respiratory Tract Infections

- Adults usually get one to six URTIs per year, and athletes are no exception, with URTIs predominating even at Olympic competition (24). They are generally viral and are transmitted by direct contact, usually hand to nose, eyes, or mouth. Transmission occasionally occurs via small-particle aerosols and large-particle droplets. Rhinovirus (10%–40%), coronavirus (20%), and respiratory syncytial virus (10%) are the most common causes (49). In closed communities, such as locker rooms, one index patient can infect 25%–70% of exposed teammates (49).

- URTI diagnosis is clinical, with symptoms including nasal congestion, sore throat, cough, and fatigue (56). Physical findings include rhinorrhea with boggy nasal mucosa and oropharyngeal erythema. Fever greater than 100.4°F is unusual (24). The incubation period is usually 1–3 days, and symptoms usually last 3–7 days. Complications include bacterial sinusitis (2.5%), asthma exacerbations (up to 40%), and lower respiratory infections (49).

- Treatment is symptomatic, including fluids, nonnarcotic pain control, and decongestants or antihistamines as needed. Saline nose rinses can improve symptoms (53). If the URTI can be traced to a specific pathogen, such as influenza, antivirals, such as oseltamivir, can be useful (9).

- Handwashing with soap and water or use of alcohol-based hand sanitizers minimizes transmission. Good nutrition, moderate exercise, good hydration, and adequate sleep contribute to good health. Symptomatic individuals should cough or sneeze on their sleeve, not on their hand, and avoid public gatherings when possible (http://www.cdc.gov/flu/protect/covercough.htm).

- Influenza vaccine has an efficacy of 70%–90% in the under 65 population, so every athlete should get immunized annually (38). One study suggested that exercise might improve response to influenza immunization (17).

- The "neck check" described later is a good rule of thumb to decide when to send an athlete back to play.

Sinusitis

- Sinusitis is inflammation of the paranasal sinuses, especially the maxillary and frontal sinuses. It is usually viral and self-limited and is a common complication of URTI, affecting 16% of U.S. adults annually (49).

- Bacterial sinusitis can be caused by *Haemophilus influenzae, Streptococcus pneumoniae, Moraxella catarrhalis, Staphylococcus aureus,* and other less common bacteria. Seventy-five percent of cases of bacterial sinusitis will spontaneously resolve within 1 month (49). Swimmers, divers, water polo players, and surfers seem to be more likely to develop sinusitis (41).

- Fever, purulent nasal discharge, maxillary toothache, sinus pain, and sinus tenderness to palpation suggest a bacterial cause (8,28). Patients who develop a URTI and improve for several days and then abruptly worsen again are more likely to have a bacterial sinus infection (24).

- The Berg Prediction Rule considers purulent rhinorrhea and sinus pain, unilateral and bilateral, in determining the likelihood of bacterial sinusitis (54).

- Bacterial sinusitis is best treated with antibiotics, such as amoxicillin or trimethoprim-sulfamethoxazole (28). Second-line agents include doxycycline, clarithromycin, or amoxicillin clavulanate. The standard course is 10–14 days, but some studies suggest that a 3-day course is sufficient (41). Treatment of viral sinusitis is symptomatic, similar to that for URTI, but saline nasal spray can dilute thick mucus and provide short-term relief (53).

- The "neck check" is a useful return-to-play guideline for sinusitis.

COUGH

Acute Bronchitis

- Acute bronchitis is characterized by inflammation of the bronchial tree with cough lasting up to 3 weeks, with or without sputum production, in the presence of URTI (2). More than 10 million office visits per year are diagnosed as acute bronchitis (36). The same viruses that cause URTI cause 90% of acute bronchitis cases, and the last 10% generally involve bacteria such as *Bordetella pertussis, Mycoplasma pneumoniae,* and *Chlamydia pneumoniae* (36). Patients with bronchitis complain of cough as the dominant symptom. Fever can be present but more likely represents influenza or pneumonia.

- Treatment is symptomatic, and antibiotics are rarely indicated. Bronchodilators may be useful to improve respiratory flow dynamics, which are often temporarily impaired (2), especially in patients with exercise-induced bronchospasm or asthma (35). Antitussive medications lack proof of effectiveness (2).

- Return to play can be complicated by postbronchitic airway inflammation. Inhaled steroids or bronchodilators may be helpful.

Pneumonia

- Pneumonia is a lower respiratory tract infection caused by viruses in 30%–50% of cases and by bacteria in the rest of cases in healthy adults (41). Community-acquired pneumonia affects about 12 people per 1,000 population per year (37), and fever, productive cough, malaise, anorexia and myalgias are common complaints. In severe cases, patients may show tachypnea, nasal flaring, intercostal and neck retractions, rales, abnormal pulse oximetry, and cyanosis. Chest x-ray (CXR) may show infiltrates, and complete blood count (CBC) may show leukocytosis with a left shift (36).

■ Clinical prediction tools such as the Pneumonia severity index (PSI) or PORT score and the CURB-65/CRB-65 can help clinicians decide on inpatient or outpatient therapy (16). The PSI/PORT score predicts severity based on the patient's demographics, comorbidities, examinations, and laboratory or radiologic findings. The CURB-65/CRB-65 predicts severity based on the patient's mental status, blood urea nitrogen, respiratory rate, blood pressure, and age.

■ Macrolides are the first choice for oral outpatient therapy. Patients with more severe disease should be hospitalized; however, even in the inpatient setting, intravenous antibiotics did not outperform oral antibiotics in patients without life-threatening illness (37). Both influenza and pneumococcal vaccines decreased the incidence of pneumonia in immunocompetent people, especially the elderly, in several studies (37).

■ Athletes should be on strict rest while symptomatic and very gradually return to play thereafter.

SORE THROAT

Pharyngitis

■ Viruses that cause URTI cause the majority of cases of pharyngitis. Symptoms and treatment are similar to those for URTI. Other infectious causes include Epstein-Barr virus (EBV), herpes simplex virus (HSV), group A beta-hemolytic streptococci (GABHS), and rarely, *Mycoplasma* and gonococcus (10,29).

■ History should include time of onset, ill contacts, presence of URTI symptoms, throat pain, and difficulty swallowing or speaking.

■ Pharyngitis is caused by GABHS in 5%–15% of cases (29). Presenting signs include bright red, swollen tonsils with overlying white exudates. Abdominal pain, fever, and headache are sometimes present, and URTI symptoms such as cough generally are not.

■ Historically, 0.1%–3% of patients, typically children, developed rheumatic fever after a case of untreated GABHS pharyngitis (6). Other potential complications include peritonsillar abscess, otitis media, and mastoiditis.

■ The modified Centor Score is a clinical decision rule that can aid in management of pharyngitis (10). It considers age, fever, tonsillar exudates, cervical lymphadenopathy, and presence or absence of cough and provides a percentage risk of GABHS. Rapid strep screening tests are up to 80%–90% sensitive in diagnosing strep throat (24).

■ Penicillin (500 mg twice a day for 10 days) is still the first-line treatment for GABHS. Azithromycin and erythromycin are good second-line choices.

■ Patients with pharyngitis who do not have GABHS should be treated symptomatically.

■ The "neck check" can be used to guide return to play.

Infectious Mononucleosis

■ Infectious mononucleosis (IM) is an acute, self-limiting disease caused by EBV. EBV is secreted in saliva and spread by direct contact, hence the moniker "kissing disease." IM incidence peaks from ages 15–25. Eventually, 95% of adults demonstrate immunity (23).

■ IM begins with a 3- to 5-day prodrome including fatigue, headache, loss of appetite, and myalgias. Sore throat, lymphadenopathy (especially posterior cervical), and fever then develop, and these classic symptoms typically last up to 4 weeks (52). Although the physical exam can be unreliable, 50%–75% of infected patients develop palpable splenomegaly, and 10%–15% develop jaundice (23,41).

■ The false-negative rate of heterophile antibody absorption tests (Monospot) is 25% during the first week of infection and 5% by the third week, so it is important to retest patients who were Monospot negative early in their course (24). Liver function tests may show a mild hepatitis, and a complete blood count (CBC) may show mild lymphocytosis and atypical lymphocytes (52).

■ IM is treated symptomatically because antibiotics and antivirals are not effective and some antibiotics can precipitate a nonallergic rash (52). Aspirin should be avoided because of the risk of Reye syndrome. Corticosteroids should only be used in patients with significant complications, such as impending airway compromise, myocarditis, hepatitis, or neurologic involvement (23).

■ Complications are infrequent but include splenic rupture, airway obstruction, thrombocytopenia, agranulocytosis, hepatic necrosis, myocarditis, pericarditis, orchitis, and hemolytic anemia. Neurologic complications include Guillain-Barré syndrome, encephalitis, myelitis, optic neuritis, and Bell palsy (41,52).

■ Splenic rupture occurs in 0.1%–0.2% of cases (24), usually in males, in the first 21 days after infection and often without trauma or even exertion. Computed tomography and ultrasound can reliably detect spleen size, but normal spleens have significant size variability, and since most athletes do not receive baseline measurements, imaging generally is not a reliable guide for return-to-play decisions (23).

■ The American Medical Society for Sports Medicine consensus statement states that athletes should avoid all exercise for 21 days after illness onset (52). After that time, athletes should slowly begin increasing their activity, starting with walking and progressing no more than 10% per week in duration and intensity. Patients are usually recovered after 2–3 months but can take longer.

OTHER COMMON HEAD, EAR, AND EYE CONDITIONS

Otitis Media and Externa

■ Over 20 million visits to providers per year are for middle ear infections, and 20% of those patients are adults (41). Thirty percent of cases of otitis media (OM) are viral and bacterial causes included *Pneumococcus, H. influenzae,* and *M. catarrhalis* (24).

■ Patients usually present with URTI symptoms and ear pain. Most cases are self-limited, and treatment is symptomatic since antibiotics typically do not affect the course in people older than 2 years (41). Antibiotics should be used in diabetics and other immunocompromised patients or if complications such as mastoiditis occur.

■ Otitis externa (OE) is often related to repetitive water exposure, preexisting allergies, and inadequate cerumen (24). *Pseudomonas aeruginosa* is the most common identifiable cause but fungi, such as *Aspergillus,* have been implicated (24). Patients present with ear pain, especially with pulling on the tragus, and purulent discharge. Preauricular or postauricular or cervical lymphadenopathy may occur. Treatment involves cleaning the debris from the auditory canal and applying topical antibiotic/corticosteroid drops if the tympanic membrane is intact (24).

■ Athletes can decrease their risk of developing OE by avoiding sticking things into the ear canal and using isopropanol drops to dry or dilute acetic acid to acidify the external ear canal. Ear plugs are controversial.

■ Patients with OM who are involved in water sports should not return to play until the tympanic membrane is intact and has normal mobility (41). Patients with OE who are involved in water sports may return to play when asymptomatic.

Conjunctivitis

■ Many factors can cause inflammation of the conjunctiva, including foreign bodies, excessive brightness, mechanical irritation from rubbing, allergens, irritant toxins, and infections. Infectious agents are usually viruses but bacterial causes include *S. aureus, Staphylococcus epidermidis, Streptococci,* and *Haemophilus* (19).

■ Presenting symptoms include injected conjunctiva, watery eyes, and discharge. Purulent discharge suggests bacterial conjunctivitis (24). Symptoms of more serious disease include loss of visual acuity or visual field defect. Mild disease is usually self-limited, but antibiotic treatment is common because infectious conjunctivitis is highly transmissible. Patients with severe symptoms should be referred for ophthalmologic care.

■ *Neisseria gonorrhoeae* and HSV are less common and more dangerous causes. *Neisseria* must be considered in any sexually active adolescent presenting with a prominent purulent discharge (41). Discharge should be Gram stained and cultured, and parenteral antibiotics are indicated if the lab is positive. Vesicular lesions on eyelids and prominent lymphadenopathy suggest HSV conjunctivitis. Immediate ophthalmologic consultation is indicated (41).

■ Infected athletes should be excluded from competition in high-contact sports (such as wrestling) until the infection has completely cleared. Because adenovirus can be transmitted in chlorinated pool water, infected water sports athletes should also be kept out of the water (41).

Meningitis

■ The meninges, the tissue layers covering the brain and spinal cord, are typically infected via local extension of infection and hematogenous spread. There are two primary categories of meningitis: septic meningitis, usually caused by bacteria such as *Pneumococcus, Neisseria meningitidis,* or *H. influenzae* B, and aseptic meningitis (4). Septic or bacterial meningitis is almost universally fatal if untreated and often has a poor outcome even with treatment. Even in developed countries with advanced medical treatment, 14% of patients recovering from bacterial meningitis have residual hearing loss, and 4% have hemiparesis (4).

■ Aseptic meningitis is much more common. It is defined as "clinical and laboratory evidence for meningeal inflammation with negative routine bacterial cultures." Enteroviruses such as coxsackie virus are responsible for 55%–70% of cases (24). Other viruses, fungi, protozoa, other bacteria (tuberculosis), *Rickettsia,* and even noninfectious causes are seen. Aseptic meningitis is most common during summer and fall, when enteroviridae, transmitted by the fecal–oral route, are most likely to be passed (41).

■ Fever, stiff neck, and headache form the "classic triad" of meningitis, but only 44% of patients present with the triad (4). Nausea, vomiting, pharyngitis, diarrhea, and photophobia are common, but focal neurologic signs and mental status changes are especially worrisome. In the presence of these more serious symptoms, the patient should be sent to emergency care.

■ Prevention is a must for this life-threatening disease. Good hand washing and avoiding shared water bottles help decrease fecal–oral transmission. Immunization against *H. influenzae* and *N. meningitidis* are important as well.

MYOCARDITIS

■ An uncommon complication of systemic infections, myocarditis usually follows infection with such viruses as coxsackie virus, adenovirus, hepatitis C virus (HCV), cytomegalovirus, influenza virus, echovirus, and EBV (36). It can also be caused by bacteria, such as *Mycoplasma* and *Chlamydia,* and even noninfectious agents, such as cocaine. Men between 20 and 40 are at the highest risk (9).

■ In animal models, strenuous exercise while febrile has been associated with the development of myocarditis. This may be true in humans as well (41).

■ The disease course usually begins with a common cold or other viral infection. Over time, chest pain, fatigue, fever, and palpitations may develop. In severe cases, the patient can develop symptoms of heart failure, including dependent edema, shortness of breath, paroxysmal nocturnal dyspnea, and orthopnea (39). Muffled heart sounds, mitral regurgitation, and a pericardial friction rub (if the pericardium is also involved) can occur on exam. Electrocardiogram may demonstrate nonspecific ST and T wave abnormalities, and echocardiogram may show globally decreased ventricular function (36).

■ Myocarditis is typically self-limiting, but rarely, patients develop dilated cardiomyopathy and heart failure. Athletes unfortunate enough to develop this complication will usually completely recover but while infected, they are at increased risk for arrhythmias and sudden cardiac death (39).

■ If myocarditis is suspected or confirmed, providers should immediately withdraw the patient from all competitive sports and avoid all strenuous activity for 6 months since becoming symptomatic. Athletes may return to exercise once their echocardiogram and electrocardiogram are completely normal, they have no arrhythmias, and they have no serum evidence of heart failure or inflammation (39).

GASTROENTERITIS

■ Spending large amounts of time in congregate settings, such as locker rooms and team buses, competitive athletes commonly share food and water, travel and live in close quarters, and share personal care items. These practices contribute to the spread of infectious disease, especially respiratory and gastrointestinal disease.

■ FoodNet reported in 2001 that an estimated 76 million cases of foodborne illness occur each year in the United States (27). After URTI, gastroenteritis is the most common infection in adolescents and young adults (43). Bacteria, such as *Escherichia coli* and *Salmonella*, and protozoa, such as *Cryptosporidium* and *Giardia lamblia*, can cause gastroenteritis, but the most common causative organisms are viruses (rotavirus, Norwalk virus). Because transmission is usually fecal–oral, good health practices can break the chain and prevent disease.

■ Athletes with acute gastroenteritis present with diarrhea, abdominal cramps, nausea, and vomiting. Myalgias and fevers commonly occur (43). If severe or untreated, significant dehydration can occur, resulting in dry mucous membranes, very dark yellow urine or low volume of urine, and tenting of the skin. Patients who are more than 3%–5% dehydrated

should receive oral rehydration fluid if they can tolerate oral intake and intravenous fluids if they cannot (15). Isotonic sports drinks can be helpful, and cool water is fine in most cases. Patients with mild or moderate dehydration can generally be rehydrated orally. Myalgias, fevers, and other symptoms are treated symptomatically, and gastroenteritis usually resolves spontaneously in 3–4 days. Antimotility drugs, such as loperamide, can help patients who must maintain their activity. "Traveler's diarrhea" can be prevented with bismuth subsalicylate or antibiotics (26).

■ Antibiotic treatment should be used judiciously in acute infectious gastroenteritis. Viral causes do not require antibiotic treatment. *Giardia lamblia* and *Entamoeba histolytica* are best treated with antiprotozoal drugs, such as metronidazole. *Campylobacter* resolves without antimicrobials, and using antimicrobials in *E. coli* infection is frequently ineffective and can increase the risk of hemolytic uremic syndrome (27). *Salmonella* rarely requires antibiotic therapy, but antibiotics shorten the course of disease in *Shigella* infections (27).

■ A well-hydrated, asymptomatic athlete should be able to gradually return to play.

BLOODBORNE INFECTIONS

■ Human immunodeficiency virus (HIV), hepatitis B virus (HBV), and HCV are transmitted through blood and other body fluids (51). Sexual contact and needle sharing are common ways to transmit these infections. Tattooing and body piercing are also high-risk activities.

■ Since the recognition of HIV infection in 1981, there has been considerable concern about transmission through athletics. There has been one highly questionable case (32), but there has never been a documented case of HIV transmission during a sporting event (3). Sexual contact, especially men having sex with men, and needle sharing, such as when athletes share needles to inject vitamins or anabolic steroids, are the most common paths of transmission. Over 1 million Americans are infected with the HIV virus, and about 21% do not know that they are infected (61). Body fluids, such as saliva and sweat, do not appear to have HIV levels high enough to efficiently transmit the disease during sports.

■ HIV-infected patients seem to benefit from moderate exercise. Progressive resistance exercise (PRE) and moderate aerobic exercise (AE) improve $\dot{V}O_{2max}$, CD4 count, and viral load (48). PRE improves body weight and limb girth, and AE enhances lipid profiles and decreases adiposity (20). Exercise training also seems to improve overall quality of life (12).

■ The Centers for Disease Control and Prevention estimated in 2007 that nearly 43,000 Americans were newly infected with HBV (59). HBV is able to survive outside the body for more than 7 days and is resistant to alcohol, drying, temperature changes, and many detergents (32). It is approximately

100 times more infectious than HIV and can be transmitted via fomites (22). Investigators reported, in a 1982 case report, that 5 of 10 members of a sumo wrestling club at a Japanese high school contracted HBV in 1 year (51). An outbreak of HBV in an American football team infected 11 of 65 players in 19 months (51). Jaundice, fatigue, nausea and vomiting, abdominal pain, dark urine, and light stool are common presenting symptoms. Evidence of liver failure, such as ascites, peripheral edema, and encephalopathy, may be the presenting complaints in severe infections. Interferon and some antivirals are effective treatments.

■ The HBV vaccine is 95% effective and is strongly recommended, especially in high-risk collision sports and for health care staff, such as team physicians and athletic trainers (3). Some patients will clear HBV, but others go on to a chronic carrier state, which in 20% of cases will result in death.

■ HCV is the most common bloodborne infection in the United States, with 3.2 million people infected (60). One case report exists of HCV transmission transmitted by sharing a bloody rag during a fist fight (9), but no cases of HCV transmission during sports have been reported. Three soccer players from an amateur club were infected with HCV from sharing needles to inject vitamin complexes (51). Symptoms are very similar to HBV, and the treatments are also similar.

■ Universal precautions should be strictly followed to minimize the risk of transmission.

■ Routine screening of athletes for HIV is not recommended (3), and asymptomatic HIV infection is not grounds for exclusion from competition (12).

■ For HBV and HCV, there are no restrictions to play as long as the athlete is in good general health (3,25).

SEXUALLY TRANSMITTED DISEASES

■ As estimated by the U.S. Centers for Disease Control and Prevention, 2.3 million U.S. civilians ages 14–39 are infected with chlamydia (57). These people are usually asymptomatic but may complain of discharge, increased urinary frequency, or pain with urination. Azithromycin and doxycycline are generally effective treatments, but failure to treat can result in pelvic inflammatory disease and permanent sterility in women. Chlamydia infection increases the likelihood of becoming infected with HIV (9). All sexually active women age 25 and younger or those with new sexual partners should be tested every year.

■ There are about 700,000 new cases of gonorrhea annually in the United States, making it one of the most common sexually transmitted diseases (58). Vaginal or urethral discharge, increased urinary frequency, and pain with urination occur, but as with chlamydia, most cases are asymptomatic. Gonorrhea can also increase the risk of HIV (9). It is readily treatable with antibiotics, such as ceftriaxone. There are no screening recommendations.

■ Human papillomavirus (HPV) is a common sexually transmitted virus that causes venereal warts and cervical cancer. The HPV vaccine dramatically decreases the risk of cancer and is recommended for nonpregnant women between ages 9 and 26 (9).

REPORTABLE DISEASES

■ HIV, hepatitis A virus (HAV), HBV, HCV, chlamydia, and gonorrhea are reportable diseases, as are meningococcus and many others.

■ Every health care facility should have a reporting mechanism. It is extremely important to be aware of and report reportable diseases.

EXERCISE IN UNUSUAL PLACES

■ In the 21st century, many are pushing the envelope in sports participation. Marathons used to be the longest running races, but ultramarathons up to 100 miles and triathlons combining marathons with swimming and bicycle racing have entered the mainstream (65). Many of these events occur in developing countries and away from areas of good sanitation and medical care.

■ Infectious disease threats, such as malaria, cholera, and dengue, rare or nonexistent in the developed world, are prevalent. Pretrip vaccinations, chemoprophylaxis, and other interventions are important. Clinicians caring for these athletes should add travel medicine to their list of skills and address the athlete's needs both before and after the trip.

IMMUNE MODULATORS

■ Because high-intensity and long-duration exercise is associated with relative immunosuppression, athletes, coaches, and sports medicine providers seek ways to keep athletes healthy and to help them win. Athletes in sports such as long-distance running, swimming, cycling, and cross-country skiing are especially prone to respiratory infectious disease.

■ A military study in 2005 found that a novel nutritional immune formula (NNIF), including vitamin C, zinc, vitamin E, folic acid, biotin, vitamin A, and selenium, improved many aspects of the immune response, including improving the delayed-type hypersensitivity response, increasing proportions of T-helper cells, improving activation of B cells, enhancing phagocytosis, and attenuating declines in certain functional populations of white blood cells (63)

■ Zinc does not seem to be able to prevent URTIs, but using zinc gluconate lozenges shortly after the onset of symptoms seems to be associated with a shorter duration and lower intensity of symptoms (41).

- Carbohydrates are important because no athlete can compete successfully without adequate energy stores, and the immune system function seems to be increased in athletes taking ample carbohydrates before, during, and after intense exercise (46). However, there is no reliable evidence that increasing carbohydrate ingestion prevents or mitigates infections.

- Vitamin C improves iron absorption in the gastrointestinal tract, and therefore is useful in iron-deficient patients. Endurance athletes, the ones most likely to develop weakened immunity as a result of their exercise, are also the ones most likely to develop iron deficiency (41). One South African study suggested that vitamin C supplementation led to fewer reports of URTI (50). However, the overall evidence that vitamin C decreases an athlete's risk of infectious disease is very weak.

- Echinacea accounts for about 10% of the total market. A few studies suggest that, if started immediately after symptom onset, it may be effective for truncating the course of viral URTIs. As with zinc gluconate, echinacea does not show promise in preventing viral URTIs. Allergic reactions and even anaphylaxis can occur, but overall, side effects are rare.

- Glutamine, a nucleoside precursor, is produced in lung, skeletal muscle, and gastrointestinal mucosa and ingested in meats and greens. It is important in synthesis of antibodies and interleukin-2 and proliferation of B and T lymphocytes. As with many other immune factors mentioned earlier, short episodes of exercise increase glutamine levels, but prolonged exercise decreases levels. Overtrained athletes often have marked glutamine depletion, and glutamine levels are a common diagnostic marker for overtraining syndrome. While adequate stores are important, it is not clear if supplementation helps prevent infection (21).

- Throat sprays: Endurance athletes often have chronic airway inflammation, and some believe that such chronic inflammation contributes to the development of URTIs. One study showed that Difflam Forte, a combination antibacterial/anti-inflammatory throat spray, decreased the incidence and severity of URTI in marathon participants (13).

- *Lactobacillus* powders: IgA is an important component of immunity at the mucosal level, but mucosal concentrations of secretory IgA decrease after intense exercise. A recent study compared the use of freeze-dried capsules of *Lacto fermentum* with placebo in a group of runners. The treatment group demonstrated a reduction in the duration and severity of URTI (14).

RETURN TO PLAY

- Physicians should adopt the "neck check" to guide return-to-play decisions (18). Athletes with symptoms only above the neck (runny nose, sore throat) may exercise at low intensity for 10 minutes. If the symptoms worsen, the athlete should stop exercise until symptoms improve. If the symptoms do not worsen, he or she can continue the workout at 50% intensity. Over time, the athlete can gradually increase to full training. Athletes with symptoms below the neck (fever, gastrointestinal symptoms, fatigue) should not exercise until all below-the-neck symptoms have resolved (18).

- When recovering from an illness, athletes should begin at no more than 50% intensity and gradually increase to preillness training levels over several days.

- Training delay serves to avoid training while systemic symptoms that limit training benefit and predispose to injury are ongoing. It allows athletes, coaches, and medical providers to grasp the true severity of the illness (18). Finally, it may prevent the spread of disease to other athletes.

- Return-to-play recommendations, especially the "neck check" and restrictions on play after mononucleosis and myocarditis, are important to know.

CONCLUSION

- Infectious disease is a major cause of morbidity in athletes, sometimes requiring them to miss important competitions and occasionally threatening their athletic career or even their lives.

- Sports medicine providers must be well versed in the epidemiology, presentation, treatment, and prevention of infectious disease in their athletes. Further, they must be aware of the risk of disease outbreaks in their sporting populations, especially with teams who live and travel in congregate settings.

- Vaccines and good public health practices are vital.

- Sports clinicians who meet the challenge will provide the best possible care for their athletes, the best chance of winning for their team, and the most professional success and satisfaction for themselves.

REFERENCES

1. Abbas AK, Lichtman AH. *Basic Immunology*. Philadelphia (PA): Saunders Elsevier; 2010. 312 p.
2. Albert RH. Diagnosis and treatment of acute bronchitis. *Am Fam Physician*. 2010;82(11):1345–50.
3. American Academy of Pediatrics Committee on Sports Medicine and Fitness. Human immunodeficiency virus and other blood borne viral pathogens in the athletic setting. *Pediatrics*. 1999;104(6):1400–3.
4. Bamberger DM. Diagnosis, initial management and prevention of meningitis. *Am Fam Physician*. 2010;82(12):1491–8.
5. Belda J, Ricart S, Casan P, et al. Airway inflammation in the elite athlete and type of sport. *Br J Sports Med*. 2008;42(4):244–8.
6. Benedek TJ. Rheumatic fever and rheumatic heart disease. In: Kiple KF, editor. *The Cambridge World History of Human Disease*. Cambridge: Cambridge University Press; 1993. p. 720.
7. Brolinson PG, Elliott D. Exercise and the immune system. *Clin Sports Med*. 2007;26(3):311–9.

8. Brukner P, Khan K. Common sports related infections. In: *Clinical Sports Medicine*. New York: McGraw Hill; 2006. p. 863–74.

9. Callahan LR, Giugliano DN. Infections in athletes. In: Madden CC, Putukian M, Young CC, McCarty EC, editors. *Netter's Sports Medicine*. Philadelphia: Saunders Elsevier; 2010. p. 197–203.

10. Choby BA. Diagnosis and treatment of streptococcal pharyngitis. *Am Fam Physician*. 2009;79(5):383–90.

11. Chubak J, McTiernan A, Sorensen B, et al. Moderate-intensity exercise reduces the incidence of colds among postmenopausal women. *Am J Med*. 2006;119(11):937–42.

12. Clem KL, Borchers JR. HIV and the athlete. *Clin Sports Med*. 2007;26(3):413–24.

13. Cox AJ, Gleeson M, Pyne DB, Saunders PU, Callister R, Pricker PA. Respiratory symptoms and inflammatory responses to Difflam throat-spray intervention in half-marathon runners: a randomized controlled trial. *Br J Sports Med*. 2010;44(2):127–33.

14. Cox AJ, Pyne DB, Saunders PU, Fricker PA. Oral administration of the probiotic Lactobacillus fermentum VRI-003 and mucosal immunity in endurance athletes. *Br J Sports Med*. 2010;44(4):222–6.

15. Divine J, Takagishi J. Exercise in the heat and heat illness. In: Madden CC, Putukian M, Young CC, McCarty EC, editors. *Netter's Sports Medicine*. Philadelphia: Saunders Elsevier; 2010. p. 136–48.

16. Ebell MH. Outpatient vs. inpatient treatment of community acquired pneumonia. *Fam Pract Manag*. 2006;13(4):41–4.

17. Edwards KM, Burns VE, Reynolds T, Carroll D, Drayson M, Ring C. Acute stress exposure prior to influenza vaccination enhances antibody response in women. *Brain Behav Immun*. 2006;20(2):159–68.

18. Eichner R. Infection, immunity, and exercise: what to tell patients. *Phys Sportsmed*. 1993;21(1):125.

19. Epling J. Clinical evidence handbook: bacterial conjunctivitis. *Am Fam Physician*. 2010;82(6):665–6.

20. Fillipas S, Cherry CL, Cicuttini F, Smirneos L, Holland AE. The effects of exercise training on metabolic and morphological outcomes for people living with HIV: a systematic review of randomized controlled trials. *HIV Clin Trials*. 2010;11(5):270–82.

21. Gleeson M. Dosing and effectiveness of glutamine supplementation in human exercise and sport training, *J Nutr*. 2008;138(10):2045S–9S.

22. Gutierrez RL, Decker CF. Blood-borne infections and the athlete. *Dis Mon*. 2010;56(7):436–42.

23. Hosey RG, Rodenberg RE. Infectious disease and the college athlete. *Clin Sports Med*. 2007;26(3):449–71.

24. Hosey RG, Rodenberg RE. Training room management of medical conditions: infectious diseases. *Clin Sport Med*. 2005;24(3):477–506, vii.

25. Johnson DL, Mair SD. The preparticipation physical exam. In: *Clinical Sports Medicine*. Philadelphia (PA): Mosby Elsevier; 2006. p. 764.

26. Juckett G. Prevention and treatment of traveler's diarrhea. *Am Fam Physician*. 1999;60(1):119–24, 135–6.

27. Karagenanes SJ. Gastrointestinal infections in the athlete. *Clin Sports Med*. 2007;26(3):433–48.

28. Kim AS. Clinical evidence handbook: sinusitis (acute). *Am Fam Physician*. 2009;79(4):320–1.

29. King OS. Infectious disease and boxing. *Clin Sports Med*. 2009;28(4):545–60, vi.

30. Klentrou P, Cieslak T, MacNeil M, Vintinner A, Plyley M. Effect of moderate exercise on salivary IgA. *Eur J Appl Physiol*. 2002;87(2):153–8.

31. Klosner D. Appendix D, NCAA banned drugs. In: *2010–2011 NCAA Sports Medicine Handbook*. 21st ed. Indianapolis: National Collegiate Athletic Association; 2010.

32. Kordi R, Wallace WA. Blood borne infections in sport: risks of transmission, methods of prevention, and recommendations for hepatitis B vaccination. *Br J Sports Med*. 2004;38(6):678–84.

33. Kostka T, Drygas W, Jegier A, Praczko K. Physical activity and upper respiratory tract infections. *Int J Sports Med*. 2008;29(2):158–62.

34. Kostka T, Praczko K. Interrelationship between physical activity, symptomatology of upper respiratory tract infections, and depression in elderly people. *Gerontology*. 2007;53(4):187–93.

35. Kovan JR, Moeller JL. Respiratory system. In: McKeag DB, Moeller JL, editors. *ACSM's Primary Care Sports Medicine*. Philadelphia: Lippincott Williams & Wilkins; 2007. p. 165.

36. Kruse RJ, Cantor CL. Pulmonary and cardiac infections in athletes. *Clin Sports Med*. 2007;26(3):361–82.

37. Loeb M. Community-acquired pneumonia. *Am Fam Physician*. 2002;66(1):135–7.

38. Luke A, d'Hemecourt P. Prevention of infectious diseases in athletes. *Clin Sports Med*. 2007;26(3):321–44.

39. Maron BJ, Ackerman MJ, Nishimura RA, Pyeritz RE, Towbin JA, Udelson JE. Task Force 4: HCM and other cardiomyopathies, mitral valve prolapse, myocarditis, and Marfan syndrome. *JACC*. 2005;45(8):1340–5.

40. Matthews CE, Ockene IS, Freedson PS, Rosal MC, Merriam PA, Hebert JR. Moderate to vigorous physical activity and risk of upper-respiratory tract infection. *Med Sci Sports Exerc*. 2002;34(8):1242–8.

41. McGrew CA. Acute infections. In: McKeag DB, Moeller JL, editors. *ACSM's Primary Care Sports Medicine*. Philadelphia: Lippincott Williams & Wilkins; 2007. p. 251–60.

42. McKune AJ, Smith LL, Semple SJ, Mokethwa B, Wadee AA. Immunoglobulin responses to a repeated bout of downhill running. *Br J Sports Med*. 2006;40(10):844–9.

43. Natarajan B. Gastrointestinal problems. In: Madden CC, Putukian M, Young CC, McCarty EC, editors. *Netter's Sports Medicine*. Philadelphia: Saunders Elsevier; 2010. p. 204–8.

44. National Sporting Goods Association [Internet]. Ten-year history of sports participation; [cited 2011 Feb 23]. Available from: http://www.nsga.org/files/public/Ten-Year_History_of_Sports_Participation_4web_100521.pdf.

45. Neiman D. Is infection risk linked to exercise workload? *Med Sci Sports Exerc*. 2000;32(7)(suppl):S406–11.

46. Neiman D. Nutrition, exercise and immune system function. *Clin Sport Med*. 1999;18(3):537–48.

47. Novas AD, Rowbottom DG, Jenkins DG. Tennis, incidence of URTI and salivary IgA. *Int J Sports Med*. 2003;24(3):223–9.

48. O'Brien K, Nixon S, Tynan AM, Glazier RH. Effectiveness of aerobic exercise in adults living with HIV/AIDS: systematic review. *Med Sci Sports Exerc*. 2004;36(10):1659–66.

49. Page CL, Diehl JJ. Upper respiratory tract infections in athletes. *Clin Sports Med*. 2007;26(3):345–59.

50. Peters EM, Goetzsche JM, Grobbelaar B, Noakes TD. Vitamin C supplementation reduces the incidence of postrace symptoms of upper respiratory tract infection in ultramarathon runners. *Am J Clin Nutr*. 1993;57(2):170–4.

51. Pirozzolo JJ, LeMay DG. Blood-borne infections. *Clin Sports Med*. 2007;26(3):425–31.

52. Putukian M, O'Connor FG, Stricker PR, et al. Mononucleosis and athletic participation: an evidence-based review. *Clin J Sport Med*. 2008;18(4):309–15.

53. Rabago D, Zgierska A. Saline nasal irrigation for upper respiratory conditions. *Am Fam Physician*. 2009;80(10):1117–9.

54. Scheid DC, Hamm RM. Acute bacterial rhinosinusitis in adults: part I. Evaluation. *Am Fam Physician*. 2004;70(9):1685–92.

55. Shephard RJ, Kavanagh T, Mertens DJ, Qureshi S, Clark M. Personal health benefits of Masters athletics competition. *Br J Sports Med*. 1995;29(1):35–40.

56. Simasek M, Blandino DA. Treatment of the common cold. *Am Fam Physician*. 2007;75(4):515–20.

57. U.S. Centers for Disease Control and Prevention. Chlamydia [Internet]. 2010 [cited 2011 Jan 14]. Available from: http://www.cdc.gov/std/chlamydia/STDFact-Chlamydia.htm.

58. U.S. Centers for Disease Control and Prevention. Gonorrhea: CDC Fact Sheet [Internet]. 2010 [cited 2011 Jan 14]. Available from: http://www.cdc.gov/std/gonorrhea/STDFact-gonorrhea.htm.

59. U.S. Centers for Disease Control and Prevention. Hepatitis B information for health professionals [Internet]. 2008–2009 [cited 2011 Jan 14]. Available from: http://www.cdc.gov/hepatitis/HBV/HBVfaq.htm#overview.

60. U.S. Centers for Disease Control and Prevention. Hepatitis C information for health professionals [Internet]. 2010 [cited 2011 Jan 14]. Available from: http://www.cdc.gov/hepatitis/HCV/index.htm.

61. U.S. Centers for Disease Control and Prevention. HIV in the United States [Internet]. 2010 [cited 14 Jan 2011]. Available from: http://www.cdc.gov/hiv/resources/factsheets/us.htm.

62. West NP, Pyne DB, Kyd JM, Renshaw GM, Fricker PA, Cripps AW. The effect of exercise on innate mucosal immunity. *Br J Sports Med*. 2010;44(4):227–31.

63. Wood SM, Kenedy JS, Arsenault JE, et al. Novel nutritional formula maintains host defense mechanisms. *Mil Med*. 2005;170(11):975–85.

64. Yamamoto Y, Nakaji S, Umeda T, et al. Effects of long-term training on neutrophil function in male university judoists. *Br J Sports Med*. 2008;42(4):255–9.

65. Young CC, Niedfeldt MW, Gottschlich LM, Peterson CS, Gammons MR. Infectious disease and the extreme sport athlete. *Clin Sport Med*. 2007;26(3):473–87.

34 Endocrinology and Sports

J. Andrew McMahon and William W. Dexter

■ The endocrine system is a complex framework of glands and hormones that takes input and provides feedback to the hypothalamic–pituitary axis. The hormones are often ubiquitous and ultimately govern many key physiologic functions, such as metabolism, growth, and muscle function. Hormones are responsible for the machinery that allows us to exercise, and when deficient, provides a management challenge to both the athlete and the sports medicine physician. This chapter will review some of the key components of the endocrine system and the implications of disease of this system in sports.

PANCREATIC HORMONES

■ Insulin and glucagon are secreted by the islet cells in the pancreas. *Glucagon* is a catabolic hormone secreted as a counter balance to insulin through its stimulation of gluconeogenesis.

■ *Insulin* is an anabolic hormone that regulates glucose channels and insulin receptors, stimulates protein and glycogen synthesis, and generally inhibits catabolism. When it is absent, lipolysis produces fatty acids and ketones as the primary fuel source, resulting in a metabolic acidosis. Insulin is also involved in development through its numerous interactions with other mediators of growth-like growth hormone (GH) and insulin-like growth factor-1 (IGF-1) (20).

■ During exercise, insulin levels decrease while glucagon and catecholamines drive hepatic glycogenolysis and free fatty acid production to provide glucose to stressed cells. In this state, active muscles use glucose through insulin-independent means and potentiate the action of residual insulin through adaptations in the affinity for and quantity of insulin receptors.

■ After exercise, insulin production and sensitivity are increased in response to elevated blood sugars. Insulin drives replenishment of glycogen and protein stores and downregulates counterregulatory hormones.

■ **Diabetes and exercise**
  ■ Because insulin is administered exogenously in diabetics, this cascade relies heavily on proper management. Insulin in excess prior to exercise inhibits catecholamines, suppressing the liver's ability to mobilize fuel while muscles continue to use circulating glucose. Hypoglycemia, with blood sugars < 70 mg $\cdot$ dL^{-1}, ensues.

■ **Hypoglycemic emergencies** arise as the counterregulatory hormones are inhibited by the exogenous insulin. Following exercise, enhanced glucose uptake and insulin sensitivity predisposes the insulin-dependent diabetic to hypoglycemia for as much as 12–24 hours.

  ■ Pallor, diaphoresis, confusion, headache, shakiness, irritability, and a change in mental status are common presentations and may progress to syncope, seizure, or coma if left untreated.

  ■ Athletes with long-standing diabetes have a blunted stress response and may not exhibit these warning signs, which are the result of sympathetic activation. Fatigue, hunger, and irritability may be the only clues (22).

  ■ **Treatment**, if alert, is oral replacement with 15 g of glucose.
    ❏ Repeat blood sugar every 15 minutes until euglycemic.
    ❏ If obtunded, administer glucagon 1 mg intramuscularly (IM)/subcutaneously (SC) if > 100 lb or 0.5 mg if < 100 lb.
      ■ Glucagon has a short half-life and should be continuously supplemented with additional carbohydrates until sugars normalize (7).

■ **Hyperglycemia** can also be problematic for athletes when insufficient insulin is present during exercise. When control is poor prior to exercise, athletes may have high blood glucose and subsequent polyuria resulting in dehydration. Without insulin's inhibitory effect on lipolysis, ketogenesis contributes to the deteriorating metabolic state.

  ■ Counterregulatory hormones are normally active in the stressed state but in this setting, will contribute detrimentally to the hyperglycemia. Diabetic ketoacidosis may be the end result. These athletes need urgent supplemental insulin and hydration.

■ **Therapeutic use exemption (TUE)**
  ■ No TUE is needed for insulin.

■ **Return to play**
  ■ Athletes with routine hypoglycemia can return to play when repeat blood sugars have stabilized. Blood sugars in excess of 250 mg $\cdot$ dL^{-1} or ketonuria is a relative contraindication to play. Athletes with sugars between 180 and 249 mg $\cdot$ dL^{-1} should be monitored closely but can continue to play.

PARTICIPATION GUIDELINES

- **Preseason**
  - Assess athlete's disease literacy.
    - ❏ Nutrition, carbohydrate counting
    - ❏ Ability to monitor blood sugars with appropriate frequency
    - ❏ Recognizes the symptoms of hypoglycemia and hyperglycemia
    - ❏ Knows how to treat diabetic emergencies, sick day plan
    - ❏ Medical alert bracelet
  - Screen for long-term complications of diabetes.
    - ❏ Recent hemoglobin A1c, blood pressure, lipid profile, creatinine, microalbumin
    - ❏ Screen for peripheral neuropathy, foot care education
    - ❏ Screen for retinopathy, if present, no heavy lifting
    - ❏ Consider screening for coronary artery disease
    - ❏ Graded exercise testing if older than 35 or 25 with > 15 years of diabetes
  - Create plan with sports medicine staff for diabetic emergencies.
  - Athlete should experiment in preseason with insulin regimens.
    - ❏ Start season conditioning to minimize changes in insulin needs that develop with fitness.
    - ❏ Experiment with injection site and effects of exercise and climate on absorption (38).
- **Before exercise**
  - Estimate intensity, duration, and energy demand of event.
  - Reduce SC insulin based on intensity and duration of exercise.
    - ❏ Reduce premeal insulin by 20%–75%.
    - ❏ Reduce by 70%–80% if > 90 minutes in duration (38).
  - Insulin pump users should reduce basal rate by 50% 1 hour prior to sport.
    - ❏ May remove pump for up to 1 hour for sport, especially water or contact sports
    - ❏ Frequent glucose checks
    - ❏ Contingency plan for extended events (36)
  - Check blood sugars prior to exercise.
    - ❏ If blood glucose < 100 mg · dL^{-1}, ingest 15 g of carbohydrate. Wait 15 minutes, and recheck blood sugar. Repeat as needed.
    - ❏ If blood glucose is between 180 and 249 mg · dL^{-1}, increase frequency of blood sugar checks. Hold carbohydrate intake pending clinical course.
    - ❏ If blood glucose > 250 mg · dL^{-1}, postpone exercise, measure urine ketone, and administer insulin.

- **During exercise**
  - Add 15 g of carbohydrate for the first 30–60 minutes of exercise.
    - ❏ During events of longer duration, 30–60 g · h^{-1} carbohydrate should be ingested every 15–30 minutes.
  - Hydration
  - Monitor glucose levels at least hourly.
- **Postexercise**
  - Meal within 30 minutes of activity and increased caloric intake for 12–24 hours after activity
  - Continued blood glucose surveillance, especially overnight
    - ❏ Watch for late-onset hypoglycemia.
    - ❏ Adjust insulin as needed.
  - Proper foot care
  - Hydration

THE ADRENAL GLAND

Adrenal Cortex

- Adrenocorticotropin (ACTH), synthesized in the anterior pituitary, is secreted under control of corticotropin-releasing factor (CRF) and vasopressin. ACTH stimulates the adrenal glands to secrete glucocorticoids, mineralocorticoids, and weak androgens.
- *Glucocorticoids* provide negative feedback to the hypothalamus when steroid levels are adequate, downregulating the axis.
- Superficially, the *zona glomerulosa* produces mineralocorticoids (*e.g.*, aldosterone). Mineralocorticoids help maintain blood volume by governing a sodium channel in the kidney under direction of the renin–angiotensin system and in response to fluctuations in potassium and blood pressure (39).
- In the *zona fasciculata*, glucocorticoids (*e.g.*, cortisol) are produced diurnally, with the highest concentrations secreted in the morning. The key functions of cortisol are to increase blood sugar through gluconeogenesis and glycolysis. Cortisol is a potent anti-inflammatory, decreases bone formation, strengthens cardiac muscle contractions, and causes water retention. Glucocorticoids are secreted in response to stress and hypoglycemia under direction of ACTH and catecholamines (39).
- The deepest layer is the *zona reticularis* where weak androgens are produced. They are secreted with cortisol in response to stress and in a diurnal fashion. Please refer to the section on androgens for more details (39).

Adrenal Insufficiency

- Insufficiency results when the adrenal glands, or the hypothalamic–pituitary axis, fail to produce steroids. Patients present with weakness, nausea, abdominal pain, or hypovolemia with orthostatic hypotension. Myalgias and paralysis secondary to hyperkalemia are not uncommon (25).

■ **Diagnosis** is suggested by hypoglycemia, hyponatremia, and hyperkalemia on routine fasting metabolic profile.

  ■ Cortisol and ACTH levels are a reasonable first step in diagnosis.

  ■ A fasting morning basal cortisol level $< 3 \ \mu g \cdot dL^{-1}$ is diagnostic.

  ■ The diagnosis is unlikely in an otherwise healthy individual with a level $> 10 \ \mu g \cdot dL^{-1}$ (25).

■ **Treatment** includes hydrocortisone (25–30 mg orally divided 3 times a day).

  ■ Fludrocortisone (0.1–0.2 mg every day) may be needed for additional mineralocorticoid activity.

  ■ Long-acting prednisone or dexamethasone may also be used (25).

Acute Adrenal Crisis

■ In those treated with exogenous steroids, an *acute adrenal crisis* may be precipitated by extreme stresses (surgery, infection, dehydration) or rapid withdrawal of long-term glucocorticoid therapy. Chronic prednisone administration results in corticotrophic cell atrophy and a subsequent inability to sustain the adrenal axis when the exogenous source is removed.

  ■ These individuals may present with shock, an "acute" abdomen, or high fever, or be comatose.

  ■ Normal exercise does not require stress doses of corticosteroids, but a fracture, moderate blood loss, or vomiting may precipitate an emergency.

■ **Treatment** includes 100 mg of injectable Solu-Cortef or 4 mg of dexamethasone.

  ■ Medication should be available at all times.

  ■ The athlete and sports medicine staff should be educated about how and when to use these rescue medications.

  ■ Attention to blood glucose levels and volume resuscitation with normal saline should be a priority.

  ■ Athletes with hypotension or hypoglycemia need to be transferred urgently to the nearest medical facility for volume resuscitation, intravenous steroids, and close monitoring of vitals and electrolytes (25).

■ **TUE**

  ■ For primary adrenal insufficiency, a TUE is granted for a term of 4 years (and often lifetime).

  ■ It is subject to yearly review by an endocrinologist.

  ■ A plan for adrenal crisis in times of high stress should be integrated into the TUE.

  ■ The athlete should report use of stress doses on the doping control form at time of testing.

  ■ A TUE for functional adrenal insufficiency resulting from glucocorticoid withdrawal can be granted for a period of 4–12 weeks.

  ■ Given the controversy surrounding the efficacy of and need for dehydroepiandrosterone (DHEA) supplementation, an independent expert should consulted (40).

■ **Return to play**

  ■ With adequate therapy and a TUE, there are no restrictions.

Adrenal Medulla

■ The adrenal medulla is a collection of postganglionic neurons under direct control of the central nervous system through autonomic preganglionic fibers. The medulla secretes catecholamines into the blood under direct stimulation of the autonomic nervous system in response to stress and exercise.

■ Catecholamines, which include norepinephrine and epinephrine, act at adrenergic receptors located throughout the body, activating the sympathetic division of the nervous system. They increase heart rate, cardiac output, and arterial pressure through the α-adrenergic receptors. Catecholamines also cause bronchodilation, vasodilatation, and mydriasis.

■ Ephedra alkaloids are weak sympathomimetic agents with actions similar to epinephrine. They are perceived as agents that improve competitiveness and focus and reduce tiredness. There are currently no data supporting the ergogenic benefit of ephedra alkaloids for power, endurance, strength, or speed. High doses of the compound can cause anxiety, delirium, irritability, aggression, and convulsions, although the most dangerous side effects are hypertension and tachyarrhythmia (3).

■ **TUE**

  ■ Ephedrine and stimulants, in general, are banned during competition. There is no TUE available.

  ■ There are a number of other agents acting on the adrenergic axis that are prohibited by the World Anti-Doping Agency (WADA); please refer to a current prohibited substances list for details.

THYROID HORMONE

■ Thyroid hormone (TH), produced by the thyroid gland under direction of the hypothalamic–pituitary axis, is secreted in response to elevated thyroid-stimulating hormone (TSH) when TH levels are low. When there is adequate hormone, negative feedback shuts down the axis.

■ TH helps govern fat mobilization, gluconeogenesis, and glycogenolysis and plays a key role in physical and neurologic development. It is responsible for maintaining body temperature through complex thermogenic mechanisms (15).

■ TH upregulates β-adrenergic receptors, resulting in an increased sensitivity to circulating catecholamine and has multiple responsibilities in muscle function. TSH and thyroxine (T_4) have been shown to increase proportionally with exercise and, when preserved within normal physiologic parameters, appear to improve muscle efficiency with exercise and play a key role in physical and metabolic function (15).

Hypothyroidism

- Manifestations are that of a slowed metabolic state that includes fatigue, slowed movement, cold intolerance, constipation, weight gain, delayed relaxation of deep tendon reflexes, and bradycardia.

- In athletes, however, the complaint may be as simple as a decrease in performance or fatigue. This is a challenging and infrequent diagnosis in young athletes. In a 2007 study of 50 athletes with fatigue, only 6% were found to have abnormal thyroid function assays (8).

- Cakir et al. (4) noted that 30%–80% of patients with hypothyroidism present with muscular complaints, including cramps, weakness, stiffness, and poor exercise tolerance.
  - Exercise intolerance is likely a result of mitochondrial dysfunction and loss of β-adrenergic receptors affecting many metabolic pathways that supply active muscles.
  - In extreme cases, this may cause rhabdomyolysis or a polymyositis-like weakness (4).
  - Carpal tunnel syndrome is also a common manifestation (4).

- Function of the cardiovascular system is greatly affected by hypothyroidism. Both systolic function and diastolic function are reduced, and the relaxation of vascular smooth muscles is impaired, increasing systemic vascular resistance (16).

- In children, TH is a key component in bone and muscle development, brain maturation, and onset of puberty. Thus, a young athlete with hypothyroidism may present with stunted growth, delayed onset of puberty, or cognitive impairment (31).

- **Diagnosis**
  - A high TSH and a low free T_4 are suggestive of primary hypothyroidism.

- **Treatment**
  - Replacement is with levothyroxine at 25–50 $\mu g \cdot d^{-1}$ with subsequent increases every 4–6 weeks by 25–50 μg until the patient responds (15).

- **TUE**
  - A TUE is not required for thyroid replacement (40).

- **Return to play**
  - Return to play is largely based on symptoms; there are no particular restrictions.

Hyperthyroidism

- Hyperthyroidism is a hypermetabolic condition, often the result of autoimmune disease, which results in excess TH (15).

- Symptoms may include unexplained weight loss despite an increased appetite, anxiety, sweating, hyperactivity, and palpitations, all signs of sympathetic activation. Like hypothyroid individuals, however, their only complaint may be a decrease in performance.
  - Thyrotoxicosis should be included in the differential diagnosis of any well-trained athlete with resting tachycardia.

- Females athletes may have oligomenorrhea and accelerated bone resorption, but there does not appear to a risk for premature osteoporosis in women of reproductive age (9).

- Exogenous thyroid use has historically been a tool of many weight loss clinics in an effort to produce a hypermetabolic state in hopes of enhancing weight loss.
  - Haluzik et al. (12) found decreased abdominal adipose tissue believed secondary to a hyperadrenergic state.
  - Locker et al. (19) noted that factitious TH use is linked to myocardial infarction and other overt characteristics of thyrotoxicosis.

- **Diagnosis**
  - TSH is the best initial test and is typically undetectable in true thyrotoxicosis.
  - Elevated free T_4 and total triiodothyronine (T_3) support the diagnosis (29).

- **Treatment**
  - Antithyroid medications, which include methimazole and propylthiouracil, are often first line in combination with steroids and β-blockers.

- **TUE**
  - β-blockers are banned during competition for a number of sports requiring concentration. Prednisone requires a TUE. Please refer to WADA guidelines (40).

- **Return to play**
  - As with hypothyroidism, there are no restrictions on return to play. However, any athlete with ongoing thyrotoxicosis is at risk for tachyarrhythmia and should be encouraged to avoid exercise until the disease is stabilized.

GROWTH HORMONE

- GH is produced in the anterior pituitary, under direction of GH-releasing hormone in a very complex interaction with many peripheral inputs. GH secretion occurs in response to hypoglycemia, androgens, sleep, fasting and eating, and exercise. Inhibitors include glucocorticoids, hyperglycemia, and fatty meals.

- GH is produced in a pulsatile manner throughout the day but peaks an hour after sleep begins. GH promotes protein synthesis, lipolysis, and epiphyseal growth. However, it seems to exert a majority of its effect through IGF-1.

- IGF-1 is produced in the liver and promotes cell proliferation. It inhibits apoptosis, causing skeletal muscle hypertrophy and activation of chondrocytes and osteocytes (24).

GH Deficiency (GHD)

- A pure GHD is rare in adults and may not be an obvious syndrome. It is commonly diagnosed in the setting of multiple anterior pituitary deficiencies and other hormone deficiencies that produce recognizable patterns of disease.

- GHD results in increased intra-abdominal visceral fat and an increase in the waist-to-hip ratio. Lean muscle mass is lost, and hypertension, hyperlipidemia, and systolic dysfunction are additional features.
- Bone mineralization is reduced, and an athlete may present with osteopenia or a pathologic fracture (35).
- In children, GHD typically presents at ages 2–3 years when stunted growth, poor dental development, and abdominal obesity are recognized (27).

- **Diagnosis**
  - GH levels are often not helpful.
  - A low serum IGF-1 concentration is only suggestive of GHD (34).

- **Treatment**
  - In adults, human GH is given at a starting dose of 0.1–0.2 mg · d^{-1} SC every night and is titrated based on serial IGF-1 levels.
  - In children, dose is 25–50 μg · kg^{-1} · d^{-1} SC, and efficacy is based on tracking growth and serial IGF-1 levels (35).

- **TUE**
  - In adults, treatment of partial GH deficiency remains debatable, and for WADA purposes, only documented severe GH deficiency is eligible for TUE.
  - An independent reviewer is recommended, given potential controversy surrounding GH supplementation.
  - In children, a TUE is granted in most instances (40).

- **Return to play**
  - There are no restrictions on return to play with GHD.

Doping and GH

- Historically, athletes and trainers have felt that GH increases lean body mass and strength in highly trained athletes. It has been an intriguing substance to athletes given its ability to augment lean muscle mass and strength and because there have been limited methods to detect GH abuse.
  - WADA reports that, despite testing, no professional or Olympic athlete has ever tested positive for factitious GH use (40).
- The merits of GH as a performance-enhancing substance were challenged in a review of 252 studies by Liu et al. (18) who found a near significant increase in "lean muscle mass," but these results are questionable given limited means to distinguish solid tissue from simple fluid.
  - The papers reviewed failed to show an increase in measurable strength despite an increase in muscle mass, potentially supporting the theory that fluid retention is involved.
  - A subsequent study found that 2 mg · d^{-1} of GH may increase sprint capacity and anaerobic work capacity on a cycle ergometer when given alone and in combination with testosterone (23).

- **Detection**
  - IGF-1 and N-terminal extension peptide of procollagen type III, which are markers of GH activity, are being used. Powrie et al. (26) noted that these markers were elevated in subjects receiving exogenous GH for 4 weeks.
  - GH isoforms are also being used to detect GH abuse. Normal GH secretion from the pituitary includes a variety of isoforms, including varies configurations of both 22- and 20-kd forms.
    - Exogenous GH has only a 22-kd monomer, which downregulates the production of natural forms through negative feedback. This skews the normal ratio of isoforms that are detected by immunoassays (23).

PARATHYROID HORMONE

- The parathyroid gland is located on the poles of the thyroid gland and secretes parathyroid hormone (PTH), which plays a role in governing serum calcium and phosphorous. Calcium and phosphorus are key mediators of bone health, blood coagulation, muscle contraction, and nerve function. PTH responds to low serum calcium and increases bone resorption, through a complex interaction with osteoclasts, mobilizing calcium and increasing phosphate excretion.
- Hypercalcemia inhibits the secretion of PTH. *Calcitonin* opposes PTH and is secreted in response to hypercalcemia (Ca$^+$ > 9.5 mg · dL^{-1}). It subsequently inhibits bone resorption and encourages calciuria (20). A hyperactive gland results in hypercalcemia, causing bone pain, weakness, myalgias, cognitive impairment, and osteoporosis.

VITAMIN D

- Vitamin D is produced in the skin from cholesterol by the stimulation of sunlight, forming vitamin D$_3$. Vitamin D$_3$ is 25-hydroxylated in the liver to 25-hydroxycholecalciferol [25(OH)D] and then is 1α-hydroxylated in the kidney, creating the more active metabolite, 1,25-dihydroxycholecalciferol.
- Vitamin D is responsible for the transport of Ca^{2+} and PO$_4^{3-}$ from the intestine and inhibits calciuria. It also is a stimulant of osteoblasts and plays a role in appropriate bone mineralization. Vitamin D is loosely regulated but appears to be inhibited by hypercalcemia (41).

Vitamin D Deficiency

- Deficiency results in defective calcification of the bone matrix and is implicated in a number of disease states.
  - Ruohola et al. (30) studied military recruits in Finland and found an increased risk of stress fractures with vitamin D deficiency. Vitamin D also appears to be important in the expression of genes that contribute to muscle growth and

- can result in atrophy of fast-twitch fibers and decreased muscle performance (17).
  - ▪ Athletes at risk include those who train indoors, in northern latitudes, with sunscreen, or at dusk and dawn (17).
  - ▪ Osteomalacia is seen in adults with inadequate amounts of vitamin D and is characterized by softening of the bones due to defective bone mineralization.
  - ▪ Patients present with bone pain and lumbar back pain and occasionally have pathologic fractures and proximal muscle weakness.
  - ▪ The disease is the result of inadequate calcium absorption and common in malabsorptive states and those with eating disorders (41).
- ▪ Diagnosis
  - ▪ Vitamin D insufficiency is defined by 25(OH)D levels less than 20 ng $\cdot$ mL^{-1}, and deficiency is defined as 25(OH)D levels between 20 and 30 ng $\cdot$ mL^{-1} (6).
  - ▪ There are no recommendations to universally screen for vitamin D deficiency. For most, it is likely more efficient to ensure adequate intake through supplementation than it is to pursue laboratory testing (6).
- ▪ Treatment
  - ▪ The recommended daily intakes of calcium and vitamin D are 1,200 mg of elemental calcium and 800 IU of vitamin D daily for most adults.
  - ▪ Those with insufficiency can be treated with 50,000 units of vitamin D$_3$ every week for 12 weeks initially.
  - ▪ Currently, the treatment for those with vitamin D deficiency is very controversial. It appears to be reasonable to treat these individuals with 800–1,000 IU of vitamin D$_3$ daily, although some argue for the weekly high-dose regimen (6,14).
- ▪ Return to play
  - ▪ There are currently no WADA restrictions on therapy and no rules governing return to play (40).

POSTERIOR PITUITARY HORMONES

- ▪ The posterior pituitary is a collection of axons that extend from the hypothalamus producing, among other hormones, antidiuretic hormone (ADH).
- ▪ ADH plays an important role in salt and water homeostasis, maintaining serum osmolality between 280 and 295 mOsm $\cdot$ kg^{-1} H$_2$O. Secretion of ADH is initiated by changes in both serum osmolality and plasma volume.
- ▪ Nausea, stress, pain, hypoxia, and a large number of medications, including nonsteroidal anti-inflammatory drugs (NSAIDs), which sensitize the kidneys to ADH are also commonly implicated in stimulation of ADH secretion (28).
- ▪ ADH acts on antidiuretic receptors in the collecting duct of the kidney, causing an increase in permeability of the plasma membrane. A number of clinical conditions result in a condition of vasopressin excess, otherwise known as the syndrome of inappropriate antidiuretic hormone (SIADH).
- ▪ With this excess, a surplus of free water results, leading to hyponatremia and subsequent neurologic and metabolic disturbances.

Exercise-Associated Hyponatremia (EAH)

- ▪ With the growing popularity of endurance sports, such as marathons, EAH has become more common. The pathogenesis of EAH is poorly understood.
- ▪ The current practice of aggressive fluid replacement with water or hypotonic sports drinks in excess of typical and insensible fluid loss seems to play a role.
- ▪ Almond et al. (1) looked at 488 runners in the 2002 Boston Marathon and found that 13% had a serum sodium of < 135 mmol $\cdot$ L^{-1} and 0.6% had a value of $< 120 \cdot$ mmol L^{-1}.
- ▪ Speedy et al. (37) looked 330 ultramarathoners and found that 18% were hyponatremic and 11% had a serum sodium of < 130 mmol $\cdot$ L^{-1}.
- ▪ A common denominator among athletes with hyponatremia is weight gain or maintenance during an endurance event. What separates those who overhydrate and do not develop hyponatremia from those that do is not clear.
  - ▪ SIADH has also been implicated.
  - ▪ Freund et al. (11) discovered that exercise at levels above 60% of maximal oxygen consumption stimulated the secretion of vasopressin.
  - ▪ A net loss of 5%–10% of body weight will also stimulate vasopressin secretion, but most athletes do not have this level of volume depletion (33).
  - ▪ Almond et al. (1) and Sharwood et al. (33) both found that hyponatremia was far more common in women than men.
  - ▪ It has been hypothesized that smaller body size or differences in pain processing plays a role in this distinction.
  - ▪ Several studies suggest that higher levels of interleukin-6, a secretagogue of ADH, are produced in women in response to muscle damage, explaining this difference (28).
- ▪ When sodium is rapidly lowered, water crosses the blood–brain barrier seeking to equilibrate tonicity across the membrane. The resulting influx of water causes swelling and an increased cerebral pressure, which explains many of the neurologic symptoms accompanying hyponatremia. Given enough time, typically 24 hours, the brain is able to shunt water and electrolytes to the cerebrospinal fluid, restoring balance.
  - ▪ When the influx is rapid, this mechanism is overwhelmed, and the swelling and subsequent symptoms can be severe; seizure, cerebral edema, and coma may result.
- ▪ Many athletes with hyponatremia are asymptomatic, whereas others look pale and have weakness, dizziness, headache, nausea, irritability, and subtle changes in mental status. In one review, 30% of athletes with postexertional syncope were found to have hyponatremia (28).

■ **Treatment**
- ■ Asymptomatic athletes should be fluid restricted and observed.
- ■ Normal saline should be avoided.
- ■ Severe hyponatremia is a medical emergency, and these patients should be transferred to the nearest medical facility. These individuals often need 3% saline to rapidly correct a portion of the sodium deficit in the setting of life-threatening neurologic disorders.
- ■ Currently, there is insufficient evidence to support the suggestion that ingestion of sodium prevents or decreases the risk for EAH.
- ■ Hypotonic sports drinks will not prevent EAH (28).
- ■ The American College of Sports Medicine® (ACSM) recommends 0.5–0.7 g sodium $\cdot$ L^{-1} of water as the appropriate level of sodium intake to replace the sodium that is lost in sweat during endurance events (2).

■ **Return to play**
- ■ There are no strict rules governing return to play following EAH. Clearly, a more appropriate fluid management strategy and close monitoring should be employed in subsequent events.

SEX HORMONES

Estrogen

- ■ Estrogens are a group of steroid hormones that are manufactured in the ovaries and, in small amounts, in the male testes and the adrenal glands, brain, and fat.
- ■ Luteinizing hormone (LH) stimulates the production of androstenedione from cholesterol, which is then converted to estrogen directly. Estrogen is also created through aromatization, under the direction of follicle-stimulating hormone (FSH), converting androgens to estrogens. Estrogen plays a role in the menstrual cycle, reduces bone resorption, accelerates metabolism, reduces muscle mass, and increases fat stores (13). Please refer to Chapter 115, The Female Athlete for more details.

Testosterone

- ■ Testosterone is primarily a male sex hormone that is primarily produced in Leydig cells of the testicle and is regulated by LH and FSH.
- ■ DHEA and androstenedione are precursors to testosterone and have a weak androgenic effect. Testosterone increases muscle mass and strength, as well as bone density, and encourages bone maturation.
- ■ Hypogonadism refers to a decrease in one or both of the major functions of the testes: sperm production or testosterone production. Testosterone deficiency prior to puberty results in underdeveloped genitals. Muscle weakness, osteoporosis, impotence, infertility, and depression are manifestations of untreated hypogonadism in adults and adolescents (35).

■ **Diagnosis**
- ■ Total testosterone (8 a.m. laboratory draw), LH and FSH, and TSH are reasonable first steps in making the diagnosis. For the purpose of WADA and a TUE, interpretation and evaluation by an endocrinologist are required.

■ **Treatment**
- ■ Testosterone can be given as an injection 100–200 mg IM every 2 weeks, applied daily to skin in gel form (5–10 mg), or applied as a 2.5- to 5-mg daily patch. Serial total testosterone levels are needed to monitor efficacy (34).

■ **TUE**
- ■ A TUE for testosterone replacement is required in the setting of appropriately diagnosed and managed hypogonadism.
- ■ TUE is subject to yearly review.
- ■ Given the potential controversy associated with the use of testosterone, management by an endocrinologist and the opinion of an independent expert are strongly recommended (40).

■ **Return to play**
- ■ There are no restrictions on return to play.

■ **Testosterone abuse**
- ■ A large Centers for Disease Control and Prevention survey found that 4% of adolescents in high school reported taking androgenic steroids without a doctor's prescription (10). It can be challenging to determine which athletes are using these drugs.
- ■ With testosterone, especially at supratherapeutic doses, there is an increase in lean body mass through hypertrophy of existing muscle fibers and through growth of new fibers. This is accomplished through enhanced protein synthesis, interactions with GH, and inhibition of cortisol's catabolic actions (21).
- ■ There is some suggestion that testosterone supplementation may make the athlete more aggressive, and it also appears to positively affect oxygen utilization and systolic function.
- ■ Androstenedione and DHEA are precursors to testosterone. There is little evidence suggesting that androstenedione has a measurable physiologic benefit. DHEA has been marketed heavily recently as an antiaging drug given its theoretical ability to burn fat and build muscle. There is a paucity of data to support this claim. It is available over the counter and commonly used by athletes but may result in feminization when it is aromatized. Studies have had mixed results on the efficacy of DHEA (36).

■ **Side effects of androgen abuse**
- ■ Gynecomastia, virilization, hirsutism, male pattern baldness, acne, deepening of the voice, and clitoral enlargement are some of the cosmetic complications of testosterone.

- Testicular atrophy is a result of the inhibition of natural testosterone production by high exogenous concentrations through negative feedback. Some will try to mask this by using human chorionic gonadotropin (21).
- Coagulopathy, hyperlipidemia, hepatotoxicity, and potentially hemorrhagic liver cysts have also been described.
- In young athletes, testosterone may stimulate premature epiphyseal fusion, resulting in short stature.
- A number of psychiatric issues have been described, but the data are largely anecdotal (36).

- **Drug testing**
  - Androgens other than testosterone can be detected by gas chromatograph.
  - It is not currently possible to distinguish between exogenous and endogenous testosterone. The conventional method is to determine the urinary ratio of testosterone to epitestosterone glucuronide (T/E ratio), which is typically 3:1 (36).
    - ❏ Supplemented testosterone will increase the ratio to 6:1 or higher (5).
    - ❏ However, this test is skewed by genetic differences in testosterone metabolism (32).
  - The method currently used to confirm testosterone abuse is determination of the ratio of carbon 13 to carbon 12 in urinary metabolites of testosterone (36).

REFERENCES

1. Almond CS, Shin AY, Fortescue EB, et al. Hyponatremia among runners in the Boston Marathon. *N Engl J Med.* 2005;352(15):1550–6.
2. American College of Sports Medicine, Sawka MN, Burke LM, et al. American College of Sports Medicine: exercise and fluid replacement (position stand). *Med Sci Sports Exerc.* 2007;39(2):377–90.
3. Avois L, Robinson N, Saudan C, Baume N, Mangin P, Saugy M. Central nervous system stimulants and sport practice. *Br J Sports Med.* 2006; 40(suppl 1):i16–20.
4. Cakir M, Samanci N, Balci N, et al. Musculoskeletal manifestations in patients with thyroid disease. *Clin Endocrinol (Oxf).* Aug 2003;59(2): 162–7.
5. Catlin DH, Cowan DA. Detecting testosterone administration. *Clin Chem.* 1992;38(9):1685–6.
6. Dawson-Hughes B. Treatment of vitamin D deficient states. In: Drezner MK, editor. *UpToDate.* Waltham: UpToDate; 2010.
7. Draznin MB. Managing the adolescent athlete with type 1 diabetes mellitus. *Pediatr Clin North Am.* 2010;57(3):829–37.
8. Du Toit C, Locke S. An audit of clinically relevant abnormal laboratory parameters investigating athletes with persistent symptoms of fatigue. *J Sci Med Sport.* 2007;10(6):351–5.
9. Duhig TJ, McKeag D. Thyroid disorders in athletes. *Curr Sports Med Rep.* 2009;8(1):16Y19.
10. Eaton DK, Kann L, Kinchen S, et al. Youth risk behavior surveillance–United States, 2005. *MMWR Surveill Summ.* 2006;55(5):1–108.
11. Freund BJ, Shizuru EM, Hashiro GM, Claybaugh JR. Hormonal, electrolyte and renal responses to exercise are intensity dependent. *J Appl Physiol.* 1991;70(2):900–906.

12. Haluzik M, Nedvidkova J, Bartak V, et al. Effects of hypo- and hyperthyroidism on noradrenergic activity and glycerol concentrations in human subcutaneous abdominal adipose tissue assessed with microdialysis. *J Clin Endocrinol Metab.* 2003;88(2):5605–8.
13. Hewitt SC, Korach KS. Molecular biology and physiology of estrogen action. In: Snyder PJ, editor. *UpToDate.* Waltham: UpToDate; 2010.
14. Institute of Medicine. Dietary reference intakes for calcium and vitamin D. [Internet] [cited 2010 Dec]. Available from: http://www.iom.edu/Reports/2010/Dietary-Reference-Intakes-for-Calcium-and-Vitamin-D.aspx.
15. Jameson JL, Weetman A. Disorders of the thyroid gland. In: Kasper DL, Fauci AS, Longo DL, Braunwald E, Hauser SL, Jameson JL, editors. *Harrison's Principles of Internal Medicine.* 16th ed. New York: McGraw-Hill; 2005. p. 2104.
16. Klein I. Cardiovascular effects of hypothyroidism. In: Ross DS, editor. *UpToDate.* Waltham: UpToDate; 2010.
17. Larson-Meyer DE, Willis KS. Vitamin D and athletes. *Curr Sports Med Rep.* 2010;9(4):220–6.
18. Liu H, Bravata DM, Olkin I, et al. Systematic review: the effects of growth hormone on athletic performance. *Ann Intern Med.* 2008;148(10): 747–58.
19. Locker GH, Kotzmann H, Frey B, et al. Factitious hyperthyroidism causing acute myocardial infarction. *Thyroid.* 1995;5(6):465–7.
20. Mantzoros C, Shanti S. Insulin action. In: Nathan D, editor. *UpToDate.* Waltham: UpToDate; 2010.
21. McDevitt ER, Brown DE. Mechanism of action and efficacy of anabolic-adrenergic steroids. In: DeLee JC, editor. *DeLee and Drez's Orthopaedic Sports Medicine.* 3rd ed. St. Louis: W.B. Saunders; 2009. p. 414.
22. McVean JJF, David AB. Diabetes mellitus. In: DeLee JC, editor. *DeLee and Drez's Orthopaedic Sports Medicine.* 3rd ed. St. Louis: W.B. Saunders; 2009. p. 172–9.
23. Meinhardt U, Nelson AE, Hansen JL, et al. The effects of growth hormone on body composition and physical performance in recreational athletes: a randomized trial. *Ann Intern Med.* 2010;152(9):568–77.
24. Melmed S. Physiology of growth hormone. In: Snyder PJ, editor. *UpToDate.* Waltham: Uptodate; 2010.
25. Nieman LK. Treatment of adrenal insufficiency in adults. In: Lacroix A, editor. *UpToDate.* Waltham: UpToDate; 2010.
26. Powrie JK, Bassett EE, Rosen T, et al. Detection of growth hormone abuse in sport. *Growth Horm IGF Res.* 2007;17(3):220–6.
27. Rogol AD. Treatment of growth hormone deficiency in children. In: Kirkland JL, editor. *UpToDate.* Waltham: UpToDate; 2010.
28. Rosner MH, Kirven J. Exercise-associated hyponatremia. *Clin J Am Soc Nephrol.* 2007;2(1):151–61.
29. Ross DS. Diagnosis of and screening for hypothyroidism In: Cooper DS, editor. *UpToDate.* Waltham: UpToDate; 2010.
30. Ruohola JP, Laaksi I, Ylikomi T, et al. Association between serum 25(OH)D concentrations and bone stress fractures in Finnish young men. *J Bone Miner Res.* 2006;21(9):1483–8.
31. Salerno M, Oliviero U, Lettiero T, et al. Long-term cardiovascular effects of levothyroxine therapy in young adults with congenital hypothyroidism. *J Clin Endocrinol Metab.* 2008;93(7):2486–91.
32. Schulze JJ, Lundmark J, Garle M, et al. Doping test results dependent on genotype of uridine diphospho-glucuronosyl transferase 2B17, the major enzyme for testosterone glucuronidation. *J Clin Endocrinol Metab.* 2008;93(7):2500–6.
33. Sharwood K, Collins M, Goedecke J, Wilson G, Noakes T. Weight changes, sodium levels, and performance in the South African Ironman Triathlon. *Clin J Sport Med.* 2002;12(6):391–9.
34. Snyder PJ. Growth hormone deficiency in adults. In: Cooper DS, editor. *UpToDate.* Waltham: UpToDate; 2010.

35. Snyder PJ. Clinical features and diagnosis of male hypogonadism. In: Basow DS, editor. *UpToDate*. Waltham: UpToDate; 2010.

36. Snyder PJ. Use of androgens and other performing enhancing drugs by athletes. In: Matsumoto AM, O'Leary MP, editors. *UpToDate*. Waltham: UpToDate; 2010.

37. Speedy DB, Noakes TD, Rogers IR, et al. Hyponatremia in ultradistance triathletes. *Med Sci Sports Exerc*. 1999;31(6):809–15.

38. Toni S, Reali MF, Barni F, et al. Managing insulin therapy during exercise in type 1 diabetes mellitus. *Acta Biomed*. 2006;77(suppl 1):34–40.

39. Williams GH, Dluhy RG. Disorders of the adrenal cortex. In: Kasper DL, Fauci AS, Longo DL, Braunwald E, Hauser SL, Jameson JL, editors. *Harrison's Principles of Internal Medicine*. 16th ed. New York: McGraw-Hill; 2005. p. 2127.

40. World Anti-Doping Agency [Internet]. [cited 2010 July 13]. Available from: http://www.wada-ama.org/Documents/World_Anti-Doping_Program/ WADP-Prohibited-list/WADA_Prohibited_List_2010_EN.pdf.

41. Zalman AS. Metabolism of vitamin D. In: Drezner MK, editor. *UpToDate*. Waltham: UpToDate; 2010.

Hematology in the Athlete

William B. Adams

INTRODUCTION

■ Athletes as a group tend to be healthier, but they are still susceptible to the same hematologic diseases as nonathletes. However, symptoms from hematologic disturbances may manifest earlier and at lower severity, often presenting as impaired physical performance (12,14).

■ Maximal or prolonged exertion efforts typically cause transient changes in several hematologic indices (4,7,9,19,25,31,37,41). Regular endurance and altitude training generally results in more sustained alterations of hematologic parameters (2,34). Dietary inadequacies, not uncommon in athletes, may cause hematologic problems because of a deficit of calories or critical nutrients (2,18,29,32).

ANEMIA

■ Anemia is a deficiency of total red blood cell (RBC) mass that manifests as RBC volume (hematocrit [Hct]) or hemoglobin (Hb) concentration below normal values. Symptoms and physical manifestations depend on reduction in RBC volume, the decrement in oxygen delivery to tissues, the rate at which these changes occur, and compensatory capacity of the cardiopulmonary system (23,24).

  ■ Prevalence in U.S. males: 2.9% overall, 0.7% in those ages 19–40, but 9.4% in men older than 60 (15).

  ■ Prevalence in U.S. women of all ages is 7.5%, with a higher proportion (24%) of black women having anemia. Prevalence in all women ages 19–40 is 8% (6,15).

  ■ Anemia arises from either excessive loss or inadequate production of RBCs or a combination of both (13,23,24).

  ■ Athletes trying to restrict weight or follow special diets that are deficient in iron, vitamins, or calories may have a higher prevalence of anemia (4,29,34).

ATHLETIC PSEUDOANEMIA

■ Regular consistent aerobic or endurance-level training causes an increase in both RBC production and plasma volume;

however, plasma volume expansion typically exceeds the increase in RBC mass, causing a slight reduction in Hb and Hct in the resting state. This condition, common in athletes, is not a true anemia but rather a physiologic adaptation that promotes increased cardiac output and enhanced oxygen delivery to tissues and protects against hyperviscosity (8,11,14,34).

■ Plasma volume can decrease 5%–20% with endurance exercise (sweat losses and intravascular fluid shifts) (34).

■ Conditioned endurance athletes tend to have greater transient reductions in plasma volume as a result of greater sweat losses.

■ Hb values typically run $0.5 \text{ g} \cdot \text{dL}^{-1}$ lower for athletes regularly pursuing moderate-intensity training and $1.0 \text{ g} \cdot \text{dL}^{-1}$ lower for elite-level athletes (8).

■ Diagnosis may be confirmed by the following:

  ❏ Retesting the athlete after several days of rest from training as the hemodilution of conditioning reverses within days of terminating endurance-level training (34).

  ❏ Inferred from laboratory testing yielding are the following:

    ▪ Normal RBC indices and reticulocyte distribution width (RDW) on complete blood count (CBC)

    ▪ Normal reticulocyte count

    ▪ Normal serum ferritin level

IRON DEFICIENCY ANEMIA

■ Deficiency of iron in the body is the most common cause of true anemia in the athlete, as in the nonathlete (8,11). It may arise from inadequate dietary intake, excess losses through blood loss, or a combination of both.

  ■ Occurs more often in female athletes mostly because of menstrual losses coupled with inadequate consumption of meat or other sources of iron (5,11).

  ■ Laboratory testing reveals a low Hb and Hct with low mean corpuscular volume (MCV) and mean corpuscular hemoglobin (MCH).

  ■ RDW is increased, unless iron deficiency is longstanding.

  ■ Peripheral smear reveals hypochromic microcytic cells with a low to normal reticulocyte count.

- Serum ferritin levels are low, typically $< 12\ \mu g \cdot L^{-1}$ (note, however, that ferritin levels of $12–35\ \mu g \cdot L^{-1}$ may reflect inadequate iron stores with associated decrement in athletic performance without anemia manifesting) (29,31).
- Total iron binding capacity (TIBC) tends to be elevated.
- Transferrin saturation (serum iron $\times$ 100/TIBC) tends to be low (particularly $< 16\%$) (23,24).
- In evaluation of iron deficiency anemia, it is imperative to determine the cause of the deficiency in order to choose the best therapy and to avoid overlooking potentially serious conditions. Iron replacement should continue until 6–12 months after anemia has resolved (35).

ANEMIA FROM BLOOD LOSS

- Anemia may arise from acute bleeding or massive hemolysis, as well as chronic cumulative losses from insidious bleeding or persistent accelerated destruction of RBCs. Acute hemorrhage is typically obvious from history or examination findings of gross blood, melena, or manifestations of hypovolemia. Bleeding contained within tissues or the body cavity may be less obvious, particularly in the retroperitoneal space. Characteristics of rapid blood loss include the following:
  - Hb and Hct (both concentration values) are initially normal in the absence of any fluid administration (22,23).
  - Platelet counts initially drop with hemorrhage but become elevated within 1 hour if hemorrhage stops (22,23).
  - Hb and Hct values decline over the ensuing days with plasma volume expansion.
  - RBC indices are initially normal. After 3–5 days, MCV and RDW start to increase because of reticulocyte response (22,23).
  - Bilirubin levels are normal unless bleeding is internal. Similar to hemolysis, internal bleeding causes a rise in unconjugated bilirubin and lactate dehydrogenase (LDH) but without evidence of hemolysis on peripheral smear.
- If blood loss is slow and insidious, as in chronic low-grade gastrointestinal (GI) bleeding or menstrual blood loss in women, anemia may not manifest until iron stores are depleted. This situation may be revealed by a reticulocytosis with concomitant increase in RDW well before iron stores are depleted and MCV becomes low.
- **GI blood loss:** GI bleeding is a very common and often serious cause of anemia. It may arise from peptic ulcer disease, vascular anomalies, inflammatory bowel diseases, ischemic bowel syndromes, infection, diverticula, or tumors. Thus, stool occult blood testing is indicated in any anemia evaluation (28). Note that it is not uncommon for athletes to manifest mild transient GI bleeding from marathons and similar endurance events (exercise-associated GI bleeding).
- Features of exercise-associated GI bleeding include the following:
  - Occurs exclusively with prolonged endurance events and is low grade (5,34,35).
  - Source of bleeding is seldom detectable; it is theorized to arise from acute transient ischemia or mechanical contusion (e.g., cecal slap syndrome) (5,34,35).
  - In the absence of this or other pathology, bleeding is seldom significant enough to cause anemia (14).
- Note that regular use of nonsteroidal anti-inflammatory drugs (NSAIDs) is common among athletes. In addition to NSAID-induced acute GI bleeding, chronic use may cause enough insidious blood loss over time to impact RBC mass (5,34,35). All GI bleeding warrants thorough investigation to rule out serious causes.
- **Menstrual blood loss:** Menstrual bleeding with concomitant loss of iron coupled with inadequate iron replacement are common causes of anemia in women. When evaluating any woman for anemia, the provider should estimate the volume of menstrual blood loss and adequacy of iron replacement. Treatment is focused on reduction of menstrual flow if excessive and enhancing iron replacement. Clues for significant iron losses through menstruation include the following:
  - Heavy and/or frequent menses
  - Twelve or more soaked pads throughout menses
  - Passage of clots beyond the first day
  - Flow greater than 7 days
  - More than one episode of menstrual flow per month
  - Diet inadequate to compensate for cumulative menstrual losses (e.g., low intake of dietary iron sources) (18,24)
- **Exertional hemolysis (i.e., footstrike hemolysis):** Intravascular destruction of RBCs may occur in association with various exertional activities. Originally described as "march hemoglobinuria" in foot soldiers in the late 1800s, it was thought to arise from the footstrike causing compression of capillaries and rupturing RBCs; however, it is also seen in swimmers, rowers, and weightlifters, although usually to a much lesser degree (8,11,34). It is now hypothesized that intravascular turbulence, acidosis, and elevated temperature in muscle tissues may be causative factors as well (8).
  - Typically hemolysis is not significant enough to affect CBC parameters (8,11,34).
  - Reticulocyte count, RDW, and MCV may be elevated (8,11,34).
  - Haptoglobin levels may be reduced if there is enough cumulative hemolysis (8,11,34).
  - Transient hemoglobinuria may occur if hemolysis exceeds binding capacity of serum haptoglobin (approximately 20 cc of blood) (8,11,34).
- Generally no treatment is necessary; reducing impact forces to the feet (e.g., improved shoe cushioning, softer running terrain) may benefit some, particularly distance runners (8).

SICKLE CELL TRAIT

- Sickle cell trait (SCT), the heterozygous state where Hb S is present with Hb A in RBCs, is a common condition. It typically does not cause anemia and causes little impairment of athletic performance (10,14).
  - Present in 8% of blacks in the United States.
  - May confer heightened risk of complications with exercise at altitude: Sickling may be provoked in hypoxic environments, particularly altitudes above 10,000 ft, and cause a clinical picture similar to sickle cell anemia. Vigorous exertion at altitudes of 5,000 ft or more may result in enough hypoxic and metabolic stress to induce sickling and its sequelae (10,20).
  - Epidemiologically associated with increased risk of sudden death in heat stress environments and settings of rapid accelerated conditioning and sustained maximal exertion efforts (20).
  - May manifest mild microscopic hematuria independent of physical exertion, which is rarely significant (10).
  - May confer higher risk of exertion-related rhabdomyolysis, particularly in heat stress conditions (10).

ERYTHROCYTHEMIA (POLYCYTHEMIA)

- RBC mass may be increased as a physiologic response to hypoxic stress, disease processes, or drug use. Smoking, carbon monoxide exposure (*e.g.*, ice rinks), and training at altitude may also increase RBC mass in athletes. A spurious erythrocytosis may also arise from transient plasma volume contraction (*e.g.*, exercise, dehydrated status) (30). True polycythemia arises from conditions of excess RBC production, either as part of a hyperplastic marrow response (polycythemia vera) or secondary response to excess erythropoietin production (secondary polycythemia).

ETIOLOGIES OF ERYTHROCYTOSIS

- **Pseudoerythrocytosis:** Patient in a dehydrated state when phlebotomy is performed.
- **Polycythemia vera:** A myeloproliferative disorder involving trilineage marrow hyperplasia. RBC mass increase is associated with leukocytosis and thrombocytosis. Erythropoietin levels are low, with markedly elevated Hct. These patients require regular phlebotomy to prevent a hyperviscosity state (27).
- **Secondary erythrocytosis:** Results from intrinsic elevated erythropoietin or excess erythrocyte production (30).
  - Hypoxic stress
  - Endogenous conditions of excessive erythropoietin production

  - Endogenous conditions of isolated excess erythrocyte production
- **Blood doping**
  - Transfusion (phlebotomy later followed with autologous blood transfusion).
  - Exogenous erythropoietin characterized by elevated RBC and erythropoietin levels with normal white blood cell (WBC) and platelet counts (30,36). Erythropoietin produced by recombinant DNA techniques (rEPO) is identical to endogenous human erythropoietin, making detection difficult (42).

WBC LINE ABNORMALITIES

- Strenuous or prolonged vigorous exercise may acutely produce profound transient perturbations of WBC populations. This effect, however, resolves with rest and is not typically associated with persistent abnormalities of WBC lines. Various drugs may either elevate or depress WBC production, as may infection. Persistent leukopenia may be indicative of human immunodeficiency virus infection or marrow disorders. Some populations (*e.g.*, black males) may manifest a mild neutropenia that is nonpathologic (19).
- If blood work indicates a pathologic alteration of the WBC population, examination should include a thorough assessment of lymphatic and hematologic systems with investigation for infectious, toxic, or oncologic causes.
- Readily treatable etiologies, such as infection, are addressed as indicated. Otherwise, referral to a hematologist for bone marrow assessment may be necessary, particularly if there is profound leukopenia, leukocytosis, or disturbances of other cell lines suggestive of malignancy (38).

ABNORMALITIES OF PLATELETS AND COAGULATION

- The effects of exercise, particularly endurance activities, seem to have a net neutral effect on platelets and coagulation. Athletes manifesting petechiae, unusual bruising, or bleeding problems should undergo prompt investigation for causes of these disorders. Longstanding history of mild prolonged bleeding, slow clotting, or bruising problems may indicate von Willebrand disease or mild factor VIII or IX deficiency. Some medications such as aspirin-containing compounds, often a component in analgesics, directly or indirectly impair platelet or clotting activity. Disseminated intravascular coagulation (DIC) may be induced by autoimmune disorders, infections, certain drugs, toxins, malignancies, and other conditions, resulting in thrombocytopenia ranging from mild to severe. Diets deficient in green vegetables may manifest coagulopathy because of impairment of vitamin K-dependent factors (38).

- Evaluation of platelet and coagulation disorders focuses on assessment for causative conditions as listed earlier. Laboratory assessment should start with a CBC with peripheral smear looking for abnormalities in all hematologic cell lines. Coagulation studies (prothrombin time [PT], partial thromboplastin time [PTT], and international normalized ratio [INR]) should be conducted as well. If the clinical picture suggests DIC (low platelets, fragmented RBCs, and prolonged coagulation times), confirmatory testing to include fibrinogen, fibrin split products, and D-dimer should be added (38).

- Thrombocytosis is often a transient condition, typically a manifestation of an acute response to physiologic stress. Transient isolated thrombocytosis is rarely of significance. Persistent thrombocytosis should prompt investigation for infection, inflammatory disorders, malignancies, or other hyperproliferative disorders (*e.g.*, polycythemia vera, myeloproliferative diseases) (27).

OTHER DISORDERS CAUSING ANEMIA/ CELL LINE ABNORMALITIES

- Anemia and other cell line abnormalities may result from several other conditions, such as inherited disorders (*e.g.*, thalassemia), or as a consequence of various disease processes. These may manifest in the form of accelerated cell destruction or hemolysis or through impaired erythropoiesis. Details regarding diagnosis and evaluation of these conditions may be found in hematology reference books (1,26).

EXERTIONAL RHABDOMYOLYSIS

- Rhabdomyolysis is a condition of skeletal muscle breakdown with release of myocyte contents into the circulation. Exertional rhabdomyolysis is the term applied to rhabdomyolysis precipitated by exercise or exertion. It is most frequently seen in running or prolonged exertion activity, particularly in settings of accelerated physical training. Often, it occurs with exertional heat illness (3,16,17,39). Biochemically, muscle injury causes a release of myoglobin and muscle enzymes — creatine phosphokinase (CPK), LDH, and transaminases. Severe states with a large volume of muscle damage typically cause electrolyte disturbances (potassium, phosphate, and calcium) plus extracellular fluid shifts into injured tissues. Various extrinsic and intrinsic factors may enhance susceptibility to rhabdomyolysis. (3,16,17,39). These include the following:
    - Drug or toxin exposure (*e.g.*, stimulants, antihistamines, alcohol, ephedra, and statin drugs)
    - Infection
    - Heat stroke
    - Dehydration
    - Excessive muscle overload activities (especially eccentric loading)
    - Genetic muscle diseases/enzyme deficiencies
    - Metabolic diseases or disorders (diabetes, thyroid disease, chronic electrolyte disorders, or acidosis)
    - SCT
    - Autoimmune disorders (*e.g.*, polymyositis)
    - Deconditioned state (especially with rapidly accelerated physical training)

- Exertional rhabdomyolysis is a spectrum condition. Manifestations range from mild muscle injury with negligible symptoms or systemic effects to fulminate cases with large muscle mass injury, severe metabolic derangements, DIC, and death (3,16,17,39). Myoglobin release may cause nephrotoxicity, but occurrence may not directly correlate with degree of muscle enzyme elevation or severity of metabolic disturbance. Severity of rhabdomyolysis is gauged initially by magnitude of symptoms and early perturbations of blood chemistries. Collapse short of a finish line, severe pain with inability to walk, and early sustained acidosis are ominous indicators. Alternately, symptoms may start off relatively mild but progressively worsen in subsequent hours or days. Muscle enzyme levels following insult may be deceptively low early on but subsequently rise and peak 1–3 days after the injury (if there is no persistent or recurrent muscle insult).

- Management of rhabdomyolysis requires a high index of suspicion to allow for early recognition, initiation of interventions appropriate to degree of injury, and monitoring for progression. Initial laboratory studies should include basic electrolyte panel including creatinine (Cr), CPK, transaminases, LDH, uric acid, CBC, and urinalysis with microscopy. In more severe cases, calcium, phosphate, PT, PTT, fibrinogen, and fibrin split products should be added (17).

- Urinalysis demonstrating positive Hb with no RBCs is used to infer presence of myoglobinuria because results of myoglobin tests in most settings are not available quickly enough to be of value in acute management (3,17,33). Muddy casts indicate heavy myoglobin load and likely renal toxicity (39).

MILD RHABDOMYOLYSIS

- Mild muscle soreness that typically resolves within 1–2 days; otherwise no complaints.

- On examination, patient has mild soreness to palpation and minimal to no soreness with passive muscle stretch.

- Laboratory studies reveal isolated CPK elevation (generally $< 3,000 \text{ mg} \cdot \text{L}^{-1}$ but may be up to $5,000 \text{ mg} \cdot \text{L}^{-1}$); transaminases may peak slightly above normal in 1–2 days (generally less than 3 times normal values).

- Treat with oral hydration and avoidance of strenuous exertion for 1–2 days.

- Monitor for escalation or recurrence of symptoms; educate patient regarding preventive measures.
- Patient may return to activity the next day after becoming asymptomatic and after laboratory studies improved.

MODERATE RHABDOMYOLYSIS

- Symptoms of moderate muscle soreness or stiffness.
- On examination, patient has moderate muscle soreness to palpation with pain toward extremes of passive stretch.
- Moderate elevation of CPK in first few hours with mild increase in Cr ($1.5-2$ mg $\cdot$ L^{-1}), LDH, aspartate aminotransferase (AST), and alanine aminotransferase (ALT) (3 times normal or more) several hours to 1 day after injury, with CPK peak typically $< 30,000$ mg $\cdot$ L^{-1}; uric acid and electrolyte studies remain normal.
- Initial treatment is 2 L of intravenous (IV) isotonic fluids and assessment of response (symptoms and studies):
  - No worsening of symptoms and laboratory studies improved: oral hydration and reevaluate in 12–24 hours.
  - Symptoms improved but laboratory studies little changed: Assess need for further hydration; reassess every 4–6 hours until laboratory studies improve or refer for hospitalization if studies worsen or do not improve.
  - Symptoms not improving and laboratory studies rising: Refer to hospital for continued IV hydration and monitoring (watch for progression to severe or fulminant state).
  - If urine is positive for myoglobin or strongly positive for hemoglobin on urine dipstick testing, and not improving, continuous IV fluid therapy is needed (typically in hospital) for treatment of myoglobinuria.

SEVERE RHABDOMYOLYSIS

- Severe rhabdomyolysis has marked muscle soreness and pain with any muscle activity.
- Examination reveals tight muscles that are painful to palpation and limited passive stretch.
- Laboratory studies reveal transient acidosis, elevated uric acid, and minor electrolyte alterations that resolve with hydration; Cr is elevated typically > 2 mg $\cdot$ L^{-1}; and CPK progressively rises well above $30,000$ mg $\cdot$ L^{-1}; LDH, AST, and ALT progressively rise, peaking above 3 times normal at 2–3 days after insult.
- Treatment is IV fluids (2 L bolus); arrange for continued IV fluid therapy ($150-200$ cc $\cdot$ h^{-1}). Repeat laboratory studies after fluid bolus and then again after next 3–4 hours of IV fluid therapy.
  - Symptoms and laboratory studies improved: oral hydration and evaluate response over next 12–24 hours.

- Symptoms improved but laboratory studies little changed: Assess adequacy of hydration and need for additional measures (*e.g.*, compartment pressure testing); reassess every 4–6 hours.
- Symptoms not improving and laboratory studies rising: Transfer to intensive care unit (ICU) addressing comorbid issues of electrolyte disturbances, myoglobinuria, and compartment syndrome.
- If urine is positive for myoglobin or strongly positive for hemoglobin on urine dipstick testing, and not improving, continuous IV fluid therapy is needed at $150-200$ cc $\cdot$ h^{1} for treatment of myoglobinuria.
- In subacute setting (presenting days after injury), if symptoms and labs are stable or improving, condition may be managed as moderate rhabdomyolysis with particular assessment for renal injury and exclusion of myoglobinuria.

FULMINANT RHABDOMYOLYSIS

- Patient often presents with collapse and sometimes with early to delayed obtundation. Extreme muscle tightness and pain with weakness and extreme difficulty moving involved muscle(s).
- Often associated with findings typical of heat stroke, shock, and dehydration (16).
- May manifest as progressively escalating symptoms refractory to less aggressive interventions.
- On examination, involved muscles are tense, very tender, and extremely painful to any passive stretch.
- Initial laboratory studies collected near time of collapse typically manifest acidosis, hypokalemia, hypocalcemia, elevated uric acid, and/or decreased phosphate. Initial CPK levels may be deceptively low. In subsequent hours, serum chemistries manifest persistent acidosis with a shift to hyperkalemia, hypercalcemia, and hyperphosphatemia with rapidly rising CPK, LDH, AST, and ALT (39).
- Treatment necessitates cardiac monitoring for dysrhythmias in setting with advance life support capability, aggressive IV fluid hydration, and transfer to ICU for management of the metabolic derangements (3,8).
- Consult orthopedic surgeon for fasciotomy evaluation. Mild to moderate increased compartment pressures perpetuate muscle necrosis and condition improves with early fasciotomy of involved muscle areas (21,40).

RHABDOMYOLYSIS OF AN ISOLATED MUSCLE OR MUSCLE GROUP

- Typically occurs with excessive overload in weightlifting or excessive repetition of a calisthenic exercise.
- CPK levels may become elevated into the tens of thousands.

■ Typically this is self-limited, rarely manifesting systemic effects beyond the involved muscle, although sometimes myoglobinuria may be significant enough to require treatment.

RHABDOMYOLYSIS FOLLOW-UP

■ Healthy individuals with **uncomplicated** mild to moderate rhabdomyolysis may return to activity in a graduated manner after resolution of symptoms and 3 consecutive days of decline in muscle enzymes (particularly transaminases) below 50% of peak value or level back to near normal. Graduation of activity should be limited by fatigue or provocation of soreness or tightness in affected muscles. Recurrent bouts of rhabdomyolysis and any severe or fulminant episodes warrant investigation for an underlying disease process, muscle enzyme deficiencies, or underlying myopathy (16,17,20).

CONCLUSION

■ With the exception of athletic pseudoanemia, it is uncommon to encounter significant persistent hematologic alterations from exercise. Although high intensity and prolonged endurance training may result in alterations of several hematologic parameters and occasional lysis of RBCs, rarely are these of pathologic significance. However, signs and symptoms of hematologic disease may manifest at an earlier state in the athlete because of physiologic demands that require maximal hematologic system performance.

■ The condition of exertional rhabdomyolysis may occasionally manifest in athletes advancing training too rapidly but may also appear in a conditioned athlete in association with underlying disease states or as a consequence of severe overexertion or exertional heat illness. Identification and early treatment of those with myoglobin release or severe myocyte injury are crucial to preclude serious complications.

REFERENCES

1. Abramson SD, Aramson N. "Common" uncommon anemias. *Am Fam Physician.* 1999;59(4):851–8.

2. Akabas SR, Dolins KR. Mironutrient requirements of physically active women: what we can learn from iron? *Am J Clin Nutr.* 2005;81(5): 1246S–51S.

3. Baggaley PA. Rhabdomyolysis [Internet]. 1995 [cited 2011 Feb 27]. Available from: http://members.tripod.com/~baggas/rhabdo.html.

4. Bourey RE, Santuro SA. Interaction of exercise, coagulation, platelets and fibrinolysis—a brief review. *Med Sci Sports Exer.* 1988;20(5):439–46.

5. Cook JD. The effect of endurance training on iron metabolism. *Semin Hematol.* 1994;31(2):146–54.

6. Cusick SE, Mei Z, Freedman DS, et al. Unexplained decline in the prevalence of anemia among US children and women between 1988–1994 and 1999–2002. *Am J Clin Nutr.* 2008;88(6):1611–7.

7. Drygas WK. Changes in platelet function, coagulation, and fibrinolytic activity in response to moderate, exhaustive and prolonged exercise. *Int J Sports Med.* 1998;9(1):67–72.

8. Eichner ER. Anemia and blood doping. In: Sallis RE, Massimino F, editors. *Essentials of Sports Medicine.* St. Louis: Mosby; 1997. 672 p.

9. Eichner ER. Infection, immunity, and exercise: what to tell patients. *Phys Sportsmed.* 1993;21(1):125–35.

10. Eichner ER. Sickle cell trait, heroic exercise and fatal collapse. *Phys Sportsmed.* 1993;21(7):51–64.

11. Eichner ER. Sports anemia, iron supplements and blood doping. *Med Sci Sports Exerc.* 1992;24(9)(suppl):S315–8.

12. Eichner ER, Scott WA. Exercise as disease detector. *Phys Sportsmed.* 1998;26(3):41–52.

13. Elghetany MT, Banki K. Erythrocytic disorders. In: McPherson RA, Pincus MR, editors. *Henry's Clinical Diagnosis and Management by Laboratory Methods.* 21st ed. St. Louis: Saunders; 2007. p. 504–44

14. Fields KB. The athlete with anemia. In: Fields KB, Fricker PA, editors. *Medical Problems in Athletes.* Malden: Blackwell Science; 1997.

15. Ganji V, Kafai MR. Hemoglobin and hematocrit values are higher and prevalence of anemia is lower in the post–folic acid fortification period than in the pre–folic acid fortification period in US adults. *Am J Clin Nutr.* 2009;89(1):363–71.

16. Gardner JW, Kark JA. Clinical diagnosis, management, and surveillance of exertional heat illness. In: *Textbook of Military Medicine: Medical Aspects of Harsh Environments.* Vol 1. Washington: Department of the Army, Office of the Surgeon General, Borden Institute; 2002.

17. Gardner JW, Kark JA. Heat-associated illness. In: Srickland GT. *Hunter's Tropical Medicine.* 8th ed. Philadelphia: W.B. Saunders; 2000.

18. Harris SS. Helping active women avoid anemia. *Phys Sportsmed.* 1995; 23(5):35–48.

19. Jandl JH. Blood cell formation. In: Jandl JH, editor. *Blood. Textbook of Hematology.* New York: Little Brown; 1996.

20. Kark JA, Ward FT. Exercise and hemoglobin S. *Semin Hematol.* 1994; 31(3):181–225.

21. Kuklo TR, Tis JE, Moores LK, Schaefer RA. Fatal rhabdomyolysis with bilateral gluteal, thigh, and leg compartment syndrome after the Army Physical Fitness Test. A case report. *Am J Sports Med.* 2000; 28(1):112–6.

22. Lee GR. Acute posthemorrhagic anemia. In: Greer JP, Foerester J, Rogers GM, et al., editors. *Wintrobe's Clinical Hematology.* 10th ed. Baltimore: Lippincott Williams & Wilkins; 1999.

23. Lee GR. Anemia: a diagnostic strategy. In: Greer JP, Foerester J, Rogers GM, et al., editors. *Wintrobe's Clinical Hematology.* 10th ed. Baltimore: Lippincott Williams & Wilkins; 1999.

24. Lee GR. Anemia: general aspects. In: Greer JP, Foerester J, Rogers GM, et al., editors. *Wintrobe's Clinical Hematology.* 10th ed. Baltimore: Lippincott Williams & Wilkins; 1999.

25. Lee GR. Granulocytes – neutrophils. In: Lee GR, Bithell TC, Foerster J, Athens JW, Lukens JN, editors. *Wintrobe's Clinical Hematology.* 9th ed. Philadelphia: Lea & Febiger; 1993.

26. Lee GR. Hemolytic disorders: general considerations. In: Greer JP, Foerester J, Rogers GM, et al., editors. *Wintrobe's Clinical Hematology.* 10th ed. Baltimore: Lippincott Williams & Wilkins; 1999.

27. Levine SP. Thrombocytosis. In: Greer JP, Foerester J, Rogers GM, et al., editors. *Wintrobe's Clinical Hematology.* 10th ed. Baltimore: Lippincott Williams & Wilkins; 1999.

28. Little DR. Ambulatory management of common forms of anemia. *Am Fam Physician.* 1999;59(6):1598–604.

29. Lukaski HC. Vitamin and mineral status: effects on physical performance. *Nutrition.* 2004;20(7–8):632–44.

30. Means RT. Polycythemia: erythrocytosis. In: Greer JP, Foerester J, Rogers GM, et al., editors. *Wintrobe's Clinical Hematology.* 10th ed. Baltimore: Lippincott Williams & Wilkins; 1999.

31. Nieman DC, Nehlsen-Cannarella SL. The immune response to exercise. *Semin Hematol.* 1994;31(2):166–79.

32. Rodriguez NR, Dimarco NM, Langley S. American Dietetic Association position statement: nutrition and athletic performance: vitamins and minerals [Internet]. [cited 2010]. Available from: http://www.medscape.com/viewarticle/717046.

33. Saad EB. Rhabdomyolysis and myoglobinuria. *Intensive Care* [Internet]. 1997 [cited 2011 Mar 31]. Available from: http://www.medstudents.com.br/terin/terin3.htm.

34. Selby G. When does an athlete need iron? *Phys Sportsmed.* 1991; 19(4):96–102.

35. Selby GB, Eichner ER. Hematocrit and performance: the effect of endurance training on blood volume. *Semin Hematol.* 1994;31(2):122–7.

36. Simon TL. Induced erythrocythemia and athletic performance. *Semin Hematol.* 1994;31(2):128–33.

37. Streiff M, Bell WR. Exercise and hemostasis in humans. *Semin Hematol.* 1994;31(2):155–65.

38. Tenglin R. Chapter 23: hematologic abnormalities. In: Lillegard WA, Butcher JD, Rucker KS, editors. *Handbook of Sports Medicine: A Symptom-Oriented Approach.* 2nd ed. Boston: Butterworth-Heinemann; 1999.

39. Visweswaran P, Guntupalli J. Rhabdomyolysis. *Crit Care Clin.* 1999; 15(2):415–28, ix–x.

40. Wise JJ, Fortin PT. Bilateral exercise induced thigh compartment syndrome diagnosed as exertional rhabdomyolysis. A case report and review of the literature. *Am J Sports Med.* 1997;25(1):126–9.

41. Woods JA, Davis M, Smith JA, Nieman DC. Exercise and cellular innate immune function. *Med Sci Sports Exerc.* 1999;31(1):57–66.

42. World Anti-Doping Agency. World anti-doping code: athlete biological passport operating guidelines and compilation of required elements (version 2.1) [Internet]. 2010 [cited 2011 Mar 31]. Available from: http://www.uci.ch/Modules/BUILTIN/getObject.asp?MenuId=&ObjTypeCode=FILE&type=FILE&id=NjA2NzM&LangId=142.

36 Neurology

Joel Shaw

INTRODUCTION

- Concussion is a common injury seen by sports medicine physicians and is often a difficult scenario due to the athlete's desire to return to play, coaches' desire to have their athletes available, and the social pressure of parents and media. Due to the potential sequelae of injury, it is important to understand how to evaluate the patient initially looking for potentially dangerous symptoms and to be comfortable in how to safely return an athlete to sports.

- Due to the frequency of headaches in athletes and the general population and the potential to limit activity, it is important to understand how to diagnose the type of headache and how to treat each type to enable an athlete to return to activity.

- The history of limiting athletes with epilepsy from participation has led to many unwanted effects, including obesity and its health effects, social isolation, depression, and anxiety. It is important for the long-term health of patients with epilepsy to increase their ability to participate in sports.

CONCUSSIONS

Definition

- Concussion is defined as a complex pathophysiologic process affecting the brain, induced by traumatic biomechanical forces. Concussion can be caused either by a direct blow to the head and face or by transmitted forces from contact to another part of the body. This usually results in a rapid onset of impairment that resolves spontaneously.

- The symptoms are primarily caused by a functional disturbance in the brain without structural damage. In most patients, the symptoms resolve in a sequential pattern, although in rare cases, the postconcussion symptoms may be prolonged.

- Concussions do not result in changes on typical neuroimaging studies. As originally discussed in the Prague guidelines, the majority of concussions (80%–90%) resolve quickly (7–10 days), with a possible extended resolution period in children and adolescents (21).

CONCUSSION EVALUATION

Signs and Symptoms

- In evaluating a patient with presumed concussion, the medical evaluation should include an extensive injury history, clinical symptoms, physical signs, behavior, balance, and cognition. Symptoms may include but are not limited to headache, a sensation of fogginess, drowsiness, and lability.

- Physical signs include amnesia and possible loss of consciousness (LOC). Cognitive impairment may include slowed reaction times, irritability, anxiety, or depressed mood. It is important to remember that, in some cases, the symptoms may not appear until several hours after the injury.

Sideline Evaluation

- When a patient shows any potential features of a concussion, the athlete should initially be evaluated by emergency procedures including the ABCs (airway, breathing, and circulation) of emergency care, with a special emphasis on evaluating for a possible cervical spine injury. The disposition based on emergency protocol should be determined by the treating health care provider. A stable patient should next be evaluated by a sideline tool designed for concussion evaluation, such as the Sports Concussion Assessment Tool (SCAT2). After diagnosis of a concussion, a player should not be left alone, with serial monitoring for several hours after the injury. Based on the Zurich consensus, an athlete should not be allowed to return to competition on the same day as the injury (22).

- One essential part of sideline evaluation is testing of cognitive function. Standard orientation questions (*e.g.*, time, place, and person) have been shown to be ineffective in sideline evaluations compared to memory assessment (19).

- Brief tests for attention and memory function have been shown to be effective, including the Maddocks questions (19) and the Standardized Assessment of Concussion (SAC) (20). These tests are effective for rapid sideline evaluation, but in questions of more subtle, persistent changes, they are not able to replace the effectiveness of comprehensive neuropsychological testing.

Advanced Outpatient Testing

- The use of neuroimaging studies is still not effective for the standard evaluation of concussions. Brain computed tomography (CT) and magnetic resonance imaging (MRI) are normal in concussive injuries but should still continue to be used when there are symptoms suspicious for possible intracerebral structural lesions. These situations include prolonged disturbance in consciousness, focal neurologic deficits, or worsening symptoms.

- Newer studies, including perfusion and diffusion MRIs, functional MRI, positron emission tomography, and magnetic resonance spectroscopy, show some future promise but are still limited by minimal published studies and inability to compare to preinjury imaging.

- Objective balance assessment can provide additional information in concussed patients. Studies consistently show, whether by sophisticated force plate testing or clinical balance tests, that postural stability deficits persist for about 72 hours. These tests are useful tools to evaluate the motor portion of neurologic function.

- Neuropsychological testing (NP) gives critical information that can be valuable in concussion evaluation and recovery. In some cases, cognitive recovery and symptom recovery follow the same pattern, but studies have demonstrated that frequently cognitive recovery lags behind symptom recovery. In these cases, NP testing would be beneficial in determining which patients are not fully recovered functionally. It is important to recognize that NP assessment should not be used singularly to make return-to-play decisions, but that it is effective as an addition to clinical decision making. Based on the data from several studies, NP testing is best used in return-to-play decisions after the patient is asymptomatic (4).

Concussion Management

- The main tenet of treatment for concussion is physical and cognitive rest. Complete rest should be encouraged until the symptoms have completely resolved. This includes all physical activity and any activities that involve concentration and attention, including school work, videogames, and texting. All these activities have the potential to exacerbate symptoms and delay recovery. With complete rest, the majority of symptoms will resolve spontaneously within several days.

- When symptoms have resolved, the next step is a gradual return to activity. A graduated return-to-play protocol is listed in Table 36.1. The athlete needs to remain asymptomatic to continue along the stepwise progression. Each stage should last for 24 hours. If any postconcussion symptoms develop, the patient should return to the previous asymptomatic stage. The Zurich committee discussed the possibility of some high-level athletes returning on the day of injury. This should only occur in a small population, described as adult athletes in a setting with team physicians experienced in concussion management and access to immediate

Table 36.1	Return-To-Play Protocol
Rehabilitation Stage	**Functional Exercise**
1. No activity	Complete physical and cognitive rest
2. Light aerobic exercise	Walking, swimming, or stationary cycling keeping intensity < 70% maximum predicted heart rate; no resistance training
3. Sport-specific exercise	Skating drills in ice hockey, running drills in soccer; no head impact activities
4. Noncontact training drills	Progression to more complex training drills, *e.g.*, passing drills in football and ice hockey; may start progressive resistance training
5. Full-contact practice	Following medical clearance, participate in normal training activities
6. Return to play	Normal game play

neurocognitive assessment. This is based on a National Football League (NFL) study showing safe same-day return in some NFL athletes (27). This does not include high school or college-age athletes, because multiple studies have shown that athletes in this age group often continue to show NP deficits despite being asymptomatic on the sidelines and are more likely to have delayed onset of symptoms (6,7).

- There are several factors that should cause the physician to consider a more deliberate approach to return to play. One controversial factor is LOC. Although prior guidelines that were primarily based on presence or absence of LOC have been shown to be less helpful, LOC is still an importance indicator of severity. If LOC lasts greater than a minute, that is an indicator of a more severe concussion that will likely require longer recovery time. Presence of amnesia is still difficult to interpret but may correlate with prolonged recovery. Athletes with multiple concussions should be given more time to recover. Athletes with repeated concussions occurring with progressively less impact are likely to require a longer period of recovery.

- Several populations require a more vigilant approach to provide effective care. Child and adolescent athletes tend to recover at a slower pace, with a more deliberate resolution of symptoms and return to baseline cognition. The Zurich guidelines were determined to be applicable to athletes 10 years and older. In younger athletes, the symptoms are often interpreted and described differently. It is often helpful to seek input from parents and teachers about concussion effects. It remains important for young athletes to be completely symptom free prior to return to sport, and this often takes a longer period in the developing brain. Cognitive rest is an important emphasis in this age group with the frequent use of computers, videogames, and texting. Students may also benefit from time off from school, studies, and school activities. Due to the prolonged recovery, in many cases, it is beneficial to extend the length of asymptomatic time until return to sport or to extend the length of each stage of the return-to-play plan. Although females are more prone to concussion, the experts at the Zurich conference determined that there is no need to adjust the evaluation and treatment of female athletes.

- Second impact syndrome is one reason for the graduated return to play. This occurs in an athlete who returns to contact before resolution of the symptoms and physiologic changes associated with concussion. A second traumatic event results in loss of cerebral vasomotor control. This results in uncontrollable cerebral edema and increasing intracranial volume and pressure. This often leads to neurologic collapse and death.

Postconcussion Syndrome

- Postconcussion syndrome is a poorly defined entity. It can be defined as persistence of cognitive, physical, or emotional symptoms of concussion lasting longer than what is normally expected. The time frame is not well defined but usually refers to symptoms lasting more than a couple weeks. The cause of persistent symptoms is controversial, but appears to be a combination of psychogenic and physiologic changes. The condition is a clinical diagnosis made by an intensive history with minimal changes on physical exam and no benefit of current imaging techniques.

- There are several symptoms and historical factors that correlate with increased likelihood of persistent symptoms. Amnesia is connected with risk of symptoms lasting past 5 days but not necessarily for longer periods (8). Migraine symptoms (17) and noise sensitivity (11) are connected with increased risk of prolonged symptoms. Several studies show that athletes with several previous concussions are more likely to develop postconcussion syndrome (7,24). The pre-existence of psychiatric issues also appears to correlate with prolonged symptoms.

- The effect of previous concussions has been well documented. One study confirmed significant increase in cognitive deficits in professional football players with previous history of at least 3 concussions (15). Other studies have shown similar results in younger athletes with cumulative effects from less violent hits. Athletes with prior concussions require longer recovery time and are at increased risk for future head injuries.

- The symptoms include the typical cognitive and physical symptoms of concussion, but especially headache, distractibility, and poor concentration. Other common symptoms include depression, anxiety, personality changes, irritability, and apathy.

- Treatment of postconcussion syndrome is controversial. There are several options to try for the cognitive deficits. Dopaminergic agents, including amantadine, levodopa, and bromocriptine, have some evidence supporting their

beneficial effect on cognitive deficits. Due to the similarities with Alzheimer disease, there has been an effort to treat cholinergic dysfunction with physostigmine and donepezil with some effect. The mood disorders associated with this syndrome are best treated with psychiatric counseling. Selective serotonin reuptake inhibitors (SSRIs) and buspirone are effective in treatment of mood disorders, including anxiety and depression. Trazodone is beneficial for the associated sleep disturbances. Benzodiazepines and antipsychotics should be avoided because they may exacerbate cognitive changes.

HEADACHES

Classification

- Classification of exercise-associated headaches is difficult due to minimal studies related to exercise-associated headaches. The International Headache Society groups exertional headaches in the category of "miscellaneous headaches unassociated with structural lesion." In evaluating the athlete, especially on the sideline, it is most important to initially triage the patient to an appropriate treatment plan.

- The first responsibility is to determine the severity of the headache. Severe headaches require immediate in-depth evaluation and treatment. Neurologic symptoms require a more intensive initial evaluation. An athlete who describes a "thunderclap headache" should be taken seriously. An athlete with a traumatic headache that is rapidly increasing in severity or associated with neurologic symptoms should be evaluated with further imaging to look for cerebral hemorrhage or infarct. Neurologic symptoms that should be evaluated further include mental status changes, nausea, vomiting, increased neck stiffness, or focal neurologic findings. It is important to look for these abnormalities because one study found that 10% of patients with exertional headache had an organic lesion as the cause of headache.

- Exertional headaches are the most common type of headache in athletes. These headaches are often preceded by prodromal migraine symptoms. These symptoms may include scotomata, photopsia, vertigo, aphasia, ataxia, or paresthesias. The auras usually occur 10–20 minutes prior to the headache and cease prior to the headache. Generally, the headache is bilateral and throbbing in nature. It will last between 5 minutes and 24 hours. It usually occurs with high-intensity exertion. The associated increased intracranial pressure appears to be the cause. According to one study, patients who suffer from recurrent headaches are more likely to have myofascial trigger points and postural abnormalities associated with cervical and thoracic dysfunction. It is important to remember to treat the associated musculoskeletal abnormalities that may lead to recurrent headaches.

- Weightlifter's headache is one type of exertional headache. It most commonly occurs during power lifting or maximal lifts. The presumed mechanism is breath holding during lifting associated with Valsalva maneuver. The increase in intracranial pressure leads to headache in the posterior occipital region. The headache begins as sharp and intense, often incapacitating. Symptoms often last at least several days, lasting longer than the other benign headaches. If these headaches become more severe or recurrent, then further evaluation looking for Arnold-Chiari malformation or aneurysm becomes necessary.

- Effort headaches occur in endurance activities, such as long-distance running or triathlons. The headaches tend to be similar to migraines, often unilateral with associated nausea, vomiting, and visual aura. Beside endurance, these headaches appear to occur in relation to heat, humidity, altitude, dehydration, or poor nutrition. The best treatment for this type of headache is preventative, including hydration, proper conditioning, and avoidance of altitude changes.

Treatment

- Treatment of migraines should be multifactorial. In order to most effectively treat migraines, it is important to have an accurate diagnosis. There are three main stages of treatment to include prevention, acute treatment, and in some cases prevention.

- Prevention is the most effective form of treatment. A healthy lifestyle is essential to limit headaches, including a healthy, well-balanced diet, adequate sleep (8 hours a day), and good hydration. According to several studies, the use of riboflavin 200 mg twice a day and magnesium citrate 200 mg twice a day is beneficial. The riboflavin improves mitochondrial energy and the magnesium decreases neurologic hyperexcitability. Proper warm-up and breathing techniques will help to limit the effects of breath holding and Valsalva maneuver.

- Acute treatment of headaches is most commonly treated with typical nonsteroidal anti-inflammatory drugs (NSAIDs), including ibuprofen and naproxen. When the pattern is more typical of migraines, 5-hydroxytryptamine blockers, such as sumatriptan or ergotamines, are effective. Prophylactic treatment may include medications such as indomethacin or other NSAIDs, amitriptyline, and SSRIs. For difficult-to-manage patients, several alternative treatments have been shown to be effective. Botulinum toxin type A is effective and safe as prophylaxis for chronic headaches (3). A randomized controlled trial showed that acupuncture improves quality of life and decreases headache pain (5).

EPILEPSY

- There is a long history of controversy involving epileptic patients and their safety to participate in athletics and exercise. For the past several decades, the concerns of parents, administrators, and coaches have led to restrictions on athletic involvement for epileptic patients. Medical recommendations

for a long period supported the exclusion of these patients and have only recently made some progress in allowing participation. Until 1974, organizations such as the American Medical Association (AMA) and the American Academy of Pediatrics (AAP) recommended significant restrictions in activity due to fear of injury and induction of seizure activity. Articles published in 1973 argued both for and against participation for epileptic patients (18,23). This discussion led to a change in the recommendations of the AMA in 1974 allowing participation in contact sports in some cases to assist in adjustment to school, social interactions, and the diagnosis of seizure disorder (9). In 1983, the AAP adjusted their recommendation to allow participation in most sports, including contact sports, as long as seizures were adequately controlled and supervision was available.

- Epilepsy is present in 1%–2% of the population. Seventy-five percent of these patients have their first seizure by the age of 20 (10), and 30%–40% of patients who have an initial seizure will have a recurrent episode and then are likely to have repetitive episodes in the future. Despite this frequency, based on a study in 1997, 80% of patients are well controlled on 2 or fewer antiepileptic medications (2). This should reassure patients and physicians that these patients would benefit from exercise. Multiple studies confirm the connection of decreased exercise and activity in epileptic patients with decreased self-esteem, increased anxiety and depression, and diseases associated with poor physical fitness, such as obesity, heart disease, and diabetes. For this reason, the psychosocial and psychological benefits of physical activity should be used to encourage patients with well-controlled epilepsy to be involved frequently in physical activity, athletics, and exercise.

Classification

- Partial seizures are localized to 1 area of the brain with activation of a smaller number of neurons. Partial seizures are further classified as simple or complex in reference to the effect on consciousness. Seizures with no LOC are termed partial seizures but may include motor, sensory, or autonomic symptoms. Seizures associated with altered consciousness, which may include diminished responsiveness, staring, lip smacking, and repetitive swallowing, are termed complex seizures.

- Generalized seizures are seizures associated with bilateral discharges on electroencephalography (EEG) and involve the entire cortex. Generalized seizures can be either convulsive or nonconvulsive. Nonconvulsive generalized seizures include absence and myoclonic seizures.

Risks of Participation

- It is important for patients and physicians to understand the things that may make participation in sports dangerous or unsafe. First, we need to understand factors that may precipitate seizures. These may include fatigue, emotional stress, fever, hormonal changes of the menstrual cycle, alcohol, caffeine, heat, humidity, and sleep deprivation. These factors vary depending on the patient and should be individualized. There are rare cases when exercise may be a trigger for a specific patient. In 2 separate studies, only 1%–2% of patients had identified exercise as a trigger for seizure activity (13,26). Hypoglycemia and hyponatremia are also common abnormalities that may lower the seizure threshold. The concern for an increased risk of injury with sports participation is unfounded in most sports (1), although there are certain activities that are connected with higher risk and will be discussed in a later section.

Benefits of Exercise

- As stated before, epileptic patients have a higher rate of obesity, body mass index, and body fat ratio (28). To counteract this medical risk, according to a study by Eriksen et al. (12), an active exercise program decreased cholesterol levels and increased aerobic performance. This same study showed that a regular exercise program reduces sleep problems and fatigue, improves psychosocial functioning, and increases sense of well-being. There are multiple studies, including the study by Eriksen et al., that show decreased seizure risk in patients who follow a regular exercise program. Two studies showed improved EEG results, including a decrease in occurrence of epileptiform discharge, normalization of EEG changes, and lowering of the seizure threshold (14,25).

Sports Participation

- Based on these benefits of athletic participation, it is important to support epileptic patient participation whenever possible and safe. Because of the potential risk, it is important to do everything possible to make participation safe, including controlling risk when possible and using protective equipment when available. The first standard is to have adequate control of seizure activity prior to participation. There is no consensus or standard on what is adequate control of seizures. The most definitive statement is by the International League Against Epilepsy, which states that a patient controlled without a seizure for the past year should be cleared from most restrictions in activity (16). Other recommendations for risk reduction include adequate rest, proper hydration, and a well-balanced diet to decrease the risk of hypoglycemia or other abnormalities that may lower the seizure threshold. It is also important to follow medication levels and restrict activity when the levels are not well controlled.

Sports-Specific Participation

Contact and Collision Sports

- There are no recommendations or studies to support restricting the participation of epileptic patients in contact or collision sports. Any current restrictions in sports should be based only on risk to the athlete or other participants if a seizure occurs during the sporting activity. According to the AMA and AAP, there should be no restrictions for well-controlled epileptics to participate in football, hockey, rugby, soccer, basketball, or baseball. Boxing is the only collision sport without specific recommendations by the AMA, AAP, or the American Academy of Neurology (AAN). In the case of boxing, because there are no studies or consensus statements to allow or restrict participation, the decision to allow participation should be done on an individual basis with full disclosure of potential risk to the patient.

Swimming and Water Sports

- Obviously, the main concern with swimming is the risk of drowning if a seizure occurs while in the water. One study showed a fourfold increase in the risk of drowning or near drowning from submersion in epileptic patients. The general consensus is that epileptic patients with good control of seizure activity may participate in water competition and swimming if there is direct visual supervision by someone adequately trained in rescue and resuscitation techniques. This should only be done in events with clear water. Obviously patients with poor control and frequent seizures should be restricted from swimming. Scuba diving is much more restricted due to the risk of dislodging the regulator, the poor airway protection during an emergency rapid ascent increasing the risk of aspiration of "the bends," and the potential for injury to the rescue partner. Any patient with poor control of seizures should not be allowed to dive, and even allowing the well-controlled epileptic to scuba dive should only happen after significant deliberation and consideration.

Sports from Heights

- Sports in which a fall could cause serious injury require more serious consideration of seizure control and the benefit or participation for the athlete. Gymnastics requires appropriate planning and preparation for each individual. When seizures are well controlled, close observation and assistance by coaches and trainers are essential. In some cases, the use of safety harnesses may be beneficial. Horseback riding and harnessed rock climbing may be possible with good seizure control and the assistance of a partner who can provide first aid and has the ability to contact emergency personnel, as long as the patient has full understanding of the risks. Hang gliding, parachuting, and free climbing should not be recommended for any epileptic.

Motor Sports

- The risk of injury to the driver, other drivers, or spectators in motor sports due to the high speed and force of collision is severe. For this reason, any effort to reduce the frequency of accidents and the risk of severe injury is essential. The general recommendation is that all epileptic patients should avoid participation in motor sports.

Medical Treatment of Epilepsy

- Medical treatment of epilepsy is difficult in the athletic population due to the frequent side effects from these medications that may affect the performance of athletes. We will discuss side effects of several medications that may impact athletic performance, but the main point is that each patient must be treated individually for better seizure control with reduction of side effects.

- **Gabapentin** is well tolerated compared to most antiepileptic medications, with minimal side effects or drug interactions.
- **Lamotrigine** has the potential to cause dizziness, movement disorders, sedation, and headaches.
- **Valproate** is known to cause increased appetite, resulting in weight gain and tremors. Sedation and cognitive impairment are much less common.
- **Carbamazepine** may cause sedation, ataxia, nausea, and dizziness.
- **Phenytoin** is known to result in sedation, depressed cognitive function, and depressed activity.

REFERENCES

1. Aisenson MR. Accidental injuries in epileptic children. *Pediatrics.* 1948;2(1):85–8.
2. Baker GA, Jacoby A, Buck D, Stalgis C, Monnet D. Quality of life of people with epilepsy: a European study. *Epilepsia.* 1997;38(3): 353–62.
3. Blumenfeld A. Botulinum toxin type A as an effective prophylactic treatment in primary headache disorders. *Headache.* 2003;43(8): 853–60.
4. Broglio SP, Macciocchi SN, Ferrara MS. Sensitivity of the concussion assessment battery. *Neurosurgery.* 2007;60(6):1050–7.
5. Coeytaux RR, Kaufman JS, Kaptchuk TJ, et al. A randomized controlled trial of acupuncture for chronic daily headache. *Headache.* 2005;45(9):1113–23.
6. Collins M, Field M, Lovell M, et al. Relationship between postconcussion headache and neuropsychological test performance in high school athletes. *Am J Sports Med.* 2003;31(2):168–73.
7. Collins M, Grindel S, Lovell M, et al. Relationship between concussion and neuropsychological performance in college football players. The NCAA Concussion Study. *JAMA.* 1999;282(10):964–70.
8. Collins M, Iverson GL, Lovell MR, McKeag DB, Norwig J, Maroon J. On-field predictors of neuropsychological and symptom deficit following sports-related concussion. *Clin J Sport Med.* 2003;13(4): 222–9.
9. Corbitt RW, Cooper DL, Erickson DJ, Kriss FC, Thornton ML, Craig TT. American Medical Association Committee on Medical Aspects of Sports: epileptics and contact sports. *JAMA.* 1974;229(7):820–1.
10. Daniel JC, Nassiri JD, Wilckens J, Land BC. The implementation and use of the standardized assessment of concussion at the U.S. Naval Academy. *Mil Med.* 2002;167(10):873–6.
11. Dischinger PC, Ryb GE, Kufera JA, Auman KM. Early predictors of postconcussive syndrome in a population of trauma patients with mild traumatic brain injury. *J Trauma.* 2009;66(2):289–96.
12. Eriksen HR, Ellertsen B, Grønningsaeter H, Nakken KO, Løyning Y, Ursin H. Physical exercise in women with intractable epilepsy. *Epilepsia.* 1994;35(6):1256–64.
13. Frucht MM, Quigg M, Schwaner C, Fountain NB. Distribution of seizure precipitants among epilepsy syndromes. *Epilepsia.* 2000; 41(12):1534–9.
14. Götze W, Kubicki S, Munter M, Teichmann J. Effect of physical exercise on seizure threshold. *Dis Nerv Syst.* 1967;28(10):664–7.
15. Guskiewicz KM, Marshall SW, Bailes J, et al. Recurrent concussion and risk of depression in retired professional football players. *Med Sci Sport Exerc.* 2007;39(6):903–9.
16. ILAE Commission report. Restrictions for children with epilepsy. Commission of Pediatrics of the International League Against Epilepsy. *Epilepsia.* 1997;38(9):1054–6.
17. Lau B, Lovell MR, Collins MW, Pardini J. Neurocognitive and symptom predictors of recovery in high school athletes. *Clin J Sport Med.* 2009;19(3):216–21.
18. Livingston S, Berman W. Participation of epileptic patients in sports. *JAMA.* 1973;224(2):236–8.
19. Maddocks DL, Dicker GD, Saling MM. The assessment of orientation following concussion in athletes. *Clin J Sport Med.* 1995;5(1):32–5.
20. McCrea M. Standardized mental status assessment of sports concussion. *Clin J Sport Med.* 2001;11(3):176–81.
21. McCrory P, Johnston K, Meeuwisse W, et al. Summary and agreement statement of the 2nd International Conference on Concussion in Sport, Prague 2004. *Br J Sports Med.* 2005;39(4):196–204.
22. McCrory P, Weeuwisse W, Johnston K, et al. Consensus Statement on Concussion in Sports 3rd International Conference on Concussion in Sport held in Zurich, November 2008. *Clin J Sport Med.* 2009;19(3):185–200.
23. McLaurin RL. Epilepsy and contact sports: factors contraindicating participation. *JAMA.* 1973;225(3):285–7.
24. Moser RS, Schatz P, Jordan BD. Prolonged effects of concussion in high school athletes. *Neurosurgery.* 2005;57(2):300–6.
25. Nakken KO, Løyning A, Løyning T, Gløersen G, Larsson PG. Does physical exercise influence the occurrence of epileptiform EEG discharges in children? *Epilepsia.* 1997;38(3):279–84.
26. Nakken KO. Physical exercise in outpatients with epilepsy. *Epilepsia.* 1999;40(5):643–51.
27. Pellman EJ, Viano DC, Casson IR, Arfken C, Feuer H. Concussion in professional football: players returning to the same game—part 7. *Neurosurgery.* 2005;56(1):79–90; discussion, 2.
28. Steinhoff BJ, Neusüss K, Thegeder H, Reimers CD. Leisure time activity and physical fitness in patients with epilepsy. *Epilepsia.* 1996;37(12):1221–7.

37 Gastroenterology

David L. Brown, Chris G. Pappas, and Courtney A. Dawley

INTRODUCTION AND EPIDEMIOLOGY

- From a gastrointestinal (GI) perspective, long-distance runners have been the most scrutinized group, but recent studies have looked at the GI symptoms of long-distance walkers, cyclists, triathletes, and weightlifters. Upper and lower GI tract symptoms occur with equal prevalence in cyclists. Lower GI symptoms predominate nearly 2 to 1 over upper GI symptoms in endurance runners. Whether running or riding, these same patterns also hold true in triathletes (24). In low-intensity long-distance walking, the overall occurrence of GI symptoms is much lower than in other sports studied. The most common symptoms are flatulence and nausea, which occur at similar rates to those of the baseline population (only 5% of walkers) (25).

- Symptomatic gastroesophageal reflux is extremely common in athletes. Cyclists have the lowest esophageal acid exposure, followed closely by runners. Weightlifters have the highest rates of reflux. All groups have increased reflux when exercising postprandially. Cyclists have a modest increase in reflux after eating, whereas weightlifters nearly double and runners triple their reflux (8).

- Peptic ulcer disease (PUD) is associated with the primary risk factors of *Helicobacter pylori* infection and nonsteroidal anti-inflammatory drug (NSAID) use. *H. pylori* is associated with 65%–95% of gastric ulcers and 75% of duodenal ulcers. The estimated risk of a clinically significant NSAID-induced event, including bleeding and perforation, is 1%–4% per year for nonselective NSAID. Either of these factors alone increases ulcer risk 20-fold. When both risk factors are present, an individual is 61 times more likely to develop ulcer disease (31).

- The primary lower GI condition of athletes is runner's diarrhea, affecting up to 26% of marathon runners (14). Runner's diarrhea is not typically associated with bleeding; however, studies in marathon runners showed that 20% of runners completing a marathon had occult blood in their stools, another 6% had bloody diarrhea, and 17% had frank hematochezia while in training (20).

UPPER GI DISEASES

Gastroesophageal Reflux Disease

- The most common presenting complaints for gastroesophageal reflux disease (GERD) are heartburn and acid regurgitation. The classic presentation is retrosternal burning, exacerbated by meals, intense workouts, and recumbency, with resolution on antacids. Symptoms are typically more common during initial training periods with improvement as the athlete becomes more conditioned (22). Atypical symptoms include nausea, excessive salivation (water brash), bloating, and belching (27). Extraintestinal complaints include sore throat, exertional dyspnea, cough, or wheezing (Table 37.1).

- GERD pathophysiology involves retrograde movement of gastric acid and the proteolytic enzyme pepsin, which causes irritation of the esophageal epithelium. Reflux alone is insufficient to explain why individuals become symptomatic because affected patients have reflux rates similar to healthy individuals (11). The critical factor in symptom development appears to be that the contact time between refluxed material and the epithelium is so excessive that the normal gastric contents overwhelm the epithelial protective mechanisms. Alternatively, symptoms may develop when normal contact time occurs in the face of insufficient protective mechanisms.

- Symptomatic reflux episodes during exercise are likely multifactorial but correlate best with transient lower esophageal sphincter relaxations (TLESRs). This vagally mediated reflex facilitates lower esophageal sphincter (LES) relaxation and gas venting in response to gaseous stomach distention. The decrease in LES tone and reflux associated with TLESRs last longer and are not accompanied by a swallow-induced peristaltic sweep, leading to prolonged acid exposure. Supine or forward-flexed posture during particular modes of exercise increases intra-abdominal pressure, overcoming the mechanical protection of the LES and negating bolus acid clearance achieved by gravity. Increasing exercise intensity is associated with increased reflux episodes and duration of acid exposure (28).

Table 37.1	GERD Symptom Patterns	
Classic Symptoms	**Atypical Symptoms/Signs**	**Red Flag Symptoms**
Heartburn	**Pulmonary**	Chronic untreated symptoms
Acid regurgitation	Asthma	Dysphagia
Nonspecific Symptoms	Chronic cough	Weight loss
Nausea	**ENT**	Hematemesis
Dyspepsia	Dental erosions	Melena
Bloating	Halitosis	Odynophagia
Belching	Lingual sensitivity	Vomiting
Indigestion	Chronic pharyngitis	Early satiety
Hypersalivation/ water brash	Hoarseness Rhinitis/sinusitis Globus **Cardiac** Atypical chest pain	

ENT, ear, nose, and throat; GERD, gastroesophageal reflux disease.

As exercise intensity increases, the frequency, duration, and amplitude of esophageal contractions progressively decrease. High-intensity exercise also reduces splanchnic blood flow, which may inhibit restoration of acid-base balance and deprive the epithelium of the oxygen and nutrients needed for damage repair.

- If the history and physical raise red flags, symptoms are particularly severe, or the diagnosis is unclear, the athlete should be referred for gastroenterology evaluation (Fig. 37.1). In patients with extraintestinal manifestations or atypical GERD symptoms, providers can consider an initial therapeutic trial. If empiric therapy fails, it is important not only to consult gastroenterology, but also the specialty that would evaluate for extraintestinal complications (Fig. 37.2).

- Behavioral and training interventions may improve symptoms such as decreasing the intensity of training briefly, then gradually increasing intensity as tolerated. Other interventions include avoiding postprandial exercise or waiting to exercise for at least 3 hours after a meal. Avoiding high-calorie meals and fatty foods prior to exercise may also help symptoms (22).

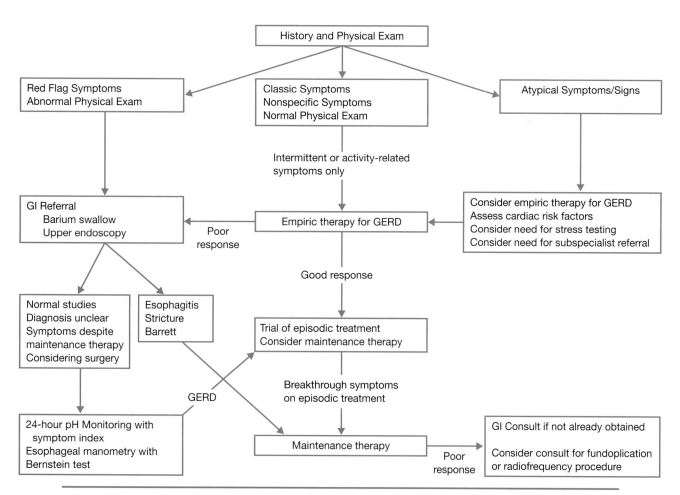

FIGURE 37.1: Evaluation of gastroesophageal reflux disease (GERD). GI, gastrointestinal. Adapted with permission from O'Connor FG. Gastrointestinal problems in runners. In: O'Connor FG, Wilder R, editors. *Textbook of Running Medicine.* 1st ed. New York: McGraw-Hill; 2001. p. 307–314.

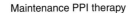

| Maintenance PPI therapy |
| Maintenance H₂RA therapy or consider episodic PPI** |
| Pre-exercise/competition Antacids or H₂RA* |

Lifestyle modifications

Avoid exercise or recumbency within 3 hours of meals
Avoid restrictive clothing
Weight loss

Review Medications
Alpha Blockers
Anticholinergics
Barbiturates
Beta-blockers
Ca²⁺ Blockers
Demerol
Morphine
Progesterone
Theophylline
Valium

Smoking cessation
Elevate head of bed 4–8 inches
Moderation of food/drink triggers
Citric or tomato juices
Chocolate
Alcohol
Coffee (both regular & decaf)
Peppermint
Onions/garlic
Fats

*H₂RA = histamine 2 receptor antagonist   **PPI = proton pump inhibitor

FIGURE 37.2: Therapeutic pyramid for exercise-related gastroesophageal reflux disease. Adapted with permission from O'Connor FG. Gastrointestinal problems in runners. In: O'Connor FG, Wilder R, editors. *Textbook of Running Medicine.* 1st ed. New York: McGraw-Hill; 2001. p. 307–314.

■ Persistent symptoms despite behavioral interventions warrant medical therapy. Episodic complaints are treated with over-the-counter (OTC) antacids, as needed, or antireflux medication, such as histamine 2 receptor antagonists (H₂RAs) or standard-dose proton pump inhibitors (PPIs) (22). This can be advanced to prescription-strength antireflux (H₂RA or PPI) therapy if control is insufficient. Should symptoms continue after 6 weeks of H₂RA therapy, neither continuing therapy nor increasing the dose is likely to achieve control (13). It was previously common practice to consider add-on therapy to prescription-dose H₂RA with a prokinetic agent to improve LES tone, gastric emptying, and peristalsis. These agents all have side effects that make them undesirable for use in athletes. Bethanechol has generalized cholinergic effects. Metoclopramide has a high incidence of fatigue, restlessness, tremor, and tardive dyskinesia, making it a poor choice for anything more than sporadic use. Cisapride, formerly the prokinetic agent of choice, was found to be associated with arrhythmia development, especially with concomitant use of macrolides, imidazoles, or protease inhibitors (34). This discovery led to severe prescribing restrictions in the United States.

■ In individuals who fail to respond to H₂RAs, PPIs are the treatment of choice. PPIs provide more rapid relief of symptoms (2) and are more likely than H₂RAs to heal and prevent recurrence of erosive esophagitis (7). The agents in this class are equally efficacious in controlling heartburn and have similar healing and relapse rates (5). Because reported differences in initial bioavailability and antisecretory potency are not clinically significant with longstanding use, 1 PPI cannot be recommended over another (33). If the response to episodic treatment is generally favorable but symptoms are occurring on a more chronic basis, maintenance therapy is beneficial. Because their efficacy is dosedependent, PPI therapy can be stepped up to control symptoms. Failure to respond to high-dose PPI therapy requires gastroenterologist evaluation to rule out complications of GERD. In the absence of findings consistent with reflux disease, further GI testing will be necessary to confirm GERD and assess for other esophageal disorders.

■ More invasive treatments are available for patients with an established diagnosis of GERD who respond poorly to PPIs, who are intolerant of medical therapy, or who desire a permanent solution to potentially eliminate their need for medication. Laparoscopic antireflux surgery has been shown to provide a 96% improvement in primary symptoms and 96% long-term satisfaction rate; however, 2% of patients were worse after surgery and 14% still required medication (1). Other endoscopic therapies, including suturing, radiofrequency ablation, injection therapy, and bulking therapy, are preformed in certain patient populations and are still being looked at in terms of long-term efficacy.

Peptic Ulcer Disease

■ Epigastric pain is the hallmark of PUD. Both gastric and duodenal ulcers typically present with deep burning or gnawing pain, sometimes with radiation to the back. Duodenal ulcer symptoms usually develop 2–3 hours after meals and are relieved with food or antacids. Gastric ulcer symptoms develop sooner after meals but are less consistently relieved with food or antacids. Food ingestion can actually precipitate gastric ulcer pain in some individuals. Most PUD patients have associated anorexia and weight loss. Some patients, particularly with duodenal ulcers, experience hyperphagia and weight gain, presumably because of the mitigating effects of food. Not uncommonly, the initial presentation of PUD can be life-threatening upper GI hemorrhage or perforation (29).

■ Peptic ulcers are erosions in the surface of the stomach or duodenum that extend down to the muscularis mucosa. *H. pylori* induces ulcers by both direct and indirect mechanisms. Bacterial phospholipases weaken the protective mucus barrier, allowing the toxic compounds created from its breakdown of urea to directly damage the epithelium. The same urease enzyme that promotes this direct cell damage acts as a potent antigenic stimulator of immune cells. By inciting an exuberant host inflammatory response, *H. pylori* produces indirect epithelial damage as well (21).

■ NSAID inhibition of prostaglandins affects multiple layers of the GI tract's protective barrier. With increasing concentration, NSAIDs diminish mucosal blood flow and penetrate the epithelial cells, eventually leading to mitochondrial oxidative uncoupling and cell death (16). There are no studies directly relating NSAID use to upper GI symptoms or bleeding specifically in athletes. Nevertheless, the increased mucosal permeability and decreased splanchnic blood flow that occurs with prolonged exercise may magnify the effects of *H. pylori* and the NSAIDs.

■ Athletes should be questioned regarding any relationship of symptom onset with NSAID use. Laboratory analysis should assess for occult GI bleeding and anemia. If any alarm signs or symptoms are present or if an individual has new-onset dyspepsia after the age of 45 or has a family history of gastric cancer, early gastroenterology referral is recommended.

■ If NSAID use is discovered, it should be discontinued if possible. If analgesic therapy is crucial, replacing a nonselective NSAID with acetaminophen or a cyclooxygenase-2 (COX-2) inhibitor would be prudent. Upper GI safety and tolerability studies have shown that COX-2 inhibitors have a 46% lower rate of medication withdrawal for adverse events, a 71% lower risk of ulcers on endoscopy, and a 39% lower incidence of symptoms because of ulcers, perforations, bleeding, or obstruction compared to nonselective NSAIDs (9).

■ If symptoms are not predominantly GERD related, there are no markers for severe disease, and medication-induced disease is eliminated, consensus recommendations support a "test and treat" approach in adults under the age of 55 with persistent dyspepsia that has not been worked up. These patients should have a noninvasive test for *H. pylori* infection. Urea breath analysis is the favored test, with the stool antigen assay and whole blood or serum serology as alternatives. Those who are *H. pylori* negative should receive short-term H_2RA or PPI therapy (4–6 weeks). If they fail empiric antisecretory therapy or symptoms recur upon cessation of treatment, they should have endoscopy. Symptomatic individuals who test positive for *H. pylori* require eradication therapy. Triple therapy with twice-daily PPI,

Table 37.2	Regimens For Treatment of *Helicobacter Pylori* Infection	
Regimen		**Eradication Rate***
PPI bid		
Amoxicillin 1,000 mg bid Clarithromycin 500 mg bid		96.4%
PPI bid		
Bismuth subsalicylate 525 mg qid Tetracycline 500 mg qid Metronidazole 250 mg qid		85%–90%
PPI bid		
Metronidazole 500 mg bid Clarithromycin 500 mg bid		89.8%
PPI bid		
Amoxicillin 1,000 mg bid Metronidazole 500 mg bid		79.0%

bid, twice a day; PPI, proton pump inhibitor; qid, four times a day.
*All eradication rates are based on a 7-day regimen. Although European data suggest 7 days are adequate; this has not been confirmed by U.S. studies. Thus, a full 14-day treatment course is recommended.
SOURCE: O'Connor FG. Gastrointestinal problems in runners. In: O'Connor FG, Wilder R, editors. *Textbook of Running Medicine.* 1st ed. New York: McGraw-Hill; 2001, p. 307–314; with permission.

clarithromycin (500 mg twice daily), and amoxicillin (1,000 mg twice daily) should be used as first-line therapy (6). Metronidazole can be substituted for amoxicillin in penicillin-allergic patients. Subsequent second-line therapy should be with a PPI, bismuth, tetracycline, and metronidazole (Table 37.2). All patients should be retested for evidence of a cure no sooner than 4 weeks after therapy. The athlete should be off any antisecretory medication, especially PPIs, for a minimum of 1 week prior to retesting. Urea breath analysis is the posttreatment diagnostic test of choice. Stool antigen testing can be used if urea breath testing is unavailable. Individuals who fail second-line therapy and those with persistent dyspepsia should be referred to gastroenterology for further evaluation (19).

LOWER GI DISEASES

Runner's Diarrhea

■ Lower GI symptoms occur more frequently in endurance athletes and more frequently affect women than men (12). Runner's diarrhea is a spectrum of exertional or immediately postexertional lower GI symptoms. Complaints range from abdominal cramping and fecal urgency to diarrhea and frank incontinence. Often, runner's diarrhea occurs in association with increases in training mileage or with particularly strenuous training sessions and competitions. An individual may be able to endure an episode by transiently reducing their pace. When symptoms are more severe, it may be necessary to suspend their workout and quickly seek relief.

- While the true etiology of runner's diarrhea remains unknown, several physiologic mechanisms have been proposed. Increased parasympathetic output during moderate exercise may intensify peristalsis, leading to cramping and rapid bowel transit. Alternatively, heightened sympathetic tone during more intense exercise could lead to increased bowel activity by increasing the release of hormones, such as gastrin and motilin (4). Strenuous exercise may lead to rapid shifts in intestinal fluid and electrolytes, causing colonic irritability (26). Another hypothesis is that the 70%–80% reduction in splanchnic blood flow with vigorous exercise may lead to an ischemic enteropathy. Poor tissue perfusion maintained over the length of the exercise session could cause mucosal ischemia, leading to fluid shifts and diarrhea. This theory could explain the high prevalence of GI bleeding in marathon runners (3).

- In addition to the basics, the history should document any recent travel, unusual food ingestion, or exposure to sick contacts to determine a potential infectious etiology. Diarrhea not associated with training should prompt a more intensive investigation. A focused lab assessment includes fecal occult blood testing and a complete blood count to look for anemia. In the presence of severe diarrhea, serum electrolytes should be drawn. Liver enzymes and pancreatic enzymes can be considered. If the history is suggestive of an infectious process, the stool should be examined for leukocytes, ova, parasites, and stool cultures.

- Treatment starts with a temporary reduction in training intensity and duration for 1–2 weeks. In most cases, this alone is enough to abolish symptoms (10). During this time, cross-training with low-impact or nonimpact activities at a level that does not trigger symptoms can be used to maintain the athlete's aerobic capacity. Any dietary or fluid replacement triggers should be eliminated. If a specific trigger is not identified, individuals with ongoing symptoms may benefit from dietary manipulation. A diet low in fiber can be helpful. Although not an adequate regimen for the control of chronic symptoms, some individuals may benefit from a complete liquid diet on the day prior to competition or scheduled intense exercise session. Once the diarrhea is under control, a full return to high-intensity exercise can be achieved by gradually increasing training as symptoms tolerate. Antidiarrheal medication should be used sparingly and with great caution. Antispasmodics, such as loperamide, are generally safe; however, anticholinergic medications, such as diphenoxylate with atropine (Lomotil), are to be avoided because of the increased heat injury risk secondary to their effect on sweating. Consult GI for unresolved symptoms despite conservative therapy or for red flag symptoms.

Abdominal Pain — "Side Stitch"

- In the young, active population, abdominal pain with exertion is common. The conditions previously discussed notwithstanding, the "side stitch," or exercise-related transient abdominal pain (ETAP), is the most common cause of this in athletes. Typically seen in runners, with 33% reporting abdominal pain, it presents as a somewhat pleuritic aching sensation, usually in the right upper abdominal quadrant. Of the athletes who report experiencing ETAP, 90% will complain of pain described as sharp, stabbing, cramping, aching, or pulling (30,32). It is often seen in deconditioned individuals starting an exercise program but can also be observed in athletes intensifying their training. Exercise in the postprandial period is a frequent exacerbating factor. Side stitches usually stop immediately on ceasing exercise. As an individual gains aerobic fitness, the frequency and severity of attacks tend to subside.

- Although their true etiology remains elusive, they are most likely caused by hypoxia-induced diaphragmatic muscle spasm (23). Other potential etiologies include pleural irritation, hepatic capsule irritation, symptomatic abdominal adhesions, and right colonic gas pain (15).

- The management involves using the history to rule out not only the other GI diseases discussed in this chapter but also other exertional pain syndromes, especially angina. Fortunately, other serious causes of abdominal pain with exercise, such as mesenteric ischemia, bowel infarction, omental infarction, and hepatic vein thrombosis, are rare; however, in the setting of unremitting pain, especially with signs of systemic illness or shock, these conditions need to be considered in the differential and patients referred for potential surgical evaluation.

- Athletes with the typical features of a side stitch should be reassured that this is a benign process and will get better as their conditioning improves. They should be advised against exercise immediately after eating. If an episode of pain does occur, temporarily stopping exercise, stretching the right arm over their head, and exhaling through pursed lips can help abort it quickly (29).

Elevated Liver Enzymes

- Liver enzyme elevations observed in otherwise asymptomatic long-distance runners and other athletes are usually incidental findings. The suspected etiology is an ischemic insult secondary to reduced splanchnic blood flow and oxygen tension during vigorous exercise (17). Observed increases in alanine aminotransferase (ALT), aspartate aminotransferase (AST), alkaline phosphatase, creatinine phosphatase, and lactate dehydrogenase are confounded by the fact that these enzymes can be elevated in response to musculoskeletal injury. Hepatocellular injury can be confirmed by measuring glutamate dehydrogenase and γ-glutamyltransferase (GGT), enzymes more specific to the liver (18).

- Because these asymptomatic enzyme abnormalities are often discovered in the convalescent setting, the history and physical should focus on recent training sessions and environmental exposure, evaluating for evidence of a missed heat injury or episode of exertional rhabdomyolysis. The athlete should be questioned regarding any history of chronic liver disease or alcohol dependence and their medication list reviewed for any potentially hepatotoxic agents. With the nearly ubiquitous use of nutritional supplements, it is crucial to investigate this often overlooked area.

■ The majority of athletes can be reassured that this is a benign process and the enzyme abnormalities usually revert to normal within just 1 week after abstaining from exercise. The first step in the laboratory evaluation is to obtain a repeat liver enzyme panel after abstaining from NSAIDs, alcohol, and exercise for 1 week. If the liver enzymes are elevated at that time, they can be rechecked in 1 month. If the liver enzyme abnormalities persist on serial examinations, further evaluation should start with an iron panel, total iron-binding capacity, and hepatitis serologies to look for viral hepatitis or hemochromatosis. Second-tier tests include antinuclear antibody titer, antismooth muscle antibody, ceruloplasmin, α_1-antitrypsin, and serum protein electrophoresis, which would look for other causes for elevated aminotransferases, such as muscle disorders, Wilson disease, or thyroid disease. A right upper quadrant ultrasound is useful to evaluate for fatty liver, cholelithiasis, or other obstruction. GI referral should occur for abnormal lab testing, mildly elevated liver enzymes for over 6 months despite a negative evaluation, significantly elevated AST or ALT (> 150) without improvement for 2 months, or signs of evolving hepatic insufficiency (18).

REFERENCES

1. Bammer T, Hinder RA, Klaus A, Klingler PJ. Five-to eight-year outcome of the first laparoscopic Nissen fundoplications. *J Gastrointest Surg*. 2001; 5(1):42–8.

2. Bardhan KD, Müller-Lissner S, Bigard MA, et al. Symptomatic gastro-oesophageal reflux disease: double-blind controlled study of intermittent treatment with omeprazole or ranitidine. The European Study Group. *BMJ*. 1999;318(7182):502–7.

3. Bounous G, McArdle AH. Marathon runners: the intestinal handicap. *Med Hypotheses*. 1990;33(4):261–4.

4. Cammack J, Read NW, Cann PA, Greenwood B, Holgate M. Effect of prolonged exercise on the passage of a solid meal through the stomach and small intestine. *Gut*. 1982;23(11):957–61.

5. Caro JJ, Salas M, Ward A. Healing and relapse rates in gastroesophageal reflux disease treated with the newer proton-pump inhibitors lansoprazole, rabeprazole, and pantoprazole compared with omeprazole, ranitidine, and placebo: evidence from randomized clinical trials. *Clin Ther*. 2001;23(7):998–1017.

6. Chey WD, Wong BC; Practice Parameters Committee of the American College of Gastroenterology. American College of Gastroenterology guideline on the management of *Helicobacter pylori* infection. *Am J Gastroenterol*. 2007;102(8):1808–25.

7. Chiba N, De Gara CJ, Wilkinson JM, Hunt RH. Speed of healing and symptom relief in grade II to IV gastroesophageal reflux disease: a meta-analysis. *Gastroenterology*. 1997;112(6):1798–810.

8. Collings KL, Pierce Pratt F, Rodriguez-Stanley S, Bemben M, Miner PB. Esophageal reflux in conditioned runners, cyclists, and weightlifters. *Med Sci Sports Exerc*. 2003;35(5):730–5.

9. Deeks JJ, Smith LA, Bradley MD. Efficacy, tolerability, and upper gastrointestinal safety of celecoxib for treatment of osteoarthritis and rheumatoid arthritis: systematic review of randomized controlled trials. *BMJ*. 2002;325(7365):619–23.

10. Fogoros RN. Runner's trots. Gastrointestinal disturbances in runners. *JAMA*. 1980;243(17):1743–4.

11. Hirschowitz BI. A critical analysis, with appropriate controls of gastric acid and pepsin secretion in clinical esophagitis. *Gastroenterology*. 1991; 101(5):1149–58.

12. Ho GW. Lower gastrointestinal distress in endurance athletes. *Curr Sports Med Rep*. 2009;8(2):85–91.

13. Kahrilas PJ, Fennerty MB, Joelsson B. High- versus standard-dose ranitidine for control of heartburn in poorly responsive acid reflux disease: a prospective, controlled trial. *Am J Gastroenterol*. 1999;94(1):92–7.

14. Keeffe EB, Lowe DK, Goss JR, Wayne R. Gastrointestinal symptoms of marathon runners. *West J Med*. 1984;141(4):481–4.

15. Lauder TD, Moses FM. Recurrent abdominal pain from abdominal adhesions in an endurance triathlete. *Med Sci Sports Exerc*. 1995;27(5):623–5.

16. Lichtenstein DR, Syngal S, Wofe MM. Nonsteroidal anti-inflammatory drugs and the gastrointestinal tract. The double-edged sword. *Arthritis Rheum*. 1995;38(1):5–18.

17. Lijnen P, Hespel P, Fagard R, et al. Indicators of cell breakdown in plasma in men during and after a marathon race. *Int J Sports Med*. 1988;9(2):108–13.

18. Liver enzyme elevation referral guideline [Internet]. [cited 1999]. Available from: http://www.mamc.amedd.army.mil/referral/guidelines.

19. Malfertheiner P, Mégraud F, O'Morain C, et al. Current concepts in the management of *Helicobacter pylori* infection—the Maastrict 2-2000 Consensus Report. *Aliment Pharmacol Ther*. 2002;16(2):167–80.

20. McCabe ME 3rd, Peura DA, Kadakia SC, Bocek Z, Johnson LF. Gastrointestinal blood loss associated with running a marathon. *Dig Dis Sci*. 1986;31(11):1229–32.

21. Nilius M, Malfertheiner P. Helicobacter pylori enzymes. *Aliment Pharmacol Ther*. 1996;10(suppl 1):65–71.

22. Parmelee-Peters K, Moeller JL. Gastroesophageal reflux in athletes. *Curr Sports Med Rep*. 2004;3(2):107–11.

23. Pate R. Principles of training. In: Kulund D, editor. *The Injured Athlete*. Philadelphia: JB Lippincott; 1988.

24. Peters HP, Bos M, Seebregts L, et al. Gastrointestinal symptoms in long-distance runners, cyclists, and triathletes: prevalence, medication, and etiology. *Am J Gastroenterol*. 1999;94(6):1570–81.

25. Peters HP, Zweers M, Backx FJ, et al. Gastrointestinal symptoms during long-distance walking. *Med Sci Sports Exerc*. 1999;31(6):767–73.

26. Rehrer N, Janssen GM, Brouns F, Saris WH. Fluid intake and gastrointestinal problems in runners competing in a 25-km marathon. *Int J Sports Med*. 1989;10(suppl 1):S22–25.

27. Richter JE. Typical and atypical presentations of gastroesophageal reflux disease. The role of esophageal testing in diagnosis and management. *Gastroenterol Clin North Am*. 1996;25(1):75–102.

28. Soffer EE, Merchant RK, Duethman G, Launspach J, Gisolfi C, Adrian TE. Effect of graded exercise on esophageal motility and gastroesophageal reflux in trained athletes. *Dig Dis Sci*. 1993;38(2):220–4.

29. Spechler JS. Peptic ulcer disease and its complications. In: Feldman M, Friedman LS, Sleisinger MH, editors. *Sleisenger and Fordtran's Gastrointestinal and Liver Disease*. 7th ed. Philadelphia: Saunders; 2002.

30. Stamford B. A "stitch" in the side. *Phys Sportsmed*. 1985;13(5):187.

31. Tytgat G, Langenberg W, Rauws E, et al. Campylobacter-like organism (CLO) in the human stomach. *Gastroenterology*. 1985;88:1620.

32. Viola T. Evaluation of the athlete with exertional abdominal pain. *Curr Sports Med Rep*. 2010;9(2):106–10.

33. Williams MP, Sercombe J, Hamilton MI, Pounder RE. A placebo-controlled trial to assess the effects of 8 days of dosing with rabeprazole versus omeprazole on 24-hour intragastric acidity and plasma gastrin concentrations in young healthy male subjects. *Aliment Pharmacol Ther*. 1998;12(11):1079–89.

34. Wysowslci KD, Bacsanyi J. Cisapride and fatal arrhythmia. *N Engl J Med*. 1996;335(4):290–1.

38 Pulmonary

Carrie A. Jaworski

INTRODUCTION

- Patients with pulmonary disorders can benefit greatly from exercise when their disease process is under proper control.
- Awareness of when and when not to participate and the ability to use pharmacologic agents and environmental controls greatly enhance one's ability to participate safely.

ASTHMA

- Asthma is a chronic pulmonary disorder characterized by varying degrees of airflow obstruction, bronchial hyperresponsiveness, and underlying chronic inflammation (42).
- Approximately, 22 million adults and 6 million children in the United States have chronic asthma (42).
- The National Heart, Lung, and Blood Institute (NHLBI) has set forth guidelines on the diagnosis and management of asthma in an effort known as the National Asthma Education and Prevention Program (NAEPP). This program is evidence based and routinely updates its recommendations based on the newest research. The third edition was completed in 2007; the latest recommendations can be found at the NHLBI Web site: http://www.nhlbi.nih.gov/ (21).
- While in the past, asthmatics were discouraged from exercise, today it is recognized that regular exercise can reduce airway reactivity and decrease medication use (8). Current data support this trend, with decreased numbers of asthmatics reporting limitations in their activity (5,42).

Diagnosis of Asthma

- History or presence of episodic symptoms of airflow obstruction, such as wheezing, chest tightness, shortness of breath, or cough. Absence of symptoms at time of examination does not exclude diagnosis.
- Airflow obstruction needs to be at least partially reversible demonstrated through the use of spirometry. First, establish airflow obstruction: forced expiratory volume in 1 second (FEV_1) < 80% predicted and FEV_1/forced vital capacity (FVC) ratio < 70% or below the lower limit of normal. Then establish reversibility by an FEV_1 increase of ≥ 12% from baseline or ≥ 10% of predicted FEV_1 after using a short-acting inhaled β_2-agonist (41).
- Must exclude other diagnoses, such as vocal cord dysfunction, vascular rings, and reflux disease, if spirometry is normal.
- Classification of asthma severity is based on history and spirometry (Table 38.1).
- Management should focus on patient education, environmental control, and objective monitoring.
- **Patient education:** Patients and their families should understand signs and symptoms of an asthma exacerbation, the chronicity of the disease, and potential triggers of an attack. A written plan should be reviewed, and instruction on proper use of inhaled medications and peak flow monitoring should be provided.
- **Environmental control:** Avoidance of exposure to precipitating factors is paramount. Potential triggers include pollen, mold, ozone, exercise, and cold air. Athletes should exercise indoors on bad weather days or use measures, such as masks, to decrease chance of attack. Indoor swimming is considered an excellent option secondary to the warm, moist environment at the pool. Some asthmatics are susceptible to aspirin and nonsteroidal anti-inflammatory drugs, so judicious use must be exercised (33).
- **Monitoring:** Athletes need to be monitoring their peak flows on a daily basis to recognize decline in function, as well as response to treatment. Formal spirometry is recommended for initial diagnosis, after treatment and peak flows have stabilized, and then every 1–2 years when asthma is stable, or more often when unstable (42).
- Pharmacologic therapy should be instituted to control inflammation and treat episodes of bronchoconstriction. Use a stepwise approach to treatment as outlined in Table 38.2.

Medication Classes

The two main classes of asthma medications are long-term control medications that are used to treat and control the persistent symptoms of asthma and short-acting agents that provide quick relief of symptom exacerbations.

Table 38.1 | Severity Classification

	Components of Control	Classification of Asthma Control (Youth ≥ 12 years of age and adults)		
		Well Controlled	**Not Well Controlled**	**Very Poorly Controlled**
Impairment	Symptoms	≤ 2 days a week	> 2 days a week	Throughout the day
	Nighttime awakening	≤ 2× a month	1–3× a week	≥ 4× a week
	Interference with normal activity	None	Some limitation	Extremely limited
	Short-acting β_2-agonist use for symptom control (not prevention of EIB)	≤ 2 days a week	> 2 days a week	Several times per day
	FEV_1 or peak flow	> 80% predicted/ personal best	60%–80% predicted/ personal best	< 60% predicted/ personal best
	Validated questionnaires			
	ATAQ	0	1–2	3–4
	ACQ	≤ 0.75*	≥ 1.5	N/A
	ACT	≥ 20	16–19	≤ 15
Risk	Exacerbations	0–1 a year	≥ 2 a year (see note)	
		Consider severity and interval since last exacerbation		
	Progressive loss of lung function	Evaluation requires long-term follow-up care		
	Treatment-related adverse effects	Medication side effects can vary in intensity from none to very troublesome and worrisome. The level of intensity does not correlate to specific levels of control but should be considered in the overall assessment of risk.		

* ACQ values of 0.76–1.4 are indeterminate regarding well-controlled asthma.

ACQ, Asthma Control Questionnaire; ACT, Asthma Control Test; ATAQ, Asthma Therapy Assessment Questionnaire; EIB, exercise-induced bronchospasm; FEV_1, forced expiratory volume in 1 second.

LONG-TERM CONTROLLERS

- **Corticosteroids:** Mechanism is to block late-phase reaction to allergens, decrease airway hyperresponsiveness, and inhibit inflammatory cell actions. Inhaled corticosteroids (ICSs) are the mainstay of treatment in the long-term control of asthma. ICSs are considered to be the most potent and consistently effective anti-inflammatory asthma medication (10,25,37,42,44). ICSs must be taken on a regular basis; therefore, they are not useful as a rescue medication. Side effects can include local irritation, dysphonia, and oral candidiasis. Systemic forms may be needed in asthma flares and cases recalcitrant to inhaled glucocorticoids.

- **Khellin derivatives:** Cromolyn sodium (Intal) and nedocromil sodium (Tilade) act to stabilize mast cells, thus preventing the release of inflammatory mediators. Both are inhaled medications with a strong safety profile and can be considered as an alternative to ICSs but not a preferred therapy. Cromolyn is approved for children of all ages, while nedocromil is approved in children older than age 6. Both take about 2 weeks to demonstrate a therapeutic response.

- **Leukotriene modifiers:** Zileuton (Zyflo), a 5-lipo oxygenase inhibitor, blocks the synthesis of leukotrienes, whereas zafirlukast (Accolate) and montelukast (Singulair), leukotriene receptor antagonists (LTRAs), block the effects of leukotrienes after they are formed. All 3 medications decrease airway inflammation and offer another alternative to ICSs. Montelukast and zafirlukast are approved in children, have a favorable safety profile, and are taken orally every day or twice a day. Less desirable is zileuton, which is not approved in children < 12 years old and requires dosing 4 times a day and monitoring of hepatic function.

- **Long-acting β_2-agonists (LABAs)** are bronchodilators that last up to 12 hours after 1 dose. Examples include salmeterol and formoterol. LABAs are the recommended medication to be used in combination with ICSs for management of moderate to severe asthma (3,4,43). Concern regarding the use of LABA as monotherapy and an increased risk of asthma exacerbations and asthma-related deaths has caused a black box warning to be placed on all preparations containing a LABA (16,22). An expert panel recommends weighing the benefit of LABA use in uncontrolled asthmatics versus the small increased risk (42).

- **Immune modulators:** Omalizumab is a monoclonal antibody that prevents binding of immunoglobulin (Ig) E to mast cells and basophils. It can be used as adjunctive therapy in patients older than 12 years with allergies and severe

Table 38.2	Treatment: Stepwise Approach

Intermittent Asthma	Persistent Asthma: Daily Medication Consult with asthma specialist if step 4 care or higher is required. Consider consultation at step 3.					
Step 1	Step 2	Step 3	Step 4	Step 5	Step 6	
Preferred: SABA PRN	*Preferred:* Low-dose ICS *Alternative:* Cromolyn, LTRA, nedocromil, or theophylline	*Preferred:* Low-dose ICS + LABA OR Medium-dose ICS *Alternative:* Low-dose ICS + either LTRA, theophylline, or zileuton	*Preferred:* Medium-dose ICS + LABA *Alternative:* Medium-dose ICS + either LTRA, theophylline, or zileuton	*Preferred:* High-dose ICS + LABA AND Consider Omalizumab for patients who have allergies	*Preferred:* High-dose ICS + LABA + oral corticosteroid AND Consider Omalizumab for patients who have allergies	Step up if needed (first check adherence, environmental control, and comorbid conditions) *Assess control* Step down if possible (and asthma is well controlled at least 3 months)

Each step: Patient education, environmental control, and management of comorbidities.
Steps 2–4: Consider subcutaneous allergen immunotherapy for patients who have allergic asthma (see notes).

Quick-Relief Medication for All Patients
• **SABA as needed for symptoms. Intensity of treatment depends on severity of symptoms: up to 3 treatments at 20-minute intervals as needed. Short course of oral systemic corticosteroids may be needed.**
• **Use of SABA > 2 days a week for symptom relief (not prevention of EIB) generally indicates inadequate control and the need to step up treatment.**

Alphabetical order is used when more than 1 treatment option is listed within either preferred or alternative therapy.
EIB, exercise-induced bronchospasm; ICS, inhaled corticosteroid; LABA, inhaled long-acting β$_2$-agonist; LTRA, leukotriene receptor antagonist; PRN, as needed; SABA, inhaled short-acting β$_2$-agonist.

asthma. It is for those with severe persistent asthma not controlled with a combination of high-dose ICS and LABA (14).

■ **Methylxanthines:** Sustained-release theophylline is a bronchodilator with mild anti-inflammatory effects that is an alternative, but not preferred, adjunctive therapy with ICS. It requires monitoring of blood levels.

SHORT-ACTING AGENTS

■ **Short-acting β$_2$-agonists (SABAs):** Inhaled albuterol is the main rescue medication for acute bronchoconstriction and prevention of exercise-induced asthma. Inhaled forms have a good safety profile with primarily mild central nervous system (CNS) side effects. Medication has an immediate effect and is, therefore, subject to overuse. Chronic use can also lead to decreases in efficacy and increased bronchial hyperreactivity. Oral forms are not approved for use by the International Olympic Committee or National Collegiate Athletic Association (NCAA).

■ **Anticholinergics:** Ipratropium bromide (Atrovent) is a bronchodilator used more often in patients with chronic obstructive pulmonary disease (COPD). It can be an adjunct for patients who have an inadequate response to β$_2$-agonists. The duration of action is 3–4 hours with an onset of 30–90 minutes.

ASTHMA MANAGEMENT

■ The goal of therapy is to maintain control of asthma with the least amount of medication necessary. Use a stepwise approach while minimizing impairment and risk (42). See Table 38.2.

■ Use caution when prescribing medications to collegiate, professional, and elite athletes. Always check with the sport's governing body in regard to banned substances. The U.S. Olympic Committee has an up-to-date list available through their Web site (http://www.usantidoping.org), or you can call their drug control hotline at 1-800-233-0393.

■ Once asthma is well controlled, exercise should be encouraged. Studies have demonstrated decreased numbers of exacerbations, less medication use, and fewer missed days of work or school in asthmatics who exercised (42).

■ The exercise prescription should include a preexercise assessment to document control. FEV$_1$ should be ≥ 80% of expected levels (8). The exercise goal should be consistent with the American College of Sports Medicine's recommendation to exercise on most days of the week for 20–30 minutes (11). The type of exercise can be anything that the patient enjoys but should provide aerobic benefit, as well as strength and flexibility conditioning.

■ Advise caution on risky activities, such as exercising outside on a cold day, when wheezing or when peak flows suggest a decline in lung function because exercise can trigger symptoms of bronchoconstriction. (See next section.)

EXERCISE-INDUCED ASTHMA/BRONCHOSPASM

■ Exercise-induced asthma (EIA) is defined as the transitory increase in airway resistance that typically occurs following vigorous exercise in a patient with chronic asthma. Exercise-induced bronchospasm (EIB) refers to those individuals with no symptoms outside of exercise. It is important to understand that some asthmatics will only mount symptoms with exercise, so ensuring that no symptoms or reductions in pulmonary function exist at rest is paramount in guiding treatment (41).

■ Ninety percent of patients with chronic asthma will have EIA, and 40% of patients with allergic rhinitis or atopic dermatitis will have EIB (9).

■ The prevalence of EIA/EIB in athletes varies by sport with ranges between 12% and 55% (15), and EIA/EIB occurs in amateur to elite level athletes. Higher risk sports include those with high-minute ventilation, such as basketball, track, and soccer, as well as those done in cool, dry air, such as cross-country skiing, ice skating, and hockey.

■ The pathophysiology of EIB remains debatable. Two main theories exist.
  ■ The *water loss theory* attributes EIB to the loss of water through the bronchial mucosa as the body tries to warm rapidly inhaled air during exercise. This dries the mucosa and causes local changes in pH, osmolarity, and the temperature of the airway, which may trigger bronchoconstriction (35).
  ■ The *thermal expenditure theory* holds that EIB is the result of respiratory heat loss that occurs during exercise. The increased ventilation of exercise causes a cooling of the airways. Once exercise ceases, the blood vessels dilate and engorge to rewarm the epithelium, which may lead to rebound hyperemia and bronchoconstriction (35).

■ Some studies demonstrate that the presence of inflammatory mediators are also involved in EIB (1,2,6).

Presentation

■ Clinical symptoms may include coughing, wheezing, chest tightness, or shortness of breath during or minutes after intense exercise. Symptoms usually peak 5–10 minutes after exercise and last for 20–30 minutes. Atypical symptoms can include stomach cramps, chest pain, nausea, headache, or feeling out of shape. Examination during an attack may demonstrate increased respiratory rate, prolonged expiration, decreased breath sounds, and wheezing. Some athletes may describe a late response 6–8 hours after the onset of exercise.

Diagnosis

■ The diagnosis of EIA/EIB is often based on history and self-reported symptoms. Numerous studies have demonstrated that this approach is unreliable and can both underdiagnose, as well as overdiagnose the condition (26,38,40). Parsons et al. (26) found that 36% of athletes with a positive eucapnic voluntary hyperventilation (EVH) test did not report any symptoms and that only 35% of athletes with symptoms were found to have positive tests. More reliable diagnosis is based on pulmonary function testing after a thorough history and physical examination has ruled out any other explanation of the symptoms.

■ Office spirometry should be done at rest to rule out underlying chronic asthma in anyone suspected of having EIB. A normal resting test with suspicion of EIB warrants a bronchoprovocation test. Many physicians will give a trial of a prophylactic bronchodilator if classic history and mild symptoms exist.

■ Normal testing with no response to medication should prompt consideration of vocal cord dysfunction as the diagnosis. Gastroesophageal reflux and cardiac disorders need to be considered as well.

■ Options for confirming EIB include indirect and direct challenge tests. (See Chapter 24, Exercise-Induced Bronchoconstriction Testing, for detailed discussion.)

INDIRECT CHALLENGE TESTS

Exercise Challenge Test

■ Performed either in a laboratory or in the field, this test seeks to simulate the athlete's sport in order to provoke EIB. Formal pulmonary function tests are done, with FEV_1 being the index most often measured in the lab versus peak expiratory flow rate (PEFR) in the field. Solitary EIB will have a preexercise baseline FEV_1 or PEFR between 80% and 100% of normal predicted values. The exercise is most commonly free or treadmill running for 5–8 minutes at a high intensity ($\geq$ 85%–90% maximum predicted heart rate). FEV_1 or PEFR is measured at 1-, 3-, 5-, 10-, and 15-minute intervals. Positive test = a decrease in FEV_1 or PEFR of 15%. Mild EIB = 15%–25% decrease. Moderate EIB = 25%–40% decrease. Severe EIB = a decrease of > 40% (31).

■ Field testing offers the advantage of more closely mimicking actual sport, but it can be difficult to control environmental factors and hard to control/monitor rate of exertion.

■ Laboratory testing is more costly and eliminates possible contributing environmental triggers. It offers the advantages of controlled cardiovascular workload and ability to monitor pulmonary and cardiovascular function during exercise (28).

■ Other indirect challenge tests include the EVH challenge test, the hyperosmolar saline challenge test, and the mannitol challenge test. EVH testing is considered the "gold standard" by many; however, it is not readily available other than at research centers (13).

DIRECT CHALLENGE TESTS

■ Direct challenge testing involves administration of increasing doses of a pharmacologic agent, such as methacholine, to cause bronchoconstriction. These tests are highly sensitive but have a poor specificity for EIB.

Treatment

■ Good long-term control of chronic asthma should allow participation in athletics without any EIA symptoms. If symptoms are occurring, adjustment to the treatment needs to be made (Table 38.2). A variety of agents are available to treat EIB. Treatment should be tailored to the individual athlete and his or her sport.

PHARMACOLOGIC TREATMENTS (ALSO SEE LONG-TERM CONTROLLERS SECTION)

■ SABAs: First-line therapy is usually with an inhaled SABA, such as albuterol, 2–4 puffs taken 15–30 minutes prior to activity. Albuterol's onset of action is ≤ 5 minutes and duration of effect is ~2–6 hours. It will prevent EIB in > 80% of patients (42). All athletes with EIA/EIB should carry an SABA inhaler with them during exercise to relieve acute exacerbations that occur despite prophylaxis.

■ LABAs can be protective for up to 12 hours and should be considered in athletes involved in endurance/all-day events, as well as in children where activity is unpredictable. When used daily, shortening of duration of action occurs (30). Frequent use of LABAs for EIA/EIB is not recommended because it may disguise poorly controlled persistent asthma (42).

■ Cromolyn or nedocromil can be used as an alternative to SABAs, but they are not as effective. Both should be administered as 2–4 puffs 20 minutes prior to exercise. The duration of action is ~2 hours. They are not to be used to treat acute symptoms but are useful for repeated bouts of exercise because they have minimal/no side effects. Combining cromolyn with SABA can be helpful (32).

■ LTRAs offer the advantage of oral administration and long duration of action. Attenuation of EIB symptoms occurs in up to 50% of patients (42). Montelukast is administered at 10 mg daily in adults and 5 mg in 6- to 14-year-old children. It has a 3- to 4-hour onset of action and a duration of 24 hours. Zafirlukast is administered at 20 mg twice a day in adults and 10 mg twice a day in children 5–11 years old. It has an onset of action of 30 minutes and duration of 12 hours.

■ ICSs are not effective as prophylaxis prior to exercise but need to be considered in patients refractory to the aforementioned medications; patients should also be reevaluated for chronic asthma.

NONPHARMACOLOGIC TREATMENTS

■ The use of masks or scarves to decrease the amount of heat and water lost with exercise in cold weather may diminish EIB.

■ Aerobic conditioning may reduce severity of EIB by improving rate of ventilation during exercise, but there is no proof it prevents EIB (13).

■ Appropriate cooldowns help decrease EIB. Cooling down helps by allowing gradual rewarming of the airways, which decreases vascular dilation and edema.

■ **Refractory period:** Defined as the time after spontaneous recovery from an episode of EIB where > 50% of athletes will not experience another episode of bronchoconstriction with exercise. Effect is usually 1–2 hours in duration. It can benefit athletes who experience this effect in that they can induce a refractory period prior to their actual competition to lessen the severity of EIB during their event. Various methods exist to induce the effect, including 20–30 minutes of low-intensity exercise or seven 30-second sprints separated by short intervals (8,13). Studies demonstrate that a continuous low-intensity warm-up is more beneficial than interval training to decrease risk of EIB (18). Studies also demonstrate that this effect is inhibited with use of nonsteroidal anti-inflammatories (24). Athletes should be counseled to still use their prescribed EIB medications because effect is partial for most people (36).

CHRONIC OBSTRUCTIVE PULMONARY DISEASE

■ COPD is a progressive disease that primarily refers to emphysema and chronic bronchitis. It is a condition of slowly deteriorating pulmonary function whereby expiratory airflow obstruction leads to dyspnea and deconditioning. While exercise cannot reverse the process, it can provide improvements in quality of life and decreased disability (19).

■ Estimated worldwide prevalence is 7%–19%, but COPD is largely underdiagnosed (17). Death rates from COPD continue to rise, and it is the fourth leading cause of death in the United States.

■ The primary cause is chronic tobacco use, but other etiologies, such as α_1-antitrypsin deficiency and environmental exposures, do play a role.

■ The pathophysiology of COPD is multifactorial. Airway hyperreactivity and/or increased respiratory secretions lead to chronic obstruction. This results in air trapping and respiratory muscle dysfunction, which, over time, causes generalized deconditioning. Additionally, the emphysematous component causes destruction of alveolar capillary membranes, which leads to hypoxemia. Chronic hypoxemia results in pulmonary hypertension and right ventricular failure (31).

- Severe limitations in respiratory function and chronic hypoxemia cause great fear and anxiety in COPD patients, including a fear of exercise and thus further deconditioning (7).

- Our role as sports medicine physicians is to enable COPD patients to exercise comfortably and safely.

- **Evaluation:** Prior to providing an exercise prescription, patients must have an assessment of their current status through a physical examination and pulmonary function testing. One can expect reductions in FEV_1 and increased ventilatory muscle effort.

- A careful assessment of cardiac risk and exercise capacity, including exercise testing, is recommended for all patients. Many protocols exist for both treadmill and stationary cycle testing. Exercise testing can help to determine safe levels of exercise to prevent arrhythmias and hypoxemia, the amount of supplemental oxygen needed during exercise, and any need for bronchodilators.

- **Management:** The care of the COPD patient is aimed at maintaining, or improving, the functional capacity through a multidisciplinary approach.

- **Exercise:** Studies demonstrate that exercise improves dyspnea, provides an aerobic training response, reduces ventilation, and improves overall exercise tolerance (27). No evidence exists that exercise lengthens life expectancy in the COPD patient, but it provides immense physical and psychological benefits.

- Supervised exercise through a pulmonary rehabilitation program is warranted if patient has significant disease. Most can graduate to independent exercise within 6 weeks (19).

- Independent exercise goal should be to exercise 3 days a week at 60%–80% of maximal heart rate for 20–30 minutes. Type of exercise will vary based on patient's ability and comorbidities. Stationary cycling is useful initially because many patients are unsteady on their feet, and arm ergometry can be used for those with lower extremity limitations. These goals may take months to reach, if at all. Start with several minutes of exercise and progress at a rate appropriate for the individual (27,34).

- Exercise aids can include supplemental oxygen and medications. Bronchodilators and anticholinergics are the mainstay of pharmacologic therapy in COPD and should be used aggressively. Mucolytics can assist with excessive secretions. ICS can also assist in decreasing airway inflammation. Oral corticosteroids are reserved for more severe cases, and theophylline remains a controversial therapy.

- Bronchopulmonary toilet and pursed lip breathing are two other mechanical techniques that can aid COPD patients in achieving activity goals.

- Careful attention to preventive health care, such as influenza and polyvalent pneumococcal immunizations, can help COPD patients avoid setbacks in their exercise programs and enhance overall well-being.

CYSTIC FIBROSIS

- Cystic fibrosis (CF) is an autosomal recessive disorder that affects multiple organ systems, including the pulmonary, gastrointestinal, reproductive, and skeletal systems, as well as the sweat glands. Chronic pulmonary disease is the leading cause of morbidity and mortality because the thick mucus found with CF leads to infection and inhibits pulmonary function. Aerobic exercise has been shown to aid in the clearance of secretions and improve quality of life in patients with CF.

- Diagnosis of CF is made by an abnormal sweat chloride test. Prenatal screening is now available and should be offered to couples at higher risk, particularly those of Northern European descent. Pulmonary function tests are similar to an asthmatic but also demonstrate a decreased FVC.

- Management of CF is dependent on the extent of disease. A goal of preventing recurrent respiratory infections is attempted through chest physiotherapy, bronchodilators, and antibiotics. Corticosteroids, oxygen, recombinant deoxyribonuclease I, and possibly lung transplantation in advanced cases may also be warranted.

- Exercise can augment mobilization of secretions when combined with chest physiotherapy (39). A study also demonstrated less loss of FVC compared to controls (29). In mild forms of CF, athletes should be allowed to participate as their pulmonary function allows. Moderate to severe cases of CF benefit from more formal rehabilitation programs where the need for supplemental oxygen can be tracked.

- All athletes with CF need to be counseled on safe exercise in the heat because they are subject to increased sodium and chloride losses in their sweat when compared to those without CF.

RESPIRATORY INFECTIONS

- Respiratory tract infections are one of the most common medical problems encountered in the care of athletes. Upper respiratory tract infections (URIs) comprise the majority of these infections.

- Immune function affects avoidance and occurrence of URIs. Studies demonstrate that moderate exercise can protect against URIs, whereas intense exercise can decrease immunity and increase the risk of URIs (23).

- Prevention of URIs can be augmented through avoidance of overtraining, adequate sleep, proper nutrition, and limiting stress. Influenza vaccination of athletes in winter sports should be considered.

- Treatment of URIs is primarily symptomatic. Nasal ipratropium bromide and oral/topical decongestants can be helpful in the short term. Caution must be exercised with antihistamines in athletes because they can impair temperature regulation and cause sedation. Inhaled β-agonists can help with URI-associated coughs. Antibiotics are only indicated if progression to a secondary bacterial infection occurs. Zinc and vitamin C may reduce the duration of URI symptoms (12,20).

- Athletes with a common cold can continue to participate to a lesser degree provided no fever is present. Care should be taken to increase hydration and cease activity if constitutional symptoms occur, such as fever, myalgias, productive cough, vomiting, or diarrhea.

- Progression to diseases, such as pneumonia and complicated bronchitis, warrant up to 10–14 days of rest before resuming full activity.

REFERENCES

1. Anderson SD. Single-dose agents in the prevention of exercise-induced asthma: a descriptive review. *Treat Respir Med.* 2004;3(6):365–79.

2. Anderson SD, Brannan JD. Long-acting beta2-adrenoceptor agonists and exercise-induced asthma: lessons to guide us in the future. *Paediatr Drugs.* 2004;6(3):161–75.

3. Bateman ED, Bantje TA, João GM, et al. Combination therapy with single inhaler budesonide/formoterol compared with high dose of fluticasone propionate alone in patients with moderate persistent asthma. *Am J Respir Med.* 2003;2(3):275–81.

4. Bateman ED, Boushey HA, Bousquet J, et al. Can guideline-defined asthma control be achieved? The Gaining Optimal Asthma Control study. *Am J Respir Crit Care Med.* 2004;170(8):836–44.

5. Bundgaard A. Exercise and the asthmatic. *Sport Med.* 1985;2(4):254–66.

6. Carlsen KH, Carlsen KC. Exercise-induced asthma. *Paediatr Respir Rev.* 2002;3(2):154–60.

7. Casaburi R. Exercise training in chronic obstructive lung disease. In: Casaburi R, Petty TL, editors. *Principles and Practice of Pulmonary Rehabilitation.* Philadelphia: Saunders; 1993. p. 204–24.

8. Disabella V, Sherman C. Exercise for asthma patients: little risk, big rewards. *Phys Sportsmed.* 1998;26(6):75–84.

9. Feinstein RA, LaRussa J, Wang-Dohlman A, Bartolucci AA. Screening adolescent athletes for exercise-induced asthma. *Clin J Sport Med.* 1996;6(2):119–23.

10. Garcia Garcia ML, Wahn U, Gilles L, Swern A, Tozzi CA, Polos P. Montelukast, compared with fluticasone, for control of asthma among 6- to 14-year-old patients with mild asthma: the MOSAIC study. *Pediatrics.* 2005;116(2):360–9.

11. Haskell WL, Lee IM, Pate RR, et al. Physical activity and public health: updated recommendation for adults from the American College of Sports Medicine and the American Heart Association. *Med Sci Sports Exerc.* 2007;39(8):1423–34.

12. Hemilä H. Does vitamin C alleviate the symptoms of the common cold?—a review of current evidence. *Scand J Infect Dis.* 1994;26(1):1–6.

13. Holzer K, Brukner P, Douglass J. Evidence-based management of exercise-induced asthma. *Curr Sports Med Rep.* 2002;1(2):86–92.

14. Humbert M, Beasley R, Ayres J, et al. Benefits of omalizumab as add-on therapy in patients with severe persistent asthma who are inadequately controlled despite best available therapy (GINA 2002 step 4 treatment): INNOVATE. *Allergy.* 2005;60(3):309–16.

15. Langdeau JB, Boulet LP. Prevalence and mechanism of development of asthma and airway hyperresponsiveness in athletes. *Sports Med.* 2001;31(8):601–16.

16. Mann M, Chowdhury B, Sullivan E, Nicklas R, Anthracite R, Meyer RJ. Serious asthma exacerbations in asthmatics treated with high-dose formoterol. *Chest.* 2003;124(1):70–4.

17. Mannino DM, Homa DM, Akinbami LJ, Ford ES, Redd SC. Chronic obstructive pulmonary disease surveillance: United States, 1971–2000. *MMWR Surveill Summ.* 2002;51(6):1–16.

18. McKenzie DC, McLuckie SL, Stirling DR. The protective effects of continuous and interval exercise in athletes with exercise-induced asthma. *Med Sci Sports Exerc.* 1994;26(8):951–6.

19. Mink BD. Exercise and chronic obstructive pulmonary disease: modest fitness gains pay big dividends. *Phys Sportsmed.* 1997;25(11):43–52.

20. Mossad SB, Macknin ML, Medendorp SV, Mason P. Zinc gluconate lozenges for treating the common cold. A randomized, double-blind, placebo-controlled study. *Ann Intern Med.* 1996;125(2):81–8.

21. National Institute of Health. *Highlights of the Expert Panel Report 3: guidelines for the diagnosis and management of asthma, National Institutes of Health publication.* Bethesda (MD): National Institutes of Health, National Heart, Lung, and Blood Institute; 2007.

22. Nelson HS, Weiss ST, Bleecker ER, Yancey SW, Dorinsky PM, SMART Study Group. The Salmeterol Multicenter Asthma Research Trial: a comparison of usual pharmacotherapy for asthma or usual pharmacotherapy plus salmeterol [published correction appears in *Chest.* 2006;129(5):1393]. *Chest.* 2006;129(1):15–26.

23. Nieman DC. Is infection risk linked to exercise workload? *Med Sci Sports Exerc.* 2000;32(7)(suppl):S406–11.

24. O'Byrne PM, Jones GL. The effect of indomethacin on exercise-induced bronchoconstriction and refractoriness after exercise. *Am Rev Respir Dis.* 1986;134(1):69–72.

25. Ostrom NK, Decotiis BA, Lincourt WR, et al. Comparative efficacy and safety of low-dose fluticasone propionate and montelukast in children with persistent asthma. *J Pediatr.* 2005;147(2):213–20.

26. Parsons JP, Kaeding C, Phillips G, Jarjoura D, Wadley G, Mastronarde JG. Prevalence of exercise-induced bronchospasm in a cohort of varsity college athletes. *Med Sci Sports Exerc.* 2007;39(9):1487–92.

27. Ries AL, Bauldoff GS, Carlin BW, et al. Pulmonary rehabilitation: Joint ACCP/AACVPR Evidence-Based Clinical Practice Guidelines. *Chest.* 2007;131(5)(suppl):4S–42S.

28. Rundell KW, Wilber RL, Szmedra L, Jenkinson DM, Mayers LB, Im J. Exercise-induced asthma screening of elite athletes: fields versus laboratory exercise challenge. *Med Sci Sports Exerc.* 2000;32(2):309–16.

29. Schneiderman-Walker J, Pollock SL, Corey M, et al. A randomized controlled trial of a 3-year home exercise program in cystic fibrosis. *J Pediatr.* 2000;136(3):304–10.

30. Simons FE, Gerstner TV, Cheang MS. Tolerance to the bronchoprotective effect of salmeterol in adolescents with exercise-induced asthma using concurrent inhaled glucocorticoid treatment. *Pediatrics.* 1997;99(5):655–9.

31. Smith BW, MacKnight JM. Pulmonary. In: Safran MR, McKeag DB, VanCamp SP, editors. *Manual of Sports Medicine.* Philadelphia: Lippincott-Raven; 1998. p. 244–54.

32. Spooner CH, Spooner GR, Rowe BH. Mast-cell stabilising agents to prevent exercise-induced bronchoconstriction. *Cochrane Database Syst Rev.* 2003;4:CD002307.

33. Stevenson DD, Szczeklik A. Clinical and pathologic perspectives on aspirin sensitivity and asthma. *J Allergy Clin Immunol.* 2006;118(4):773–86; quiz 787–8.

34. Storer TW. Exercise in chronic pulmonary disease: resistance exercise prescription. *Med Sci Sports Exerc.* 2001;33(7)(suppl):S680–92.

35. Storms WW. Exercise-induced asthma: diagnosis and treatment for the recreational or elite athlete. *Med Sci Sports Exerc.* 1999;31(1)(suppl):S33–8.

36. Storms WW, Joyner DM. Update on exercise-induced asthma: a report of the olympic exercise asthma summit conference. *Phys Sportsmed.* 1997;25(3):45–55.

37. Szefler SJ, Phillips BR, Martinez FD, et al. Characterization of within-subject responses to fluticasone and montelukast in childhood asthma. *J Allergy Clin Immunol.* 2005;115(2):233–42.

38. Thole RT, Sallis RE, Rubin AL, Smith GN. Exercise-induced broncho-spasm prevalence in collegiate cross-country runners. *Med Sci Sports Exerc.* 2001;33(10):1641–6.

39. Thomas J, Cook DJ, Brooks D. Chest physical therapy management of patients with cystic fibrosis: a meta-analysis. *Am J Respir Crit Care Med.* 1995;151(3, pt 1):846–50.

40. Tikkanen HO, Peltonen JE. Asthma-cross-country skiing. *Med Sci Sports Exerc.* 1999;31(5)(suppl):S99.

41. U.S. Department of Health and Human Services. *EPR-2. Expert panel report 2: guidelines for the diagnosis and management of asthma* (EPR-2 1997). NIH Publication No. 97-4051. Bethesda (MD): U.S. Department of Health and Human Services, National Institutes of Health, National Heart, Lung, and Blood Institute, National Asthma Education and Prevention Program.

42. U.S. Department of Health and Human Services. *EPR-3. Expert panel report 3: guidelines for the diagnosis and management of asthma–full report* [Internet]. [cited 2007]. Available from: http://www.nhlbi.nih.gov/guidelines/asthma/asthgdln.pdf

43. U.S. Department of Health and Human Services. *EPR-Update 2002. Expert panel report: guidelines for the diagnosis and management of asthma. Update on selected topics 2002* (EPR-Update 2002). NIH Publication No. 02-5074. Bethesda (MD): U.S. Department of Health and Human Services, National Institutes of Health, National Heart, Lung, and Blood Institute, National Asthma Education and Prevention Program.

44. Zeiger RS, Szefler SJ, Phillips BR, et al. Response profiles to fluticasone and montelukast in mild-to-moderate persistent childhood asthma. *J Allergy Clin Immunol.* 2006;117(1):45–52.

39

Allergic Diseases in Athletes

David L. Brown, Nathan P. Falk, and Linda L. Brown

INTRODUCTION

- Allergic rhinitis alone affects over 60 million Americans (2). It is the fifth most common chronic disease and the most prevalent in patients under 18 years of age, affecting up to 40% of children (2,16).
- Urticaria and angioedema affect 20%–30% of the population during their lifetime (9).
- Approximately 20,000–50,000 patients with anaphylaxis present for medical care in the United States each year. Annual mortality figures are difficult to quantify, but available estimates indicate anaphylaxis causes up to 1,000 deaths each year (15).

ALLERGIC RHINITIS

- Allergic rhinitis occurs when an individual develops immunoglobulin (Ig) E sensitization to aeroallergens. Inhalation of the aeroallergens leads to mast cell activation and release of histamine and other chemical mediators of inflammation.
- Common symptoms include rhinorrhea, postnasal drip, congestion, sneezing, cough, and pruritus of the nose and soft palate. Patients may complain of generalized irritability and fatigue. Eye pruritus, injection, irritation, and watery discharge may indicate coexisting allergic conjunctivitis.
- Symptoms recur on exposure to any aeroallergen to which a patient is sensitized.
- Spring and early summer exacerbations occur with tree and grass pollination. Late summer and fall symptoms are usually because of weeds and mold. Indoor flares suggest sensitivity to cockroach, dust mites, pet dander, or molds. Perennial symptoms may be sensitive to a combination of these allergens or indicate nonallergic rhinitis.

NONALLERGIC RHINITIS

- The etiology of nonallergic rhinitis is unknown.
- The prominent complaint is nasal congestion. Nasal, eye, and soft palate pruritus are usually absent. Symptoms are often perennial and triggered by strong odors or smoke. Seasonal air temperature, humidity, and barometric pressure changes may lead to exacerbations, making it difficult to distinguish from allergic rhinitis.

Evaluation

- The history should focus on isolating an allergen exposure. A personal or family history of asthma, allergies, and eczema leads to a higher suspicion for allergic rhinitis.
- Physical examination will not distinguish allergic and nonallergic rhinitis.
  - The nasal mucosa in allergic rhinitis is classically pale or bluish, but can be red or edematous or appear normal. Postnasal drip of any etiology causes posterior pharyngeal cobblestoning. "Allergic shiners" from infraorbital venous congestion are also nonspecific.
  - Findings suggestive of allergic rhinitis include an accentuated transverse nasal crease (seen in children who repeatedly rub their nose because of pruritus), atopic stigmata, such as eczema, and wheezing on auscultation.

Management

- Allergen avoidance is essential in managing allergic rhinitis.
  - Avoidance of animal dander is always best. Exclusion of the pet from the bedroom and high-efficiency particulate air (HEPA) filter use may provide some benefit.
  - For dust mite allergy, use occlusive covers on the pillows, mattress, and box springs. Frequent washing of bed linens and blankets in hot water is helpful. Dehumidifiers and removing carpet may help. HEPA filters are ineffective because dust mite products are not airborne for an extended period of time.
  - Mold allergen can be difficult to control, but dehumidifiers and scrupulous cleaning can be beneficial.

Medical Therapy

- Medical therapy is initiated in a stepwise fashion (Fig. 39.1). Available medications include nasal corticosteroids, antihistamines, decongestants, cromolyn, leukotriene receptor blockers, and nasal ipratropium bromide.
- Nasal corticosteroids are the most effective therapy for persistent or severe symptoms (3). Several days of treatment are

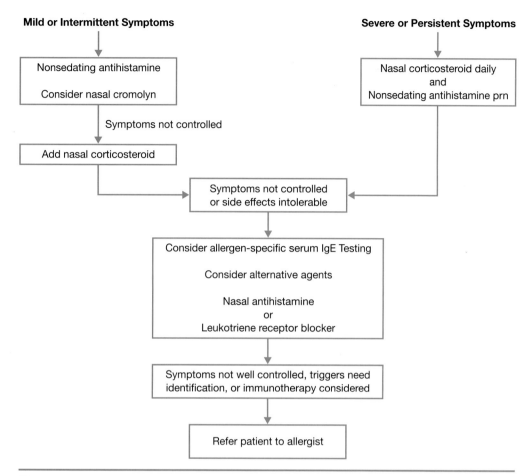

Figure 39.1: Suggested therapeutic strategy for allergic rhinitis in athletes. IgE, immunoglobulin E; prn, as needed.

usually necessary for maximal effectiveness. They can be used periodically for an athlete's allergy season, but once initiated, the steroid needs regular administration for optimal efficacy (Table 39.1). Side effects are low and include irritation, burning, sneezing, and bloody nasal discharge.

Table 39.1	Nasal Corticosteroids	
Nasal Corticosteroid	**Dose: Sprays per Nostril**
Flonase, Veramyst (fluticasone)	Age ≥ 12: 2 daily Age 4–11: Same but start at 1 daily
Nasonex (mometasone furoate)	Age ≥ 12: 2 daily Age 2–11: 1 daily
Rhinocort Aqua (budesonide)	Age ≥ 12: 1–4 daily Age 6–11: 1–2 daily
Omnaris (ciclesonide)	Age ≥ 6: 2 daily
Nasarel (flunisolide)	Age ≥ 15: 2 bid to tid Age 6–14: 1 tid or 2 bid
Nasacort AQ (triamcinolone)	Age ≥ 12: 2 daily Age 6–11: 1–2 daily
Beconase and Vancenase AQ (beclomethasone)	Age ≥ 12: 1–2 bid Age 6–11: 1 bid

bid, twice a day; tid, three times a day.

- Chronic nasal steroids, when used properly, are not associated with significant adrenal suppression, nasal or pharyngeal candidiasis, cataracts, or glaucoma (4,5,12). Studies using mometasone furoate and fluticasone in children showed no difference in growth compared to placebo (1,17,19).

- Oral antihistamines relieve sneezing, itching, and rhinorrhea in allergic rhinitis. Their efficacy is roughly equivalent to nasal cromolyn but less than nasal steroids. They provide little relief of nasal obstruction and are generally ineffective in the treatment of nonallergic rhinitis. First-generation antihistamines can cause significant sedation, decreased alertness, and performance impairment, making them undesirable for most competitive athletes. These effects can exist without an individual's awareness and can be present even with nighttime-only dosing. Second-generation antihistamines are at least as effective as first-generation antihistamines and possess much lower rates of sedation (Table 39.2). Antihistamines can decrease heat dissipation by their anticholinergic effects on sweat glands and should be used with caution in athletes.

- Nasal antihistamines can be beneficial in both allergic and nonallergic rhinitis. Side effects include drowsiness and an unpleasant aftertaste. While nasal steroids provide greater relief of nasal symptoms, nasal antihistamines can be

Table 39.2 | **Second-Generation Oral Antihistamines**

Second-Generation Oral Antihistamine	Dose	Sedation
Fexofenadine (Allegra)	Age ≥ 12: 180 mg daily or 60 mg bid Age 2–11: 30 mg bid	No different than placebo
Cetirizine (Zyrtec)	Age ≥ 6: 5–10 mg daily Age 2–5: 2.5–5 mg daily (syrup)	Slightly higher than placebo but less than first generation
Levocetirizine (Xyzal)	Age ≥ 12: 5 mg daily Age 6–11: 2.5 mg daily Age 2–5: 1.25 mg daily (syrup)	Slightly higher than placebo but less than first generation
Loratadine (Claritin)	Age ≥ 6: 10 mg daily Age 2–5: 5 mg daily	No different than placebo at 10 mg; sedating at higher doses
Desloratadine (Clarinex)	Age ≥ 12: 5 mg daily Age 6–11: 2.5 mg daily Age 2–5: 1.25 mg daily	No different than placebo*

bid, twice a day.
* Seven percent of population may have sedation because of decreased metabolism of the drug.

considered as an alternative when the response to an oral antihistamine and a nasal steroid is inadequate (24).

- Oral decongestants relieve congestion in allergic and non-allergic rhinitis. In allergic rhinitis, they are most effective when combined with an oral antihistamine (21). Side effects include insomnia, irritability, tachycardia, and palpations. Because they decrease heat dissipation via peripheral vasoconstriction, they should be avoided during training or competition in the heat. Athletes must be aware of the rules of their particular sport. Governing bodies for competitive sports have individual guidelines that may ban certain decongestants (see later section, Athlete-Specific Medication Issues).

- Topical nasal decongestants are for short-term control of severe congestion. Their use should not exceed 3 days. If used for more than 5–7 days, they can cause severe rebound congestion and rhinorrhea.

- Cromolyn, a topical mast cell stabilizer, provides modest improvement in the sneezing, itching, and rhinorrhea associated with allergic rhinitis and has a low potential for toxicity. It is useful when given prior to allergen exposure but often requires dosing up to 4–6 times daily to be effective.

- Leukotriene receptor antagonists (LRAs) provide mild improvement in allergic rhinitis with efficacy similar to second-generation antihistamines (14). Their side effect profile is no different than placebo. They should be considered when nasal steroids and/or antihistamines fail or have intolerable side effects. Patients with concomitant asthma may also benefit from LRA therapy.

- Ipratropium bromide 0.03% nasal spray is effective for treating rhinorrhea, particularly vasomotor-induced rhinorrhea triggered by cold air or exercise. It has no effect on pruritus or congestion. Side effects include occasional epistaxis and nasal dryness but no systemic anticholinergic or rebound effects. It is effective when dosed 30 minutes prior to exercise or exposure.

- When treatments fail, consider medication inadequacy and noncompliance, as well as the possibility of other diagnoses, such as anatomic or physical obstruction and/or chronic sinusitis.

Athlete-Specific Medication Issues

- Because restrictions on over-the-counter and prescription medications can change, an athlete should discuss a medication's status with the governing body for their particular sport or level of competition prior to its use. This would include the National Collegiate Athletic Association (NCAA) and the World Anti-Doping Agency (WADA).

- The NCAA has no restrictions on any allergy-related products with the exception that any products containing ephedrine are banned.

- The WADA standards are more stringent. Ephedrine and pseudoephedrine are both banned. However, the urinary concentration of pseudoephedrine associated with normal therapeutic use typically falls below the WADA limit of 150 $\mu g \cdot mL^{-1}$. Oral glucocorticoids are also banned. Injected epinephrine (EpiPen) for emergency use requires a therapeutic use exemption (TUE). Antihistamines, cromolyn, and leukotriene receptor blockers, as well as topical and nasal steroids, are not banned and do not require a TUE. The WADA releases a new list of banned substances each year and requires review by participants and medical staff to ensure compliance (23).

ALLERGY TESTING

- In patients with a history suggestive of allergic rhinitis, indications for referral for skin testing include targeting allergens for avoidance, as well as institution of immunotherapy when medical therapy is failing. Allergy consultation is recommended prior to drastic environmental interventions, such as pet elimination, taking up carpets, or purchasing new mattresses, bedding, dust mite covers, and the like.

■ Antihistamines should be stopped 1 week prior to testing, so as not to blunt the cutaneous response to skin testing.

■ Allergy testing is contraindicated in the setting of severe lung disease or poorly controlled asthma with a forced expiratory volume in 1 second (FEV_1) of less than 70%.

■ Skin testing is preferred over in vitro allergen-specific serum IgE testing with radioallergosorbent testing (RAST) or ImmunoCAP because it is more sensitive. Serum testing is a reasonable alternative when skin testing cannot be performed and is helpful for validating the diagnosis and supporting environmental controls.

ALLERGEN IMMUNOTHERAPY

■ Allergen immunotherapy (AIT) is effective for allergic rhinitis and allergic asthma. Advantages include long-lasting symptom remission and a reduction in the risk of developing new allergies and asthma in children (13). Notable symptom relief usually takes several months of treatment. Three to 5 years of AIT are required to sustain symptom remission. Any individual who cannot fully commit to treatment, has poorly controlled asthma, or is on a β-blocker should not receive AIT. It should be prescribed and administered by a board-certified allergist to ensure a thorough discussion of the benefits and potential risks of therapy and to provide ongoing follow-up.

ALLERGIC CONJUNCTIVITIS

■ Etiology is the same as for allergic rhinitis. Symptoms occur on inoculation of the allergen onto the mucosa of the eyes.

■ Symptom control can be achieved with the same measures as discussed for allergic rhinitis. Persistent eye symptoms may require targeted ocular medications (Table 39.3).

Combination of mast cell blocker and antihistamine topical therapy is very effective. Other options include topical mast cell blockers or antihistamine alone, topical decongestants, and topical mast cell stabilizers. Topical decongestants should be reserved for short-term use because rebound hyperemia occurs with chronic application. Topical corticosteroids are associated with significant complications and should only be used after consultation with an ophthalmologist.

URTICARIA AND ANGIOEDEMA

Pathophysiology

■ Urticaria is caused by mast cell degranulation in the superficial dermis and is characterized by pruritic, erythematous, cutaneous elevations that blanch with pressure. Hives may appear anywhere on the body, but occur primarily on the trunk and extremities. Mast cell mediators involved include histamine, prostaglandins, leukotrienes, platelet-activating factor, anaphylatoxins, bradykinin, and Hageman factor. All cause blood vessel dilation and tissue edema.

■ Angioedema is similar to urticaria but occurs in the deeper dermis and subcutaneous tissues. It is more painful and burning than pruritic and often involves the face.

■ Acute urticaria is defined as new-onset symptoms of less than 6 weeks in duration. If symptoms persist more than 6 weeks, it is considered chronic urticaria.

■ In chronic urticaria, 75% have symptoms for over 1 year, 50% have symptoms for over 5 years, and 20% have symptoms for decades. Urticaria occurs at any age but is most common in children and young adults. Approximately 50% of patients at presentation have both urticaria and angioedema, 40% have urticaria only, and 10% have angioedema only (22).

■ Most cases are idiopathic, but potential triggers are medications, insect stings, infections, and foods and food additives. Table 39.4 lists the most common known triggers.

Table 39.3	Allergic Conjunctivitis Topical Medications	
Topical Agent	**Mechanism of Action**	**Dose**
Patanol (olopatadine)	Mast cell blocker/antihistamine	Age ≥ 3: 1 drop bid
Zaditor (ketotifen)	Mast cell blocker/antihistamine	Age ≥ 3: 1 drop 2–3 times daily
Alomide (lodoxamide)	Mast cell blocker	Age ≥ 2: 1–2 drops qid
Alamast (pemirolast)	Mast cell blocker	Age ≥ 3: 2 drops qid
Livostin (levocabastine)	Antihistamine	Age ≥ 12: 1 drop qid
Alocril (nedocromil)	Inhibits activation and mediator release from inflammatory cells	Age > 3: 1–2 drops bid
Emadine (emedastine)	Antihistamine	Age ≥ 3: 1 drop qid
Optivar (azelastine)	Antihistamine	Age ≥ 3: 1 drop bid
Crolom (cromolyn)	Mast cell blocker	Age > 4: 1–2 drops qid
Naphcon-A, Opcon-A, Visine-A	Antihistamine/decongestant	Age ≥ 6: 1 drop up to 4 times daily

bid, twice a day; qid, four times a day.

Table 39.4 | Common Triggers for Urticaria

Medications
   Antibiotics
   β-Lactams
   Sulfa compounds
   NSAIDs
   Progesterone
   Local anesthetics
   Opioid analgesics

Physical Contacts
   Latex
   Nickel
   Plants and plant resins
   Fruits/vegetables
   Raw fish
   Animal saliva

Insect Stings

Foods and Food Additives
   Milk
   Egg
   Peanut
   Nuts
   Soy
   Wheat
   Fish/shellfish
   Sulfites

Infections
   Coxsackie A and B
   Hepatitis A, B, and C
   HIV
   Ebstein-Barr virus
   Herpes simplex
   Intestinal parasites
   Dermatophyte infections

HIV, human immunodeficiency virus; NSAIDs, nonsteroidal anti-inflammatory drugs.

■ Physical stimuli can also cause urticaria. Physical urticarias represent 20% of chronic urticaria cases and are important to consider in athletes because they are triggered by conditions occurring during practice and competition (7). (See Table 39.5 for their evaluation and management) (6).

   ▪ Cholinergic urticaria, from elevation in core body temperature, is precipitated by exercise or use of hot tubs. Classically, patients develop small, punctate wheals with prominent erythematous flare. Symptoms usually occur within 2–30 minutes of exposure and last up to 90 minutes.

   ▪ Cold urticaria is precipitated by contact with cold air or objects. Within 2–5 minutes, the exposed area develops swelling and pruritus. Symptoms generally worsen as the area rewarms and last up to 2 hours. Patients with cold urticaria should avoid swimming and diving because this condition carries a risk of anaphylaxis during rewarming if patients have a significant drop in core body temperature.

   ▪ Aquagenic urticaria, which is extremely rare, is caused by contact with water itself. For athletes in water sports, this condition could be confused with cholinergic or cold urticaria. Aquagenic urticaria differs from cholinergic urticaria because it occurs even in cool water and even if the athlete is not exercising while in the water. Unlike cold urticaria, aquagenic urticaria will not be precipitated by application of a cold object that is not water-based.

   ▪ Solar urticaria occurs with exposure to ultraviolet light. Anaphylaxis could occur if large body areas are exposed.

   ▪ Pressure urticaria (angioedema) is precipitated by direct pressure on the skin. Skin pressure is followed 3–12 hours later by localized hives, fever, malaise, and leukocytosis. It can be precipitated by running, clapping, sitting, or using hand equipment. Symptoms can last up to 24 hours.

Table 39.5 | Physical Urticarias

Type	Precipitant	Evaluation	Treatment
Cholinergic urticaria	Elevation in core temperature; exercise, hot tubs, etc.	History and classic pencil eraser-sized punctate wheals	Premedicate with nonsedating antihistamine prior to exercise
Cold urticaria	Contact with cold object	Place cold object on skin for 15 minutes	Nonsedating antihistamines as needed; avoidance of swimming and diving sports because of risk of anaphylaxis
Aquagenic urticaria	Water contact	History; expose skin to water	Nonsedating antihistamines
Solar urticaria	Ultraviolet light exposure	Expose small, unprotected patch of skin to sunlight	Limit sun exposure; protective clothing and sunscreen use
Pressure urticaria/ angioedema	Direct pressure on skin. Running, prolonged sitting, clapping, etc.	Place 15-lb weight on patient for 20 minutes and look for skin changes; test for fever and leukocytosis 3–12 hours later	Avoidance of precipitants; nonsedating antihistamines and NSAIDs; consider steroid burst/taper if symptoms severe
Symptomatic dermatographism	Stroking or rubbing skin; areas where clothing or equipment abrades skin	Look for linear, pruritic wheal 2–5 minutes after rubbing the skin	Loose fitting clothing; treatment usually not necessary; nonsedating antihistamines only for severe symptoms

NSAIDs, nonsteroidal anti-inflammatory drugs.

- Symptomatic dermatographism is another type of physical urticaria. Patients develop linear, pruritic wheals 2–5 minutes after an area of skin is stroked.

Evaluation

- In the acute setting, providers should assess for symptoms indicating anaphylaxis rather than isolated urticaria or angioedema (8). (See later section, Anaphylactic and Anaphylactoid Reactions.)
- Although in most cases the precipitant remains unknown, a detailed history may isolate the cause. Searching for a trigger is more beneficial in acute urticaria as compared to chronic urticaria where the cause is found in less than 10% of cases. For known causes, drug hypersensitivity is most common. Individuals should be asked about any recent prescription medication, over-the-counter medication, or supplement use. Food and food additives rarely cause isolated urticaria, but the relationship to food inhalation, contact, and consumption should be documented. It is important to document physical triggers, occupational exposures, insect envenomations, and recent illnesses. A thorough review of systems will help rule out any disease associations, such as an acute bacterial or viral illness, parasitic infection, autoimmune/collagen vascular disease, serum sickness, endocrine disease, or malignancy (20).
- The physical examination is especially helpful in the acute setting when skin manifestations are present. It can help document whether urticaria and angioedema are occurring together or in isolation and whether there are any signs of anaphylaxis. The examination should also look for evidence of other diseases that are rarely associated with urticaria and angioedema.
- The use of laboratory and imaging studies should be targeted by the history and physical.
- Consider the following tests: Monospot or Epstein-Barr virus antibody titers if acute mononucleosis is suspected; hepatitis A, B, and C panel; and human immunodeficiency virus (HIV) testing given the right clinical setting. The association of urticaria with other viral infections remains unclear, and routine testing for other viral pathogens is not recommended.
- If a significant travel history is discovered and the complete blood count shows eosinophilia, stool studies should be obtained looking for intestinal parasites. Progressive weight loss and/or the presence of lymphadenopathy or hepatosplenomegaly on examination would warrant an evaluation for an underlying lymphoreticular malignancy.
- If enlargement or nodularity of the thyroid is present, a thyroid function panel, thyroid autoantibodies, thyroid ultrasound, and nuclear medicine thyroid studies should be considered.
- Testing for C1 esterase inhibitor deficiency should be considered for any athlete presenting with recurrent isolated angioedema.

- A skin biopsy for vasculitis is indicated when individual urticarial lesions last longer than 24 hours or are associated with purpura, pain, hyperpigmentation, or systemic symptoms (10).
- If the history and physical examination are unrevealing, a limited laboratory evaluation consisting of a complete blood count with differential, urinalysis, erythrocyte sedimentation rate, thyroid-stimulating hormone, and liver panel is reasonable to screen for occult conditions.

Management

- After the initial evaluation, the management of urticaria and angioedema becomes primarily symptomatic. Known triggers should be avoided if possible. Mild symptoms can be controlled with a low-sedating antihistamine (Table 39.2). Athletes with exercise-induced symptoms only, such as cholinergic urticaria, can take the antihistamine 1–2 hours prior to exercise. Those who exercise regularly and those with chronic symptoms often require daily medication to prevent exacerbations. For moderate or poorly controlled symptoms, the antihistamine dose should be maximized prior to considering add-on therapy. Additive therapies include leukotriene antagonists, H_2 blockers, and nighttime doxepin. For periods of moderate to severe symptoms, prednisone therapy can be helpful, but chronic use should be avoided because of the risk of long-term side effects.
- Because food and food additives are a rare cause of chronic urticaria and angioedema, elimination diets are unnecessary unless the history pinpoints a specific food.
- Referral to an allergist is recommended when there is suspicion of an allergic component precipitating symptoms, when symptoms are not well controlled with treatment, when there is a history of respiratory distress and hypotension suggesting anaphylaxis, or when there is severe angioedema. The athlete should be referred to dermatology for skin biopsy if urticarial vasculitis is suspected.

ANAPHYLACTIC AND ANAPHYLACTOID REACTIONS

Pathophysiology

- Anaphylaxis is an acute, life-threatening, systemic reaction mediated through IgE antibodies and their receptors. It requires previous sensitization and subsequent reexposure to an allergen.
- Anaphylactoid reactions are clinically indistinguishable from true anaphylaxis. Both are caused by massive release of potent chemical mediators from mast cells and basophils. The differences are that IgE antibodies do not mediate anaphylactoid reactions, they do not require prior sensitization, and they are less commonly associated with severe hypotension and cardiovascular collapse. Both are managed with the same treatment measures discussed here.

■ Anaphylaxis includes cutaneous signs or symptoms accompanied by obstructive respiratory symptoms and/or hemodynamic changes. Additional features include gastrointestinal complaints and experiencing a "sense of impending doom" (Table 39.6). The onset of symptoms typically begins seconds to minutes after the inciting cause. More rarely, symptoms may be delayed for up to 2 hours.

■ Approximately 80% of anaphylaxis cases have a uniphasic course with abrupt onset of symptoms. In the most fulminant cases, symptoms can be followed by death within minutes despite treatment. Up to 20% of patients have a biphasic presentation with a 1- to 8-hour asymptomatic period following the acute phase. After the symptom-free period, a late-phase reaction ensues with recurrence of severe symptoms. The late phase can be protracted, persisting for several hours in 28% of individuals (11).

Evaluation

■ The diagnosis of anaphylaxis is affected by variability in the standard case definition. Obtaining as much information from the affected athlete and any witnesses will define the time course, severity of the reaction, and potential cause.

■ Anaphylaxis triggers include food, medications, and insect stings (Table 39.7). Any food exposure prior to the onset of

symptoms should be documented. Of special concern would be exposure to the most common food allergens, which include eggs, peanut, cow's milk, nuts, fish, soy, shellfish, and wheat. Several medications have been known to cause anaphylaxis, with the most common being β-lactam antibiotics. Documenting exposure to prescription medications, as well as over-the-counter medications and supplements, is important. Bee-sting sensitivity should be suspected in any athlete with a reaction that occurs outdoors, even if the patient does not recall being stung.

■ Exercise-induced anaphylaxis is a rare condition associated with exercising within 2–4 hours after food ingestion. It is characterized by the usual manifestations of anaphylaxis beginning within 5–30 minutes of exercise and lasting up to 3 hours. The medical history should explore the relationship of symptom onset to physical exercise to assess for this rare trigger.

■ The physical manifestations of anaphylaxis involve multiple sites, including the skin, upper airway, lower airway, and cardiovascular system. The physical examination should start by evaluating upper airway patency by listening for inspiratory stridor and looking for oral or pharyngeal edema. The

Table 39.6	Symptoms and Signs of Anaphylaxis

Psychological
  "Sense of impending doom"

Cutaneous
  Tingling/pruritus
  Generalized erythema
  Urticaria
  Angioedema

Upper Airway
  Nasal congestion
  Rhinorrhea
  Sneezing
  Globus sensation
  Throat tightness
  Dysphonia
  Dysphagia

Lower Airway
  Dyspnea
  Wheezing
  Cough

Cardiovascular
  Lightheadedness
  Syncope
  Palpitations
  Shock

Gastrointestinal
  Abdominal cramps
  Bloating
  Nausea/vomiting

Table 39.7	Causes of Anaphylaxis

Idiopathic

Medications

Antibiotics

Intravenous and local anesthetics

Aspirin/NSAIDs

Chemotherapeutic agents

Opiates

Vaccines

Allergy immunotherapy sera

Radiographic contrast media

Blood products

Latex

Hymenoptera envenomation

Foods

Eggs

Peanut

Cow's milk

Nuts

Seafood

Soy

Wheat

Exercise

NSAIDs, nonsteroidal anti-inflammatory drugs.

athlete's work of breathing and accessory muscle use can be used to assess their respiratory status. Auscultation may reveal wheezing, indicating acute bronchospasm. A set of vital signs is critical to patient management, looking for any evidence of cardiovascular or respiratory compromise. Once the ABCs (airway, breathing, and circulation) are assessed and secured, the skin can be examined for the presence of generalized erythema, urticaria, and angioedema.

Acute Management

■ Initial management of anaphylaxis should always start with 0.2–0.5 mL epinephrine (1:1,000) intramuscular (IM) or subcutaneous (SC), even if symptoms are mild. The IM route is preferred, especially in children, because SC injection may delay absorption. Doses may be repeated every 10–15 minutes if symptoms persist. Intravenous (IV) epinephrine at 1 $\mu g \cdot min^{-1}$ of 1:10,000 (10 $\mu g \cdot mL^{-1}$) can be considered for symptoms resistant to repeated SC or IM administration. The IV dosage can be increased to 2–10 $\mu g \cdot min^{-1}$ for severe reactions. Patients on β-blockers may not respond to epinephrine. In these cases, glucagon 2–5 mg IM/SC is beneficial. Supportive therapy includes oxygen for hypoxemia, recumbent positioning and IV fluids for hypotension, and inhaled β-agonists or racemic epinephrine for bronchospasm. Antihistamines (diphenhydramine 1–2 $mg \cdot kg^{-1}$ or 25–50 mg IV or orally) may provide additional benefit. Corticosteroids (prednisone 0.5–2.0 $mg \cdot kg^{-1}$ up to 125 mg) should also be considered to help prevent late-phase reactions. Neither antihistamines nor steroids should be used as substitutes for epinephrine. Their onset of action is much slower, and they are insufficient to prevent or treat more severe anaphylaxis with respiratory or cardiovascular involvement.

■ Mild anaphylaxis cases should be observed a minimum of 3 hours after symptoms have resolved. Severe reactions should be observed at least 6 hours, and hospitalization should be strongly considered to monitor for late-phase reactions.

Long-Term Management

■ All patients with anaphylaxis need an action plan to include allergen identification, symptom recognition, and appropriate treatment. A provider knowledgeable in allergic disease should provide education on allergen avoidance, hidden allergens, and cross-reacting substances. All individuals should have an epinephrine autoinjector with them at all times and be educated on the indications and proper technique for its use. The trainer and coach should be familiar with anaphylaxis recognition and epinephrine use as well. The athlete should wear a medical alert bracelet at all times, indicating their condition and allergy if known.

■ Because there are no measures proven to prevent exercise-induced anaphylaxis, affected athletes should never exercise alone. Pretreatment with antihistamines is not effective. The primary preventative strategy is to avoid eating for 4 hours prior to exercise. Other measures that may limit attacks are to avoid nonsteroidal anti-inflammatory drugs and aspirin prior to exercise and to avoid outdoor exercise during periods of high humidity, temperature extremes, and the individual's allergy season (18). Occasionally, skin testing can identify a specific food that the patient can avoid, but often the results are inconclusive. Athletes should carry an epinephrine autoinjector on their person when they do not have immediate access to their gear bag. They should discontinue exercise at the first sign of symptoms and self-administer epinephrine.

■ Indications for allergy referral include when further testing is necessary for an unclear diagnosis or an unknown inciting agent, when reactions are recurrent and difficult to control, or when desensitization is required, such as for stinging insects or antibiotic administration. Allergists also serve as an important resource for athletes, parents, and coaches needing education on allergen avoidance, as well as institution or reinforcement of an individual's action plan.

REFERENCES

1. Allen DB, Meltzer EO, Lemanske RF Jr, et al. No growth suppression in children treated with the maximum recommended dose of fluticasone propionate aqueous nasal spray for one year. *Allergy Asthma Proc.* 2002;23(6):407–13.

2. American Academy of Allergy, Asthma and Immunology. The allergy report [Internet]. 2010 [cited 2010 Oct 8]. Available from: http://www.aaaai.org/.

3. Benninger M, Farrar JR, Blaiss M, et al. Evaluating approved medication to treat allergic rhinitis in the United States: an evidence-based review of efficacy for nasal symptoms by class. *Ann Allergy Asthma Immunol.* 2010;104(1):13–29.

4. Boner AL. Effects of intranasal corticosteroids on the hypothalamic-pituitary-adrenal axis in children. *J Allergy Clin Immunol.* 2001;108 (1)(suppl):S32–9.

5. Bruni FM, De Luca G, Venturoli V, Boner AL, et al. Intranasal corticosteroids and adrenal suppression. *Neuroimmunomodulation.* 2009; 16(5):353–62.

6. Casale TB, Sampson HA, Hanifin J, et al. Guide to physical urticarias. *J Allergy Clin Immunol.* 1988;82(5, pt 1):758–63.

7. Fernando S, Broadfoot A. Chronic urticaria—assessment and treatment. *Aust Fam Physician.* 2010;39(3):135–8.

8. Frigas E, Park MA. Acute urticaria and angioedema: diagnostic and treatment considerations. *Am J Clin Derm.* 2009;10(4):239–50.

9. Kaplan AP. Clinical practice. Chronic urticaria and angioedema. *N Engl J Med.* 2002;346(3):175–9.

10. Kaplan AP. Urticaria and angioedema. In: Middleton E Jr, Reed CE, Ellis EF, et al., editors. *Allergy: Principles and Practice.* St. Louis: Mosby; 1993. p. 1553–80.

11. Kemp SF. Current concepts in the pathophysiology, diagnosis, and management of anaphylaxis. *Immunol Allergy Clin North Am.* 2001; 21(4):611–34.

12. Krahnke J, Skoner D. Benefit and risk management for steroid treatment in upper airway diseases. *Curr Allergy Asthma Rep.* 2002;2(6):507–12.

13. Ledford DK. Efficacy of immunotherapy. *Immunol Allergy Clin North Am.* 2000;20(3):503–25.

14. Nayak A, Langdon RB. Montelukast in the treatment of allergic rhinitis: an evidence-based review. *Drugs.* 2007;67(6):887–901.

15. Neugut AI, Ghatak AT, Miller RL. Anaphylaxis in the United States: an investigation into its epidemiology. *Arch Intern Med.* 2001;161(1):15–21.

16. Public Health Service. *U.S. Department of Health and Human Services Publication (PHS) 93-1522.* Washington (DC): Public Health Service; 1997.

17. Schenkel EJ, Skoner DP, Bronsky EA, et al. Absence of growth retardation in children with perennial allergic rhinitis after one year of treatment with mometasone furoate aqueous nasal spray. *Pediatrics.* 2000;105(2):E22.

18. Shadick NA, Liang MH, Partridge AJ, et al. The natural history of exercise-induced anaphylaxis: survey results from a 10-year follow-up study. *J Allergy Clin Immunol.* 1999;104(1):123–7.

19. Skoner DP, Rachelefsky GS, Meltzer EO, et al. Detection of growth suppression in children during treatment with intranasal beclomethasone dipropionate. *Pediatrics.* 2000;105(2):E23.

20. Stafford CT. Urticaria as a sign of systemic disease. *Ann Allergy.* 1990; 64(3):264–70.

21. Sussman GL, Mason J, Compton D, Stewart J, Richard N. The efficacy and safety of fexofenadine HCL and pseudoephedrine alone and in combination in seasonal allergic rhinitis. *J Allergy Clin Immunol.* 1999;104(1):100–6.

22. Tharp MD. Chronic urticaria: pathophysiology and treatment approaches. *J Allergy Clin Immunol.* 1996;98(6)(pt 3):S325–30.

23. World Anti-Doping Agency. *The 2011 Prohibited List: International Standard* [Internet]. 2010. Available from: http://www.wada-ama.org/ Documents/World_Anti-Doping_Program/WADP-Prohibited-list/ To_be_effective/WADA_Prohibited_List_2011_EN.pdf.

24. Yáñez A, Rodrigo GJ. Intranasal corticosteroids versus topical H1 receptor antagonists for the treatment of allergic rhinitis: a systematic review with meta-analysis. *Ann Allergy Asthma Immunol.* 2002;89(5):479–84.

Overtraining Syndrome

40

Elizabeth Gannon and Thomas M. Howard

INTRODUCTION

- Overtraining has been described and has been well known to athletes and trainers for decades. In 1923, Dr. Parmenter described overtraining as "a condition difficult to detect and still more difficult to describe. Evaluation should focus on training load, nutrition, sleep, rest, competition stress, and psychological state" (14).

- There are multiple hypotheses on the cause of overtraining. There continues to be research on overtraining to further define the condition and pathophysiology and identify markers for diagnosis, treatment, and prevention.

- Overtraining, if left unrecognized or untreated, can result in injury, poor performance, and early retirement.

- Overtraining syndrome is a condition that arises along a continuum of fatigue.

- The diagnosis of overtraining syndrome is one of exclusion and often requires an extensive workup of the athlete.

- Treatment of overtraining syndrome is rest; however, it often requires a multidisciplinary approach involving the physician, trainers, nutritionist, and often, a sports psychologist.

DEFINITIONS

- **Training:** A series of stimuli or displacement of homeostasis to provide stimulation for adaptation. A progressive overload in an effort to improve performance.

- **Adaptation:** A physiologic response to stress that results in an adjustment in function.

- **Recovery:** Period of time following a training stimulus when adaptation occurs, resulting in supercompensation to allow better performance in the future (*i.e.,* the training effect). Recovery includes hydration, nutritional replenishment, sleep/rest, stretching, relaxation, and emotional recovery.

- **Periodization:** Planned sequencing of increased training loads and recovery periods within a training program.

- **Overreaching:** A short-term decrement in performance after a period of overload (intensity or volume). This acute phase is thought to last 1–2 weeks. Some authors even consider overreaching to represent normal physiologic fatigue to overload training (2).

- **Overtraining syndrome:** This syndrome is defined as prolonged decrease in sport-specific performance, usually > 2 weeks. It is manifested by premature fatigability, emotional and mood changes, lack of motivation, sleep disorders, pronounced vegetative somatic complaints, overuse injuries, and immune dysfunction (2,8,9). It is the result of prolonged heavy exercise over an extended period of time with inadequate recovery time between training sessions.

PHYSIOLOGIC CHANGES WITH TRAINING

Immunologic

- Decreased salivary immunoglobulin A (IgA)

- Increased white blood cells (WBCs), lymphocytes, natural killer cells, and polymorphonuclear cell (PMN) activity

- Transient decrease in T helper/T suppressor (Th/Ts) ratio

- Decreased serum glutamine

Endocrine

- Increased testosterone proportional to exercise intensity and muscle mass stimulating glycogen regeneration and protein synthesis (anabolism).

- Transient increase in cortisol relative to the duration and intensity of exercise. The stress response (catabolism).

- The ratio of free testosterone to cortisol (FTCR) represents the balance of catabolism and anabolism. A 30% decrease in this ratio may suggest inadequate recovery or overreaching (5).

- Norepinephrine increases before exercise (anticipation) and early in exercise, stimulating lipolysis.

- Epinephrine increases proportional to exercise intensity.

- Decreased sex hormone binding globulin (SHBG) production with intense exercise.

- Suppression of pulsatile secretion of gonadotropin-releasing factor (GnRH), probably affected by stress and poor nutrition.

- Growth hormone peak secretion at night and with exercise ~50% $\dot{V}O_{2max}$, blunted response with intense exercise.

EPIDEMIOLOGY

- Overtraining affects 5%–15% of elite athletes at any one time and as much as two-thirds of runners during an athletic career. It may also be seen in amateur athletes.
- More commonly seen in endurance events, such as swimming, cycling, or running. Overtraining in powerlifters is probably different.
- Susceptible athletes include highly motivated, goal-oriented individuals; athletes who design exercise programs by themselves; and athletes that tend to be focused, conventional, and conservative.

HYPOTHESES

- **Glycogen depletion:** Chronic nutritional deficiency and extensive periods of heavy training lead to glycogen depletion in muscles, resulting in peripheral fatigue. Central fatigue is interrelated to changes in branched-chain amino acids (BCAAs); see central fatigue hypothesis (18).
- **Central fatigue hypothesis/BCAA hypothesis:** Peripheral fatigue and nutrient depletion lead to the consumption of BCAAs with subsequent change in the BCAA to free tryptophan ratio in plasma. This favors transport of tryptophan into the central nervous system. Tryptophan is a precursor for serotonin 5-hydroxytryptamine, which causes central fatigue (1,6).
- **Autonomic imbalance:** An increase in sympathetic activity from stress and overloaded target organs and increased catabolism leading to decreased sympathetic intrinsic activity. Chronically increased catecholamine levels causes downregulation of receptors and fatigue (12).
- **Glutamine hypothesis/immune dysfunction:** Overload training leads to depressed glutamine production from stressed muscle tissue. Glutamine deficiency, as well as acute exercise stress on the immune system, creates an immunologic open window leading to repeated minor infections and systemic stress (19).
- **Cytokine hypothesis:** Incomplete recovery of locally damaged tissue causes a local inflammatory response that becomes systemic with elevated proinflammatory cytokines interleukin (IL)-1β, tumor necrosis factor-α, and IL-6. These cytokines cause central nervous system fatigue (17).

CATEGORIES OF OVERTRAINING

- **Sympathetic overtraining:** Probably represents early overtraining. It is manifested by increased resting heart rate (HR) and blood pressure, loss of appetite, loss of lean body mass (LBM), irritability, sleep disturbances, and fatigue (5).

- **Parasympathetic overtraining:** Probably represents more chronic state, prolonged overtraining. It is manifested by low resting HR and blood pressure, sleep disturbances, depressed mood, and fatigue (5).

Physical Findings

- Elevated resting HR (usually > 10 beats per minute [bpm] over baseline)
- Decreased LBM
- Depressed mood on various evaluation tools
- Otherwise normal physical exam

Differential Diagnosis

Common Causes

- Caffeine withdrawal, environmental allergies, exercise-induced bronchospasm, infectious mononucleosis, insufficient sleep, iron deficiency with or without anemia, overtraining, performance anxiety, mood disorder (anxiety, depression, adjustment reaction), psychosocial stress, and upper respiratory infection

Less Common Causes

- Dehydration, diabetes mellitus, eating disorder, hepatitis (A, B, or C), hypothyroidism, inadequate carbohydrate or protein intake, lower respiratory infection, medication side effect (antidepressants, antihistamines, anxiolytics, β-blockers), postconcussive syndrome, pregnancy, and substance abuse

Relatively Rare Causes, but Important

- Adrenocortical insufficiency or excess, congenital or acquired heart disease, arrhythmia, bacterial endocarditis, congestive heart failure, coronary heart disease, human immunodeficiency virus, malabsorption, lung disease, Lyme disease, malaria, malignancy, neuromuscular disorder, renal disease, and syphilis

Evaluation (Fig. 40.1)

First Visit

- A thorough history focusing on chief complaint, training program, diet, medications, nutrition, illness, review of systems (ROS), and an assessment of the goals of the athlete's training program.
- Initial lab studies to consider: complete blood count (CBC), erythrocyte sedimentation rate (ESR), metabolic panel, thyroid-stimulating hormone (TSH), ferritin, serum β-human chorionic gonadotropin (β-hCG), monospot, and other specifically indicated tests based on history, ROS, and examination.
- Prescribe decrease in intensity or even absolute rest for 2 weeks. During that time, consider cross-training for enjoyment and evaluation of other confounding stressors.

Second Visit

- Review lab results, training over the past 2 weeks, and symptoms.
- If improved, consider the diagnosis of physiologic fatigue (overreaching) and focus on adjustments to the training

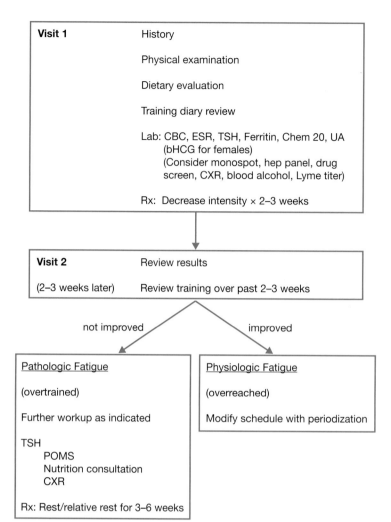

Visit 1

History

Physical examination

Dietary evaluation

Training diary review

Lab: CBC, ESR, TSH, Ferritin, Chem 20, UA
    (bHCG for females)
    (Consider monospot, hep panel, drug
    screen, CXR, blood alcohol, Lyme titer)

Rx: Decrease intensity × 2–3 weeks

Visit 2

(2–3 weeks later)

Review results

Review training over past 2–3 weeks

not improved   improved

Pathologic Fatigue

(overtrained)

Further workup as indicated

TSH
    POMS
    Nutrition consultation
    CXR

Rx: Rest/relative rest for 3–6 weeks

Physiologic Fatigue

(overreached)

Modify schedule with periodization

FIGURE 40.1: Algorithm for evaluation of fatigue in the athlete. bHCG, β-human chorionic gonadotropin; CBC, complete blood count; CXR, chest x-ray; ESR, erythrocyte sedimentation rate; Hep, hepatitis; POMS, Profile of Mood States; TSH, thyroid-stimulating hormone; UA, urinalysis.

schedule with periodization, cross-training, and addressing the other stressors identified.

■ If no improvement, consider the diagnosis of pathologic fatigue or overtraining. Patients will require prolonged relative rest from intense training and further workup. Consider consulting with a sports psychologist and dietician and further evaluation to work through the differential diagnosis.

TREATMENT

■ The first line of treatment should be prevention. To try to prevent overtraining syndrome, review the athlete's training schedule and concepts of cross-training and emphasize adequate rest and minimization of coexisting life stressors.

■ When prevention fails, the treatment is rest. There is no quick fix. An initial rest period of 2–4 weeks should be considered.

■ Life stressors should be reviewed in depth, as well as a review of the athlete's diet, sleep schedule, and training and competition schedules.

■ A multidisciplinary approach is recommended. Consultation with a nutritionist and sports psychologist can be beneficial.

■ Close monitoring of the athlete is recommended. Upon return to practice and competition, the athlete should pay careful attention to sleep, nutrition, social stress, and competition stress with slow advancement of training. The sequence of advancing activity should focus on frequency, then duration, and finally the intensity of the sessions.

MONITORING

■ Poor markers for overtraining include body mass, hemoglobin, ferritin, and creatine phosphokinase.

■ Indicators of inadequate recovery, but not necessarily overtraining, include FTCR ratio decrease > 30%, a decrease in SHBG, and a glutamine-to-glutamate level < 3.58 (7,16).

■ Psychiatric indicators generally change before biologic markers.

■ **Good markers for monitoring:** Athletes, trainers, and coaches often use baseline HR. An increase of > 10 bpm from baseline is considered abnormal. This rise represents an imbalance between sympathetic and parasympathetic systems with heightened sympathetic tone (3). In the past, this was not considered to be a great monitoring tool because of considerable confounding factors.

■ Increase in HR variability also indicates inadequate recovery (15).

■ Monitor performance in time trials and standard exercise challenges.

■ Foster (4) described a "session RPE," or rating of perceived exertion, as the athlete's self-described intensity of the training session multiplied by the duration of the session. Daily mean load and standard deviated (SD) can be calculated to quantitative monotony (daily mean/SD) and strain (weekly load × monotony) (4).

■ **Psychological tools:** Profile of Mood States (POMS) — 65 questions assessing 5 negative mood states (tension, depression, anger, fatigue, and confusion) and 1 positive mood state (vigor) (13).

■ Total Quality Recovery (TQR) action and RPE scales (11).

   ■ Action: A total score in 4 major areas of recovery

     ❑ Nutrition/hydration: 10 points
     ❑ Sleep/rest: 4 points
     ❑ Relaxation/emotional support: 3 points
     ❑ Stretching/active rest: 3 points

   ■ Perceived: A reverse Borg RPE scale of perceived recovery (Table 40.1)

■ Recovery-Stress Questionnaire for Athletes (RESTQ-Sport) (10): 90-question survey tool answered on a Likert-type scale to assess training stress and recovery

PREVENTION

■ Individualized and variable training programs
■ Coaching and supervised training
■ Periods of "time out"
■ Cross-training
■ Reasonable goal setting (short- and long-term)
■ Relaxation and visualization techniques or use of a sports psychologist

REFERENCES

1. Davis MJ, Bailey SP. Possible mechanism of central nervous system fatigue during exercise. *Med Sci Sports Exerc.* 1997;29(1):45–57.
2. Derman W, Schwellnus MP, Lambert MI, et al. The 'worn-out athlete': a clinical approach to chronic fatigue in athletes. *J Sports Sci.* 1997;15(3):341–51.
3. Dressendorfer RH, Hansen AM, Timmis GC. Reversal of runner's bradycardia with training overstress. *Clin J Sport Med.* 2000;10(4):279–85.
4. Foster C. Monitoring training in athletes with reference to overtraining syndrome. *Med Sci Sports Exerc.* 1998;30(7):1164–8.
5. Fry AC, Kraemer EJ. Resistance exercise overtraining and overreaching. Neuroendocrine responses. *Sports Med.* 1997;23(2):106–29.
6. Gastmann UA, Lehmann MJ. Overtraining and the BCAA hypothesis. *Med Sci Sports Exerc.* 1998;30(7):1173–8.
7. Halson SL, Lancaster GI, Jeukendrup AE, Gleeson M. Immunological response to overreaching in cyclists. *Med Sci Sports Exerc.* 2003;35(5):854–61.
8. Hawley CJ, Schoene RB. Overtraining syndrome: a guide to diagnosis, treatment and prevention. *Phys Sportmed.* 2003;31(6):25–31.
9. Hendrickson CD, Verde TJ. Inadequate recovery from vigorous exercise: recognizing overtraining. *Phy Sportsmed.* 1994;22:56–64.
10. Kellman M, Günther KD. Changes in stress and recovery in elite rowers during preparation for the Olympic Games. *Med Sci Sports Exerc.* 2000;32(3):676–83.
11. Kenttä G, Hassmén P. Overtraining and recovery. A conceptual model. *Sports Med.* 1998;26(1):1–16.
12. Lehmann M, Foster C, Dickhuth HH, Gastmann U. Autonomic imbalance hypothesis and overtraining syndrome. *Med Sci Sports Exerc.* 1998;30(7):1140–5.
13. McNair DM, Lorr M, Dropplemen L. *EdITS for the Profile of Mood States (POMS).* San Diego (CA): Educational & Industrial Testing Service; 1971.
14. Parmenter DC. Some medical aspects of the training of college athletes. *Boston Med Surg J.* 1923;189:45–50.
15. Pichot V, Busso T, Roche F, et al. Autonomic adaptations to intensive and overload training periods: a laboratory study. *Med Sci Sports Exerc.* 2002;34(10):1660–6.
16. Smith LL. Cytokine hypothesis of overtraining: a physiological adaptation to excessive stress? *Med Sci Sports Exerc.* 2000;32(2):317–31.
17. Smith DJ, Norris SR. Changes in glutamine and glutamate concentrations for tracking training tolerance. *Med Sci Sports Exerc.* 2000;32(3):684–9.
18. Synder AC. Overtraining and glycogen depletion hypothesis. *Med Sci Sports Exerc.* 1998;30(7);1146–50.
19. Walsh NP, Blannin AK, Robson PJ, Gleeson M. Glutamine, exercise, and immune function. *Sports Med.* 1998;26(3):177–91.

Table 40.1	Total Quality Recovery Action

Rating of Perceived Exertion	Total Quality Recovery
6	6
7 Very, very light	7 Very, very poor recovery
8	8
9 Very light	9 Very poor recovery
10	10
11 Faintly light	11 Poor recovery
12	12
13 Somewhat hard	13 Reasonable recovery
14	14
15 Hard	15 Good recovery
16	16
17 Very hard	17 Very good recovery
18	18
19 Very, very hard	19 Very, very good recovery
20	20

Exercise and Chronic Disease

41

Karl B. Fields, Wes Bailey, Kenneth P. Barnes, Catherine R. Rainbow, and Shane Hudnall

INTRODUCTION

- Medical problems lead to approximately 70% of the visits that athletes make to doctors.
- Many athletes, particularly those older than age 35, have chronic medical problems.
- In recent decades, obesity, diabetes, hypertension, and asthma have increased in frequency in youth and adolescents.
- This chapter provides an overview of principles of healthy exercise in athletic individuals who have some of the more common chronic diseases.

OBESITY

- According to data from the National Health and Nutrition Examination Survey (NHANES) obtained in 2007–2008, approximately 32.2% of men and 35.5% of women in the United States are obese. Overall, 68.0% of Americans are either overweight or obese (body mass index [BMI] > 25.0) (34)
- In 2007–2008, an estimated 16.9% of children and adolescents between ages 2 and 19 were obese — an increase from 5.0% in 1971–1974 and 10.0% from 1988–1994 data (85). (NHANES data)
- Obesity contributes to excess morbidity and mortality from hypertension, Type 2 diabetes, coronary artery diseases, stroke, gallbladder disease, sleep apnea, and osteoarthritis. Cancers with an increased frequency in obese individuals include endometrial, breast, prostate, and colon cancers (82,91).
- Centripetal obesity in which the waist-to-hip ratio is high indicates a subset of individuals at much higher risk of cardiovascular diseases (91). Generally a waist circumference of > 35 inches in women and > 40 inches in men is considered high risk (82).
- Some over weight athletes have achieved high levels of sports success. In sports, including football, weight throws in track and field, heavyweight wrestling, and power lifting, excessive weight has generally been considered advantageous.
- Athletes often pursue strategies that lead to dietary excess and pose health risks when they are trying to gain excessive weight. These may include diets with excessive high fat and high glycemic foods.

- Obesity has direct consequences in sport, for example, a much greater risk of heat illness during competition (50).
- The odds of sustaining a musculoskeletal injury increase with BMI. Overweight individuals are 15% more likely and those with Class III Obesity (BMI > 40) are 48% more likely to have an exercise-related injury (33).
- Highly competitive athletes may need to consume 1,500–2,000 excess calories daily during intense training. Dietary calorie consumption appears to be a learned behavior and appetite often does not decline with a reduction in activity levels in the off-season or after retirement (56). This can quickly lead to obesity.
- All forms of muscular activity burn calories, but aerobic activity generally serves as the backbone of a weight-loss program. Individuals on a strength-training program or on a mixed exercise program may show comparable weight loss with a well-designed, vigorous program.
- Most weight loss occurs with decreased caloric intake, but sustained physical activity is important in maintenance of weight loss (82).
- A combination of a reduced calorie diet and increased physical activity has strong evidence as an effective way to achieve weight loss (80) (based on meta-analysis of 15 randomized controlled trials [RCTs])
- Nonathletes have trouble losing weight on an exercise program alone perhaps because effective weight loss through exercise requires a consistent moderate-to-high level of activity.
- Epidemiologists note that we have seen a dramatic gain in weight of Americans in the last 2 decades; a period with a modest increase in calorie consumption but a dramatic decline in physical activity.

DIABETES

- As of 2007, 23.6 million Americans had diabetes with an approximate 5.7 million of those undiagnosed (22).

Cardiovascular Benefits

- Diabetes mellitus is considered a cardiac equivalent because of the strong association of this disease with cardiovascular problems. Maintaining a good fitness level lowers the risk of cardiac death and is associated with longevity (11).

■ In a large group of diabetics, walking at least 2 hours a week lowered cardiovascular mortality rates. This level of walking prevented 1 death per year for every 61 patients (41). A similar study demonstrated patients who performed moderate-to-vigorous exercise had a 40% lower risk of cardiovascular disease than those who did not exercise (47).

■ Aerobic exercise mildly lowers systolic and diastolic blood pressure (119). Aerobic exercise may also delay or prevent the development of hypertension. Good control of blood pressure (BP) lessens the risk of complications in diabetic patients.

■ Aerobic exercise improves lipid profiles. In a meta-analysis of > 4 weeks aerobic exercise, high-density lipoprotein (HDL) was shown to increase 9% and triglycerides to decrease by 11% — other effects were not statistically significant (54). A focused meta-analysis in diabetics (220 patients) revealed a statistically significant reduction of 5% in LDL with more than 8 weeks of aerobic exercise (53).

■ Diabetics are encouraged to perform 30–60 minutes of moderate-intensity exercise most days of the week.

Improved Metabolic Control

■ A meta-analysis of 14 studies (12 aerobic and 2 resistance) demonstrated exercise leads to a statistically significant reduction in hemoglobin A1c levels (13).

■ Another meta-analysis showed all types of exercise lead to statistically significant reductions in hemoglobin A1c levels (109).

■ Exercise improves insulin sensitivity in liver, muscle, and fat cells (117).

■ A single exercise session has been shown to increase insulin sensitivity for 16 hours (59).

■ A strong benefit of exercise may help individuals with impaired glucose tolerance and lead to prevention of diabetes (23,114).

Reduced Morbidity and Mortality

■ An epidemiologic study following male with Type 1 diabetics for 20 years shows those who participated in high school or college sports had lower mortality and lower incidence of macrovascular disease than sedentary counterparts (63).

Improved Self-Esteem

■ Exercise has a positive effect on the self-esteem of diabetic patients and allows many to cope better with physical and emotional stress.

Scientific Consensus on Exercise Activity for Type 2 Diabetes

■ The American College of Sports Medicine® (ACSM) and the American Diabetes Association have concurred that physical activity has major benefits for individuals with Type 2 diabetes.

■ Physical activity coupled with diet helps lessen risk of developing Type 2 diabetes in obese individuals by as much as 58%.

■ Physical activity now has strong evidence for benefits of management in almost all target areas that complicate diabetic care (23).

HYPERTENSION

■ The National High Blood Pressure Education Program recommends the evaluation of BP using percentiles based on age, height, and gender for children and adolescents (81).

■ Prehypertensive values are systolic or diastolic pressures between the ninetieth and ninety-fifth percentiles or if BP exceeds 120 mm Hg systolic or 80 mm Hg diastolic.

■ BP above the ninety-fifth percentile for age-adjusted norms is considered hypertension (79). BPs above the ninety-ninth percentile of age-adjusted norms are considered severe hypertension.

■ For adults, any levels above 140 systolic or 90 diastolic indicate hypertension.

■ BP is a product of cardiac output multiplied by peripheral resistance. Peripheral resistance must fall dramatically during exercise or else BP rises excessively since increasing physical activity requires a higher cardiac output than rest.

■ In patients whose BP rises too dramatically during dynamic exercise, the relative risk of subsequent hypertension is higher (112,120).

■ Heavy-resistance exercise particularly weight lifting can cause dramatic rises in BP that are transient (66).

■ A meta-analysis of 54 clinical trials of aerobic exercise showed reductions of systolic and diastolic BP in both hypertensive and normotensive individuals (119).

■ The Osaka Health Survey demonstrated that a daily walk of 20 minutes or more reduced the risk of hypertension in men. In fact, for every 26 men who walked, 1 case of hypertension was prevented (42). Vigorous exercise for as little as 30 minutes, just once weekly, also reduced risk.

■ Endurance exercise lowers BPs of hypertensives by 5–7 mm Hg after an exercise session or following a period of exercise training (92). BP can remain reduced for up to 22 hours following a bout of endurance exercise. The greatest decreases occur in those with severe hypertension.

■ The ACSM recommends performance of low-to-moderate exercise (*e.g.*, walking), at 40%–59% of oxygen reuptake reserve (VO_2R), 4–7 days per week, for a total of at least 30 minutes daily (92).

■ Most resistance exercise seems to benefit hypertensive athletes, although maximal resistance efforts pose theoretical risks. Resistance exercise can supplement endurance activities (92).

■ The ACSM recommends that resistance training in hypertensive patients be mixed with aerobic activity (92).

CORONARY ARTERY DISEASE

■ Patients with known coronary artery disease (CAD) can reduce their risk of coronary events by maintaining high fitness levels (76).

■ Moderate exercise is recommended for individuals with CAD, and the individual's exercise capacity should be measured by exercise tolerance testing.

■ Formal cardiac rehabilitation programs help coronary artery disease patients get started on a therapeutic exercise regimen.

■ Patients with CAD who develop the fitness to achieve a 10.7 metabolic equivalent (MET) level workload have a normal age adjusted mortality rate (76).

■ Recent research suggests that exercise lowers C-reactive protein (CRP) levels. Athletes, such as swimmers and runners, have significantly lower CRP levels than the average individual and the more intensely they train, the greater the decline in their CRP level. Speculation centers as to whether this may be one of the mechanisms by which exercise lowers the risk of cardiovascular disease (122).

■ The American Heart Association and the American College of Cardiology recommend 30 minutes of moderate intensity aerobic exercise per day, 5–7 days per week (107). Resistance training can supplement these exercises 2 days per week.

■ High-risk patients (*e.g.,* those with recent acute coronary syndrome or revascularization or heart failure) should be medically supervised during exercise (107).

EXERCISE POSTCEREBRAL VASCULAR ACCIDENT

■ Exercise is important in primary and secondary prevention of cardiovascular and stroke risk. A study of over 16,000 men found an inverse relationship between cardiovascular fitness and stroke mortality (65).

■ Poststroke patients often suffer from weakness, paralysis, sensory loss, and decrease overall exercise capacity. A study by Mackay-Lyons revealed in less than 1 month after stroke, patients developed a significant compromise in exercise capacity (67).

■ Poststroke patients who increase activities of daily living (ADL), showed a significant increase in peak oxygen intake (39). Additionally, poststroke patients' training on treadmills showed significant improvements of VO_{2max}, gait and overall functional mobility, balance, and muscular activity (64,68). A supervised exercise program for stroke survivors

with multiple comorbidities is effective at improving fitness while potentially decreasing risk of further disease and disability (100).

■ Strength training can safely be used in most poststroke rehabilitation to improve muscle strength and overall balance (100). Caution should be used in patients with uncontrolled hypertension, as well as avoidance of excessive weight and Valsalva.

■ The oxygen cost of exercise in hemiplegic patients is up to 2 times that of controls. This can lead to inactivity and secondary deconditioning, atrophy, osteoporosis, and impaired leg circulation (87,118).

■ Role for exercise during immediate poststroke period is limited by increased risk of recurrent stroke and secondary cardiac complications.

■ Exercise becomes increasingly important beyond the first several months to increase aerobic capacity and sensorimotor function (43,68,96,106).

■ Aerobic conditioning can enhance glucose regulation, mobilization of fat stores, BP, CRP, triacylglycerol (TG), total cholesterol (TC), low-density lipoprotein (LDL), and high-density lipoprotein (HDL) (36).

■ There is inconclusive data relating exercise to prevention of secondary strokes.

■ Role and timing of exercise stress testing poststroke is controversial.

■ RCT of 88 men with CAD and disability (two-thirds were stroke victims) who completed a 6-month home exercise training program showed significant increases in peak left ventricular ejection fraction and HDL cholesterol and decreases in resting heart rate and total serum cholesterol.

■ Six months of treadmill aerobic exercise allowed patients to perform ADL at submaximal energy expenditure (68).

■ RCT of 42 hemiparetic stroke survivors demonstrated that they could increase their fitness by a magnitude similar to that of healthy controls in similar programs. Aerobic training 3 times weekly for 10 weeks improved peak oxygen consumption, workload, submaximal blood pressure response, exercise time, and sensorimotor function.

■ Fewer than 50% of patients reliably have their risk factors assessed, treated, or controlled (24).

■ Exercise trainability may be comparable to that of age-matched controls (16,35,68,96,100).

■ Aerobic exercise can help improve risk factors.

■ Recommended exercise strategies involve large muscle activities, such as walking, treadmill, stationary cycle, arm-leg ergometry, arm ergometry, seated stepper for 20–60 minutes sessions, 3–7 days per week at 40%–70% peak oxygen uptake/heart rate reserve, or 50%–80% of maximum heart rate or rating of perceive exertion of 11–14 (40).

■ Flexibility stretches 2–3 days per week can help prevent contractures and improve range of motion.

■ Coordination and balance activities 2–3 days weekly can improve safety during performance of ADL.

RENAL DISEASE IN ATHLETES

Kidney Problems Associated With Exercise

- Dehydration, hyperpyrexia, hyperkalemia, and rhabdomyolysis may all occur as a result of exercise and may lead to renal damage (32).
- Rhabdomyolysis, especially in untrained athletes, can lead to renal ischemia and nephrotoxins (86).
- Subsets of athletes, such as those with sickle cell trait, may have higher risk for rhabdomyolysis and renal failure.
- Cardiovascular disease accounts for most deaths in patients with end stage renal disease (ESRD) (115).
- $\dot{V}O_2$ peak (peak oxygen uptake) has been purported to strongly predict survival in ESRD patients (105). Patients with CKD (chronic kidney disease) have significantly reduced $\dot{V}O_2$ peaks in comparison to age and gender matched controls. Moderate exercise ($< 60\%$ $\dot{V}O_2$ peak) for 10–20 minutes can produce modest improvements, although CKD patients do not reach predicted $\dot{V}O_2$ peak.
- CKD negatively affects skeletal muscle function, including atrophy, derangement, and abnormal mitochondria (39).
- Resistance training can increase muscle size and strength on a low-protein diet (20).
- Combined cardiovascular and resistance training helps improve cardiovascular function, strength, endurance, and muscle size. This exercise regimen produced greater increases in $\dot{V}O_2$ peak likely via effects of resistance training on skeletal muscle function, which thereby improved $\dot{V}O_2$ peak (10).
- Contraindications to exercise in CKD include systolic BP > 200 mm Hg, diastolic pressure over 110 mm Hg, electrolyte abnormalities, recent myocardial infarction, or recent change in the electrocardiogram (10).

Prevention of Renal Disease

- Adequate hydration is important in minimizing muscle damage, promoting myoglobin elimination, and maintaining renal blood flow.
- Athletes reduce the risk of rhabdomyolysis and secondary renal failure through adequate fluid intake, avoidance of excessive heat stress, not exercising at the time of febrile illness, appropriate carbohydrate intake to avoid glycogen depletion, and exercising within the limits of their muscular tolerance.

THYROID DISEASE IN ATHLETES

Hypothyroidism

- Hypothyroidism and subclinical hypothyroidism are associated with decreased exercise tolerance (19,70).
- Patients often develop muscle weakness, cramps, and fatigue, which is worse in elderly patients (52).

- This exercise intolerance is due to increased systemic vascular resistance, which decreases blood flow to exercising muscles leading to reduced oxygen delivery and blood-borne substrate availability (52).
- Replacement of thyroxin is the mainstay of treatment.
- Exercise is safe when adequate replacement is maintained.

Hyperthyroidism

- Hyperthyroidism is associated with decreased exercise tolerance (70).
- Higher blood lactate, depletion of glycogen, and relative hyperthermia may all contribute to decreased performance that is due to mitochondrial dysfunction (52,83).
- Patients with hyperthyroidism have an increased heart rate, blood volume, left ventricular stroke volume, ejection fraction, and cardiac output, as well as decreased systemic vascular resistance at rest (52).
- They have an overall increased preload and decreased afterload (52).
- When patients with hyperthyroidism exercise, they have an impaired inotropic and chronotropic response to incremental exercise leading to a plateau in exercise capacity (52).
- Patients with hyperthyroidism reach anaerobic threshold faster than controls showing a lower increase in heart rate from baseline (which is elevated at baseline) to the anaerobic threshold, as well as increased respiratory rate when compared to controls (51).
- β-blockers can be helpful in the treatment of hyperthyroidism but may have a negative effect on performance and are banned for specific sports under Olympic regulations.
- Exercise is safe after appropriate treatment and close supervision.

OSTEOPOROSIS

- Approximately 10 million people in the United States have osteoporosis with several million more having osteopenia. Eighty percent of people with osteoporosis are women. One out of every 2 women and 1 in 4 men older than 50 will break a bone in their lifetime due to osteoporosis (2).
- Exercise at an early age is important to develop adequate bone density. Multiple studies on young men and women have shown that both resistance and endurance exercise programs can lead to site-specific increases in bone mineral density (BMD) (38,108). BMD is reported to be higher in athletic young adults than in their sedentary peers (57).
- A Cochrane meta-analysis of 18 RCTs demonstrated aerobics, weight bearing, and resistance exercises were effective at increasing the BMD of the spine. Walking increased the BMD of the hip and aerobic exercise increased the BMD of the wrist (12).

- Exercise appears to lower risk of fractures in addition to increasing BMD. In a prospective study of 61,200 women, moderate levels of activity (walking > 4 hours a week) were associated with substantially lower risk of hip fracture in postmenopausal women (compared to < 1 hour a week) (31).

- It is recommended that women with osteoporosis exercise 3–5 times a week at moderate to high intensity for 30–60 minutes a day. Exercise should comprise weight-bearing activities 3–5 times a week and resistance exercise 2–3 times a week (1,2).

- Exercise goals for individuals with osteoporosis include reducing pain, increasing mobility, improving muscle endurance, balance, and stability in order to improve the quality of life and reduce the risk of falling.

- Exercise should not take the place of other treatments for osteoporosis (*i.e.*, bisphosphonates) if medically necessary. It should instead be a component of osteoporotic therapy.

EPILEPSY

- Older data estimated that less than 5% of individuals with epilepsy participate in a regular exercise program (77). Parents, coaches, physicians, and epileptics themselves often limit participation in exercise for fear of uncontrolled seizures, embarrassment, or because of ignorance about the disease. Education and improved medical control allow more patients with epilepsy to participate in sports.

- Exercise helps to reduce overall seizure susceptibility, reduce anxiety and depression, and lead to improvements in quality of life and integration into society (8).

- Possible causes of decreased seizures with exercise are β-endorphin release, lowered blood pH after lactic acid release, increased *gamma-aminobutyric acid* (GABA) concentration, or increased mental alertness and attention.

- Some studies have shown that seizure frequency can increase in the postexercise period (46,77).

- In general, in a patient with regular seizures, the following activities should be avoided: scuba diving, boxing, auto racing, gliding, aviation, parachuting, archery, and riflery. Other water sports should be performed with direct supervision (7). Athletes who are well controlled can generally participate in all sports (including contact and collision sports).

- Exercise improves self-esteem and the overall sense of well-being in epileptics (77,78). In a population where isolation and depression are common, participation in exercise may improve self-worth and social integration.

CEREBRAL PALSY (CP)

- In patients with CP and other chronic neuromuscular syndromes, physical therapy is a mainstay in treatment. Therapy enhances motor development and minimizes the development of contractures. Emphasis is generally placed on range of motion, both passive and active. Neuromuscular electric stimulation has been added to improve mobility, control muscular movements, increase strength, and to decrease spasticity. The effectiveness of physical therapy, however, is uncertain.

- Strength training has been avoided in cerebral palsy owing to a theory that it can lead to increased spasticity in antagonist muscles; however, multiple studies have shown that in mild-moderate spastic CP, strength training can improve motor skills and strength without decreased range of motion or increased spasticity (28). In addition, strength training may lessen the amount of bone loss that frequently occurs in less mobile CP patients (28).

- Aerobic exercise has been studied minimally in CP patients; and, studies show that many patients with cerebral palsy do not participate in aerobic activities (25). Horseback riding and swimming are often activities offered for patients with cerebral palsy. Aerobic exercise in CP has been shown to increase fitness level and $\dot{V}O_{2max}$. while also improving patient's social skills, behavioral and emotional problems, and overall sense of well-being (101).

- Caution must be used in planning an exercise program for patients with CP. Scoliosis, contractures, chronic arthritis, and risk of hip subluxation can limit patient's physical ability. Likewise, patients often suffer from sensory defects, such as poor vision. Lastly, behavioral and emotional maladjustments may require special accommodations (121).

EXERCISE-INDUCED ASTHMA (EIA) / EXERCISE-INDUCED BRONCHOCONSTRICTION (EIB)

- EIA describes those with persistent or chronic asthma who also get bronchospasm with exercise (4,89,90).

- EIB refers to the phenomenon of transient airway narrowing that occurs during or after physical exertion in those patients who have bronchospasm with exercise with no previous history of asthma (4,48,89,90).

- As many as 90% of known asthmatics exhibit some form of exercise-induced airway compromise, or EIA (72,90). EIB occurs in 10% of patients without known asthma or atopy (55).

- Symptoms include wheezing, cough, chest pain, shortness of breath, and/or chest tightness (60,61,69,102,111).

- EIB is defined as a decrease in lung function, usually greater than a 10% fall in FEV_1, occurring within 30 minutes after vigorous exercise, at a power output, which elicits 85% or more of maximal O_2 consumption for 4- to 10-minute periods (69,95,102,103).

- The exact pathogenesis of EIB is poorly understood.

- There are 2 prevailing hypotheses:
- The "water loss theory" proposes that hyperventilation associated with strenuous exercise leads to loss of water through the epithelium of the bronchial mucosa. Water loss leads to changes in intracellular osmolarity, pH, and temperature, producing inflammation and bronchoconstriction (5,6,95,111).
- The "respiratory heat exchange theory" suggests that heat is transferred from the bronchiolar blood vessels in the pulmonary vascular bed, with heat loss during exercise. After exercise, rewarming causes dilatation and hyperemia of the vessels with fluid leakage causing vascular engorgement with resultant inflammation and airway constriction (71,72,95,111).
- Exercise challenge testing can be performed in a lab setting; however, sport-specific field testing has been shown to be superior. This consists of 6–8 minutes of vigorous exercise sufficient enough to raise the heart rate to 85% of age-predicted maximum (103).
- Baseline spirometry before exercise is followed by postexercise measurements every 5 minutes for up to 30 minutes following exercise termination (44,45,100,102,103).
- A fall of > 10% in FEV_1 is considered abnormal, and > 15% is considered diagnostic of EIB (44,45,100,102,103).
- Traditional methacholine challenge has low sensitivity for diagnosing EIB and should not be used (44,100).
- The International Olympic Committee (IOC) recommends eucapnic voluntary hyperpnea (EVH) challenge test to diagnose EIB, which involves stimulation of ventilation with carbon dioxide, oxygen, and nitrogen. Specificity is very high (45,102).
- Although inexpensive and easy to standardize, EVH is lab dependent and available in specialized referral centers and may not be practical for most collegiate and high school athletic centers (45).
- Treatment should incorporate both nonpharmacological and pharmacological regimens.
- Nonpharmacologic options include induction of a relative refractory period prior to the exercise event and controlling the climatic conditions. This is generally performed at 40%–80% of maximum intensity for 15 minutes about 1 hour prior to the athletic event and has been shown to attenuate the EIB response (26,45,73).
- Pharmacological options include (a) short-acting β2-agonists (*i.e.*, albuterol) with 2 puffs 5–15 minutes prior to exercise providing up to 80% protection for up to 2 hours, (b) long-acting β2-agonists (*i.e.*, salmeterol) given 30–60 minutes prior to exercise provide similar efficacy, lasting up to 12 hours, (c) chromoglycans (*i.e.*, nedocromil, cromolyn sodium) provide 50%–60% protection for 1–2 hours but are not bronchodilators and are not effective in the acute setting, and (d) leukotriene-modifying agents (*i.e.*, montelukast, zafirlukast) also provide 50%–60% protection up to 24 hours but are also not effective in treatment of acute bronchospasm. Theophylline

and short-acting anticholinergics (*i.e.*, ipratropium) have also been used (61,95,111,113).
- All medications should be initiated and their use monitored under the supervision of a physician.
- Although only applicable to a small percentage of elite athletes, on January 1, 2010, World Anti-Doping Agency (WADA) implemented a number of significant changes in their policy for therapeutic use exception (TUE) (116).
- The key change to the policy concerns the TUE procedure for inhaled β2-agonists in asthma and EIB.
- All β2-agonists are prohibited except inhaled salbutamol and inhaled salmeterol, which only require a declaration of use (116).

CHRONIC LUNG DISEASE IN CHILDREN

Cystic Fibrosis

- Patients with cystic fibrosis are often refrain from physical activity due to fatigue and shortness of breath, which are believed to be caused by deficits in skeletal muscle aerobic and anaerobic capacity, muscle strength deficits, as well as decreased pulmonary function (104).
- Short- and long-term studies suggest that both aerobic and anaerobic training have a positive effect on exercise capacity, strength, and lung function (58).
- Strength and aerobic training both increased physical work capacity and patient weight (88).
- Decreased breathlessness allows greater mobility and participation with peers in social and sporting activities, improves confidence and self-esteem, and creates a greater pleasure in life for the individual patient (15).
- Limitations in exercise performance appear related to the extent of lung disease and compromised nutritional status (97).
- Oxygen therapy during exercise improves oxygenation but causes a mild hypercapnia, which may not be clinically significant. Patients are able to exercise longer while using oxygen (29).

Bronchopulmonary Dysplasia

- There is limited information concerning the exercise performance of long-term survivors of bronchopulmonary dysplasia.

Bronchiectasis

- A systematic review, which included only 2 studies, found evidence of the benefits of inspiratory muscle training, which improved endurance exercise capacity and quality of life measured on chronic respiratory questionnaire (15).

- There was no evidence of the effect of other types of physical training (including pulmonary rehabilitation) in bronchiectasis (15).
- According to 1 study, left ventricular diastolic functions are affected in bronchiectasis, although the performance of patients is dependent on their pulmonary status.

CHRONIC OBSTRUCTIVE PULMONARY DISEASE (COPD) IN ADULTS

- Exercise training and pulmonary rehabilitation should be considered for all patients who experience exercise intolerance despite optimal medical therapy (14).
- Before prescribing an exercise program, patients with COPD require careful evaluation to assess cardiac risk and exercise capacity (75).
- The 3 medical determinations that would preclude patients with COPD from exercising include corpulmonale, resting hypercapnea, and dyspnea at rest (32).
- Studies consistently demonstrate that peripheral muscles are weak in patients with COPD exhibiting effort-dependent strength scores that are 70%–80% of these measures in age-matched healthy subjects (110).
- In COPD patients, up to 40% of total oxygen intake during low-level exercise is devoted to the respiratory muscles, compared to 10%–15% in healthy persons (75).
- Exercise tolerance may improve following exercise training because of gains in aerobic fitness, peripheral muscle strength, enhanced mechanical skill, efficiency of exercise, improvements in respiratory muscle function, breathing pattern, and lung hyperinflation while decreasing anxiety, fear, and dyspnea associated with exercise (14).
- Pulmonary rehabilitation improves symptoms of dyspnea and health-related quality of life while decreasing the number of hospital days, hospital admissions, and other healthcare utilization (98,99).
- Exercise training of the muscles of ambulation is highly recommended as a component of pulmonary rehabilitation (99).
- Both low- and high-intensity exercise training leads to clinical benefits for patients with COPD. Strength training also increased muscle strength and mass (99).
- Unsupported endurance training of the upper extremities is beneficial for patients with COPD, even though this type of exercise leads to faster fatigue (99).
- There is insufficient evidence to suggest that exercise improves survival (99).
- Oxygen should be used during exercise in patients who develop severe exercise-induced hypoxemia but can also be used in patients without exercise-induced hypoxemia to improve endurance (84,99).
- Short-acting bronchodilators have little effect on exercise capacity while long-acting bronchodilators reduce dyspnea associated with moderate exercise intensity (3).

OSTEOARTHRITIS

- Patients with arthritis have substantially worse health-related quality of life than those without arthritis (21).
- The Centers for Disease Control and Prevention advocate physical activity for patients with arthritis recommending 150 minutes of moderate-intensity aerobic activity or 75 minutes of vigorous activity in addition to muscle strengthening activities at least 2 days per week in all adults (93).
- There are limited high-quality studies that have reviewed long-term outcomes on exercise therapy and osteoarthritis (74).
- Systematic reviews of exercise for hip osteoarthritis are very limited but suggest that exercise programs may reduce pain slightly but may not improve physical function (37).
- There is high-quality level of evidence that land-based exercise has short-term benefits for patients with osteoarthritis of the knee by reducing pain and improving physical function (37).
- Patients with osteoarthritis of the knee benefit from both high- and low-intensity aerobic exercise training, which significantly improves their functional status, gait, pain, and aerobic capacity (17).
- Both high- and low-resistance training improves muscle strength, as well as self-reported measures of pain and physical function for knee osteoarthritis (49,62).
- Strength training of the whole body appears to be more beneficial than limiting work to the muscles around the affected joint (27).
- Aquatic exercises may have some beneficial short-term effects for patients with hips and or knee osteoarthritis. However, no long-term effects have been studied to date (9).
- The benefits of exercise therapy do not appear to be sustained in the long-term (> 6 months) for knee and hip osteoarthritis unless the patient continues to exercise (94).
- Data from the Fitness Arthritis and Seniors Trial suggested that beneficial effects of exercise on functional capacity in osteoarthritis patients are independent of exercise type (30).
- High-impact activities that include running and jumping may be detrimental for established osteoarthritis of lower extremity joints (18).

REFERENCES

1. ACSM Position Stand: osteoporosis and exercise. *Med Sci Sports Exerc.* 1995;27(4):i–vii.
2. ACSM Position Stand: physical activity and bone health. *Med Sci Sports Exerc.* 2004;36(11):1985–96.
3. Aguilaniu B. Impact of bronchodilator therapy on exercise tolerance in COPD. *Int J Chron Obstruct Pulmon Dis.* 2010;5:57–71.
4. Allen TW. Return to play following exercise-induced bronchoconstriction. *Clin J Sports Med.* 2005;15(6):421–5.
5. Anderson S. Is there a unifying hypothesis for exercise-induced asthma? *J Allergy Clin Immunol.* 1984;73(5, pt 2):660–5.

6. Anderson SD, Daviskas E. The mechanism of exercise induced asthma is. . .. *J Allergy Clin Immunol.* 2000;106(3):453–9.

7. Arida RM, Cavalheiro EA, da Silva AC, Scorza FA. Physical activity and epilepsy: proven and predicted benefits. *Sports Med.* 2008;38(7):607–15.

8. Arida RM, Scorza FA, Gomes da Silva S, Schachter SC, Cavalheiro EA. The potential role of physical exercise in the treatment of epilepsy. *Epilepsy Behav.* 2010;17(4):432–5.

9. Bartels EM, Lund H, Hagen KB, Dagfinrud H, Christensen R, Danneski-old-Samsøe B. Aquatic exercise for the treatment of knee and hip osteoarthritis. *Cochrane Database Syst Rev.* 2009;4:CD005523.

10. Beekley MD. Exercise and chronic kidney disease [Internet]. [cited 2007 Sep 20]. Available from: http://www.medscape.com/viewarticle/561596_print.

11. Blair SN, Khol HW 3rd, Paffenbarger RS Jr, Clark DG, Cooper KH, Gibbons LW. Physical fitness and all-cause mortality. A prospective study of healthy men and women. *JAMA.* 1989;262(17):2395–401.

12. Bonaiuti D, Shea B, Iovine R, et al. Exercise for preventing and treating osteoporosis in postmenopausal women. *Cochrane Database Syst Rev.* 2002;3:CD000333.

13. Boulé NG, Haddad E, Kenny GP, Wells GA, Sigal RJ. Effects of exercise on glycemic control and body mass in type 2 diabetes mellitus: a meta-analysis of controlled clinical trials. *JAMA.* 2001;286(10):1218–27.

14. Bourjeily G, Rochester CL. Exercise training in chronic obstructive pulmonary disease. *Clin Chest Med.* 2000;21(4):763–81.

15. Bradley JM, Moran F, Greenstone M. Physical training for bronchiectasis. *Cochrane Database Syst Rev.* 2002;3:CD002166.

16. Brinkmann JR, Hoskins TA. Physical conditioning and altered self-concept in rehabilitated hemiplegic patients. *Phys Ther.* 1979;59(7):859–65.

17. Brosseau L, MacLeay L, Robinson V, et al. Intensity of exercise for the treatment of osteoarthritis. *Cochrane Database Syst Rev.* 2003;2:CD004259.

18. Buckwalter JA, Lane NE. Aging, sports, and osteoarthritis. *Sports Med Arthros Rev.* 1996;4(3):276–87.

19. Caraccio N, Natali A, Sironi A, et al. Muscle metabolism and exercise tolerance in subclinical hypothyroidism: a controlled trial of levothyroxine. *J Clin Endocrinol Metab.* 2005;90(7):4057–62.

20. Castaneda C, Gordon PL, Uhlin KL, et al. Resistance training to counteract the catabolism of a low-protein diet in patients with chronic renal insufficiency. *Ann Intern Med.* 2001;135(11):965–76.

21. Centers for Disease Control and Prevention. Health-related quality of life among adults with arthritis—behavioral risk factor surveillance system, 11 states, 1996–1998. *MMWR Morb Mortal Wkly Rep.* 2000;49(17):366–9.

22. Centers for Disease Control and Prevention. National diabetes fact sheet, 2007 [Internet]. Available from: http://www.cdc.gov/diabetes/pubs/pdf/ndfs_2007.pdf.

23. Colberg SR, Albright AL, Blissmer BJ, et al. Exercise and type 2 diabetes: American College of Sports Medicine and the American Diabetes Association: joint position statement. *Med Sci Sports Exerc.* 2010;42(12):2282–303.

24. Cooper R, Cutler J, Desvigne-Nickens P, et al. Trends and disparities in coronary disease, stroke, and other cardiovascular diseases in the United States: findings of the national conference on cardiovascular disease prevention. *Circulation.* 2000;102(25):3137–47.

25. Darrah J, Wessel J, Nearingburg P, O'Connor M. Evaluation of a community fitness program for adolescents with cerebral palsy. *Pediatr Phys Ther.* 1999;11:18–23.

26. de Bisschop C, Guenard H, Desnot P, Vergeret J. Reduction of exercise-induced asthma in children by short repeated warm ups. *Br J Sports Med.* 1999;33(2):100–4.

27. DiNubile NA. Strength training. *Clin Sports Med.* 1991;10(1):33–62.

28. Dodd KJ, Taylor NF, Damiano DL. A systemic review of the effectiveness of strength-training programs for people with cerebral palsy. *Arch Phys Med Rehabil.* 2002;83(8):1157–64.

29. Elphick HE, Mallory G. Oxygen therapy for cystic fibrosis. *Cochrane Database Syst Rev.* 2009;1:CD003884.

30. Ettinger WH Jr, Burns R, Messier SP, et al. A randomized trial comparing aerobic exercise and resistance exercise with a health education program in older adults with knee osteoarthritis. The Fitness Arthritis and Seniors Trial (FAST). *JAMA.* 1997;277(1):25–31.

31. Feskanich D, Willett W, Colditz G. Walking and leisure-time activity and risk of hip fracture in postmenopausal women. *JAMA.* 2002;288(18):2300–6.

32. Fields KB, Fricker PA. *Medical Problems in Athletes.* Malden (MA): Blackwell Science; 1997. p. 209–15.

33. Finkelstein EA, Chen H, Prabhu M, Trogdon JG, Corso PS. The relationship between obesity and injuries among U.S. adults. *Am J Health Promot.* 2007;21(5):460–8.

34. Flegal KM, Carroll MD, Ogden CL, Curtin LR. Prevalence and trends in obesity among US adults. 1999–2008. *JAMA.* 2010;303(3):235–41.

35. Fletcher BJ, Dunbar SB, Felner JM, et al. Exercise testing and training in physically disabled men with clinical evidence of coronary artery disease. *Am J Cardiol.* 1994;73(2):170–4.

36. Franklin BA, Sanders W. Reducing the risk of heart disease and stroke. *Phys Sportsmed.* 2000;28(10):19–26.

37. Fransen M, McConnell S, Hernandez-Molina G, Reichenback S. Exercise for osteoarthritis of the hip. *Cochrane Database Syst Rev.* 2009;3:CD007912.

38. Friedlander AL, Genant HK, Sadowsky S, Byl NN, Glüer CC. A two-year program of aerobics and weight training enhances bone mineral density of young women. *J Bone Miner Res.* 1995;10(4):574–85.

39. Fujitani J, Ishikawa T, Akai M, Kakurai S. Influence of daily activity on changes in physical fitness for people with post-stroke hemiplegia. *Am J Phys Med Rehabil.* 1999;78(6):540–4.

40. Gordon NF, Gulanick M, Costa F, et al. Physical activity and exercise recommendations for stroke survivors: an American Heart Association scientific statement from the Council on Clinical Cardiology, Subcommittee on Exercise, Cardiac Rehabilitation, and Prevention; the Council on Cardiovascular Nursing; the Council on Nutrition, Physical Activity, and Metabolism; and the Stroke Council. *Circulation.* 2004;109(16):2031–41.

41. Gregg EW, Gerzoff RB, Caspersen CJ, Williamson DF, Narayan KM. Relationship of walking to mortality among US adults with diabetes. *Arch Intern Med.* 2003;163(12):1440–7.

42. Hayashi T, Tsumura K, Suematsu C, Okada K, Fujii S, Endo G. Walking to work and the risk for hypertension in men: the Osaka Health Survey. *Ann Intern Med.* 1999;131(1):21–6.

43. Hesse S, Bertelt C, Jahnke MT, et al. Treadmill training with partial body weight support compared with physiotherapy in nonambulatory hemiparetic patients. *Stroke.* 1995;26(6):976–81.

44. Holzer K, Anderson S, Douglass J. Exercise in the elite summer athletes: challenges for diagnosis. *J Allergy Clin Immunol.* 2002;110(3):374–80.

45. Holzer K, Bruckner P. Screening of athletes for exercise-induced bronchoconstriction. *Clin J Sport Med.* 2004;14(3):134–8.

46. Horyd W, Gryziak J, Niedzielska K, Zielin;aaski JJ. Effect of physical exertion in the EEG of epilepsy patients. *Neurol Neurochir Pol.* 1981;15(5–6):545–52.

47. Hu FB, Stampfer MJ, Solomon C, et al. Physical activity and risk for cardiovascular events in diabetic women. *Ann Intern Med.* 2001;134(2):96–105.

48. Hull JH, Hull PJ, Parsons JP, Dickinson JW, Ansley L. Approach to the diagnosis and management of suspect exercise-induced bronchoconstriction by primary care physicians. *BMC Pulm Med.* 2009;29(9):1–7.

49. Jan MH, Lin JJ, Liau JJ, Lin YF, Lin DH. Investigation of clinical effects of high- and low-resistance training for patients with knee osteoarthritis: a randomized controlled trial. *Phys Ther.* 2008;88(4):427–36.

50. Jones BH, Bovee MW, Harris JM 3rd, Cowan DN. Intrinsic risk factors for exercise-related injuries among male and female army trainees. *Am J Sports Med.* 1993;21(5):705–10.

51. Kahaly G, Hellermann J, Mohr-Kahaly S, Treese N. Impaired cardiopulmonary exercise capacity in patients with hyperthyroidism. *Chest.* 1996;109(1):57–61.

52. Kahaly G, Kampmann C, Mohr-Kahaly S. Cardiovascular hemodynamics and exercise tolerance in thyroid disease. *Thyroid.* 2002;12(6):473–81.

53. Kelley GA, Kelley KS. Effects of aerobic exercise on lipids and lipoproteins in adults with type 2 diabetes: a meta-analysis of randomized-controlled trials. *Public Health.* 2007;121(9):643–55.

54. Kelley GA, Kelley KS, Franklin B. Aerobic exercise and lipids and lipoproteins in patients with cardiovascular disease: a meta-analysis of randomized controlled trials. *J Cardiopulm Rehabil.* 2006;26(3):131–9.

55. King C, Moores LK. Clinical asthma syndromes and important asthma mimics. *Respir Care.* 2008;53(5):568–80.

56. King NA, Tremblay A, Blundell JE. Effects of exercise on appetite control: implications for energy balance. *Med Sci Sports Exerc.* 1997;29(8):1076–89.

57. Kirchner EM, Lewis RD, O'Conner PJ. Effect of past gymnastic participation on adult bone mass. *J Appl Physiol.* 1996;80(1):226–32.

58. Klijn PH, Oudshoorn A, van der Ent CK, van der Net J, Kimpen JL, Helders PJ. Effects of anaerobic training in children with cystic fibrosis: a randomized controlled study. *Chest.* 2004;125(4):1299–305.

59. Landry GL, Allen DB. Diabetes mellitus and exercise. *Clin Sports Med.* 1992;11(2):403–18.

60. Langdeau JB, Boulet LP. Is asthma over- or under-diagnosed in athletes? *Respir Med.* 2003;97(2):109–14.

61. Langdeau JB, Boulet LP. Prevalence and mechanisms of development of asthma and airway hyperresponsiveness in athletes. *Sports Med.* 2001;31(8):601–16.

62. Lange AK, Vanwanseele B, Fiatarone Singh MA. Strength training for treatment of osteoarthritis of the knee: a systematic review. *Arthritis Rheum.* 2008;59(10):1488–94.

63. LaPorte RE, Dorman JS, Tajima N, et al. Pittsburg Insulin-Dependent Diabetes Mellitus Morbidity and Mortality Study: physical activity and diabetic complications. *Pediatrics.* 1986;78(6):1027–33.

64. Laufer Y, Dickstein R, Chefez Y, Marcovitz E. The effect of treadmill training on the ambulation of stroke survivors in the early stages of rehabilitation: a randomized study. *J Rehabil Res Dev.* 2001;38(1):69–78.

65. Lee CD, Blair SN. Cardiorespiratory fitness and stroke mortality in men. *Med Sci Sports Exerc.* 2002;34(4):592–5.

66. MacDougall JD, Tuxen D, Sale DG, Moroz JE, Sutton JR. Arterial blood pressure response to heavy resistance exercise. *J Appl Physiol.* 1985;58:785–90.

67. MacKay-Lyons MJ, Makrides L. Exercise capacity early after stroke. *Arch Phys Med Rehabil.* 2002;83(12):1697–702.

68. Macko RF, Smith GV, Dobrovolny CL, Sorkin JD, Goldberg AP, Silver KH. Treadmill training improves fitness reserve in chronic stroke patients. *Arch Phys Med Rehabil.* 2001;82(7):879–84.

69. Mannix ET, Farber MO, Palange P, Galassetti P, Manfredi F. Exercise-induced asthma in figure skaters. *Chest.* 1996;109(2):312–5.

70. McAllister RM, Sansone JC Jr, Laughlin MH. Effects of hyperthyroidism on muscle blood flow during exercise in the rats. *Am J Physiol.* 1995;268(1, pt 2):H330–5.

71. McFadden ER Jr. Exercise-induced asthma. Assessment of current etiologic concepts. *Chest.* 1987;91(6)(suppl):151S–7S.

72. McFadden ER Jr, Gilbert IA. Exercise-induced asthma. *N Engl J Med.* 1994;330(19):1362–7.

73. McKenzie DC, McLuckie SL, Stirling DR. The protective effect of continuous and interval exercise in athletes with exercise-induced asthma. *Med Sci Sports Exerc.* 1994;26(8):951–6.

74. McNair PJ, Simmonds MA, Boocock MG, Larmer PJ. Exercise therapy for the management of osteoarthritis of the hip joint: a systematic review. *Arthritis Res Ther.* 2009;11(3):R98.

75. Mink BD. Exercise and chronic obstructive pulmonary disease: modest fitness gains pay big dividends. *Phys Sportsmed.* 1997;25(11):42–52.

76. Myers J, Prakash M, Froelicher V, Do D, Parlington S, Atwood JE. Exercise capacity and mortality among men referred for exercise testing. *N Engl J Med.* 2002;346(11):783–801.

77. Nakken KO, Bjørholt PG, Johannessen SI, Løyning T, Lind E. Effect of physical training on aerobic capacity, seizure occurrence and serum level of antiepileptic drugs in adults with epilepsy. *Epilepsia.* 1990;31(1):88–94.

78. Nakken KO, Løyning T, Taubøll O. Epilepsy and physical fitness. *Tidsskr Nor Laegeforen.* 1985;105(16):1136–8.

79. National Heart, Lung, and Blood Institute. The seventh report of the Joint National Committee on Prevention, Detection, Evaluation, and Treatment of High Blood Pressure (JNC VII) [Internet]. NIH Publication No. 04-5230, 2004 Aug. Available from: http://www.nhlbi.nih.gov/guidelines/hypertension/.

80. National Heart, Lung, and Blood Institute. Clinical guidelines on the identification, evaluation, and treatment of overweight and obesity in adults [Internet]. NIH Publication No. 98-4083. 1998 Sep. Available from: http://www.ncbi.nlm.nih.gov/books/NBK2003/.

81. National High Blood Pressure Education Program Working Group on High Blood Pressure in Children and Adolescents. The fourth report on the diagnosis, evaluation, and treatment of high blood pressure in children and adolescents. *Pediatrics.* 2004;114(2)(suppl 4th Report):555–76.

82. National Institutes of Health. The practical guide identification, evaluation and treatment of overweight and obesity in adults [Internet]. NIH Publication No. 02-4084. 2000. Available from: http://www.nhlbi.nih.gov/guidelines/obesity/ob_home.htm.

83. Nazar K, Chwalbin;aaska-Moneta J, Machalla J, Kaciuba-Us;aaciłko H. Metabolic and body temperature change during exercise in hyperthyroid patients. *Clin Sci Mol Med.* 1978;54(3):323–7.

84. Nonoyama ML, Brooks D, Lacasse Y, Guyatt GH, Goldstein RS. Oxygen therapy during exercise training in chronic obstructive pulmonary disease. *Cochrane Database Syst Rev.* 2007;2:CD005372.

85. Ogden CL, Carroll MD. Prevalence of obesity among children and adolescents: United States, trends 1963–1965 through 2007–2008 [Internet]. CDC. 2010 June. Available from: http://www.cdc.gov/nchs/data/hestat/obesity_child_07_08/obesity_child_07_08.pdf.

86. Olerud JE, Homer LD, Carrol HW. Incidence of acute exertional rhabdomyolysis. Serum myoglobin and enzyme levels as indicators of muscle injury. *Ann Emerg Med.* 1994;23:1301–6.

87. Olney SJ, Griffin MP, Monga TN, McBride ID. Work and power in gait of stroke patients. *Arch Phys Med Rehabil.* 1991;72(5):309–14.

88. Orenstein DM, Hovell JF, Mulvihill M, et al. Strength vs aerobic training in children with cystic fibrosis: a randomized controlled trial. *Chest.* 2004;126(4):1204–14.

89. Parsons J, Kaeding C, Phillips G, Jarjoura D, Wadley G, Mastronarde JG. Prevalence of exercise-induced bronchospasm in a cohort of varsity college athletes. *Med Sci Sports Exerc.* 2007;39(9):1487–92.

90. Parsons JP, Mastronade JG. Exercise-induced bronchoconstriction in athletes. *Chest.* 2005;128(6):3966–74.

91. Perry AC, Applegate EB, Allison MD, Jackson ML, Miller PC. Clinical predictability of waist-to-hip ratio in assessment of cardiovascular disease risk factors in overweight, premenopausal women. *Am J Clin Nutr.* 1998;68(5):1022–7.

92. Pescatello L, Franklin B, Fagard R, et al. American College of Sports Medicine position stand. Exercise and hypertension. *Med Sci Sports Exer.* 2004;36(3):533–53.

93. Physical Activity Guidelines Advisory Committee. *Physical Activity Guidelines for Americans. Center for Disease Control and Prevention, 2008.* Washington (DC): U.S. Department of Health and Human Services; 2008.

94. Pisters MF, Veenhof C, van Meeteren NL, et al. Long-term effectiveness of exercise therapy in patients with osteoarthritis of the hip or knee: a systematic review. *Arthritis Rheum.* 2007;57(7):1245–53.

95. Pope JS, Koenig SM. Pulmonary disorders in the training room. *Clin Sports Med.* 2005;24(3):541–64.

96. Potempa K, Lopez M, Braun LT, Szidon JP, Fogg L, Tincknell T. Physiological outcomes of aerobic exercise training in hemiparetic stroke patients. *Stroke.* 1995;26(1):101–5.

97. Prasad SA, Cerny FJ. Factors that influence adherence to exercise and their effectiveness: application to cystic fibrosis. *Pediatr Pulmonol.* 2002;34(1):66–72.

98. Puhan MA, Gimeno-Santos, E, Scharplatz M, et al. Pulmonary rehabilitation following exacerbations of chronic obstructive pulmonary disease. *Cochrane Database Syst Rev.* 2010;11:CD005305.

99. Ries AL, Bauldoff GS, Carlin BW, et al. Pulmonary rehabilitation: joint ACCP/AACVPR evidence-based clinical practice guidelines. *Chest.* 2007;131(5)(suppl):4S–42S.

100. Rimmer JH, Riley B, Creviston T, Nicola T. Exercise training in a predominately African-American group of stroke survivors. *Med Sci Sport Exerc.* 2000;32(12):1990–6.

101. Rogers A, Furler BL, Brinks S, Darrah J. A systematic review of the effectiveness of aerobic exercise interventions for children with cerebral palsy: an AACPDM evidence report. *Dev Med Child Neurol.* 2008;50(11):808–14.

102. Rundell KW, Slee JB. Exercise and other indirect challenges to demonstrate asthma or exercise-induced bronchoconstriction in athletes. *J Allergy Clin Immunol.* 2008;122(2):238–46.

103. Rundell KW, Wilber RL, Szmedra L, Jenkinson DM, Mayers LB, Im J. Exercise induced asthma screening of elite athletes: field versus laboratory challenge. *Med Sci Sports Exerc.* 2000;32(2):309–16.

104. Shoemaker MJ, Hurt H, Arndt L. The evidence regarding exercise training in the management of cystic fibrosis: a systematic review. *Cardiopulm Phys Ther J.* 2008;19(3):75–83.

105. Sietsema KE, Amato A, Adler SG, Brass EP. Exercise capacity as a predictor of survival among ambulatory patients with end-stage renal disease. *Kidney Int.* 2004;65(2):719–24.

106. Smith GV, Silver KHC, Goldberg AP, Macko RF. "Task-oriented" exercise improves hamstring strength and spastic reflexes in chronic stroke patients. *Stroke.* 1999;30(10):2112–8.

107. Smith SC Jr, Benjamin EJ, Bonow RO, et al. AHA/ACC guidelines for secondary prevention for patients with coronary and other atherosclerotic vascular disease: 2006 update: endorsed by the National Heart, Lung, and Blood Institute. *J Am Coll Cardiol.* 2006;47(10):2130–9.

108. Snow-Harter C, Bouxsein ML, Lewis BT, Carter DR, Marcus R. Effects of resistance and endurance exercise on bone mineral status of young women: a randomized exercise intervention trial. *J Bone Miner Res.* 1992;7(7):761–9.

109. Snowling NJ, Hopkins WG. Effects of different modes of exercise training on glucose control and risk factors for complications in type 2 diabetic patients: a meta-analysis. *Diabetes Care.* 2006;29(11):2518–27.

110. Storer TW. Exercise in chronic pulmonary disease: resistance exercise prescription. *Med Sci Sports Exerc.* 2001;33(7)(suppl):S680–92.

111. Storms W. Exercise-induced asthma: diagnosis and treatment for the recreational or elite athlete. *Med Sci Sports Exerc.* 1999;31(1):S33–8.

112. Tanji JL, Champlin JJ, Wong GY, Lew EY, Brown TC, Amsterdam EA. Blood pressure recovery curves after submaximal exercise: a predictor of hypertension at ten-year follow-up. *Am J Hypertens* 1989;2(3, pt 1):135–8.

113. Truwit J. Pulmonary disorders and exercise. *Clin Sports Med.* 2003;22(1):161–80.

114. Tuomilehto J, Lindström J, Eriksson JG, et al. Prevention of type 2 diabetes mellitus by changes in lifestyle among subjects with impaired glucose tolerance. *N Engl J Med.* 2001;344(18):1343–50.

115. United States Renal Data System. *USRDS 2003 Annual Data Report: Atlas of End-Stage Renal Disease in the United States.* Bethesda (MD): National Institutes of Health, National Institute of Diabetes and Digestive and Kidney Diseases; 2003. 560 p.

116. Vessey J. *Primary Care of the Child with a Chronic Condition.* 2nd ed. Philadelphia (PA): Mosby Year Book; 1996. 880 p.

117. Wallberg-Henriksson H. Exercise and diabetes mellitus. *Exerc Sports Sci Rev.* 1992;20:339–68.

118. Waters RL, Yakura JS. The energy expenditure of normal and pathologic gait. *Crit Rev Phys Rehabil Med.* 1989;1:183–209.

119. Whelton SP, Chin A, Xin X, He J. Effect of aerobic exercise on blood pressure: a meta-analysis of randomized, controlled trials. *Ann Intern Med.* 2002;136(7):493–503.

120. Wilson MF, Sung BH, Pincomb GA, Lovallo WR. Exaggerated pressure response to exercise in men at risk for systemic hypertension. *Am J Cardiol.* 1990;66(7):731–6.

121. World Anti-Doping Agency [Internet]. Available from: www.wada-ama.org/Documents/Science_Medicine/Medical_info_to_support_TUECs/WADA_Med_info_Asthma_v2.2_Nov2009_EN.pdf.

122. Zebrack JS, Anderson JL. Role of inflammation in cardiovascular disease: how to use C-reactive protein in clinical practice. *Prog Cardiovasc Nurs.* 2002;17(4):174–85.

42

Environmental Injuries: Hypothermia, Frostbite, Heat Illness, and Altitude Illness

Brian V. Reamy

HYPOTHERMIA

Definition

- Hypothermia occurs when the body's core temperature drops below 35°C (95°F).

Epidemiology

- Individuals younger than 2 years of age and older than 60 years of age are most at risk.
- Increasing homelessness and sports activities in inclement environments have contributed to an increased incidence of hypothermia in the past decade.
- Risk factors include the use of intoxicants, psychiatric illness, medical illnesses, sleep deprivation, dehydration, malnutrition, and trauma. Impaired judgment resulting from psychiatric illness or the use of ethanol is the most common predisposing factor (8).

Pathophysiology

- The body combats the fall in core temperature through shivering thermogenesis and increased gluconeogenesis. When the core temperature drops below 35°C, the victim becomes poikilothermic and cools to the ambient temperature.
- Central nervous system (CNS) function is directly depressed by the cold. The electroencephalogram (EEG) becomes abnormal below at temperature of 33.5°C (92.5°F) and silent at 19°C (66°F) (4).
- Initial reflex tachypnea continues until core temperature falls below 30°C (86°F). Failure of brainstem control of respiratory drive and the freezing of the thoracic musculature eventually lead to a cessation of breathing.
- Cold triggers peripheral vasoconstriction and tachycardia.
- Below 34°C (93°F), bradycardia, hypotension, decreased cardiac output, and a lengthening of cardiac electrical conduction ensue. A J-wave (Osborn hypothermic hump) may be noted at the QRS–ST junction. The myocardium becomes increasingly irritable, and spontaneous atrial and ventricular dysrhythmias can occur (4).
- Below 28°C (82°F), ventricular fibrillation can develop with minor stimuli, such as removing a patient's wet clothing or ambulance transport.

Clinical Features

- Nonspecific symptoms and signs predominate and mimic the effects of mild dementia or ethanol intoxication. The CNS effects of cold lead to impaired memory and judgment, slurred speech, and decreased alertness. Paradoxic bradycardia and hypoventilation occur despite hypotension. Multiple cardiac dysrhythmias develop as the core temperature falls. A cold-induced ileus, abdominal spasm, and rigidity can mimic an acute abdomen.

Diagnosis

- An accurate core temperature is crucial and is ideally obtained with a rectal thermistor probe. At a minimum, a rectal temperature obtained with a thermometer scaled for hypothermia is required. Oral and ear temperatures are grossly inaccurate. A core temperature above 35°C can rapidly exclude hypothermia.
- Hypothermia is classified as mild, moderate, or severe based on the core temperature (Table 42.1).
- Common laboratory findings include a falsely elevated hematocrit caused by dehydration, a low leukocyte count caused by sequestration, hyperamylasemia resulting from pancreatic injury, an aberrant coagulation profile, hypokalemia, and hypoglycemia caused by glycogen depletion. Below 30°C, insulin is rendered inactive, and a paradoxic hyperglycemia can ensue.

Treatment

- Field treatment should focus on *gentle handling* of the victim, so as to not cause cardiac dysrhythmias. Wet clothing should

Table 42.1 | Hypothermia Severity and Treatment

Temperature	Clinical Features	Treatment
Mild		
35°C/95°F	Maximum shivering	Passive external
33°C/91°F	Ataxia, apathy, tachypnea	Rewarming Passive external Warming
Moderate		
32°C/90°F	Stupor, shivering stops	Active core rewarming (± active external rewarming)
Severe		
28°C/82°F	Decreased ventricular fibrillation threshold, hypoventilation	Active core rewarming
14°C/57°F	Lowest adult accidental hypothermia survival	Active core rewarming
9°C/48°F	Lowest therapeutic survival	Active core rewarming

be removed and dry clothing or a blanket applied. Massage of cold-injured limbs should be avoided; it can damage fragile, frozen parts and trigger dysrhythmias. Traumatic injuries to the spine or limbs should be stabilized.

- An airway should be maintained and cardiac monitoring begun **if available**. If the skin is frozen, needle electrodes should be used or can be fashioned by passing a 20-gauge needle through an electrode pad into the frozen skin. If the patient is alert, warm, noncaffeinated beverages can be provided. Fluid resuscitation with intravenous (IV) 5% dextrose in normal saline (D5NS) should be started. Lactated Ringer's should be avoided because of problems with the metabolism of lactate by a cold-injured liver.

- Emergency room treatment should focus on rewarming of the patient. Defibrillation is generally limited to 1 countershock until the core temperature is raised above 30°C (86°F) (level of evidence [LOE] B, nonrandomized clinical trials; Emergency Cardiovascular Care Guidelines of the American Heart Association [AHA], 2010) (3). It may also be reasonable to perform defibrillation attempts concurrent with rewarming regardless of core temperature (Class IIb, LOE C, AHA advanced cardiac life support [ACLS] guidelines, 2010) (3). Medications may be less effective with severe hypothermia, but it is not unreasonable to consider use of vasopressors according to standard ACLS algorithms (Class IIb, LOE C, AHA ACLS guidelines, 2010) (3).

- Passive external rewarming (PER) by covering the victim with a blanket or wrap is ideal in an alert patient whose core temperature is greater than 32°C (90°F).

- Below 90°F, rewarming should proceed with active core rewarming (ACR) concurrent with active external rewarming

(AER). ACR can be accomplished with IV D5NS warmed to 40–42°C (104–108°F) or the inhalation of humidified oxygen warmed to 104–108°F. More invasive techniques include peritoneal lavage with dialysate warmed to 104–108°F, thoracic lavage with normal saline at 104–108°F, or warming of the gastrointestinal tract with gastric/colonic lavage (LOE C).

- AER (fires, hot water bottles, and heating pads) should be employed when ACR has already begun to avoid the life-threatening risk of core temperature afterdrop. This devastating process occurs when sudden exposure of vasoconstricted cool extremities to AER causes peripheral vasodilatation, a drop in central blood pressure, and a sudden influx of cool blood from the periphery to the core that can trigger dysrhythmias and shock (4). Table 42.1 provides an overview of hypothermia severity and ideal treatment modalities (4).

Prevention

- Good conditioning, proper nutrition, experienced leadership in backcountry environments, normal hydration, avoidance of ethanol or tobacco and habituation to the cold environment (both physiologic and behavioral), and the use of proper clothing help prevent hypothermia (6).
- Clothing choice centers on the 3 Ls: layered, loose, and lightweight. A waterproof outer layer is key. If exercise is occurring in a temperature of < 0°F, three-layered hand and footwear are optimal for the prevention of frostbite.

FROSTBITE

Definition

- Frostbite is freezing of tissues leading to damage. Frostnip is the formation of superficial ice crystals and causes *no tissue damage*. Chilblains is an *autoimmune* lymphocytic vasculitis, common in women, which leads to localized nodules or ulcers on the extremities 12 hours after cold exposure.

Epidemiology

- Frostbite is most common in active individuals from 30–49 years of age. High-risk outdoor activities in inclement environments account for a large percentage of injuries.
- Risk factors for frostbite are shown in Table 42.2. Ethanol and psychiatric problems underlie up to 70% of most cases of frostbite. The need for amputation correlates more with the *duration* of cold exposure rather than the *lowness* of the temperature. This explains why the impaired judgment resulting from ethanol use and psychiatric illness account for such a large percentage of injuries.
- Anatomic sites of injury include the following, in order of most common occurrence: feet and hands (90% of all frostbite), ears, nose, cheeks, and the penis (a particular concern for runners).

Table 42.2	Risk Factors for Frostbite

Predisposing Factors	
Behavioral	**Organic**
Ethanol use	Prior cold injury
Psychiatric illness	Wound infection
Motor vehicle problems	Atherosclerosis
Homelessness	Diabetes mellitus
Smoking	Fatigue
Improper clothing	
High-risk outdoor activities (back-country skiing/ mountaineering)	

Pathophysiology

- There are 3 synchronous pathways that lead to tissue damage in frostbite: tissue freezing, hypoxia, and the release of inflammatory mediators. Each pathway multiplies and catalyses the damage caused by the other pathways. Freezing leads to denaturation of the membrane lipid–protein matrix and cellular disruption. Hypoxia occurs from cold-induced vasoconstriction that triggers acidosis, increased viscosity, microthrombosis, and vessel endothelial damage. Inflammatory mediators (prostaglandin $F_2\alpha$, thromboxane A_2) are released from damaged endothelium, which triggers more vasoconstriction, platelet aggregation, thrombosis, hypoxia, and cell death. The same prostaglandins are found in the blister fluid of heat and frostbite-damaged skin (17–19).

- The release of these prostaglandins peaks during rewarming; *therefore, cycles of recurrent freezing and rewarming must be avoided to lessen the extent of injury* (17–19).

Clinical Features

- Symptoms include numbness, clumsiness, tingling, and throbbing pain after rewarming.

- The signs of frostbite were classically divided into first through fourth degrees. This scheme is not prognostically useful. It is better to distinguish between 2 types of injury: superficial and deep frostbite. Superficial injury is characterized by normal skin color, large blisters filled with clear or milky fluid, intact pinprick sensation, and skin that will indent with pressure. Deep frostbite shows small blood-filled dark blisters, nonblanching cyanosis, and skin that is wooden to the touch and will not indent with pressure.

Diagnosis

- Tissue viability is not ultimately determined until 22–45 days after injury. The primary utility of diagnostic tests is to help define tissue viability at an earlier time.

- Doppler flow studies and angiography can determine tissue viability and predict the need for surgical intervention as early as 7 days after injury. Technetium-99m scintigraphy can be employed as soon as 72 hours from injury to assess tissue viability with a positive predictive value (PPV) of 0.84 for viable tissue. A scan on day 7 raises the PPV to 0.92 (LOE A, randomized clinical trial) (7).

- Magnetic resonance imaging/magnetic resonance angiography (MRI/MRA) may emerge as the optimal modality for early tissue assessment.

Treatment

- Field warming should not be instituted until refreezing can be prevented. The injured part should be protected with a loose bulky splint during transport for definitive care. Hypothermia should be treated first; smoking, ethanol, and massage of the frozen part should be avoided. Definitive emergency department care is outlined in Table 42.3. It is based on the work of Heggers et al. (14) and McCauley et al. (17). Adjuvant therapies with heparin, warfarin, steroids, dextran, vitamin C, and hyperbaric oxygen have not been proven to be helpful. Pentoxifylline (Trental) has been shown to be useful in pedal frostbite (13).

HEAT ILLNESS

Definitions

- Heat illness is best thought of as a continuum of disease that progresses along a spectrum from the mild (heat cramps),

Table 42.3	Stepwise Treatment of Frostbite

Treat hypothermia and any concomitant injuries.

Rapidly rewarm the affected parts in water at 40–42°C (104–108°F) until thawing is complete and the skin is pliable in texture. (Typically 15–30 minutes of rewarming).

Debride blisters filled with clear or milky fluid. Apply aloe vera (at least 70%; Dermaide aloe). Cover with a bulky dressing.

Leave hemorrhagic blisters intact.

Splint and elevate the extremity.

Administer ibuprofen orally at standard doses. (Avoid aspirin or steroids, but consider use of pentoxifylline 400 mg orally twice a day.)

Give tetanus toxoid and tetanus immune globulin if > 10 years since last booster.

Administer intravenous penicillin 500,000 units every 6 hours for 72 hours.

(Clindamycin is the recommended alternative for penicillin-allergic patients.)

Treat pain with parenteral narcotics as needed.

Begin daily hydrotherapy with hexachlorophene at 40°C for 30–60 minutes daily.

No smoking.

through the moderate (heat exhaustion), to the life-threatening (heatstroke). Heat cramps are involuntary, painful contractions of skeletal muscle typically occurring during or after prolonged exercise. Heat exhaustion is a sign of systemic vascular strain in the body's attempt to maintain normothermia; *if untreated, it may progress to heatstroke.* Heatstroke occurs when heat generation exceeds heat loss, leading to a rise in core temperature and thermoregulatory failure. Classical heatstroke is confined to individuals without access to cool environments or debilitated by medical illness. Exertional heatstroke is the form most common in athletes and is defined by a rectal temperature > 40°C with CNS changes (LOE B, American College of Sports Medicine® [ACSM] 2007) (1).

Epidemiology

- Frequency of heat illness correlates with the wet bulb globe temperature (WBGT). WBGT = (wet bulb temp × 0.7) + (dry bulb × 0.1) + (black globe × 0.2), where the wet bulb represents the humidity, the dry bulb the air temperature, and the black globe the radiant heat.

- Risk factors for exertional heatstroke include obesity, low physical fitness, dehydration, fatigue, recent episode of heat illness, concomitant febrile illness, sleep deprivation, wear of impermeable garments, lack of acclimatization, and use of medicines or supplements that decrease sweating and increase thermogenesis (antihistamines, ephedra, caffeine, diuretics) (15).

Pathophysiology

- The cause of heat cramps is unclear. Heat illness occurs when heat storage outpaces heat loss that leads to deleterious changes at the cellular level. Core temperature > 41°C leads to a release of many inflammatory mediators to include interleukin 1 (IL-1), interleukin 6 (IL-6), and tumor necrosis factor (TNF). These cytokines amplify cellular and endothelial damage that triggers systemic vascular collapse and multiorgan failure.

Clinical Features

- Symptoms of heat exhaustion and heatstroke overlap. The diagnosis of heatstroke rests not on absolute temperature criteria; rather, it is due to the presence of an altered mental status and the progression of disease despite first-line treatments. Initial symptoms include headache, dizziness, fatigue, irritability, anxiety, chills, nausea, vomiting, and heat cramps. Seizures and disordered thoughts are evidence of heatstroke (15).

- Signs include a core temperature greater than 40°C, tachycardia, hyperventilation, hypotension, and syncope. A lack of spontaneous cooling with cessation of exertion and profuse sweating that *ceases* despite an elevated core temperature are both ominous signs that point toward heatstroke.

Diagnosis

- The diagnosis hinges on an elevated core temperature *combined* with the presence of the symptoms and signs noted earlier. Ideally, this temperature should be rectal. Any collapse during exertion should include heat illness in the differential, and early core temperature measurement is crucial. Of note, healthy athletes can raise their core temperature to 39°C simply from exertion alone and be asymptomatic.

- Laboratory tests are normal until heatstroke is present. Lab alterations, such as increased liver function tests, disordered coagulation profile, leukocytosis, electrolyte disturbances, and evidence of acute renal failure are nonspecific and similar to other shock states.

Treatment

- The key is to not delay treatment while trying to determine where on the continuum of heat illness a particular patient is located. Immediate treatment increases the likelihood of the body's return to normal thermoregulation and prevents progression to heatstroke.

- Field treatment should involve cessation of activity; removal to a shaded, cool environment; fluid replacement beverages; and fanning after spraying the patient with a cool mist. Heat cramps can be treated with passive stretching of the affected muscles (16).

- In case of altered mental status, seizures, or a core temperature greater than 104°F, heatstroke should be presumed; **immediate whole body cooling with cold water immersion is the key to a successful outcome, and the patient should be cooled prior to being evacuated** (10). If the patient responds to field treatment, he or she should avoid exertion for at least 24–48 hours to avoid a transient, but increased risk of recurrent heat illness.

- Heatstroke treatment involves the 9 steps shown in Table 42.4. Concerns that ice water immersion would increase seizures or trigger shivering thermogenesis have been allayed by recent studies (LOE A, ACSM 2007 Position Stand: Exertional Heat Illness) (1).

Five Keys to Prevention

- *Acclimatization* to high heat and humidity for 10–14 days prior to competition is ideal. The first 4–5 days are when 2 key physiologic changes occur: changes in sweat composition and an increase in the ability of the body to rapidly dissipate heat.

- *Clothing* should be light colored, lightweight, and offer sun protection.

- *Medications* that impair heat loss should be stopped or changed, for example, change antihistamines to nasal steroids to treat allergic rhinitis and stop ephedra compounds.

- *Activity planning or reduction* should be based on the WBGT scale: < 65, low risk for heat illness; 65–72, high-risk individuals

Table 42.4	Treatment of Heatstroke

Immediate cooling. Ice water immersion is best. If not, fanning after misting the patient should be undertaken. Cool until rectal temperature reaches 39°C (102.2°F).

Avoid antipyretics. The hypothalamic set point is normal! Antipyretics can aggravate hepatic or renal injury.

Avoid alcohol baths. Vasodilated skin can lead to systemic absorption.

Monitor core temperature until it is < 38°C (100.5°F).

Consider diazepam (5 mg) or lorazepam (2 mg) to control shivering and as prophylaxis against seizures.

Monitor renal function closely. Early dialysis is indicated.

Correct *persistent* electrolyte abnormalities.

Check coagulation profile at admission and serially until 72 hours have passed.

Use fresh frozen plasma (FFP) and/or platelets as needed.

Rehydrate vigorously; monitor for fluid overload and hyponatremia.

should be monitored or told not to compete; 72–78, risk rises for all; 78–82, high-risk individuals should not exercise; 82–86, unacclimated or unfit athletes should stop; 86–90, exercise should be limited for even fit and acclimated individuals; and > 90, all activities should stop (ACSM 2007) (1).

■ *Prehydration and hydration per ACSM recommendations.* These can be summarized for patients as follows: drink 16 oz of water or sports beverages several hours before exercise. The goal of drinking is to prevent a greater than 2% body weight loss and should be customized to the activity and the athlete. Approximately 400–800 mL (13–27 oz) per hour is a reasonable amount of fluid consumption to recommend. After exercise, replace each kilogram of weight lost with approximately 1.5 L of fluids (2).

ALTITUDE ILLNESS

Definitions and Clinical Syndromes

■ Rapid ascent past 8,000 ft leads to the onset of the physiologic effects of decreased oxygen concentration at altitude. These effects are most pronounced for those attempting exercise at altitude. Several clinical syndromes exist.

■ High altitude headache (HAH) is the first symptom of altitude exposure. It may or may not progress to acute mountain sickness.

■ Acute mountain sickness (AMS) is a syndrome that includes HAH and at least 1 of 4 symptoms: nausea/vomiting, fatigue/lassitude, dizziness, or insomnia. The Lake Louise Acute Mountain Sickness Scoring System (LLS) can be used as a tool to screen for AMS. High altitude cerebral edema (HACE) is the clinical progression of AMS, so that severe CNS symptoms develop, such as ataxia, altered consciousness, confusion, drowsiness, stupor, or coma.

■ High altitude pulmonary edema (HAPE) is the most common cause of altitude-related death. It is characterized by classic signs of pulmonary edema: wet cough, dyspnea at rest, weakness, and orthopnea.

Epidemiology

■ Altitude illness is most common in the unacclimatized, regardless of fitness level, who ascend rapidly past 8,000 ft. The severity is linked to the rate of ascent, altitude attained, sleeping altitude, length of altitude exposure, level of exertion, and an individual's inherent physiologic susceptibility that remains static despite reexposure.

Pathophysiology

■ A rapid rate of ascent, an inappropriately slowed hypoxic ventilatory response to ambient hypoxia and hypercarbia, fluid retention, and vasogenic edema are the initial pathologic changes. Days later, cerebral edema, pulmonary hypertension, and alveolar leakage lead to death if untreated (11,12).

■ Maximal oxygen uptake ($\dot{V}O_{2max}$) falls 10% for each 3,281 ft of altitude gained over 5,000 ft. $\dot{V}O_{2max}$ at sea level is *not* predictive of performance at altitude. Many of the world's elite mountaineers have average sea level $\dot{V}O_{2max}$ values. Past performance and personal problems with altitude illness are the best predictors of future performance and the need for aggressive preventive interventions (12).

Differential Diagnosis

■ Any of the symptoms of AMS on ascent past 8,000 ft should trigger suspicion for altitude illness. Key differential diagnostic considerations include dehydration, hypothermia, and a viral infection. Dehydration can be differentiated by response to a fluid challenge. Hypothermia can be distinguished by a low core temperature and improvement with exertion/increased body temperature. Altitude illness worsens with exertion. Although viral syndromes have similar symptoms, they are typically accompanied by fever, myalgia, or diarrhea and are more subacute in onset than AMS. Dyspnea at rest, worsening of symptoms after sleeping, and gait disturbance point toward altitude illness. Abnormal tandem gait is a sensitive examination finding for severe AMS progressing to HACE. Improvement with descent confirms the diagnosis.

Treatment

■ Initial field treatment involves stopping the ascent and rest. A lack of improvement in 12 hours should lead to a descent in altitude. Typically, descending 1,000–3,000 ft is sufficient. Acetazolamide (125–250 mg twice a day) should be given. If available, low-flow oxygen and portable hyperbaric bags are helpful. Additional useful medications are ibuprofen or aspirin for headache and promethazine (25–50 mg) or prochlorperazine (5–10 mg) for nausea and vomiting (5,9).

Table 42.5	**Prevention of Altitude Illness**
Begin exertion below 8,000 ft. Spend 2–3 nights sleeping between 8,000 and 10,000 ft before ascending above 10,000 ft.
Sleep no more than 1,500 ft higher each day above 10,000 ft.
Avoid alcohol or sedatives.
Avoid dehydration or hypothermia.
Consider acetazolamide 125–250 mg orally twice a day beginning the day before ascent: for any individual with a prior history of acute mountain sickness (AMS), when climbing above 11,400 ft, or when acclimatization is not possible. (Continue until after 48 hours at maximum altitude.)
If Lake Louise AMS score of 3 or higher, do not ascend. Descend if symptoms do not improve in 12 hours.
Reserve dexamethasone (4 mg every 6 hours) for the treatment of severe AMS or high-altitude cerebral edema.

- Treatment of HACE or HAPE should include *immediate* descent and evacuation. Dexamethasone (4 mg oral/intramuscular every 6 hours) for HACE and nifedipine (10 mg orally once followed by 30 mg of the extended-release tablet twice a day) should be instituted for HAPE (LOE B, nonrandomized clinical trial) (5).

- Hospital treatment will also include high-flow oxygen or hyperbaric oxygen and loop diuretics for pulmonary edema. Mechanical ventilation is only required in cases of coma.

Prevention

- Altitude illness can be prevented by proper acclimatization. Physiologic changes of hyperventilation, tachycardia, erythropoiesis, and a variety of cellular changes take from minutes to months to reach their peak. Recommendations for the prevention of altitude illness are provided in Table 42.5.

REFERENCES

1. American College of Sports Medicine, Armstrong LE, Casa DJ, et al. American College of Sports Medicine position stand. Exertional heat illness during training and competition. *Med Sci Sports Exerc.* 2007;39(3):556–72.

2. American College of Sports Medicine, Sawka MN, Burke LM, et al. American College of Sports Medicine position stand. Exercise and fluid replacement. *Med Sci Sports Exerc.* 2007;39(2):377–90.

3. American Heart Association. 2010 Guidelines for Cardiopulmonary Resuscitation and Emergency Cardiovascular Care. *Circulation.* 2010; 122(suppl 3).

4. Auerbach PS, editor. Chapters 1, 5, 8, and 11. *Wilderness Medicine.* 5th ed. St. Louis (MO): Mosby; 2007.

5. Bärtsch P, Maggiorini M, Ritter M, Noti C, Vock P, Oelz O. Prevention of high-altitude pulmonary edema by nifedipine. *N Engl J Med.* 1991;325(18):1284–9.

6. Castellani JW, Young AJ, Ducharme MB, et al. American College of Sports Medicine position stand: prevention of cold injuries during exercise. *Med Sci Sports Exerc.* 2006;38(11):2012–29.

7. Cauchy E, Marsigny B, Allamel G, Verhellen R, Chetaille E. The value of technetium 99 scintigraphy in the prognosis of amputation in severe frostbite injuries of the extremities: a retrospective study of 92 severe frostbite injuries. *J Hand Surg Am.* 2000;25(5): 969–78.

8. Danzl DF, Pozos RS. Accidental hypothermia. *N Engl J Med.* 1994; 331(26):1756–60.

9. Fiore DC, Hall S, Shoja P. Altitude illness: risk factors, prevention, presentation and treatment. *Am Fam Physician.* 2010;82(9):1103–10.

10. Gaffin SL, Gardner JW, Flinn SD. Cooling method for heatstroke victims. *Ann Intern Med.* 2000;132(8):678.

11. Graham CA, McNaughton GW, Wyatt JP. *Wilderness Environ Med.* 2001; 12(4):232–5.

12. Hackett PH, Roach RC. High-altitude illness. *N Engl J Med.* 2001; 345(2):107–14.

13. Hayes DW Jr, Mandracchia VJ, Considine C, Webb GE. Pentoxifylline. Adjunctive therapy in the treatment of pedal frostbite. *Clin Podiatr Med Surg.* 2000;17(4):715–22.

14. Heggers JP, Robson MC, Manavalen K, et al. Experimental and clinical observations on frostbite. *Ann Emerg Med.* 1987;16(9):1056–1062.

15. Herring SA, Bernhardt DT, Boyajian-O'Neil L, et al. Selected issues in injury and illness prevention and the team physician: a consensus statement. *Med Sci Sports Exerc.* 2007;39(11):2058–68.

16. Markenson D, Ferguson JD, Chameides L, et al. Part 17: first aid: 2010 American Heart Association and American Red Cross Guidelines for First Aid. *Circulation.* 2010;122(18)(suppl 3):S934–46.

17. McCauley RL, Hing DN, Robson MC, Heggers JP. Frostbite injuries: a rational approach based on pathophysiology. *J Trauma.* 1983;23(2): 143–7.

18. Murphy JV, Banwell PE, Roberts AH, McGrouther DA. Frostbite: pathogenesis and treatment. *J Trauma.* 2000;48(1):171–8.

19. Reamy BV. Frostbite: review and current concepts. *J Am Board Fam Pract.* 1998;11(1):34–40.

Head Injuries

43

Carlos M. Alvarado and Dennis A. Cardone

- Head injuries are the most frequent direct cause of death in athletic competition (31).
- There were greater than 400,000 sports-related head injuries requiring emergency room visits in 2009 alone. Cycling, football, and baseball were the activities associated with the highest number of head injuries per 100,000 emergency room visits in 2009 (32).
- Injury to the head takes on a singular importance when we realize the brain is capable of neither regeneration nor, unlike many other body parts and organs, transplantation. Every effort must be made to protect the athlete's head during competition because even minor injuries have been demonstrated to have lifelong cognitive effects (17).
- Football-related head injuries contribute more to fatalities than any other organized sport at approximately 3.4 per 100,000 athletes (22).
- The injury rate among football players has been shown to increase with level of play, player age, and player experience (39).
- Brain injury is the most common direct cause of death among National Football League (NFL) players with 497 brain injury–related fatalities during a period from 1945 to 1999. Subdural hematoma (SDH) was responsible for 86% of deaths (8).
- Most brain injury-related fatalities involved an SDH sustained by high school football players while either tackling or being tackled in a game (8).
- Per 100,000 participants, American football is less likely to result in a fatal head injury when compared to horseback riding, skydiving, or car or motorcycle racing (1,2,21,33).
- Football has about the same risk of a fatal head injury as gymnastics and ice hockey (11,15).
- Other sports historically have been shown to have a high rate of head injury, including boxing, the martial arts, and rugby football, although a fatal head injury in rugby is rare (10,14,25,28,29,36,41).

CEREBRAL CONCUSSION

- Concussion comes from the Latin word *concutere*, which means to shake violently.
- According to the Consensus Statement on Concussion in Sport from 2008 (28), concussion is defined as a complex pathophysiologic process affecting the brain, induced by traumatic biomechanical forces. Several common features that incorporate clinical, pathologic, and biomechanical injury constructs that may be used in defining the nature of the concussive head injury include the following:
  - May be caused by direct blow to head or indirect blow with impulsive force transmitted to head.
  - Typically rapid onset of short-lived impairment of neurologic function with spontaneous resolution.
  - Clinical symptoms largely reflect functional disturbance rather than a structural injury.
  - Concussion results in a graded set of clinical symptoms that may or may not involve loss of consciousness.
  - Resolution of clinical and cognitive symptoms typically follows a sequential course.
  - Postconcussive symptoms may be prolonged in a small percentage of cases.
  - No abnormality on standard structural neuroimaging studies is seen in concussion.
- According to Centers for Disease Control and Prevention, there are approximately 300,000 sports-related concussions annually.
- Rates of concussion in several popular sports are listed in Table 43.1 (9).
- Concussion represents 8.9% of all high school athletic injuries and 5.8% of collegiate athletic injuries (9).
- National Football League Players Association injury report from 2011 demonstrated a concussion rate of 5.8%; this is increased from 2.5% in 2002.
- These rates may be grossly underestimated because approximately 50% of concussions sustained by high school athletes go unreported, making accurate determination of incidence difficult (27).
- The risk of sustaining a concussion in football is 4–6 times greater for the player who has sustained a previous concussion (12,42).
- Diagnosis of acute concussion involves an assessment of clinical symptoms, physical signs, behavior, balance, sleep, and cognition.
  - List of signs and symptoms are included in Table 43.2.
  - The **Sports Concussion Assessment Tool 2 (SCAT2)** is a standardized tool used to evaluate athletes for possible

Table 43.1	Concussion Rates Among U.S. High School and Collegiate* Athletes, High School Sports-Related Injury Surveillance Study, and National Collegiate Athletic Association Injury Surveillance System, United States, 2005–2006 School Year (13)

| | | | | Rates per 1,000 Athlete Exposures | | | Overall Rate Comparison Collegiate Versus High School | | |
Sport	Division	No. of Concussions	National Estimates†	Practice	Competition	Overall	Rate Ratio	95% Confidence Interval	*P* Value
Football	High school	201	55,007	0.21	1.55	0.47	N/A‡	N/A	N/A
	Collegiate	245	—	0.39	3.02	0.61	1.31	1.09, 1.58	≤ 0.01
Boys' soccer	High school	33	20,929	0.04	0.59	0.22	N/A	N/A	N/A
	Collegiate	42	—	0.24	1.38	0.49	2.26	1.43, 3.57	≤ 0.01
Girls' soccer	High school	51	29,167	0.09	0.97	0.36	N/A	N/A	N/A
	Collegiate	57	—	0.25	1.80	0.63	1.76	1.21, 2.57	≤ 0.01
Volleyball	High school	6	2,568	0.05	0.05	0.05	N/A	N/A	N/A
	Collegiate	14	—	0.21	0.13	0.18	3.63	1.39, 9.44	≤ 0.01
Boys' basketball	High school	16	3,823	0.06	0.11	0.07	N/A	N/A	N/A
	Collegiate	33	—	0.22	0.45	0.27	3.65	2.01, 6.63	≤ 0.01
Girls' basketball	High school	40	12,923	0.06	0.60	0.21	N/A	N/A	N/A
	Collegiate	49	—	0.31	0.85	0.43	1.98	1.31, 3.01	≤ 0.01
Wrestling	High school	30	5,935	0.13	0.32	0.18	N/A	N/A	N/A
	Collegiate	15	—	0.35	1.00	0.42	2.34	1.26, 4.34	.01
Baseball	High school	9	1,991	0.03	0.08	0.05	N/A	N/A	N/A
	Collegiate	12	—	0.03	0.23	0.09	1.88	0.79, 4.46	.22
Softball	High school	10	3,558	0.09	0.04	0.07	N/A	N/A	N/A
	Collegiate	15	—	0.07	0.37	0.19	2.61	1.17, 5.82	.03
Boys' sports total	High school	289	87,685	0.13	0.61	0.25	N/A	N/A	N/A
	Collegiate	347	—	0.30	1.26	0.45	1.78	1.52, 2.08	≤ 0.01
Girls' sports total	High school	107	48,216	0.07	0.42	0.18	N/A	N/A	N/A
	Collegiate	135	—	0.23	0.74	0.38	2.04	1.59, 2.64	≤ 0.01
Overall total	High school	396	135,901	0.11	0.53	0.23	N/A	N/A	N/A
	Collegiate	482	—	0.28	1.02	0.43	1.86	1.63, 2.12	≤ 0.01

*Collegiate data for the 2005–2006 school year were provided by the National Collegiate Athletic Association Injury Surveillance System.
†National estimates for the National Collegiate Athletic Association data were not available.
‡Indicates not applicable.
SOURCE: Gessel LM, Fields SK, Collins CL, Dick RW, Comstock RD. Concussions among United States high school and collegiate athletes. *J Athl Train.* 2007;42(4):495–503.

Table 43.2	Signs and Symptoms That may Suggest Concussion		
Physical	**Cognitive**	**Emotional**	**Sleep**
Headache	Feeling mentally "foggy"	Irritability	Drowsiness
Nausea	Feeling slowed down	Sadness	Sleeping more than usual
Vomiting	Difficulty concentrating	More emotional	Sleeping less than usual
Balance problems	Difficulty remembering	Nervousness	Difficulty falling asleep
Visual problems	Forgetful of recent information		
Fatigue	Confused about recent events		
Sensitivity to light	Answers questions slowly		
Sensitivity to noise	Repeats questions		
Dazed			
Stunned			

SOURCE: Halstead M, Walter K, Council on Sports Medicine and Fitness. American Academy of Pediatrics. Clinical repost—sport-related concussion in children and adolescents. *Pediatrics.* 2010;126(3):597–615.

concussion. It can be used in all athletes 10 years of age and older. In addition, it can be used to monitor recovery and assist in determining return to play (RTP). The complete SCAT2 is included in Table 43.3.

- **On-Field Evaluation**
  - Standard emergency medicine procedures should be observed, including ABCs (airway, breathing, and circulation) and cervical spine precautions.
  - If there is no health care provider available, the player should be removed from practice or game and urgent referral arranged.
  - Once medical issues have been addressed, concussive injury should be assessed using SCAT2.
  - Player should not be left alone after injury, and serial monitoring for deterioration is essential over the initial few hours following injury.
  - Athletes diagnosed with concussion should not be allowed to RTP the same day as injury.
- **RTP:** This is done using a stepwise progression. The athlete should proceed to the next level in the graduated RTP protocol only if asymptomatic at current level. Each step should take 24 hours, so an athlete will take 1 week to proceed through full rehabilitation protocol. If any symptoms occur during rehabilitation, the athlete should drop

Table 43.3	Pocket SCAT2

Concussion should be suspected in the presence of **any 1 or more** of the following: symptoms (such as headache) or physical signs (such as unsteadiness) or impaired brain function (such as confusion) or abnormal behavior.

1. Symptoms

Presence of any of the following signs and symptoms may suggest a concussion:

■ Loss of consciousness	■ Feeling slowed down
■ Seizure or convulsion	■ Feeling like "in a fog"
■ Amnesia	■ "Don't feel right"
■ Headache	■ Difficulty concentrating
■ "Pressure in head"	■ Difficulty remembering
■ Neck pain	■ Fatigue or low energy
■ Nausea or vomiting	■ Confusion
■ Dizziness	■ Drowsiness
■ Blurred vision	■ More emotional
■ Balance problems	■ Irritability
■ Sensitivity to light	■ Sadness
■ Sensitivity to noise	■ Nervous or anxious

2. Memory function

Failure to answer all questions correctly may suggest a concussion.

"At what venue are we at today?"

"Which half is it now?"

"Who scored last in this game?"

"What team did you play last week/game?"

"Did your team win the last game?"

3. Balance testing

Instructions for tandem stance:

*"Now stand heel-to-heel with your **nondominant** foot in back. Your weight should be evenly distributed across both feet. You should try to maintain stability for 20 seconds with your hands on your hips and your eyes closed. I will be counting the number of times you move out of this position. If you stumble out of this position, open your eyes and return to the start position and continue balancing. I will start timing when you are set and have closed your eyes."*

Observe the athlete for 20 seconds. If they make more than 5 errors (such as lift their hands off their hips; open their eyes; lift their forefoot or heel; step, stumble, or fall; or remain out of the start position for more than 5 seconds), then this may suggest a concussion.

Any athlete with a suspected concussion should be IMMEDIATELY REMOVED FROM PLAY, urgently assessed medically, should not be left alone, and should not drive a motor vehicle.

SCAT2, Sport Concussion Assessment Tool 2.
SOURCE: McCrory P, Meeuwisse W, Johnston K, et al. Consensus statement on concussion on sport—the 3rd International Conference on concussion in sport, held in Zurich, November 2008. *J Clin Neurosci.* 2009;16(6):755–63.

Table 43.4	Graduated Return-to-Play Protocol

Step	Activity
1. Light: conditioning exercises (Goal: Increase heart rate)	Begin with sport-specific warm-up. Do 15- to 20-minute workout: stationary bicycle, fast paced walking or light jog, rowing, or freestyle swimming.
2. Moderate general conditioning and sport-specific skill work; individually. (Goal: add movement, individual skill work)	Sport-specific warm-up. Slowly increase intensity and duration of workout to 20–30 minutes. Begin sport-specific skill work within the workout. No spins, dives, or jumps.
3. Heavy general conditioning, skill work; individually and with teammate. NO CONTACT. (Goal: Add movement, teammate skill work)	Continue with general conditioning up to 60 minutes. Increase intensity and duration. Begin interval training. ■ Continue individual skill work. ■ Begin skill work with a partner but with no contact. Continue with individual skill work as per Step 2. ■ Begin beginner-level spins, dives, and jumps.
4. Heavy general conditioning, skill work, and team drills. No live scrimmages. VERY LIGHT CONTACT.	Resume regular conditioning and duration of practice. ■ Increase interval training and skill work as required. ■ Gradually increase skill level of spins, dives, and jumps. ■ Review team plays with no contact. ■ Very light contact and low intensity on dummies.
5. Full team practice with body contact	Participate in a full practice. ■ If a full practice is completed with no symptoms, return to competition is appropriate. Discuss with the coach about getting back in the next game.

SOURCE: Canadian Academy of Sport Medicine Concussion Committee. Guidelines for assessment and management of sport-related concussion. *Clin J Sport Med.* 2000; 10(3):209–11.

back to the previous level and progress again after a 24-hour period of rest.

- ▨ Graduated RTP protocol is provided in Table 43.4.
- ▨ Prior to RTP, concussed athletes should be completely symptom free and should not be taking any pharmacologic agents that may mask symptoms.
- ■ Concussion management
  - ▨ Physiologic and cognitive rest until symptoms resolve.
  - ▨ Once complete resolution of symptoms, then proceed with graduated program of exertion.
  - ▨ After successful completion of graduated program of exertion, the athlete may be medically cleared for competition.
  - ▨ In athletes with multiple concussions, prolonged recovery time, or progressively less force required to cause concussion, strong consideration should be given to changing position or sport to one with less risk of head injury (35).

Table 43.5	Head Injury Red Flags

Seizure	Poor awakening
Severe headache	Slurred speech
Focal neurologic deficit on exam	Poor orientation to person, place, or time
Repeated emesis	Neck pain
Significant drowsiness	

SOURCE: U.S. Department of Health and Human Services, Centers for Disease Control and Prevention. Heads up: facts for physicians about mild traumatic brain injury (MTBI). Available at: www.cdc.gov/NCIPC/pub-res/tbi_toolkit/physicians/mtbi/mtbi.pdf.

- ■ Neuroimaging
  - ▨ Routine computed tomography (CT) and magnetic resonance imaging (MRI) are rarely necessary in concussion management.
  - ▨ Rarely, concussions may be associated with intracranial hemorrhage, cervical spine injuries, and skull fractures (19).
  - ▨ CT is the test of choice for detecting skull fractures and intracranial bleeding within the first 24–48 hours (30,39).
  - ▨ Table 43.5 includes a list of signs and symptoms indicative of further neuroimaging.
  - ▨ Any patient with worsening symptoms should undergo neuroimaging.
  - ▨ Patients with loss of consciousness for 30 seconds or more are at higher risk for intracranial bleeding and should undergo neuroimaging (11).
  - ▨ A normal imaging study acutely after injury does not rule out a chronic SDH or future neurobehavioral abnormalities, so continued observation and management may still be required (20).

POSTCONCUSSION SYMPTOMS

- ■ A second late effect of concussion is the postconcussion syndrome. This syndrome, consisting of headache (especially with exertion), dizziness, fatigue, irritability, and especially impaired memory and concentration, has been reported in football players, but its true incidence is not known.
- ■ The persistence of these symptoms reflects altered neurotransmitter function and usually correlates with the duration of posttraumatic amnesia.
- ■ When these symptoms persist, the athlete should be evaluated with a CT scan and neuropsychiatric tests. Return to competition should be deferred until all symptoms have abated and the diagnostic studies are normal.
- ■ Mental health issues:
  - ▨ Retired professional football players with history of concussion have higher rates of major depression (17).

- Caregivers and family members should be vigilant of this increased risk of depression.
- There is concern for development of chronic traumatic encephalopathy in athletes who have sustained multiple concussions.

INTRACRANIAL HEMORRHAGE

- The leading cause of death from athletic head injury is intracranial hemorrhage. There are 4 types of hemorrhage: epidural, subdural, subarachnoid, and intracerebral, to which the examining trainer or physician must be alert in every instance of head injury.
- Because all 4 types of intracranial hemorrhage may be fatal, a rapid and accurate initial assessment, as well as an appropriate follow-up, is mandatory after an athletic head injury.
- The most common type of intracranial hemorrhage is SDH.
- Clinical presentation can be variable.
- Outcomes are equally variable and can range from death to asymptomatic return to competition (7).

POSTTRAUMATIC SEIZURE

- If a seizure occurs in an athlete with a head injury, it is important to logroll the patient onto his or her side. By this maneuver, any blood or saliva will roll out of the mouth or nose and the tongue cannot fall back and obstruct the airway.
- These events are usually dramatic, last several minutes, and then cease. They are usually benign and require no further treatment other than treatment of the underlying injury (28).

MALIGNANT BRAIN EDEMA

- This condition is found in athletes in the pediatric age range and consists of rapid neurologic deterioration from an alert conscious state to coma and sometimes death minutes to several hours after head trauma (34,38).
- Pathology studies show diffuse brain swelling with little or no brain injury (38). Rather than true cerebral edema, Langfitt and colleagues have shown that the diffuse cerebral swelling is the result of a true hyperemia or vascular engorgement (23,24).
- Prompt recognition is extremely important because there is little initial brain injury, and the seriousness of fatal neurologic outcome is secondary to raised intracranial pressure with herniation.
- Prompt treatment with intubation, hyperventilation, and osmotic agents has helped to reduce the mortality (3,4).

SECOND IMPACT SYNDROME

- The syndrome occurs when an athlete who sustains a head injury — often a concussion or worse injury, such as a cerebral contusion — sustains a second head injury before symptoms associated with the first have cleared (6,8,37).
- The vulnerability of the brain after injury is thought to be due to altered cerebral metabolism that occurs after injury and may last approximately 10 days involving decreased protein synthesis and reduced oxidative capacity (19).
- The second blow may be remarkably minor, perhaps only involving a blow to the chest that jerks the athlete's head and indirectly imparts accelerative forces to the brain.
- Usually within seconds to minutes of the second impact, the athlete — conscious yet stunned — quite precipitously collapses to the ground, semicomatose with rapidly dilating pupils, loss of eye movement, and evidence of respiratory failure.
- The pathophysiology of second impact syndrome is due to the precarious metabolic environment of the injured brain. The sublethal second impact results in complete loss of the brain's ability to autoregulate intracranial and cerebral perfusion pressures (26). This may lead to cerebral edema followed by herniation.
- Prevention is accomplished by strict adherence to RTP guidelines outlined previously.
- Overall incidence is unknown because it is very rare, with 35 documented cases among American football players from 1980 to 1993 (5).
- Mortality rate approaches 100%; prevention is key.

DIFFUSE AXONAL INJURY

- This condition results when severe shearing forces are imparted to the brain and axonal connections are literally severed, in the absence of intracranial hematoma.
- The patient is usually deeply comatose with a low Glasgow Coma Scale score and a negative head CT, and immediate neurologic triage for treatment of increased intracranial pressure is indicated.

MANAGEMENT GUIDELINES

- **Immediate treatment:** With a head injury, the ABCs of first aid must be followed. Before a neurologic examination is undertaken, the treating physician must determine if the airway is adequate and the circulation is being maintained. Thereafter, attention may be directed to the neurologic examination. It is important to understand that all players who have had a concussion must be removed from competition.

- **Definitive treatment:** Definitive treatment of severe concussions as well as of the second impact syndrome and intracranial hematoma should take place at a medical facility where neurosurgical and neuroradiologic capabilities are present.

- **What tests to order and when:** After a concussion, observation alone may be all that is indicated. In instances of a more severe concussion, however, a CT scan or MRI of the brain is recommended. Please see Table 43.5 for a list of red flags that would be an indication for further imaging studies.

- **When to refer:** More severe head injuries should be referred for neurologic or neurosurgical evaluation following removal of the athlete from the contest.

- **Appropriate time course for resolution:** In cases of head injury, the RTP guidelines outlined in this chapter may be used as a reference. Each case needs to be considered on an individual basis.

CONCLUSION

- While head injuries may always be a part of athletic competition, we must continue to strive to decrease their effect on athletes and their incidence overall. Great strides have been made, including increased recognition and appropriate treatment at athletic competitions and strict regulations regarding RTP criteria at all levels of sport. We must continue to move in this direction by instating rules that continue to respect the nature of competition while not putting athletes in harm's way.

REFERENCES

1. Barber HM. Horse-play: survey of accidents with horses. *Br Med J.* 1973;3(5879):532–4.
2. Barclay WR. Equestrian sports. *JAMA.* 1978;240(17):1892–3.
3. Bowers SA, Marchall LF. Outcome in 200 consecutive cases of severe head injury treated in San Diego County: a prospective analysis. *Neurosurgery.* 1980;6(3):237–42.
4. Bruce DA, Schut L, Bruno LA, Wood JH, Sutton LN. Outcome following severe head injuries in children. *J Neurosurg.* 1978;48(5):679–88.
5. Cantu RC. Second-impact syndrome. *Clin Sports Med.* 1998;17(1):37–44.
6. Cantu RC. Second impact syndrome: immediate management. *Phys Sports Med.* 1992;20:55–66.
7. Cantu RC, Mueller FO. Brain injury-related fatalities in American football, 1945–1999. *Neurosurgery.* 2003;52(4):846–52.
8. Cantu RC, Voy R. Second impact syndrome—a risk in any contact sport. *Phys Sportsmed.* 1995;23:27–34.
9. Dick RW. A summary of head and neck injuries in collegiate athletes using the NCAA injury surveillance system. In: Hoerner EF, editor. *Head and Neck Injuries in Sports.* Philadelphia: American Society for Testing and Materials; 1994.
10. Erlanger D, Cantu R, Barth J, Kaushki T, Kroger H. Loss of consciousness, anterograde memory dysfunction, and history of concussion: implications of return-to-play decision making. *JAMA.* 2002. (Submitted)
11. Fekete JF. Severe brain injury and death following rigid hockey accidents. The effectiveness of the "safety helmets" of amateur hockey players. *Can Med Assoc J.* 1968;99(25):1234–9.
12. Gerberich SG, Priest JD, Boen JR, Straub CP, Maxwell RE. Concussion incidences and severity in secondary school varsity football players. *Am J Public Health.* 1983;73(12):1370–5.
13. Gessel LM, Fields SK, Collins CL, Dick RW, Comstock RD. Concussions among United States high school and collegiate athletes. *J Athl Train.* 2007;42(4):495–503.
14. Gibbs N. Common rugby league injuries. Recommendation for treatment and preventative measures. *Sports Med.* 1994;18(6):438–50.
15. Goldberg MJ. Gymnastic injuries. *Orthop Clin North Am.* 1980;11(4):717–26.
16. Guidelines for assessment and management of sport-related concussion. Canadian Academy of Sport Medicine Concussion Committee. *Clin J Sport Med.* 2000;10(3):209–11.
17. Guskiewicz KM, Marshall SW, Bailes J, et al. Association between recurrent concussion and late-life cognitive impairment in retired professional football players. *Neurosurgery.* 2005;57(4):719–26.
18. Halstead ME, Walter KD, Council on Sports Medicine and Fitness. American Academy of Pediatrics. Clinical report—sport-related concussion in children and adolescents. *Pediatrics.* 2010;126(3):597–615.
19. Kawamata T, Katayama Y, Hovda DA, Yoshino A, Becker DP. Administration of excitatory amino acid antagonists via microdialysis attenuates the increase in glucose utilization seen following concussive brain injury. *J Cereb Blood Flow Metab.* 1992;12(1):12–24.
20. Kelly JP, Nichols JS, Filley CM, Lillehei KO, Rubinstein D, Kleinschmidt-DeMasters BK. Concussion in sports. Guidelines for the prevention of catastrophic outcome. *JAMA.* 1991;266(20):2867–9.
21. Kiel FW. Parachuting for sport. Study of 100 deaths. *JAMA.* 1965;194(3):264–8.
22. Kirkwood MW, Yeates KO, Wilson PE. Pediatric-sport related concussion: a review of clinical management of an oft-neglected population. *Pediatrics.* 2006;117(4):1359–71.
23. Langfitt TW, Kassell NF. Cerebral vasodilations produced by brainstem stimulation: neurogenic control vs. autoregulation. *Am J Physiol.* 1968;215(1):90–7.
24. Langfitt TW, Tannanbaum HM, Kassell NF. The etiology of acute brain swelling following experimental head injury. *J Neurosurg.* 1966;24(1):47–56.
25. Lindberg R, Freytag E. Brainstem lesions characteristics of traumatic hyperextension of the head. *Arch Pathol.* 1970;90(6):509–15.
26. Maroon JC, Lovell MR, Norwig J, Podell K, Powell JW, Hartl R. Cerebral concussion in athletes: evaluation and neuropsychological testing. *Neurosurgery.* 2000;47(3):659–69.
27. McCrea M, Hammeke T, Olsen G, Leo P, Guskiewicz K. Unreported concussion in high school football players: implications for prevention. *Clin J Sport Med.* 2004;14(1):13–7.
28. McCrory P, Meeuwisse W, Johnston K, et al. Consensus statement on concussion in sport—the 3rd International Conference on concussion in sport, held in Zurich, November 2008. *J Clin Neurosci.* 2009;16(6):755–63.
29. McLatchie GR, Davies JE, Culley JH. Injuries in karate—a case for medical control. *J Trauma.* 1980;20(11):956–8.
30. McQuillen JB, McQuillen EN, Morrow P. Trauma, sports and malignant cerebral edema. *Am J Forensic Med Pathol.* 1988;9(1):12–5.
31. Mueller FO, Blyth CS. Survey of catastrophic football injuries: 1977–1983. *Phys Sports Med.* 1985;13:75–81.
32. National Electronic Injury Surveillance System. [cited 2011 Feb 10]. Available from: www.cpsc.gov/library/neiss.html

33. Petras AF, Hoffman EP. Roentgenographic skeletal injury patterns in parachute jumping. *Am J Sports Med*. 1983;11(5):325–8.

34. Pickles W. Acute general edema of the brain in children with head injuries. *N Engl J Med*. 1950;242(16):607–11.

35. Purcell L, Carson J. Sports-related concussion in pediatric athletes. *Clin Pediatr (Phila)*. 2008;47(2):106–13.

36. Ryan JM, McQuillan R. A survey of rugby injuries attending an accident and emergency department. *Ir Med J*. 1992;85(2):72–3.

37. Saunders RL, Harbaugh RE. Second impact in catastrophic contact-sports head trauma. *JAMA*. 1984;252(4):538–9.

38. Schnitker MT. A syndrome of cerebral concussion in children. *J Pediatr*. 1949;35(5):557–60.

39. Stuart MJ. Gridiron football injuries. *Med Sport Sci*. 2005;49:62–85.

40. U.S. Department of Health and Human Services, Centers for Disease Control and Prevention [Internet]. Heads up: facts for physicians about mild traumatic brain injury (MTBI). Available from: http://www.cdc.gov/NCIPC/pub-res/tbi_toolkit/physicians/mtbi/mtbi.pdf.

41. Van Allen MW. The deadly degrading sport. *JAMA*. 1983;249(2):250–1.

42. Zemper E. Analysis of cerebral concussion frequency with the most common models of football helmets. *J Athl Train*. 1994;29(1):44–50.

44 Cervical Spine

Gerard A. Malanga, Garrett S. Hyman, Jay E. Bowen, and Ricardo J. Vasquez-Duarte

BACKGROUND

- Sports-related cervical spine injuries, while relatively uncommon, can be season ending, career ending, life altering, or even life ending.
- The majority of neck injuries are ligament sprains, muscle strains, or contusions (2).
- The sports medicine physician can take steps to help prevent catastrophic neck injuries in athletes. The training of physicians who wish to care for athletes, therefore, should impart an understanding of the mechanisms and management of cervical spine injuries.
- The majority of athletic cervical spine injuries in the United States occur in football players, partly related to the large numbers of participants in the sport. As a result, most of the sports literature has examined the epidemiology and pathomechanics of cervical spine injuries in football players. Regardless of the sport, the principles for management of athletic cervical spine injuries remain constant.

EPIDEMIOLOGY

- Athletes sustain 10% of the 10,000 cervical spinal cord injuries that occur each year.
- Sports with a greater risk of cervical spine injuries include diving, football, rugby, surfing, skiing, boxing, ice hockey, wrestling, and gymnastics (16).
- While the prevalence of sports-related cervical spine injuries has not been adequately researched, it is estimated that 10%–15% of football players may experience a soft tissue or neurologic injury of the cervical spine that results in time loss from sport (10).
- In football, those most at risk play defensive positions, that is defensive backs, linemen, and linebackers (4,5).
- The prevalence of the stinger or burner (*i.e.*, neurapraxic injury to the nerve root or brachial plexus) is reported to be ≥ 50% in football players (7).
- Helmets have decreased fatalities but may have increased the risk of nonfatal cervical spine injury due to the emergence of spear tackling and by imparting a sense of invincibility to the athlete in his "armor" (15).

FUNCTIONAL ANATOMY

- There are seven cervical vertebrae and eight exiting nerve roots.
- The cranium articulates with C1 at the atlantooccipital joint, where approximately 50% of all flexion and extension occur (the "yes" joint). The first and second cervical vertebrae form the atlantoaxial joint and are uniquely designed to allow for 50% of all cervical rotatory motion (the "no" joint).
- Lateral bending occurs coupled with rotation via motion from C3 to C7.
- Intervertebral discs between C2 and C7 serve to dissipate and transmit compressive or axial loads.
- The discs are thicker anteriorly and this design contributes to the normal cervical lordosis.
- Normal sagittal diameter of the cervical spinal canal between C3 and C7 is ≥ 15 mm, and spinal stenosis is suggested and may be present below 13 mm. Functional spinal stenosis refers to the loss of protective cushioning from cerebrospinal fluid around the spinal cord as documented on magnetic resonance imaging (MRI), computed tomography (CT), or myelography (3).
- Each nerve root occupies between 25% and 33% of the neural foramen, which is bordered by the uncovertebral joints anteromedially, the intervertebral disc medially, the zygapophyseal or facet joints posterolaterally, and superiorly/inferiorly by the pedicles of adjoining vertebrae. Degenerative arthritic changes of any of the structures that form or border the foramina may contribute to nerve root compression.
- From C2 to C7, the nerve roots exit above their corresponding numbered vertebral body, whereas C1 exits between the occiput and atlas, and C8 exits between the C7 and T1 vertebrae (8).
- The cervical spine depends on both static (*i.e.*, osseocartilaginous and ligamentous) and dynamic (*i.e.*, musculotendinous) stabilizing factors to absorb and/or dissipate forces.
- Pain in the cervical spine is mediated by free nerve endings in the outer one-third of the annulus fibrosus of each intervertebral disc, in the zygapophyseal (facet) joints, in the ligaments (*i.e.*, posterior longitudinal ligament, ligamentum flavum, interspinous and supraspinous ligaments), and in the supporting musculature.

SPORT-SPECIFIC BIOMECHANICS

- The cervical spine is normally able to absorb significant multidirectional external forces by virtue of several supportive mechanisms.

- The cervical lordosis aids in dissipating axial loads through the intervertebral discs, facet joints, interspinous ligaments, and paraspinal muscles. Tucking the chin during a tackle or before an impact can lead to reversal of the normal lordosis and impairs the mechanism for dissipating axial loads.

- Axial loading has been shown to be the mechanism of catastrophic cervical spine injury in all National Football League cases that were documented well enough to allow detailed analysis (13).

- Hyperflexion or hyperextension of the cervical spine in an athlete with a congenitally or developmentally narrowed canal may cause neurologic injury by a *pincer* mechanism (12).

- External forces that cause a combination of lateral bending and extension may lead to neuroforaminal compression and the neurologic injury commonly called a stinger or burner.

- A second proposed mechanism for the stinger or burner is flexion or extension combined with lateral bending and ipsilateral shoulder depression resulting in a traction injury to the cervical nerve roots.

- Acceleration/deceleration forces, such as those that occur in whiplash injuries, occur commonly in contact/collision sports and commonly cause injury to the muscular or ligamentous supports (cervical strain/sprain) or the cervical facet joints.

CLINICAL FEATURES

Differential Diagnosis of Neck Pain in the Athlete

- Cervical muscle strain or ligament sprain
- Herniated nucleus pulposus
- Burner/stinger (*i.e.*, cervical nerve root, brachial plexus, or peripheral nerve neurapraxia)
- Cervical radiculopathy
- Brachial plexopathy
- Fracture or dislocation
- Facet arthropathy
- Medical causes of neck pain, such as cardiovascular (myocardial infarction), endocrine (thyroid), pulmonary (pneumomediastinum), or infection (osteomyelitis or diskitis)

History

- Sideline physicians at an athletic event should keep in mind that most cervical spine injuries in athletes are cervical sprains or strains, followed by the stinger or burner. Fortunately, fracture-dislocation injuries are rare (14).

- That said, the sports medicine physician must err on the side of caution. Neck pain in any downed athlete is treated as an unstable cervical spine injury until proven otherwise.

- The stinger or burner (cervical nerve root, brachial plexus, or peripheral nerve neurapraxia) typically involves the C5 and C6 innervated muscles (*i.e.*, deltoid, biceps, and rotator cuff), and so the athlete may complain of an inability to raise the arm (6).

- Head injuries frequently occur concomitantly with spinal injuries. An athlete with both a suspected concussion and neck pain should be considered to have a cervical spine injury until proven otherwise.

- Immobilize the spine-injured athlete immediately to prevent further neurologic deterioration. Manipulating an individual with an unstable cervical spine injury may worsen the neurologic outcome (9).

- The examiner should always inquire about the following:
  - Neck, shoulder, arm, and leg pain
  - Arm or leg numbness, tingling, or weakness
- Rule of thumb (simple guidelines):
  - Symptoms in one arm → peripheral nerve injury
  - Symptoms in two arms or in one or both legs → spinal cord injury
  - Signs of head injury such as headache, blurred vision, dizziness, and disorientation
  - Previous head or neck injuries
  - Bowel or bladder dysfunction
  - Prior treatments and functional status (if not seen acutely)
- Athletes with Down syndrome (trisomy 21) and rheumatoid arthritis may be at increased risk for rupture of the transverse and/or alar ligaments and atlantoaxial instability. Minor trauma in such persons may cause complete atlantoaxial dissociation.

Physical Examination

- Inspection for the normal spinal curvature, ecchymosis, laceration, and obvious deformity.
- Palpation for deformity or step-off and bony or soft tissue tenderness.
- Range of motion (ROM), including flexion, extension, lateral bending, and rotation.
- Strength examination via manual muscle testing.
- Sensation testing in all cervical dermatomes.
- Reflex assessment of the C5 (biceps), C6 (brachioradialis), C6/7 (pronator), and C7 (triceps), as well as the L4 (patellar), L5 (medial hamstring), and S1 (Achilles) myotomes.
- Pathologic reflex testing (Hoffman and Babinski).
- Special tests such as the Spurling and Lhermitte signs.

ON-SITE ACUTE MANAGEMENT

- A physician and/or certified athletic trainer with skills in the acute management of cervical spine injuries should always be on site at collision sporting events. The aim of acute care is to prevent further neurologic deterioration, immobilize the spine, and safely transport the athlete to a trauma center for definitive evaluation and treatment. An emergency care plan should be in place and rehearsed *before* the opportunity arises to put it into action.

DIAGNOSTIC STUDIES

Imaging

- Plain radiographs are appropriate if osseoligamentous disruption is a concern or in cases of recurrent stingers or burners or cervical cord neurapraxia. Anterior-posterior, lateral, and open-mouth views should always be obtained. Flexion and extension views may be indicated to rule out abnormal segmental motion.

- Studies of intact cadaver cervical spine segments have shown that horizontal movement of one vertebra on the next does not normally exceed 3.5 mm, and the angular displacement of one vertebral body on another is always ≤ 11 degrees. These measurements may be made with lateral neutral or flexion/extension radiographs. One caveat, however, is that younger athletes are more likely to demonstrate ligamentous laxity, and these criteria may not always be applicable (1,2,17).

- The Torg–Pavlov ratio compares the diameter of the spinal canal to that of the vertebral body. A ratio of less than 0.8 is used to predict cervical stenosis and has been found commonly in persons with an episode of transient cervical cord neurapraxia. The ratio has been found, however, to have low positive predictive value for determining future injury. It is not, therefore, a recommended screening tool.

- A diagnosis of "spear tackler's spine" constitutes an absolute contraindication to participation in collision sports. It is identified as follows:
  - Developmental cervical canal stenosis
  - Reversal of the normal cervical lordosis on lateral radiographs
  - Preexisting posttraumatic radiographic abnormalities of the cervical spine
  - Documentation of the athlete having used spear tackling techniques
- Advanced imaging such as a CT scan is recommended to investigate a clinically suspected fracture when plain radiographs are unrevealing or equivocal. CT scan with myelography is a sensitive measure of spinal stenosis.

- MRI is used to evaluate soft tissues for ligamentous disruption or herniated nucleus pulposus and can also demonstrate spinal cord contusions. T2-weighted images may be used to determine the extent of *functional* reserve, the protective cushioning of cerebrospinal fluid around the spinal cord.

Electrodiagnostics

- Electromyography and nerve conduction studies may be useful in evaluating an athlete after neurologic insult with persistent motor or sensory abnormalities. Such testing can help delineate whether the lesion is at the level of the nerve root, brachial plexus, or peripheral nerve.

TREATMENT

- Sideline management of any athlete with neck pain or tenderness and neurologic symptoms, excluding those with a clear diagnosis of a stinger or burner, includes immobilizing the athlete on a spine board and emergent transport to a trauma center for evaluation by a spine specialist. The helmet should *not* be removed. Trainers and physicians should be trained in equipment to remove the athlete's facemask.

- Fractures should be referred to an orthopedic spine specialist for definitive treatment.

- Cervical sprains or strains are generally self-limited injuries managed with relative rest, icing, nonsteroidal anti-inflammatory medications for pain and inflammation, and early mobilization and strengthening in a pain free ROM.

- There is no benefit to using a soft cervical collar for cervical sprains or strains other than perhaps providing a sense of security and local warmth. In fact, the use of a collar can delay recovery by causing a decrease in cervical spine ROM.

- Stingers or burners are generally self-limited, with symptom resolution in minutes to hours. Once an athlete's neurologic examination has normalized, a tailored rehabilitation program should be instituted to prevent recurrence.

- Unresolved neurologic symptoms should be observed closely for progression.

REHABILITATION

- Rehabilitation is the cornerstone of ensuring prompt return of an athlete to competition and for preventing recurrent injury. Alternative methods of conditioning should be used while the athlete is kept out of play.

- The sports rehabilitation paradigm is as follows:
  - Decrease pain and inflammation.
  - Restore pain-free, full cervical spine ROM.
  - Optimize head and neck posture.
  - Strengthen the cervical spine musculature (dynamic stabilizers), scapular stabilizers, upper extremities, and trunk.

■ Maintain cardiovascular endurance according to the demands of the sport.

■ Direct sport-specific training.

■ Review and refine specific techniques such as tackling skills. Determine, if possible, the issues surrounding the initial injury.

■ Optimize use of well-fitted protective gear (*e.g.*, pads, collars).

RETURN-TO-PLAY GUIDELINES

■ Several authors have published guidelines to assist clinicians in determining when an athlete should be allowed to return to collision sports following a cervical spine injury (2,11,14). All of these guidelines are based on expert opinion (Table 44.1).

■ In general, return to play may be contemplated when the athlete:

■ Demonstrates full and pain-free ROM.

■ Displays a normal neurologic examination including strength, sensation, and reflexes.

■ Does not have an osseous or unstable ligamentous injury.

■ Controversy exists over returning an athlete to sport after sustaining an episode of cervical cord neurapraxia (transient quadriparesis).

PREVENTION

■ Reductions in the numbers of cervical spine injuries in sport can be made by the following:

■ Rule changes: In the National Football League, for instance, rule changes in 1976 eliminated the head as an initial contact area for blocking and tackling. Coaches are encouraged to instruct players to block and tackle with their head up. Spearing with the head has been banned.

■ Conditioning exercises to strengthen the neck and sports-specific training.

■ Prohibiting spewing or tackling using the head as a battering ram or grabbing the facemask.

■ Strict enforcement of the rules by officials and intolerance of illegal play.

■ Understand that football players playing defensive positions are more likely to sustain a catastrophic injury, so safe blocking and tackling techniques should be reinforced and stressed.

■ Ensuring that equipment properly fits.

■ Expert on-site medical care. A certified athletic trainer, and if possible, a sports medicine physician should be available at the playing field. A plan for managing a catastrophic neck injury must be rehearsed and be in place.

Table 44.1	Torg and Ramsey-Emrhein Collision Sport Participation Guidelines

NO CONTRAINDICATION

Congenital

Spina bifida occulta

Type II Klippel-Feil at C3 and below

Developmental

Torg–Pavlov ratio < 0.8

Nondisplaced stable healed fracture at compression or endplate, no posterior involvement; or clay shoveler's fracture

Healed herniated nucleus pulposus

One-level fusion

RELATIVE CONTRAINDICATION

Developmental

Torg–Pavlov ratio < 0.8, with motor and/or sensory neurapraxia

Previous episodes of neurapraxia

Two- or three-level fusions

Healed but displaced stable fracture C3–C7 at posterior ring or compression fracture

Healed, nondisplaced stable fracture C1–C2

Instability < 3.5 mm or 11 degrees

Healed herniated nucleus pulposus with residual facet instability

ABSOLUTE CONTRAINDICATION

Congenital

Odontoid (C2) abnormalities such as odontoid agenesis, odontoid hypoplasia, or os odontoideum

Atlantooccipital fusion

C1–C2 anomaly or fusion

Klippel-Feil anomaly with congenital fusion of one or more vertebral segments and a loss of segmental motion or instability

Developmental

Spear tackler's spine

Residual pain or limited range of motion

Acute fracture or central herniated nucleus pulposus

Recurrent cervical cord neurapraxia

Fracture or ligamentous laxity at C1–C2

Acute or chronic hard disc

C1–C2 fusion

Instability > 3.5 mm or 11 degrees

Body fracture with sagittal compression, arch fracture, ligament injury, fragmentation at canal

Lateral mass fracture with facet incongruity

> Three level fusion

SOURCE: Malanga GA. The diagnosis and treatment of cervical radiculopathy. *Med Sci Sports Exerc.* 1997;29(7)(suppl):S236–S245; Torg JS, Guille JT, Jaffe S. Current concepts review—injuries to the cervical spine in American football players. *J Bone Joint Surg Am.* 2002;84–A(1):112–122.

- Any athlete with a suspected head or neck injury should be managed as if he or she has an unstable cervical spine fracture until proven otherwise. The player should be instructed not to move, the head and neck should be immobilized, and trained professionals should coordinate safe transfer onto a spine board and referral to a trauma center.

- When possible, identifying congenital anomalies of the spine through a thorough preparticipation history and physical examination.

REFERENCES

1. Albright JP, Moses JM, Feldick HG, Dolan KD, Burmeister LF. Nonfatal cervical spine injuries in interscholastic football. *JAMA.* 1976;236(11):1243–5.

2. Cantu RC. Cervical spine injuries in the athlete. *Semin Neurol.* 2000; 20(2):173–8.

3. Cantu RC, Bailes JE, Wilberger JE Jr. Guidelines for return to contact or collision sport after a cervical spine injury. *Clin Sports Med.* 1998;17(1):137–46.

4. Cantu RC, Mueller FO. Catastrophic football injuries: 1977–1998. *Neurosurgery.* 2000;47(3):673–5.

5. Castro FP Jr, Ricciardi J, Brunet ME, Busch ME, Busch MT, Whitecloud TS III. Stingers, the Torg ratio, and the cervical spine. *Am J Sports Med.* 1997;25(5):603–8.

6. Feinberg JH. Burners and stingers. *Phys Med Rehabil Clin N Am.* 2000; 11(4):771–84.

7. Levitz CL, Reilly PH, Torg JS. The pathomechanics of chronic, recurrent cervical nerve root neurapraxia. The chronic burner syndrome. *Am J Sports Med.* 1997;25(1):73–6.

8. Malanga GA. The diagnosis and treatment of cervical radiculopathy. *Med Sci Sports Exerc.* 1997;29(7)(suppl):S236–45.

9. McAlindon RJ. On field evaluation and management of head and neck injured athletes. *Clin Sports Med.* 2002;21(1):1–14.

10. Meyer SA, Schulte KR, Callaghan JJ, et al. Cervical spinal stenosis and stingers in collegiate football players. *Am J Sports Med.* 1994;22(2): 158–66.

11. Morganti C, Sweeney CA, Albanese SA, Burak C, Hosea T, Conolly PJ. Return to play after cervical spine injury. *Spine.* 2001;26(10):1131–6.

12. Penning L. Some aspects of plain radiography of the cervical spine in chronic myelopathy. *Neurology.* 1962;12:513–9.

13. Torg JS, Guille JT, Jaffe S. Current concepts review—injuries to the cervical spine in American football players. *J Bone Joint Surg Am.* 2002; 84–A(1):112–22.

14. Torg JS, Ramsey-Emrhein JA. Management guidelines for participation in collision activities with congenital, developmental, or postinjury lesions involving the cervical spine. *Clin J Sports Med.* 1997;7(4): 273–91.

15. Torg JS, Vesgo JJ, Sennett B, Das M. The National Football Head and Neck Injury Registry. 14-Year report on cervical quadriplegia, 1971 through 1984. *JAMA.* 1985;254(24):3439–43.

16. Vaccaro AR, Watkins B, Albert TJ, Pfaff WL, Klein GR, Silber JS. Cervical spine injuries in athletes: current return-to-play criteria. *Orthopedics.* 2001;24(7):699–703.

17. White AA III, Johnson RM, Panjabi MM, Southwick WO. Biomechanical analysis of clinical stability in the cervical spine. *Clin Orthop Relat Res.* 1975;(109):85–96.

Thoracic and Lumbar Spine

45

Reginald S. Fayssoux

INTRODUCTION AND EPIDEMIOLOGY

- Back pain is a frequent complaint and source of morbidity among athletes in all sports, with low back pain accounting for 5%–8% of injuries (10).

- Nearly 15% of spinal injuries (cervical, thoracic, and lumbar) in the United States relate to participation in a sport or recreational activity. Depending on the mechanisms of applied load, different patterns of spinal injury are possible; thus, certain sports are predisposed to certain injury patterns.

- Musculoligamentous injuries of the paraspinal musculature are common to all sports that involve trunk rotation (*e.g.*, golf, baseball, tennis), contact (*e.g.*, basketball, football, soccer), or repetitive injury mechanisms (*e.g.*, gymnastics, swimming, diving, volleyball).

- Full-contact collision sports, such as American football, ice hockey, and rugby, are a common cause of spinal injury. The most common injuries involve the cervical spine. Thoracic and lumbar injuries occur less frequently. A classic example is spondylolysis in linemen resulting from repeated lumbar hyperextension.

- High-speed sports such as downhill skiing and snowboarding are relatively common causes of spine injury. Impact speeds are typically much higher than in other sports. Risk factors for injury include poorly groomed slopes, equipment failure, unfavorable weather conditions, overcrowding, skier error, and skier loss of control (1). The reported incidence of spine injuries among snowboarders is three to four times higher than among skiers. Jumping is responsible for as many as 80% of spine injuries among snowboarders and typically affects the thoracolumbar region (7).

- With the aging population being more and more active, spinal injuries are occurring in older patients with preexisting degenerative spinal changes, resulting in evaluation and treatment challenges. Decisions regarding return to play are especially complex in these patients, especially when surgery has been done or is being considered.

ANATOMY

- The spinal column allows for controlled spinal motion while protecting the enclosed neural elements.

Osseous Anatomy

- The spinal column is the foundation of the axial skeleton, extending from the base of the skull to the pelvis with articulations to the rib cage.

- The spinal column is composed of 7 cervical, 12 thoracic, 5 lumbar, 5 sacral, and 4–5 coccygeal vertebral segments. The cervical, thoracic, and lumbar vertebrae are separated by intervertebral discs.

- Normally, the spine positions the head directly over the pelvis in the coronal and sagittal planes (*i.e.*, coronal and sagittal balance). In the coronal plane, the spine is straight. In the sagittal plane, the cervical and lumbar regions are lordotic, whereas the thoracic region is kyphotic. These sagittal curvatures in conjunction with the intervertebral discs, provides resiliency to applied loads.

- Vertebrae are comprised of a thin cortical bony shell surrounding trabecular cancellous bone.

- The wedged shape of the thoracic vertebrae is responsible for normal thoracic kyphosis.

- The lumbar vertebrae are rectangular in shape. Thus it is the intervertebral discs that are responsible for normal lumbar lordosis. Loss of disc height as a result of disc degeneration results in loss of the normal lumbar lordosis and, subsequently, loss of resiliency to axial load.

- The vertebrae increase in size as one moves caudally as they become progressively more involved in load bearing.

- The sacrum forms the base of the spinal column and also functions as the keystone of the pelvic ring, transferring load from the spinal column to the lower extremities.

- Each vertebra has a bony ring posteriorly that contributes to the anatomy of the spinal canal, as well as multiple processes that serve as lever arms for the ligamentous and muscular attachments (*e.g.*, spinous process, transverse process).

- The intervertebral foramina are the lateral openings between adjacent pedicles through which the spinal nerves exit the spinal canal.

- The thoracic spine is inherently more stable than the cervical and lumbar spines due to the stabilizing effects of the rib cage and sternum.

- The thoracolumbar junction is a transition zone between the relatively rigid thoracic spine and the relatively flexible lumbar segments and thus is at higher risk for injury.

Articular Anatomy

- The posterior zygapophyseal/facet joints are additional paired linkages that, with the intervertebral disc, are responsible for controlled intersegmental motion of the vertebral bodies.

- Facet joint orientation plays a role in directing allowable spinal motion. In the thoracic spine where the facet joints are more coronally oriented, rotation is the predominant allowable motion. In the upper lumbar spine where the facet joints are more sagittally oriented, flexion and extension predominate. Finally, at the thoracolumbar and lumbosacral transition zones, the transitioning orientation of the facet joints (coronal to sagittal at the thoracolumbar junction and sagittal to coronal at the lumbosacral junction) allow for limited multiplanar motion.

- Because of the lumbar facet joints' dorsolateral relationship to the thecal sac and nerve roots, they can contribute to root compression (in conjunction with disc protrusion), classically in degenerative lumbar stenosis associated with facet joint hypertrophy.

- The costovertebral joints are synovial joints located between the vertebral bodies and the ribs.

- The costotransverse joints are also synovial joints located between the rib and the transverse processes of the vertebra of the same level.

- The costochondral joints are articulations that lie between the rib and its connection with the sternum.

Intervertebral Disc Anatomy

- The outer portion of the disc is the annulus fibrosis, composed of concentric rings of fibrocartilaginous tissue.

- The inner portion of the disc is the nucleus pulposus, gelatinous material consisting of loose, randomly oriented collagen embedded in a matrix of glycosaminoglycans, water, and salt.

- With age, the amount of water within the disc decreases, and therefore, the height of the disc decreases.

- The vertebral endplates are composed of hyaline cartilage.

- The blood supply to the disc is obliterated within the first three decades of life. Thereafter, the discs must rely on diffusion from the endplate and the annulus for nutrition.

Musculoligamentous Anatomy

- The vertebral motion segments are stabilized by the strong anterior longitudinal ligament (ALL) ventral to the vertebral bodies, the weaker posterior longitudinal ligament (PLL) dorsal to the vertebral bodies, and the posterior ligamentous complex (PLC).

- The anatomic structures of the PLC include the supraspinous ligament, interspinous ligament, ligamentum flavum, and facet joint capsules. The PLC plays a critical role in protecting the spine and spinal cord against excessive flexion, rotation, translation, and distraction. Some have likened it to a posterior tension band that restricts excessive motion. If disrupted, the ligamentous structures demonstrate poor healing ability, which often results in the need for stabilization of the involved vertebrae to prevent progressive kyphotic collapse.

- Because of narrowing of the PLL, the lumbar region tends to be more susceptible to disc herniations because there is an inherent weakness in the posterolateral aspect of the intervertebral disc.

- The ligamentum flavum lies dorsal to the thecal sac between the lamina. It is continuous with the anterior capsule of the zygapophyseal joint and helps to resist flexion. With loss of disc height, the ligamentum flavum can buckle into the spinal canal, resulting in neural compression.

- The back muscles are innervated by dorsal rami of the spinal nerve roots and are divided into layers.
  - Superficial layer: trapezius, latissimus dorsi, and lumbodorsal fascia.
  - Superficial middle layer: levator scapulae, and the major and minor rhomboids.
  - Deep middle layer: erector spinae muscle group consisting of the spinalis, semispinalis, longissimus, and iliocostalis.
  - Deep layer: multifidi, rotatores, and intertransversarii.

Nervous System

- The ventral and dorsal spinal nerve roots exit the spinal canal via the intervertebral foramen, form the spinal nerve proper, and then divide into the ventral and dorsal rami.

- The ventral rami form the lumbosacral plexus innervating the lower extremity musculature.

- The dorsal rami form the cutaneous and muscular innervation to the back, erector spinae, fascia, ligaments, and facet joints.

- The sinuvertebral nerve, a branch originating distal to the dorsal root ganglion, supplies the PLL, posterior annulus, and posterior vertebral body. It is thought to be one of the nerves responsible for conveying signals responsible for the experience of back pain.

- In the thoracic spine, the nerve root passes through the center of the foramen.

- In the lumbar spine, the nerve root hugs the inferior border of the pedicle. Thus, posterolateral disc herniations do not compress the exiting root because it has already exited the foramen. Involvement of the traversing root is more typical (*i.e.*, a posterolateral L5–S1 disc herniation tends to affect the S1 nerve root since the L5 nerve root has already exited the spinal canal through the foramen, cranial to the L5–S1 disc protrusion.)

INITIAL EVALUATION

- On the field management of the injured athlete with suspected spinal trauma is discussed more comprehensively elsewhere in this text. Briefly, when a spine injury occurs during sports, the primary goal is to prevent additional damage (11). One should have a high index of suspicion for

Table 45.1 | Historical Information to Obtain When Evaluating a Patient with Low Back Pain

General health of the patient aids risk–benefit analysis of treatment options

- Age
- Comorbidities

Sport activity level of the patient aids return-to-play decision making

- Recreational vs. competitive vs. professional athlete

Mechanism of injury suggests diagnosis and treatment options (activity modification)

- Repetitive injury vs. acute injury
- Blunt trauma
- Axial load
- Hyperflexion
- Hyperextension
- Rotation

Location of symptoms can aid in diagnosis

- Back – spinal vs. musculoligamentous
- Buttocks – spinal vs. sacroiliac vs. tendinitis/bursitis (*e.g.*, at the ischial tuberosity)
- Groin – hip joint vs. spinal
- Hips – spinal vs. trochanteric pain syndromes
- Radiating leg pain that does not go past the knee – spinal vs. sacroiliac
- Radiating leg pain past the knee – radicular pain

Severity of symptoms aids selection of treatment options

Neurologic symptoms narrow differential to spinal, plexus, or peripheral nerve involvement

- Anesthesia
- Paresthesia
- Dysesthesia
- Weakness

Character of symptoms can suggest neurologic etiology

- Burning, stabbing

Aggravating and alleviating factors suggest possible diagnoses

- Pain worse with certain motions – mechanical pain
- Pain improves with recumbency – mechanical pain
- Night pain, rest pain – fracture, infection, tumor
- Groin or buttock pain worse with hip motion (putting on socks) – hip pathology
- Radiating chest or leg pain worse with Valsalva maneuver – radicular pain
- Chest pain worse with inspiration, expiration – costochondritis, rib fracture
- Back pain worse when sitting (lumbar spine flexed) – disc herniation
- Buttock or leg pain worse when sitting – disc herniation, ischial bursitis, proximal hamstring injury
- Back or leg pain worse when standing (lumbar spine extended) – spinal stenosis, facet joint pathology

Knowledge of complicating factors aids risk–benefit analysis of treatment options

- Prior spinal surgery
- Secondary gain

unstable spinal injuries when an appropriate mechanism for injury exists. Patients with acute complaints of severe neck or back pain, patients with neurologic symptoms, and all unconscious patients should be treated as if they have an unstable spinal injury until proven otherwise. Early recognition and institution of appropriate management protocols for spinal trauma by emergency medical services have resulted in improved outcomes in spine-injured patients. These same algorithms should be used for the injured athlete.

- In the office, the assessment of an injured athlete with complaints potentially referable to the spine should be thorough and requires a broad understanding of spinal column anatomy and biomechanics and the relevant sports-specific considerations. The timing of the onset of symptoms to the traumatic event does not necessarily presume causality; consequently, the practitioner should keep a broad differential diagnosis in mind.

- See Tables 45.1, 45.2, and 45.3 for *history*, *red flags*, and *physical examination*, respectively.

- The benefit of any planned intervention should be weighed against its specific risks to the patient taking into consideration the patient's comorbidities. Thus, in order to appropriately analyze the risk–benefit ratio, it is critical to understand the general health of the patient being treated and what risks the patient is willing to accept.

Imaging

- Plain radiographs of the thoracic and lumbar spine are useful for initial evaluation. Flexion and extension views are useful for evaluating for radiographic signs of instability (*i.e.*, listhesis). Radiographs can help to identify fractures, dislocations, degenerative spondylosis, spondylolysis, spondylolisthesis, and scoliosis.

- Computed tomography (CT) allows better visualization of bony detail. CT is most useful for identifying impinging osteophytes, for evaluating facet joint arthrosis, and for evaluating fracture orientation and alignment. For patients with neurologic symptoms who are unable to undergo magnetic resonance imaging (MRI), CT myelogram is a useful study to evaluate for neural compression.

- MRI allows for a detailed assessment of the soft tissues and is especially helpful for identifying pathology of the neural elements, intervertebral discs, and ligaments. Given the high prevalence of abnormal MRI findings in asymptomatic individuals, however, one should be cautious in interpreting MRI results (2). In asymptomatic patients younger

Table 45.2 | Red Flags

Age > 50, significant trauma, rest pain, night pain, history of cancer, unexplained weight loss, steroid usage, fever, intravenous drug use, failure to improve with appropriate treatment, bowel or bladder dysfunction

Table 45.3	Physical Examination Findings To Elicit When Evaluating A Patient With Low Back Pain

General health of the patient aids risk–benefit analysis of treatment options.

- General appearance
- Body mass index (BMI)

Neurologic signs can narrow differential to spinal, plexus, or peripheral nerve involvement.

- Sensory deficits (dermatomal vs. peripheral nerve distribution)
- Motor weakness (myotomal vs. peripheral nerve distribution)
- Reflex testing
- Presence of pathologic reflexes (*e.g.*, Babinski) suggests upper motor neuron (*e.g.*, myelopathy)

Range of motion (ROM)

- Decreased ROM in the back can predispose the patient to back injury.
- Decreased flexibility in the lower extremities (*i.e.*, hips, knees, ankles) may result in increased load transfer to the lumbar spine with the potential for injury (*e.g.*, increased lumbar torsional strains during the golf swing in a patient with inflexible hips).

Provocative maneuvers can aid in diagnosis.

- Straight leg raise test, Lasegue maneuver (worsening of pain with ankle dorsiflexion), and the femoral nerve stretch test, when positive, suggest radiculopathy.
- Fortin finger test (points to pain within 1 inch of posterior superior iliac spine), flexion-abduction-external rotation (FABER) of the hip, Gaenslen's maneuver (hip extension with contralateral hip flexion), and sacroiliac joint thrust/compression, when positive, suggest sacroiliac joint dysfunction.
- Flexion-adduction-internal rotation of the hip suggests intra-articular labral pathology.
- Hip pain with single leg squat may result from trochanteric pain syndrome.

Gait can suggest diagnosis.

- Sciatic list, foot drop, foot slap, and steppage gait suggest neurologic involvement.
- Trendelenburg gait may be evident in patients with hip pathology.

Waddell signs can suggest a nonorganic component to pain. Three or more signs suggest symptom magnification, *not* malingering.

- Superficial or nonanatomic tenderness
- Pain with axial loading or simulated rotation
- Distracted straight leg raise
- Nonanatomic sensory change or breakaway weakness
- Overreaction

than 60 years of age, 20% will have MRI evidence of disc herniation. In patients older than 60 years of age, nearly 40% of patients will have MRI evidence of disc herniation and 20% will have MRI evidence of spinal stenosis.

- Bone scan and single-photon emission computed tomography (SPECT) studies are useful to identify areas of bone activity that may correlate with relevant pathology (*e.g.*, "hot" facet joint).
- Electrodiagnostic testing can be useful in patients with neurologic symptoms, especially when trying to distinguish neuropathy from radiculopathy. These studies can also be used to follow neurologic recovery and determine chronicity.

Laboratory

- A comprehensive evaluation may also include a complete blood count (CBC) with differential, erythrocyte sedimentation rate, and urinalysis, as well as other specific tests as indicated.
- Using laboratory diagnostics is appropriate when infection, malignancy, and inflammatory arthropathy are in the differential diagnosis.

CLINICAL SYNDROMES

Musculoligamentous Injuries

- Thoracolumbar musculoligamentous injuries are common and typically present as "back strain."
- These injuries result from significant rotational and bending forces to the trunk and commonly occur in full-contact sports and high-speed events.
- The onset of pain is typically delayed from the time of injury, presumably because of the timing of the inflammatory cascade.
- Examination may reveal tenderness within the musculature and paravertebral muscle spasm. Pain with resisted motion may help isolate a specific muscle. Range of motion (ROM) is often limited due to protective guarding. Tenderness of the facet joints may suggest facet capsular injury. No neurologic signs or symptoms should be evident.
- Radiographs may show loss of normal lumbar lordosis. It is important to avoid missing a fracture in a persistently symptomatic patient. While radiographs are a useful screening study, CT and MRI are more sensitive for traumatic injury.
- Treatment initially is directed at managing pain and inflammation. The mainstay of therapy is to avoid injury-provoking activity. Ice is useful in the acute setting to reduce inflammation; subsequently, moist heat may be used for muscle relaxation. When the pain is tolerable, ROM and strengthening exercises aid in the return to normal flexibility and strength.
- Formal physical therapy with attention to postural biomechanics may be useful as symptoms improve and active participation becomes possible. Core conditioning focuses on strengthening of the abdominal, paraspinal, and gluteal musculature in order to improve the stability and control during

sports participation because studies have demonstrated the importance of pelvic stabilization in training (6,9).

- Nonsteroidal anti-inflammatory drugs (NSAIDs) and muscle relaxants are useful adjuncts to treatment.
- Bracing can be useful for back support in the acute setting, but long-term use should be discouraged and stretching and core strengthening encouraged in its place.
- Older patients with arthritic facets that are overloaded in a traumatic event may develop symptoms that mimic musculoligamentous back pain. In select patients, facet blocks may be useful.
- The prognosis of musculoligamentous injury typically is good but depends on the extent of injury. Return to play is allowed when the patient is asymptomatic and has a normal ROM, typically within 1–2 weeks.

Disc Herniation

- Disc herniations are infrequent in sports but can result in significant morbidity. Patients can present with isolated back pain, radiculopathy, or, in rare circumstances, injury to the spinal cord or cauda equina.
- Disc herniation occurs in the lumbar spine in athletes through a mechanism of axial loading and rotation of the flexed lumbar spine. Lumbar disc herniations are more common in obese athletes because of their increased risk for premature disc degeneration.
- Back pain is typically acute in onset in contrast to musculoligamentous injury. Radiculopathy may develop as inflammation of the nerve root occurs.
- Cauda equina syndrome and conus medullaris syndrome should be ruled out because these require urgent/emergent intervention. These patients typically present with bilateral leg pain and/or bowel and bladder dysfunction.
- Plain films may show loss of disc height but typically are negative. MRI is best at identifying acute traumatic herniations, but the prevalence of abnormal MRI findings in asymptomatic individuals should be recognized (2).
- Management consists of conservative measures as previously described with judicious use of epidural steroid injections for refractory pain.
- Operative intervention is reserved for failure of nonoperative management or severe or progressive neurologic symptoms.
- Return to play after conservative management of lumbar disc herniation averaged 5 months in one study (5). Single-level lumbar disc surgery did not appear to limit or compromise sporting activities in young people in at least one study (12).

Fracture, Subluxation, and Dislocation

- Vertebral fracture, subluxation, and dislocation type injuries range from benign spinous and transverse process fractures to thoracolumbar fracture-dislocations with complete spinal cord injury. The management of the majority of these injuries is beyond the scope of this chapter.

Osteoporotic Thoracic Vertebral Compression Fractures in the Elderly

- The incidence of these fractures is increasing with the aging of the population and the increasing participation of older individuals in athletic activity.
- In younger patients (*i.e.*, under 60 years of age), although the fracture may appear similar radiographically, a heightened index of suspicion for either pathologic bone or more extensive injury (*e.g.*, burst fracture) is needed.
- The thoracolumbar junction is most commonly affected because there is a naturally occurring stress riser there where the relatively rigid thoracic spine transitions into the relatively flexible lumbar spine.
- Patients typically present after an injury resulting in axial load or hyperflexion.
- Tenderness of the affected vertebral body when percussed suggests an acute/subacute fracture.
- The diagnosis can be established by radiographs, MRI, CT scan, and/or bone scan.
- Treatment may include relative rest, pain medications, and therapy using an extension-based program. Intranasal calcitonin and bisphosphonate therapy has been shown to improve pain scores. Vertebroplasty and kyphoplasty are reserved for failure of nonoperative treatment
- It is critical that patients be evaluated and treated for osteoporosis, including its secondary causes, to minimize the chances of recurrence.
- In the young female athlete with a compression fracture, evidence for the female athlete triad of amenorrhea, osteoporosis, and anorexia needs to be a part of the evaluation.

Spondylolysis and Spondylolisthesis

- Lumbar spondylolysis is typically an acquired bony defect of the pars interarticularis, the anatomic bony bridge between the inferior articular facet and the rest of the vertebral body.
- Spondylolysis is thought to be caused by repetitive microtrauma during growth caused by repetitive lumbar hyperextension (8).
- It is more common in certain high-risk sports activities associated with repetitive lumbar hyperextension, such as a football block, military press, tennis serve, baseball pitch, gymnastic back walkover, and the butterfly swim stroke.
- Athletes who participate in these high-risk sports may be five times more likely to have an unfavorable outcome than those who participate in low-risk sports (3).
- Adolescent patients typically present with localized back pain refractory to conservative management. Radiculopathy can result from foraminal compression secondary to callus from the healing pars defect, which forms one of the boundaries of the foramen.
- Rarely, traumatic bilateral spondylolysis can result in anterior slippage (*i.e.*, traumatic isthmic spondylolisthesis) of the vertebral body on the caudal vertebral body.

- More commonly, isthmic spondylolisthesis is a preexisting developmental radiographic finding in the adolescent patient presenting with back pain. Thus, children and adolescents who present with back pain and an isthmic spondylolisthesis should have alternative causes for back pain ruled out prior to initiation of treatment.

- On physical examination, there is localized tenderness that worsens with lumbar hyperextension. In the presence of spondylolisthesis, there is often an associated loss of normal lumbar lordosis with hamstring tightness.

- Lateral and oblique lumbar spine radiographs may demonstrate the pars defect. L5 is most commonly affected.

- MRI is preferred in the growing child. CT, SPECT, or bone scan may be useful when MRI is nondiagnostic.

- Nonoperative treatment of spondylolysis consists of rest, management of inflammation, activity restriction, physical therapy, and, on occasion, bracing. Injection of the pars defect may be diagnostic and possibly therapeutic. Surgical repair of the pars defect is an option in selected individuals.

- Spondylolisthesis is treated similarly. Spondylolisthesis more commonly is associated with radiculopathy and may require epidural steroid injections for symptomatic relief. Surgical treatment requires fusion and consequently is avoided if possible.

Facet Joint Syndrome

- With facet joint syndrome, pain is generally localized to the spine but can radiate into the buttock and upper thigh.

- The pain is typically exacerbated by extension and improves with activity.

- Physical therapy should be the initial treatment for this condition in conjunction with a comprehensive exercise program with attention toward postural biomechanics.

- Additional treatment may include relative rest, weight control, analgesics, nonsteroidal anti-inflammatories, flexion-based exercise therapies, lumbosacral support, facet injections, and radiofrequency neurotomy in refractory episodes.

Sacroiliac Joint Dysfunction

- Typically results from direct impact but can result from repetitive motion.

- Pain is localized to the sacroiliac joint but can radiate posteriorly down the leg to the knee.

- Multiple positive provocative maneuvers suggest the diagnosis. Sacroiliac joint injection is diagnostic and potentially therapeutic.

- Sacroiliac joint braces may be helpful in patient with the appropriate body habitus to accommodate the brace.

- Sacroiliac joint fusion for refractory cases is possible but has long been avoided because of the surgical morbidity. Recently developed minimally invasive sacroiliac joint fusion is a promising option, but long-term results are lacking.

Rib Syndromes

Costochondritis (Tietze Syndrome)

- Costochondritis involves a painful inflammatory process of the costal cartilage.

- The second rib is most commonly affected (4).

- Palpation of the chest wall often reproduces the pain and is important in distinguishing this syndrome from a cardiac source of pain.

- Bone scan may help confirm the diagnosis and the extent of involvement.

- Treatment often consists of anti-inflammatory medications or, in refractory cases, a corticosteroid injection.

Costovertebral Joint Pain

- Costovertebral joint pain is a result of osteoarthritic changes and most commonly involves the ribs that are single articulations with the vertebral bodies (ribs 1, 11, and 12) and the ribs that are the longest (ribs 6–8).

- Pain is often unilateral and may be described as achy, burning, or radiating.

- Palpation of the costovertebral junction may reproduce pain, as can manipulation of the rib.

- The diagnosis may be confirmed with an injection of a local anesthetic.

- Treatment may include a corticosteroid injection or surgical excision of the affected joint in refractory cases.

Lower Rib Pain Syndromes (Rib-Tip Syndrome)

- These syndromes involve pain that radiates, generally from the lower four ribs, from anterior to posterior.

- The pain is often reproducible with palpation.

- Treatment often consists of anti-inflammatory medications or, in refractory cases, a corticosteroid injection (4).

RETURN-TO-PLAY GUIDELINES

- The decision as to when an athlete may safely return to play after an injury to their spine is complex.

- The desire and motivation of the athlete to return to play is beneficial in that they tend to comply with physician recommendations with regard to treatment. However, that same desire leads them to be less apt to comply with recommendations regarding duration of abstinence from sporting activity.

- There is a wide variation in opinion regarding return-to-play criteria and, unfortunately, no strong evidence to guide clinical decision making.

- Most physicians agree on the basic criteria for normal strength, painless ROM, a stable vertebral column, and adequate space for neurologic elements prior to return to play.

- Considerations in the decision to return an athlete to play include, but are not limited to, the type of injury and the typical duration required for healing, anatomic factors that could potentially predispose to further injury, the posttraumatic injury status, the particular sport or recreational activity and the potential for reinjury, the degree of skill of the athlete (*e.g.*, a professional golfer needs to wait longer prior to returning to golf after a back injury because the torques golfers generate are much higher than those of recreational golfers), the dependency of the athlete on the sport or recreational activity for income (*e.g.*, recreational vs. professional), and the amount of risk tolerable to the patient and physician.

REFERENCES

1. Boden BP, Jarvis CG. Spinal injuries in sports. *Neurol Clin.* 2008; 26(1):63–78, viii.

2. Boden SD, Davis DO, Dina TS, Patronas NJ, Wiesel SW. Abnormal magnetic-resonance scans of the lumbar spine in asymptomatic subjects. A prospective investigation. *J Bone Joint Surg Am.* 1990;72(3):403–8.

3. d'Hemecourt PA, Zurakowski D, Kriemler S, Micheli LJ. Spondylolysis: returning the athlete to sports participation with brace treatment. *Orthopedics.* 2002;25(6):653–7.

4. Errico TJ, Stecker S, Kostuik JP. Thoracic pain syndromes. In: Frymoyer JW, editor. *The Adult Spine: Principles and Practice.* 2nd ed. Philadelphia: Lippincott-Raven; 1997. p. 1623–37.

5. Iwamoto J, Takeda T, Sato Y, Wakano K. Short-term outcome of conservative treatment in athletes with symptomatic lumbar disc herniation. *Am J Phys Med Rehabil.* 2006;85(8):667–74.

6. Jeng S. Lumbar spine stabilization exercise. *Hong Kong J Sport Med Sports Sci.* 1999;8:59–64.

7. Levy AS, Smith RH. Neurologic injuries in skiers and snowboarders. *Semin Neurol.* 2000;20(2):233–45.

8. Morita T, Ikata T, Katoh S, Miyake R. Lumbar spondylolysis in children and adolescents. *J Bone Joint Surg Br.* 1995;77(4):620–5.

9. Pollock ML, Leggett SH, Graves JE, Jones A, Fulton M, Cirulli J. Effect of resistance training on lumbar extension strength. *Am J Sports Med.* 1989;17(5):624–9.

10. Stanish W. Low back pain in athletes: an overuse syndrome. *Clin Sports Med.* 1987;6(2):321–44.

11. Swartz EE, Boden BP, Courson RW, et al. National athletic trainers' association position statement: acute management of the cervical spine-injured athlete. *J Athl Train.* 2009;44(3):306–31.

12. Watkins RG IV, Williams LA, Watkins RG III. Microscopic lumbar discectomy results for 60 cases in professional and Olympic athletes. *Spine J.* 2003;3(2):100–5.

46 Magnetic Resonance Imaging in the Upper Extremity

Courtney T. Tripp and John F. Feller

SHOULDER

- High sensitivity and specificity for diagnosis of both labral and rotator cuff abnormalities have been demonstrated with magnetic resonance imaging (MRI) on 1.5-T scanners, with even greater sensitivity and specificity demonstrated recently with higher strength 3.0-T scanners (10,14,15,39). Although some authors advocate the routine use of magnetic resonance arthrography (MRA) for evaluation of the labrum and partial-thickness rotator cuff tears (37), the increasing availability of 3.0-T MRI may obviate the need to perform MRA in the future.

- Traumatic shoulder dislocation/subluxation is a common athletic injury, and MRI can provide valuable information regarding the integrity of the capsulolabral, cartilaginous, and osseous structures, which may be injured.

- The normal glenoid labrum on MRI is a uniformly hypointense ovoid rim of fibrocartilage at the margin of the glenoid and is triangular in shape on cross-sectional imaging. The joint capsule, along with multiple band-like regions of capsular thickening known as glenohumeral ligaments, attaches directly to the glenoid labrum.

- The most common injury associated with traumatic shoulder dislocation is a Bankart lesion, a detachment of the anteroinferior labrum and capsule from the glenoid rim, first described by Bankart in 1923 (2) (Fig. 46.1). A number of "Bankart variants" have subsequently been described, all of which involve injury of the anteroinferior capsulolabral complex and are associated with clinical shoulder instability (19) (Fig. 46.2). A tear (detachment) of the glenoid labrum is diagnosed on MRI as abnormal morphology of the labrum and/or curvilinear hyperintensity traversing the labrum or between the base of the labrum and glenoid rim.

- A Hill-Sachs lesion is an osseous impaction injury of the posterolateral humeral head, which is often seen on MRI subsequent to anterior shoulder dislocation (Fig. 46.3). An osseous avulsion of the anteroinferior glenoid, which is

important to surgical management, can also be seen and is known as a "bony Bankart" lesion.

- Superior labral tear from anterior to posterior (SLAP) lesions of the glenoid labrum are common injuries in athletes and represent tears of the superior labrum that extend in an anterior to posterior direction (Fig. 46.4). Four types of SLAP lesions were originally described by Snyder and colleagues and have been demonstrated to be accurately diagnosed on high-resolution noncontrast MRI (10,23) and MRA (16,35):
  - Type 1 lesions are characterized by degenerative fraying of the free edge of the superior labrum.
  - Type 2 tears are unstable lesions with avulsion of the superior labrum and biceps anchor from the glenoid.
  - Type 3 lesions constitute a bucket handle tear of the superior labrum with an intact biceps anchor.
  - Type 4 lesions constitute a bucket handle tear of the superior labrum with extension into the biceps anchor (30).

- The classification of SLAP lesions has been expanded further into several additional types, which principally represent combinations of the most common form, SLAP type 2 lesion, with other associated injuries of the labrum and capsular structures (18). However, the original Snyder classification remains the most widely used (37).

- Tendinosis of the proximal long head of the biceps tendon occurs frequently in association with impingement syndrome and rotator cuff tears (usually subscapularis or leading edge of supraspinatus). Biceps instability, manifest on MRI with medial subluxation/dislocation of the biceps tendon at the level of the intertubercular groove, is associated with injury to the structures of the rotator interval (coracohumeral ligament, superior glenohumeral ligament, superior subscapularis tendon, and anterior supraspinatus tendon) (21).

- Impingement syndrome (IS) of the shoulder is a clinical diagnosis and constitutes a range of pathology affecting the rotator cuff beginning with mild tendinosis and progressing to partial- and full-thickness rotator cuff tear (RCT) and finally rotator cuff arthropathy.

- Although IS is a clinical syndrome, MRI can provide supportive diagnostic confidence by revealing any number of findings that are highly associated with IS, including a type

The opinions and assertions expressed herein are those of the authors and should not be construed as reflecting those of the Department of Defense.

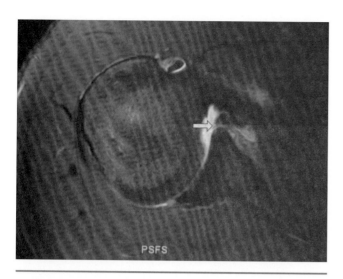

Figure 46.1: Axial fat suppression intermediate-weighted MRI demonstrating evidence of prior unidirectional anterior instability with a torn anterior labrum (Bankart lesion) (*arrow*).

III acromion process, a subacromial enthesophyte, tendinosis and/or partial- or full-thickness tears of the rotator cuff, rotator cuff muscle atrophy with fatty infiltration, and subacromial subdeltoid bursal fluid.

■ Normal tendons appear as uniformly hypointense curvilinear bands on all MRI sequences.

■ Tendinosis is seen as either abnormal morphology and/or abnormal hyperintense signal of a tendon, but not fluid-like signal intensity; findings are true for all tendons imaged on MRI.

■ Tendon tears demonstrate abnormal morphology and hyperintense fluid-like signal intensity of the tendon with partial or complete focal tendinous discontinuity. MRI has been demonstrated to be highly accurate for diagnosis of rotator cuff tendon tears (91% sensitivity and 88% specificity for all tears in a study conducted by Zlatkin et al. [39], and 95% and 84% accurate for full- and partial-thickness tears, respectively, in a study by Raffii et al. [26]). Fluid distention of the subacromial subdeltoid bursa is a secondary sign often seen associated with RCT.

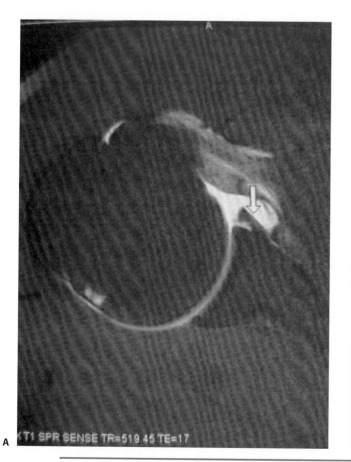

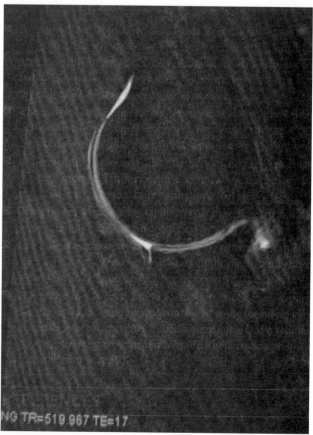

A   B

Figure 46.2: **A:** Axial fat suppression intermediate-weighted MRI of the shoulder demonstrating an anterior labral tear, a Bankart variant lesion (Perthes lesion) with an intact scapular periosteum (*arrow*). **B:** Abduction-external rotation (ABER) fat suppression intermediate-weighted MRI of the same shoulder further demonstrating the Bankart variant lesion (Perthes lesion) with an intact scapular periosteum (*arrow*).

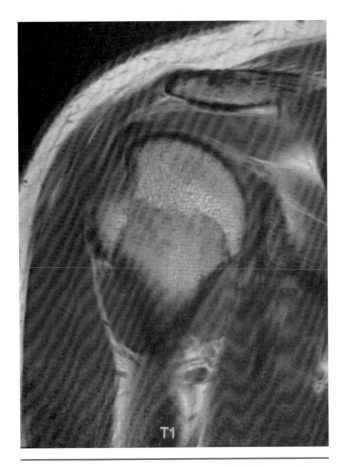

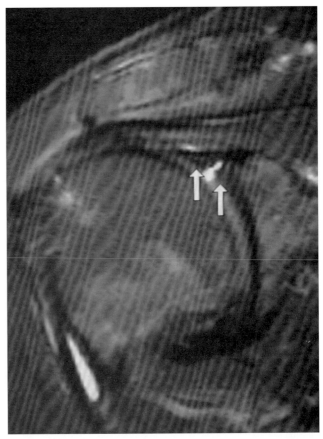

Figure 46.3: Coronal T1 MRI of the same shoulder demonstrating a Hill-Sachs deformity of the posterosuperior humeral head; further evidence of prior unidirectional anterior instability.

Figure 46.4: Coronal fat suppression intermediate-weighted MRI demonstrating a superior labral anterior to posterior (SLAP) type 2 lesion of the superior labrum. Arrows denote torn and separated portions of the labrum, with intervening bright fluid signal seen.

■ In the case of full-thickness RCT, the degree of tendon retraction and muscle atrophy/fatty infiltration should be noted because these findings portend poorer postsurgical functional outcomes and can significantly influence clinical management (8,36). On MRI, muscle atrophy is diagnosed as fatty infiltration of the muscle (linear/streaky T1 hyperintense signal throughout the muscle) and decreased overall muscle bulk.

■ The use of abduction-external rotation (ABER) positioning sequences in shoulder MRI can aid in detection of intra-articular pathology. Tirman et al. (32) found increased detection rates of partial-thickness articular surface RCTs with imaging in the ABER position on MRA in overhead-throwing athletes, and Cvitanic et al. (7) found increased accuracy in detection of anteroinferior labral injuries with imaging in the ABER position.

■ Internal posterosuperior impingement (PSI) of the shoulder occurs commonly in overhead movement (throwing, tennis) athletes when the posterior glenoid labrum and rotator cuff tendons (supraspinatus and infraspinatus) are repeatedly wedged between the humeral head and posterosuperior glenoid rim during maximal cocking of the arm in abduction

and external rotation. MRI findings of PSI include partial articular-sided tearing of the supraspinatus and infraspinatus tendons, posterosuperior labral abnormalities and glenoid degenerative changes, and cystic changes in the superolateral humeral head (6) (Fig. 46.5).

■ The clinical syndrome of adhesive capsulitis ("frozen shoulder"), manifest as shoulder pain and stiffness, can be suggested on MRI and typically confirmed on direct MRA with findings of capsular thickening and reduced capsular volume (especially in the axillary recess) and hypointense granulation/fibrous tissue within the rotator interval (Fig. 46.6). The essential abnormal lesion involves a pathologically rigid and inelastic coracohumeral ligament (17,21).

■ MRI allows imaging evaluation of injuries to the pectoralis major musculotendinous unit, an injury often found in weightlifters, and can accurately identify high-grade partial and complete tears, which have better outcomes with surgical repair shortly after time of injury. Clinical examination shortly after injury is often difficult due to localized swelling and pain, limiting accurate evaluation of the musculotendinous integrity (5,13).

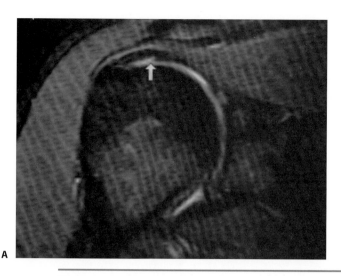
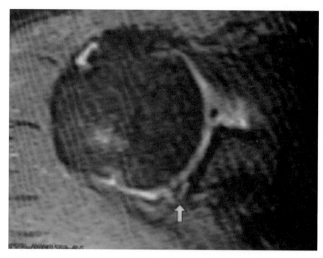

Figure 46.5: **A:** Coronal fat suppression intermediate-weighted MRI demonstrating evidence of internal posterosuperior impingement (PSI) with a delaminating partial-thickness tear of the supraspinatus tendon articular surface (*arrow*). **B:** Axial fat suppression intermediate-weighted MRI of the same shoulder demonstrating further evidence of internal PSI with a posterosuperior quadrant labral tear (*arrow*).

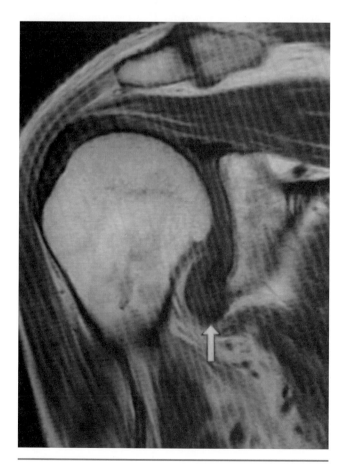

Figure 46.6: Coronal T1 MRI demonstrating a finding that can be seen in the clinical syndrome of adhesive capsulitis with abnormal capsular thickening in the region of the axillary pouch of the glenohumeral joint (*arrow*).

- Acromioclavicular (AC) joint separations are classified into six types (Rockwood classification) (27). Type I consists of partial disruption of the AC joint capsule. Type II consists of disruption of the AC joint capsule and partial disruption of the coracoclavicular (CC) ligament. Type III through VI injuries all result from double disruption of the suspensory ligaments of the shoulder (AC and CC ligaments) and may be treated surgically. MRI can help establish disruption or integrity of these suspensory ligaments, especially in cases wherein radiographic and clinical findings are confounding (especially differentiating between types II and III) (1).

- MRI has been shown to be accurate for cartilage evaluation and, with appropriate sequences, is useful for evaluating chondral injuries and postoperative changes (24,29).

ELBOW

- Most sports-related elbow injuries are adequately evaluated with noncontrast MRI. Triplanar imaging of the elbow should be performed with some combination of T1, T2, or STIR (water-sensitive) sequences, and high-resolution cartilage-sensitive sequences. Imaging can be performed with the elbow either at the patient's side or with the arm positioned overhead. MRA is generally unnecessary, although it may be helpful for loose body evaluation.

- Evaluation for epicondylitis, while typically a clinical diagnosis, is a common indication for MRI. An advantage of MRI includes characterization of severity of tendinosis and partial- or full-thickness tendon tears and evaluation and/or exclusion of other possible causes of elbow pain.

- The term epicondylitis implies that inflammation is present and is a misnomer. The preferred term of tendinosis (of the elbow) more accurately describes the histology of mucoid degeneration and vascular hyperplasia that exists within the diseased tendon (12).

- Tendinosis of either the common flexor-pronator tendon or extensor tendons about the elbow is seen as thickening and abnormal hyperintensity within the tendon origin. Partial- or full-thickness tears can be seen as fluid-like signal intensity within the tendon origin, an important finding directing patient treatment (33).

- Lateral epicondylitis (tennis elbow) commonly affects tennis players, although it is more common in nonathletic populations; it occurs with activities involving repetitive pronation and supination of the forearm with the elbow in extension. The tendinosis principally affects the extensor carpi radialis brevis tendon portion of the common extensor tendon with tenderness over the lateral epicondyle. When MRI is used to evaluate lateral epicondylitis, imaging findings of tendinosis and degree of tear correlate well with surgical findings (33).

- Medial epicondylitis (golfer's elbow), although less common than lateral epicondylitis, is mainly seen in athletes. The tendinosis principally involves the flexor carpi radialis and pronator teres tendons at the medial condylar origin and shows MRI findings of tendinosis and/or tearing as described previously (34).

- Distal biceps complete tendon rupture occurs almost exclusively in men and is the result of a single traumatic event with sudden forceful extension. Tears may be accurately characterized on MRI as partial or complete and typically occur at the insertion site of the tendon into the radial tuberosity. Complete tears are seen as focal discontinuity of the tendon, and tendon retraction can also be characterized (33).

- MRI is useful in evaluating partial or complete sprains of the collateral ligaments about the elbow.

- Repetitive or excessive valgus stress of the elbow, as can be encountered in throwing athletes, may result in partial or complete rupture of the anterior band of the ulnar collateral ligament, which normally is a thin dark strand at the medial capsular margin of the elbow joint. Most tears of the ulnar collateral ligament are full thickness and involve the anterior bundle (11).

- Lateral ulnar collateral ligament tears are typically the result of an elbow dislocation in young individuals and caused by a varus extension stress injury without dislocation in adults. Typically tears are full thickness, occur at the proximal attachment to the lateral epicondyle, and manifest as a focal disruption on MRI (Fig. 46.7). Disruption of the lateral ulnar collateral ligament is closely associated with posterolateral rotary instability of the elbow (20,25).

- MRI is extremely useful for detecting occult fractures and osteochondral injuries of the elbow. Subtle nondisplaced fractures of the radial head and supracondylar/epicondylar regions in children are readily diagnosed on MRI with linear low signal fracture lines with surrounding perifocal marrow edema.

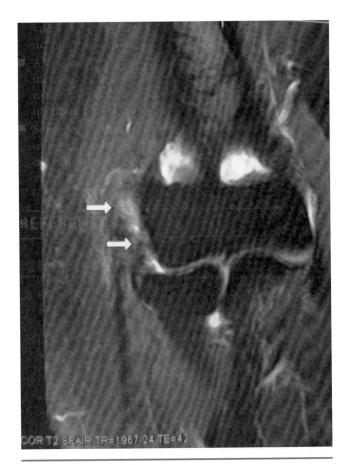

Figure 46.7: Coronal fat suppression T2 MRI demonstrating both a full-thickness lateral ulnar collateral ligament tear (*lower arrow*) and partial-thickness common extensor tendon tear (*upper arrow*).

- Osteochondral abnormalities, such as traumatic osteochondral injuries, osteochondritis dissecans in the adolescent, and osteochondrosis of the capitellum (Panner disease) in children, are well characterized with MRI. Osteochondral lesions can be characterized as stable or unstable with MRI evaluation with unstable fragments circumscribed by high T2 signal (fluid equivalent) between the fragment and the parent bone (28). Chondral surface irregularities and intra-articular loose bodies should also be commented upon.

- An apophyseal stress injury of the medial epicondyle apophysis (little leaguer's elbow) can be seen in children involved as throwing athletes. MRI may be useful in revealing linear fluid signal at the synchondrosis and associated perifocal marrow edema.

WRIST AND HAND

- MRI evaluation of the wrist and hand is commonly obtained for evaluation of intrinsic ligament tears, tears or degeneration of the triangular fibrocartilaginous complex, ganglion cysts, carpal tunnel evaluation, and tendon abnormalities.

- MRI technique of the wrist and hand should include triplanar imaging with high-resolution sequences, using small dedicated surface coils and small fields of view. T1 and high-resolution intermediate-weighted sequences provide excellent anatomic detail, whereas T2-weighted (water-sensitive) sequences are useful for visualizing most pathologic conditions.

- All normal tendons of the hand and wrist are uniformly low signal intensity tubular-shaped structures.

- The main flexor tendons of the digits contained within the carpal tunnel, which are clearly evaluated on axial sequences, include the flexor digitorum superficialis, flexor digitorum profundus, and flexor pollicis longus tendons.

- The median nerve is also within the carpal tunnel, is seen as an intermediate-intensity tubular structure with visible internal fascicles, and is located adjacent to the flexor retinaculum. Compression of the median nerve within the carpal tunnel may occur by space-occupying lesions such as soft tissue masses or ganglion cysts, which contribute to the clinical entity of carpal tunnel syndrome.

- de Quervain disease refers to tendinopathy and stenosing tenosynovitis of the first dorsal extensor compartment tendons, composed of the abductor pollicis longus and extensor pollicis brevis tendons (9). Although often idiopathic, de Quervain disease occurs often in athletes involved in racket sports and golfing. MRI findings include thickening and abnormal hyperintense signal of the first compartment tendons and tenosynovial effusion (tenosynovitis) (3).

- With respect to the dorsal extensor tendons of the wrist, tenosynovitis is only common involving the extensor carpi ulnaris (ECU) tendon, which frequently is associated with instability of the tendon with a tendency to ulnar subluxation during supination. MRI findings of tenosynovitis and tendinosis of the ECU parallel that of other tendons with abnormal tendon signal and thickening and tenosynovial effusion (3).

- The intrinsic ligaments of the wrist are important stabilizers of the wrist and can be accurately evaluated with high-resolution MRI (38). Scapholunate instability, the result of a full-thickness scapholunate ligament tear, is the most common carpal instability. The scapholunate ligament has a variable appearance on MRI, with a more uniform low signal intensity appearance at its thick dorsal band and more intermediate signal intensity of its volar band. MRI sensitivity for scapholunate ligament tears is better than for lunotriquetral ligament tears. Complete tears are seen as a focal discontinuity of the ligament or complete absence of the ligament. Some advocate the use of MRA, which may have slightly increased sensitivity of detection of intrinsic ligamentous tears (3).

- Triangular fibrocartilaginous complex (TFCC) is a complex structure whose main components are composed of a thin central disc, volar and dorsal radial ulnar ligaments, the ulnar collateral ligament, and the ECU tendon sheath. Various avulsions or perforations of the components of the TFCC may occur due to traumatic or degenerative tearing, the exact locations of which can be verified on MRI to direct further treatment (22). TFCC tears are associated with ulnar-sided wrist instability and pain.

- Ulnar impaction syndrome is a clinical entity with associated imaging findings of positive ulnar variance, degenerative tears of the TFCC, and degenerative arthritic changes involving the distal ulna and ulnar aspect of the lunate and triquetrum. MRI can demonstrate these findings as well as earlier findings of ulnar aspect lunate chondromalacia, which may direct earlier treatment (40) (Fig. 46.8).

- "Gamekeeper's thumb" or "skier's thumb" is a common ulnar collateral ligament injury of the metacarpal-phalangeal joint of the thumb typically occurring in skiers, which is generally apparent on physical examination. MRI plays a role in confirmation of the diagnosis and in further evaluation of a possible complication termed a Stener lesion, wherein the torn and retracted ulnar collateral ligament is positioned abnormally superficial to the adjacent adductor pollicis aponeurosis. On MRI, the retracted ligament appears as a tiny balled-up mass of tissue superficial to the aponeurosis (31). This is an important finding because surgical intervention of this ligament is usually reserved for Stener lesions (40).

- Nondisplaced carpal bone fractures can be occult and poorly recognized on conventional radiographs. MRI is clearly useful in identifying such fractures, especially with use of water-sensitive sequences to detect bone marrow edema. MRI is particularly useful in identification of occult carpal fractures of the scaphoid and hook of the hamate.

- MRI is extremely sensitive for bone marrow abnormalities and hence useful for evaluation of avascular necrosis in the scaphoid and lunate bones. MRI for assessment of osseous fragment vascularity in avascular necrosis–affected carpal bones is best achieved with gadolinium-enhanced MRI sequences (38).

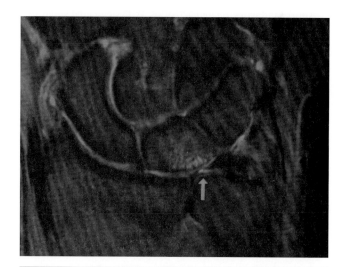

Figure 46.8: Coronal fat suppression intermediate-weighted MRI of the wrist demonstrating the sequela of ulnocarpal abutment. There is chondromalacia and subchondral cyst formation of the proximal ulnar -aspect of the lunate at the ulnolunar articulation. In addition, a full-thickness central disc tear of the triangular fibrocartilage complex is present (*arrow*).

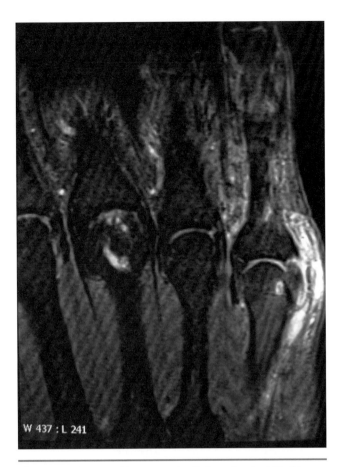

W 437 : L 241

Figure 46.9: Coronal fat suppression T2 fast spin echo MRI of the hand demonstrating a full-thickness tear of the ulnar collateral ligament and capsular disruption of the small finger.

■ Finger injuries are a common traumatic injury in both sports and work-related activities. With dedicated small surface coils and high-resolution imaging sequences, MRI of the finger can accurately evaluate the integrity of the flexor and extensor tendons, collateral ligaments, and pulley system of the fingers (Fig. 46.9). Lesions caused by hyperextension are those most frequently seen in sports medicine practice. Commonly torn or avulsed structures include the volar plate, flexor tendons, or annular pulleys. Injuries common to the athletic population include both a "mallet finger" deformity resulting from avulsion of the terminal extensor tendon from the base of the distal phalanx and the "jersey finger" deformity resulting from avulsion of the flexor digitorum profundus tendon from the volar distal phalanx (4).

REFERENCES

1. Alyas F, Curtis M, Speed C, Saifuddin A, Connell D. MR imaging appearances of acromioclavicular joint dislocation. *Radiographics.* 2008;28(2):463–79; quiz 619.

2. Bankart AS. Recurrent or habitual dislocation of the shoulder-joint. *Br Med J.* 1923;2(3285):1132–3.

3. Bencardino JT, Rosenberg ZS. Sports-related injuries of the wrist: an approach to MRI interpretation. *Clin Sports Med.* 2006;25(3):409–32.

4. Clavero JA, Alomar X, Monill JM, et al. MR imaging of ligament and tendon injuries of the fingers. *Radiographics.* 2002;22(2):237–56.

5. Connell DA, Potter HG, Sherman MF, Wickiewicz TL. Injuries of the pectoralis major muscle: evaluation with MR imaging. *Radiology.* 1999;210(3):785.

6. Cowderoy GA, Lisle DA, O'Connell PT. Overuse and impingement syndromes of the shoulder in the athlete. *Magn Reson Imaging Clin N Am.* 2009;17(4):577–93, v.

7. Cvitanic O, Tirman PF, Feller JF, Bost FW, Minter J, Carroll KW. Using abduction and external rotation of the shoulder to increase the sensitivity of MR arthrography in revealing tears of the anterior glenoid labrum. *AJR Am J Roentgenol.* 1997;169(3):837–44.

8. Gladstone JN, Bishop JY, Lo IK, Flatow EL. Fatty infiltration and atrophy of the rotator cuff do not improve after rotator cuff repair and correlate with poor functional outcome. *Am J Sports Med.* 2007;35(5):719–28.

9. Glajchen N, Schweitzer M. MRI features in de Quervain's tenosynovitis of the wrist. *Skeletal Radiol.* 1996;25(1):63–5.

10. Gusmer PB, Potter HG, Schatz JA, et al. Labral injuries: accuracy of detection with unenhanced MR imaging of the shoulder. *Radiology.* 1996;200(2):519–24.

11. Kijowski R, Tuite M, Sanford M. Magnetic resonance imaging of the elbow. Part II: abnormalities of the ligaments, tendons, and nerves. *Skeletal Radiol.* 2005;34(1):1–18.

12. Kraushaar BS, Nirschl RP. Tendinosis of the elbow (tennis elbow). Clinical features and findings of histological, immunohistochemical, and electron microscopy studies. *J Bone Joint Surg Am.* 1999;81(2):259–78.

13. Lee J, Brookenthal KR, Ramsey ML, Kneeland JB, Herzog R. MR imaging assessment of the pectoralis major myotendinous unit: an MR imaging-anatomic correlative study with surgical correlation. *AJR Am J Roentgenol.* 2000;174(5):1371–5.

14. Magee T, Williams D. 3.0-T MRI of the supraspinatus tendon. *AJR Am J Roentgenol.* 2006;187(4):881–6.

15. Magee TH, Williams D. Sensitivity and specificity in detection of labral tears with 3.0-T MRI of the shoulder. *AJR Am J Roentgenol.* 2006;187(6):1448–52.

16. Magee T, Williams D, Mani N. Shoulder MR arthrography: which patient group benefits most? *AJR Am J Roentgenol.* 2004;183(4):969–74.

17. Mengiardi B, Pfirrmann CW, Gerber C, Hodler J, Zanetti M. Frozen shoulder: MR arthrographic findings. *Radiology.* 2004;233(2):486–92.

18. Mohana-Borges AV, Chung CB, Resnick D. Superior labral anteroposterior tear: classification and diagnosis on MRI and MR arthrography. *AJR Am J Roentgenol.* 2003;181(6):1449–62.

19. Murray PJ, Shaffer BS. Clinical update: MR imaging of the shoulder. *Sports Med Arthrosc.* 2009;17(1):40–8.

20. O'Driscoll SW, Bell DF, Morrey BF. Posterolateral rotatory instability of the elbow. *J Bone Joint Surg.* 1991;73(3):440–6.

21. Petchprapa CN, Beltran LS, Jazrawi LM, Kwon YW, Babb JS, Recht MP. The rotator interval: a review of anatomy, function, and normal and abnormal MRI appearance. *AJR Am J Roentgenol.* 2010;195(3):567–76.

22. Potter HG, Asnis-Ernberg L, Weiland AJ, Hotchkiss RN, Peterson MG, McCormack RR Jr. The utility of high-resolution magnetic resonance imaging in the evaluation of the triangular fibrocartilage complex of the wrist. *J Bone Joint Surg Am.* 1997;79(11):1675–84.

23. Potter HG, Birchansky SB. magnetic resonance imaging of the shoulder: a tailored approach. *Techn Shoulder Elbow Surg.* 2005;6(1):43–56.

24. Potter HG, Black BR, Chong le R. New techniques in articular cartilage imaging. *Clin Sports Med.* 2009;28(1):77–94.

25. Potter HG, Weiland AJ, Schatz JA, Paletta GA, Hotchkiss RN. Postero-lateral rotatory instability of the elbow: usefulness of MR imaging in diagnosis. *Radiology*. 1997;204(1):185–9.

26. Rafii M, Firooznia H, Sherman O, et al. Rotator cuff lesions: signal patterns at MR imaging. *Radiology*. 1990;177(3):817–23.

27. Rockwood C, Green D, Bucholz R. *Rockwood and Green's Fractures in Adults*. 5th ed. Baltimore (MD): Lippincott Williams & Wilkins; 2001.

28. Rosenberg ZS, Blutreich SI, Schweitzer ME, Zember JS, Fillmore K. MRI features of posterior capitellar impaction injuries. *AJR Am J Roentgenol*. 2008;190(2):435–41.

29. Shindle M, Foo L, Kelly B, et al. Magnetic resonance imaging of cartilage in the athlete: current techniques and spectrum of disease. *J Bone Joint Surg Am*. 2006;88(suppl 4):27–46.

30. Snyder SJ, Karzel RP, Del Pizzo W, Ferkel RD, Friedman MJ. SLAP lesions of the shoulder. *Arthroscopy*. 1990;6(4):274–9.

31. Stener B. Skeletal injuries associated with rupture of the ulnar collateral ligament of the metacarpophalangeal joint of the thumb. *Acta Chir Scand*. 1963;125:583–6.

32. Tirman P, Bost F, Steinbach L, et al. MR arthrographic depiction of tears of the rotator cuff: benefit of abduction and external rotation of the arm. *Radiology*. 1994;192(3):851–6.

33. Tuite MJ, Kijowski R. Sports-related injuries of the elbow: an approach to MRI interpretation. *Clin Sports Med*. 2006;25(3):387–408, v.

34. Van Hofwegen C, Baker CL III, Baker CL Jr. Epicondylitis in the athlete's elbow. *Clin Sports Med*. 2010;29(4):577–97.

35. Waldt S, Burkart A, Lange P, Imhoff A, Rummeny E, Woertler K. Diagnostic performance of MR arthrography in the assessment of superior labral anteroposterior lesions of the shoulder. *AJR Am J Roentgenol*. 2004;182(5):1271.

36. Williams MD, Ladermann A, Melis B, Barthelemy R, Walch G. Fatty infiltration of the supraspinatus: a reliability study. *J Shoulder Elbow Surg*. 2009;18(4):581–7.

37. Woertler K, Waldt S. MR imaging in sports-related glenohumeral instability. *Eur Radiol*. 2006;16(12):2622–36.

38. Zanetti M, Saupe N, Nagy L. Role of MR imaging in chronic wrist pain. *Eur Radiol*. 2007;17(4):927–38.

39. Zlatkin M, Iannotti J, Roberts M, et al. Rotator cuff tears: diagnostic performance of MR imaging. *Radiology*. 1989;172(1):223.

40. Zlatkin M, Rosner J. MR imaging of ligaments and triangular fibro-cartilage complex of the wrist. *Magn Reson Imaging Clin N Am*. 2004;12(2):301.

47

Shoulder Instability

Thomas M. DeBerardino and Robert A. Arciero

CLASSIFICATION

- Instability of the shoulder is a common problem. The incidence of shoulder instability has a broad variability based on sports-specific demands, mechanism of traumatic injury, and patient age and gender; therefore, a specific incidence rate for all athletes is impossible to determine. There are three basic categories of instability. Instability should be considered as a spectrum of pathology. Unidirectional traumatic instability is on one end of the spectrum, and acquired instability and atraumatic multidirectional instability (MDI) are at the other end (32).

Traumatic

- Traumatic instability is further classified by the direction the humerus subluxates or dislocates in relationship to the glenoid.
- **Anterior:** Fall with the arm in an abducted and externally rotated position or an anterior force with the arm in abduction and external rotation (arm tackling in football, falling while snow skiing).
- **Posterior:** Posterior directed force with the arm forward elevated and adducted (motor vehicle accident or pass blocking in football). Grand mal seizure or electrical shock can also produce a traumatic posterior dislocation.

Acquired

- **Microinstability:** Subtle instability associated with pain in a throwing athlete or associated with rotator cuff tendinosis/dysfunction. This instability can occur from repetitive stretching of shoulder ligaments from daily activity or sports participation.

Atraumatic

- **Multidirectional:** These patients have symptomatic glenohumeral subluxation or dislocations in more than one direction. Many patients will present with severe pain as an initial complaint and not overt instability. For treatment purposes, it is important to differentiate by patient history and physical examination the primary direction of instability.
  - Primary anterior: Pain associated with the arm in an abducted, externally rotated position

  - Primary posterior: Pain with pushing open a heavy door
  - Primary inferior: Pain associated with carrying heavy objects at the side
- Shoulder instability can be further classified:
  - Degree of instability: Dislocation, subluxation, apprehension
  - Chronology of instability: Congenital, acute, chronic, recurrent
  - Direction of instability: Anterior, posterior, inferior, superior
  - Laxity is not instability: Laxity refers to translation of the humerus within the glenoid fossa. Many individuals are extremely lax but are asymptomatic. Instability refers to the symptomatic complaint of instability and dysfunction.

PATHOLOGY OF INSTABILITY

- The primary pathologic entity for traumatic instability is disruption of the anterior inferior labrum from the glenoid (Bankart lesion) combined with concomitant but variable damage to the capsule. The primary pathology for MDI is a loose, redundant capsule.

Dynamic Restraints

- This is a term that refers to the stability provided by contraction of the rotator cuff (supraspinatus, infraspinatus, subscapularis, and teres minor) and scapular stabilizers (serratus anterior, trapezius, and levator scapulae). The long head of the biceps can stabilize when contracting as well as the acromial arch (coracoacromial ligament and conjoined tendon).

Static Restraints

- These restraints comprise bony, ligamentous, and labral anatomy that restrains translation statically and is independent of muscle contraction. It is important to recognize that the shoulder capsule only stabilizes the joint at the end ranges of motion similar to a checkrein.
  - The labrum provides stability to the humeral head like a chock block for a tire. It is a fibrocartilaginous structure attached to both the capsule and the glenoid. It surrounds the entire glenoid and is tightly attached in the anterior inferior quadrant, has a variable attachment in the superior quadrant, and is generally less prominent posteriorly.

- The glenohumeral ligaments represent thickenings of the shoulder capsule. These are checkreins for stability. They are best visualized arthroscopically on the inside of the capsule but are difficult to distinguish on the outside as with open surgery.
- Negative pressure, adhesion/cohesion
- Finite joint volume limits end ranges of motion.
- Joint conformity is increased with an intact capsulolabral complex that provides concavity to an otherwise flat glenoid.

Congenital Factors

- Individual collagen laxity
- Bone configuration (small glenoid, retroverted glenoid)
- Age

CLINICAL PRESENTATION (PHYSICAL EXAMINATION)

- **Examination:** A careful and complete vascular and neurologic examination is essential. The frequency of axillary nerve injuries increases with age, with incidence of 5%–35% (6).

Traumatic Dislocation

- **Anterior:** This patient is in acute distress. Arm is held in slight abduction and internal rotation. There is a loss of deltoid contour, and there will be a prominence of the acromion (2).
- **Posterior:** Associated either with a high-energy event with a posterior directed force or a subluxation. Arm is held in significant internal rotation. An anterior dimple can be appreciated. A hallmark physical examination feature is inability to externally rotate the arm with the humerus lodged behind the posterior edge of the glenoid.

Atraumatic Multidirectional

- These patients present with complaints of pain and multiple subluxation events. A hallmark physical examination feature is generalized ligamentous laxity and a sulcus sign. These patients may or may not have global joint laxity and, due to pain and spasm, sometimes do not have significant glenohumeral translation (25).

Radiographic Examination

- It is essential to obtain at least three views of the shoulder to determine direction of dislocation and also to ascertain the involvement of other bony pathology. It is important to obtain at least two orthogonal views to avoid missing a dislocation.
  - **Anteroposterior (AP):** The arm is held in slight internal rotation. This view will assist in identification of greater tuberosity fractures. The glenoid in profile or an AP with the beam angled perpendicular to the glenohumeral joint will allow more accurate identification of glenoid rim fractures.
  - **West point:** This is a special view taken with the patient prone and the beam directed inferiorly. It is a view that allows visualization of the anterior glenoid with no other overlying bone involvement. A traditional axillary view is also very useful for evaluating direction of dislocation and fractures of the glenoid.
  - **Supraspinatus outlet view, scapular lateral view, or Y view:** This is a lateral view of the shoulder that can provide information on direction of dislocation as well as angulation of proximal humerus fractures.
  - **Stryker notch:** This is a view taken to evaluate the humeral head. A Hill-Sachs lesion is an impression fracture of the humeral head and, if large enough, can impact on clinical outcome. The patient is supine with the shoulder and elbow flexed and the beam directed through the axilla.

IMAGING

- Various imaging technology is used to quantify the amount of capsular labral damage as well as evaluate the articular surface, rotator cuff, and bony architecture.
- **Computed tomography arthrography:** This study allows axial cuts to evaluate glenoid morphology (amount of excess retroversion or anteversion) with size and shape of glenoid fracture fragment.
- **Magnetic resonance imaging (MRI):** The MRI allows visualization of the articular cartilage and rotator cuff. It also allows visualization of the glenolabral structures and capsule and can indicate whether there is a humeral avulsion of the glenohumeral ligaments (HAGL), which would predicate a much different operative course.
- **Magnetic resonance arthrography (intra-articular gadolinium):** Shown to have the best sensitivity, specificity, and accuracy when compared to computed tomography arthrography and MRI for documenting glenolabral pathology (10).

METHODS OF REDUCTION

- After a complete history, physical examination, and radiographic evaluation, reduction should be completed as quickly as possible.
  - **Rockwood (traction/counter-traction) method:** An assistant provides counter-traction with a sheet draped around the torso stabilizing the chest. The caregiver then applies counter-traction of the dislocated extremity distally. Slight internal and external rotation may be used to "free" up the engaged humeral head (26).
  - **Stimson method:** The patient is placed in a prone position with the thorax supported by the table. Five

to 10 lb of weight are applied to the wrist with the arm straight. In time, the muscle will relax and the shoulder will be reduced (21).

- **Westin method:** Stockinette is placed around the proximal forearm flexed at 90 degrees, and the patient is sitting. A foot is placed in the loop created by the stockinette and a gentle force applied with internal and external rotation (33).
- **Scapula manipulation technique:** The patient is placed prone with the arm flexed, hanging over the gurney or table, and 5–15 lb of traction are placed at the elbow. The scapula is rotated medially by pushing medially on the inferior tip and rotating the superior aspect of the scapula outward.
- **Milch technique:** The patient is supine, and the arm is elevated slowly to 90 degrees. It is then abducted with external rotation, and thumb pressure is used to gently reduce the shoulder (24).
- **Kocher technique:** The arm is flexed to 90 degrees, and traction is applied in the line of the humerus. The arm is then fully externally rotated and then adducted across the chest. The arm is then internally rotated until the hand is placed on the opposite shoulder. This has been associated with proximal humerus fractures in the elderly (26).

POSTREDUCTION CARE

- It is paramount to examine and document neurovascular status before and after reduction. A sling can be provided for comfort, and pendulum exercises should be taught to the patient. Follow-up evaluation should be in 10–14 days when spasm and pain have subsided. Rehabilitation can then be employed to establish full strength and range of motion (ROM) (2).
- **Rotator cuff injury:** In patients over 40 years, tears of the rotator cuff can occur with an incidence of 15% (27). In patients over 50, there is a 63% incidence of rotator cuff pathology or proximal humerus fractures (29).
- **Axillary nerve injury:** This complication has been reported to be between 1% and 7%. At 4 weeks postreduction, if active abduction cannot be established, an electromyogram (EMG) may be necessary to diagnose and follow an axillary nerve injury. Full functional and EMG recovery is typically documented 3–6 months after this complication (2).
- **Proximal humerus fractures:** Fractures of the greater tuberosity have been observed in up to 40% of patients older than the age of 50. Displacement of 1 cm may require surgical treatment.
- *Note:* Associated injuries involving the rotator cuff, proximal humerus fractures, and axillary nerve injuries increase with age at time of dislocation.

NATURAL HISTORY AND NONOPERATIVE TREATMENT

- **Traumatic anterior:** Recurrence rates after primary dislocation:
  - 65%–95% in patients younger than 20 years depending on the author
  - 60% in patients 20–40 years old
  - 10% in patients older than 40 years old
- Early research demonstrated that immobilization had little effect on outcome (17,23,30). There are new, recent data that arm position with immobilization may play a role in nonoperative treatment. Immobilization of the arm in 35 degrees of external rotation better approximates the labrum to the glenoid than the traditional position of internal rotation (15,19).
- **Posterior:** Posterior subluxation patients responded better to nonoperative treatment than anterior subluxation patients (9).
- **Multidirectional instability (MDI):** The natural history of MDI patients involves a much larger spectrum of pathology. Eighty percent of patients diagnosed with MDI respond favorably to nonoperative treatment (9).

REHABILITATION

- Rehabilitation for instability involves activation of the dynamic stabilizers of the shoulder to aide in the overall stabilization. There are three main components — ROM, strengthening, and brace wear.
- **ROM:** Full external, internal, abduction, and forward elevation should be established. This is obtained by passive, active assisted, and finally active ROM. A trained therapist is critical for accuracy of movement, safety, and motivation.
- **Strengthening:** This begins with isometric contractions within a ROM that is comfortable for the patient. Once this is established, dynamic exercise band exercises can begin. Finally, isokinetic and isotonic strengthening with a complete arc of motion complete the program. Strengthening of the rotator cuff and scapular stabilizers is critical. Scapular dyskinesis is often a byproduct of instability and must be corrected to maintain shoulder stability.
- **Brace:** Braces are used to limit the "at-risk" position for return to sports.
  - Shoulder Subluxation Inhibitor (SSI) brace (Boston Brace International): Limits motion and protects against blows.
  - The SAWA Shoulder Orthosis (Brace International) provides anterior support and adds a checkrein.
  - The Duke–wire harness–lace up corset
  - The SSI brace was the most effective in limiting anterior shoulder subluxation, whereas the SAWA was considered to be the most comfortable (13).

OPERATIVE TREATMENT OPTIONS

- **Recurrent traumatic anterior**: Recurrence rates in the young athletic population after nonoperative treatment are unpredictable (65%–95%). Surgical stabilization should be considered in a young athlete who desires return to sport. Arthroscopic surgery has the advantage of creating less morbidity and allowing a more detailed examination of the shoulder. Although controversial, acute stabilization in the high-demand patient has been very successful and should be considered in the correct setting (3,7,14,20).

  - **Arthroscopic results:** Arthroscopic techniques have evolved over the last 35 years. The literature is replete with methods involving staples, transglenoid sutures, cannulated implants, and suture anchors. In the last 3–5 years, arthroscopic techniques have evolved to the level where they mimic the open technique. This involves plication of redundant inferior capsule, reattachment of the anterior inferior labrum directly to bone with suture anchors, and closure of the rotator interval. Recent reports place the recurrent dislocation event after surgery at 5%–15% (4). In high-demand patients, the risk of a recurrent subluxation event was 15% (2 of 13 patients), with one requiring surgery (22).

  - **Open results:** Historically, many procedures have been described for glenohumeral instability. Many of these did not repair the labral lesion, and high rates of instability were still found. Only the open Bankart suture repair and coracoid process transfers (Bristow and Laterjet) are currently being performed by almost all orthopedic surgeons.

    - Magnuson-Stack — muscle transposition of the subscapularis
    - Putti-Platt — shortening of the subscapularis and capsule
    - Bristow — transfer of the coracoid process
    - Weber — osteotomy of the proximal humerus
    - Meyer-Burgdorff — osteotomy of glenoid
    - Gallie — reconstruction with fascia lata
    - Nicola — biceps tendon through humeral head
    - Du Toit — staple repair of labrum
    - Bankart — suture repair of labrum
    - Laterjet transfer of the coracoid process

  - **Open versus arthroscopic results:** A recent systematic review identified over 60 studies reporting results of arthroscopic procedures for chronic anterior shoulder instability or comparisons between arthroscopic and open surgery. The failure rates of older arthroscopic techniques using staples or transglenoid suture techniques were significantly higher than failure rates for open or arthroscopic stabilization using suture anchors or bioabsorbable tacks. The meta-analysis concluded that arthroscopic stabilization using newer techniques had a similar rate of failure compared to open stabilization after 2 years (16).

  - Another recent systematic review comparing arthroscopic with open stabilization procedures concluded that further research is needed. Randomized controlled trials that are sufficiently powered, use validated outcome measures, and have long-term follow-up are required (28).

- Bankart lesions (tears of the anterior inferior labrum) were found in 84% of patients with continued instability after surgery. Stability was restored in 92% with repair of labrum. Uncorrected capsular redundancy was also a reason for failure in over 80% of patients (31).

  - **Bone reconstruction:** There are instances where the anterior inferior glenoid has a large fracture or is deficient secondary to impaction or chronic instability. In these instances soft tissue procedures are not adequate, and bone graft may be required.

    - **Glenoid deficiency:** A 21% glenoid defect caused instability and limited ROM after Bankart repair (18). For large defects, two procedures exist:
      - **Laterjet/Bristow:** Coracoid bone transferred to the glenoid (8).
      - **Extracapsular iliac crest:** Iliac crest autograft placed extracapsular with 3.5-mm screws; 20 of 21 patients with excellent results after chronic instability (11).

    - **Hill-Sachs lesion:** If the humeral head lesion is large ($> 33\%$) or engages the glenoid in a functional ROM, then various procedures can be considered (8).
      - Humeral head allograft
      - Open capsular shift
      - Lesser tuberosity transfer with subscapularis tendon
      - Rotational osteotomy of the humerus

- **Recurrent traumatic posterior:** This is a less frequent multifactorial condition with several modes of presentation.

  - **Open capsular posterior shift:** Associated with a posterior Bankart lesion and good success. Posterior capsule is shifted superiorly and laterally through a posterior approach (5).

  - **Arthroscopic:** Suture anchor or bioabsorbable tack fixation arthroscopically of the posterior Bankart lesion; associated with an 8% reoperation rate for failure (34).

  - **Acquired microinstability:** This is a condition that exists in the throwing or overhead athlete. Subtle anterior instability may lead to an impingement of the articular supraspinatus/infraspinatus tendons against the posterior superior labrum termed internal impingement.

- **Multidirectional:** Open inferior shift: This procedure, first reported by Neer and Foster (25), has been successful. Reports of 2%–8% failure rates in MDI patients (12,25).

REFERENCES

1. Anderson D, Zvirbulis R, Ciullo J. Scapular manipulation for reduction of anterior shoulder dislocations. *Clin Orthop Relat Res.* 1982;164:181–3.

2. Arciero RA. Acute anterior dislocations. In: Warren RF, Craig EV, Altchek DW, editors. *The Unstable Shoulder.* Philadelphia: Lippincott-Raven; 1999. p. 159–75.

3. Arciero RA, Wheeler JH, Ryan JB, McBride JT. Arthroscopic Bankart repair versus nonoperative treatment for acute, initial anterior shoulder dislocations. *Am J Sports Med.* 1994;22(5):589–94.

4. Bacilla P, Field LD, Savoie FH III. Arthroscopic Bankart repair in a high demand patient population. *Arthroscopy.* 1997;13(1):51–60.

5. Bigliani LU, Pollock RG, McIlveen SJ, Endrizzi DP, Flatow EL. Shift of the posterior inferior aspect of the capsule for recurrent posterior glenohumeral instability. *J Bone Joint Surg Am.* 1995;77(7):1011–20.

6. Blom S, Dahlbäck LO. Nerve injuries in dislocations of the shoulder joint and fractures of the neck of the humerus. A clinical and electromyographical study. *Acta Chir Scand.* 1970;136(6):461–6.

7. Bottoni CR, Smith EL, Berkowitz MJ, Towle RB, Moore JH. Arthroscopic versus open shoulder stabilization for recurrent anterior instability: a prospective randomized clinical trial. *Am J Sports Med.* 2006;34(11):1730–7.

8. Burkhart SS, De Beer JF. Traumatic glenohumeral bone defects and their relationship to failure of arthroscopic Bankart repairs: significance of the inverted–pear glenoid and the humeral engaging Hill Sachs lesion. *Arthroscopy.* 2000;16(7):677–94.

9. Burkhead WZ Jr, Rockwood CA Jr. Treatment of instability of the shoulder treated with an exercise program. *J Bone Joint Surg Am.* 1992;74(6):890–6.

10. Chandnani VP, Yeager TD, DeBerardino TM, et al. Glenoid labral tears: prospective evaluation with MR imaging, MR arthrography, and CT arthrography. *AJR Am J Roentgenol.* 1993;161(6):1229–35.

11. Churchill R, Moskal M, Lippitt S, et al. Extracapsular anatomically contoured anterior glenoid bone grafting for complex glenohumeral instability. *Tech Shoulder Elbow Surg.* 2001;2(3):210–8.

12. Cooper RA, Brems JJ. The inferior capsular shift procedure for multidirectional instability of the shoulder. *J Bone Joint Surg Am.* 1992;74(10):1516–21.

13. DeCarlo M, Malone K, Geric J, Hucker M. Evaluation of shoulder instability braces. *J Sports Rehabil.* 1996;5:143–50.

14. Fabbriciani C, Milano G, Demontis A, Fadda S, Ziranu F, Mulas PD. Arthroscopic versus open treatment of Bankart lesion of the shoulder: a prospective randomized study. *Arthroscopy.* 2004;20(5):456–62.

15. Finestone A, Milgrom C, Radeva-Petrova DR, et al. Bracing in external rotation for traumatic anterior dislocation of the shoulder. *J Bone Joint Surg Br.* 2009;91(7):918–21.

16. Hobby J, Griffin D, Dunbar M, Boileau P. Is arthroscopic surgery for stabilisation of chronic shoulder instability as effective as open surgery? A systematic review and meta-analysis of 62 studies including 3044 arthroscopic operations. *J Bone Joint Surg Br.* 2007;89(9):1188–96.

17. Hovelius L, Augustini BG, Fredin H, Johansson O, Norlin R, Thorling J. Primary anterior dislocation of the shoulder in young patients. A ten-year prospective study. *J Bone Joint Surg Am.* 1996;78(11):1677–84.

18. Itoi E, Lee S, Berglund L, Berge LL, An KN. The effect of a glenoid defect on anteroinferior stability of the shoulder after Bankart repair: a cadaveric study. *J Bone Joint Surg Am.* 2000;82(1):35–46.

19. Itoi E, Sashi R, Minigawa H, Shimizu T, Wakabayashi I, Sato K. Position of immobilization after dislocation of the glenohumeral joint. A study with use of magnetic resonance imaging. *J Bone Joint Surg.* 2001;84–A(5):661–7.

20. Kirkley A, Griffin S, Richards C, Miniaci A, Mohtadi N. Prospective randomized clinical trial comparing the effectiveness of immediate arthroscopic stabilization versus immobilization and rehabilitation in first traumatic anterior dislocations of the shoulder. *Arthroscopy.* 1999; 15(5):507–14.

21. Matsen FA, Thomas SC, Rockwood CA Jr. Anterior glenohumeral instability. In: Rockwood CA Jr, Matsen FA, editors. *The Shoulder. Vol. 2.* 2nd ed. Philadelphia: Saunders; 1998. p. 669–72.

22. Mazzocca AD, Brown FM Jr, Carreira DS, Hayden J, Romeo AA. Arthroscopic anterior shoulder stabilization of collision and contact athletes. *Am J Sports Med.* 2005;33(1):52–60.

23. McLaughlin HL, MacLellan DI. Recurrent anterior dislocation of the shoulder. II. A comparative study. *J Trauma.* 1967;7(2):191–201.

24. Milch H. Treatment of dislocation of the shoulder. *Surg.* 1938;3:732–40.

25. Neer CS II, Foster CR. Inferior capsular shift for involuntary inferior and multidirectional instability of the shoulder. A preliminary report. *J Bone Joint Surg Am.* 1980;62(6):879–908.

26. Neer CS, Rockwood CA Jr. Fractures and dislocations of the shoulder. In: Rockwood CA Jr, Green DP, editors. *Fractures in Adults. Vol. 1.* 4th ed. Philadelphia: JB Lippincott; 1996.

27. Neviaser RJ, Neviaser TJ, Neviaser JS. Concurrent rupture of the rotator cuff and anterior dislocation of the shoulder in the older patient. *J Bone Joint Surg Am.* 1988;70(9):1308–11.

28. Pulavarti RS, Symes TH, Rangan A. Surgical interventions for anterior shoulder instability in adults. *Cochrane Database Syst Rev.* 2009;7(4): CD005077.

29. Ribbans WJ, Mitchell R, Taylor GJ. Computerised arthrotomography of primary anterior dislocation of the shoulder. *J Bone Joint Surg Br.* 1990;72(2):181–5.

30. Rowe CR. Prognosis in dislocation of the shoulder. *J Bone Joint Surg Am.* 1956;38-A(5):957–77.

31. Rowe CR, Zarins B, Ciullo JV. Recurrent anterior dislocation of the shoulder after surgical repair. Apparent causes of failure and treatment. *J Bone Joint Surg Am.* 1984;66(2):159–68.

32. Thomas SC, Matsen FA III. An approach to the repair of avulsion of the glenohumeral ligaments in the management of traumatic anterior glenohumeral instability. *J Bone Joint Surg Am.* 1989;71(4):506–13.

33. Westin CD, Gill EA, Noyes ME, Hubbard M. Anterior shoulder dislocation. A simple and rapid method for reduction. *Am J Sports Med.* 1995;23(3):369–71.

34. Williams RJ III, Strickland S, Cohen M, Altchek DW, Warren RF. Arthroscopic repair for traumatic posterior shoulder instability. *Am J Sports Med.* 2003;31(2):203–9.

Rotator Cuff Pathology

Patrick St. Pierre

48

HISTORY

- John Gregory Smith published the first detailed series of rotator cuff ruptures, describing seven cases obtained by grave robbing, in a letter to the editor of the London Medical Gazette in 1834. Muller and Perthes were the first to perform repairs in the late 1800s. Codman and later McLaughlin were pioneers in the early 1900s, describing their approach to the shoulder and detailing rotator cuff repair techniques that have been followed until today (9).

- In 1972, Charles Neer II (33) first proposed the phrase "impingement syndrome" for pain involving the subacromial bursa and superior rotator cuff. He described the clinical presentation of the painful shoulder and proposed a mechanism for how the pathology developed. He noted that many of these patients had a hooked acromion, and his hypothesis was that the bursa and rotator cuff were impinged between the humeral head and acromion with elevation of the arm. This would usually start as mild inflammation of the tendon, would progress to fibrosis and tendonitis, and eventually could lead to full-thickness rotator cuff tear.

IMPINGEMENT OR ROTATOR CUFF SYNDROME (33,34)

- Stage I, as described by Neer, included edema and hemorrhage in the tendon. Tendinosis of the supraspinatus and, less frequently, the infraspinatus or subscapularis is involved.

- Stage II consisted of fibrosis and tendonitis in the subacromial space. This is a secondary process resulting from the underlying etiology.

- Stage III resulted in the development of spurs and eventually tendon rupture.

- The long head of the biceps tendon may also be involved with pathology ranging from inflammation to rupture (12). Dislocation of the biceps tendon from the bicipital groove is pathognomonic for a tear of the upper border of the subscapularis muscle from its humeral insertion (17,18).

- Pain will often occur along the anterior-lateral acromion, in the infraspinatus fossa, or distally at the deltoid insertion on the humerus. This pain is likely to be referred pain from the inflamed bursa, which irritates the deep deltoid. Pain referring proximally to the neck usually originates from the acromioclavicular (AC) joint (10,39,41,46).

- There have been several other etiologies proposed for shoulder pain emanating from the subacromial space following Dr. Neer's initial description (23,24,40). These different etiologies may or may not lead to actual impingement of the cuff by the acromion. Because multiple pathologies are often factors in this condition, including tendinosis and bursitis, the best global term to describe this condition is rotator cuff syndrome, reserving impingement syndrome for cases of true external impingement caused by AC arthritis or from the development of a coracoacromial (CA) ligament spur. Specific etiologies, as discussed later, may also be used.

PATHOPHYSIOLOGY

Rotator Cuff Syndrome

- Historically, patients will occasionally remember a direct blow or some other form of trauma. There may be history of a traction injury or a fall directly on a patient's shoulder.

- Overuse injury is also a frequent cause of this syndrome. Patients will often not recall a specific injury but may have carried luggage all weekend, cleaned out their attic, or worked on their car. Frequently, repetitive overhead activity such as tennis, softball, or swimming is the causative factor.

- These conditions occur primarily because of injury to the rotator cuff causing tendinosis and rotator cuff dysfunction. The subacromial impingement occurs chronically with the development of subacromial spurs and superior humeral head migration due to lower rotator cuff inhibition or fatigue.

Secondary Impingement

- Subtle shoulder instability can lead to rotator cuff dysfunction and thus to rotator cuff syndrome. Jobe and colleagues described this as secondary or internal impingement syndrome (23,24). This condition was originally noted in overhead-throwing athletes, but should be suspected in all younger athletes who complain of "impingement"-type pain. Treatment of this condition must address the underlying instability and not just the secondary pathology in the subacromial space.

Posterosuperior Glenoid Impingement

- This condition, as described by Walch et al. (40), has also been proposed as an etiology occurring in patients who play repetitive overhead sports such as baseball, tennis, and swimming. Walch did not find the anterior instability described by Jobe in his patients, but rather noted an impingement of the supraspinatus and infraspinatus tendons between the posterosuperior glenoid labrum and the humeral head.

- These internal impingement syndromes are characterized by partial tears of the articular surface of the rotator cuff, in distinction to the external compression described by Neer (29).

- Whatever the etiology, weakness of the rotator cuff results, especially the lower cuff, and superior humeral head migration occurs. The humeral head then compresses the bursa and tendon into the acromion, leading to impingement. This causes more bursitis, more tendinosis, and eventually more weakness. Often with chronic injury, shoulder mechanics will change, leading to abnormal scapulothoracic motion. Physical therapy will need to include rehabilitation of the scapular stabilizing musculature as well as the lower rotator cuff muscles (25).

- Any subacromial changes such as lateral hooking, CA ligament calcification, or AC joint arthritis (inferior spurs), will cause the condition to get worse and will more likely need operative intervention than when the acromion is flat.

- Calcific tendinitis
  - The etiology of calcific tendinitis remains unknown. Degenerative changes and relative hypoxia have been suggested as possible explanations. Conservative treatment similar to that for rotator cuff syndrome is reported as successful in 60%–90% of patients (13,20,31). Repetitive needling and injection of local anesthetic have also been successful in relieving symptoms and often result in disappearance of the calcified mass. Infrequently, the patient's symptoms will persist, and the patient will require operative intervention. The mass is localized within the substance of the tendon while viewing in the subacromial space. The calcified substance is then evacuated and debrided. Some argue that a repair of the tendon is not necessary, but the surgeon should evaluate the cuff after debridement in each case to determine if repair is necessary.

EXAMINATION (44)

- Inspection should focus on normal alignment of chest wall, shoulders, and clavicle. Have the patient perform active range of motion (ROM) in forward flexion, abduction, adduction, external rotation, and internal rotation. Look from the back and front for asymmetric motion or atrophy. Often patients will have a painful arc of motion over 120 degrees of elevation.

- Palpate the AC and sternoclavicular joints, the anterior and lateral acromion edges, and the infraspinatus fossa. Tenderness at the AC joint should lead you to further evaluation and treatment of AC joint arthrosis. Cross-arm adduction is often painful with AC arthrosis. However, this test is not very specific and is often positive with rotator cuff syndrome.

- Palpation of the long head of the biceps tendon within the bicipital groove is helpful to determine biceps involvement. O'Brien active compression test, Speed test, and Yergason test are also used to determine biceps involvement and are covered in Chapter 50.

- Strength testing should involve the deltoid, biceps, and triceps muscles. Although there is no way to totally isolate each of the rotator cuff muscles, the tests that have shown to be most specific are the following (26):
  - Supraspinatus: Active elevation against resistance with the elbow in extension and the arm elevated to 90 degrees and externally rotated to 45 degrees. The hand should be supinated to neutral as if holding a full can of soda.
  - Infraspinatus/teres minor: Active external rotation with arm at the side and elbow flexed to 90 degrees.
  - Subscapularis: Active internal rotation with elbow flexed to 90 degrees and hand placed behind the back. This is often referred to as the Gerber lift-off test (17–19). In patients who are unable to internally rotate their hand behind their back, a belly press test or "Napoleon's test" is performed. The patient places their hand on their belly and presses hard into their abdomen while bringing their elbow forward in the sagittal plane. Subscapularis tear or dysfunction is indicated if they are unable to do this maneuver and the elbow stays close to the side (42).

- Lag tests are also often used to detect rotator cuff tears. The hornblower's sign, external rotation lag, and internal rotation lag tests were described by Gerber and Hertel and are helpful to determine subtle weakness (18,22).

- Special tests include the Neer impingement sign and test and Hawkins sign.
  - The Neer impingement sign is similar to the supraspinatus testing described earlier, except the arm is held in maximal internal rotation as if pouring out a can of soda. This rotates the greater tuberosity under the acromion to elicit a painful response if the bursa or tendons are injured. A positive Neer test is when a subacromial injection of local anesthetic relieves the pain elicited prior to the injection (33,34).
  - The Hawkins test forward flexes the arm to 90 degrees and applies maximum internal rotation to the flexed elbow. If one supplies downward pressure at the elbow while the patient resists, the sensitivity of the exam increases (21,39).
  - The accuracy of these and many other tests in the shoulder have been called into question, however they remain the standard as the initial baseline test. Clinical history, examination and diagnostic testing must all be used together to make an accurate diagnosis (27).

- A cervical spine examination should be performed if there is any concern of radicular symptoms as a factor in diagnosis. This is particularly useful in patients older than 50 years of age and if painful symptoms radiate distal to the elbow.

RADIOGRAPHIC EXAMINATION

- Standard radiographs include anteroposterior (AP), axillary, and supraspinatus outlet views. These views will allow you to determine if there is degenerative joint disease in the AC or glenohumeral joints, spurring from the acromion or calcification within the tendon (calcific tendonitis). Chronic rotator cuff tears will often result in superior humeral head migration secondary to atrophy of the lower rotator cuff. A true scapular AP view will allow better examination of the glenoid, and internal and external rotation view will allow better assessment of the humeral head for defects or impression fractures.

- Special radiographs are indicated in certain conditions. A supraspinatus outlet view is often obtained to evaluate the morphology of the acromion in rotator cuff or impingement syndrome. A West Point view is helpful in evaluating the anterior glenoid for bony deficiency in cases of instability.

- Magnetic resonance imaging (MRI) is an excellent tool for determining rotator cuff pathology but is often overused and/or obtained too soon.

- Certain signal characteristics are indicative of full tears versus partial tears versus AC arthritis. An MRI can determine labral pathology (Bankart lesions or superior labral anterior to posterior [SLAP] tears), bursitis, acromial morphology, and articular cartilage condition. More details about MRI for upper extremity injuries can be found in Chapter 46.

- An MRI does not need to be obtained immediately if the patient has full ROM and only complains of pain and weakness. These patients can be started on the nonoperative treatment described in the next section, and the vast majority will improve. An MRI can be obtained after the next visit if the patient's symptoms have not resolved with therapy.

- The MRI is useful in determining the extent of the tear and for preoperative planning. In larger, chronic tears, the MRI is useful for determining atrophy of the muscles and efficacy of repair.

NONOPERATIVE TREATMENT

- Rotator cuff strengthening is essential for recovery, and many patients improve after surgical intervention because they finally commit themselves to the rehab.

- The focus of rehabilitation should be to reduce inflammation (usually bursal), restore motion, and strengthen muscles to help stabilize the scapula and humerus. Therapists will start with anti-inflammatory modalities, work on ROM, and begin periscapular strengthening to stabilize the scapula (25,43).

- Nonsteroidal anti-inflammatory drugs (NSAIDs) are usually helpful to decrease the bursitis and reduce the pain. They are not curative in themselves, but decrease pain so the patient can do therapy. In rare instances, the pain is severe enough for a short course of narcotics.

- A subacromial injection can be performed as a diagnostic test or as part of the treatment plan. When the Neer sign is positive, an injection is made into the subacromial space using a local anesthetic. The patient is retested after 3–5 minutes, and the Neer test is positive if the pain is relieved. Many physicians who are certain of their diagnosis will proceed with a therapeutic injection of 2–3 mL of an injectable corticosteroid at the same time. Others will inject a second time if the initial injection relieves the patient's symptoms.

- If there is a diagnostic dilemma between whether the AC joint is the cause of pain or the bursa, injections can be performed in one location and then the second to determine the source. The subacromial injection should be done first because with AC pathology, the capsule is often disrupted and an AC injection is likely to go into the bursa as well. The reader is referred to Chapter 72 on injections for more information.

- Once the pain is reduced and the ROM restored, more aggressive strengthening exercises are instituted. Internal and external rotation exercises using rubber tubing or resistance bands are very useful, and the patient progresses to heavier tubing as he or she gets stronger. Supine or lateral decubitus exercises with small weights are also started at this time.

- Core strengthening exercises to help stabilize the scapula are also instituted. These exercises are very important and often neglected. Simple exercises such as squeezing the shoulder blades together or scapular rows are often effective. Progress is monitored by observing normal scapulothoracic motion with elevation. If scapular winging is severe or fails to improve with treatment, further workup for other etiologies such as trapezius or long thoracic nerve palsy should occur.

- Deltoid strengthening should include isolated training of all 3 parts of the deltoid.

- Strengthening of the supraspinatus is not instituted immediately because it will aggravate symptoms. Supraspinatus strengthening should be started when ROM is restored and lower cuff strength is sufficient to allow overhead motion without pain.

- Most patients' symptoms resolve with this program. Injections are usually limited to 3, but each patient treatment is individualized. Many practitioners are concerned about the effects of corticosteroids on the damaged tendon and either forego this step or limit the number of injections. Patients who have developed subacromial spurs and AC arthritis are less likely to improve due to fixed impingement and may require surgery. However, a younger patient with normal radiographs may get more injections and physical therapy prior to surgical intervention.

SURGICAL INTERVENTION

- Subacromial decompression:
  - Originally described by Neer as an open operation to remove anterior and lateral spurs on the acromion, to

remove the inflamed bursa, and for resection or release of the CA ligament (33).

■ Many believe the development of spurs is a secondary process and is not causative in nature as once thought by Neer (35). The spurs are usually anterior and medial and due to calcification of the CA ligament. Inspection of the acromion and CA ligament should be performed, with the removal of bone only if abnormal ossification has occurred. Frequently an acromioplasty and CA ligament resection are not necessary. This is especially true for articular-sided tears caused by intrinsic pathology.

■ Arthroscopy has led to a less invasive approach to decompression, and the operative goal is usually to convert the acromion to a so-called type I acromion. A bursectomy and inspection of the cuff are included.

■ Pathology of the long head of the biceps tendon is often a part of this syndrome. A thorough inspection of the biceps tendon intra-articularly and into the bicipital groove is necessary. Treatment of these conditions is described in Chapter 50.

■ AC joint surgery (also discussed in Chapter 49):

■ Originally described as an open operation by Mumford (2), 1.5–2.0 cm of the distal clavicle is removal for treatment of AC joint arthritis (10).

■ This surgery relies on the coracoclavicular ligaments providing stabilization of the clavicle. The AC ligaments are repaired at closure.

■ Arthroscopic surgeons have found that resection of 8–10 mm is all that is necessary for adequate decompression and pain relief.

■ Often neglected is medial spurring on the acromion at the AC joint. This should also be resected with either an open or arthroscopic procedure.

■ Rotator cuff repair

■ The indications and necessity of rotator cuff repair remain controversial. The fact that many patients with a full-thickness rotator cuff tear are asymptomatic indicates that the mere presence of a hole in the supraspinatus tendon does not necessitate surgical repair. Many patients also do well with a simple lower rotator cuff rehabilitation program to strengthen and balance the anterior and posterior forces providing humeral head depression (7). This is especially true of chronic tears that present with insidious onset as opposed to those that are traumatic in nature (7). Some surgeons advocate subacromial decompression alone without repair of the rotator cuff (3).

■ On the other hand, Yamaguchi et al. (45) have shown that many tears will progress, leading to a dysfunctional shoulder. Once these tears are large, the muscles will atrophy and undergo fatty degeneration, making a functional repair impossible. A recent study following nonoperative treatment of rotator cuff tears by MRI (28)

revealed that progression of the tear was predicted by age > 60 years, presence of a full-thickness tear, and fatty infiltration of the rotator cuff muscles. Another study in Europe (48) revealed that if initial nonoperative treatment of massive rotator cuff tears was effective, progression of degenerative joint changes occurred over 4 years and often led to reparable tears becoming irreparable.

■ Therefore, most shoulder surgeons will repair rotator cuff tears whenever possible. Burkhart has shown us that balancing the forces of the infraspinatus and subscapularis, without necessarily a "water-tight closure," is often sufficient for a successful repair (4–6,8,47). However, for large, massive tears, many advocate decompression alone or tendon transfers to restore some function of the lower rotator cuff (15). The use and technique of tendon transfer for rotator cuff deficiency are beyond the scope of this book.

❏ Open rotator cuff repair: Open repair of the rotator cuff to the tuberosities of the humerus has been the gold standard for many years (11,30). This requires detachment of a portion of the deltoid off of the acromion. The risk of postoperative deltoid detachment leads some surgeons to take off a sliver of bone to enhance healing. The fear of deltoid failure or detachment has led surgeons to develop less invasive techniques. This has almost completely been abandoned for less invasive techniques.

❏ Mini-open repair (2): Development of shoulder arthroscopy methods has allowed surgeons to perform subacromial decompression by burscoscopy. This allows visualization of the rotator cuff and the ability to address subacromial bursitis, AC joint pathology, and acromial changes such as the development of spurs or ossification of the CA ligament. The mini-open repair takes advantage of this preparation and utilizes a deltoid split to access the rotator cuff tear and perform an open repair (2). The advantage is that the deltoid is preserved (barring overretraction and iatrogenic deltoid detachment); however, large tears are difficult to address with this approach.

❏ Arthroscopic rotator cuff repair: Further development of arthroscopic suture management, arthroscopic knot tying, and use of arthroscopically delivered suture anchors has led to the ability to perform rotator cuff repairs arthroscopically. It is estimated that over 70% of rotator cuff repairs today are done arthroscopically (38). This percentage is increasing, and arthroscopic repair has become standard of care. The ability to preserve cortical bone enhances the strength of fixation while maintaining the ability of the tendon to heal to bone (37). These techniques require a significant amount of practice and skill at arthroscopic techniques. Newer techniques and instruments are being developed, and this procedure now can be done as effectively as open repair (14,16,32,38,44).

❑ Augmentation techniques: Investigators are using platelet-rich plasma (PRP) preparations to enhance healing at the tendon–bone interface. Studies to date have been equivocal, with some studies showing effectiveness (36) and others equivalence (1). Further investigations are pending for the use of PRP as well as stem cells to enhance the biologic milieu and influence healing.

POSTOPERATIVE REHABILITATION

Subacromial Decompression/ Distal Clavicle Resection

■ Following surgery, a good rehabilitation program should be instituted to ensure optimal recovery (43). This may be done with formal physical therapy or with a physician-directed program.

■ Following arthroscopic subacromial decompression, a sling is used for a few days for comfort, and active motion may be resumed immediately. Once motion is achieved, strengthening exercises are started.

■ Strengthening should focus on lower rotator cuff strength and scapular stabilization.

■ Pool therapy is often very effective for shoulder rehabilitation for regaining proper motion and allowing protected use of the shoulder muscles in the recovery period.

■ Return to sports is recommended when full painless motion is recovered following surgery.

Rotator Cuff Repair

■ Following rotator cuff repair, the recovery is slower to allow the cuff to heal to the tuberosities. Histologic studies have shown that this can take up to 12–16 weeks (37).

■ The surgeon will direct postoperative ROM based on the size of the tear and the stability of the repair at the time of surgery.

■ Many surgeons are following a much more conservative rehabilitation program to allow the rotator cuff to start healing before starting motion.

■ Passive motion may be started early, with active motion being delayed for at least 6 weeks.

■ Forward elevation should be delayed as the motion will cause stress on the repair.

■ Formal rehabilitation is often not started for 6 weeks, and some surgeons are using a home-directed rehabilitation program for independent and motivated patients.

■ This will differ for each patient; however, 6–8 weeks are usually sufficient for decompression alone, and 4–6 months are sufficient for rotator cuff repair.

CONCLUSION

■ Rotator cuff pathology is a frequent cause of pain in active patients in all stages of life. It is seen in younger patients participating in throwing or racquet sports, in the weekend athlete developing overuse injuries, and in the elderly patient throwing a baseball with his grandson; the proper diagnosis and treatment of this condition can lead to resolution of symptoms and return the patient to a more functional and usually normal use of their arm.

REFERENCES

1. Barber FA, Hrnack SA, Snyder SJ, Hapa O. Rotator cuff repair healing influenced by platelet-rich plasma construct augmentation. *Arthroscopy*. 2011;27(8):1029–35.

2. Blevins FT, Warren RF, Cavo C, et al. Arthroscopic assisted rotator cuff repair: results using a mini-open deltoid splitting approach. *Arthroscopy*. 1996;12(1):50–9.

3. Burkhart SS. Arthroscopic debridement and decompression for selected rotator cuff tears: clinical results, pathomechanics, and patient selection based on biomechanical parameters. *Orthop Clin North Am*. 1993;24(1):111–23.

4. Burkhart SS. Arthroscopic repair of massive rotator cuff tears: concept of margin convergence. *Tech Shoulder Elbow Surg*. 2000;1:232–9.

5. Burkhart SS. Arthroscopic treatment of massive rotator cuff tears. *Clin Orthop Relat Res*. 2001;(390):107–18.

6. Burkhart SS. Partial repair of massive rotator cuff tears: the evolution of a concept. *Orthop Clin North Am*. 1997;28(1):125–32.

7. Burkhart SS, Esch JC, Jolson RS. The rotator crescent and rotator cable: an anatomic description of the shoulder's "suspension bridge." *Arthroscopy*. 1993;9(6):611–6.

8. Burkhart SS, Nottage WM, Ogilvie-Harris DJ, Kohn HS, Pachelli A. Partial repair of irreparable rotator cuff tears. *Arthroscopy*. 1994;10(4):363–70.

9. Burkhead WZ, Habermeyer P. The rotator cuff: a historical review of our understanding. In: Burkhead WZ Jr, editor. *Rotator Cuff Disorders*. Baltimore: Williams & Wilkins; 1996. p. 3–18.

10. Chen AL, Rokito AS, Zuckerman JD. The role of the acromioclavicular joint in impingement syndrome. *Clin Sports Med*. 2003;22(2):343–57.

11. Cordasco FA, Bigliani LU. The rotator cuff: large and massive tears. Techniques of open repair. *Orthop Clin North Am*. 1997;28(2):179–93.

12. Crenshaw AH, Kilgore WE. Surgical treatment of bicipital tenosynovitis. *J Bone Joint Surg Am*. 1966;48(8):1496–502.

13. DePalma AF, Kruper JS. Long-term study of shoulder joints afflicted with and treated for calcific tendinitis. *Clin Orthop*. 1961;20:61–72.

14. Ellman H, Kay SP, Wirth M. Arthroscopic treatment of full-thickness rotator cuff tears: 2- to 7-year follow-up study. *Arthroscopy*. 1993;9(2):195–200.

15. Gartsman GM. Massive, irreparable tears of the rotator cuff. Results of operative debridement and subacromial decompression. *J Bone Joint Surg Am*. 1997;79(5):715–21.

16. Gartsman GM, Khan M, Hammerman SM. Arthroscopic repair of full-thickness tears of the rotator cuff . *J Bone Joint Surg Am*. 1998; 80(6):832–40.

17. Gerber C, Hersche O, Farron A. Isolated rupture of the subscapularis tendon. Results of operative repair. *J Bone Joint Surg Am*. 1996; 78(7):1015–23.

18. Gerber C, Krushell RJ. Isolated rupture of the tendon of the subscapularis muscle. Clinical features in 16 cases. *J Bone Joint Surg Br.* 1991;73(3):389–94.

19. Greis PE, Kuhn JE, Schultheis J, Hintermeister R, Hawkins R. Validation of the lift-off test and analysis of subscapularis activity during maximal internal rotation. *Am J Sports Med.* 1996;24(5):589–93.

20. Harmon PH. Methods and results in the treatment of 2,580 painful shoulders, with special reference to calcific tendinitis and the frozen shoulder. *Am J Surg.* 1958;95(4):527–44.

21. Hawkins RJ, Kennedy JC. Impingement syndrome in athletes. *Am J Sports Med.* 1980;8(3):151–8.

22. Hertel R, Ballmer FT, Lombert SM, Gerber C. Lag signs in the diagnosis of rotator cuff rupture. *J Shoulder Elbow Surg.* 1996;5(4):307–13.

23. Jobe FW, Jobe CM. Painful athletic injuries of the shoulder. *Clin Orthop Relat Res.* 1983;(173):117–24.

24. Jobe FW, Kvitne RS, Giangarra CE. Shoulder pain in the overhand or throwing athlete: the relationship of anterior stability and rotator cuff impingement. *Orthop Rev.* 1989;18(9):963–75.

25. Jobe FW, Moynes DR. Delineation of diagnostic criteria and a rehabilitation program for rotator cuff injuries. *Am J Sports Med.* 1982; 10(6):336–9.

26. Kelly BT, Kadrmas WR, Kirkendall DT, Speer KP. Optimal normalization tests for shoulder muscle activation: an electromyographic study. *J Orthop Res.* 1996;14(4):647–53.

27. MacDonald PB, Clark P, Sutherland K. An analysis of the diagnostic accuracy of the Hawkins and Neer subacromial impingement signs. *J Shoulder Elbow Surg.* 2000;9(4):299–301.

28. Mamar E, Harris C, White L, Tomlinson G, Shashank M, Boynton E. Outcome of nonoperative treatment of symptomatic rotator cuff tears monitored by magnetic resonance imaging. *J Bone Joint Surg Am.* 2009;91(8):1898–906.

29. McFarland EG, Hsu CY, Neira C, O'Neil O. Internal impingement of the shoulder: a clinical and arthroscopic analysis. *J Shoulder Elbow Surg.* 1999;8(5):458–60.

30. McLaughlin HL. Lesions of the musculotendinous cuff of the shoulder. The exposure and treatment of tears with retraction. *Clin Orthop Relat Res.* 1944;(304):3–9.

31. Moseley HF. The results of nonoperative and operative treatment of calcified deposits. *Surg Clin North Am.* 1963;43:1505–6.

32. Murray TF Jr, Lajtai G, Mileski RM, Snyder SJ. Arthroscopic repair of medium to large full-thickness rotator cuff tears: outcome at 2- to 6-year follow-up. *J Shoulder Elbow Surg.* 2002;11(1):19–24.

33. Neer CS II. Anterior acromioplasty for the chronic impingement syndrome in the shoulder: a preliminary report. *J Bone Joint Surg Am.* 1972;54(1):41–50.

34. Neer CS II. Impingement lesions. *Clin Orthop Relat Res.* 1983;(173):70–7.

35. Nirschl RP. Rotator cuff tendinitis: basic concepts of pathoetiology. *Instr Course Lect.* 1989;38:439–45.

36. Randelli P, Arrigoni P, Rangone V, Aliprandi A, Ciapitza P. Platelet rich plasma in arthroscopic rotator cuff repair: a prospective RCT study, 2-year follow-up. *J Shoulder Elbow Surg.* 2011;20(4):518–28.

37. St Pierre P, Olson EJ, Elliott JJ, O'Hair KC, McKinney LA, Ryan J. Tendon-healing to cortical bone compared with healing to a cancellous trough. A biomechanical and histological evaluation in goats. *J Bone Joint Surg.* 1995;77(12):1858–66.

38. Tauro JC. Arthroscopic rotator cuff repair: analysis of technique and results at 2- and 3-year follow-up. *Arthroscopy.* 1998;14(1):45–51.

39. Valadie AL III, Jobe CM, Pink MM, Ekman EF, Jobe FW. Anatomy of provocative tests for impingement syndrome of the shoulder. *J Shoulder Elbow Surg.* 2000;9(1):36–46.

40. Walch G, Boileau P, Noel E, Donnell ST. Impingement of the deep surface of the supraspinatus tendon on the posterosuperior glenoid rim: an arthroscopic study. *J Shoulder Elbow Surg.* 1992;1(5):238–45.

41. Warner JJ, Higgins L, Parsons IM IV, Dowdy P. Diagnosis and treatment of anterosuperior rotator cuff tears. *J Shoulder Elbow Surg.* 2001; 10(1):37–46.

42. Warner JJP, Allen AA, Gerber C. Diagnosis and management of subscapularis tendon tears. *Techn Orthop.* 1994;9(2):116–25.

43. Wilk KE, Arrigo C. Current concepts in the rehabilitation of the athletic shoulder. *J Orthop Sports Phys Ther.* 1993;18(1):365–78.

44. Wilson F, Hinov V, Adams G. Arthroscopic repair of full-thickness tears of the rotator cuff: 2- to 14-year follow-up. *Arthroscopy.* 2002;18(2):136–44.

45. Yamaguchi K, Tetro AM, Blam O, Evanoff BA, Teefey SA, Middleton WD. Natural history of asymptomatic rotator cuff tears: a longitudinal analysis of asymptomatic tears detected sonographically. *J Shoulder Elbow Surg.* 2001;10(3):199–203.

46. Yocum LA. Assessing the shoulder. History, physical examination, differential diagnosis, and special tests used. *Clin Sports Med.* 1983;2(2):281–9.

47. Yoo JC, Ahn JH, Koh KH, Lim KS. Rotator cuff integrity after arthroscopic repair for large tears with less-than-optimal footprint coverage. *Arthroscopy.* 2009;25(10):1093–100.

48. Zingg PO, Jost B, Sukthankar A, Buhler M, Pfirrmann CW, Gerber C. Clinical and structural outcomes of nonoperative management of rotator cuff tears. *J Bone Joint Surg Am.* 2007;89(9):1928–34.

Sternoclavicular, Clavicular, and Acromioclavicular Injuries

49

Nicholas A. Bontempo and Augustus D. Mazzocca

INTRODUCTION

- Injuries to the clavicle and its articulations are very common.

- High-energy injuries have been seen in increasing frequency as more people participate in higher risk sports such as mountain biking and rollerblading.

- Because man is an upper extremity–dependant animal, these injuries can lead to significant disabilities and limitations.

STERNOCLAVICULAR JOINT

- Injury to the sternoclavicular (SC) joint is very uncommon. In one large study conducted by Rowe and Marble, out of 1,603 shoulder girdle injuries, there was only a 3% incidence of SC joint injuries (65). This is in comparison to an 85% incidence of glenohumeral injuries and 12% incidence of acromioclavicular (AC) dislocations. That being said, it has also been commented that SC joint dislocations are not as rare as posterior glenohumeral dislocations.

- The SC joint is the only true joint connecting the axial skeleton to the shoulder girdle (Fig. 49.1).

- Despite having such an important role, the SC joint lacks inherent bony stability and relies solely on ligamentous and capsular attachments.

Anatomy and Biomechanics

- The SC joint represents the articulation of the proximal end of the clavicle with the sternum and is a diarthrodial joint.

- Although the clavicle is the first long bone in the body to ossify during the fifth intrauterine week, the medial clavicular epiphysis is the last epiphysis to close. Closure of the medial clavicular epiphysis typically begins at age 18 and is usually fused to the clavicular shaft by age 25. It has even been documented in autopsy studies that complete union of the medial clavicular epiphysis may not occur until age 31 (25).

- Similar to the AC joint, the SC joint has an intra-articular disc, or meniscal homologue. Unlike the AC joint, however, the articular surface of the medial clavicle of the SC joint is covered with fibrocartilage.

- The SC joint is incongruous as the medial clavicle is enlarged, bulbous, and saddle-shaped, whereas the clavicular notch of the sternum is concave. Because there is such a large discrepancy in shape and size of the clavicle with the sternum, there is relatively little to no bony stability of the joint. In fact, less than half of the medial clavicle actually articulates with the sternum. It has been shown that in 2.5% of patients, the inferior aspect of the medial clavicle actually articulates with the superior aspect of the first rib (42).

- The SC joint articulation is held in place by the SC capsular ligaments, the costoclavicular ligaments, and the infraclavicular ligaments (Fig. 49.2).

- There are two parts of the capsular ligament: the anterior and posterior portions. The capsular ligaments help to support and reinforce the anterosuperior and posterior SC joint. Of the ligaments surrounding the SC joint, the capsular ligament is the strongest and most important structure preventing upward displacement of the medial clavicle (62).

- The intra-articular disc ligament arises from the junction of the sternum and first rib and attaches on the superior and posterior aspects of the medial clavicle, after passing directly through the SC joint. The fibers of the intra-articular disc ligament blend into the fibers of the capsular ligaments and help to separate the SC joint into medial and lateral compartments. It prevents medial displacement of the clavicle with compression.

- The costoclavicular ligament consists of an anterior and posterior fasciculus with an interpositional bursa (62). The anterior and posterior fasciculi cross over one another, which helps to provide rotational stability of the SC joint during overhead elevation (67). The anterior fasciculus helps to resist upward rotation and lateral displacement of the medial clavicle. The fibers of the posterior fasciculus resist downward rotation and medial displacement of the medial clavicle.

- Connecting the two clavicles is the interclavicular ligament, which connects the superomedial aspect of the clavicles and the

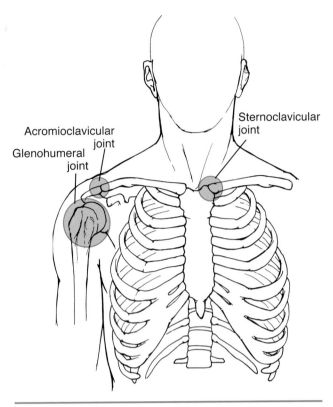

Figure 49.1: Anterior view of the bones and joints of the shoulder complex.

capsular ligaments. The purpose of this ligament is to maintain "shoulder poise," by holding the clavicle and shoulder up (67).

■ Despite the presence of the ligaments and capsule stabilizing the SC joint, a relatively large amount of motion is still seen. There is approximately 30–35 degrees of upward elevation, 35 degrees of translation in the anterior to posterior plane, and 50 degrees of rotation around the longitudinal axis of the clavicle (12,20).

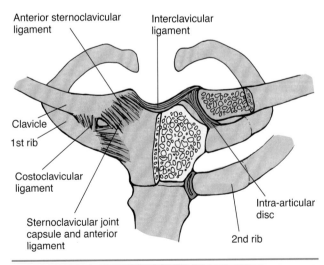

Figure 49.2: Sternoclavicular joint.

Classification

■ The SC joint can be dislocated anteriorly or posteriorly and be the result of traumatic or atraumatic injury (Fig. 49.3). Anterior and posterior dislocations are described based on the location of the medial clavicle with respect to the sternum. Of the 2 types of dislocations, anterior dislocations are far more common.

■ Atraumatic instability of the SC joint can either be acquired or congenital in etiology. The SC joint may subluxate or dislocate with overhead motion in patients who have systemic ligamentous laxity. Typically, atraumatic instability is not associated with pain.

■ Traumatic injury to the SC joint is the most common etiology. Motor vehicle collisions and sports participation are the top two causes of traumatic SC joint injury (43–45). Traumatic SC joint injuries have been classified into 3 types.

   ■ Type 1: mild sprain, SC joint is stable and ligaments are intact

   ■ Type 2: moderate sprain, SC joint subluxates and there is partial disruption of ligaments and capsule

   ■ Type 3: severe sprain, SC joint is dislocated and ligaments and capsule are completely disrupted

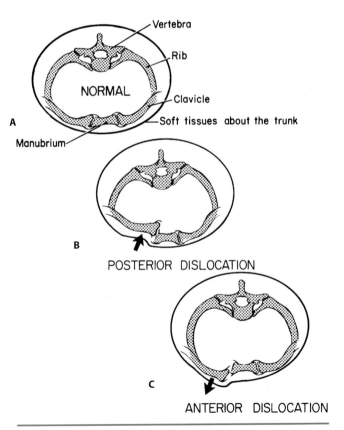

Figure 49.3: Cross sections through the thorax at the level of the SC joint. **A:** Normal anatomical relations. **B:** Posterior dislocation of the SC joint. **C:** Anterior dislocation of the SC joint.

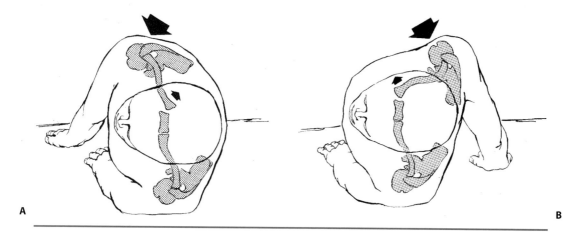

Figure 49.4: Mechanisms that produce anterior or posterior dislocations of the SC joint. **A:** If the patient is lying on the ground and a compression force is applied to the posterolateral aspect of the shoulder, the medial end of the clavicle will be displaced posteriorly. **B:** When the lateral compression force is directed from the anterior position, the medial end of the clavicle is dislocated anteriorly.

Mechanism of Injury

■ Posterior dislocations of the SC joint typically occur as the result of a direct force to the anteromedial clavicle, as can happen during a motor vehicle collision, as a result of the steering wheel hitting the clavicle, or a direct kick to the chest (Figs. 49.4 and 49.5).

■ Anterior dislocations, on the other hand, rarely occur as a result of direct trauma. Instead, anterior dislocations can occur when an anterolateral force is applied to the clavicle and the shoulder is rolled backward. In three separate studies looking at SC joint dislocations, an indirect force was the most common mechanism of injury (9,26).

■ Rockwood describes a common mechanism of indirect SC joint dislocation — a pile-up during a football game (26). One player usually falls to the ground with the ball. Other players begin to jump and fall on top of the first player.

Physical Examination

■ Often with an acute dislocation, either anterior or posterior, palpable step-off at the SC junction can be appreciated (Fig. 49.6).

■ Posterior dislocations, although rare, have more significant symptoms and implications.

　■ Posterior dislocations can be associated with venous congestion present in the neck or ipsilateral upper extremity from compression on the subclavian vessels (Fig. 49.7).

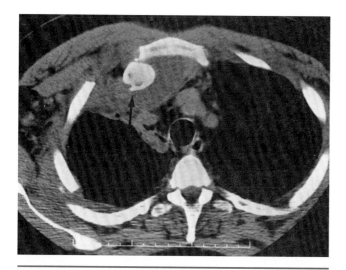

Figure 49.5: Axial CT of a posterior SC joint dislocation that occurred when the driver's chest impacted the steering wheel during a motor vehicle accident. The vehicle was totaled, and the steering wheel was fractured from the driving column.

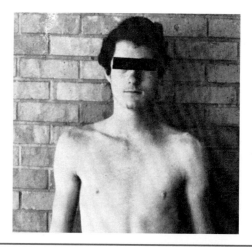

FIGURE 49.6: Clinical view of a patient with a left posterior SC joint dislocation. Notice the difference in appearance of the SC joint from the uninjured (right) side.

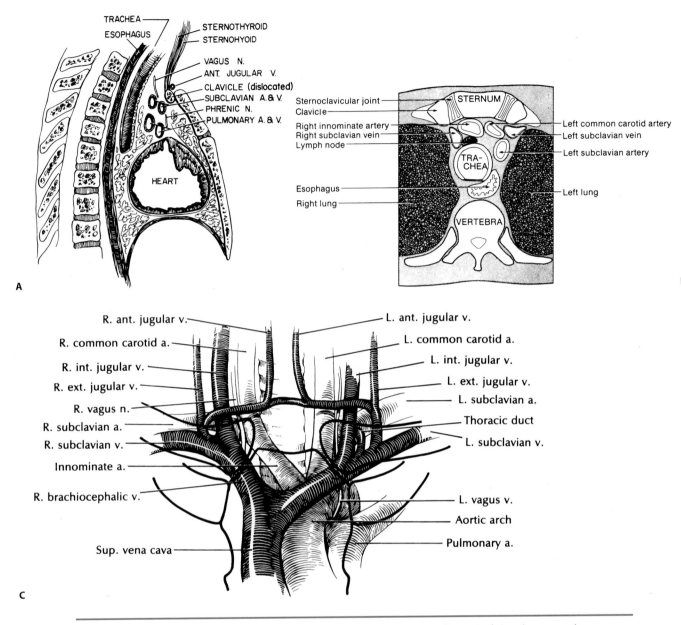

Figure 49.7: Applied anatomy of the vital structures posterior to the SC joint. **A and B:** Sagittal views in cross section demonstrating the structures posterior to the SC joint. **C:** A diagram demonstrating the close proximity of the major vessels posterior to the SC joint.

- ▪ The posteriorly displaced clavicle can also compress the trachea or esophagus (Fig. 49.8).
- ▪ As such, patients may complain of dyspnea, a choking sensation, difficulty swallowing, or a tight feeling in the throat.
- ▪ In the most severe cases, the posterior dislocation can result in complete shock or a pneumothorax.
- ▪ For patients with a type 1 injury (mild sprain), there is usually mild to moderate pain associated with movement of the upper extremity. Instability is usually absent, but the SC joint may be tender to palpation and slightly swollen. With this injury, the ligaments remain intact so the joint should not be unstable.

- ▪ Type 2 injuries (moderate sprain) are associated with partial disruption of the ligaments. There may be some instability or subluxation when the joint is manually stressed, but it is not grossly dislocated or dislocatable. These patients usually have more swelling and pain than patients with type 1 injuries, and the SC joint is more tender to palpation.
- ▪ Type 3 (severe sprain) injury results in complete dislocation, either anterior or posterior, of the SC joint. Patients with this injury present with severe pain that is exacerbated by any movement of the upper extremity. The ipsilateral shoulder may appear protracted in comparison to the contralateral uninjured shoulder. Patients will often hold the affected

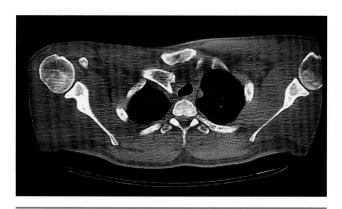

Figure 49.8: Axial CT image showing a posterior SC joint dislocation with compression of the trachea.

arm across the chest in an adducted position and support it with the contralateral arm. The head may be tilted toward the side of the injured clavicle. Examination of the patient lying supine on the examining table will lead to a worsening of symptoms, and the involved shoulder will not lie flat on the table.

Radiologic Evaluation

- A standard anteroposterior (AP) x-ray of the chest or SC joint may suggest an injury to the SC joint; however, this is not the best view for visualizing the joint.

- The serendipity view is the best view to visualize the SC joint. It is taken by tilting the x-ray tube 40 degrees cephalad and centered on the sternum (Fig. 49.9).

- Computed tomography (CT) scan of the chest should include a special note to the radiology technician to do views of the bilateral SC joint for comparison. With a CT scan, axial sections

can be viewed of both the injured and uninjured sides on one image. Subtle differences from side to side can be picked up more easily by the physician looking at the axial views.

Nonoperative Treatment

- Type 1 and 2 injuries are often treated nonoperatively. Nonoperative treatment consists of a short period of immobilization in a sling, anti-inflammatory medication, and ice.

- After a short period of immobilization, the patient can gradually return back to activities based on his or her own level of comfort.

- As in type 2 injuries where the clavicle is subluxated, the joint can be reduced by retracting the shoulders in a figure-of-eight brace. This treatment modality can be incorporated whether the subluxation is anterior or posterior.

- When the SC joint is completely dislocated, as seen in a type 3 injury, an attempt can be made at closed reduction.

- For an anterior dislocation, the patient should be placed supine with a roll in the center of the back between the shoulder blades (Fig. 49.10).
  - This positioning allows the scapula to assume a retracted position and pull the clavicle laterally.
  - A gentle pressure can then be applied to the anteromedial clavicle in order to reduce.
  - Anterior dislocations are often easy to reduce; however, they are usually unstable and will dislocate once the pressure is released.
  - If, however, the SC joint maintains reduction after closed means, the patient should be immobilized in a soft figure-of-eight brace for a period of 6 weeks.

- Prior to any attempt at closed reduction of posteriorly displaced clavicle, injury to local vessels, heart, and lung need to be ruled out.

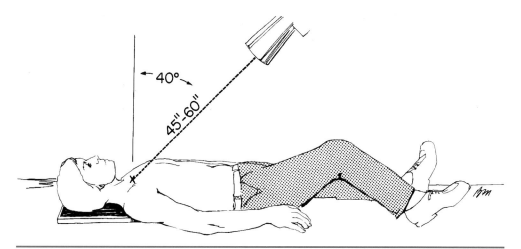

40°

45"–60"

Figure 49.9: Serendipity view. Positioning of the patient to take the "serendipity" view of the SC joints. The x-ray tube is tilted 40 degrees from the vertical position and aimed directly at the manubrium. The nongrid cassette should be large enough to receive the projected images of the medial halves of both clavicles. In children, the tube distance from the patient should be 45 inches; in thicker-chested adults, the distance should be 60 inches.

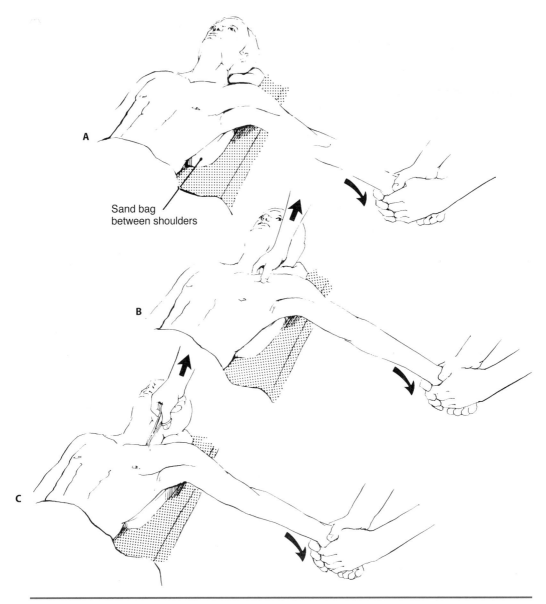

Sand bag
between shoulders

Figure 49.10: Technique for closed reduction of the sternoclavicular joint. **A:** The patient is positioned supine with a sandbag placed between the two shoulders. Traction is then applied to the arm against countertraction in an abducted and slightly extended position. In anterior dislocations, direct pressure over the medial end of the clavicle may reduce the joint. **B:** In posterior dislocations, in addition to the traction, it may be necessary to manipulate the medial end of the clavicle with the fingers to dislodge the clavicle from behind the manubrium. **C:** In stubborn posterior dislocations, it may be necessary to sterilely prepare the medial end of the clavicle and use a towel clip to grasp around the medial clavicle to lift it back into position.

■ Closed reduction of a posterior dislocation should be done in the operating room with the patient under general anesthesia (Fig. 49.11).

  ▪ Similar to an anterior dislocation, the patient should lay supine with a roll between the scapula.

  ▪ Traction should then be applied to the abducted arm while it is slowly extended. Often the joint will reduce with this maneuver; if not, the clavicle can be manipulated with fingers or a towel clip.

■ The towel clip can be used to grasp the medial clavicle under sterile conditions and pull it anteriorly in order to achieve reduction.

■ Posterior dislocations are usually stable once reduced.

■ It is important to have a vascular surgeon available if the patient is taken to the operating room for an attempted closed reduction because of the potential complications that may arise as a result of the injury or the attempt at reduction.

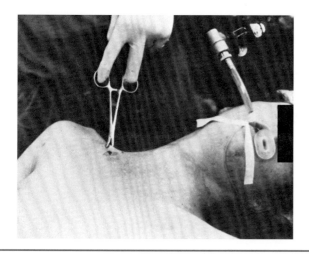

Figure 49.11: Posterior dislocation of the right SC joint can be reduced in the operating room under general anesthesia. A rolled towel should be applied between the patient's shoulder blades. A towel clip can be applied to the medial aspect of the clavicle and the clavicle can be pulled anteriorly.

■ The patient with a reduced SC joint should then be placed in a figure-of-eight brace for 4–6 weeks while the ligaments heal.

Operative Treatment

■ Most SC joint dislocations are best managed nonoperatively and either left unreduced or attempted to be closed reduced.

■ Surgical stabilization of the clavicle is not recommended by most authors (28,61). In most cases, the benefits of surgery are outweighed by the risks.

■ Numerous complications have been reported in the literature, including infection, recurrence, poor cosmesis, and hardware migration.

■ If patients develop symptomatic SC joint instability, then several surgical options exist.

■ Good long-term outcomes have been reported in patients who have medial clavicle excision or SC joint reconstruction for SC joint instability (50).

■ In a biomechanical analysis of reconstructions for SC joint instability, Spencer and Kuhn tested three SC joint fixation methods in a cadaveric study (68). They concluded that figure-of-eight semitendinosus reconstruction provided superior biomechanical properties to subclavius tendon reconstruction and intramedullary ligament reconstruction.

■ Cautiously recommended in the recent literature is a 2-stage approach for SC joint instability (77).

■ The first stage involves fixation of the medial clavicle to the sternum with a concomitant midclavicle osteotomy to offload the fixation at the SC joint.

■ The second stage, usually performed 4 months after the first, involves removal of the hardware at the SC joint and plate osteosynthesis at the osteotomy site.

■ Any surgery being performed for a posterior SC joint dislocation should be done with a cardiothoracic surgeon present due to risk of injury to surrounding structures.

CLAVICLE

■ The clavicle grows through intramembranous ossification like the skull and scapula.

■ Ossification begins at the fifth week of gestation, and it is the first bone to ossify.

■ It is also the last bone to finish growing as the medial physis closes at age 23–25 years.

Anatomy and Biomechanics

■ The clavicle is a subcutaneous double S-shaped bone that articulates with the sternum and the scapula via the SC and AC joints, respectively (Fig. 49.12).

■ The acromial end of the clavicle is more broad and flat than the sternal end.

■ The undersurface of the acromial end has bony projections called the conoid tubercle and trapezoid line. These projections mark the attachment sites of the conoid and trapezoid ligaments, respectively, of the coracoclavicular ligament complex.

■ The trapezius, sternocleidomastoid, and sternohyoid muscles insert on the posterior-superior border of the clavicle (Figs. 49.13 and 49.14).

■ The deltoid, clavicular head of the pectoralis major, and subclavius muscles originate from the anterior inferior surface of the clavicle.

■ The clavicle acts as a strut that connects the upper limb to the trunk and allows the arm to hang freely.

■ The clavicle also functions to protect the neurovascular structures running from the neck to the arm.

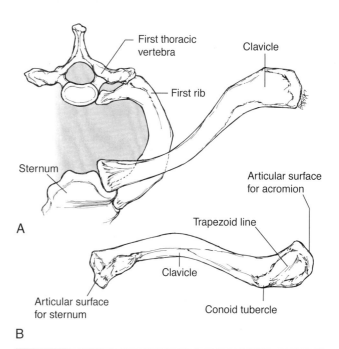

Figure 49.12: View of the superior surface **(A)** and inferior surface **(B)** of the clavicle.

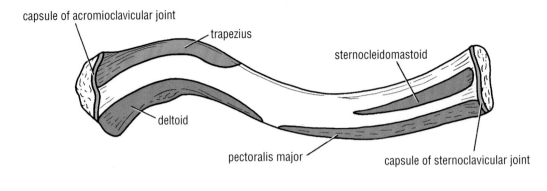

superior surface

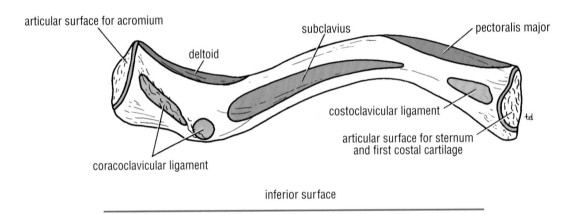

inferior surface

Figure 49.13: Important muscular and ligamentous attachments to the right clavicle.

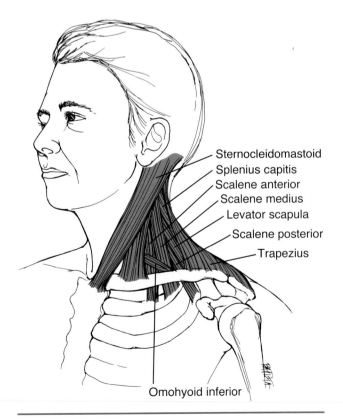

Figure 49.14: Muscles between the clavicle and the scapula.

Clavicle Fractures

■ Clavicle fractures are very common fractures, accounting for nearly 5%–15% of all fractures

■ Classification

   ■ Allman (3) created the classification system that is still used today (Fig. 49.15).

      ❏ Type I – middle third clavicle fractures

      ❏ Type II – lateral third clavicle fractures

      ❏ Type III – medial third clavicle fractures

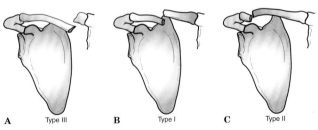

Figure 49.15: A: Fracture of the medial third of the clavicle. **B:** Fracture of the middle third of the clavicle. **C:** Fracture of the lateral third of the clavicle. From Bucholz RW, Heckman JD, Court-Brown C, et al., editors. *Rockwood and Green's Fractures in Adults.* 6th ed. Philadelphia (PA): Lippincott Williams & Wilkins; 2006. 2400 p.

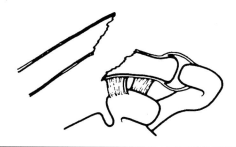

Figure 49.16: Lateral clavicle fracture with intact coracoclavicular ligaments. From Rockwood CA Jr, Green DP, Bucholz RW, Heckman JD, editors. *Rockwood and Green's Fractures in Adults.* 4th ed. Vol. 1. Philadelphia (PA): Lippincott-Raven; 1996. 1118 p.

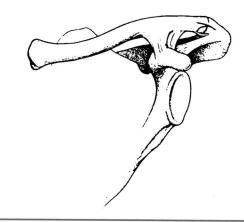

Figure 49.18: Intra-articular lateral clavicle fracture involving the AC joint, but coracoclavicular ligaments remain intact. From Rockwood CA Jr, Green DP, Bucholz RW, Heckman JD, editors. *Rockwood and Green's Fractures in Adults.* 4th ed. Vol. 1. Philadelphia (PA): Lippincott-Raven; 1996. 1118 p.

- In 1968, Neer (54) further divided lateral clavicle fractures into three types.
  - ❏ Type I – lateral clavicle fracture with intact coracoclavicular ligaments (Fig. 49.16)
  - ❏ Type II – lateral clavicle fracture with torn coracoclavicular ligaments (Fig. 49.17)
  - ❏ Type III – intra-articular lateral clavicle fracture involving the AC joint, but coracoclavicular ligaments remain intact (Fig. 49.18)
- Of all clavicle fractures, 80% involve the middle third of the clavicle, and 10%–15% involve the lateral third of the clavicle.
- Clavicle fractures most commonly result from a fall on the lateral aspect of the shoulder, but can also result from a direct blow (Fig. 49.19).
- Traditionally, clavicle fractures have been treated nonoperatively with a reported healing rate of 99% (53,70). More recent studies have shown that the clavicle fracture nonunion rate is actually higher than previously reported, at around 15%–25% (22,34,57,58).
- With midshaft clavicle fractures, the medial fragment is displaced superomedially due to the pull of the sternocleidomastoid and sternohyoid muscles. The lateral fragment is displaced inferolaterally due to gravity and the pull of the deltoid, trapezius, and pectoralis major muscles (Fig. 49.20).

Physical Examination

- Typically, patients present with a clear history of falling on the lateral aspect of their shoulder or having a direct blow to the clavicle.
- It is important to assess the quality of the skin over the clavicle to make sure that the skin is not ischemic, open, or compromised in any way.
- A complete neurovascular exam is important in order to ensure that there has been no injury to the subclavian vessels or brachial plexus.
- Fractures of the clavicle may occur in isolation, but be sure to assess the scapula, humerus, and ribs for other fractures that may be concomitantly present.

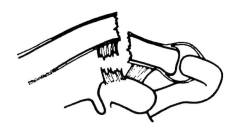

Figure 49.17: Lateral clavicle fracture with torn coracoclavicular ligaments. From Rockwood CA Jr, Green DP, Bucholz RW, Heckman JD, editors. *Rockwood and Green's Fractures in Adults.* 4th ed. Vol. 1. Philadelphia (PA): Lippincott-Raven; 1996. 1118 p.

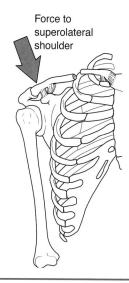

Force to superolateral shoulder

Figure 49.19: The most common mechanism of clavicle fracture is a fall on the superolateral shoulder. Since the SC ligaments are extremely strong, the force exits the clavicle in the midshaft.

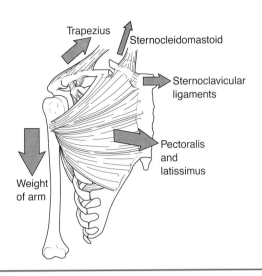

Figure 49.20: The displacing forces on a midshaft clavicle fracture.

Radiologic Evaluation

- Like other fractures, in order to unders and the displacement and angulation of the fracture, views in two different planes are needed (Fig. 49.21). Obtaining an AP of the clavicle and a 45-degree cephalic tilt AP usually suffice (8). Also a bilateral Zanca view can be helpful for side-to-side comparison (Fig 49.22).

- If there is any confusion regarding the fracture pattern and displacement, a CT scan can be ordered.

- An axillary view is often helpful in lateral third clavicle fractures to assess posterior displacement of the medial fragment.

Treatment

- Traditionally clavicle fractures have been treated nonoperatively, regardless of the amount of shortening or displacement.

- Surgical treatment of clavicle fractures of all types has been increasing given recent literature findings supporting better functional outcomes (16).

- Certain cases where surgery is indicated include:
  - Open fractures
  - Tenting of the skin, when the skin integrity is compromised
  - Neurovascular injury that is present or is getting progressively worse
  - Floating shoulder injuries where there is an unstable scapula fracture including the glenoid along with a fracture of the clavicle
  - Polytrauma patient where traditional methods of immobilization are difficult

- A relative indication for midshaft clavicle fractures is > 100% displacement and ≥ 2 cm of shortening (16).

- Other relative indications are for patients who are unhappy with the cosmetic appearance of their deformity or patients who cannot tolerate immobilization due to underlying medical issues such as neurologic conditions, parkinsonism, and seizure disorders.

Nonoperative Treatment

- Nonoperative care still remains the treatment of choice for most fractures of the clavicle shaft, especially those that are minimally displaced or nondisplaced.

- Other instances where these fractures should be treated nonoperatively are in the elderly, patients with significant medical comorbidities, or noncompliant patients.

- There is no technique available to successfully close reduce and maintain position of a clavicle fracture.

- Options for immobilization for clavicle fractures include sling, sling and swathe, or figure-of-eight brace (Fig. 49.23).

- Studies have shown that there is no difference in terms of functional outcomes of fractures with any of the previously

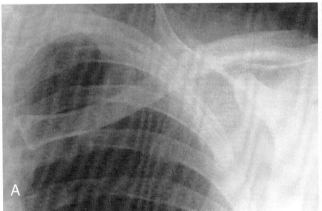
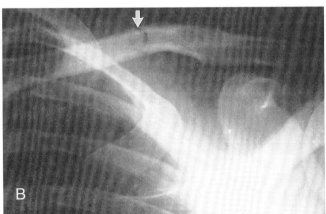

Figure 49.21: A: Nonangulated AP clavicle. Note that no fracture line is visible on this view. **B:** Angulated clavicle. Observe that with 15-degree cephalad tube angulation, the fracture line is clearly evident (*arrow*). *Comment*: In evaluation of clavicular trauma, specific clavicle projections must be obtained to demonstrate fractures, particularly through the midportion of the clavicle. (Courtesy of Kenneth E. Yochum, DC, St. Louis, Missouri.)

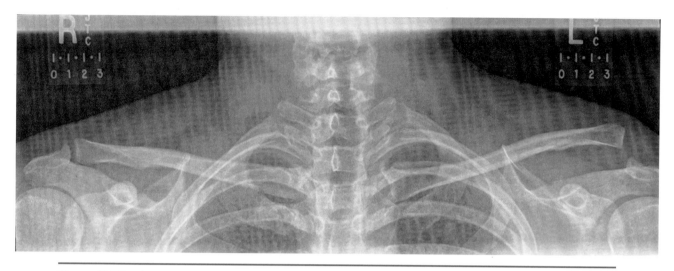

Figure 49.22: Bilateral Zanca view is an important view for making side to side comparisons of the AC joints, SC joints, and clavicles.

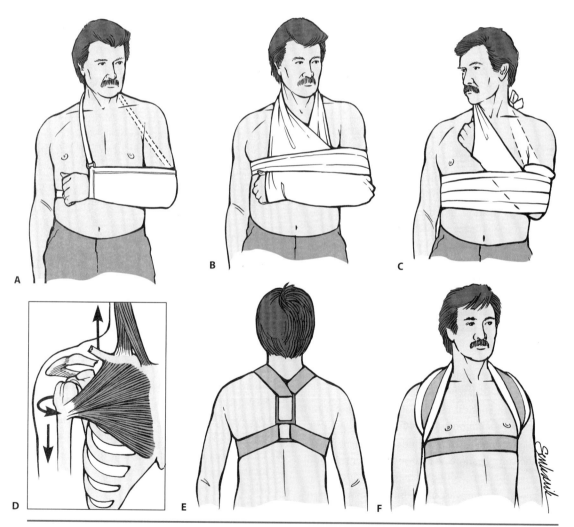

Figure 49.23: Immobilization bandages: used for clavicle fractures: **(A)** commercial sling and swathe, **(B)** conventional sling and swathe, and **(C)** stockinette Velpeau and swathe; **(D)** used for fractures of the clavicle: **(E)** clavicular strap, posterior view, and **(F)** clavicular strap, anterior view.

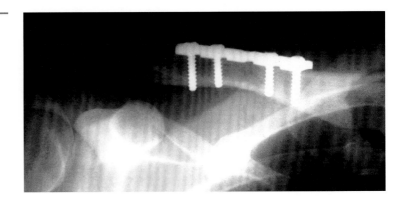

Figure 49.24: Midshaft clavicle fracture fixed with a four-hole plate. A minimum of 6 cortices on each fracture segment must be purchased for adequate fixation.

mentioned forms of immobilization. Overall patients are more satisfied with a sling compared with the other options (4).

- Patients treated with a sling should wear the sling only as needed for comfort and begin shoulder motion as soon as it is comfortable for them.
- The nonunion rate with nonoperative treatment has been reported to be from 15%–30%, with many of the nonunions being symptomatic (36).
- Patients treated nonoperatively often complain of a short, sagging, asymmetric shoulder with functional and cosmetic issues (13,36,58).

Operative Treatment

- Operative treatment is usually of one or two types: plate and screw fixation or intramedullary pin fixation (Fig. 49.24).
- Intramedullary pin fixation has been described and promoted because of less soft tissue disruption. Disadvantages include difficulty inserting a straight intramedullary pin in a curved bone, inability to control rotation, and the potential of migration of the pin in the lung or surrounding neurovascular structures (10,17,31,40).
- In a multicenter prospective clinical trial, 132 patients with a displaced midshaft fracture of the clavicle were randomized to either operative treatment with plate fixation or nonoperative treatment with a sling. Patients treated with surgery had improved functional and subjective outcomes at 1 year compared to patients treated nonoperatively (16).
- Patients treated with surgical plate fixation also have a reported lower rate of malunion and nonunion (16,49,64,79).
- Potential problems with surgery include prominent hardware, soft tissue complications, neurovascular injuries, and often need for a second procedure for hardware removal.
- Lateral third clavicle fractures are often difficult to treat given the location of the fracture. Distal clavicle locking plates have become an option for fixation as have hook plates that hook underneath the acromion. Most surgeons prefer fixation of the clavicle to the coracoid with either a screw or cerclage technique, with excision or saving the lateral clavicle fragment at the surgeon's discretion.

- Lateral third clavicle nonunions often require, in addition to distal clavicle excision, reconstruction of the coracoclavicular ligaments with an autograft or allograft.

ACROMIOCLAVICULAR JOINT

- Injuries of the AC joint represent 9% of all shoulder girdle injuries. It has been previously reported that 43.5% of AC joint injuries occur in patients in their 20s.
- AC joint injuries are five times more common in men and are twice as likely to be incomplete versus complete (65).
- AC joint separations have been found to be the third most common in jury in Division I college hockey teams, and account for as many as 40% of the shoulder injuries seen in National Football League (NFL) quarterbacks (25,42).

Anatomy and Biomechanics

- The articulation of the acromion and the distal clavicle represents a diarthrodial joint.
- There are four planes of motion at this articulation: anterior/posterior and superior/inferior.
- Similar to most joints, the AC joint is surrounded by a capsule, has intra-articular synovium, and has an articular cartilage interface.
- There is a meniscal homologue present within the joint that has a large variation in both shape and size.
- The average size of the adult AC joint is 9 mm by 19 mm, but tremendous variation has been documented (12).
- The true articular portion of the distal clavicle varies in both location and size. Articular cartilage can cover the entire distal clavicle or it can cover a smaller percentage, which can complicate the fixation and treatment of AC joint injuries.
- In the frontal plane, the AC joint line can have 20–50 degrees of lateral inclination (20) (Fig. 49.25).
- Motion at the AC joint is facilitated by the clavicle, which allows up to 20–30 degrees of motion in the vertical, horizontal, and frontal planes (43,45).

■ Rockwood et al. (65) have reported that, with full overhead elevation, the clavicle can rotate up to 40–50 degrees. Most of this motion, however, is achieved with scapular rotation rather than at the AC joint itself.

■ Only about 5–8 degrees of motion have been found to occur at the AC joint with forward elevation and abduction to 180 degrees (65).

■ Motion at the AC joint is necessary for full shoulder range of motion (ROM) due to the coupling of clavicle rotation with scapular motion and arm elevation.

■ Stability at the AC joint is achieved through a combination of both static and dynamic stabilizers.

■ The coracoclavicular, AC, and coracoacromial ligaments comprise the static stabilizers. The dynamic stabilizers include the deltoid and trapezius muscles (Fig. 49.26)

■ For added stability at the AC joint, the superior fibers from the AC ligament blend with the fascia of the deltoid and trapezius muscles.

■ There are four AC ligaments: superior, inferior, anterior, and posterior.

■ The AC joint capsule and the AC ligaments resist movement of the distal clavicle primarily in the horizontal plane (anterior to posterior direction) with respect to the scapula (26).

■ Resistance to posterior translation is important because instability of the distal clavicle in the posterior direction can lead to abutment with the spine of the scapula (44). In sectioning studies where the AC ligaments were serially sectioned, the superior ligament was found to contribute to 56% resistance of posterior clavicle displacement, whereas the posterior ligament contributed to 25%.

■ The fibers of the superior AC ligament coalesce with the dynamic AC joint stabilizers (deltoid and trapezius).

■ The coracoclavicular ligament complex is the primary restraint to vertical (superior to inferior) translation at the AC joint, but it has significant influence in the horizontal plane as well. This complex is comprised of the conoid and trapezoid ligaments.

■ In addition to stabilizing the AC joint in the vertical plane, the coracoclavicular ligaments also strengthen the AC articulation and mediate scapulohumeral motion by attaching the clavicle to the scapula.

■ The conoid ligament is cone shaped, with the apex attaching at the posteromedial side of the base of the coracoid. The base of the conoid ligament attaches posterior to the conoid tubercle on the undersurface of the clavicle.

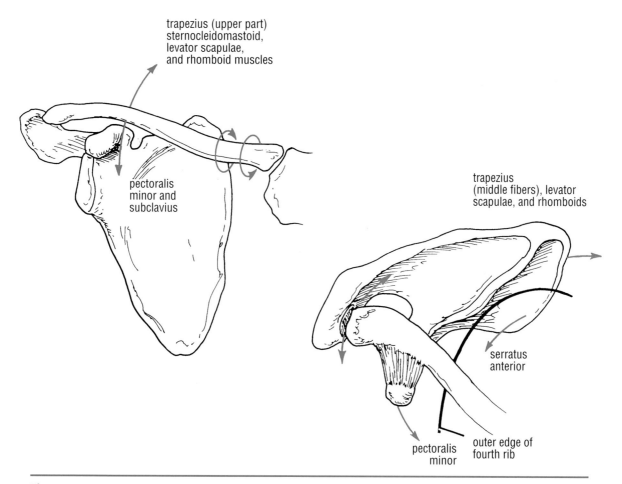

Figure 49.25: The wide range of movements possible at the SC and AC joints gives great mobility to the clavicle and the upper limb.

Anterior view

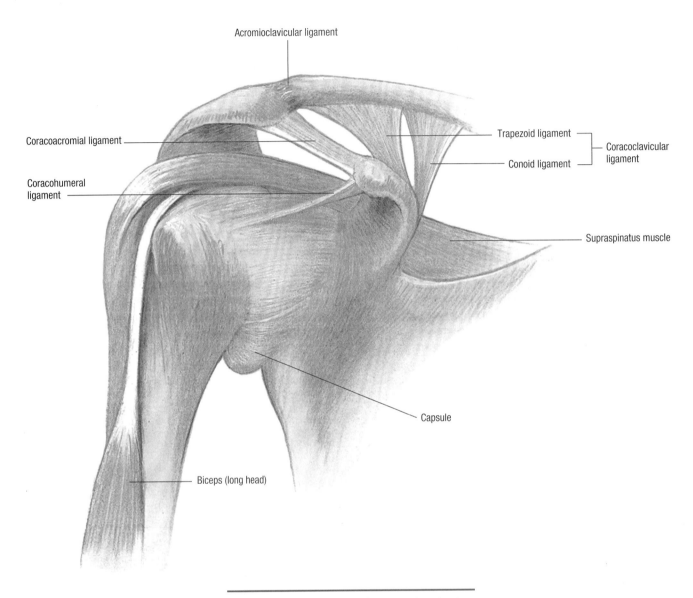

Acromioclavicular ligament

Trapezoid ligament

Coracoclavicular ligament

Conoid ligament

Coracoacromial ligament

Coracohumeral ligament

Supraspinatus muscle

Capsule

Biceps (long head)

Figure 49.26: Shoulder joint ligaments. Anterior view.

■ The trapezoid ligament arises anterior to the conoid ligament at the base of the coracoids and inserts laterally to the conoid ligament on the undersurface of the clavicle.

■ The radiographic anatomic distance between the coracoid and the clavicle has been found to range between 1.1 and 1.3 cm (9). This anatomic distance is important when reviewing radiographs of a suspected AC joint injury and when trying to restore normal functional anatomy during repair or reconstruction of the coracoclavicular ligaments.

■ The bilateral Zanca view is used to compare the coracoclavicular distance of the injured side to the contralateral uninjured side.

Classification

■ The radiographic classification of AC joint injuries represents a continuum of increased soft tissue injury (Fig. 49.27).

  ■ Type I: AC ligament sprain with the AC joint intact

  ■ Type II: AC ligament tear with coracoclavicular ligament intact and AC joint subluxed

  ■ Type III: AC and coracoclavicular ligaments torn and 100% dislocation in joint

  ■ Type IV: complete dislocation with posterior displacement of distal clavicle into or through the trapezius muscle

  ■ Type V: exaggerated superior dislocation of between 100% and 300% dislocation of the joint increasing the

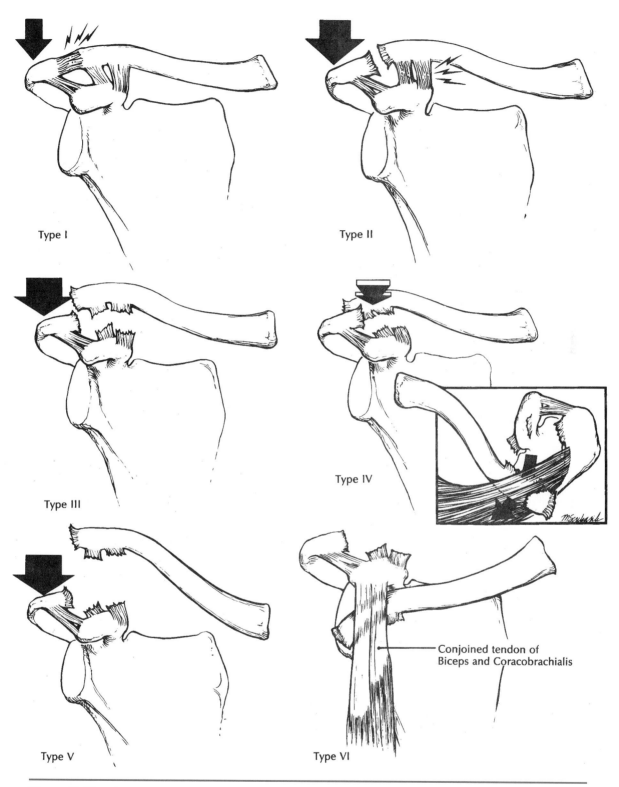

Type I

Type II

Type III

Type IV

Type V

Type VI

Conjoined tendon of
Biceps and Coracobrachialis

Figure 49.27: Schematic drawings of the classification of ligamentous injuries to the AC joint. *Top left:* In the type I injury, a mild force applied to the point of the shoulder does not disrupt either the AC or the coracoclavicular ligaments. *Top right:* A moderate to heavy force applied to the point of the shoulder will disrupt the AC ligaments, but the coracoclavicular ligaments remain intact (type II). *Center left:* When a severe force is applied to the point of the shoulder, both the AC and the coracoclavicular ligaments are disrupted (type III). *Center right:* In a type IV injury, not only are the ligaments disrupted, but the distal end of the clavicle is also displaced posteriorly into or through the trapezius muscle. *Bottom left:* A violent force applied to the point of the shoulder not only ruptures the AC and coracoclavicular ligaments but also disrupts the muscle attachments and creates a major separation between the clavicle and the acromion (type V). *Bottom right:* This is an inferior dislocation of the distal clavicle in which the clavicle is inferior to the coracoid process and posterior to the biceps and coracobrachialis tendons. The AC and coracoclavicular ligaments are also disrupted (type VI).

coracoclavicular ligament distance two to three times including disruption of the deltotrapezial fascia
- Type VI: complete dislocation with inferior displacement of distal clavicle into a subacromial or subcoracoid position

Mechanism of Injury

- Two common mechanisms account for AC joint injury: direct and indirect (Fig. 49.28).
  - The most common mechanism is a result of a direct force to the AC joint. A direct injury occurs when a person falls onto the AC joint with their arm at their side in an adducted position. This is commonly seen in collision sports such as hockey, football, rugby, and karate.
  - An indirect injury to the AC joint can also occur as the result of a fall on an outstretched hand. The fall typically drives the humeral head superiorly into the acromion. In this mechanism of injury, energy is only referred to the AC ligaments, as the coracoclavicular interspace is decreased during loading.

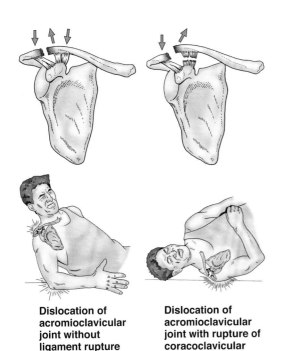

Dislocation of acromioclavicular joint without ligament rupture

Dislocation of acromioclavicular joint with rupture of coracoclavicular ligament

Figure 49.28: Although its extrinsic (coracoclavicular) ligament is strong, the AC joint itself is weak and easily injured by a direct blow. In contact sports such as football, soccer, and hockey, it is not uncommon for dislocation of the AC joint to result from a hard fall on the shoulder with the impact taken by the acromion or from a fall on the outstretched upper limb. Dislocation of the AC joint also can occur when a hockey player is driven violently into the boards. The AC injury, often called a "shoulder separation," is severe when both the AC and coracoclavicular ligaments are torn. When the coracoclavicular ligament tears, the shoulder separates (falls away) from the clavicle because of the weight of the upper limb. Dislocation of the AC joint makes the acromion more prominent, and the clavicle may move superior to this process.

Radiologic Evaluation

- One of the most important things to remember when obtaining an x-ray for evaluation of an AC joint injury is to reduce the penetration by one-third to one-half of that used for a standard glenohumeral x-ray. Failure to do so will result in an over-penetrated (dark) film, which prevents the ability to see small or subtle fractures.
- AP, supraspinatus outlet, and axillary views are the standard views necessary for examining the shoulder.
- As previously mentioned, the axillary view is particularly helpful in visualizing a type IV AC joint injury with a posteriorly displaced distal clavicle.
- When there is a normal coracoclavicular interspace but a complete dislocation of the AC joint, a coracoid fracture should be suspected.
- The best view to visualize a coracoid fracture is the Stryker notch view, which is taken with the patient supine and the palm on their affected side placed on their head. The x-ray beam is then tilted 10 degrees cephalad (Fig. 49.29).
- The Zanca view is the most accurate view to visualize the AC joint.
  - This view is achieved by tilting the x-ray beam 10–15 degrees cephalad and using one-half of the standard penetrance (Fig. 49.30).
  - Because of the significant variation in AC joint anatomy from one side to another, a bilateral Zanca view is recommended to visualize both AC joints on a single x-ray cassette while maintaining the same orientation of the x-ray beam.
  - By visualizing both AC joints on the same cassette, the coracoclavicular distance can be compared from side to side (Fig. 49.31).
- Basmania (7) has described a cross-arm adduction view of the AC joint. This view is taken with the arm forward elevated to 90 degrees and adducted across the body. If the clavicle overrides the acromion on this view, the injury is considered unstable.
- AP stress views are obtained by hanging 5–10 lb of weight from both of the patient's wrists with wrist straps. The use of wrist straps, as opposed to having the patient hold the weight, encourages full muscle relaxation.
  - Coracoclavicular distance is measured and compared between the injured and uninjured sides.
  - Stress x-rays are most useful to differentiate between type II and type III injuries.
  - Literature has shown that the added cost, time, and patient discomfort associated with stress views is not outweighed by their utility.
  - Patients who have complete dislocations (type II, IV, V, or VI) most often have evidence of coracoclavicular widening on standard AP x-rays.
- On standard x-rays, it has been reported by Zanca that the AC joint space is between 1.0 and 3.0 mm (77). This width decreases with age and has been found to be as small as 0.5 mm

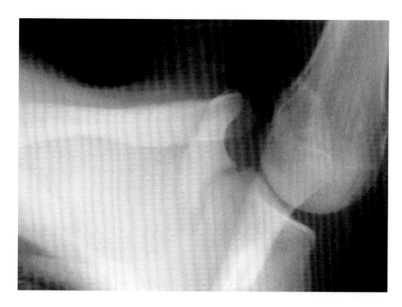

Figure 49.29: A fracture of the base of the coracoid is best seen on a Stryker notch view.

by age 60 (62). As previously mentioned, the coracoclavicular interspace has been found to be between 1.1 and 1.3 cm. Bearden et al. (9) reported that an increase in this interspace by 25%–50%, when compared to the uninjured side, indicates complete disruption of the coracoclavicular ligament.

History and Physical Examination

- Pathology of the AC joint is identified by a reproducible triad of point tenderness at the AC joint, pain with cross-arm adduction, and relief of symptoms by injection of a local anesthetic.

- The cross-arm adduction test creates pain at the AC joint because compression forces at the joint are generated with this maneuver. This test is performed with the arm elevated and internally rotated to 90 degrees and the elbow flexed to 90 degrees. The arm is then slowly adducted across the body.

- In addition, patients with AC joint pathology will complain of pain in the superior anterior aspect of the shoulder. This can be explained, in part, by the innervations of the AC joint and superior glenohumeral joint.

  - Gerber et al. (27) studied the patterns of pain produced by irritation of the AC joint and the subacromial space.

  - They found that irritation of the AC joint was referred to the anterolateral neck in the region of the anterolateral deltoid.

  - Conversely, irritation of the subacromial space resulted in pain referred to the lateral acromion and lateral deltoid; no pain was referred to the neck or trapezius.

  - Impingement of the lateral pectoral nerve is referred anteriorly, and impingement of the suprascapular nerve is referred posteriorly.

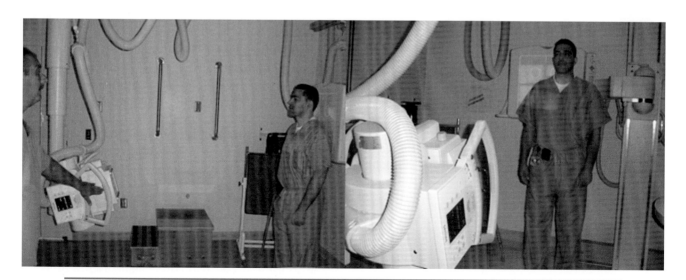

Figure 49.30: A bilateral Zanca view is achieved by tilting the x-ray beam 10–15 degrees cephalad and using one-half of the standard penetrance.

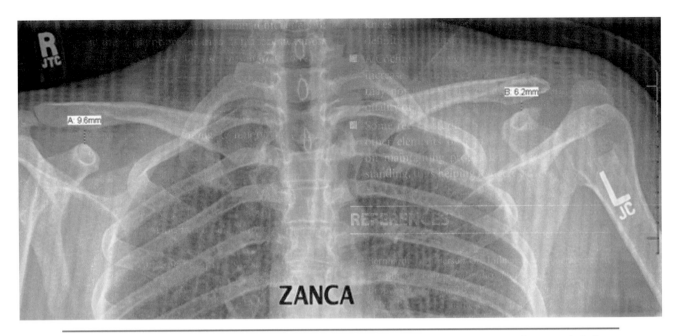

Figure 49.31: An example of a bilateral Zanca view. By visualizing both AC joints on the same cassette, the coracoclavicular distance can be compared from side to side.

- Patients with a type V injury, however, may have pain in the neck or trapezius due to the disruption of the deltotrapezial fascia.
- Examination of the patient with a suspected AC injury should be done with the patient standing or sitting, which allows the weight of the arm to stress the AC joint and exaggerate any deformity (Fig. 49.32).
- The O'Brien test results in active compression across the AC joint.
  - The test is performed by having the patient extend the elbow, fully pronate the forearm (resulting in obligate

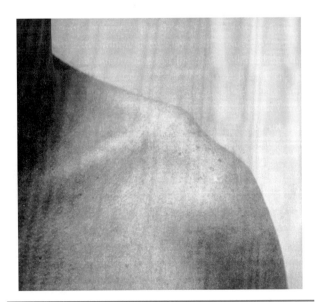

Figure 49.32: Clinical photograph of a patient with a type V AC joint dislocation sitting in an upright position. The weight of the upper extremity exaggerates the deformity.

internal rotation of the humerus), elevate the arm to 90 degrees, and adduct it approximately 10–15 degrees. The patient is then asked to resist a downward force applied by the examiner.

- AC joint pathology is localized to the superior aspect of the shoulder and confirmed by palpation of the examiner over the AC joint.
- If, however, pain is referred to the anterior glenohumeral joint, then labral or biceps pathology should be suspected.
- The O'Brien test is helpful in differentiating AC joint pathology from intra-articular labral pathology.
- Other conditions that have been associated with AC joint pain are pseudogout and synovial chondromatosis.
- In patients with Crohn disease, an aseptic inflammation has been described.
- Patients who have glenohumeral arthritis have been found to have AC joint cysts.
- Distal clavicle osteolysis is a pathologic process resulting in resorption of subchondral bone in the distal clavicle. The condition results from repetitive microtrauma and is commonly seen in weightlifters from bench pressing (Fig. 49.33).

Physical Examination and Radiographic Correlation

- Type I injuries result in minimal to moderate tenderness and swelling over the AC joint.
  - There is no palpable displacement of the joint itself.
  - Patients typically only have minimal pain with movement of the arm.
  - Both the AC and coracoclavicular ligaments are intact, and x-ray examination is normal.

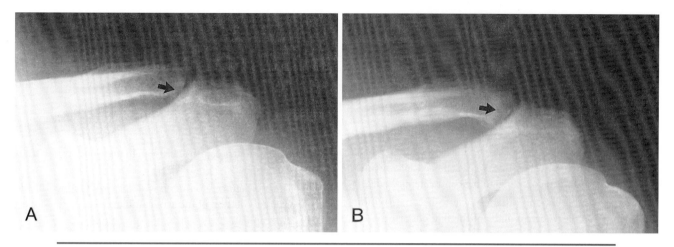

Figure 49.33: A. AC joint. Note that 2 months after trauma to the shoulder, a cystic rarefaction (*arrow*) is present at the inferior aspect of the distal articular surface of the clavicle. B. AP AC joint. Note that there has been extension of the area of rarefaction in the distal clavicle involving the entire distal surface (*arrow*). Observe the smooth and regular articular margins of the acromial surface, differentiating it from inflammatory joint diseases (rheumatoid arthritis and septic arthritis).

- There may be mild soft tissue swelling on x-ray, but there is no widening, separation, or deformity at the AC joint.
- Type II injuries are characterized by moderate to severe pain at the AC joint.
  - The distal end of the clavicle may be palpated to be slightly superior to the acromion, and shoulder motion produces more pain at the AC joint.
  - The distal clavicle is also found to be unstable in the horizontal plane if grasped and moved anteriorly to posteriorly.
  - The AC ligaments are disrupted, but the coracoclavicular ligaments are not.
  - X-rays may demonstrate that the distal clavicle is slightly elevated, but stress x-rays do not show 100% displacement of the clavicle from the acromion.
  - Stress x-rays also demonstrate that the coracoclavicular interspace is the same in both the injured and uninjured shoulders.

- Type III injuries present with the upper extremity in a supported adducted and elevated position to help relieve pain. The distal clavicle may be prominent enough to tent the skin.
  - These patients have a severe amount of pain with tenderness to palpation at the AC joint.
  - Any movement of the arm, especially abduction, creates pain and discomfort, especially for the first 1–3 weeks.
  - The distal clavicle is unstable in both the vertical and horizontal planes because both the AC and coracoclavicular ligaments are disrupted, but the deltoid and trapezial fascia are intact.
  - Both plain and stress x-rays reveal that the distal clavicle is 100% displaced superiorly in relation to the acromion. In actuality, the position of the clavicle is not altered by the injury. The weight of the upper extremity causes the acromion to displace inferiorly in relation to the horizontal plane of the lateral clavicle (Fig. 49.34).

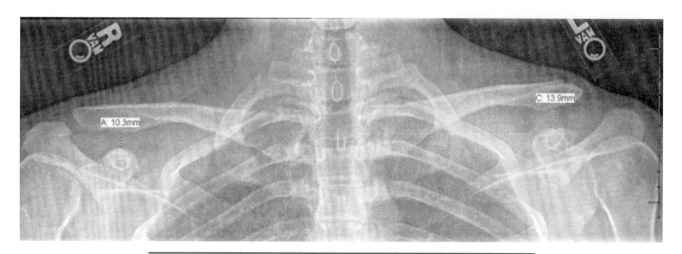

Figure 49.34: Bilateral Zanca view showing superior displacement of the left clavicle.

- A shrug test has been described to differentiate a type III injury from a type V injury. If when the patient shrugs their shoulders the joint reduces, then the deltotrapezial fascia is intact and a type V injury can be ruled out.
- Type IV injuries are characterized by complete dislocation with posterior displacement of the distal clavicle into or through the fascia of the trapezius.
  - Physical examination of these patients is very similar to patients with type III, but examination of the seated patient from above will reveal that the distal clavicle is inclined posteriorly when compared to the contralateral shoulder.
  - It is possible for the distal clavicle to become "button-holed" in the trapezius and tent the skin posteriorly.
  - With a type IV injury, it is also important to examine the SC joint for a concomitant anterior dislocation.
  - The posteriorly displaced clavicle is best appreciated on an axillary x-ray of the shoulder (Fig. 49.35).
- Type V injuries represent a greater degree of soft tissue damage, with the deltoid and trapezial fascia being stripped off the acromion and the clavicle.
  - These injuries present as a more severe type III injury with more pain and a greater amount of displacement at the AC joint.
  - The distal end of the clavicle appears to be grossly displaced superiorly toward the neck.
  - The scapula gets translated anteriorly and inferiorly as it migrates around the thorax.

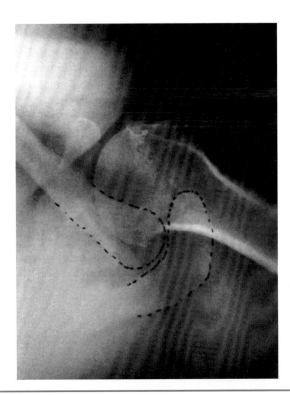

Figure 49.35: Type IV posterior dislocation of the AC joint. Axillary view with the distal clavicle and acromion outlined.

- On x-ray, there is 100%–300% increase in the coracoclavicular interspace.
- Type VI injuries are inferior AC joint dislocations. Three cases have been described by Gerber and Rockwood, and other cases have been described by Patterson, McPhee, and Schwartz (28,50,61,68).
  - None of the cases described in the literature had accompanying vascular injuries.
  - Type VI injuries are usually seen in high-energy polytrauma patients.
  - The mechanism of injury is extreme hyperabduction and external rotation of the arm combined with retraction of the scapula.
  - The distal end of the clavicle can displace either subcoracoid or subacromial. In a subcoracoid dislocation, the clavicle gets stuck behind the conjoined tendon. As such, the acromion is very prominent with a palpable inferior step-off to the superior surface of the coracoids.
  - Associated injuries include clavicle and upper rib fractures and upper root brachial plexus injuries.
  - It is not uncommon for these patients to have transient paresthesias that subside after reduction.

Treatment

- The goal of treatment for AC joint injuries is pain-free shoulder movement with full ROM and stability.
- Most type I and type II injuries are successfully treated nonoperatively with sling, ice, and a 3- to 7-day period of immobilization, although some can become painful later on.
- Type IV, V, and VI AC joint injuries are usually treated operatively due to the morbidity associated with a chronically dislocated joint and soft tissue disruption.
- Controversy exists over the appropriate treatment of type III injuries. There has been a trend to treat these injuries nonoperatively, and if nonoperative management fails, then an operative intervention could be pursued.
- Rockwood has previously reported that in patients who participate in contact sports (football, hockey, soccer, and lacrosse) where the risk of reinjury is high, nonoperative treatment is recommended. In the small group of patients who have persistent pain and are unable to return to work or sports after nonoperative treatment, surgical stabilization is encouraged.
- A meta-analysis report supports nonoperative treatment of type III dislocations (63). This analysis included 1,172 patients; 88% of those who underwent surgery and 87% of those treated nonoperatively had satisfactory outcomes. Complications included the need for further surgery (59% operative vs. 6% nonoperative), infection (6% vs. 1%), and deformity (3% vs. 37%). Pain and ROM were not significantly affected. The authors did not recommend surgery for type III AC joint injuries in young patients.
- A survey of Major League Baseball team physicians regarding treatment modalities for a type III injury in a pitcher was

conducted by McFarland et al. (48) in 1997. Of the physicians surveyed, 69% reported that they would recommend nonoperative treatment for their players. Within the study, 32 pitchers with type III injuries were evaluated. Twenty pitchers were treated nonoperatively and 12 were treated operatively. Eighty percent of the pitchers treated nonoperatively and 91% of those treated operatively had achieved pain relief and normal function.

Nonoperative Treatment

- Nonoperative treatment is typically indicated in type I and type II injuries. Type III injuries are evaluated on a case-by-case basis with regard to treatment.

- The goal of treatment, whether operative or not, is to restore the patient back to their preinjury activity level with a painless shoulder.

- Most nonoperative treatment is centered around a brief period of immobilization in a sling accompanied by ice and oral anti-inflammatory medication if tolerated.

- Particularly in patients with type III injuries, surgery may be indicated if pain persists for 6–8 weeks. However, it is important to remember that at the 2-year follow-up, nonoperatively versus operatively treated type III injuries show no difference in strength (73).

- A specific rehabilitation protocol for athletes has been previously described by Gladstone et al. (29). Their rehabilitation protocol consists of 4 phases:
  - Pain control, immediate protective ROM, and isometric exercises.
  - Strengthening exercises using isotonic contractions.
  - Unrestricted functional participation to increase strength, power, endurance, and neuromuscular control.
  - Return to activity with sports-specific functional drills.

Operative Treatment

- There are four basic types of surgical procedures that have been described for treatment of these injuries. These include:
  - Primary repair of the AC joint with pins, screws, or rods
  - Distal clavicle excision with soft tissue reconstruction (Weaver-Dunn)
  - Anatomic coracoclavicular reconstruction (ACCR)
  - Arthroscopic suture fixation

Primary AC Joint Repair

- AC ligament repair was first advocated by Sage and Salvatore (66) in 1963, who also recommended reinforcement of the superior AC ligament with joint meniscus. Supplementation of this repair with transarticular smooth or threaded pins was subsequently advocated by many surgeons (1,5,6, 9,15,19,23,37,51,52,56,59,78).

- Eskola et al. (21) then did a comparative study of smooth pins, threaded pins, and a cortical screw. Of the 86 patients available for follow-up, 13 had osteolysis, and 8 of the 13 patients were among the 25 patients who were initially treated with a Bosworth screw.

- Treatment with a plate or pins across the AC joint has been described by several other authors, with good to excellent results ranging from 60% to 94% (14,33,35,74).

- Broos et al. (14) compared the Wolter plate to the Bosworth screw and found no significant difference in outcome.

Distal Clavicle Excision with Soft Tissue Reconstruction

- Distal clavicle excision with soft tissue reconstruction was initially described in 1972 as the Weaver-Dunn technique (76). The original description of the procedure involved resection of the distal clavicle followed by release of the coracoacromial ligament from its attachment on the acromion. The detached end of the ligament was then attached to the distal clavicle to help hold it in a reduced position. Although the original description involved a distal clavicle excision, the procedure has also been described without one.

- Arguments have been made that the aforementioned technique for the Weaver-Dunn leads to an obligate anterior displacement of the clavicle based on the location of the coracoid.

- Various other techniques have since been described that include detaching the coracoacromial ligament with a piece of bone attached for transfer. Transfer of the conjoined tendon has most recently been described in 2007, where the lateral half of the tendon is transferred to the distal clavicle (39). After transfer of the conjoined tendon, additional coracoclavicular fixation is achieved through the use of a double loaded Ethibond suture anchor.

- It has been proposed that transfer of the conjoined tendon is superior to the original Weaver-Dunn technique because the functioning coracoacromial ligament is left intact.

Anatomic Coracoclavicular Ligament Reconstruction

- Coracoclavicular ligament repair was first introduced by Bosworth in 1941 through the placement of a percutaneous screw suspension procedure (11). Bearden and Albrecht described reconstruction of the coracoclavicular ligaments through the use of wire loops around the clavicle and coracoids (2,9). Various other materials have also been reported in the literature for use as a loop around the clavicle and coracoids (24,30,41,55,60,71).

- Based on these data, the ACCR was developed with the use of free grafts (46).
  - The ACCR procedure begins with a diagnostic shoulder arthroscopy.
  - Two drill holes are made in the clavicle at the origins of the conoid and trapezoid ligaments.

- A gracilis or semitendinosus autograft or allograft is then looped underneath the coracoid and through two drill holes in the clavicle.
  - The graft is then tied to itself in a figure-of-eight fashion or fixed to the clavicle with interference screws.
- Several biomechanical studies have been completed that illustrate that ACCR more closely approximates the stiffness of the coracoclavicular ligament complex and produces less anterior to posterior translation at the AC joint as compared to the Weaver-Dunn procedure (18,32,47,72).

Arthroscopic Suture Fixation

- Recently in the literature, 2 techniques for restoring the coracoclavicular ligaments without a graft have been described.
  - The first technique involves using 2 suture anchors through four drill holes in the clavicle for fixation (69). The suture anchors are fixed in the coracoid and tied over a bone bridge in the clavicle. As part of this procedure, the coracoacromial ligament is transferred as well.
  - Previously a technique was described using a single suture anchor (38). In a controlled laboratory study on cadaveric shoulders, two tightrope devices were used to reconstruct the coracoclavicular ligaments through 2 single tunnels in the clavicle and coracoid. Both studies report anatomic restoration of the AC joint with favorable biomechanical results (69,75).

Postoperative Care

- During the first 6–8 weeks, the patients wear a brace that provides support and protects the surgical repair against the force of gravity such as the Lerman Shoulder Brace (DJO Inc., Vista, CA) or a Gunslinger Shoulder Orthosis (Hanger Prosthetics & Orthotics, Inc., Bethesda, MD).
- At 8 weeks, the repair has achieved enough stability that upright ROM exercises may be started.
- By 12 weeks, pain-free ROM and strengthening exercises can be started.
- Weight training may begin at 3–5 months postoperatively, and full-contact sports may be resumed at 6 months.

REFERENCES

1. Ahstrom JP Jr. Surgical repair of complete acromioclavicular separation. *JAMA.* 1971;217(6):785–9.
2. Albrecht F, Kohaus H, Stedtfeld HW. [The Balser plate for acromioclavicular fixation]. *Chirurg.* 1982;53(11):732–4.
3. Allman FL Jr. Fractures and ligamentous injuries of the clavicle and its articulation. *J Bone Joint Surg Am.* 1967;49(4):774–84.
4. Andersen K, Jensen PO, Lauritzen J. Treatment of clavicular fractures. Figure-of-eight bandage versus a simple sling. *Acta Orthop Scand.* 1987;58(1):71–4.
5. Augereau B, Robert H, Apoil A. [Treatment of severe acromioclavicular dislocations. A coraco-clavicular ligamentoplasty technique derived from Cadenat's procedure (author's transl)]. *Ann Chir.* 1981;35(9, pt 1):720–2.
6. Bartoníček J, Jehlicka D, Bezvoda Z. [Surgical treatment of acromioclavicular luxation]. *Acta Chir Orthop Traumatol Cech.* 1988;55(4):289–309.
7. Basmania C. *Boston Shoulder Course.* Boston (MA); 2009.
8. Basmania CJ, Rockwood CA Jr. Fractures of the clavicle. In: Rockwood CA Jr, Matsen FS III, editors. *The Shoulder.* Philadelphia: Saunders; 2003.
9. Bearden JM, Hughston JC, Whatley GS. Acromioclavicular dislocation: method of treatment. *J Sports Med.* 1973;1(4):5–17.
10. Boehme D, Curtis RJ Jr, DeHaan JT, Kay SP, Young DC, Rockwood CA Jr. Non-union of fractures of the mid-shaft of the clavicle. Treatment with a modified Hagie intramedullary pin and autogenous bonegrafting. *J Bone Joint Surg Am.* 1991;73(8):1219–26.
11. Bosworth BM. Acromioclavicular separation: new method of repair. *Surg Gynecol Obstet.* 1941;73:866–71.
12. Bosworth BM. Complete acromioclavicular dislocation. *N Engl J Med.* 1949;241(6):221–5.
13. Brinker MR, Edwards TB, O'Connor DP. Estimating the risk of nonunion following nonoperative treatment of a clavicular fracture. *J Bone Joint Surg Am.* 2005;87(3):676–7; author reply 677.
14. Broos P, Stoffelen D, Van de Sijpe K, Fourneau I. [Surgical management of complete Tossy III acromioclavicular joint dislocation with the Bosworth screw or the Wolter plate. A critical evaluation]. *Unfallchirurgie.* 1997;23(4):153–9; discussion 160.
15. Bundens WD Jr, Cook JI. Repair of acromioclavicular separations by deltoid-trapezius imbrication. *Clin Orthop.* 1961;20:109–15.
16. Canadian Orthopaedic Trauma Society. Nonoperative treatment compared with plate fixation of displaced midshaft clavicular fractures. A multicenter, randomized clinical trial. *J Bone Joint Surg Am.* 2007;89(1):1–10.
17. Chuang TY, Ho WP, Hsieh PH, Lee PC, Chen CH, Chen YJ. Closed reduction and internal fixation for acute midshaft clavicular fractures using cannulated screws. *J Trauma.* 2006;60(6):1315–20; discussion 1320–1.
18. Costic RS, Labriola JE, Rodosky MW, Debski RE. Biomechanical rationale for development of anatomical reconstructions of coracoclavicular ligaments after complete acromioclavicular joint dislocations. *Am J Sports Med.* 2004;32(8):1929–36.
19. Dannöhl C. [Angulation osteotomy of the clavicle in old luxations of the acromioclavicular joint]. *Aktuelle Traumatol.* 1984;14(6):282–4.
20. DePalma A. *Surgery of the Shoulder.* 3rd ed. Philadelphia (PA): J.B. Lippincott; 1983.
21. Eskola A, Vainionpää S, Korkala O, Rokkanen P. Acute complete acromioclavicular dislocation. A prospective randomized trial of fixation with smooth or threaded Kirschner wires or cortical screw. *Ann Chir Gynaecol.* 1987;76(6):323–6.
22. Eskola A, Vainionpää S, Myllynen P, Pätiälä H, Rokkanen P. Outcome of clavicular fracture in 89 patients. *Arch Orthop Trauma Surg.* 1986;105(6):337–8.
23. Fama G, Bonaga S. [Safety pin synthesis in the cure of acromioclavicular luxation]. *Chir Organi Mov.* 1988;73(3):227–35.
24. Fleming RE, Tornberg DN, Kiernan H. An operative repair of acromioclavicular separation. *J Trauma.* 1978;18(10):709–12.
25. Flik K, Lyman S, Marx RG. American collegiate men's ice hockey: an analysis of injuries. *Am J Sports Med.* 2005;33(2):183–7.
26. Fukuda K, Craig EV, An KN, Cofield RH, Chao EY. Biomechanical study of the ligamentous system of the acromioclavicular joint. *J Bone Joint Surg Am.* 1986;68(3):434–40.

27. Gerber C, Galantay RV, Hersche O. The pattern of pain produced by irritation of the acromioclavicular joint and the subacromial space. *J Shoulder Elbow Surg*. 1998;7(4):352–5.

28. Gerber C, Rockwood CA Jr. Subcoracoid dislocation of the lateral end of the clavicle. A report of three cases. *J Bone Joint Surg Am*. 1987;69(6):924–7.

29. Gladstone J, Wilk K, Andrews J. Nonoperative treatment of acromioclavicular joint injuries. *Op Tech Sports Med*. 1997;5(2):78–87.

30. Goldberg JA, Viglione W, Cumming WJ, Waddell FS, Ruz PA. Review of coracoclavicular ligament reconstruction using Dacron graft material. *Aust N Z J Surg*. 1987;57(7):441–5.

31. Grassi FA, Tajana MS, D'Angelo F. Management of midclavicular fractures: comparison between nonoperative treatment and open intramedullary fixation in 80 patients. *J Trauma*. 2001;50(6):1096–100.

32. Grutter PW, Petersen SA. Anatomical acromioclavicular ligament reconstruction: a biomechanical comparison of reconstructive techniques of the acromioclavicular joint. *Am J Sports Med*. 2005;33(11):1723–8.

33. Habernek H, Weinstabl R, Schmid L, Fialka C. A crook plate for treatment of acromioclavicular joint separation: indication, technique, and results after one year. *J Trauma*. 1993;35(6):893–901.

34. Harris RI, Wallace AL, Harper GD, Goldberg JA, Sonnabend DH, Walsh WR. Structural properties of the intact and the reconstructed coracoclavicular ligament complex. *Am J Sports Med*. 2000;28(1):103–8.

35. Henkel T, Oetiker R, Hackenbruch W. [Treatment of fresh Tossy III acromioclavicular joint dislocation by ligament suture and temporary fixation with the clavicular hooked plate]. *Swiss Surg*. 1997;3(4):160–6.

36. Hill JM, McGuire MH, Crosby LA. Closed treatment of displaced middle-third fractures of the clavicle gives poor results. *J Bone Joint Surg Br*. 1997;79(4):537–9.

37. Inman V, McLaughlin H, Neviaser JS. Treatment of complete acromioclavicular dislocation. *J Bone Joint Surg Am*. 1962;44:1008–11.

38. Jerosch J, Filler T, Peuker E, Greig M, Siewering U. Which stabilization technique corrects anatomy best in patients with AC-separation? An experimental study. *Knee Surg Sports Traumatol Arthrosc*. 1999;7(6):365–72.

39. Jiang C, Wang M, Rong G. Proximally based conjoined tendon transfer for coracoclavicular reconstruction in the treatment of acromioclavicular dislocation. *J Bone Joint Surg Am*. 2007;89(11):2408–12.

40. Jubel A, Andermahr J, Schiffer G, Tsironis K, Rehm KE. Elastic stable intramedullary nailing of midclavicular fractures with a titanium nail. *Clin Orthop Relat Res*. 2003;(408):279–85.

41. Kappakas GS, McMaster JH. Repair of acromioclavicular separation using a Dacron prosthesis graft. *Clin Orthop Relat Res*. 1978;(131):247–51.

42. Kelly BT, Barnes RP, Powell JW, Warren RF. Shoulder injuries to quarterbacks in the national football league. *Am J Sports Med*. 2004;32(2):328–31.

43. Kent BE. Functional anatomy of the shoulder complex. A review. *Phys Ther*. 1971;51(8):947.

44. Klimkiewicz JJ, Williams GR, Sher JS, Karduna A, Des Jardins J, Iannotti JP. The acromioclavicular capsule as a restraint to posterior translation of the clavicle: a biomechanical analysis. *J Shoulder Elbow Surg*. 1999;8(2):119–24.

45. Lucas DB. Biomechanics of the shoulder joint. *Arch Surg*. 1973;107(3):425–32.

46. Mazzocca AD, Arciero RA, Bicos J. Evaluation and treatment of acromioclavicular joint injuries. *Am J Sports Med*. 2007;35(2):316–29.

47. Mazzocca AD, Santangelo SA, Johnson ST, Rios CG, Dumonski ML, Arciero RA. A biomechanical evaluation of an anatomical coracoclavicular ligament reconstruction. *Am J Sports Med*. 2006;34(2):236–46.

48. McFarland EG, Blivin SJ, Doehring CB, Curl LA, Silberstein C. Treatment of grade III acromioclavicular separations in professional throwing athletes: results of a survey. *Am J Orthop*. 1997;26(11):771–4.

49. McKee MD, Seiler JG, Jupiter JB. The application of the limited contact dynamic compression plate in the upper extremity: an analysis of 114 consecutive cases. *Injury*. 1995;26(10):661–6.

50. McPhee IB. Inferior dislocation of the outer end of the clavicle. *J Trauma*. 1980;20(8):709–10.

51. Mikusev IE, Zainullin RV, Skvortsov AP. [Treatment of dislocations of the acromial end of the clavicle]. *Vestn Khir Im I I Grek*. 1987;139(8):69–71.

52. Moshein J, Elconin K. Repair of acute acromioclavicular dislocation utilizing the coracoacromial ligament. *J Bone Joint Surg Am*. 1969;51:812.

53. Neer CS II. Nonunion of the clavicle. *J Am Med Assoc*. 1960;172:1006–11.

54. Neer CS II. Fractures of the distal third of the clavicle. *Clin Orthop Relat Res*. 1968;58:43–50.

55. Nelson C. Repair of acromioclavicular separations with knitted Dacron graft. *Clin Orthop*. 1979;143:289.

56. Neviaser JS. Acromioclavicular dislocation treated by transference of the coraco-acromial ligament. A long-term follow-up in a series of 112 cases. *Clin Orthop Relat Res*. 1968;58:57–68.

57. Nowak J. *Clavicular Factures: Epidemiology, Union, Malunion, Nonunion*. Uppsala, Sweden: Acta Universitatis Upsalaiensis; 2002. 80 p.

58. Nowak J, Holgersson M, Larsson S. Can we predict long-term sequelae after fractures of the clavicle based on initial findings? A prospective study with nine to ten years of follow-up. *J Shoulder Elbow Surg*. 2004;13(5):479–86.

59. O'Donoghue D. *Treatment of Injuries in Athletes*. Philadelphia (PA): WB Saunders Company; 1970.

60. Park JP, Arnold JA, Coker TP, Harris WD, Becker DA. Treatment of acromioclavicular separations. A retrospective study. *Am J Sports Med*. 1980;8(4):251–6.

61. Patterson WR. Inferior dislocation of the distal end of the clavicle. A case report. *J Bone Joint Surg Am*. 1967;49(6):1184–6.

62. Petersson CJ. Degeneration of the acromioclavicular joint. A morphological study. *Acta Orthop Scand*. 1983;54(3):434–8.

63. Phillips AM, Smart C, Groom AF. Acromioclavicular dislocation. Conservative or surgical therapy. *Clin Orthop Relat Res*. 1998;(353):10–7.

64. Poigenfürst J, Rappold G, Fischer W. Plating of fresh clavicular fractures: results of 122 operations. *Injury*. 1992;23(4):237–41.

65. Rockwood CA Jr, Williams GR, Young D. Disorders of the acromioclavicular joint. In: Rockwood CA Jr, Matsen F, editors. *The Shoulder*. Philadelphia: Saunders; 1998. p. 483–553.

66. Sage FP, Salvatore JE. Injuries of the acromioclavicular joint: a study of results in 96 patients. *South Med J*. 1963;56:486–95.

67. Salter EG Jr, Nasca RJ, Shelley BS. Anatomical observations on the acromioclavicular joint and supporting ligaments. *Am J Sports Med*. 1987;15(3):199–206.

68. Schwarz N, Kuderna H. Inferior acromioclavicular separation. Report of an unusual case. *Clin Orthop Relat Res*. 1988;(234):28–30.

69. Shin SJ, Yun YH, Yoo JD. Coracoclavicular ligament reconstruction for acromioclavicular dislocation using 2 suture anchors and coracoacromial ligament transfer. *Am J Sports Med*. 2009;37(2):346–51.

70. Stanley D, Trowbridge EA, Norris SH. The mechanism of clavicular fracture. A clinical and biomechanical analysis. *J Bone Joint Surg Br*. 1988;70(3):461–4.

71. Tagliabue D, Riva A. Current approaches to the treatment of acromioclavicular joint separation in athletes. *Ital J Sports Traumatol*. 1981;3:15–24.

72. Tauber M, Gordon K, Koller H, Fox M, Resch H. Semitendinosus tendon graft versus a modified Weaver-Dunn procedure for acromioclavicular joint reconstruction in chronic cases: a prospective comparative study. *Am J Sports Med.* 2009;37(1):181–90.

73. Tibone J, Sellers R, Tonino P. Strength testing after third-degree acromioclavicular dislocations. *Am J Sports Med.* 1992;20(3):328–31.

74. Voigt C, Enes-Gaiao F, Fahimi S. [Treatment of acromioclavicular joint dislocation with the Rahmanzadeh joint plate]. *Aktuelle Traumatol.* 1994;24(4):128–32.

75. Walz L, Salzmann GM, Fabbro T, Eichhorn S, Imhoff AB. The anatomic reconstruction of acromioclavicular joint dislocations using 2 TightRope devices: a biomechanical study. *Am J Sports Med.* 2008;36(12): 2398–406.

76. Weaver JK, Dunn HK. Treatment of acromioclavicular injuries, especially complete acromioclavicular separation. *J Bone Joint Surg Am.* 1972;54(6):1187–94.

77. Zanca P. Shoulder pain: involvement of the acromioclavicular joint. (Analysis of 1,000 cases). *Am J Roentgenol Radium Ther Nucl Med.* 1971;112(3):493–506.

78. Zaricznyj B. Late reconstruction of the ligaments following acromioclavicular separation. *J Bone Joint Surg Am.* 1976;58(6):792–5.

79. Zlowodzki M, Zelle BA, Cole PA, Jeray K, McKee MD, Evidence-Based Orthopaedic Trauma Working Group. Treatment of acute midshaft clavicle fractures: systematic review of 2144 fractures: on behalf of the Evidence-Based Orthopaedic Trauma Working Group. *J Orthop Trauma.* 2005;19(7):504–7.

Shoulder Superior Labrum Anterior and Posterior Tears and Biceps Tears

50

Jeffrey S. Abrams

INTRODUCTION

- Superior labrum anterior to posterior (SLAP) tears can be a cause of shoulder pain following repetitive extension or traction injuries.

- The increased number of postoperative complications following surgical repair have raised questions about patient selection and treatment.

- Successful return to preinjury throwing activities has not been as successful as was once thought.

SUPERIOR LABRUM

- SLAP tears may be an isolated etiology for shoulder pain or in combination with other pathology.

- The superior labrum is the part of the cartilaginous ring that extends anterior and posterior to the biceps insertion. The labrum contributes to depth of the shallow glenoid, increasing humeral head contact and stability. Capsular ligaments and the long head of the biceps attach to the labrum and to the adjacent glenoid. Disruption of the labrum affects the attached ligaments and long head of the biceps (28).

- Superior labral tears have been described, as shoulder arthroscopy experience has increased (41). Arthrotomy with division of the subscapularis did not allow visualization of this anatomy, and little has been mentioned in the literature prior to 1985 (5).

- Anatomic variants and developmental changes with age can initiate tissue failure (14). The greatest success with surgical treatment is following traumatic instability events.

- Overhead sports, as in baseball pitching, may place additional stresses on the superior labrum. As sports participation and injury recognition increase, so does the experience in treatment of injuries to the superior labrum (2,5,8,16).

Superior Labrum Anatomy

- The labrum is a cartilaginous ring surrounding the perimeter of a shallow glenoid, contributing to depth and humeral head contact (23). Superior labrum lesions can occur alone or can extend to create anterior or posterior labral avulsions.

- The superior labrum consists of dense fibrocartilage and elastin that connects the superior and middle capsular ligaments and long head of the biceps to the glenoid.

- Normal variants include a fovea, a Buford complex, and a peel-back labrum. The fovea is an incomplete anterior superior labral attachment to the glenoid with a hole or thin fibrous tissue between the labrum and the glenoid (11). A Buford complex is a thickened middle glenohumeral ligament band that inserts at the biceps labral junction with an absent anterior superior labrum (44). A large fovea or superior labral absence may mistakenly resemble an avulsion injury. The posterior superior labrum may be attached to the glenoid neck rather than to the articular margin (9). Variations of labral attachment can be normal embryonic variants or repetitive activity adaptations.

- Arthroscopic evaluation along the undersurface of the labrum and adjacent articular cartilage should demonstrate abnormal wear, suggesting instability of the superior labrum in pathologic settings (37).

- Superior labral tears (SLAP tears) have been classified by Snyder as type I degenerative, type II avulsion, type III bucket-handle tears, and type IV combined labral tear and biceps insertion split (40). Expanded classification includes extension of Bankart lesions (20,38).

- Superior labral tears can allow extraarticular collection of synovial fluids encapsulating as paralabral cysts. These cysts, often recognized on magnetic resonance imaging (MRI) or ultrasound exam, can create pressure on adjacent structures (25).

- The anatomy can be visualized arthroscopically in a static and dynamic exam. The peel-back labrum can be seen arthroscopically as loss of posterior superior, glenoid contact when the shoulder is placed in abduction and external rotation (9). An otherwise normal finding may increase with repetitive stresses, potentially leading to a painful condition.

Superior Labrum Function

- Superior labrum contributes to superior, anteroinferior, inferior, and posterior glenohumeral stability. Superior humeral head translation can be reduced with secure attachment of the superior labrum and its biceps and capsular attachments. Investigators have increased anteroinferior translation after creating superior labral tears (34,39). In addition, arthroscopists have noted SLAP tears associated with some patients with posterior and multidirectional shoulder instability (1).

- The rotator cuff interval plays a role in stabilizing the adducted shoulder (22). This interval consists of the superior labrum, superior glenohumeral ligament, middle glenohumeral ligament, and coracohumeral ligament. Reduction of an enlarged interval has decreased inferior translation or sulcus, reduced anterior translation, and external rotation and can be used to augment anterior stabilization.

- Superior translation of the humeral head can be limited with an intact superior labrum and biceps anchor with the humerus in external rotation (2). The long head of the biceps attaches to the superior labrum and glenoid tubercle. When the shoulder is in the cocked throwing position (abduction, external rotation, and extension), the head is translated posteriorly (24). Capsular changes and tears in the superior labrum may alter these relationships.

- The superior labrum may contribute to articular lesions on the undersurface of the rotator cuff. Internal impingement is a common pathologic finding in overhead throwers with shoulder pain. Excessive contact of the posterosuperior labrum with the supraspinatus and infraspinatus during early acceleration can create partial-thickness rotator cuff tears. Subscapularis tendons can abrade on the anterosuperior labrum with flexion and internal rotation.

Superior Labral Pathologic Conditions

- SLAP tears can be a source of pain and disability either in isolation or coexistent with other shoulder pathology (26,31). SLAP tears have been associated with instability, rotator cuff pathology, and ganglion cysts.

- SLAP tears can result from a single traumatic event. A fall on an outstretched arm or elbow can create a superior humeral translation that can avulse or tear the superior labrum. Shoulder hyperextension, as in an arm tackle or seat belt restraint or lifting injuries, can place traction on the biceps and capsular attachments avulsing the superior labrum. Large Bankart lesions can include the superior labrum and biceps anchor. SLAP avulsion can increase inferior translation of the shoulder contributing to shoulder instability.

- SLAP tears often coexist with other shoulder pathology as a result of overuse. Baseball pitchers develop upper extremity velocity by placing the arm in maximum extension as they externally rotate and abduct. Torso forward projection places additional contact forces on the undersurface of the rotator cuff against the superior labrum. Internal impingement occurs when excessive compressive forces occur and may be associated with rotator cuff tears, superior labral tears, posterior capsular changes, and scapular dyskinesia.

- Juxta-articular ganglions adjacent to the glenohumeral joint have been diagnosed with increasing frequency since MRI of the shoulder has been used. Ganglions often originate from the joint space and communicate with the ganglion with a defect or tear in the superior or posterosuperior labrum (43). Ganglions may be asymptomatic or cause neurologic dysfunction due to peripheral pressure on the suprascapular nerve prior to the supraspinatus innervation at the scapular notch or adjacent to the scapular spine prior to the infraspinatus innervation.

Superior Labral Diagnosis

- Patients most often complain of pain in provocative positions. A painful click may occasionally be reproducible, especially when associated with instability.

- The mechanism of injury can be traumatic and overuse. Traumatic events include a fall on an outstretched arm, hyperextension injury, and seat belt injury. The body torso projects forward as the shoulder and arm are restrained. Overuse injuries, as in baseball pitching, accentuate internal impingement contact forces. Forced inferior translation may create superior labral avulsions due to traction on the biceps and capsular attachments.

- Degenerative changes are commonly found in the superior labrum, and their significance has not been established.

- Physical examination has had variable results (26,30,31). Examination of the biceps with provocative testing has been helpful in anterior tears (Speed, Yergason tests). Translation test (load and shift, jerk tests) and provocative position (relocation test) testing can produce pain but are often associated with common complaints exterior to the shoulder (i.e., the acromioclavicular joint). Some SLAP lesions are not diagnosed preoperatively, but rather at the time of arthroscopic surgery.

- Imaging tests can be helpful. MRI without contrast can identify ganglion cysts adjacent to the shoulder. MRI with articular contrast may illustrate superior labral tear. Anatomic variants may contribute to abnormal imaging findings.

Superior Labral Treatment

- Most common treatment for intrasubstance tears of the superior labrum is debridement (type I and III) (4).

- Type II tears in young active individuals associated with shoulder instability, rotator cuff pathology, and ganglion origin and as isolated source of pain are considered for repair (15). These repairs may be done in combination with capsulorrhaphies, cuff repairs, ganglion decompression, and subacromial decompressions.

- Surgical indication is continued symptoms after an appropriate rest and rehabilitation period (12). Focus of rehabilitation should be scapular stabilization and rotator cuff strengthening.

- Superior labral repairs are most commonly performed with suture anchors (35). An anchor is inserted along the articular margin of an abraded glenoid neck. Sutures are advanced through the labrum and tied as mattress or simple sutures. Anterior labral repairs should not close naturally occurring fovea. Posterosuperior SLAP repairs may need accessory portals to properly place anchors along the glenoid to secure the labrum (31).

- Treatment of symptomatic SLAP tears should be individualized (3). Options include debridement, SLAP repair, or biceps tenotomy or tenodesis. Due to a higher complications rate of shoulder stiffness following a SLAP suture anchor repair, biceps tenodesis has been popularized (7). The best indications for a suture anchor repair are shoulder instability, shoulder hyperlaxity, overhead throwers with hypermobility of the biceps labral complex, and ganglion resection. Many patients with stable shoulders can achieve satisfactory pain relief with biceps tenodesis or tenotomy.

- Postoperative management should include immobilization (3–4 weeks) and regulated movement, followed by strengthening. Return to demanding activities takes 3–6 months.

BICEPS (SHOULDER)

- The long head of the biceps is susceptible to injury in multiple locations in the shoulder. The articular portion of the biceps has a twisted pathway before attaching to the superior labrum and glenoid. As the shoulder is positioned in abduction and external rotation, additional stresses are placed on these attachments (9).

- The articular portion of the tendon exits the shoulder and enters the tuber groove between the humeral tuberosities. Tendinosis may develop due to repetitive humeral movements, friction between the tuberosities with humeral elevation and rotation, impingement below the subacromial arch, and compromised blood supply.

- Instability of the long head of the biceps may occur when pulley ligaments or rotator cuff tendons are disrupted. Patients perceive clicking as the humerus is rotated, which may reproduce these findings in a painful shoulder.

- Tendinopathies and instability of the biceps are most often associated with additional injuries of the shoulder. Rotator cuff pathology and impingement syndromes are common coexistent pathologies.

Biceps Anatomy

- The biceps has 2 proximal origins and inserts below the elbow on the tubercle of the proximal radius. It traverses both the shoulder and the elbow and plays a role in shoulder flexion, elbow flexion, and forearm supination. From a shoulder perspective, the long head of the biceps is the most susceptible to injury. The short head originates from the coracoid process.

- The musculocutaneous nerve (C5, C6, and C7) innervates the biceps. The nerve can be seen to enter the short head inferior to the coracoid. The second portion is innervated more distally, prior to this nerve becoming a cutaneous nerve along the anterolateral aspect of the forearm. Injury to this nerve can result from anterior surgical approaches from surgical retractors.

- The long head of the biceps originates from the glenoid tubercle and superior labrum (21). This tendon changes direction as it exits the shoulder. Capsular ligaments act as a pulley as the tendon exits the articular space and traverses under the transverse ligament (33). Extraarticularly, it runs within a groove between the greater and lesser tuberosities. The muscle tendon junction is adjacent to the inferior border of the pectoralis major tendon. Anatomic variations, including attachments to the rotator cuff and absence of glenoid attachment, may be rarely found and are nonproblematic.

- Biceps pathology involving the elbow will be discussed in the appropriate section.

Biceps Function

- The role of the normal biceps in the shoulder includes arm elevation and humeral head stabilization when positioned in external rotation most commonly located (10).

- Due to 2 proximal attachment sites, the long head may rupture and not severely impact shoulder functions if the rotator cuff or short head attachments can compensate for this tear (29).

- During the throwing motion, the biceps is positioned with the arm in abduction, extended, and externally rotated. A complex change in pull occurs as the shoulder changes from cocking to acceleration (20). In addition to shoulder stresses, elbow extension occurs simultaneously, placing additional eccentric tension on the proximal anatomy (2,5).

Biceps Pathologic Conditions

- Shoulder biceps tears can be located adjacent to the superior labrum, along the articular portion, beneath the transverse ligament, within the groove, or at the muscle tendon junction.

- Biceps tendinosis is most commonly located adjacent to the location where the tendon has a directional change as it exits the shoulder. Because the shoulder abducts and adducts, these tears extend proximally and distally and can be seen arthroscopically during the articular and bursal exams as it exits above the bicipital groove (13).

- Biceps tendon subluxation can occur when the supporting capsular ligaments are disrupted (42). This can occur when the superior portion of the subscapularis is detached from the lesser tuberosity (36). Capsular pulley and coracohumeral ligament injury can allow medial subluxation without significant tendon tear (33). Lateral subluxation can occur if the supraspinatus tears and dorsal interval ligaments are disrupted (27).

- Tears at the muscle tendon junction can result from traumatic events. Abrupt eccentric contraction may create a tear (18).

- Biceps long head tendinosis can be coexistent with rotator cuff pathology in the impingement syndrome (32). The tendon is aligned along the leading edge of the supraspinatus. During forward flexion, these structures can be impinged by the acromion and the coracoacromial ligament.

Biceps Complaints and Findings

- The most common complaint is pain along the anteromedial aspect of the shoulder. Some patients can demonstrate a click with rotation of the humerus.

- The impingement test is not specific but can be sensitive to biceps pathology. Localized tenderness along the groove can help distinguish this from supraspinatus tendinosis.

- A Speed test is performed by an examiner applying resistance to arm flexion while the arm is supinated. A Yergason sign reproduces pain while palpating the tendon while applying resistance against supinating a flexed forearm. Pain and weakness caused by pain can be reproduced with these maneuvers (10,13).

- Muscular biceps examination is done with elbow flexion and the arm in neutral and supination. Additional testing can be performed with resistive elbow flexion or supination while the shoulder is in the overhead throwing position (6).

- Disruptions of the long head of the biceps may produce a "biceps Popeye muscle" if the tendon retracts distally beyond the transverse ligament. A tear at the muscle tendon junction can create a similar deformity. This appears as a bulging muscle located distal to the contralateral side. There is often ecchymosis initially, and it is commonly associated with a rotator cuff tear (32).

- Biceps imaging can be best accomplished with MRI without enhancement. The sagittal views can demonstrate the articular portion, and the transverse cuts demonstrate the extraarticular portions. Rotator cuff tears in the coronal view may raise suspicion of associated pathology. Transverse cuts may demonstrate the biceps medial to the bicipital groove. An important coexistent pathology to recognize is disruption of the subscapularis insertion.

Biceps Tendon Tear Treatment

- Biceps pathology is often coexistent with rotator cuff problems. Tendinosis and impingement can coexist with supraspinatus tears. Biceps instability following trauma can be associated with a subscapularis tear. Diagnosing rotator cuff tears is important in determining treatment options.

- Traditionally, treatment has been divided into biceps tears involving up to 50% of the tendon or greater than 50% of the tendon (13). More mild tears are debrided, and larger tears are considered for tenotomy or tenodesis. This concept is controversial, and sports physicians have individualized treatment rather than relying on degree of tendon involvement (19).

- Biceps tendon debridement can be done arthroscopically or through an open approach. The articular part of the tendon can be easily debrided arthroscopically. To visualize the extraarticular portion, the tendon needs to be drawn into the articular viewing area or has to be visualized on the bursal side after the supporting capsule has been divided.

- Current controversy exists between cutting the damaged biceps tendon (tenotomy) (19) versus reattachment of the biceps tendon in a different location (tenodesis) (13,17). Generally, older individuals who are less active are comfortable with tenotomy supported by a minimal postoperative recovery. Younger and high-demand individuals may wish to avoid a possible biceps muscle deformity that may be created by completing the tear of the biceps and prefer a tenodesis. Functional deficits from a long-head rupture or iatrogenic division of the long head of the biceps are usually temporary (29). Patients' concerns and options should be discussed preoperatively.

- Biceps tenodesis can be performed after dividing the tendon adjacent to the superior labrum. The biceps can be fastened to the proximal humerus or to adjacent soft tissue. Tenodesis to bone can be performed with suture anchors, bone tunnels, or interference screw fixation. Soft tissue repairs can be created with sutures, tendon to tendon, or tendon to capsule.

- Patients can be categorized as rotator cuff intact with biceps tear or coexistent cuff and biceps tears. In the latter, the arthroscopic or open suture anchor repair can be used to create a secure tendon-to-bone repair of both the cuff and the biceps. Patients with an intact cuff may have tenodesis performed but will need postoperative activity restriction during the initial healing period to protect the biceps attachment. Resistive exercises are generally delayed to 8 weeks postoperatively.

- Subpectoral open tenodesis repairs have been popularized when extensive tendon involvement includes the extraarticular portion. This allows for excision of the diseased portion prior to tendon-to-humerus reattachment. The muscle tendon junction is aligned along the inferior border of the pectoralis major tendon.

REFERENCES

1. Abrams JS. Arthroscopic treatment of posterior instability. In: Tibone JE, Savoie FH III, Shaffer BS, editors. *Shoulder Arthroscopy*. New York: Springer-Verlag; 2003. p. 97–103.

2. Abrams JS. Special shoulder problems in the throwing athlete: pathology, diagnosis and nongenerative management. *Clin Sports Med*. 1991; 10(4):839–61.

3. Alpert JM, Wuerz TH, O'Donnell TF, Carroll KM, Brucker NN, Gill TJ. The effect of age on the outcomes of arthroscopic repair of type II superior labral anterior and posterior lesions. *Am J Sports Med.* 2010;38(11):2299–303.

4. Altchek DW, Warren RF, Wickiewicz TL, Ortiz G. Arthroscopic labral debridement: a three-year follow-up study. *Am J Sports Med.* 1992;20(6):702–6.

5. Andrews JR, Carson WG Jr, McLeod WD. Glenoid labrum tears related to the long head of the biceps. *Am J Sports Med.* 1985;13(5):337–41.

6. Bell RH, Noble JS. Biceps disorders. In: Hawkins RJ, Misamore GW, editors. *Shoulder Injuries in the Athlete.* New York: Churchill Livingstone; 1996. p. 267–82.

7. Boileau P, Parratte S, Chuinard C, Roussane Y, Shia D, Bicknell R. Arthroscopic treatment of isolated type II SLAP lesions: biceps tenodesis as an alternative to reinsertion. *Am J Sports Med.* 2009;37(5):929–36.

8. Brockmeier SF, Voos JE, Williams RJ 3rd, et al. Outcomes after arthroscopic repair of type-II SLAP lesions. *J Bone Joint Surg Am.* 2009; 91(7):1595–603.

9. Burkhart SS, Morgan CD. The peel-back mechanism: its role in producing and extending posterior type II SLAP lesions and its effect on SLAP repair rehabilitation. *Arthroscopy.* 1998;14(6):637–40.

10. Burkhead WZ Jr, Arcand MA, Zeman C, et al. The biceps tendon. In: Rockwood CA Jr, Matsen FA, editors. *The Shoulder.* 2nd ed. Philadelphia: W.B. Saunders; 1998; p. 1009–63.

11. Cooper DE, Arnoczky SP, O'Brien SJ, Warren RF, DiCarlo E, Allen AA. Anatomy, histology, and vascularity of the glenoid labrum. An anatomical study. *J Bone Joint Surg Am.* 1992;74(1):46–52.

12. Cordasco FA, Steinmann S, Flatow EL, Bigliani LU. Arthroscopic treatment of glenoid labral tears. *Am J Sports Med:* 1993;21(3):425–30; discussion 430–1.

13. Curtis AS, Snyder SJ. Evaluation and treatment of biceps tendon pathology. *Orthop Clin North Am.* 1993;24(1):33–43.

14. Davidson PA, Rivenburgh DW. Mobile superior glenoid labrum: a normal variant or pathologic condition? *Am J Sports Med.* 2004;32(4): 962–6.

15. Franceschi F, Longo UG, Ruzzini L, Rizzello G, Maffulli N, Denaro V. No advantages in repairing a type II superior labrum anterior and posterior (SLAP) lesion when associated with rotator cuff repair in patients over age 50: a randomized controlled trial. *Am J Sports Med.* 2008;36(2): 247–53.

16. Friel NA, Karas V, Slabaugh MA, Cole BJ. Outcomes of type II superior labrum, anterior to posterior (SLAP) repair: prospective evaluation at a minimum two-year follow-up. *J Shoulder Elbow Surg.* 2010;19(6): 859–67.

17. Frost A, Zafar MS, Maffulli N. Tenotomy versus tenodesis in the management of pathologic lesions of the tendon of the long head of the biceps brachii. *Am J Sports Med.* 2009;37(4):828–33.

18. Garrett WE Jr, Safran MR, Seaber AV, Glisson RR, Ribbeck BM. Biomechanical comparison of stimulated and nonstimulated skeletal muscle pulled to failure. *Am J Sports Med.* 1987;15(5):448–54.

19. Gill TJ, McIrvin E, Mair SD, Hawkins RJ. Results of biceps tenotomy for treatment of pathology of the long head of the biceps brachii. *J Shoulder Elbow Surg.* 2001;10(3):247–9.

20. Glousman R, Jobe F, Tibone J, Moynes D, Antonelli D, Perry J. Dynamic electromyographic analysis of the throwing shoulder with glenohumeral instability. *J Bone Joint Surg Am.* 1988;70(2):220–6.

21. Habermeyer P, Walch G. The biceps tendon and rotator cuff disease. In: Burkhead WZ Jr, editor. *Rotator Cuff Disorders.* Baltimore: Williams & Wilkins; 1996. p. 142–59.

22. Harryman DT 2nd, Sidles JA, Harris SL, Matsen FA 3rd. The role of the rotator interval capsule in passive motion and stability of the shoulder. *J Bone Joint Surg Am.* 1992;74(1):53–66.

23. Howell SM, Galinat BJ. The glenoid labral socket. A constrained articular surface. *Clin Orthop Relat Res.* 1989;(243):122–5.

24. Howell SM, Galinat BJ, Renzi AJ, Marone PJ. Normal and abnormal mechanics of the glenohumeral joint in the horizontal plane. *J Bone Joint Surg Am.* 1988;70(2):227–32.

26. Kim TK, Quele WS, Cosgarea AJ, McFarland EG. Clinical features of different types of SLAP lesions: an analysis of one hundred and thirty-nine cases. *J Bone Joint Surg Am.* 2003;85-A(1):66–71.

27. Lafosse L, Reiland Y, Baier GP, Toussaint B, Jost B. Anterior and posterior instability of the long head of the biceps tendon in rotator cuff tears: a new classification based on arthroscopic observations. *Arthroscopy.* 2007;23(1):73–80.

28. Maffet MW, Gartsman GM, Moseley B. Superior labrum biceps tendon complex lesions of the shoulder. *Am J Sports Med.* 1995;23(1):93–8.

29. Mariani EM, Cofield RH, Askew LJ, Li GP, Chao EY. Rupture of the tendon of the long head of the biceps brachii. Surgical versus nonsurgical treatment. *Clin Orthop Relat Res.* 1988;(228):233–9.

30. McFarland EG, Kim TK, Savino RM. Clinical assessment of three common tests for superior labral anterior-posterior lesions. *Am J Sports Med.* 2002;30(6):810–5.

31. Morgan CD, Burkhart SS, Palmieri M, Gillespie M. Type II SLAP lesions: three subtypes and their relationships to superior instability and rotator cuff tears. *Arthroscopy.* 1998;14(6):553–65.

32. Neer CS II, Bigliani LU, Hawkins RJ. Rupture of the long head of the biceps related to the subacromial impingement. *Orthop Trans.* 1977;1:114.

34. Pagnani MJ, Deng XH, Warren RF, Torzilli PA, Altchek DW. Effects of lesions of the superior portion of the glenoid labrum on glenohumeral translation. *J Bone Joint Surg Am.* 1995;77(7):1003–10.

35. Panossian VR, Mihata T, Tibone JE, Fitzpatrick MJ, McGarry MH, Lee TQ. Biomechanical analysis of isolated type II SLAP lesions and repair. *J Shoulder Elbow Surg.* 2005;14(5):529–34.

36. Peterson CJ. Spontaneous medial dislocation of the tendon of the long biceps brachii. *Clin Orthop Relat Res.* 1986;(211):224–7.

37. Pfahler M, Haraida S, Schulz C, Anetzberger H, Refior HJ, Bauer GS, Bigliani LU. Age-related changes of the glenoid labrum in normal shoulders. *J Shoulder Elbow Surg.* 2003;12(1):40–52.

38. Powell SE, Nord KD, Ryu RKN. The diagnosis, classification, and treatment of SLAP lesions. *Oper Tech Sports Med.* 2004;12(2):99–110.

39. Rodosky MW, Harner CD, Fu FH. The role of the long head of the biceps muscle and superior glenoid labrum in anterior stability of the shoulder. *Am J Sports Med.* 1994;22(1):121–30.

40. Snyder SJ, Banas MP, Karzel RP. An analysis of 140 injuries to the superior glenoid labrum. *J Shoulder Elbow Surg.* 1995;4(4):243–8.

41. Snyder SJ, Karzel RP, Del Pizzo W, Ferkel RD, Friedman MJ. SLAP lesions of the shoulder. *Arthroscopy.* 1990;6(4):274–9.

42. Walch G, Nové-Josserand L, Boileau P, Levigne C. Subluxations and dislocations of the tendon of the long head of the biceps. *J Shoulder Elbow Surg.* 1998;7(2):100–8.

43. Westerheide KJ, Karzel RP. Ganglion cysts of the shoulder: technique of arthroscopic decompression and fixation of associated type II superior labral anterior to posterior lesions. *Orthop Clin North Am.* 2003;34(4): 521–8.

44. Williams MM, Snyder SJ, Buford D Jr. The Buford complex — the "cord-like" middle glenohumeral ligament and absent anterosuperior labrum complex: a normal anatomic capsulolabral variant. *Arthroscopy.* 1994;10(3):241–7.

51 The Throwing Shoulder

James P. Sostak, II and Carlos A. Guanche

INTRODUCTION

Throwing Motion

- Throwing in baseball has been analyzed extensively, with the specific maneuvers being broken down into 6 phases (6). While the analysis of the baseball throw is the best understood and most studied, other throwing, racquet, and overhand sports have also been evaluated. The mechanics of a baseball throw are transferable, for the most part, to other sports with some modifications depending on the size of the ball or the maneuver being analyzed. The baseball throw, by virtue of its speed and frequency, however, is the most traumatic to the shoulder.

- The phases of throwing are summarized as follows:
  - Wind up
    - Readying phase
    - Minimal shoulder stress
    - Ground, legs, and trunk are force generators
  - Early cocking
  - Late cocking
    - Scapular retraction for stable throwing base
    - Maximal external rotation
    - Posterior translation of the humeral head as a result of abduction/external rotation (ABER)
    - Shear force across anterior shoulder of 400 newtons
    - Compressive force of 650 newtons generated by cuff
  - Acceleration
    - Transition from eccentric to concentric forces anteriorly (vice versa posteriorly)
    - Rotation occurs at 7,000–9,000 degrees per second
    - Only one-third of the kinetic energy leaves with the ball (the remainder is dissipated through the extremity)
  - Deceleration
    - Most violent phase (responsible for dissipation of energy not imparted to ball)
    - Distractive forces generated by the acceleration phase are countered by violent contraction of posterior rotator cuff and scapular stabilizers

- Largest joint loads
  - Posterior shear force of 400 newtons
  - Inferior shear forces of > 300 newtons
  - Compressive forces of > 1000 newtons
  - Adduction torque > 80 newton-meter; horizontal abduction torque of 100 newton-meter
- Follow-through
  - Rebalancing phase
  - Compressive forces of 400 newtons
  - Inferior shear of 200 newtons
- The entire motion takes less than 2 seconds with most of the time (1.5 seconds) taken up by the early phases (wind up and cocking).
  - Three critical points in the motion:
    - Cocking: Point in process where full external rotation/abduction is achieved, shear force on labrum is maximum, biceps vector shifts posteriorly, and the energy generated by trunk/legs is transferred to shoulder; leads to potential injury situation for the shoulder at risk (2,3).
    - Acceleration: The body falls ahead of the shoulder while the internal rotators are maximally contracting and the angular velocity exceeds 7,000 degrees per second.
    - Deceleration: Scapular stabilizers and posterior rotator cuff contract violently to counter the distractive force of acceleration and lessen the load on the posterior inferior glenohumeral ligament (PIGHL).

Kinetic Chain of Throwing

- The forces needed to propel the ball and generate the velocity of the throw require contributions from all body segments (4). These contributions help to minimize joint stress and allow for the forces to be passed to distal segments as the motion progresses.
- The kinetic chain includes
  - Force generators – ground, legs, trunk
  - Force regulator – shoulder
  - Force delivery – arm

Dead Arm

- Any pathologic shoulder condition in which the thrower is unable to throw with preinjury velocity and control because of a combination of pain and subjective unease in the shoulder (4).

Glenohumeral Internal Rotation Deficit (GIRD)

- Basic definition: Loss of glenohumeral internal rotation in the throwing shoulder compared to the nonthrowing shoulder.
- What constitutes a clinically significant amount of GIRD is debated.
- Acceptable level of GIRD, as defined by Burkhart et al. (2–4), is less than 20 degrees or less than 10% of the total rotation measured in the nonthrowing shoulder.
- Clinical significance may occur when internal rotation loss exceeds external rotation gain in the throwing athlete.
- GIRD can also be seen in asymptomatic throwers and, in this case, may be related to increased humeral retroversion (21).

PATHOPHYSIOLOGY

Current Theory

- Centers around GIRD, caused by contracted PIGHL, as the essential problem in pathology of the thrower's shoulder.
- Previously, anterior capsular laxity due to repetitive microtrauma of the throwing motion had been suggested as the essential problem (9).
- Recent basic science suggests that the thrower's shoulder pathology may be the result of posterior capsular/ligament tightness rather than increased anterior laxity. There was a trend toward a less inferior position of the humeral head in the late cocking position when a posterior capsular contracture was simulated (7).

The Pathologic Cascade (2,3)

Primary event — posterior cuff and scapular stabilizer weakness; patient often asymptomatic

Muscle weakness leads to PIGHL overload as a static stabilizer, which leads to PIGHL fibrosis and contracture, clinically manifested as GIRD.

- Posterior superior shift of humeral head on the glenoid occurs in the ABER position (late cocking phase) due to posterior ligament contracture. Can lead to excessive internal impingement beyond the physiologic level, excessive labral shear forces, and excessive posterior biceps vector, thus leading to painful shoulder
- Posterior type II superior labrum anterior to posterior (SLAP) tear occurs next as labrum gives way due to increased

shear stress combined with increased peel-back force from posterior biceps vector.
- Undersurface posterior rotator cuff tears follow due to increased tensile, torsional, and compressive forces.
- Tertiary event of the cascade is anterior capsular failure with resultant instability. This is often limited to veteran throwers, who despite proceeding through the previous points in the cascade over many years have been able to compensate, continuing to throw at an elite level, and only present once the instability tips them over the edge.

Labral Tears (SLAP)

Traction Mechanism

- During deceleration, biceps muscle contraction is strong as both elbow extension and glenohumeral distractions occur. The biceps muscle has been shown to be essential to limiting torsional forces to the shoulder in the ABER position (17). By this mechanism, the effect on the superior labrum would be one of failure either by tension or direct compression.

Peel-Back Mechanism

- Tension overload develops in the ABER extremity (16) based on three observations:
  - A posterior type II SLAP, or thrower's SLAP, lesion can cause anterior pseudolaxity. Essentially, a transfer anterior of the posterior lesion.
  - ABER causes peel back of posterior superior labrum that becomes pathologic when the posterior band of the inferior glenohumeral ligament (IGHL) is contracted and shifts the humeral head posterior superior.
  - Posterior inferior capsule tightens in overhand throwers due to muscle stabilizer weakness. Axis of rotation of humeral head is shifted posterior superior, external rotation increases, and the biceps vector shifts posterior; result is increased internal impingement and maximized peel-back forces.

Rotator Cuff

- Supraspinatus, infraspinatus, and teres minor tire in late cocking to move to maximal external rotation, followed by eccentric firing in deceleration.
- Tensile and torsional stress develops in cuff muscles as external rotation becomes excessive with posterior IGHL tightness.
- These stresses may speed normal degeneration.
- Factors of stressful loading, distraction, and excessive internal and external rotation can cause acute inflammatory responses early (internal impingement) or tendon failure in the later stages (rotator cuff tears).
- Stresses on cuff can also be increased with scapular dyskinesis and a protracted scapula (secondary impingement).

Capsular

External Rotation Excess

Instability Theory

- Excessive external rotation, from repetitive throwing, leads to soft tissue adaptive changes (anterior capsular stretching) and subsequent instability (11).
- Attention must be made to the full arc of motion. Throwers may create a new set point with increased external rotation. The lack of internal rotation may be compensated by increased external rotation and may not represent true GIRD.
- Thought to possibly lead to increased internal impingement
- Secondary posterior capsular tightness also occurs.

Hyperexternal Rotation Theory (18)

- Stretching of the anterior structures is on the basis of hyperexternal rotation/hyperhorizontal abduction and not a true anterior instability pattern.
- More important is the loss of internal rotation in abduction, which far exceeds external rotation gain.

Internal Impingement

- Rotator cuff impinges on the posterosuperior rim of the glenoid in ABER (9).
- Causes pain in ABER position and correlates with positive apprehension (posterior pain) and relocation maneuvers (22).
- Etiology: 2 theories
  - Physiologic phenomenon occurring in all individuals that can cause labral and cuff tearing with overuse type/repetitive activity.
  - Secondary internal impingement occurs as a result of the excessive external rotation that developed from repetitive throwing.
- Analysis of rotator cuff contact in throwing and nonthrowing extremities has revealed contact in both arms when in ABER position, lending credence to the theory of physiologic impingement, which develops problems as a result of repetitive trauma (8).
- In addition, physiologic impingement can also be worsened by the posteroir superior shift of the humeral head that occurs with a tight PIGHL and GIRD.

Bony Changes

- Bennett lesion: bony reactive changes at the posterior glenoid margin (1)
- Symptom complex includes pain in posterior deltoid in follow-through phase.
  - Exostosis is typically at the posterior inferior glenoid margin.
  - Size of lesion is not correlated with symptoms.
  - Symptoms may occur gradually or acutely.
- Changes are not always clinically symptomatic.

- Symptomatic exostoses usually respond to rest and occasional steroid injections.
- Excision is performed through either an arthroscopic or posterior open approach (14,15).

MANAGEMENT OF SPECIFIC INJURIES

SLAP Lesions

- Variable amounts of detachment encountered. The established classification system defines the clinically unstable lesions as those that involve the biceps anchor (19).
- Type II SLAP lesions in the throwing athlete tend to be located from the biceps anchor extending posterior and less often involve the anterior superior labrum.
- Conservative management in an established SLAP lesion does not fare well in throwers.
- Attempts at rehabilitation center around stretching out the PIGHL to correct GIRD, management of scapulothoracic dyskinesia, and strengthening of the rotator cuff.
- Surgical management is arthroscopic stabilization with the use of suture anchors. If GIRD is greater than 20 degrees with exam under anesthesia, a posterior inferior capsular release should be considered (2,3).
- Rehabilitation after surgery should include PIGHL stretching and strengthening of scapula stabilizers to help correct primary problem.

Rotator Cuff Tears

- Partial-thickness tearing is most common. Partial tears result from the excessive tension/torsion developed within fibers, as well as internal impingement that occurs in the hyperexternally rotated position.
  - Intra-articular partial tears are most common.
  - Diagnosis is done via magnetic resonance imaging with intra-articular gadolinium.
    - Assess arm in ABER position.
    - Highly suspicious of diagnosis in high-level throwers.
  - Surgical indications:
    - A complete arthroscopic evaluation of joint is important due to the high incidence of labral lesions and partial cuff tears.
    - Debridement is considered with lesions less than 50% thickness and in those with normal preoperative strength.
    - Repair is considered in those lesions greater than 50% of tendon thickness.
    - Consider acromioplasty and/or coracoacromial ligament release if there are signs of primary impingement on exam. Usually not needed because impingement in throwers is often secondary due to scapular protraction and will improve with rehabilitation.

Impingement

Primary

- Rare as an isolated entity.
- High incidence of intra-articular pathology.
- A complete diagnostic arthroscopy is indicated in all patients to assess for additional pathology. An isolated subacromial decompression is seldom the answer in a thrower with shoulder pain.
- In 1 study, only 43% of patients with surgical decompression returned to preinjury level of competition (20).
- If performing decompression, it should be a conservative resection.
- Do not resect a type I acromion.

Secondary

- Due to scapular dyskinesia, which results from weak scapular stabilizers. This leads to protracted scapula and impingement in ABER position.
- With specialized scapular rehabilitation program, this pain generator will resolve.
- This problem needs to be corrected, in addition to intra-articular pathology, or the pathology will recur.

Rehabilitation Issues

Scapulothoracic Articulation

- Often the cause of secondary impingement.
- The scapula has 5 specific functions that have implications in throwers (10).
  - Stable part of the glenohumeral articulation, where rotation of the glenohumeral joint allows maximal concavity and compression
  - Retracts and protracts the shoulder complex along the thoracic wall
  - Acromial elevation to avoid impingement with arm elevation
  - Base for muscular attachments
  - Energy transfer from the legs, back, and trunk

Scapulothoracic Dyskinesia

- Abnormal set of motions and positions affecting the relative position of the scapula and the proximal humerus.
  - Etiologies include nerve or muscle injury, muscle inhibition, and glenohumeral stiffness or laxity.
  - Mechanical dysfunction may result in impingement and insufficient translation of energy from the lower body.
    - Excessive stress results in overuse injuries.
    - Clinical picture is confusing as a result of secondary impingement and capsular changes that may occur as a result of the adaptations to scapular malalignment.

Proprioception (12)

- Excessive joint laxity associated with capsuloligamentous injury and resulting microtrauma cause damage to the neural receptors and lead to deafferentation.

- Neuromuscular deficits impair reflexive muscular stabilization, predisposing the shoulder to episodes of functional instability.
  - Diminished joint position sense, kinesthetic awareness, and abnormal humeroscapular firing patterns (13).
  - Abnormal firing patterns documented on electromyography studies in throwers with glenohumeral instability (5).
  - After surgical reconstruction, joint position sense and reproduction of passive positioning improve to baseline levels (13).
- Restoration of functional stability.
  - Traditional strengthening exercises do not address neuromuscular deficits.
  - Four elements are necessary to restore functional stability (13):
    - Peripheral somatosensory: including visual and vestibular
    - Spinal reflexes: sudden alteration in joint position that requires reflex muscular stabilization
    - Cognitive programming: appreciation of joint position
    - Brainstem
- All 4 elements need to be addressed in order to fulfill the objective of stimulating all subsystems:
  - Dynamic stabilization:
    - Promotes coactivation of force couples
    - Centers humeral head.
  - Joint position sensibility:
    - Restore through conscious and unconscious pathways.
  - Reactive neuromuscular control:
    - Reflexive muscular stabilization induced by sudden alterations in joint position.
    - Eccentric activities useful.
  - Functional motor patterns:
    - Progression to the actual throwing activity.
    - Analyze direction of force, amount of loading, and resultant muscle action to incorporate functional progression.

REFERENCES

1. Bennett GE. Elbow and shoulder lesions of baseball players. *Am J Surg.* 1959;98:484–92.

2. Burkhart SS, Morgan CD, Kibler WB. The disabled throwing shoulder: spectrum of pathology. Part I: pathoanatomy and biomechanics. *Arthroscopy.* 2003;19(4):404–20.

3. Burkhart SS, Morgan CD, Kibler, WB. The disabled throwing shoulder: spectrum of pathology. Part II: evaluation and treatment of SLAP lesions in throwers. *Arthroscopy.* 2003;19(5):531–9.

4. Burkhart SS, Morgan CD, Kibler, WB. The disabled throwing shoulder: spectrum of pathology. Part III: the SICK scapula, scapular dyskinesis, the kinetic chain, and rehabilitation. *Arthroscopy.* 2003;19(6):641–61.

5. Glousman R, Jobe FW, Tibone J, Moynes D, Antonelli D, Perry J. Dynamic electromyographic analysis of the throwing shoulder with glenohumeral instability. *J Bone Joint Surg Am.* 1988;70(2):220–6.

6. Gowan ID, Jobe FW, Tibone JE, Perry J, Moynes DR. A comparative electromyographic analysis of the shoulder during pitching. Professional versus amateur pitchers. *Am J Sports Med.* 1987;15(6):586–90.

7. Grossman MG, Tibone JE, McGarry MH, Schneider DJ, Veneziani S, Lee TQ. A cadaveric model of the throwing shoulder: a possible etiology of superior labrum anterior-to-posterior lesions. *J Bone Joint Surg Am.* 2005;87(4):824–31.

8. Halbrecht JL, Tirman P, Atkin D. Internal impingement of the shoulder: comparison of findings between throwing and nonthrowing shoulders of college baseball players. *Arthroscopy.* 1999;15(3):253–8.

9. Jobe CM, Sidles J. Evidence for a superior glenoid impingement upon the rotator cuff: anatomic, kinesiologic, MRI and arthroscopic findings (Abstract). In: *5th International Conference on Surgery of the Shoulder.* 1992 Jul 12–15: Paris (France). 1992.

10. Kibler WB. The role of the scapula in athletic shoulder function. *Am J Sports Med.* 1998;26(2):325–37.

11. Kvitne RS, Jobe FW. The diagnosis and treatment of anterior instability in the throwing athlete. *Clin Orthop Relat Res.* 1993;(291):107–23.

12. Lephart SM, Henry TJ. Restoration of proprioception and neuromuscular control of the unstable shoulder. In: Lephart SM, Fu FH, editors. *Proprioception and Neuromuscular Control in Joint Stability.* New York (NY): Human Kinetics; 2000. p. 405–13.

13. Lephart SM, Henry TJ. The physiological basis for open and closed kinetic chain rehabilitation for the upper extremity. *J Sport Rehab.* 1996;5(1):71–87.

14. Lombardo SJ, Jobe FW, Kerlan RK, Carter VS, Shields CL Jr. Posterior shoulder lesions in throwing athletes. *Am J Sports Med.* 1977;5(3):106–10.

15. Meister K, Andrew JR, Batts J, Wilk K, Baumgarten T. Symptomatic thrower's exostosis. Arthroscopic evaluation and treatment. *Am J Sports Med.* 1999;27(2):133–6.

16. Morgan CD, Burkhart SS, Palmeri M, Gillespie M. Type II SLAP lesions: three subtypes and their relationships to superior instability and rotator cuff tears. *Arthroscopy.* 1998;14(6):553–65.

17. Rodosky MW, Harner CD, Fu FH. The role of the long head of the biceps muscle and superior glenoid labrum in anterior stability of the shoulder. *Am J Sports Med.* 1994;22(1):121–30.

18. Rubenstein DL, Jobe FW, Glousman RE, et al. Anterior capsulolabral reconstruction of the shoulder in athletes. *J Shoulder Elbow Surg.* 1992;1:229–37.

19. Snyder SJ, Karzel RP, Del Pizzo W, Ferkel RD, Friedman MJ. SLAP lesions of the shoulder. *Arthroscopy.* 1990;6(4):274–9.

20. Tibone JE, Jobe FW, Kerlan RK, et al. Shoulder impingement syndrome in athletes treated by anterior acromioplasty. *Clin Orthop Relat Res.* 1985;(198):134–40.

21. Tokish JM, Curtin MS, Kim YK, Hawkins RJ, Torry MR. Glenohumeral internal rotation deficit in the asymptomatic professional pitcher and its relationship to humeral retroversion. *J Sports Sci Med.* 2008;7:78–83.

22. Walch G, Boileau P, Noel E, Donell ST. Impingement of the deep surface of the supraspinatus tendon on the posterior glenoid rim: an arthroscopic study. *J Shoulder Elbow Surg.* 1992;1(5):238–45.

Elbow Instability

Scott P. Steinmann

52

INTRODUCTION

- The elbow is a congruent, complex hinge joint.
- Although constrained by bony architecture at the extremes of flexion and extension with ligamentous stability in the mid-range of motion, it accounts for 20% of all dislocations (5).
- Most instabilities result from either a single trauma (straight posterior or posterolateral rotatory instability) or chronic overuse in the overhead athlete (valgus instability). Varus instability can also occur and is frequently associated with a anteromedial coronoid fracture.

FUNCTIONAL ANATOMY

- The elbow joint comprises the radiocapitellar, ulnohumeral, and proximal radioulnar joints.
- The lateral portion of the distal humerus, the capitulum, articulates with the radial head. The medial portion of the humerus, the trochlea, articulates with the trochlear notch or "greater sigmoid notch" of the ulna. The radial notch of the ulna articulates with the radial head (7).
- The ulnohumeral joint affords flexion and extension of the elbow while the proximal radioulnar joint affords pronation and supination. The radiocapitellar joint moves in both rotation and flexion/extension.
- The primary restraints of the elbow are the osseous ulnohumeral articulation, particularly at the extremes of flexion and extension, and the ligamentous structures medially and laterally (9).
- The medial (or ulnar) collateral ligament (MCL) is the main constraint to valgus instability. It originates on the antero-inferior medial epicondyle and consists of an anterior band inserting on the sublime tubercle of the coronoid process (and provides most stability at all arcs of flexion) and the posterior band inserting on the medial margin of the semilunar notch of the ulna (and provides stability at 90 degrees of flexion). An injury pattern of valgus force tends to rupture the MCL off of the humeral origin.
- The lateral collateral ligament (LCL) complex originates from the lateral epicondyle and consists of 4 parts: (a) the radial collateral ligament; (b) the lateral ulnar collateral ligament (LUCL), which provides most lateral stability; (c) the annular ligament, which encircles the radial head; and (d) the accessory LCL. A common injury pattern is an avulsion of the complex from the humeral origin.

HISTORY (MCL)

- MCL injuries are most common in overhead-throwing athletes (2).
- The most common complaint is pain typically felt during late cocking and early deceleration of the throwing motion. Throwing velocity may also be diminished.
- Athletes do not complain of symptoms of elbow instability, such as popping, locking, or clicking; however, associated abnormalities, such as synovitis, plica, or loose bodies, may present with these symptoms. Most athletes if rested for a significant period of time or retired from overhead throwing will recover painless function, but few are willing to undergo nonoperative treatment for many months.
- It is rare to have an acute rupture of the MCL during an athletic event. Catastrophic tearing of the MCL occasionally can be seen, but patients often have had recurrent symptoms prior to ligament failure.
- Acute rupture of the MCL is most commonly seen in a full dislocation of the elbow, which may also avulse the origin of the flexor-pronator group.
- Patients may also have neuritis of the ulnar nerve, with numbness and tingling in the ulnar digits, as well as loss of strength in the finger intrinsic muscles. This may occur due to inflammatory changes along the medial side of the elbow and rarely requires isolated ulnar nerve decompression.

HISTORY (LUCL)

- Injury to the LCL complex is usually the result of trauma causing a dislocation or fracture-dislocation, such as a fall on an outstretched hand. An occasional iatrogenic cause may occur secondary to previous lateral tennis elbow surgery, especially if a full release was performed instead of a partial resection. Tennis elbow releases that stray posterior to the midportion of the capitellum may detach the LCL complex.

- Insufficiency of the LUCL is the essential lesion leading to lateral elbow instability.
- A constellation of injuries called "the terrible triad" of radial head fracture, coronoid fracture, and elbow dislocation is a common cause of lateral ligament instability.
- The main complaint of athletes with instability is popping and clicking of the elbow and a sensation of giving way. Push-ups or pushing oneself up from a chair may be painful or bring on symptoms of instability or giving way.
- The LUCL is stressed in activities of daily living (*e.g.*, lifting milk out of the refrigerator or shifting a manual transmission in a car), so unlike an MCL tear, patients will complain of pain and/or instability during normal activities, not just sports (3).

PHYSICAL EXAMINATION (MCL)

- Athlete may be tender to palpation over the MCL. This is more easily appreciated when palpation is done concurrently with valgus stress.
- A flexor-pronator origin avulsion can also present with tenderness just distal to the medial epicondyle. This can be seen in golfers who strike the ground hard accidentally with the club after a missed shot. A magnetic resonance imaging (MRI) can help distinguish between MCL avulsion and flexor pronator avulsion.
- "Golfer's elbow" is a term used to describe medial elbow pain and tenderness in a patient without a traumatic history and minimal findings on MRI.
- The patient may present with tenderness over the ulnar nerve in the cubital tunnel.
- Valgus stability is tested with the elbow flexed between 25 and 40 degrees to minimize the effect of bony restraints, and a valgus stress is applied while the examiner supports the elbow (11).

PHYSICAL EXAMINATION (LUCL)

- The lateral pivot shift test can be used for diagnosis. As originally described by O'Driscoll et al. (8), the patient is supine with the shoulder at 90 degrees of flexion with the elbow flexed 90 degrees overhead. The examiner gently supinates the forearm, and a valgus moment is applied. The arm is brought from near extension to flexion. The athlete should have apprehension during the beginning of the test, with further flexion causing a reduction of subluxation and diminution of the apprehension. The test can also be performed from flexion to extension as the elbow moves from reduced to subluxed.
- The lateral pivot shift test is rarely positive in the awake patient unless there is gross instability. Frank palpable subluxation and reduction is rare, unless the patient is under general anesthesia.

- A useful test in the clinic setting is to gently hold the patient's elbow at 90 degrees while the patient is relaxed in the sitting position. With the examiner's thumb over the radiocapitellar joint, the forearm is passively rotated into full supination. Subtle increased displacement of the radial head represents lateral ligament laxity. This can be compared to the contralateral side.

IMAGING STUDIES

- Plain radiographs may reveal associated intra-articular loose bodies, osteophytes, or calcification of the MCL (5). A shallow ulnohumeral joint may be evident on the lateral view.
- Stress views under fluoroscopy or ultrasound with a valgus or varus force can show a side-to-side difference, confirming MCL or LUCL insufficiency.
- MRI can show damage to ligaments on either side and can be useful when the diagnosis is in doubt or for preoperative planning. Injection of gadolinium dye may enhance the MRI.
- It is important to remember that in an active overhead athlete who has been competing for several years, the MRI is almost never "normal," and results should be interpreted in light of the physical examination.

TREATMENT (NONOPERATIVE)

- Document the neurovascular examination before and after any interventions.
- Immediate treatment of a frank elbow dislocation is reduction followed by splinting in 90 degrees of flexion, with postreduction x-rays to look for associated fractures (coronoid, radial head, olecranon).
- Reduction is best accomplished with sedation and gradual movement from extension to flexion with the examiner's thumbs pushing the tip of the olecranon distally and traction applied along the axis of the forearm in order to translate the coronoid over the trochlea and gently reduce the joint.
- Once the joint is reduced, it is placed through a full range of motion to assess how stable the articulation is. In most simple dislocations, the elbow should be stable from full flexion to extension. Applying a varus or valgus force to test the ligaments is not helpful because they are almost always torn and will show increased laxity, which does not warrant operative treatment.
- If the elbow dislocates as the elbow approaches extension, then options include immobilization at 90 degrees or more for 7–10 days.
- It is still possible to subluxate in a splint or cast, so radiographs should be obtained in several days to confirm continued reduction.
- For MCL injuries, a trial of nonoperative treatment with modalities to reduce swelling and medial-sided flexor-pronator strengthening is usually sufficient.

■ For LUCL injuries, avoidance of varus stress with use of a splint or brace can be helpful. Range of motion exercises in the supine position with the arm overhead allow avoidance of varus stress.

TREATMENT (OPERATIVE)

■ For MCL injuries, the indications for surgery are a failure of a quality rehabilitation regimen and the athlete's desire to return to previous level of activity. The surgical treatment consists of a tendon graft approximating the attachments of the MCL (6). Graft choices include autograft or allograft. The original reconstruction described by Jobe et al. (4) requires 5 bone tunnels with a tendon weave. Newer techniques, such as the docking procedure (10), use 2 or 3 bone tunnels (1). Results of primary repair of the MCL (without reconstruction with a graft) have been disappointing and are usually reserved for patients with a bony avulsion at the MCL origin or insertion (11).

■ For LUCL injuries, the indications are pain and dysfunction, either in activities of daily living or with athletics. Surgical treatment consists of either repair of the LUCL to the humeral origin or surgical reconstruction of the LUCL with a tendon graft (8). Similar to MCL reconstruction, newer techniques use either 2 or 3 bone tunnels and either an allograft or autograft.

REFERENCES

1. Ahmad CS, Lee TQ, El Attrache NS. Biomechanical evaluation of a new ulnar collateral ligament reconstruction technique with interference screw fixation. *Am J Sports Med.* 2003;31(3):332–7.
2. Conway JE, Jobe FW, Glousman RE, Pink M. Medial instability of the elbow in throwing athletes. Treatment by repair or reconstruction of the ulnar collateral ligament. *J Bone Joint Surg Am.* 1992;74(1):67–83.
3. Hotchkiss RN, Yamaguchi K. Elbow reconstruction. *Ortho Knowledge Update: Sports Medicine 7.* 2002;31:317–27.
4. Jobe FW, Stark H, Lombardo SJ. Reconstruction of the ulnar collateral ligament in athletes. *J Bone Joint Surg Am.* 1986;68(8):1158–63.
5. Josefsson PO, Johnell O, Gentz CF. Long-term sequelae of simple dislocation of the elbow. *J Bone Joint Surg Am.* 1984;66(6):927–30.
6. Morrey BF. Acute and chronic instability of the elbow. *J Am Acad Orthop Surg.* 1996;4(3):117–28.
7. Netter FH. Upper limb. In: *The CIBA Collection of Medical Illustrations.* Vol. 8. Summit: CIBA-GEIGY; 1987. p. 42–3.
8. O'Driscoll SW, Bell DF, Morrey BF. Posterolateral rotatory instability of the elbow. *J Bone Joint Surg Am.* 1991;73(3):440–6.
9. O'Driscoll SW, Jupiter JB, King GJW, Hotchkiss RN, Morrey BF. The unstable elbow. *J Bone Joint Surg Am.* 2000;82A(5):724–8.
10. Rohrbough JT, Altchek DW, Hyman J, Williams RJ 3rd, Botts JD. Medial collateral ligament reconstruction of the elbow using the docking technique. *Am J Sports Med.* 2002;30(4):541–8.
11. Williams RJ, Altchek DW. Atraumatic injuries of the elbow. *Ortho Knowledge Update: Sports Medicine 2.* 1999;23:229–36.

53 Elbow Articular Lesions and Fractures

Edward S. Ashman

INTRODUCTION

- Elbow articular lesions and fractures are not uncommon in the athlete. Seven percent of all fractures occur in the elbow (5). It is important for the sports physician to become familiar with patterns of injury and treatment options for athletic injuries of the elbow.

- The elbow's high degree of bony congruity, soft tissue aspects, and high potential for stiffness make the elbow uniquely challenging to treat after athletic injury. A common theme of elbow injuries is that early motion is important to minimize stiffness and to nourish the joint. Range of motion (ROM) required for activities of daily living is defined as 30–130 degrees of flexion and 50 degrees of supination and pronation (6). However, athletic activities may require far more motion than this.

- Pediatric and adult elbow fractures differ considerably and will be discussed separately.

PEDIATRIC FRACTURES

Radiographic Evaluation

- Physicians evaluating pediatric elbow fractures must be familiar with normal developmental anatomy, as well as secondary ossification centers about the elbow.

- When obtaining radiographs, it is often helpful to obtain contralateral comparison view for comparison to differentiate between normal ossification centers and fractures.

- The proximal radius should point to the capitellum in all views. The long axis of the ulna should line up with or be slightly medial to the long axis of the humerus on a true anteroposterior (AP) view. The anterior humeral line should bisect the capitellum on the lateral view. The humeral-capitellar (Baumann) angle should be within the range of 9–26 degrees of valgus (11).

- A posterior fat pad sign is always considered to be an abnormal radiographic finding and represents an elbow fracture 76% of the time (9).

- An anterior fat pad sign represents a superficial part of anterior fat pad and should be in front of the coronoid fossa. In normal elbow, the anterior fat pad should be barely visualized.

- Look for small radiolucent area between bony rim and moderate opaque shadows of brachialis.

- With joint effusion, there will be anterior and superior displacement of anterior fat pad (9).

Ossification Centers of the Elbow

- Capitellum (appears at age 1–2 years)
- Radial head (appears at age 2–4 years)
- Medial epicondyle (appears at age 4–6 years)
- Trochlea (appears at age 8–11 years)
- Olecranon (appears at age 9–11 years)
- Lateral epicondyle (appears at age 10–11 years) (11)
- A well-known, but ribald, mnemonic exists to remember this order but will not be repeated here. (So sue me; just remember: you *Can't Resist My Team Of Lawyers*.)

Supracondylar Fractures

- Extraarticular supracondylar fractures are the most common elbow fracture in the pediatric population and represent 10% of all pediatric fractures. Most occur due to a fall on the hand or elbow. Extension pattern is far more common (98%) (11).

- Performance of a careful neurovascular examination is crucial. Any of the neurovascular structures crossing the elbow joint may be at risk. Radiographs are mandatory. The pulseless, poorly perfused hand is a true emergency. It is important to rule out vascular injury. Vascular injuries are more commonly associated with posterolateral displacement and higher grade injuries. The medial spike may tether the brachial artery. One must perform frequent rechecks of the radial pulse to document its presence, as well as its quality. An intimal arterial injury may not be initially apparent but may develop over hours. Compartment syndromes must be treated emergently, and a high degree of clinical suspicion for this complication must be maintained, as a missed compartment syndrome may lead to catastrophic results (8).

- The anterior interosseous (AI) nerve is the most frequently injured nerve, but most recover spontaneously within 6 months. The AI nerve can be checked by having the patient make an "OK" sign. With posteromedial displacement, the lateral spike of proximal fragment may tether the radial nerve (4).

- Clinical signs include the "dimple sign" that occurs when the fracture ends are caught in the brachialis and subcutaneous soft tissues. The olecranon and the 2 epicondyles should form a straight line in the extended position and a triangle when the elbow is flexed to 90 degrees. This relationship is unchanged in a supracondylar fracture but is altered by an elbow dislocation (3).

- Treatment is defined by stability of fracture pattern as defined by Gartland classification. Type I is nondisplaced, and type II exhibits anterior gapping, limited rotational malalignment, and an intact posterior hinge. Type III fractures have no cortical continuity and are totally unstable. Type I may be treated with splinting; types II and III require reduction and most require operative intervention to maintain stability while in a 90-degree position of flexion (3).

- Following reduction, it is crucial to perform a repeat neurovascular examination and again check radiographs.

- Potential long-term sequelae of the supracondylar fracture include the following:

  - Cubitus varus is the most common complication following supracondylar humerus fracture. It is primarily a cosmetic deformity and does not usually create a loss of function. Previously, cubitus varus was thought to be created by growth disturbance, but it is now believed to be due to imperfect fracture reduction. It is extremely important to have perfect fracture rotation.

  - Volkmann contracture can be caused by brachial artery injury leading to a severe compartment syndrome, muscle necrosis, and degeneration. This was often a result of maintaining the arm in severe flexion in order to maintain a reduction. A closed reduction should be maintained with the arm in 90 degrees of flexion. If more flexion is needed to maintain the reduction, percutaneous pinning should be considered. Treatment options are focused on restoring vascular flow and reducing compartment pressure. It is usually too late to avoid severe morbidity. It is imperative to avoid this complication with proper fracture care and neurovascular monitoring.

  - Arterial injury occurs in approximately 5% of children with supracondylar fractures. Arteriography is indicated if the pulse is decreased following reduction. If no pulse is present before and after reduction, emergent surgery is required, and a delay for arteriography is contraindicated.

  - Nerve injuries are usually AI or radial nerve injuries and can be quite common (up to 50% AI injury with type III fractures). Most nerve palsies resulting from supracondylar fractures are neurapraxias and will resolve spontaneously within 3–6 months.

Lateral Epicondyle Fracture

- This fracture is exceedingly rare in adults (as is the medial epicondyle fracture) and is essentially a pediatric fracture. Intra-articular fractures must be considered as potentially unstable. Magnetic resonance imaging (MRI) or computed tomography (CT) may be needed to appreciate intra-articular component of fracture. Even benign-appearing injuries may develop displacement and high complication rates. Potential complications include nonunion, delayed union, and tardy ulnar nerve palsy secondary to progressive cubital valgus (12).

- If there is less than 2 mm of displacement, the fracture may be treated with cast immobilization but must be followed closely with serial radiographs. Any displacement greater than 2 mm must be surgically reduced and fixed (10,12).

Medial Epicondyle Fracture

- More common in young throwing athletes (*i.e.*, pitchers) that subject their elbows to high valgus stress. If chronic, the condition is termed "little leaguer's elbow."

- Must perform careful neurologic examination, as ulnar nerve may be involved (12).

- Must test for signs of instability, as it is possible that elbow is dislocated and spontaneously reduced because youths have less inherent stability than adults (2). Valgus instability should be assessed at 25 degrees of flexion. Also, the gravity stress test may be used. With the patient lying supine, externally rotate and abduct the shoulder to 90 degrees, flex the elbow to 20 degrees, and observe for pain and laxity. Stress x-ray views may also be performed (11).

- Even minimally displaced fractures may be well tolerated in the nonathlete (12). However, in the young athlete who is expected to have valgus stress on the elbow (throwers), operative intervention is more likely necessary. Surgical indications include the following (12):

  - Displacement greater than 10 mm may cause loss of strength of the flexor mass and should be fixed.

  - Ulnar neuropathy with displaced fracture

  - Valgus instability, as determined earlier

  - Displaced fracture that blocks joint motion

Olecranon Fracture

- Occur with other elbow fractures 20% of time.

- Displacement of 5 mm and articular step-off of 2 mm are operative indications. Hardware used depends on stability of fracture pattern, with plates used for less stable injury.

- Treat nonoperatively in 20 degrees of flexion to minimize triceps pull (11).

Proximal Radius Fracture

- Radial neck fractures are more common in 8- to 12-year-olds. Treatment is determined by angulation. Less than 30 degrees of angulation of neck is accepted. Greater than 30 degrees requires reduction, and greater than 60 degrees may require the use of a wire to "joystick" the fracture into position (11).

ADULT ELBOW TRAUMA

Distal Humerus Fractures

■ These fractures are rare in the athlete. High energy is required to cause this injury in the young adult population. In the general population, these fractures represent one-third of elbow fractures or 2% of all fractures (6). All have a high propensity for stiffness. It is important to maintain a functional ROM for activities of daily living. Nonoperative treatment is used only for nondisplaced fractures.

■ Operative treatment for displaced articular fractures aims for anatomic reduction and early motion to minimize stiffness. Intra-articular distal humerus fractures tend to be extremely complicated to treat operatively, and discussion of operative techniques is beyond the scope of this book.

Capitellar Fracture

■ These fractures are rare (< 1% of all elbow fractures) (6). They are often associated with radial head fractures. Diagnosis may be difficult, and the lateral plain film must be carefully checked. A CT scan may be necessary to better delineate the fracture type. Nonoperative treatment is used for nondisplaced fractures.

■ There are 3 basic types of capitellar fractures: Hahn-Steinthal fracture includes a large portion of bone with the capitellar articular surface and usually is able to be primarily reduced and fixed operatively. The Kocher-Lorenz fragment involves a small amount of articular surface of the capitellum only and must often be excised. A third type of fracture is comminuted and is also difficult to fix.

■ Early motion is mandatory after these injuries.

Radial Head Fractures

■ Common: 20%–30% of elbow fractures (6). Adults tend to sustain radial head as opposed to neck fractures. May be isolated or associated with elbow dislocation, ulnar shaft fractures, distal radial joint injury (Essex-Lopresti lesion), or carpal fractures, as well as additional fracture patterns.

■ Must rule out associated medial collateral ligament (MCL) injury, interosseous membrane injury, and distal radioulnar joint injury.

■ Operative indications include displacement greater than 2 mm, mechanical block to motion (pain may be ruled out as cause with intra-articular lidocaine injection), > 20%–30% articular depression, or open fracture (7). Surgical options depend on fracture type as well as associated lesions and include excision, open reduction internal fixation (ORIF), or

hemiarthroplasty. The radial head should never be excised with an interosseous ligament or MCL injury.

Olecranon Fracture

■ Nondisplaced fractures < 2 mm are treated nonoperatively with long arm casting. Care must be taken to avoid prolonged immobilization and stiffness (6).

■ Displaced fracture requires ORIF, with technique dependent on fracture pattern stability. Although excision of up to 50% of olecranon has been described (6), this should only be used in very low-demand patients and not in the athletic population.

Coronoid Fractures

■ These fractures are caused by humeral hyperextension and are associated with dislocation of elbow 10%–33% of time. Coronoid-trochlear articulation provides up to 50% of elbow stability (6).

■ Treatment depends on fracture stability pattern, which is defined by amount of coronoid involved in fracture. Greater than 50% involvement requires ORIF, whereas less than 50% fracture may be treated nonoperatively if it is stable.

■ As with most elbow fractures, the basic treatment plan is to obtain stability so as to allow early motion.

OSTEOCHONDRITIS DISSECANS

■ Osteochondritis dissecans (OCD) of the capitellum occurs in adolescent and young adult athletes who are involved in repetitive upper extremity exercises.

■ Throwers, gymnasts, and weightlifters are particularly susceptible.

■ Etiology involves microtrauma, but exact cause is uncertain.

■ AP and lateral radiographs are usually sufficient for diagnosis, but MRI or CT may be helpful to further delineate extent of lesion. There may be a localized area in capitellum without rarefaction and crater formation (1).

■ Osteochondrosis of the capitellum or Panner disease occurs in children age 4–8 years and involves the *entire* ossific nucleus. It is self-limiting with conservative treatment (7).

■ OCD of the capitellum occurs in individuals age 10 years old or greater and involves a *portion* of the capitellum. It is believed to be due to valgus high-stress forces cause during the acceleration phase of throwing, when the capitellum becomes loaded. Symptoms include poorly defined lateral elbow pain, with later stages of disease showing catching and locking. Laxity of the MCL may be present. Permanent deformity may result. Patients should be strictly restricted from throwing for 8–12 weeks or until full, pain-free motion is restored for nondisplaced lesion with intact articular cartilage (7).

■ Indications for surgery include partially or completely detached fragment. Treatment options are dependent on lesion type and chronicity and include removal, reattachment, bone grafting, drilling, and debridement. Operative techniques continue to evolve (7).

REFERENCES

1. Chen FS, Diaz VA, Loebenberger M, Rosen JE. Shoulder and elbow injuries in the skeletally immature athlete. *J Am Acad Orthop Surg.* 2005;13 (3):172–85.

2. Fowles JV, Slimane N, Kassab MT. Elbow dislocation with avulsion of the medial humeral epicondyle. *J Bone Joint Surg Br.* 1990;72(1):102–4.

3. Harris IE. Supracondylar fractures of the humerus in children. *Orthopedics.* 1992;15(7):811–7.

4. Ippolito-E, Caterini R, Scola E. Supracondylar fractures of the humerus in children. Analysis at maturity of fifty-three patients treated conservatively. *J Bone Joint Surg Am.* 1986;68(3):333–44.

5. Regan WD. Acute traumatic injuries of the elbow in the athlete. In: Griffin LY, editor. *Orthopaedic Knowledge Update Sports Medicine.* Rosemont: American Academy of Orthopedic Surgeons; 1994. p. 191–204.

6. Scheling GJ. Elbow and forearm: adult trauma. In: Koval KJ, editor. *Orthopaedic Knowledge Update 7.* Rosemont: American Academy of Orthopedic Surgeons; 2002. p. 307–16.

7. Schenck RC Jr, Goodnight JM. Osteochondritis dissecans. *J Bone Joint Surg Am.* 1996;79(3):439–56.

8. Shaw BA, Kasser JR, Emans JB, Rand FF. Management of vascular injuries in displaced supracondylar humerus fractures without arteriography. *J Orthop Trauma.* 1990;4(1):25–9.

9. Skaggs DL, Mirzayan R. The posterior fat pad sign in association with occult fracture of the elbow in children. *J Bone Joint Surg Am.* 1999;81(10):1429–33.

10. Tejwani N, Phillips D, Goldstein RY. Management of lateral humeral condylar fracture in children. *J Am Acad Orthop Surg.* 2011;19(6):350–8.

11. Vitale MG, Skaggs DL. Elbow. Pediatric aspects. In: Koval KJ, editor. *Orthopaedic Knowledge Update 7.* Rosemont: American Academy of Orthopedic Surgeons; 2002. p. 299–306.

12. Wilson NI, Ingram R, Rymaszewski L, Miller JH. Treatment of fractures of the medial epicondyle of the humerus. *Injury.* 1988;19(5):342–4.

54 Elbow Tendinosis

Patrick St. Pierre and Robert P. Nirschl

INTRODUCTION

- Elbow tendinosis is a result of tendon overuse and a failure of tendon healing.
- Elbow tendinosis can affect the elbow laterally (extensor carpi radialis brevis [ECRB], extensor digitorum communis), medially (pronator teres, flexor carpi radialis), or posteriorly (triceps) (6).

SYMPTOMS/SIGNS

- Initial symptoms are activity-related pain followed by pain at rest as the condition becomes more chronic.
- Repetitive activities, such as golf, tennis, and typing, are often the inciting activities for this condition.
- Some loss of extension is common in medial elbow tendinosis, but often the patients maintain full range of motion.
- Tenderness over lateral or medial tendon origins or posterior insertion of triceps.
- Pain with provocative procedures (resisted wrist/finger extension for lateral tendinosis, wrist flexion/pronation for medial tendinosis, and elbow extension for posterior tendinosis).
- Because medial and lateral affected tendon units cross the elbow joint, pain is more severe with provocative testing with the elbow in extension. Therefore, pain with provocative testing with the elbow flexed indicates more severe involvement.
- Functional strength loss is common.

HISTOPATHOLOGY

- Histology of surgically resected tissue fails to reveal inflammatory cells. Thus, the term "tendinosis" is preferable to "tendonitis."
- The epicondyle (bone) itself is not affected in the disease process. Therefore, epicondylitis is a misnomer. However, a bony exostosis may be noted as a companion problem in 20% of lateral elbow tendinosis cases.
- Pathologic tendinosis shows disruption of normal collagen matrix by the characteristic invasion of fibroblasts and vascular granulation tissue termed "angiofibroblastic proliferation" (8).

DIFFERENTIAL DIAGNOSIS/ ASSOCIATED LESIONS

- Lateral tendinosis can be confused with the rare entity of posterior interosseous nerve (PIN) entrapment, which would have diffuse pain along the radial nerve in the extensor mass of the proximal forearm, painful resisted supination, and electromyography (EMG) changes of distal muscle groups (5).
- Lateral tendinosis can be seen in combination or association with intra-articular abnormalities, such as synovitis, plica, chondromalacia, and osteochondritis dissecans (OCD).
- Medial elbow–associated abnormalities may include degeneration/rupture of medial collateral ligament, entrapment of the ulnar nerve, and congenital subluxation of the ulnar nerve.
- Posterior elbow–associated abnormalities may include extra-articular olecranon bursitis and intra-articular olecranon fossa issues (synovitis, chondromalacia, and loose fragments).
- The mesenchymal syndrome, coined by Nirschl, has been used to describe a subset of patients with apparent decreased tissue durability who present with multiple affected areas that are often bilateral, including rotator cuffs, medial and lateral elbow tendinosis, carpal tunnel syndrome, trigger finger, de Quervain disease, plantar fasciosis, Achilles insertional tendinosis, and hip trochanteric bursitis (6).

TREATMENT CONCEPTS

- Anti-inflammatory medications can be helpful in controlling pain and can be a first-line therapy, allowing patients to comfortably proceed with curative rehabilitative exercises.
- Promotion of a tendon healing response (neovascularization and fibroblastic infiltration with collagen deposition and maturation) can be accomplished by
  - Rehabilitative exercise
  - High-voltage electrical stimulation
  - General conditioning/aerobic conditioning, which provides increased regional blood perfusion and minimization of loss of strength of adjacent tissue
  - Rest from inciting trauma

- Eccentric exercises have been shown to be useful in the rehabilitative exercise program with either medial or lateral disease. Eccentric exercises for other tendinopathies have been effective as well and should be included in the first course of treatment for tendinopathy around the elbow (14).

- Cortisone injections, when done correctly under the origin of the ECRB or flexor-pronator mass, can also be effective in relieving pain. However, cortisone injections have risks, including fat atrophy, skin pigmentation changes, and infection, especially if injected superficially.

- Autologous blood injection (ABI) and platelet-rich plasma (PRP) have been increasingly used and studied over the past 10 years (1,2,11,13). Using ABI and PRP has been shown to demonstrate effectiveness in several studies, with PRP having better results than ABI in one study (1,13).

- Physical modalities such as high-voltage electrical stimulation, ultrasound, heat/cold, and dexamethasone iontophoresis (9) also are useful in relieving pain.

- Control of force loads
  - Counterforce strap bracing to constrain key muscle groups while maintaining muscle balance
  - Improved sports technique, such as improved backhand stroke in tennis (lateral tendinosis) and less trailing arm activity in the golf swing (medial tendinosis)
  - Equipment changes in sports, such as low string tension on tennis racquets and perimeter weighting in golf clubs

INDICATIONS FOR SURGERY

- Chronic symptoms usually of at least 6 months and often exceeding 1 year in duration
- Failure of response to a good-quality rehabilitation program
- Failed permanent response to cortisone injections (up to 3)
- Unacceptable quality of life as determined by the patient

SURGICAL PRINCIPLES

- Historically, elbow tendinosis was treated by the total release of the origin of the combined tendon groups from the epicondyle
- Currently, surgical treatment is directed at resecting only the pathologic tissue and protecting all normal tissues and attachments, followed by quality postoperative rehabilitation.
- Surgical goals can be accomplished through a small incision (≤ 3 cm).
- Associated lesions, when present, such as OCD, loose bodies, and synovitis, can be addressed with a mini-arthrotomy at the time of the tendinosis resection (3).
- Arthroscopic treatment of lateral elbow tendinosis has been shown to be very effective, with satisfactory results of over 90% in several studies (4,10,12). For skilled elbow

arthroscopists, this is an effective treatment; although the mini-open technique is recommended for most surgeons.

- Ulnar nerve entrapment is associated with medial elbow tendinosis and should be evaluated by exam and possible nerve conduction study (5).

TREATMENT RESULTS

- The vast majority of patients with elbow tendinosis respond to nonoperative intervention.
- Of those that do require surgery, up to 97% will experience significant or total pain relief and return of strength with minimal complications (4,7,12).

REFERENCES

1. Creaney L, Wallace A, Curtis M, Connell D. Growth factor-based therapies provide additional benefit beyond physical therapy in resistant elbow tendinopathy: a prospective double-blind, randomised trial of autologous blood injections versus platelet-rich plasma injections. *Br J Sports Med.* 2011;45(12):966–71.
2. Edwards SG, Calandruccio JH. Autologous blood injections for refractory lateral epicondylitis. *J Hand Surg Am.* 2003;28(2):272–8.
3. Kraushaar BS, Nirschl RP, Cox W. A modified lateral approach for release of posttaumatic elbow flexion contracture. *J Shoulder Elbow Surg.* 1999;8(5):476–80.
4. Latterman C, Romeo AA, Anbari A, et al. Arthroscopic debridement of the extensor carpi radialis brevis for recalcitrant lateral epicondylitis. *J Shoulder Elbow Surg.* 2010;19(5):651–6.
5. Lubahn JD, Cermak MB. Uncommon nerve compression syndromes of the upper extremity. *J Am Acad Orthop Surg.* 1998;6(6):378–86.
6. Nirschl RP. Elbow tendinosis/tennis elbow. *Clin Sports Med.* 1992;11(4): 851–70.
7. Nirschl RP, Ashman ES. Tennis elbow tendinosis (epicondylitis). *Instr Course Lect.* 2004;53:587–98.
8. Nirschl RP, Pettrone FA. Tennis elbow. The surgical treatment of lateral epicondylitis. *J Bone Joint Surg Am.* 1979;61(6A):832–9.
9. Nirschl RP, Rodin DM, Ochiai DH, Maartmann-Moe C, DEX-AHE-01-99 Study Group. Iontophoretic administration of dexamethasone sodium phosphate for acute epicondylitis: a randomized, double-blinded, placebo-controlled study. *Am J Sports Med.* 2003;31(2):189–95.
10. Owens BS, Murphy KP, Kuklo TR. Arthroscopic release for lateral epicondylitis. *Arthroscopy.* 2001;17(6):582–7.
11. Peerbooms JC, Sluimer J, Bruijn DJ, Gosens T. Positive effect of an autologous platelet concentrate in lateral epicondylitis in a double-blind randomized controlled trial: platelet-rich plasma versus corticosteroid injection with 1-year follow-up. *Am J Sports Med.* 2010;38(2):255–62.
12. Savoie FH 3rd, VanSice W, O'Brien MJ. Arthroscopic tennis elbow release. *J Shoulder Elbow Surg.* 2010;19(2)(suppl):31–6.
13. Thanasas C, Papadimitriou G, Charalambidis C, Paraskevopoulous I, Papanikolaou A. Platelet-rich plasma versus autologous whole blood for the treatment of chronic lateral elbow epicondylitis: a randomized controlled clinical trial. *Am J Sports Med.* 2011;39(10):2130–4.
14. Woodley BL, Newsham-West RJ, Baxter GD. Chronic tendinopathy: effectiveness of eccentric exercise. *Br J Sports Med.* 2007;41(4):188–98.

55 Soft Tissue Injuries of the Wrist and Hand

D. Nicole Deal and A. Bobby Chhabra

INTRODUCTION

■ Injuries to the wrist and hand are common in sports. In the past, these injuries were frequently designated as sprains. More recently, however, the "waste basket" terms *wrist sprain* and *jammed finger* have given way to a specific diagnosis and a defined treatment plan. An understanding of wrist and hand anatomy, biomechanics, and function allows the physician to pinpoint specific pathology and treatment, thus allowing quicker return to sport for the athlete with a wrist or hand injury. Missed or misdiagnosed injuries can result in permanent deformity and loss of function. Radiographs are indicated in nearly all cases to evaluate for fracture or dislocation and to evaluate for joint incongruity or avulsion fracture in cases of joint or tendon injury.

EPIDEMIOLOGY

■ The incidence of injuries to the wrist varies according to sport. Hand and wrist injuries occur more frequently in younger athletes than adults. A study performed at the Cleveland clinic found that 9% of all athletic participants under the age of 16 sustained injuries involving the wrist (4). In another study, 35% of all injuries in adolescent football players involved the wrist (42). Ligamentous laxity is often seen in athletes. This joint hypermobility can lead to partial or complete ligament tears following a loading of the wrist or may predispose to cumulative injury after repetitive stress (48). Overuse syndromes of the wrist are also common in athletes as a result of tension failure or shear stresses (35).

DORSAL WRIST SYNDROMES

■ Chronic wrist pain on the dorsal aspect of the wrist can be a result of occult dorsal ganglion or dorsal impaction/dorsal impingement syndromes. Ganglions account for the most frequent soft tissue tumors of the wrist. Of these, 60%–70% originate from the dorsal scapholunate ligament and are extraarticular manifestations of a connection to the scapholunate joint. A history of wrist trauma is found in 15% of patients with a dorsal ganglion (2). An occult dorsal ganglion is difficult to detect on clinical examination and may only be palpable with extreme flexion (2). Symptoms are generally inversely related to the size of the ganglion, as smaller, tense ganglions produce more pain than larger, soft cysts. Patients often complain of localized tenderness, limitation of motion, and/or weakness of grip. Ultrasound or magnetic resonance imaging (MRI) can be more useful than plain radiographs. Often, the diagnosis is made by exclusion. Initial treatment should include aspiration followed by steroid injection of the dorsal capsule followed by immobilization (44). When conservative treatment has failed to relieve the symptoms, excision of the capsule and ganglion from the scapholunate ligament is performed. Results are generally favorable, with ultimate full return to competition in the majority of cases.

■ Dorsal impaction syndromes occur as a result of repetitive loading of the wrist in maximum extension and happen most frequently to gymnasts. The shear forces created by this action may lead to localized synovitis or even osteocartilaginous fractures (26). The athlete will often complain of pain and point tenderness on the middorsal aspect of the wrist, at the projection of the lunocapitate joint (14). Progression of the problem may lead to radiographic changes including a hypertrophic ridge of the dorsal rim of the scaphoid or the dorsal border of the lunate as a result of impingement with the capitate during hyperextension. Successful treatment usually results from restriction of wrist hyperextension, strengthening of the wrist flexors, and local steroid injection. Failure of relief of symptoms should be followed by immobilization and cessation from sport for 4–6 weeks. If symptoms should continue to persist, either abandonment of the activity or surgical treatment consists of limited synovectomy and cheilectomy of hypertrophic margins that impinge during hyperextension. Return to sport may not be possible in all cases, but relief of pain generally occurs following treatment.

CARPAL INSTABILITY

- Carpal instability can be seen in any athlete in a contact sport following a collision injury but may also be a result of chronic repetitive loading in noncontact sports. Carpal instability can be seen as a spectrum of injuries ranging in symptoms and functional deficit. Initial injury may present as something as innocuous as an occult dorsal or intracapsular ganglion (mentioned earlier) and progress to dynamic instability, then static instability, and ultimately to scapholunate advanced collapse (SLAC) (24). The dynamic instability is not apparent on routine radiographs but is reproduced by manipulation and seen on stress radiographs in pronated clenched fist views (8). Static instability can be seen on routine radiograph as abnormal carpal alignment (47). Carpal collapse is seen following complete disruption initially of ligaments between the scaphoid and lunate, progressing to disruption between the lunate and triquetrum and finally to the midcarpal joints. Carpal ligamentous injuries are common in athletes and require physicians, trainers, and therapists who treat and diagnose these injuries to have an understanding of the carpal anatomy and potential for progression to instability (45).

Scapholunate Dissociation

- Scapholunate instability occurs as the ligamentous support of the proximal pole of the scaphoid is disrupted and the scaphoid rotates into palmar flexion. The carpal instability associated with this injury is a dorsal intercalated segmental instability (DISI) deformity. This can be reproduced clinically during physical examination by performing the Watson maneuver (49). Radiographically, this is shown by widening of the scapholunate interval (compared to the uninjured wrist), an increase in the scapholunate angle (> 70 degrees; normal, 30–60 degrees), and a cortical *ring* sign in which the distal pole of the perpendicular scaphoid is seen end-on on the anteroposterior view of the wrist.

- Successful treatment may consist of closed reduction and percutaneous pinning if initiated within the first 3–4 weeks after injury. This may also be performed under arthroscopic guidance. In most cases, open reduction, ligamentous repair, and internal fixation with Kirschner wires is the most reliable treatment in the management of scapholunate ligament injuries in athletes. For chronic scapholunate dissociation without advanced arthritic changes, a dorsal capsulodesis and ligament reconstruction as described by Blatt (5), a Brunelli procedure using flexor carpi radialis (FCR) tunneled through the distal pole of the scaphoid (7), or when ligament reconstruction is not possible, a scaphotrapezial-trapezoidal fusion as described by Watson and Hempton (50) may be performed. Postoperatively, the wrist is immobilized in slight palmar flexion and pronation. Return to contact sports is limited after treatment for carpal instability.

Lunotriquetral Instability

- Injuries to the lunotriquetral ligaments may range from sprain to partial tear to complete tear with or without carpal malalignment. The carpal instability associated with this injury is a volar intercalated segmental instability (VISI) deformity. This complete injury occurs rarely in athletes. Symptoms consist of pain on the dorso-ulnar side of the carpus with a positive lunotriquetral ballottement test as described by Reagan et al. (37). Injection of local anesthetic to the lunotriquetral joint usually relieves symptoms and restores grip strength. Routine radiographic evaluation is able to detect static instability as evident by volar flexion of the lunate in neutral deviation. Midcarpal arthrography and MRI may demonstrate incomplete or complete tears of the lunotriquetral ligaments, or radiocarpal arthrography may detect a simultaneous injury to the triangular fibrocartilage, particularly in an ulna-positive patient. Ulnar variance has been shown to be associated with the location of injury. An ulnar minus variance is related to radial axis injury, whereas an ulnar neutral or plus variance has been linked to ulnar axis injury.

- Treatment of acute or untreated chronic injuries with no evidence of a tear consists of injection of a corticosteroid preparation followed by immobilization. Surgical treatment is considered when disabling pain continues and cessation from sport is not an alternative and consists of lunotriquetral ligament repair when possible. Arthroscopy may be valuable in staging and determining treatment and may be used to assist in reduction and pinning in both acute and chronic ligament tears without advanced collapse (52). In patients with an ulna plus variance, ulna shortening is the treatment of choice. Lunotriquetral arthrodesis has been performed but without uniform success (48) and is rarely performed in athletes (52).

ULNAR TRANSLOCATION

- Ulnar translocation is an extremely rare injury in athletes that is usually a result of a severe violent impact, such as in motor sports. In order for complete translocation to occur, complete disruption of both the volar and dorsal radiocarpal ligaments must take place. As a result, the carpus is allowed to slide along the incline of the radius in the ulnar direction. Physical examination includes severe swelling, loss of motion, and deformity. Radiographic evaluation will demonstrate translation of the carpus, rotation of the proximal carpal row into palmar flexion, and scapholunate diastasis due to ulnar displacement of the lunate.

- There is no role for nonoperative treatment in this injury. Surgical exploration reveals extensive capsular tears, frequently including the scapholunate ligament. Taleisnik (47) believes that capsular reattachment commonly results in recurrence, and if stability is achieved, it is usually at the expense of loss of motion. As a result, he recommends radiolunate arthrodesis to maintain reduction that results in a stable, pain-free wrist with satisfactory preservation of motion. This may allow an athlete to return to strenuous activity when full range of motion is not mandatory.

TRIANGULAR FIBROCARTILAGE COMPLEX INJURY

- The triangular fibrocartilage complex (TFCC) is made up of the triangular fibrocartilage (TFC), a cartilaginous disc that lies on the ulnar head and several supporting ligaments and acts as a stabilizer of the distal radioulnar joint (DRUJ). Injury to this structure may result in 2 forms, perforation of the disc (traumatic or degenerative) or avulsion (traumatic) of the disc with or without avulsion of the supporting ligaments. Avulsion of the TFCC occurs following acute dislocation or subluxation of the distal ulna relative to the radius. Degenerative tears usually occur after the third decade (29). Ulnar variance may play a role in degenerative changes of the TFC. Palmer et al. (32) found the center of the TFC to be thinner in ulna plus wrists. Lunotriquetral tears may occur following degenerative perforation of the TFC leading to carpal instability. Young athletes with ulna plus variants, who participate in repetitive loading of the wrist, may be susceptible to degenerative changes of the TFC similar to older patients (14).

- Patients with injury to the TFC frequently complain of ulnar-sided wrist pain exacerbated by forearm rotation. It is important to discern injury to TFC from injury to the DRUJ. Injury to the TFC is suspected when tenderness and crepitus are palpated between the ulna and triquetrum. Relief of pain during manual stabilization of the DRUJ during forearm rotation may be an indicator of DRUJ instability. Diagnostic evaluation may include plain radiographs, MRI, arthrography, and/or arthroscopy. Demonstration of ulna plus variance on plain radiographs adds to suspicion of TFC injury, and ulnolunate impaction "kissing" lesions are common. Arthrography may exhibit a communication between the radiocarpal and distal radioulnar joints. MRI and arthroscopy have been helpful in determining the size and location of lesion of the TFC.

- Treatment of acute injury of the TFC includes immobilization of the wrist in neutral rotation for up to 4–6 weeks. Gradual progression of activities may then begin with the use of supportive splinting. An injection into the ulnocarpal space with steroid may also be helpful and diagnostic prior to immobilization. If the athlete is unable to return to sport and symptoms persist, then surgical debridement of the perforation and/or repair of the TFCC should be performed (28). Decompression can be obtained through ulnar shortening (25), DRUJ excisional hemiarthroplasty (6), or the Kapandji procedure (12). If a peripheral tear is found in the outer 15%–20% of the TFC, a repair may be considered in conjunction with ulnar recession as needed (48). For patients with ulna plus variance and a degenerative tear of the TFC, ulnar shortening is the treatment of choice, whereas excision of the TFC and the Darrach procedure should be avoided. For patients with ulna minus variant, debridement of the TFC defect may relieve pain and will not increase load transmission providing only the central third is removed. For acute avulsions causing DRUJ instability, above elbow immobilization with the DRUJ reduced usually is successful. If instability persists, reattachment of the TFC is performed, usually at the fovea of the ulnar styloid using suture and drill holes (16).

FINGERTIP INJURIES

Subungual Hematoma

- Many crush injuries to the fingertips will damage the nail and underlying matrix, causing blood beneath the nail and throbbing pain. These injuries may also be associated with tuft fractures of the distal phalanx, which are typically open fractures because they communicate through the nail matrix disruption (18).

- Hematoma involving less than 50% of the nail matrix may be drained using a heated paperclip, an 18-gauge needle, or a battery-operated cautery to create one or multiple holes in the nail. An anesthetic digital block may be necessary prior to drainage. Soaking the finger in sterile water with peroxide will facilitate drainage. A sterile dressing should then be applied, with a Stack splint in cases involving fracture (9,18).

- Hematoma involving more than 50% of the underlying nail bed is presumed to be associated with an open fracture. Radiographs, surgical removal of the nail, thorough irrigation and debridement of the wound, repair of the nail matrix, and replacement of the nail with splinting are recommended (9).

Nail Avulsion

- If nail avulsion occurs without damage to the underlying sterile matrix, the wound should be thoroughly cleansed and dressed with a nonadherent dressing. If the proximal portion of the nail has also been avulsed from the nail fold and germinal matrix, the patient's cleansed nail or a piece of sterile gauze or foil should be slid under the eponychial fold to prevent adherence (9).

- If any part of the sterile or germinal matrix has been torn or lacerated, removal of any remaining nail fragments and repair of the nail bed injury are mandatory. Again, the eponychial fold should be splinted open (9).

Fingerpad Injuries

- Simple lacerations may be cleansed and sutured using nonabsorbable monofilament in adults or absorbable suture in children. Grossly contaminated wounds may be cleansed and left open.

- Partial amputations with soft tissue loss measuring less than 1 cm (2) will heal by secondary intention and may be treated with cleansing and serial dressing changes. Even larger defects will heal well in children. Larger wounds involving exposed bone or tendon, nail bed injury, or more proximal amputation should be emergently treated by a hand surgeon (9,18).

JOINT INJURIES OF THE FINGERS

- Dislocations are usually clinically apparent; are characterized by pain, limited movement, and digit deformity and should be radiographed prior to reduction to assess for associated fracture if there is any crepitus, bony point tenderness, or open injury.
- Other dislocations can be reduced and splinted, and a post-reduction radiograph obtained. Any irreducible dislocation or dislocation associated with an open wound requires emergent referral (34).
- Local or regional anesthesia may be necessary to obtain adequate pain relief and relaxation for reduction. Digital blocks are placed by injecting the ulnar and radial webspaces of a digit, anesthetizing the dorsal and volar digital nerves. The local anesthetic should not contain epinephrine, which could cause digital ischemia.

Distal Interphalangeal Joint

- Distal interphalangeal (DIP) joint dislocations are uncommon, almost always dorsal, and often open. These injuries are frequently associated with tendon disruption (see sections on mallet and jersey finger).
- If there is no open wound or tendon rupture and closed reduction is possible, extension splinting for 2–3 weeks is recommended.

Proximal Interphalangeal Joint

- Proximal interphalangeal (PIP) joint injuries are the most common joint injuries in sports, primarily occurring in athletes who participate in contact sports and ball handling (30,40).

DORSAL DISLOCATIONS

- These injuries are frequently seen in football and basketball. Dorsal dislocations are most common and result from hyperextension with axial load. This causes distal volar plate rupture with or without bony avulsion. A true lateral x-ray should be obtained to rule out a fracture (40).
- Reduction is usually uncomplicated. Dynamic and static stability should be assessed after reduction, including collateral ligament stability (19).

- If there is no associated fracture or ligament injury, splinting in 30 degrees of flexion for 1–2 weeks, followed by buddy taping for sports for 4–6 weeks, is effective. Recurrent dislocation is rare. Swelling and tenderness can persist for several months. Motion exercises as soon as comfort permits can help to prevent stiffness (40).

VOLAR DISLOCATIONS

- Volar dislocations of the PIP joint are less common injuries, are more difficult to reduce, and are associated with more complications than dorsal dislocations. They are caused by compression and rotation with PIP joint flexion. Pathology usually includes extensor tendon central slip avulsion, volar plate disruption, and collateral ligament tears (19,40).
- If closed reduction is successful, the PIP joint should be splinted in full extension for 3–4 weeks to protect the central slip, allowing the DIP joint to remain free, followed by night splinting for an additional 3–4 weeks. If closed reduction is not possible, open reduction and pinning are necessary (40).
- Late development of boutonnière deformity is a potential complication.

ROTARY PROXIMAL INTERPHALANGEAL JOINT SUBLUXATION

- This injury typically presents as an irreducible dislocation of the PIP joint. It involves buttonholing of 1 condyle of the proximal phalanx through a longitudinal rent in the extensor hood between the central slip and lateral band. A lateral profile of the proximal phalanx with an oblique profile of the middle phalanx is seen on lateral radiograph (19).
- If closed reduction is successful, buddy taping with full active range of motion is usually sufficient. Open reduction is often necessary to disengage the proximal phalanx condyle from the central slip and lateral band.

COLLATERAL LIGAMENT INJURIES

- Collateral ligament injuries occur as a result of radial or ulnar stress on the joint, most commonly in football, wrestling, and basketball. Disruption usually occurs at the proximal attachment, with radial collateral injury more common than ulnar collateral injury. The most commonly involved digit is the index finger (40).
- Tenderness and ecchymosis are usually present on examination. Radiographs should be obtained to rule out fracture. Examination and radiographs should be used to assess stability.

- Most collateral ligament injuries are treated with buddy taping to an adjacent finger, with continued participation in athletic activity. If the tear is associated with significant instability, the digit should be immobilized in a dorsal splint for 3–4 weeks (40).

Metacarpophalangeal Joint

- Metacarpophalangeal (MCP) dislocations are relatively rare and usually involve dorsal dislocation of the proximal phalanx on the metacarpal. Most occur in the index or small finger.
- Simple dislocations may be reduced by closed reduction, and if stable following reduction, then consider buddy taping alone and allowing immediate active motion. Complex dislocations involve buttonholing of the metacarpal head between the flexor tendon and the lumbrical with volar plate interposition into the dislocated joint. These usually require formal open reduction.

JOINT INJURIES OF THE THUMB

Interphalangeal Joint

- Thumb interphalangeal (IP) dislocations are uncommon injuries and are managed similarly to finger DIP dislocations.

Metacarpophalangeal Joint

- Dislocations of the thumb MCP joint are usually dorsal dislocations, resulting from hyperextension at the MCP joint with volar plate rupture. The metacarpal head may protrude through the volar plate, where it becomes buttonholed between the flexor pollicis longus and flexor pollicis brevis tendons (19).
- The volar plate, flexor pollicis longus, or sesamoids may be interposed and prevent reduction, but closed reduction is usually possible, with splinting recommended for 3–4 weeks after reduction.

Gamekeeper's Thumb

- Also known as *skier's thumb* in acute injury, this refers to the rupture of the ulnar collateral ligament (UCL) of the thumb MCP joint. The mechanism of injury involves a fall on an outstretched thumb with hyperabduction at the MCP joint. Patients present with tenderness and swelling over the ulnar aspect of the thumb MCP joint with instability of the UCL on radial stress. Instability should be assessed with the MCP in 30 degrees of flexion and at full extension. This can also be documented and quantified on stress radiographs (1,23,30,38).
- The injury may be associated with the Stener lesion, in which the torn end of the UCL is displaced superficially to the aponeurosis of the adductor pollicis, preventing primary healing. Gross instability or a palpable lump suggests a Stener lesion, which can sometimes also be directly visualized with

ultrasound or MRI. This lesion may be present in up to 70% of cases (19,30).
- Many injuries will do well with immobilization for 4 weeks in a thumb spica cast, followed by 2–4 months of protected splinting during athletic competition.
- Surgical intervention with reattachment of the UCL is typically required for any injury with greater than 30–35 degrees of instability in flexion, any instability in extension, a Stener lesion, or large bony avulsion (1,19,23,30).

Radial Collateral Ligament Injury

- Radial collateral ligament injury may involve proximal or distal ligament tears of the ligament.
- It is much less common than UCL injury but evaluated and treated in a similar manner. Injuries may be associated with volar subluxation of the joint and may require surgical stabilization (19,40).

TENDON INJURIES

Mallet Finger

- This injury is also known as *drop finger* or *baseball finger* and most commonly occurs in football receivers, baseball players, and basketball players. *Mallet finger* refers to a disruption of the extensor mechanism insertion into the distal phalanx, resulting from forced flexion of an actively extended DIP joint. A variably sized piece of bone may be avulsed with tendon (23,38,40).
- The patient will have a passively flexed DIP joint with full passive range of motion but inability to actively extend at the DIP joint (17).
- Preferred treatment is continuous extension splinting of the DIP joint for at least 6 weeks while allowing PIP motion, then up to 4 weeks of nighttime splinting. If there is a large bony fragment avulsed, some recommend surgical fixation with reduction and pinning. Surgical treatment may be necessary for late, chronic cases (3,23,38,40).

Boutonnière Deformity

- This injury is also known as a *buttonhole* deformity and involves rupture or avulsion of the extensor mechanism central slip at the middle phalanx. The head of the phalanx may buttonhole through the defect. The lateral bands then contract, causing late extension deformity at the DIP joint (usually appearing 1–3 weeks later) (23,40).
- This injury occurs with unrecognized palmer dislocation of the PIP joint, or more commonly, by forced flexion of the middle phalanx while the athlete is attempting to extend the joint. The patient will present with swelling and pain over the dorsal PIP joint, inability to extend the PIP, and possible hyperextension at the DIP joint (38).

- Treatment consists of extension splinting of the PIP for 6 weeks, allowing DIP motion, followed by gradual PIP motion. Chronic cases usually respond to closed treatment as well. Cases associated with large bony fragments should be surgically addressed (23,38,40).

Pseudo-boutonnière Deformity

- This injury has a similar clinical appearance to the boutonnière deformity but a distinctly different mechanism and treatment. It is caused by a hyperextension injury to the PIP joint, disrupting the volar plate and either the radial collateral ligament or UCL. Tissue contraction causes later development of progressive PIP flexion deformity. Differentiation from a boutonnière deformity is possible by absence of tenderness over the PIP central slip and equivalent active and passive ranges of motion at the PIP joint in this injury (19,23).

- Treatment is difficult and often prolonged, with splinting recommended if PIP deformity is less than 45 degrees. Surgical intervention with capsular release is often necessary for greater deformities (23).

Extensor Tendon Subluxation and Dislocation

- Extensor tendons usually subluxate or dislocate to the ulnar side of the MCP joint, usually resulting from a direct blow to the digit with forced flexion and ulnar deviation. Radial subluxation is rare. The middle finger is most commonly affected. Patients present with tenderness over the MCP joint, pain with resisted extension, inability to fully extend at the joint, and often palpable tendon subluxation or dislocation (3,38,40).

- Acute injuries (presenting within 4–6 weeks) may respond to extension splinting of the MCP joint. Chronic or recalcitrant cases often require surgical reconstruction with release of contractures and repair of the extensor hood and sagittal bands (23,38).

Boxer's Knuckles

- This injury, also known as *soft knuckles*, is caused by repetitive trauma to the dorsal MCP joints, most commonly involving the index and long digits. The injury manifests as pain and swelling over involved joints, usually improving with rest but recurring with resumed training (38).

- The anatomic basis of injury usually involves tears of the extensor hood, extensor tendon, or dorsal joint capsule. Rest or splinting is of little benefit; exploration with surgical repair of injured structures is often required (15,23,38).

Jersey Finger

- Jersey finger involves an avulsion of the flexor digitorum profundus (FDP) tendon from its insertion on the distal phalanx, commonly occurring in football and rugby players. Greater than 75% of cases involve the ring finger (22,23,40).

- Injury is caused by forced DIP extension during maximal FDP contraction, as in grabbing someone's jersey while attempting to tackle. Clinical findings include the inability to actively flex the DIP joint, with normal passive range of motion. Radiographs are usually negative unless a bony fragment is avulsed with the tendon (3,38).

- Injuries are graded and treated according to severity that depends on the degree of tendon retraction. In type I injuries, the tendon retracts into the palm. In type II injuries, the tendon retracts to the level of the PIP joint. In type III injuries, the tendon retracts only to the A4 pulley. These are nearly always associated with a large avulsed bony fragment (22,23,38).

- All require surgical intervention, but the greater the degree of retraction, the more quickly surgical intervention is required. Type I injuries should be addressed within 7–10 days, whereas type III injuries are often successfully treated up to 2–3 months later (23,40).

VASCULAR INJURY

Hypothenar Hammer Syndrome

- This syndrome is caused by repetitive impact to the hypothenar region of the hand, with trauma to the ulnar artery in the region of Guyon's canal resulting in arterial constriction, thickening, thrombosis, and possible aneurysm formation. It is most commonly seen in judo, karate, and lacrosse (39).

- Symptoms are caused by distal ischemia and include cold intolerance, pain in the palm or ulnar digits, and an abnormal Allen's test. Ulnar nerve compression and the corresponding symptoms may occur secondary to aneurysm formation.

- Treatment includes rest from inciting activities, increased padding of the hypothenar area, vasolytic agents, or surgical intervention with excision of the thrombosed segment and artery ligation or reconstruction (39).

Chronic Digital Ischemia

- Chronic compression or microtrauma to the hand and digital vasculature may cause distal ischemia. This is occasionally seen in baseball pitchers and catchers and handball players. Typical symptoms include cold intolerance, pallor, and pain in the involved digits (39,46).

- Increased padding during causative activities, use of pharmacologic agents, or surgical exploration may be appropriate treatments.

Frostbite

- Ischemic cold injury depends on the duration and severity of exposure, as well as the presence of constrictive clothes, vasospasm, and wetness. Early symptoms include erythema, burning, and itching (the chilblains). The involved part later becomes numb as injury progresses. Vesicles and ulcers may also develop (18,31).

- First-degree frostbite is a superficial injury from which full recovery is expected. Second-degree injury involves partial-thickness dermal loss. In third-degree injury, full-thickness dermal loss occurs, whereas involvement of deeper structures, including tendon and bone, indicates fourth-degree injury (18).

- Treatment involves gradual rewarming of involved digits in 40–42°C water. Advanced injuries and gangrenous areas will require surgical debridement, amputation, or skin grafting (31).

OVERUSE INJURIES

- The incidence of wrist and hand problems in athletes is extremely high. Wrist syndromes account for the most common upper extremity overuse injuries (39). Repetitive activities, such as gymnastics, racquet sports, rowing, and throwing sports, result in a high number of overuse injuries.

De Quervain Tenosynovitis

- Stenosis of the first dorsal compartment abductor pollicis long (APL) and extensor pollicis brevis (EPB) is referred as *de Quervain tenosynovitis*. It occurs in athletes who perform forceful grasp with repetitive use of the thumb and radial ulnar deviation (20). Sports that are more susceptible to this injury include racquet sports, golf (particularly the left thumb in right-handed golfers) (41), fly-fishing, javelin, and discus throwing. Athletes classically complain of pain over the radial styloid, particularly with range of motion of the thumb and ulnar deviation of the wrist. Generally, there is tenderness over the first dorsal compartment along with swelling and occasional crepitus or triggering. The Finklestein test is frequently positive with wrist ulnar deviation while the thumb is adducted and is pathognomonic for the diagnosis (39). Initial treatment includes anti-inflammatory medication, thumb spica splinting, and corticosteroid injection into the first dorsal compartment. Poor response from injection may be due to a longitudinal septum, which separates the APL and EPB in 20%–30% of cases (10), and may improve with a second more dorsal injection. If there is no improvement of symptoms, surgical treatment involves decompression of the first dorsal compartment with division of any septum when present. Complications of surgery include persistence of symptoms (possibly due to inadequate release), adhesions, injury to the superficial radial nerve, and volar tendon subluxation. Most athletes are able to return to full participation following surgical decompression in 3–4 weeks.

Intersection Syndrome

- Intersection syndrome is pain in the dorsoradial wrist where the first dorsal compartment crosses the second dorsal compartment extensor carpi radialis longus (ECRL) and extensor carpi radialis brevis (ECRB). It occurs in athletes exposed to repetitive wrist motions, such as rowers, racquet sports participants, weightlifters, and canoeists (53). It appears to be caused by tenosynovitis of the tendons in the second dorsal compartment. Athletes complain of dorsoradial pain and tenderness proximal to the wrist and may have swelling or crepitus 4–6 cm proximal to Lister's tubercle (36). Initial treatment consists of rest, splinting, anti-inflammatory medication, corticosteroid injection, and activity modification and is successful 95% of the time (36). For the rare failure of conservative treatment, surgical management includes release of the second dorsal compartment, exploration and debridement of the intersection zone and bursal tissue, and release of the fascial sheaths of the tendons in the first dorsal compartment (20). Postoperatively, the wrist is splinted for 7–10 days followed by a stretching and strengthening program, and return to sport is allowed when the patient is symptom free.

Extensor Carpi Ulnaris Tendinitis/Subluxation

- Extensor carpi ulnaris (ECU) tendonitis is the second most common stenosis tenosynovitis of the hand after de Quervain (53). It occurs in athletes involved in repetitive wrist motion, such as racquet sports, baseball, golf, and rowing. It may also happen after traumatic ECU subluxation with rupture of the fibrous sheath overlying the ECU during forced supination, flexion, and ulnar deviation of the wrist (similar to that seen in a baseball swing) (20). Athletes will typically complain of pain and swelling distal to the ulnar head, worsened by resisted wrist extension. A painful snap may be elicited as subluxation of the ECU occurs with supination and ulnar deviation of the wrist. Initial treatment includes rest, splinting, anti-inflammatory medication, corticosteroid injection, and activity modification. Patients who fail to respond to nonoperative treatment require surgical decompression of the sixth dorsal compartment with radial release of the fibro-osseous tunnel and repair of the extensor retinaculum (to prevent postoperative subluxation) (13). After surgery, the wrist is immobilized in 20 degrees of extension for 3 weeks prior to starting activity (39). Patients with acute ECU subluxation may be treated with long-arm casting with the wrist in full pronation and slight dorsiflexion (53). Acute ECU subluxation frequently fails to respond to conservative treatment and often requires stabilization of the ECU with return to sport after a minimum of 8–10 weeks.

Flexor Compartment Tendinopathies

- Inflammation of the flexor tendons most commonly occurs in the FCR and flexor carpi ulnaris (FCU) as a result of repetitive wrist motions, such as occur in golf and racquet sports (53). FCR tendonitis usually presents with pain over the volar aspect of the wrist, proximal to the wrist crease over the FCR tendon. Pain may be elicited with abrupt wrist extension or resisted wrist flexion and radial deviation. Athletes with FCU tendonitis may complain of pain and swelling just distal to the pisiform. Pain may be exacerbated with passive wrist extension or resisted wrist flexion and ulnar deviation. Initial treatment of both of these conditions includes rest, anti-inflammatory medication, splinting, corticosteroid injection, and activity modification. If symptoms persist, surgical decompression of the fibro-osseous tunnel containing the FCR is performed in the case of FCR tendonitis (11). Surgical treatment of FCU tendonitis includes FCU lengthening with or without pisiform excision (33).

Trigger Digits

■ Trigger digits involve inflammation of the flexor tendons as they pass through the digital flexor pulleys, especially the first annular (A1) pulley. Most occur secondary to chronic degenerative changes of the involved structures, but direct pressure from racquets, baseball bats, or golf clubs can also cause acute inflammation of the pulley and tendons (39).

■ The injury manifests as pain in the flexor area over the A1 pulley (metacarpal head) and may also produce catching or locking as swollen tendons attempt to pass through pulley.

■ A large percentage of trigger digits will respond to steroid injection into the tendon sheath and pulley. Surgical release of the A1 pulley may be either a first-line treatment or reserved for cases unresponsive to injection (39).

PEDIATRIC INJURY

Gymnast's Wrist

■ The number of athletes competing in competitive gymnastics has been steadily increasing. As a result, there has been a rise in the frequency of wrist pain in skeletally immature athletes (51). Mandelbaum et al. (27) found that 75% of all male and 50% of all female competitive gymnasts complained of some wrist pain. This is most likely due to repetitive axial loading across a hyperextended wrist (21). Injuries can result from either acute, high-energy trauma or chronic and repetitive stress. Physical examination of young gymnasts with wrist pain can be challenging due to difficulty in pinpointing the location of pain and fear of injury, which would preclude competition. Female gymnasts more commonly complain of ulnar-sided wrist pain, whereas males had similar frequency of radial- and ulnar-sided wrist pain (27).

■ Initial radiographic evaluation includes plain x-rays that may reveal stress-related changes of the distal radial epiphysis, including widening of the growth plate, epiphyseal cystic changes with beaking of the distal epiphysis, and metaphyseal irregularity (43). These changes may lead to premature physeal closure and ultimately a higher incidence of ulnar positive valiance. As a result, following skeletal maturity, gymnasts may present with ulnar abutment syndrome or Madelung-like deformity. MRI and technetium bone scanning may be useful in determining the presence or extent of physeal injury and assist in determining return to sports participation, especially in the face of normal plain radiographs (30).

■ It is rare that the treatment of wrist pain in a skeletally immature athlete is other than rest and withdrawal from the offending activity. Prevention may be the best form of treatment by using protective gear, spotters, proper warm-up, and preclusion of sudden changes in activity intensity. If a physeal injury is suspected or found, the athlete generally is withdrawn from activity, treated symptomatically, and allowed to return to sport when symptoms have resolved. It may also be possible to remove the gymnast from the specific event causing symptoms and allow continued competition in other events that do not exacerbate symptoms.

ACKNOWLEDGMENT

■ We would like to thank Steven B. Cohen and Michael E. Pannunzio for their contribution on this chapter.

REFERENCES

1. Abrahamson SO, Sollerman C, Lundborg G, Larsson J, Egund N. Diagnosis of displaced ulnar collateral ligament of the metacarpophalangeal joint of the thumb. *J Hand Surg Am.* 1990;15(3):457–60.
2. Angelides AC, Wallace PF. The dorsal ganglion of the wrist: its pathogenesis, gross and microscopic anatomy, and surgical treatment. *J Hand Surg Am.* 1976;1(3):228–35.
3. Aronowitz ER, Leddy JP. Closed tendon injuries of the hand and wrist in athletes. *Clin Sports Med.* 1998;17(3):449–67.
4. Bergfeld JA, Weiker GG, Andrish JT, Hall R. Soft playing splint for protection of significant hand and wrist injuries in sports. *Am J Sports Med.* 1982;10(5):293–6.
5. Blatt G. Capsulodesis in reconstructive hand surgery: dorsal capsulodesis for the unstable scaphoid and volar capsulodesis following excision of the distal ulna. *Hand Clin.* 1987;3(1):81–102.
6. Bowers WH. Distal radioulnar joint arthroplasty: the hemiresection-interposition technique. *J Hand Surg Am.* 1985;10(2):169–78.
7. Brunelli GA, Brunelli GR. A new technique for carpal instability with scapholunate dissociation. *Surg Technol Int.* 1996;5:370–4.
8. Dobyns JH, Linscheid RL, Chao EYS, et al. Traumatic instability of the wrist. *Instr Course Lect.* 1975;24:182–99.
9. Fassler PR. Fingertip injuries: evaluation and treatment. *J Am Acad Orthop Surg.* 1996;4(1):84–92.
10. Froimson AI. Tenosynovitis and tennis elbow. In: Green DP, editor. *Operative Hand Surgery.* 3rd ed. New York: Churchill Livingstone; 1992. p. 1989–2006.
11. Gabel G, Bishop AT, Wood MB. Flexor carpi radialis tendonitis. Part II: results of operative treatment. *J Bone Joint Surg Am.* 1994;76(7):1015–8.
12. Gonçalves D. Correction of disorders of the distal radio-ulnar joint by artificial pseudoarthrosis of the ulna. *J Bone Joint Surg Br.* 1974;56B(3):462–4.
13. Hajj AA, Wood MB. Stenosing tenosynovitis of the extensor carpi ulnaris. *J Hand Surg Am.* 1986;11(4):519–20.

14. Halikis MN, Taleisnik J. Soft-tissue injuries of the wrist. *Clin Sports Med.* 1996;15(2):235–59.

15. Hame SL, Melone CP Jr. Boxer's knuckle. Traumatic disruption of the extensor hood. *Hand Clin.* 2000;16(3):375–80, viii.

16. Hermansdorfer JD, Kleinman WB. Management of chronic peripheral tears of the triangular fibrocartilage complex. *J Hand Surg Am.* 1991;16(2):340–6.

17. Idler RS, Manktelow RT, Lucas G, et al. *The Hand Examination and Diagnosis.* 3rd ed. New York (NY): Churchill Livingstone; 1990.

18. Idler RS, Manktelow RT, Lucas G, et al. *The Hand Primary Care of Common Problems.* 2nd ed. New York (NY): Churchill Livingstone; 1990.

19. Kahler DM, McCue FC 3rd. Metacarpophalangeal and proximal inter-phalangeal joint injuries of the hand, including the thumb. *Clin Sports Med.* 1992;11(1):57–76.

20. Kiefhaber TR, Stern PJ. Upper extremity tendonitis and overuse syn-dromes in the athlete. *Clin Sports Med.* 1992;11(1):39–55.

21. Le TB, Hentz VR. Hand and wrist injuries in young athletes. *Hand Clin.* 2000;16(4):597–607.

22. Leddy JP. Avulsions of the flexor digitorum profundus. *Hand Clin.* 1985;1(1):77–83.

23. Leddy JP. Soft-tissue injuries of the hand in athletes. *Instr Course Lect.* 1998;47:181–6.

24. Lewis DM, Osterman AL. Scapholunate instability in athletes. *Clin Sports Med.* 2001;20(1):131–40, ix.

25. Linscheid RL. Ulnar lengthening and shortening. *Hand Clin.* 1987;3(1):69–79.

26. Linscheid RL, Dobyns JH. Athletic injuries of the wrist. *Clin Orthop Relat Res.* 1985;198:141–51.

27. Mandelbaum BR, Bartolozzi AR, Davis CA, Teurlings L, Bragonier B. Wrist pain syndrome in the gymnast. Pathogenetic, diagnostic, and therapeutic considerations. *Am J Sports Med.* 1989;17(3):305–17.

28. McAdams TR, Swan J, Yao J. Arthroscopic treatment of triangular fibro-cartilage wrist injuries in the athlete. *Am J Sports Med.* 2009;37(2):291–7.

29. Miki ZD. Age changes in the triangular fibrocartilage of the wrist join. *J Anat.* 1978;126(pt 2):367–84.

30. Morgan WJ, Slowman LS. Acute hand and wrist injuries in athletes: evaluation and management. *J Am Acad Orthop Surg.* 2001;9(6):389–400.

31. Murphy JV, Banwell PE, Roberts AH, McGrouther DA. Frostbite: patho-genesis and treatment. *J Trauma.* 2000;48(1):171–8.

32. Palmer AK, Glisson RR, Werner FW. Relationship between ulnar variance and triangular fibrocartilage complex thickness. *J Hand Surg Am.* 1984;9(5):681–2.

33. Palmieri TJ. Pisiform area pain treatment by pisiform excision. *J Hand Surg Am.* 1982;7:477–80.

34. Peterson JJ, Bancroft LW. Injuries of the fingers and thumb in the athlete. *Clin Sports Med.* 2006;25(3):527–42, vii–viii.

35. Pitner MA. Pathophysiology of overuse injuries in the hand and wrist. *Hand Clin.* 1990;6(3):355–64.

36. Plancher KD, Peterson RK, Steichen JB. Compressive neuropathies and tendinopathies in the athletic elbow and wrist. *Clin Sports Med.* 1996;15(2):331–71.

37. Reagan DS, Linscheid RL, Dobyns JH. Lunotriquetral sprains. *J Hand Surg Am.* 1984;9(4):502–14.

38. Rettig AC. Closed tendon injuries of the hand and wrist in athletes. *Clin Sports Med.* 1992;11(1):77–99.

39. Rettig AC. Wrist and hand overuse syndromes. *Clin Sports Med.* 2001;20(3):591–611.

40. Rettig AC, Coyle MP, Hunt TR. Hand and wrist problems in the athlete. In: *Am Orthop Soc Sports Med Ins & Course 108. AOSSM 28th Annual Meeting;* 2001 Jul 1: Orlando (FL).

41. Rettig AC, Patel DV. Epidemiology of elbow, forearm, and wrist injuries in the athletes. *Clin Sports Med.* 1995;14(2):289–97.

42. Roser LA, Clawson DK. Football injuries in the very young athlete. *Clin Orthop.* 1970;69:219–23.

43. Roy S, Caine D, Singer KM. Stress changes of the distal radial epiphysis in young gymnasts: a report of 21 cases and review of the literature. *Am J Sports Med.* 1985;13(5):301–8.

44. Sanders WE. The occult dorsal carpal ganglion. *J Hand Surg.* 1985;10(2):257–60.

45. Slade JF 3rd, Milewski MD. Management of carpal instability in athletes. *Hand Clin.* 2009;25(3):395–408.

46. Sugawara M, Oginot T, Minami A, Ishii S. Digital ischemia in baseball players. *Am J Sports Med.* 1986;14(4):329–34.

47. Taleisnik J. Post-traumatic carpal instability. *Clin Orthop Relat Res.* 1980;149:73–82.

48. Taleisnik J. Soft tissue injuries of the wrist. In: Strickland JW, Rettig AC, editors. *Hand Injuries in Athletes.* Philadelphia: Saunders; 1992. p. 107–27.

49. Watson HK, Dhillon HS. Intercarpal arthrodesis. In: Green DP, editor. *Operative Hand Surgery.* Vol. 1, 3rd ed. New York: Churchill Livingstone; 1993. p. 113–68.

50. Watson HK, Hempton RF. Limited wrist arthrodesis. Part I. The triscaphoid joint. *J Hand Surg.* 1980;5(4):320–7.

51. Webb BG, Rettig LA. Gymnastic wrist injuries. *Curr Sports Med Rep.* 2008;7(5):289–95.

52. Weiss LE, Taras JS, Sweet S, Osterman AL. Lunotriquetral injuries in the athletes. *Hand Clin.* 2000;16(3):433–8.

53. Wood MB, Dobyns JH. Sports related extra-articular wrist syndromes. *Clin Orthop Relat Res.* 1986;202:93–102.

Wrist and Hand Fractures

56

D. Nicole Deal and A. Bobby Chhabra

EPIDEMIOLOGY

- Wrist and hand injuries account for 25% of athletic injuries (3).
- Gymnasts have the highest level of wrist and hand injuries, with up to 43% suffering chronic injuries. In one series, 88% of elite male gymnasts complained of wrist pain and 58% required nonsteroidal anti-inflammatory drug (NSAID) therapy to continue competing (47).

DISTAL RADIUS FRACTURES

- Distal radius fractures account for 10% of all bony injuries, up to 75% of all fractures to the forearm, and 16% of all fractures treated in the emergency room (2,41,55).
- Injury often occurs during running or contact sports when the hand is planted on the ground, the wrist hyperextends, and the arm rotates. In addition to a fracture of the distal radius, injury to the triangular fibrocartilage complex (TFCC) and distal radioulnar joint (DRUJ) can result.
- On physical examination, examine for deformity (classic *silver fork* as described by Colles) (19), swelling, pain, and limited range of motion (ROM). Check the DRUJ for tenderness, dislocation, or subluxation, and examine for any loss of pronation or supination.
- Carpal tunnel symptoms may be present in up to 15% of patients, but controversy exists concerning acute versus delayed (48–72 hours) release (25,30).
- Clinical symptoms of DRUJ disruption, including pain and instability, have been found in 5%–15% of fractures (46).
- The TFCC is the major stabilizer of the DRUJ. Disruption of the TFCC and other carpal ligaments, including the scapholunate ligament, has been identified at time of arthroscopy in 45%–70% of cases (29,51). Most TFCC tears are in the central or radial portion of the complex and are treated with debridement (65).
- Anatomic reduction of intra-articular distal radius fractures is required. Two millimeters of articular step-off increases the risk for subsequent degenerative arthritis (43).

Radiographic Evaluation

- True posteroanterior (PA) and lateral views required. Oblique and fossa lateral views, traction views, and magnetic resonance imaging (MRI), computed tomography (CT) scan, bone scan, and fluoroscopy may provide critical information regarding the nature of the fracture and associated injuries when planning for fracture management (7,14,24).

Management of Distal Radius Fractures

- Most stable fractures can be treated with closed reduction and casting, whereas unstable fractures, suggested by (a) excessive fracture comminution, (b) fracture displacement, (c) radial articular surface angulation greater than 20 degrees, (d) articular surface separation or step-off greater than 2 mm, and (e) comminution of both volar and dorsal cortices, often require surgical intervention.
- **Extra-articular fractures:** Stable fracture treatment generally consists of closed reduction and placement of a well-fitted long-arm cast with a good 3-point mold and the forearm in neutral or supination to help stabilize the DRUJ and improve recovery of supination following fracture healing (52,69). Casting should be performed after acute swelling subsides. Close radiographic follow-up is required every 1–2 weeks to assure that loss of reduction and shortening does not occur. Unstable extra-articular fractures may require percutaneous pin fixation in conjunction with cast or external fixation for support.
- **Noncomminuted intra-articular fractures:** Barton fractures are the result of shear forces across either the volar or dorsal lip of the distal radius, resulting in two large fragments that extend into the joint (5). Closed reduction is usually obtained by reversal of the deformity, but maintenance of reduction usually requires surgical stabilization (42).
- **Comminuted or complex intra-articular fractures:** Highly comminuted articular fractures with dorsal comminution and subchondral bone defects frequently collapse and shorten thus requiring close radiographic observation and remanipulation if nonoperative management is chosen. Fractures with articular displacement > 2 mm often require external or internal fixation. Accuracy of reduction may be assessed with either open or arthroscopic visualization of the articular surface to ensure anatomic restoration of the

surface. Bone grafting may be required to fill bony defects especially in the subchondral region (6,29,74).

Complications

- Nonunion following distal radius fracture is a rare occurrence, whereas malunion — most commonly shortening and loss of volar tilt — is a common complication (20,35). Correction of malunion should be undertaken when there is persistent pain and loss of the functional wrist arc of motion, most commonly loss of flexion and supination.

Return to Sports

- Stable fractures treated with splint or cast immobilization should be maintained in a reduced position until fracture healing is evident (4–8 weeks). The athlete may then begin to rehabilitate the wrist using a removable thermoplastic splint for the next 4–6 weeks until full pain-free ROM and strength have been achieved. Return to sports without protection is usually not allowed until 3 months from the time of injury. Fractures treated with rigid internal fixation can be protected by a thermoplastic splint with early ROM exercises. Once radiographic evidence of healing is present, progressive strengthening exercises may be begun, but full return to sport is not permitted before 3 months. Unstable intra-articular fractures are often immobilized for 6–12 weeks, and full return to sports is discouraged until motion and strength have been restored (18,53).

SCAPHOID FRACTURES

- Scaphoid fractures are the most common carpal bone fracture (1 in 100 college football players per year) and often the result of apparently minor trauma (75).
- Fracture mechanism is forced hyperextension with ulnar deviation.
- Extraosseous vascular supply enters the scaphoid at the middle and distal poles while the proximal pole relies on retrograde flow. This results in a high rate of avascular necrosis and nonunion with proximal pole fractures.
- Patient presents with pain in the anatomic snuff box.
- Radiographs include PA, lateral, navicular, and closed fist views.
- Bone scan and MRI are useful in identifying nondisplaced fractures.
- Treatment: Nondisplaced fractures (< 1 mm of displacement) may be treated nonoperatively with immobilization versus open reduction and internal fixation (ORIF) (23,73).
- Options for immobilization include a long-arm thumb spica cast with the wrist in slight palmar flexion and radial deviation for 6 weeks followed by short-arm thumb spica cast until healing is evident on radiographs, usually within 3 months (31), versus short-arm thumb spica versus short-arm casting (73).

- If there is no evidence of healing by 3–4 months, then consider the use of bone grafting or electrical stimulation to enhance healing.
- Early operative intervention for nondisplaced fractures with percutaneous compression screw fixation is controversial but may allow the athlete to return earlier to sports and provide a lower risk of fracture displacement and rehabilitation time (28,44,66).
- Athletes with snuffbox pain and negative radiographs should be immobilized in thumb spica cast and reassessed at 1- to 2-week intervals until the pain resolves or the diagnosis is made radiographically with x-rays or MRI (28).
- Treatment: Displaced fractures most often requires ORIF to restore anatomic alignment and facilitate accurate reduction with compression screws.
- Compression screw fixation techniques have improved and permit minimal immobilization of 2–3 weeks followed by early restorative therapy and return to activities (37); however, with athletes susceptible to reinjury, a 3- to 4-month period of healing and rehabilitation may allow a safer return to sports (64).

Return to Sports

- Athletes may participate in sport with immobilization; plastic, synthetic, and silastic casts have been used effectively in contact sports (62).
- Splint protection is continued for strenuous activities for an additional 2–3 months following radiographic healing until strength and motion approach those of the contralateral side (49).

HAMATE FRACTURES

- Hook or body of the hamate fractures is present in 2%–4% of carpal bone fractures (63).

Hook of the Hamate Fractures

- Injury commonly occurs from direct force of bat, club, or racket.
- Diagnosis is often missed; chronic fractures are associated with flexor tendon rupture and ulnar nerve neuropathy.
- Pain is localized over the hamate in the hypothenar eminence.
- Carpal tunnel view and CT scans aid in diagnosis.
- Direct repair of the fracture results in high nonunion rates; therefore, treatment usually requires removal of the hook through the fracture site with early return to sports (9,59).

Body of the Hamate Fractures

- Less common than hook fractures; often associated with dislocation of fourth and fifth metacarpals (48).

- Oblique radiographs of the carpus and CT scans can assist in defining the fracture.
- Nondisplaced fractures are treated with cast immobilization for 4–6 weeks.
- Displaced fractures are treated with open reduction, Kirschner wire or screw fixation, and immobilization for 4–6 weeks.

Return to Sports

- Athletes with fractures treated by conservative measures may return to sport immediately with protection until pain free (49).
- Athletes treated with excision of the hamate hook may return to sport as tolerated; they will often have hypothenar tenderness for several months and will require the use of well-padded gloves for return to sport (28).
- Athletes with surgically treated fractures are restricted from sport until after healing is evident (4–6 weeks). Participation may resume with splint or cast protection until normal strength and ROM return (49).

CAPITATE FRACTURES

- The capitate is centered within the carpus, is well protected from injury, and accounts for only 1%–2% of all carpal fractures (28).
- Fractures often occur from either a direct blow to the dorsum of the wrist or from forced dorsiflexion or volar flexion. Capitate fractures are often associated with scaphoid fractures and perilunate dislocations (61).
- Radiographic assessment is performed with PA and lateral views, CT scan, or MRI.
- Nondisplaced fractures are treated with immobilization in short-arm cast for 6–8 weeks.
- Capitate fractures are associated with poor outcomes because the fractures are inherently unstable, and delayed union, nonunion, and avascular necrosis are common complications (61).
- Displaced fractures (2 mm of displacement) are treated with ORIF with Kirschner wires or screw fixation and immobilized in a short-arm cast for 6 weeks.

Return to Sports

- Athletes with nonoperative fractures may return to sport immediately with protective casting (49). Close follow-up must be maintained to assure that fracture displacement does not occur, obligating operative intervention.
- Athletes with surgically treated fractures are restricted from sport until after healing is evident (4–6 weeks). Participation may resume with splint or cast protection for an additional 3 months or until normal strength and ROM return (49).

PISIFORM FRACTURES

- Pisiform fractures are rare and usually occur from direct blow to the palm and account for 1%–3% of all carpal bone fractures (28).
- Patients tend to have tenderness over the hypothenar region.
- Fractures are best visualized on 30-degree oblique anteroposterior (AP) view or carpal tunnel view.
- Acute nondisplaced fractures are managed by immobilization in a short-arm cast for 3–6 weeks.
- Comminuted fractures and symptomatic nonunions are managed by excision, with care to preserve the flexor carpi ulnaris tendon, with little or no functional impairment (4).

Return to Sports

- Athletes return to sports as soon as acute pain subsides with taping, padded gloves, or casting as needed (28,49,64).
- Symptomatic nonunion may be excised after the season (49).

TRIQUETRUM FRACTURES

- Triquetrum fractures are common carpal bone fractures in sports accounting for 3%–4% of all carpal bone injuries (15).
- Fractures commonly consist of avulsion of the dorsal cortex following hyperextension injury causing impingement with the distal ulna.
- Treatment of this dorsal marginal fracture consists of immobilization in short-arm cast for 3–4 weeks (28,64).
- Isolated fractures through the body of the triquetrum are rare injuries and are often associated with scapholunate ligamentous disruption, which must be clinically assessed (28,38).

Return to Sports

- Athletes may return to sport wearing a semirigid cast as soon as acute pain resolves or without immobilization when pain does not interfere with sporting activity (39,49).

LUNATE FRACTURES

- The lunate is enclosed in the radial fossa, and fracture of the lunate is a rare entity.
- Athletes present with pain and swelling over the dorsum of the wrist.
- Lunate fractures occur through either a compressive force between the capitate and the distal radius fracturing through the body of the lunate or through traction from the ligamentous or capsular structures at the extremes of motion resulting in avulsion-type fractures (54).

- CT scan is often needed for diagnosis because the bony architecture of the lunate is difficult to visualize on standard radiographs.
- Prompt diagnosis, immobilization, and protection from further injury until union is evident are critical because there is a possible association with fracture nonunion and the development of avascular necrosis of the lunate (Kienböck disease) (8).
- Nondisplaced fractures are immobilized in a short-arm cast, with the metacarpophalangeal (MCP) joints flexed to reduce the compressive forces generated by gripping, for 6 weeks.
- Displaced fractures require ORIF versus percutaneous fixation to restore radiocarpal and midcarpal stability as well as lunate vascularity, with immobilization continuing until fracture healing is evident.

Return to Sports

- Athletes may return to sport once fracture healing is evident. Protective splinting is recommended when athletes return to competition (54).
- Close observation for signs of avascular necrosis (dorsal wrist pain and swelling) is required following fracture healing so it can be caught during the early stages when treatment options afford the best opportunity for return to competition (28,64).

TRAPEZIUM FRACTURES

- Fractures of the trapezium constitute 1%–5% of all carpal fractures (12,28).
- Trapezium fractures involve either the longitudinal ridge (the attachment site for the transverse carpal ligament) or the body.
- Ridge fractures are usually the result of direct trauma such as fall on outstretched hand or being struck by a ball.
- Body fractures are more common and result from falling on outstretched thumb with resultant splitting of the trapezium body and displacement of the thumb carpometacarpal joint (the mirror image of the Bennett fracture-dislocation).
- Fractures of the body of the trapezium can often be seen on standard AP and lateral views. A pronated PA view can help visualize the articular surface and detect any displacement. The carpal tunnel view is useful to visualize trapezial ridge fractures. A CT scan may be useful in fractures difficult to visualize with plain radiographs.
- Nondisplaced fractures of the trapezium are treated with immobilization in a thumb spica cast for 4–6 weeks. ROM and strengthening are then initiated with continued use of a removable thumb spica splint for an additional 2–4 weeks (54).
- Body fractures are unstable and subject to displacement; therefore, close follow-up must be maintained until fracture union is evident (28).

- Displaced body fractures are managed with ORIF with the use of compression screws, Kirschner wires, or a combination of both and repair of the capsular structures. Stable internal fixation allows early mobilization of the joint (21,64,70).
- Trapezial ridge fractures with minimal displacement have high rates of nonunion, and surgical excision of the fragment allows for an uncomplicated recovery and early return to sport (57).

Return to Sports

- Patients with nondisplaced fractures treated nonoperatively may return to sport with cast or splint immobilization once symptoms permit with protection continuing for up to 12 weeks or until strength and motion return (54).
- Trapezial body fractures treated operatively should be protected with cast or splint immobilization until complete healing and strength and motion have been restored.
- Patients with trapezial ridge fractures treated with excision may return to sport once soft tissue healing occurs; padded gloves are often required to minimize wound sensitivity that may last for several months (28,64).

TRAPEZOID FRACTURES

- The trapezoid is in a well-protected position anatomically and is the least commonly fractured carpal bone, involved in less than 1% of carpal fractures (68).
- Fracture of the trapezoid is the result of high-energy axially directed trauma along the index metacarpal.
- Trapezoid fractures are usually visualized on standard AP, lateral, and oblique views.
- Treatment usually requires ORIF of the trapezoid with pinning of the index metacarpal in a reduced position. The Kirschner wires can be pulled at approximately 6 weeks, followed by the initiation of hand therapy to restore motion and strength (28).

Return to Sports

- Athletes may return to sport wearing a protective splint once the Kirschner wires are removed or when soft tissues allow (28).

METACARPAL FRACTURES

- Metacarpal and phalangeal fractures are the most common fractures in the skeletal system, accounting for greater than 14% of all emergency room visits and greater than 36% of all hand fractures (17,56).
- The fractures are often the result of a direct blow or crush-type injury to the hand and can occur secondary to a fall onto the hand.

- Metacarpal fractures typically present with apex dorsal angulation secondary to deforming force of intrinsic muscles.
- Rotational deformity must be recognized and corrected in treating these fractures.
- Rotational alignment is best visualized with full flexion of the fingers.
- Fractures are best visualized with standard AP, lateral, and oblique radiographs of the hand.
- Classified as transverse, oblique, spiral, and comminuted.

TRANSVERSE FRACTURES

- Apex dorsal fracture angulation is secondary to forces applied by intrinsic muscles. These forces are neutralized by MCP joint flexion.
- Reduction is indicated for any angulation in the index and middle fingers, > 20 degrees for ring finger, and > 30 degrees for small finger (17,26,36).

Treatment

- Most stable fractures can be treated nonoperatively with cast immobilization for 2 weeks, followed by orthoplast splint immobilization of the affected digit and its neighbor for an additional 2 weeks and buddy taping and initiation of active motion at 4 weeks after injury (17).
- Rotational deformity is not acceptable; rotation is the most critical factor in evaluating metacarpal fractures.
- Treatment options for unstable fractures or fractures that fail closed treatment comprise closed reduction and percutaneous pinning, cross pinning to adjacent metacarpal, closed reduction and internal fixation, and ORIF (17).
- Stable fixation requires no protection except for sport, with light active use being permitted within 5 days postoperatively (17).

OBLIQUE AND SPIRAL FRACTURES

- Result of torsional forces to the metacarpal.
- Untreated fractures tend to shorten and rotate.
- Rotational deformity is unacceptable because 5 degrees of malrotation can lead to 1.5–2.0 cm of digital overlap (67).
- Five millimeters of shortening can be accepted without functional deficit (11).

Treatment

- Isolated, minimally displaced fractures may be treated by closed methods similar to the treatment of transverse fractures.
- Fractures that cannot be maintained with closed methods require either percutaneous pinning or ORIF.

- Interfragmentary lag screw fixation may be used if fracture length is twice the bone diameter and provides the most biomechanically stable construct. For fractures with a shorter surface, a lag screw and dorsal neutralization plate can provide stable fixation, permitting early return to sport (10).

COMMINUTED FRACTURES

- May be associated with soft tissue loss.
- Treatment often requires ORIF or external fixation to maintain length.
- May require delayed or primary bone grafting.

METACARPAL HEAD FRACTURES

- These are rare fractures that occur from axial loading or direct trauma and must be examined closely to assure that fractures are not the result of a fight bite.
- Nondisplaced fractures may be treated nonoperatively with initial splint immobilization followed by buddy taping and early ROM (58).
- Displaced fractures require ORIF to restore anatomic alignment and articular congruity with Kirschner wires, screws, mini fragment plates, or dynamic traction to allow for early motion; if early motion cannot be started, then immobilization in the intrinsic plus position should be maintained until motion can be initiated (58).
- Complications include limited motion and arthritis.

METACARPAL NECK FRACTURES

- These fractures most commonly involve the ring or small finger (boxer's fracture).
- Apex dorsal angulation and volar comminution can make it difficult to maintain reduction with cast immobilization.
- Angular deformity of 40–60 degrees may be accepted at the ring and small fingers secondary to the mobility of the fourth and fifth carpometacarpal joints. More than 15–20 degrees of angulation is unacceptable at the index or long metacarpals secondary to the lack of motion at their carpometacarpal joints (17,36). Rotational malalignment indicated by scissoring with finger flexion is unacceptable.
- Treatment for the majority of fractures comprises closed reduction by the technique described by Jahss (40) and immobilizing the fracture in a short-arm gutter splint with the fingers in the intrinsic plus position. Immobilization is continued for 2 weeks, when buddy taping and motion are initiated (16).
- Radiographs should be obtained weekly with index and long metacarpal fractures to assure that reduction is not lost.

- Surgical intervention is indicated for irreducible fractures or in fractures where reduction is lost. Operative intervention may include closed reduction and percutaneous pinning, open reduction, and internal fixation with tension band or a laterally applied minicondylar plate (17,26).
- Bouquet pinning with the insertion of multiple small intramedullary Kirschner wires down the metacarpal shaft and across the fracture into the metacarpal head can provide stable fixation and early return of unrestricted hand function in fractures that would otherwise require lengthy immobilization (17,32).
- The hand is immobilized in a splint for 2 weeks, after which motion is initiated with return to sports at preinjury level within 6 weeks.

METACARPAL BASE FRACTURES

- Metacarpal base fractures are rare fractures. They usually have a stable configuration secondary to a set of four strong interosseous ligaments.
- Index and long carpometacarpal joints have limited motion, whereas ring and small carpometacarpal joints have 15 and 30 degrees of mobility, respectively (17).
- Nondisplaced or minimally displaced fractures are treated in a short-arm cast with the MCP joints flexed and the interphalangeal joints free.
- Immobilization is often maintained for 6 weeks, followed by buddy taping for 2–3 weeks to maintain rotational control and allow initiation of motion (58).
- Displaced fractures often require closed or open reduction followed by percutaneous fixation and then by splint immobilization and the gradual restoration of motion at 6–8 weeks after injury (17,26,36,58).
- Fractures that proceed to malunion may cause weakness of grip or pain with evidence of arthritis and may be treated with arthrodesis without significantly compromising hand function (58).

Return to Sports after Metacarpal Fractures

- Most sports-related metacarpal fractures are stable and are treated initially with splint or cast immobilization. Return to sports with protection may be initiated within 1–2 weeks from injury depending on the requirements of the specific sport. Protection is usually continued for 8–12 weeks depending on the demands of the sport (1).
- Fractures treated with rigid internal fixation may allow the athlete earlier return to play than nonoperative treatment. Athletes may begin early motion with return to sports with immobilization as early as 2 weeks, and by 5–6 weeks, buddy taping or a light splint may be all that is required to permit sport-specific activities (1,13,32).

THUMB METACARPAL FRACTURES

- Thumb metacarpal fractures are unique from fractures of the other digits secondary to the thumb's critical role in hand function, especially grasp and power pinch.
- More than one-fourth of all metacarpal fractures are to the thumb metacarpal base and result from axial loading across the partially flexed thumb (27).
- Radiographic imaging requires views specifically of the thumb in AP and lateral projections.
- Joint anatomy comprises reciprocal saddle-shaped surfaces of the distal trapezium and proximal metacarpal.
- Intra-articular Bennett (partial articular) and Rolando (complete articular) fractures often have displacement dorsally and radially by pull of the abductor pollicis longus (34,45).
- Treatment is directed at minimizing posttraumatic arthritis by obtaining anatomic joint reduction.
- If less than 15%–20% of the joint surface is involved, then closed reduction and percutaneous pinning are successful (26).
- Immobilization in a short-arm thumb spica cast for 4–6 weeks is recommended followed by removal of pins and initiation of motion (45,58).
- If greater than 25%–30% of the joint surface is involved, then open reduction and stable internal fixation with screws or pins are indicated (33).
- ROM is initiated at 5–10 days postoperatively (45).
- Severely comminuted intra-articular Rolando fractures often require external fixation followed by limited ORIF with bone grafting (16).
- Immobilization is continued for a minimum of 6–8 weeks followed by the initiation of hand-based therapy to regain motion and strength.
- Extra-articular thumb metacarpal fractures usually occur toward the metacarpal base.
- Treatment often consists of closed reduction and immobilization in a thumb spica cast for 4–6 weeks followed by initiation of hand therapy.
- Twenty to 30 degrees of angulation are acceptable because of the multiple planes of thumb motion (17).
- Unstable fractures may require operative intervention with either closed reduction and percutaneous pinning or internal fixation similar to the treatment for other metacarpal fractures (17,26).

Return to Sports

- Athletes may return to sport with immobilization in thumb spica splint or cast as symptoms and sport-specific activity permit.
- Protection should be maintained until fracture healing is evident on radiographs and strength, stability, and motion are restored.

■ Operative intervention with stable fixation may allow for earlier initiation of motion and return to sports (45).

PHALANGEAL FRACTURES

Proximal and Middle Phalanx Fractures

■ These are very common fractures in athletes participating in contact sports or sports requiring catching of a ball.

■ Fracture displacement depends on mechanism of injury and deforming forces of muscles and tendons on bone.

■ Proximal phalanx fractures typically have volar angulation with proximal segment flexed by the interossei and the distal segment extended by pull of the central slip portion of the extensor mechanism (17,36).

■ Middle phalanx fractures are deformed by both the central slip and by the flexor digitorum superficialis tendon resulting in either volar or dorsal angulation depending on the location of the fracture (17,36).

■ Treatment depends on the stability of the fracture, correction of rotational deformation, and no greater than 10 degrees of angulation in any plane.

■ Nondisplaced and stable fractures can be treated with buddy taping and early ROM (17). Careful clinical and radiographic follow-up is required to detect subsequent fracture displacement.

■ Displaced fractures require closed reduction and immobilization with cast or splint and an outrigger with the affected finger held in the intrinsic-plus position including an adjacent digit to help maintain rotational alignment (17).

■ Fracture immobilization should be limited to 3 weeks prior to initiation of hand-based therapy to facilitate maximal restoration of motion, and protective splinting should be continued during sport-specific activities until healing is evident (17,60,72).

■ Intra-articular, unstable, or rotationally malaligned fractures may benefit from open or closed reduction and internal or percutaneous fixation to restore anatomic alignment and rotational control.

■ If rigid fixation is obtained, mobilization to regain ROM and edema control should begin within the first week after surgery, permitting earlier return to sport and a more predictable functional outcome (13,17).

■ Protective splinting should be maintained for 4 weeks or until fracture healing is evident. Simple buddy taping should be continued until ROM and strength are restored.

Distal Phalanx Fractures

■ These fractures account for 50% of all hand fractures, especially thumb and middle finger fractures (50).

■ Fibrous septa from skin minimize fracture displacement.

■ Must examine for evidence of nail bed injury.

■ Treatment is dictated by presence of soft tissue injury.

■ If a nail bed injury is present, the nail bed must be repaired to prevent nail deformity (71).

■ Immobilization is restricted to the distal interphalangeal joint for a period of 3–4 weeks, after which motion is initiated (17).

■ Tenderness may persist for > 6 months, requiring a program of desensitization to allow full return of function (22).

■ Mallet finger deformity can occur from loss of continuity of extensor mechanism through bony or tendinous disruption.

■ Treatment is almost always nonoperative, with continuous extension splinting of the distal interphalangeal (DIP) joint for at least 6 weeks followed by the removal of the splint several times a day for active ROM exercises for an additional 2 weeks (36,60).

Return to Sports after Phalangeal Fractures

■ Athletes with stable fractures treated nonoperatively may return to sports with rigid cast immobilization, thermoplast splint protection, or buddy taping (as sport-specific activities permit) as soon as symptoms allow, often within the first week (1).

■ Close follow-up must be maintained to ensure that loss of reduction or malrotation does not occur.

■ Protection should be maintained until radiographic evidence of complete healing is evident and functional recovery of ROM and strength is complete (60).

■ Athletes with surgically treated fractures may return to sports with protective splinting or casting once soft tissue healing allows.

■ Edema control and active motion are typically initiated at 2 weeks, and by 4 weeks, 75% of motion should have been regained and strengthening can be initiated. Protective splinting should be maintained for sport-specific activities until healing is evident (1,17,32). Buddy taping should be maintained until strength and motion have been regained.

ACKNOWLEDGMENT

■ We would like to thank Geoff Baer for his contribution on this chapter.

REFERENCES

1. Alexy C, De Carlo M. Rehabilitation and use of protective devices in hand and wrist injuries. *Clin Sports Med.* 1998;17(3):635–55.

2. Alffram PA, Bauer GC. Epidemiology of fractures of the forearm. A biomechanical investigation of bone strength. *J Bone Joint Surg Am.* 1962;44-A:105–14.

3. Amadio PC. Epidemiology of hand and wrist injuries in sports. *Hand Clin.* 1990;6(3):379–81.

4. Arner M, Hagberg L. Wrist flexion strength after excision of the pisiform bone. *Scand J Plast Reconstr Surg.* 1984;18(2):241–5.

5. Barton JR. Views and treatment of an important injury of the wrist. *Med Exam.* 1838;1:365–8.

6. Bass RL, Blair WF, Hubbard PP. Results of combined internal and external fixation for the treatment of severe AO-C3 fractures of the distal radius. *J Hand Surg.* 1995;20(3):373–81.

7. Batillas J, Vasilas A, Pizzi WF, Gokcebay T. Bone scanning in the detection of occult fractures. *J Trauma.* 1981;21(7):564–9.

8. Beckenbaugh RD, Shiver TC, Dobyns JH, Linscheid RL. Kienböck's disease: the natural history of Kienböck's disease and consideration of lunate fractures. *Clin Orthop Relat Res.* 1980;149:98–106.

9. Bishop AT, Beckenbaugh RD. Fractures of the hamate hook. *J Hand Surg Am.* 1988;13(1):135–9.

10. Black DM, Mann RJ, Constine RM, Daniels AU. Comparison of internal fixation techniques in metacarpal fracture. *J Hand Surg.* 1985;10(4):466–72.

11. Bloem JJ. The treatment and prognosis of uncomplicated dislocated fractures of the metacarpals and phalanges. *Arch Chir Neer.* 1971;23(1):55–65.

12. Botte MJ, Gelberman RH. Fractures of the carpus, excluding the scaphoid. *Hand Clin.* 1987;3(1):149–61.

13. Breen TF. Sport-related injuries of the hand. In: Pappas AM, editor. *Upper Extremity Injuries in the Athlete.* New York: Churchill Livingstone; 1995. p. 451–91.

14. Breitenseher MD, Metz VM, Gilula LA, et al. Radiographically occult scaphoid fractures: value of MR imaging in detection. *Radiology.* 1997;203(1):245–50.

15. Bryan RS, Dobyns JH. Fractures of the carpal bones other than the lunate and navicular. *Clin Orthop Relat Res.* 1980;149:107–11.

16. Buchler U, McCollam SM, Oppikofer C. Comminuted fractures of the basilar joint of the thumb: combined treatment by external fixation, limited internal fixation, and bone grafting. *J Hand Surg Am.* 1991;16(3):556–60.

17. Capo JT, Hastings H 2nd. Metacarpal and phalangeal fractures in athletes. *Clin Sports Med.* 1998;17(3):491–511.

18. Christensen OM, Christiansen TG, Krasheninnikoff M, Hansen FF. Length of immobilization after fractures of the distal radius. *Int Orthop.* 1995;19(1):26–9.

19. Colles A. On the fracture of the carpal extremity of the radius. *Edinburgh Med Surg J.* 1814;10:182–6.

20. Cooney WP III, Dobyns JH, Linscheid RL. Complications of Colles' fractures. *J Bone Joint Surg Am.* 1980;62(4):613–9.

21. Cordrey LJ, Ferrer-Torells M. Management of fractures of the greater multangular: report of five cases. *J Bone Joint Surg.* 1960;42-A:1111–8.

22. DaCruz DJ, Slade RJ, Malone W. Fractures of the distal phalanges. *J Hand Surg Br.* 1988;13(3):350–2.

23. Diaz JJ, Wildin CJ, Bhowal B, Thompson JR. Should acute scaphoid fractures be fixed? A randomized controlled trial. *J Bone Joint Surg Am.* 2005;87(10):2160–8.

24. Dóczi J, Springer G, Renner A, Martsa B. Occult distal radial fractures. *J Hand Surg.* 1995;20(5):614–7.

25. Ford DJ, Ali MS. Acute carpal tunnel syndrome: complications of delayed decompression. *J Bone Joint Surg Br.* 1986;68(5):758–9.

26. Freeland AE. *Hand Fractures: Repair, Reconstruction, and Rehabilitation.* Philadelphia (PA): Churchill Livingstone; 2000. 291 p.

27. Gedda KO. Studies on Bennett's fractures; anatomy, roentgenology, and therapy. *Acta Chir Scand Suppl.* 1954;193:1–114.

28. Geissler WB. Carpal fractures in athletes. *Clin Sports Med.* 2001;20(1):167–88.

29. Geissler WB, Freeland AE, Savoie FH, McIntyre LW, Whipple TL. Intracarpal soft-tissue lesions associated with an intra-articular fracture of the distal end of the radius. *J Bone Joint Surg Am.* 1996;78(3):357–65.

30. Gelberman RH, Szabo RM, Mortenson WW. Carpal tunnel pressures and wrist position in patients with Colles' fractures. *J Trauma.* 1984;24(8):747–9.

31. Gellman H, Caputo RJ, Carter V, Aboulafia A, McKay M. A comparison of short and long thumb-spica casts for nondisplaced fractures of the carpal scaphoid. *J Bone Joint Surg Am.* 1989;71(3):354–7.

32. Graham TJ, Mullen DJ. Athletic injuries of the adult hand. In: DeLee JC, Drez D Jr, Miller MD, editors. *DeLee & Drez's Orthopaedic Sports Medicine; Principles and Practice.* Philadelphia: Saunders; 2003. p. 1381–431.

33. Green DP. *Operative Hand Surgery.* 3rd ed. New York (NY): Churchill Livingstone; 1993.

34. Green DP, O'Brien ET. Fractures of the thumb metacarpal. *South Med J.* 1972;65(7):807–14.

35. Harper WM, Jones JM. Non-union of Colles' fracture: report of two cases. *J Hand Surg Br.* 1990;15(1):121–3.

36. Henry M. Fractures and dislocations of the hand. In: Bucholz RW, Heckman JD, editors. *Rockwood and Green's Fractures in Adults.* Philadelphia: Lippincott Williams & Wilkins; 2001. p. 655–748.

37. Herbert TJ, Fisher WE. Management of the fractured scaphoid using a new bone screw. *J Bone Joint Surg Br.* 1984;66(1):114–23.

38. Herzberg G, Comtet JJ, Linscheid RL, Amadio PC, Cooney WP, Stadler J. Perilunate dislocations and fracture dislocations: a multicenter study. *J Hand Surg Am.* 1993;18(5):768–79.

39. Höcker K, Menschik A. Chip fractures of the triquetrum: mechanism, classification and results. *J Hand Surg Br.* 1994;19(5):584–8.

40. Jahss S. Fractures of the metacarpals: a new method of reduction and immobilization. *J Bone Joint Surg.* 1938;20:178–86.

41. Jupiter JB. Current concepts review: fractures of the distal end of the radius. *J Bone Joint Surg Am.* 1991;73(3):461–9.

42. Jupiter JB, Fernandez DL, Toh CL, Fellman T, Ring D. Operative treatment of volar intra-articular fractures of the distal end of the radius. *J Bone Joint Surg Am.* 1996;78(12):1817–28.

43. Knirk JL, Jupiter JB. Intra-articular fractures of the distal end of the radius in young adults. *J Bone Joint Surg Am.* 1986;68(5):647–59.

44. Koman LA, Mooney JF III, Poehling GC. Fractures and ligamentous injuries of the wrist. *Hand Clin.* 1990;6(3):477–91.

45. Langford SA, Whitaker JH, Toby EB. Thumb injuries in the athlete. *Clin Sports Med.* 1998;17(3):553–66.

46. Lidstrom A. Fractures of the distal end of the radius. A clinical and statistical study of end results. *Acta Orthop Scand Suppl.* 1959;41:1–118.

47. Mandelbaum BR, Bartolozzi AR, Davis CA, Teurlings L, Bragonier B. Wrist pain syndrome in the gymnasts. Pathogenic, diagnostic, and therapeutic considerations. *Am J Sports Med.* 1989;17(3):305–17.

48. Marck KW, Klasen HJ. Fracture-dislocation of the hamato-metacarpal joint: a case report. *J Hand Surg Am.* 1986;11(1):128–30.

49. McCue FC III, Bruce JF Jr, Koman JD. The wrist in the adult. In: DeLee JC, Drez D Jr, Miller MD, editors. *DeLee & Drez's Orthopaedic Sports Medicine; Principles and Practice.* Philadelphia: Saunders; 2003. p. 1337–64.

50. McNealy RW, Lichtenstein ME. Fractures of the bones of the hand. *Am J Surg.* 1940;50:563–70.

51. Mohanti RC, Kar N. Study of triangular fibrocartilage of the wrist joint in Colles' fracture. *Injury.* 1980;11(4):321–4.

52. Moir JS, Wardlaw D, Maffulli N. Functional bracing of Colles' fractures. *Bull Hosp Jt Dis.* 1999;58(1):45–52.

53. Morgan WJ, Busconi BD. Injuries of the distal radius and distal radioulnar joint. In: Pappas AM, editor. *Upper Extremity Injuries in the Athlete.* New York: Churchill Livingstone; 1995. p. 393–412.

54. Morgan WJ, Reardon TF. Carpal fractures of the wrist. In: Pappas AM, editor. *Upper Extremity Injuries in the Athlete.* New York: Churchill Livingstone; 1995. p. 431–49.

55. Owen RA, Melton LJ III, Johnson KA, IIstrup DM, Riggs BL. Incidence of Colles' fracture in North American community. *Am J Public Health.* 1982;72(6):605–7.

56. Packer GJ, Shaheen MA. Patterns of hand fractures and dislocations in a district general hospital. *J Hand Surg Br.* 1993;18(4):511–4.

57. Palmer AK. Trapezial ridge fractures. *J Hand Surg Am.* 1981;6(6):561–4.

58. Palmer RE. Joint injuries of the hand in athletes. *Clin Sports Med.* 1998;17(3):513–31.

59. Parker RD, Berkowitz MS, Brahms MA, Bohl WR. Hook of the hamate fractures in athletes. *Am J Sports Med.* 1986;14(6):517–23.

60. Posner MA. Hand injuries. In: Nicholas JA, Hershman EB, Posner MA, editors. *The Upper Extremity in Sports Medicine.* St. Louis: Mosby; 1995. p. 483–569.

61. Rand JA, Linscheid RL, Dobyns JH. Capitate fractures: a long term follow-up. *Clin Orthop Relat Res.* 1982;165:209–16.

62. Reister JN, Baker BE, Mosher JF, Lowe D. A review of scaphoid fracture healing in competitive athletes. *Am J Sports Med.* 1985;13(3):159–61.

63. Rettig AC, Ryan RO, Stone JA. Epidemiology of hand injuries in sports. In: Strickland JW, Rettig AC, editors. *Hand Injuries in Athletes.* Philadelphia: Saunders; 1992. p. 37–48.

64. Rettig ME, Dassa GL, Raskin KB, Melone CP Jr. Wrist fractures in the athlete. Distal radius and carpal fractures. *Clin Sports Med.* 1998;17(3):469–89.

65. Richards RS, Roth JH. Common wrist injuries. In: Chan KM, editor. *The Hand and Upper Extremity: Sports Injuries of the Hand and Upper Extremity.* New York: Churchill Livingstone; 1995. p. 213–26.

66. Rizzo M, Shin AY. Treatment of acute scaphoid fractures in the athlete. *Curr Sports Med Rep.* 2006;5(5):242–8.

67. Rolye SG. Rotational deformity following metacarpal fracture. *J Hand Surg Br.* 1990;15(1):124–5.

68. Ruby L. Fractures and dislocation of the carpus. In: Brown BD, Jupiter JB, Levine AM, et al., editors. *Skeletal Trauma.* Philadelphia: Saunders; 1992. p. 1025–62.

69. Sarmiento A, Zagorski JB, Sinclair WF. Functional bracing of Colles' fractures: a prospective study of immobilization in supination versus pronation. *Clin Orthop Relat Res.* 1980;146:175–83.

70. Seitz WH Jr, Papandrea RF. Fractures and dislocations of the wrist. In: Bucholz RW, Heckman JD, editors. *Rockwood and Green's Fractures in Adults.* Philadelphia: Lippincott Williams & Wilkins; 2001. p. 749–813.

71. Simon RR, Wolgin M. Subungual hematoma: association with occult laceration requiring repair. *Am J Emerg Med.* 1987;5(4):302–4.

72. Strickland JW, Steichen JB, Kleinman WB, et al. Phalangeal fractures, factors influencing digital performance. *Orthop Rev.* 1982;11: 39–50.

73. Symes TH, Stothard J. A systematic review of the treatment of acute fractures of the scaphoid. *J Hand Surg Eur Vol.* 2011;36(9):802–10.

74. Trumble TE, Wagner W, Hanel DP, Vedder NB, Gilbert M. Intrafocal (Kapandji) pinning of distal radius fractures with and without external fixation. *J Hand Surg Am.* 1998;23(3):381–94.

75. Zemel NP, Stark HH. Fractures and dislocations of the carpal bones. *Clin Sports Med.* 1986;5(4):709–24.

57 Upper Extremity Nerve Entrapment

Margarete DiBenedetto and Robert Giering

GENERAL PRINCIPLES OF UPPER EXTREMITY NERVE ENTRAPMENT

Epidemiology

- The most common nerve entrapment is the carpal tunnel syndrome (CTS). Its occurrence is 3.46 cases per 1,000 person years. Female-to-male ratio is about 3.1 (23). The next highest incidence is entrapment of the ulnar nerve at the elbow. Krivickas and Wilbourn (25) studied 180 athletes with sports injuries in the electrodiagnostic (EDX) laboratory, of whom 23% had median nerve injuries, 22% stingers, 10.5% radial nerve lesions, 10.5% ulnar nerve compression syndromes, 12% axillary nerve problems, and 7.8% entrapment of the suprascapular nerve (SSN) only.

Pathophysiology

- Nerve entrapment occurs when a nerve passes through a tight space, placing it at risk for mechanical compression as well as ischemia secondary to pressure on the vasa nervorum. Persistent compression results in predictable, progressive degrees of nerve damage, as classified by Seddon: neurapraxia, axonotmesis, and neurotmesis (23).
  - Neurapraxia (conduction block) is reversible. Demyelination may result.
  - Large myelinated fibers are most vulnerable. Duration of compression determines degree of damage (may last minutes to months).
  - Axonotmesis specifies axonal damage, with endoneurium and perineurium intact. Wallerian degeneration ensues. Preservation of endoneurial tubes provide a guide for regeneration of axons. Recovery can take months.
  - Neurotmesis represents complete disruption of axons, endoneurium, and perineurium. Poor functional outcome. Surgery usually indicated.

Risk Factors

- Narrowed space in bony and/or muscular tendinous/fibrous canals/tunnels.
  - Examples: thoracic outlet, quadrilateral space, Struthers ligament, anomalous bone spurs, muscles or fibrous bands, cubital tunnel, radial tunnel, carpal tunnel, Guyon canal, excessive callous formation after (especially malunited) fracture
- Injury
  - Acute: compression, stretch, percussion
  - Chronic: repetitive motion, excessive pressure from equipment
  - Paralysis of cervical/thoracic muscles secondary to myelopathy
- **Medical conditions:** endocrine problems (pregnancy, hypothyroidism), compartment syndrome, peripheral neuropathy

Symptoms and Signs

- Pain, paresthesias, and weakness in distribution of affected nerve
- Lesions of pure motor nerves (anterior/posterior interosseous, suprascapular, and long thoracic nerves) cause weakness and/or muscle atrophy.

Evaluation

- Special tests: Tinel's, Phalen's, Spurling's, Adson's maneuver, pectoralis minor and costoclavicular maneuvers, and stress-abduction test that may or may not be positive
- Persistent minor pain due to entrapment may cause a regional pain syndrome — reflex sympathetic dystrophy (RSD).

Electrodiagnosis

- Electromyography (EMG) and nerve conduction studies (NCS) are significant factors in establishing the correct diagnosis of entrapment syndromes. Typical findings include the following.
- EMG shows decreased recruitment, increase in polyphasic waves, action potential durations and amplitudes, and in more severe cases, fibrillations and positive sharp waves. Complex repetitive discharges (CRDs) denote chronicity. EMG demonstrates the severity of the abnormality, especially if there is evidence of denervation, which has considerable impact on treatment decisions.
- Conduction delay across the site of compression; reduced amplitudes due to blocking or axonal loss (with normal duration) or secondary to demyelination (with increased duration)

Differential Diagnosis

- Major diagnoses to be ruled out with EMG and NCS are:
  - Radiculopathy
  - Peripheral neuropathy
  - Plexopathy, including neuralgic amyotrophy (brachial plexitis), myopathy, and malingering

SPECIFIC NERVE ENTRAPMENTS OF THE UPPER EXTREMITY

Radiculopathy

- Major differential diagnosis in all entrapment syndromes. However, it also is subject to its own compression and entrapment (C7 > C6 > C8).

Anatomy

- Entrapment is caused by pressure on a spinal nerve as it exits the spine. Primary anterior compression (disc herniation) may selectively affect motor fibers. It may spare the dorsal ramus, sparing sensation. Posterior compression may selectively affect sensory fibers. Compression of the nerve root can occur from any direction within the intervertebral foramen but most commonly occurs due to posterolateral disc herniation or facet degeneration.

Risk Factors

- Cervical spondylosis
- Cervical disc herniation
- Facet degeneration
- Space-occupying lesions
- Prior cervical spine trauma or surgery

Symptoms and Signs

- Sensory complaints
- Weakness and reflex changes in root distribution
- Provocative maneuvers often positive

Evaluation

- Muscle, sensory, and reflex examination
- Provocative maneuver: Spurling — pressure on laterally and posteriorly tilted head reproduces symptoms in the affected root distribution

Differential Diagnosis

- Peripheral neuropathy
- Brachial plexitis
- Entrapment neuropathies
- Neurologic disease

Treatment

- Indications for immediate surgical referral are as follows:
  - Progressive neurologic deficit, bowel or bladder dysfunction, and severe pain refractory to other approaches

- Surgery usually includes nerve root decompression, discectomy if needed, and possible cervical fusion.
- Conservative treatment
  - Pain medications, nonsteroidal anti-inflammatory drugs (NSAIDs)
  - Antispasmodics, antiepileptics, and antidepressants
- Physical therapy modalities: cervical traction
  - Strengthening exercises, biomechanical mobilization
  - Flexibility
  - Alignment techniques as indicated
  - Transcutaneous electrical nerve stimulation (TENS) and biofeedback
- Epidural steroid injections may help facilitate physical therapy.

Spinal Accessory Nerve: Cranial Nerve XI

Anatomy

- The trapezius, the major muscle supplied by the spinal accessory nerve, is a significant scapular stabilizer and thereby critical for the maintenance of efficient shoulder function (18).
- It originates on the occipital protuberance, the ligamentum nuchae, and spinous processes of C7–T12. The upper portion inserts at the lateral clavicle and the acromion (upward rotation of the scapula), the middle portion inserts in the spine of the scapula (retracts the scapula), and the lower portion inserts in the root of the spine of the scapula (depresses and upward rotates the scapula).
- Nerve supply is through the spinal component of cranial nerve (CN) XI. It originates from the anterior horn cells of the cervical spinal cord (C1–C5). Fibers enter the skull through the foramen magnum. The cranial component of the accessory nerve arises from the caudal part of the nucleus ambiguous. It is closely related to the vagus nerve (CN X). The cranial and spinal components, together with CN X, leave the skull through the jugular foramen and then separate again.
- An important fact of the central connections is that the corticobulbar tract from the midbrain eventually terminates in the brainstem, where the fibers to the trapezius muscle are crossed (therefore, central lesions cause contralateral deficit), whereas the corticobulbar fibers to the sternocleidomastoid muscle are either uncrossed or, more likely, double decussate (therefore, lesions are ipsilateral). These deficits help to locate the site of a lesion (12).
- In the neck, the spinal component of the accessory nerve passes through the posterior triangle (anterior border: sternocleidomastoid; posterior: trapezius; and inferior: clavicle). The roof is the platysma, and the floor is the splenius capitis, levator scapulae, and medial and posterior scalenus muscles.
- The triangle is subdivided by the traversing omohyoid. The superior space is the occipital triangle and below is the supraclavicular triangle.

- The contents of the occipital triangle are as follows:
  - Superior trunk of brachial plexus between scalenus anticus and medius
  - Branches of C5, C6, and C7
  - Dorsal scapular nerve (supplies levator scapulae and rhomboids)
  - Long thoracic nerve (innervates serratus anterior)
- The accessory nerve also passes through this space, after giving off a branch to supply the sternocleidomastoid muscle. It then supplies the trapezius muscle. This location is vulnerable for injury and compression. (Also space for nerve stimulation and conduction studies.)
- The contents of the supraclavicular triangle are as follows:
  - Middle trunk of brachial plexus
  - SSN (supplies the supraspinatus and infraspinatus muscles)
  - Nerve to subclavius muscle
  - Lower trunk of brachial plexus (C8)
  - Subclavian artery
  - External jugular vein descends across sternocleidomastoid muscle to drain into subclavian vein.

Risk Factors

- Intracranial: head injuries (especially basal skull fracture)
- Intraspinal cord: posttraumatic syrinx
- Cervical:
  - Percussion or compression of the accessory nerve in the posterior triangle in sports (football, ill-fitting shoulder pads)
  - Blows to the shoulder with a hockey stick
  - Backpack straps and shoulder dislocations
  - Mild to moderate (rarely severe) lesions result such as stingers/burners and occasionally involve nerve roots (26).
  - Traumatic penetrating neck injuries
  - Atraumatic, iatrogenic lesions, acute or delayed, mainly after radical neck dissections or lymph node biopsies
  - Cannulation of internal jugular vein or after carotid endarterectomies (due to hemorrhages, hematomas, malpositioned suction drainage, infection, or scarring)
  - Deep tissue massage
  - Spontaneous accessory nerve lesion (trapezius weakness) (16)
  - Tumor
  - Must rule out neuropathic or myopathic diseases

Symptoms and Signs

- **Shoulder syndrome:** consists of shoulder drooping, acromion prominence, limited lateral abduction, and impaired forward shoulder flexion
- Aberrant scapular rotation, abnormal scapulohumeral rhythm (8)
- Abnormal EDX findings

- Significant pain and tenderness over trapezius, exacerbated by shoulder movement
- Feeling of heaviness in the affected arm may be present.
- Difficulty with overhead activities, heavy lifting, prolonged writing, or driving
- Possible impingement pain secondary to inability to rotate scapula, thereby causing the greater tuberosity to abut the acromion (3)
- Late onset of pain is mostly due to adhesive capsulitis, a common sequela of spinal accessory nerve injury.

Evaluation

- Test trapezius strength by resistance to lateral abduction of the arm from about 100–180 degrees with arm internally rotated and hand pronated (18); check endurance. Isolation of trapezius must be assured since shoulder elevation can also be accomplished with the levator scapula and the rhomboids.
- Test strength of sternocleidomastoid muscles by resisting head turning, opposite to the side of the muscle tested. Also test tilting. Resistance to head flexion tests both sternocleidomastoid muscles at the same time.
- Lateral scapular winging is not as pronounced as with a long thoracic nerve lesion. The scapula is laterally translocated with medial rotation of the inferior angle. Shoulder winging caused by trapezius weakness is most pronounced by arm abduction, whereas weakness secondary to long thoracic nerve lesion is most pronounced by arm flexion (pushing upper extremity against a wall).
- EDX testing may be helpful (EMG looking for denervation or other neurogenic changes).
- NCS from posterior triangle to trapezius may be abnormal.

Differential Diagnosis

- Radiculopathy
- Posttraumatic focal shoulder elevation dystonia (9)
- Capsulitis
- Plexus lesions
- Neuralgic amyotrophy
- Motor neuron disease
- Meningitis

Treatment

- NSAIDs
- TENS
- Shoulder orthosis
- Physical therapy: range of motion (ROM) exercises to prevent contracture; resistive exercises to restore strength. If not successful, surgery may be considered if neurologic deficits are present (EMG confirmed).
  - Neurolysis
  - Nerve anastomosis
  - Graft procedures

Brachial Plexus

Anatomy

- The anterior rami (motor) and the posterior rami (sensory) of C5–T1 combine to form the brachial plexus. The C5–C6 roots together become the upper trunk, the C7 alone the middle trunk, and C8–T1 the lower trunk. Under and slightly below the clavicle, the trunks divide into three anterior and 3 posterior divisions. The anterior upper and middle divisions join to become the lateral cord, and the lower division forms the medial cord. All divisions participate to develop the posterior cord (position under the pectoralis minor). The cords divide into the major nerves of the upper extremities. (Terminal branches are median, ulnar, radial, axillary, and musculocutaneous nerves.)

Risk Factors

- Compression, stretch, or a combination of both
- Direct trauma
- Excessive pressure on the plexus after prolonged anesthesia, post-median sternotomy, coronary bypass surgery, jugular vein cannulation
- Difficult deliveries (Erb palsy)
- Shoulder dislocation

Symptoms and Signs

- Pain in shoulder and/or arm or hand
- Weakness of upper extremity, in one or multiple muscles
- Numbness, tingling, coldness
- Sensory loss
- Horner syndrome (ptosis, apparent enophthalmos, decreased sweating in affected side of face, miosis) possible with C8–T1 lesions such as tumors, radiculopathy (often root avulsion)

Evaluation

- Test ROM and strength in all muscle groups of the upper extremity
- Sensory examination (pinprick, light touch, temperature, and position sense)
- Reflex testing
- Nerve conduction tests and EMG
- If necessary, magnetic resonance imaging (MRI) or sonography

Differential Diagnosis

- Brachial plexitis
- Rotator cuff lesions
- Tendinitis
- Peripheral neuropathy
- Mononeuropathy
- Lesions secondary to radiation

Treatment

- Rest
- Temporary splinting
- Pain medication: NSAIDs; antiseizure medications (phenytoin, carbamazepine, gabapentin, tricyclic antidepressants) may be helpful to reduce stabbing pains
- ROM exercises
- After reinnervation, strengthening exercises
- If no significant progress after 6 months (mostly if root avulsion is present), surgery should be considered

Upper Trunk Plexopathy

Anatomy

- The upper trunk is formed from the combination of the C5 and C6 nerve roots/spinal nerves. From this region, the SSN and the nerve to the subclavius arise. The fibers to the musculocutaneous, axillary, median, and radial nerves pass through the upper trunk of the brachial plexus. An important landmark is **Erb point**. This location is about 2.5 cm above the clavicle, posterolateral to the sternocleidomastoid about the level of the sixth vertebra. This place is vulnerable to injury (compression, entrapment, stretch, or sharp disruption) and, in fact, is the area involved in the **stinger/burner** injury (13). At this point, the C5 and C6 roots, the SSN, and fibers of the musculocutaneous and axillary nerves can be electrically stimulated simultaneously, which can be helpful in correct diagnosis.
- The mechanisms of injury considered are (28):
  - Nerve root compression in the neural foramina (lack of protective epineurium and perineurium at that site)
  - Brachial plexus stretch (traction injury)
  - Direct blow to the plexus (percussion, compression)
  - A combination of stretch and percussion/compression

Risk Factors

- Football (highest incidence in defensive backs)
- Wrestlers
- Participants in other collision sports (ice hockey, field hockey, boxing)
- Shoulder laxity (33)
- Rugby
- Ill-fitting shoulder pads, neck rolls, or other equipment (26)
- Faulty techniques (especially during tackling)
- Carrying heavy loads for a long time including backpacks
- Foraminal stenosis (6,22)
- High-risk child birth (forceps, breech delivery)

Symptoms and Signs

- Burning pain and dysesthesia in affected arm on impact lasting seconds to hours, followed by mostly transient weakness and no sensory symptoms. At times, there is prolonged loss of strength (13).
- Occasionally, the only objective change may be seen as postural abnormality (drooping of the shoulder, especially if the accessory nerve is also involved).

- Weakness of shoulder muscles, especially supraspinatus and infraspinatus, deltoid, biceps

Evaluation

- Check for positive Tinel sign at Erb point
- Spurling test to rule in or out radiculopathy
- More severe injuries may involve the middle and lower trunk. There also may be denervation, which can be identified with EMG (earliest 2 weeks after the injury).

Differential Diagnosis

- Radiculopathy
- Cervical cord neurapraxia (CCN)
- Shoulder dislocation
- Tendinitis
- Neuralgic amyotrophy
- Rotator cuff injury

Treatment

- Only treatment is prevention of recurrences (improved techniques, appropriate shoulder pads, neck rolls, orthoses).
- In severe lesions, inactivity and slow return to strength and flexibility with gradually increasing collision work and improved tackling techniques are necessary before returning to contact sports.
- Emphasis is placed on postural exercises with cervicothoracic stabilization training and resistive exercises to shoulder muscles (when there is no evidence of denervation).
- The athlete may return to participation in contact sports on reestablishment of pain-free motion and full recovery of strength and functional status.
- Contraindication for return to play is two or more episodes of transient CCN, cervical myelopathy, evidence of neurologic deficit, decreased ROM, and/or neck pain (35).

Lower Trunk Plexopathy

Anatomy

- Position between clavicle and first rib. It carries sensory and motor fibers of C8–T1 distribution (median and ulnar nerves). The closeness of median motor and ulnar sensory fiber at this level has EDX significance.
- The best known and most debated compression syndrome is thoracic outlet syndrome.

Thoracic Outlet Syndrome

- **Anatomy**
  - **Thoracic outlet** clinically refers to the **thoracic inlet**, the anatomic structure of a bony ring (first thoracic vertebra, first pair of ribs, and the manubrium). The clavicle articulates with the manubrium, which represents the anterior border of the inlet. Several vital structures pass through that opening (brachial plexus, subclavian artery and vein). Thoracic outlet syndrome (TOS) is due to the impingement of the brachial plexus and/or subclavian

artery in the region of the scalenus muscles (anterior and medial), the first rib, and the clavicle. The subclavian vein lies on top of the scalenus anticus but joins the nerve and artery before the tight area between the clavicle and first rib. Compression/entrapment can also occur a bit more inferior (pectoralis minor syndrome).

- **TOS** is frequently caused by hyperextension injuries of the neck due to accidents, repetitive motion stress at work, and overhead activities like continued reaching for high-placed items. Muscles become tight (scar tissue has been found throughout the muscles by microscopic examination), or ligaments or bands press on the neurovascular structures, mostly just behind the collar bone.
- **Several TOS are identified by location:**
  - **Between the anterior and middle scalenus muscles**
  - **The scalenus anticus syndrome:** Nerve entrapment between the insertion of the scalenus anticus, the clavicle, and the first rib (especially in the presence of a cervical rib) (1)
  - **Costoclavicular syndrome:** Nerve entrapment in the narrowed space between clavicle and first rib; prolonged downward and backward shoulder pressure as by heavy loads on the shoulder; worse with abnormal clavicle or malunion or nonunion of clavicle fracture
  - **Pectoralis minor syndrome** (between chest wall and pectoralis minor)
- **Classification by structures involved:**
  - **Neurogenic thoracic outlet syndrome (NTOS):** most common; compression of brachial plexus (lower trunk)
  - **Venous thoracic outlet syndrome (VTOS)** (Paget-Schrötter syndrome): obstruction of the subclavian vein; presents with arm swelling, pain, and cyanosis, possible thrombosis
  - **Arterial thoracic outlet syndrome (ATOS):** 1% only; emboli arising from subclavian artery stenosis or aneurysm obstruct blood flow and cause ischemia; usually a cervical rib or anomalous first rib is present (27)
  - **Clinical TOS without objective findings** is very common. Identification as such depends on the diagnostician.
- **Risk factors**
  - Cervical rib (with fibrous bands to the first rib) (36)
  - Slim, asthenic females (with long "swan neck" and droopy shoulders)
  - Accessory nerve lesion (weak trapezius muscle causing droopy shoulders)
  - Sternotomy (at risk for pectoralis minor syndrome, especially those with premorbid impaired shoulder motion)
  - Neoplasm (*e.g.*, Pancoast tumor, bulky lymphadenopathy)
  - Radiculopathy
  - Klippel-Feil anomaly (24)
  - Swimmers and other sports using repeated overhead motion
  - Scalenus hypertrophy (1)
  - Heavy backpack

- **Symptoms and signs**
  - Vague pain and fatigue (claudication)
  - Color change (pallor and/or cyanosis)
  - Distended veins of arm and chest wall
  - Cool temperature of upper limb
  - Paresthesias along the median aspect of the affected hand and forearm
  - Pain in neck, shoulder, and arm, especially when elevating the arm
  - Thenar wasting and weakness of the abductor pollicis brevis (APB)
  - Ulnar hand intrinsics may also be weak and atrophic.
  - Confirmatory tests: arteriography, venography, and EMG
- **Evaluation**
  - **Physical examination:** Tenderness over scalene muscles, sometimes causing tingling radiating into arm; possible armpit tenderness (pectoralis minor syndrome); reduced sensation to light touch in involved hand; weakness and atrophy of APB may be present.
  - **Electrodiagnosis: NCS**
    - ❏ Median antebrachial cutaneous response amplitude decreased
    - ❏ Median motor response amplitude decreased
    - ❏ Ulnar sensory response amplitude decreased
      - EMG may show denervation.
  - **Provocative maneuvers:** unfortunately are not very reliable
    - ❏ **Adson's test:** Head turned to side, shoulders in military position, taking a deep breath. This decreases the space between clavicle and the first rib. It is positive when the radial pulse can no longer be palpated and/or the symptoms are reproduced. However, there are many false-positive and false-negative results.
    - ❏ **Upper limb tension test:** Abducting arms to 90 degrees in external rotation, which causes symptoms to appear within 60 seconds (comparable to straight leg raising test) (27).
    - ❏ **Test for costoclavicular compression:** Shoulders are placed in military position and clavicles forced downward posteriorly
    - ❏ **Hyperabduction-extension test:** Tries to reproduce symptoms experienced due to pectoralis minor syndrome
- **Differential diagnosis**
  - Brachial plexitis
  - Radiculopathy
  - Cervical myelopathy
  - Peripheral neuropathy
  - Complex regional pain syndrome
  - Fibromyalgia
  - Plexopathy after trauma or radiation
  - Pancoast tumor

- Glenohumeral instability
- Raynaud syndrome
- CTS
- Ulnar neuropathy (cubital tunnel syndrome, Guyon's canal syndrome)
- **Treatment**
  - **Physical therapy:** Physical therapy program including biomechanical retraining and shoulder and rib-cage elevation exercises that enlarge the entrapped space. Emphasis on stretching rather than strengthening. Pain should be addressed with specific agents for neuropathic pain (*e.g.,* tricyclics, anticonvulsants, Neurontin, etc.).
  - For ATOS and VTOS, urgent thrombolysis is indicated.
  - Prognosis for surgical results may be assessed by injecting Xylocaine (lidocaine) into the scalenus muscles and/or pectoralis muscle.
  - After results with anesthetic injection, a simple tenotomy may be performed (especially the pectoralis minor).
  - Newer trials at Johns Hopkins University suggest that Botox injections into the scalenus muscles may help, at least temporarily, to relieve pain.
  - **Surgical options:** Major procedures include transaxillary first rib resection, scalenectomy, and combined rib resection and scalenectomy (7), which may be indicated in cases of vascular etiology or the presence of a cervical rib or other prominent first rib bony abnormality.
  - Postsurgical complications are of concern. Recurrence through scarring is a definite possibility, despite wrapping nerves with plastic.

Long Thoracic Nerve

Anatomy

- C5/C6/C7 anterior primary rami are the origin of the long thoracic nerve. They together pierce the scalenus medius muscle forming the long thoracic nerve upper division. Together with the C7 spinal nerve, they travel between the scalenus medius and scalenus anticus muscles, located in the supraclavicular triangle. It supplies the anterior serratus muscle.

Risk Factors

- Weightlifting
- Carrying heavy loads, backpacks
- Back-stroke swimming
- Wrestling, gymnastics
- Motor vehicle accidents
- Chiropractic manipulation
- Deep massage
- Heavy labor
- Blow to shoulder or downward traction of the arm (may cause compression of the long thoracic nerve against the second rib)

- Heart surgery
- Trauma to the upper thorax and cervical region
- Infiltrating tumors
- Iatrogenic during radical mastectomy or axillary lymph node dissection
- Idiopathic entrapment

Symptoms and Signs

- Scapular winging
- Pain in shoulder, neck, arm
- Weakness in upper extremity, especially with overhead activities
- Frequently found weakness also in deltoid, biceps, supraspinatus, and infraspinatus muscles (additional cervical plexus involvement)
- Shoulder instability

Evaluation

- Test strength and ROM of shoulder. Forward flexion will be decreased to 90 degrees. Winging will be present when patient presses arms against a wall (compared to winging secondary to trapezius weakness, when abduction produces the greatest amount of winging). Measure angle of scapula plane to chest wall. Strength of the serratus muscle can be determined by distance of scapular angle to chest. More than 5 cm represents severe loss of function.
- EDX examination may reveal slow NCS and abnormal EMG.

Differential Diagnosis

- Neuralgic amyotrophy (29), also known as brachial plexitis or Parsonage-Turner syndrome (the long thoracic nerve is preferentially affected)
- Trapezius, rhomboid, suprascapular muscle lesions
- Motor neuron disease
- Poliomyelitis
- Radiculopathy
- Fracture
- Neoplasm
- Idiopathic long thoracic nerve palsy

Treatment

- Physical therapy: If denervation is present, ROM exercises are important to prevent contractures of the serratus as well as antagonist muscles (rhomboid and levator scapulae and pectoralis minor). (Stretching denervated muscles is contraindicated because of possible harm.) Muscle-strengthening exercises will begin upon reinnervation.
- Prognosis for spontaneous recovery is good (3 months–2 years), except in the case of root avulsion.
- A temporary shoulder orthosis is advised.
- If complete denervation persists after 6 months, a nerve graft may be necessary (*i.e.*, intercostal to long thoracic nerve).

Axillary Nerve

Anatomy

- The origin of the axillary nerve stems from roots C5 and C6. Fibers travel through the upper trunk of the brachial plexus. Their path continues through the posterior divisions followed by the posterior cord. The first terminal branch is the axillary nerve. It crosses the anteroinferior aspect of the subscapularis muscle, then through the quadrilateral space. It divides into a posterior trunk that supplies the teres minor and the posterior deltoid and terminates as the lateral brachial cutaneous nerve. The anterior trunk supplies the anterior and middle deltoid. The axillary nerve is the most common nerve affected in shoulder lesions. (Boundaries of the quadrilateral space are teres minor superior, teres major inferior, long head of triceps medial, and surgical neck of the humerus lateral).
- Points of possible compression/entrapment are:
    - At the origin from the posterior cord
    - At the anterior and inferior aspect of the subscapularis muscle
    - The subfascial surface of the deltoid
    - The quadrilateral space

Risk Factors

- Throwing athletes
- Football, crew, swimming, backpacking
- Direct blow to the deltoid
- Glenohumeral joint dislocation (32), humerus fractures or surgery
- Muscle hypertrophy and possibly fibrous bands
- Tumors
- Improper use of crutches (leaning on the axilla when standing)
- Inappropriate application of casts or orthoses
- Iatrogenic

Symptoms and Signs

- In quadrilateral space syndrome, there is posterior shoulder pain.
- Paresthesias over a circular location of the lateral arm
- Weakness of deltoid muscle
- Forward flexion and/or abduction and external rotation of the humerus aggravate the symptoms.
- Difficulty lifting arm above the head
- Possibly abnormal EDX studies

Evaluation

- ROM and strength testing of shoulder muscles.
- Subclavian arteriography may show compression of the posterior humeral circumflex artery with abduction and external rotation of the arm (5).
- EDX studies may be abnormal.

Differential Diagnosis

- Tendinitis
- Rotator cuff tear
- Frozen shoulder
- Radiculopathy
- Brachial plexopathy
- Parsonage-Turner syndrome

Treatment

- Many patients, especially young patients, recover full shoulder abduction even with continued denervation of the deltoid by substituting the supraspinatus for the deltoid. Throwing athletes experience difficulty. The deltoid provides 50% of the torque about the shoulder.
- With a direct blow to the deltoid, prognosis is poorer than with lesions from other causes.
- Acute injury: Rest, treatment of bony or other injuries must be taken care of. ROM and passive exercises to rotator cuff muscles, deltoid, and periscapular muscles, progressing to resistive exercises as muscles are reinnervated. Shoulder contracture must be avoided.
- Muscle retraining and/or job changes are recommended. If there is no evidence of reinnervation after 6 months, surgical exploration must be considered.
- Surgery for quadrilateral space syndrome aims to decompress by release of fascia and fibrous bands around the axillary nerve and posterior humeral circumflex vessels (5).
- For more extensive lesions, neurolysis nerve repair, nerve grafts, and/or nerve transfer are possibilities.
- If there is also root avulsion, grafting and nerve transfers are the optimal procedures to regain function (2).

Suprascapular Nerve

Anatomy

- The C5–C6 spinal nerves are the origin of the SSN. Fibers travel through the upper trunk of the brachial plexus, pass through the supraclavicular fossa, and then through the scapular notch covered by the transverse scapular ligament. Just distal to the notch, the SSN sends branches to the acromioclavicular joint and the subacromial bursa and extends to the shoulder joint. After innervating and passing through the supraspinatus muscle, the SSN bends around the spine of the scapula to innervate the infraspinatus.
- Points of possible compression/entrapment:
    - Scapular notch
    - Spinoglenoid notch
    - Fascia between the scapular and the spinoglenoid notches (15)

Risk Factors

- Traumatic:
    - Rotator cuff tear
    - Shoulder arthrodesis
    - Fracture of the scapula

- Nontraumatic:
    - Repetitive overhead loading activities
    - Volleyball
    - Weightlifting
    - Boxing
    - Basketball
    - Baseball
    - Painting
    - Backpack straps
    - Ganglion cysts at scapular notch
    - Superior glenoid labrum, spinoglenoid notch cysts

Symptoms and Signs

- Vague shoulder pains with possible radiation in suprascapular or radial nerve distribution
- Vague shoulder and/or acromioclavicular joint pain
- Weakness in supraspinatus and/or infraspinatus muscles

Evaluation

- Test ROM and muscle strength in shoulder muscles.
- Test for Tinel's sign at the scapular notch.
- Overhead activities may worsen symptoms.
- The crossed arm abduction test should exacerbate symptoms on the affected side.
- EDX studies may show abnormality.

Differential Diagnosis

- Cervical radiculopathy
- Discogenic pain
- Shoulder acromioclavicular joint pathology
- Rotator cuff tear
- Musculoskeletal pain syndromes
- Plexitis

Treatment

- Avoidance of exacerbating activities (overhead).
- Physical therapy focuses on maintaining ROM of the scapula and on improving muscle strength.
- Correct the scapulohumeral rhythm as much as possible.
- Injection of local anesthetic into the scapular notch may assist in the diagnosis and treatment.
- If no adequate response to conservative measures, consider surgery.
- Surgical decompression arthroscopically (through subacromial space or other portals) (19)

Musculocutaneous Nerve

Anatomy

- The musculocutaneous nerve is the terminal branch of the lateral cord of the brachial plexus (fibers from C5–C7). The nerve passes through the coracobrachialis, which it innervates, as well as the brachialis and biceps brachii.

In many subjects, the brachialis also receives a branch of the radial nerve.

■ Just above the elbow, the musculocutaneous motor nerve becomes the sensory nerve, lateral antebrachial cutaneous nerve, which innervates the volar and dorsal forearm along the radial aspect, but not the hand.

■ Entrapment is uncommon.

Risk Factors

■ Excessive resistive elbow extension (push-ups or arm presses in weightlifters)

■ Strenuous forearm pronation

■ Tight biceps aponeurosis (11)

■ Shoulder dislocation

■ A hypertrophic coracobrachialis muscle; the lateral antebrachial cutaneous nerve may be compressed as it enters the forearm.

Symptoms and Signs

■ Coracobrachialis entrapment: elbow flexor weakness, lateral arm pain (burning), and/or loss of sensation

■ Positive Tinel sign at areas of entrapment

■ Decreased biceps reflex possible

■ Distal entrapment may present only with forearm pain and/or sensory deficit.

Evaluation

■ Meticulous history and physical examination

■ Point of maximal tenderness is important for possible surgery.

■ Symptoms increase with elbow extension and forearm pronation.

■ Electrodiagnosis: Motor and sensory conduction may be slowed and amplitudes reduced. In severe lesions, EMG of biceps may show abnormal neurogenic findings.

Differential Diagnosis

■ Shoulder dislocation

■ Rotator cuff lesion

■ Plexitis

■ Tendinitis

■ Lateral epicondylitis

■ Cervical radiculopathy

■ Median or superficial radial nerve entrapment

Treatment

■ Rest, ROM, active assistive ROM, gentle stretching

■ Anti-inflammatory medication

■ Modalities

■ Lateral antebrachial cutaneous nerve entrapment near the cubital fossa mostly needs surgical decompression (10).

Median Nerve

■ **Anatomy:** The median nerve originates from the C6–T1 spinal roots/nerves. It traverses the upper, middle, and lower trunk; the anterior divisions; and the lateral and medial cord. It is one of the three nerves supplying all muscles of the forearm and hand.

Entrapment Site 1: Ligament of Struthers

Anatomy

■ Median and ulnar nerves and brachial artery can be entrapped by a fibrous band from a rare supracondylar process on the anterior humerus to its medial epicondyle or underneath the lacertus fibrosis.

Risk Factors

■ 2.7% of the population who have the anomaly

■ Distal humerus fracture

■ Space-occupying lesion

Symptoms and Signs

■ Tingling, numbness in median innervated area

■ Weakness in all median nerve innervated muscles.

■ Deficits in ulnar nerve distribution, if the ulnar is also entrapped.

■ Swelling of hand and forearm (brachial vein) and blanching (brachial artery)

■ Ape hand (severe involvement of the whole median nerve)

Evaluation

■ Good history and extensive physical examination are paramount.

■ Imaging of humerus to confirm the presence of a spur or osteochondroma

■ EDX studies can be helpful. Pronator maybe involved, but not in pronator syndrome.

Differential Diagnosis

■ Pronator syndrome

■ Humerus fracture

■ Humeral osteochondroma (spur oriented away from the joint in opposite to the anomalous supracondylar process, which points toward the joint)

■ Radiculopathy

Treatment

■ Reduction of aggravating activities

■ Anti-inflammatory medications may help some

■ Surgery will usually be the treatment of choice (spur excision; in absence of spur, ligament incision and lacertus fibrosis wedge removal) (30)

Entrapment Site 2: Pronator Syndrome

Anatomy

■ In the antecubital area the median nerve is located underneath the bicipital aponeurosis (lacertus fibrosis). Then it passes between the superficial and deep heads of the pronator teres, underneath the flexor digitorum superficialis.

■ Entrapment by these structures: pronator syndrome. An accessory head of the flexor pollicis longus (FPL), called Gantzer's muscle, may contribute to this syndrome as well as the anterior interosseous nerve syndrome. More entrapment syndromes are described by Tubbs et al. (31).

Risk Factors

- Enlarged median artery
- Musicians (pianists, fiddlers, harpists)
- Athletes (baseball players)
- Arm fractures can injure the brachial artery by compression, thereby preventing blood flow and causing ischemia. Resulting scarring of flexor muscles may cause flexion deformity at wrist and fingers (Volkmann contracture).
- Occupational (*e.g.*, machine milkers and dentists)

Symptoms and Signs

- Weak handgrip
- Aching pain with resisted flexion to the middle finger, increased activities
- Pain on active resistive forearm pronation
- Possible cramping of fingers (writer's cramp)
- Numbness of thumb and index finger
- Possible positive Tinel test over pronator teres muscle
- Negative Phalen's test
- Significant loss of median nerve function will cause the "Benedictine hand."

Evaluation

- Precise history and physical
- Strength test, especially pronation against resistance, elbow flexion, and resistive elbow extension
- Provocative maneuver: Paresthesias in the hand after 30 seconds or less of manual compression of the median nerve over the pronator teres muscle.
- EMG and NCS may be helpful.

Differential Diagnosis

- Tendinitis
- Entrapment under ligament of Struthers
- CTS
- Entrapment under the sublime bridge
- Plexitis

Treatment

- Rest, splinting
- Anti-inflammatory drugs
- Possible steroid injections into the area of entrapment
- If there is no improvement in 6 months, surgical exploration is recommended.
- Surgery: Release of offending structure leads to full recovery, unless severe axonotmesis is present (17).

Entrapment Site 3: Anterior Interosseous Nerve Syndrome (Kiloh-Nevin Syndrome)

Anatomy

- In the forearm, the median nerve gives off a large deep motor branch, the anterior interosseous nerve, that supplies the FPL,

the two lateral heads of the flexor digitorum profundus, and the pronator quadratus. Anterior interosseous lesions are rare.

Risk Factors

- Supracondylar humerus fracture (especially in children)
- Venipuncture
- Anatomic variants
- Tumor

Symptoms and Signs

- No sensory symptoms
- Weakness in thumb flexion, finger flexion, forearm pronation

Evaluation

- Careful examination of forearm and hand
- ROM and strength evaluation mainly of thumb and finger flexion and pronation
- Look for the "O" sign: Patients are unable to hold and resist the opening of the index finger to thumb tip-to-tip pinch; the two distal phalanges align flat against each other to hold the pinch.
- EMG is helpful to identify the involved muscles.

Differential Diagnosis

- Neuralgic amyotrophy (brachial plexitis)
- Pronator teres syndrome
- Radiculopathy

Treatment

- Conservative management; surgery may become necessary.

Entrapment Site 4: Carpal Tunnel Syndrome

Anatomy

- The carpal tunnel is formed by the arched carpal bones covered by the carpal ligament (retinaculum), which spans from the pisiform and hamate to the trapezium and scaphoid. It contains, in addition to the median nerve, arteries, and veins, tendons of nine flexor muscles: flexor digitorum superficialis (4 tendons), flexor digitorum profundus (4 tendons), and FPL (1 tendon). The flexor carpi radialis tendon has its own synovial sheath to prevent compression when passing through the radial attachment to the retinaculum. It travels with the radial artery and the palmar cutaneous branch superficial to the flexor retinaculum, underneath which the other flexor tendons are located (in the carpal tunnel).
- In the hand, the median nerve supplies the lateral two lumbricals and most of the thenar muscles, except for the deep head of the flexor pollicis brevis. Sensory fibers, after traveling through the carpal tunnel, supply the lateral three and one-half digits, and the distal one-third of the dorsal aspect of the digits' 1–3, one-half of the dorsal distal digit of the ring-finger, and the lateral palm, except for a small area over the thenar eminence. (Radial nerve supply)

Risk Factors

- Repetitive motion activities (job related, knitting, sewing, etc.)
- Low ratio of depth to width (< 0.70) of the wrist. (20)
- Hypothyroidism

- Myxedema
- Pregnancy, premenstrual swelling
- Tumor
- Other causes of excessive soft tissue swelling
- Wheelchair athletics
- Tennis
- Baseball, volleyball
- Musicians (violin and piano playing)

Symptoms and Signs

- Nocturnal numbness
- Tingling and wrist pain, increased with activities
- Patients prone to dropping things
- Sensory impairment in median nerve distribution in the hand
- Weak hand grip
- When holding a pinch against resistance, patients frequently will use the ulnar innervated deep flexor pollicis to oppose the index, instead of the APB.
- In the hand, severe median nerve loss will eventually cause an ape hand deformity because of the loss of thenar muscles and, thereby, loss of opposition and flexion of the thumb.

Evaluation

- Meticulous history and examination of muscle strength
- Sensory examination of all modalities (superficial and deep sensation, temperature, position sense, 2-point discrimination)
- Electrodiagnosis is extremely helpful in the diagnosis of CTS, especially to rule out radiculopathy and to identify CTS even when peripheral neuropathy is also present. Nerve conduction velocity across the wrist, EMG.

Differential Diagnosis

- Cervical radiculopathy
- Peripheral neuropathy
- Diabetes mellitus
- Tendinitis
- Space-occupying lesion
- Nerve injury or postsurgery complication

Treatment

- Night splints in neutral position
- Splints for activities that produce discomfort (avoiding constant wearing)
- Nonsteroidal pain medication
- Pyridoxine may help; frequently, a deficiency is present.
- TENS effectiveness was objectively confirmed with functional MRI (21)
- Steroid injections into the painful area; if no response, surgery may be considered
- Release of confining ligament.
- Endoscopic with minimal invasiveness

Entrapment Site 5: Digital Nerve Entrapment

Anatomy

- The median nerve sensory fibers in the hand are located at the medial and lateral side of digits 1–3 and on the lateral side of digit 4. They may become entrapped.

Risk Factors

- Vibration syndrome
- Athletes (baseball players, bowlers, etc.)
- Musicians
  - Flutists (lateral side of left index finger)
  - Violinists, cellists (right thumb)
  - Percussionists (left middle finger)

Symptoms and signs

- Numbness and tingling in fingers
- Pain in fingers
- Cramping, dystonia

Evaluation

- Careful history and physical, especially a meticulous sensory examination, all modalities
- Sensory nerve conduction may be of help (finger stimulation and finger recording)

Differential Diagnosis

- Radiculopathy
- Peripheral neuropathy
- Reynaud syndrome
- Dependant arm swelling

Treatment

- NSAIDs
- Splinting
- Steroid injections (last resort)
- Surgical release

Radial Nerve

- **Anatomy:** The radial nerve originates from fibers of the C5–C8/T1 nerve roots and emerges as the terminal branch of the posterior cord (brachial plexus). It runs between the medial and long heads of the triceps, along the spiral groove of the humerus, where the posterior antebrachial cutaneous nerve branches off, which supplies the skin of the extensor forearm. The radial nerve pierces the lateral intermuscular septum, travels anterior to the lateral epicondyle, and divides into superficial and deep branch in the cubital fossa. The latter continues in the radial tunnel through the arcade of Frohse, lies between the superficial and deep supinators, and becomes the posterior interosseous nerve, supplying the extensor forearm muscles (except the extensor carpi radialis longus [ECL]). The superficial branch courses laterally at the wrist. It supplies sensation to the dorsal-radial wrist and the proximal dorsal aspect of the first 3 and one-half digits.

Entrapment Site 1: Radial Nerve Proximal to Elbow — Spiral Groove

Risk Factors

- Humerus fracture: Estimated incidence of radial entrapment is 10%–18% (4). Most lesions are neurapraxic; functional return is seen in 4–5 months (23).
- Saturday night (honeymooner's) palsy: most common, due to prolonged compression of the nerve in or near the spiral groove.

Symptoms and Signs

- Weakness of forearm extensors (wrist drop)
- Slight weakness of elbow flexors if brachioradialis is involved
- Triceps may or may not be involved.
- Triceps reflex absent if triceps involved
- Pain and sensory change in posterior antebrachial cutaneous and/or distal superficial radial nerve distribution

Evaluation

- History: trauma to humerus, recent obtundation due to alcohol or other inebriation
- Physical examination: weakness in dorsiflexion of wrist, sensory loss to pinprick and/or light touch in distal radial nerve distribution
- Electrodiagnosis is recommended
- NCS: Recording radial nerve velocity and amplitude across the point of injury may demonstrate the deficit
- Needle exam — Involved muscles may show denervation.

Differential Diagnosis

- Radiculopathy
- Brachial plexitis
- Space-occupying lesion
- Musculocutaneous nerve lesion
- Extensor tenosynovitis

Treatment

- Assure bony stability in humerus fracture to prevent further nerve injury.
- Prognosis in lesion above elbow is good (neurapraxia).
- Conservative management
- If no recovery in several months or clinical decline, surgical exploration is indicated.

Entrapment 2: Radial Tunnel Syndrome

- This syndrome is controversial. Compression may occur anywhere in the tunnel. The cause of these symptoms often is a treatment resistant chronic tennis elbow. Generally, no definite neurologic deficit can be demonstrated clinically or by electrodiagnosis.

Entrapment 3: Supinator Syndrome — Arcade of Frohse

- This syndrome is a compression at the arcade of Frohse where the radial nerve pierces the supinator and becomes the purely motor posterior interosseous nerve (PIN). The supinator itself and the extensor carpi radialis longus (ECRL) are

mostly innervated by the posterior interosseous nerve before it enters the Arcade of Frohse.

Risk Factors

- Repetitive motion
- Fracture of proximal radius
- Fracture/dislocation at elbow (Monteggia fracture)
- Rheumatoid arthritis
- Lacerations, scarring
- Lipomas, other tumors

Symptoms and Signs

- Pain and/or weakness in radial distributions distal to elbow
- Partial wrist drop, radial deviation on wrist extension (ECL innervation above elbow)
- Interossei appear weak secondary to loss of wrist stabilization
- No sensory deficit

Evaluation

- Given risk factors, consider advanced imaging
- Physical examination: Forced supination with arm fully flexed will reproduce pain in lesions proximal to supinator.
- Forced extension of third digit may be weak (not in extensor tenosynovitis).
- Electrodiagnosis: most reliable is the needle examination of the radial innervated muscles. NCS are not always helpful. The technique would be as the previously described radial nerve study.
- Imaging helps demonstrate the cause.

Differential Diagnosis

- Radiculopathy
- Brachial plexitis
- Tumor (neuroma), rheumatoid arthritis (RA)
- Musculocutaneous nerve lesion
- Extensor tenosynovitis
- "Tennis elbow"

Treatment

- Conservative management
- If refractory or rapidly progressive (denervation on EMG study), consider surgical release

Entrapment Site 4: Distal Radial Nerve Lesion ("Handcuff Neuropathy" or Cheiralgia Paresthetica)

- Due to compression at the wrist and is mostly purely sensory

Risk Factors

- Prisoners
- With more severe injury, multiple nerves may be involved.

Symptoms and Signs

- Sensory deficits in distal superficial radial nerve distribution
- No weakness

Treatment

- Conservative management
- Recovery usually complete within 6–8 weeks
- It may predispose patient to complex regional pain syndrome.

Ulnar Nerve

- **Anatomy:** The ulnar nerve (C7, C8, T1) is the terminal branch of the inferior trunk and the medial cord of the brachial plexus. It accompanies the brachial artery and median nerve in a neurovascular bundle. It then travels between the coracobrachialis and triceps. At midpoint of the upper arm, the nerve enters the posterior compartment, piercing the intermuscular septum. The nerve runs along the medial head of the triceps in a tough investing fascia that comprises the arcade of Struthers. At the elbow, the nerve leaves this fascia and passes posterior to the medial epicondyle of the humerus (ulnar sulcus). It enters the cubital tunnel at the humeroulnar aponeurotic arcade (Osborne ligament), pierces the flexor carpi ulnaris (FCU), and lies between its two heads. It exits at the distal end of the cubital tunnel through the deep flexor pronator aponeurosis (DFPA). At the wrist, the nerve passes through Guyon canal (borders: medially, pisiform bone; laterally, hook of hamate; roof, tendon of FCU; and floor, carpal ligament) into the palm of the hand. In the canal, the ulnar nerve divides into a deep branch accompanied by the ulnar artery, which winds around the hook of the hamate and supplies the interossei, the third and fourth lumbricals, the adductor pollicis, the first dorsal interosseous, and the deep head of the flexor pollicis brevis. The superficial branch supplies the palmaris brevis and terminates as sensory nerve to digits 4 and 5.

Entrapment Site 1: Ligament of Struthers

Risk Factors

- Prior trauma
- Surgery (*e.g.*, ulnar transposition)

Symptoms and Signs

- Similar to those of median nerve compression at the same site
- Decreased sensation in ulnar nerve distribution proximal to wrist
- Severe lesion may involve ulnar motor innervation (FCU, medial flexor digitorum profundus)
- Weakness of the FCU will reveal radial deviation of wrist with flexion

Evaluation

- Advanced imaging (MRI or diagnostic ultrasound)
- EMG/NCS may be negative until case is advanced; motor fibers are well protected. Motor study of ulnar nerve with stimulation proximal to suspected lesion. May be difficult to discern entrapment here from tardy ulnar palsy, without clinical suspicion.

Differential Diagnosis

- Radiculopathy/myelopathy
- TOS
- Pancoast tumor

- Ulnar entrapment distally
- Double crush

Treatment

- Conservative management is usually not adequate.
- Surgery to release constriction band is often favored.

Entrapment Site 2: Ulnar Sulcus/Retrocondylar Groove (Tardy Ulnar Palsy)

- Second most common nerve entrapment of the upper extremity

Risk Factors

- Leaning on elbows
- Tight casting
- Compressive trauma
- Bony deformity
- Epicondyle fracture (nonunion)
- Wrestling without elbow pads
- Excessive flexion (as in prolonged driving)
- Repetitive motion at elbow
- Chronic subluxation
- High body mass index in women, older age in men
- Rheumatoid arthritis
- Occupational or recreational activities
- Prolonged use of vibrating tools

Symptoms and Signs

- Pain, paresthesia, and/or numbness in volar aspect of fifth and medial fourth digits and hypothenar eminence, increasing with elbow flexion
- Weakness and/or atrophy in ulnar innervated hand intrinsic muscles
- Flexion contracture of proximal interphalangeal joint of fifth digit
- Possible claw hand (partial flexion of the proximal and distal interphalangeal joints, with extension of the metacarpophalangeal joints)
- Diminished grip strength

Evaluation

- Dynamic assessment to look for chronic nerve subluxation
- Tinel's sign
- EMG/NCS may assist in the diagnosis (14)
- Consider ulnar inching study (multiple potential sites of entrapment).
- Consider diagnostic ultrasound.

Differential Diagnosis

- Ulnar entrapment distally or proximally
- Systemic disease with high incidence of mononeuropathies (*e.g.*, diabetes, alcoholism, thyroid)
- Compression: extrinsic or intrinsic, postoperative
- Valgus ligament instability

- Elbow injury and deformities
- Fractures and dislocations
- Cubitus valgus or varus
- Space-occupying lesions: ganglia, tumors, osteophytes, bursae
- Perineural adhesions
- Burns and heterotopic bone
- Osteophytes, synovitis (34)

Treatment

- Conservative management, pain control
- Correct underlying etiology if possible
- Muscle strengthening
- ROM
- Relative rest including avoiding exacerbating activities
- Padding and/or splinting around the elbow
- If neurologic symptoms progress, consider surgery (ulnar nerve release or ulnar nerve transposition)

Entrapment Site 3: Cubital Tunnel Syndrome

- Compression at the entry (Osborne ligament) or exit (DFPA)

Risk Factors

- Lesions mostly nontraumatic
- Repetitive motion injuries
- Anatomic predisposition

Symptoms and Signs

- Findings similar to tardy ulnar palsy
- Tinel sign over the cubital tunnel, not over sulcus
- Wartenberg sign (fifth digit abduction)
- Froment's sign: Patient pinches a piece of paper between first and second metacarpals. In response to a strong pull, patient contracts the FPL to substitute for weak first dorsal interosseous and adductor pollicis.

Differential Diagnosis

- Similar to entrapments sites 1–2 discussed earlier

Treatment

- Conservative
- Progressive symptoms with motor decline
- Surgery (cubital tunnel release)

Entrapment Sites 4 and 5: Guyon Canal and Palmar Entrapment

- Motor or sensory fibers, or both, may be involved depending on the location of the compression. Entrapment distal to Guyon canal (deep palmer branch) results in weakness of ulnar innervated intrinsics. Occasionally, the abductor digiti minimi is spared. In the canal, both may be compressed. The superficial branch causes sensory loss of the ulnar half of the fourth digit and the fifth digit. The dorsal sensory nerve branches off above the wrist.

Risk Factors

- Bicycling (handlebar palsy)
- Push-ups

- Flute or violin playing
- Vibrational trauma
- Scars, tumor, ganglion cyst, lipoma
- Ulnar artery aneurysm
- Fracture, especially hook of hamate

Symptoms and Signs

- Wrist/hand pain
- Weakness in grasp
- Numbness and tingling in distal ulnar nerve distribution; often worse at night

Evaluation

- History and physical
- Advanced imaging (MRI, computed tomography, ultrasound)
- Helpful electrodiagnostic studies are: NCS: Ulnar and Dorsal Ulnar Cutaneous SNAP (sensory nerve action potential) velocities and amplitudes. CMAP (Compound muscle action potentials) latency across the wrist.
- Tinel, Phalen, reverse Phalen signs

Differential Diagnosis

- See entrapment sites 1–3 discussed earlier
- Wrist flexor tendonitis

Treatment

- Conservative management
- Activity modification
- NSAIDs
- Padding
- Possible steroid injections
- If no improvement in 3 months or increased neurologic signs, consider surgery

REFERENCES

1. Baltopoulos P, Tsintzos C, Prionas G, Tsironi M. Exercise-induced scalenus anticus syndrome. *Am J Sports Med.* 2008;36(2):369–74.
2. Bhandari PS, Sadhotra LP, Bhargava P, et al. Surgical outcomes following nerve transfers in upper brachial plexus injuries. *Indian J Plast Surg.* 2009;42(2):150–60.
3. Bigliani LU, Compito CA, Duralde XA, Wolfe IN. Transfer of levator scapulae, rhomboid major, rhomboid minor for paralysis of the trapezius. *J Bone Joint Surg Am.* 1996;78(10):1534–40.
4. Bodner G, Buchberger W, Schocke M, et al. Radial nerve palsy associated with humeral shaft fracture. *Radiology.* 2001;219(3):811–16.
5. Cahill BR, Palmer RE. Quadrilateral space syndrome. *J Hand Surg Am.* 1973;8(1):65–9.
6. Castro FP Jr. Stingers, cervical cord neurapraxia, and stenosis. *Clin Sports Med.* 2003;22(3):483–92.
7. Chang DC, Rotellini-Coltvet LA, Mukherjee D, De Leon R, Freischlag JA. Surgical intervention for thoracic outlet syndrome improves patient's quality of life. *J Vasc Surg.* 2009;49(3):630–5.

8. Codman EA. Rupture of the supraspinatus tendon and other lesions on or about the subacromial bursa. In: Codman EA, editor. *The Shoulder*. Boston: Thomas Todd; 1934. p. 32–54.

9. Cossu G, Melis M, Melis G, Ferrigno P, Molari A. Persistent abnormal shoulder elevation after accessory nerve injury and differential diagnosis with post-traumatic focal shoulder-elevation dystonia: report of a case and literature review. *Mov Disord*. 2004;19(9):1109–11.

10. Dailiana ZH, Roulot E, Le Viet D. Surgical treatment of compression of the lateral antebrachial cutaneous nerve. *J Bone Joint Surg Br*. 2000;82(3):420–3.

11. Davidson JJ, Bassett FH III, Nunley JA II. Musculocutaneous nerve entrapment revisited. *J Shoulder Elbow Surg*. 1998;7(3):250–5.

12. Di Benedetto M. Cranial neuropathies. In: Zajtchuk R, editor. *Textbook of Military Medicine, Part IV, Surgical Combat Casualty Care: Rehabilitation of the Injured Combatant, Vol 1*. Washington: Department of Army; 1995. p. 279–352.

13. Di Benedetto M, Markey K. Electrodiagnostic location of traumatic upper trunk brachial plexopathy. *Arch Phys Med Rehabil*. 1984;65(1):15–17.

14. Dumitru D, Amato AA, Zwarts MJ, editors. *Electrodiagnostic Medicine*. 2nd ed. Philadelphia (PA): Hanley & Belfus; 2002. 1524 p.

15. Duparc F, Coquerel D, Ozeel J, Noyon M, Gerometta A, Michot C. Anatomical basis of the suprascapular nerve entrapment and clinical relevance of the supraspinatus fascia. *Surg Radiol Anat*. 2010;32(3):277–84.

16. Eisen A, Bertrand G. Isolated accessory nerve palsy of spontaneous origin. A clinical and electromyographic study. *Arch Neurol*. 1972;27(6):496–502.

17. Eversmann WW. Proximal median nerve compression. *Hand Clin*. 1992;8(2):307–15.

18. Ewing MR, Martin H. Disability following radical neck dissection. *Cancer*. 1952;5(5):873–83.

19. Ghodadra N, Nho SJ, Verma NN, et al. Arthroscopic decompression of the suprascapular nerve at the spinoglenoid notch and suprascapular notch through the subacromial space. *Arthroscopy*. 2009;25(4):439–45.

20. Gordon C, Johnson EW, Gatens PF, Ashton JJ. Wrist ratio correlation with carpal tunnel syndrome in industry. *Am J Phys Med Rehabil*. 1988;67(6):270–2.

21. Kara M, Ozçakar L, Gökçay D, et al. Quantification of the effects of transcutaneous electrical nerve stimulation with functional magnetic resonance imaging: a double-blind randomized placebo-controlled study. *Arch Phys Med Rehabil*. 2010;91(8):1160–5.

22. Kelly JD IV, Aliquo D, Sitler MR, Odgers C, Moyer RA. Association of burners with cervical canal and foraminal stenosis. *Am J Sports Med*. 2000;28(2):214–7.

23. Kimura J. *Electrodiagnosis in Diseases of Nerve and Muscle: Principles and Practice*. 3rd ed. New York (NY): Oxford University Press; 2001. p. 717–8.

24. Konstantinou DT, Chroni EM, Constantoyiannis C, Dougenis D. Klippel-Feil syndrome presenting with bilateral thoracic outlet syndrome. *Spine (Phila Pa 1976)*. 2004;29(9):E189–92.

25. Krivickas LS, Wilbourn AJ. Peripheral nerve injuries in athletes: a case series of over 200 injuries. *Semin Neurol*. 2000;20(2):225–32.

26. Markey KL, Di Benedetto M, Curl WW. Upper trunk brachial plexopathy. The stinger syndrome. *Am J Sports Med*. 1993;21(5):650–5.

27. Sanders RJ, Hammond SL, Rao NM. Diagnosis of thoracic outlet syndrome. *J Vasc Surg*. 2007;46(3):601–4.

28. Stracciolini A. Cervical burners in the athlete. *Pediatr Case Rev*. 2003;3(4):181–8.

29. Suarez GA, Giannini C, Bosch EP, et al. Immune brachial plexus neuropathy suggestive evidence for an inflammatory-immune pathogenesis. *Neurology*. 1996;46(2):559–61.

30. Suranyi L. Median nerve compression by Struthers ligament. *J Neurol Neurosurg Psychiatry*. 1983;46(11):1047–9.

31. Tubbs RS, Marshall T, Loukas M, Shoja MM, Cohen-Gadol AA. The sublime bridge: anatomy and implications in median nerve entrapment. *J Neurosurg*. 2010;113(1):110–2.

32. Toolanen G, Hildingsson C, Hedlund T, Knibestöl M, Oberg L. Early complications after anterior dislocation of the shoulder in patients over 40 years. An ultrasonographic and electromyographic study. *Acta Orthop Scand*. 1993;64(5):549–52.

33. Unlü MC, Kesmezacar H, Akgün I. Brachial plexus neuropathy (stinger syndrome) occurring in a patient with shoulder laxity. *Acta Orthop Traumatol Turc*. 2007;41(1):74–9.

34. Verheyden JR, Palmer AK. Triangular fibrocartilage complex injuries. *eMedicine* [Internet]. 2009 [cited 2009 June 23]. Available from: http://emedicine.medscape.com/article/1240789-overview

35. Weinberg J, Rokito S, Silber JS. Etiology, treatment and prevention of athletes "stinger." *Clin Sports Med*. 2003;22(3):493–500, viii.

36. Wilbourn AJ. Thoracic outlet syndromes. *Neurol Clin*. 1999;17(3):477–97, vi.

Magnetic Resonance Imaging in the Lower Extremity

58

Courtney T. Tripp and John F. Feller

HIP

- Hip magnetic resonance imaging (MRI) protocols in the athlete should be performed to optimize assessment for both internal and external derangements of the hip. Ideally, MRI evaluation includes a combination of large field-of-view bilateral hip and pelvic structures that aid in evaluation of extra-articular abnormalities (*i.e.*, musculotendinous injuries, osseous injuries, bursitis) and high-resolution small field-of-view unilateral imaging for intra-articular abnormalities (*e.g.*, articular cartilage and acetabular labrum injuries, femoral acetabular impingement [FAI], and loose bodies) (5).

- Although controversy exists regarding the most appropriate MRI assessment of intra-articular hip pathology, multiple studies have shown a high degree of accuracy with both noncontrast MRI and magnetic resonance (MR) arthrography for diagnosis of cartilage injuries of the hip (12,18,25). Newer novel MR mapping techniques for chondral assessment are also being developed (24).

- Intra-articular abnormalities that commonly affect the young athletic population and can be evaluated with MRI include acetabular labral tears, chondral injuries, intra-articular loose bodies, and FAI.

- Acetabular labral tears are well evaluated with MRI and diagnosed as a linear hyperintense signal contacting the labral surface either at the labral–acetabular junction or in the labrum itself (5).

- Osteochondral injuries of the hip may be due to impaction injury, hip dislocation, or subclinical chondral shearing, and most commonly are present in the superomedial femoral head. Moderate to moderately high sensitivity for detection of chondral lesions of the hips has been reported. Cartilage sensitive sequences, especially high-resolution intermediate-weighted sequences, are necessary for optimal evaluation of chondral injuries (12,31). Intra-articular loose bodies can be identified on MRI and are especially conspicuous in the presence of a joint effusion or arthrographic solution.

- FAI is increasingly recognized as a potential cause of early-onset osteoarthritis of the hip. This impingement essentially is due to reduced joint clearance with repetitive abutment between the femur and acetabular rim during terminal hip movement. Findings on MRI that are suggestive of the clinical syndrome of FAI include labral tears, especially at the labral–chondral transition zone, and loss of articular cartilage. A nonspherical shape of the femoral head with decreased femoral head offset and anterosuperior chondral loss is characteristic of camshaft (Cam)-type FAI, whereas acetabular overcoverage and posteroinferior acetabular chondral loss characterize pincer-type FAI (Fig. 58.1) (14,23).

- MRI is useful in imaging of the extra-articular regional musculotendinous structures demonstrating injuries such as traumatic muscular contusions or strains, tendinopathy, and tendon tears. Common to the athlete are musculotendinous strains of the hamstring and rectus femoris muscles, with abnormal high signal within the muscle and/or tendon on MRI. In adductor avulsion syndrome ("thigh splints"), there is periosteal hyperintensity near the insertion of the adductor muscles of the femur (3). Tendinosis, which is seen as thickening and or hyperintensity of the tendon, is commonly seen within the gluteus medius and minimus tendons near their greater trochanteric insertions.

- The term athletic pubalgia ("sports hernia") has been applied to various causes of lower abdominal wall and peripubic pain. A recent study by Zoga et al. (36) found a high correlation of clinical symptoms with MRI findings of rectus abdominis and adductor tendon insertional injuries at their pubic bone insertion.

- MRI evaluation of the osseous structures of the hip is excellent and is the imaging modality of choice for osseous stress injuries, avascular necrosis (AVN), and occult fractures. Osseous stress reaction and stress fractures common to the athletic population involve the femoral neck, the pubic bones, and the sacrum, all of which demonstrate marrow edema, and in the case of stress fracture, a low signal intensity line (Fig. 58.2).

- AVN and subchondral insufficiency fractures of the femoral head both demonstrate femoral head edema in early stages.

The opinions and assertions expressed herein are those of the authors and should not be construed as reflecting those of the Department of Defense.

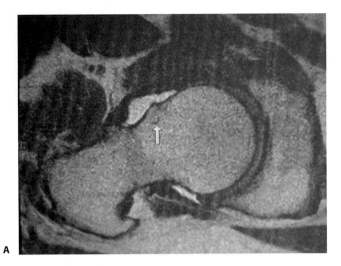

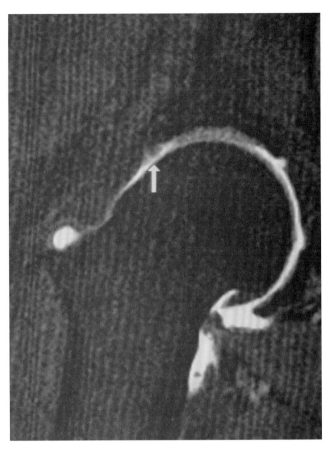

Figure 58.1: **A:** Axial oblique intermediate-weighted magnetic resonance (MR) arthrogram image of the hip demonstrating an osseous dysplastic bump at the femoral head/neck junction (*arrow*). The findings of superior labral tearing associated with an osseous dysplastic bump suggest Cam-type femoroacetabular impingement syndrome. **B:** Coronal fat suppression T1-weighted MR arthrogram image of the same hip demonstrating macerated labral tearing with abnormal imbibition of contrast into the labrum (*arrow*). Note lack of femoral head/neck offset.

Findings of AVN include a "double line sign" in nearly 80% of cases and may progress to include a subchondral fracture line and eventual articular collapse.

■ There are a few bursae in the region of the hip, notably the greater trochanteric, iliopsoas, and ischial bursa, which become inflamed by repetitive microtrauma, demonstrating fluid signal hyperintensity of the bursa on MRI.

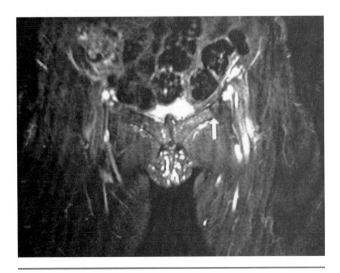

Figure 58.2: Coronal fat suppression T2 MRI demonstrating a pubic ramus stress fracture.

KNEE

■ MRI evaluation of the knee should include triplanar imaging with both high-resolution, intermediate-weighted, cartilage-sensitive sequences and water-sensitive (intermediate/T2 fat-suppressed, or STIR [short tau inversion recovery]) sequences for evaluation of marrow edema and pathology of the soft tissues.

■ In the athletic population, accurate evaluation of cartilage injury is crucial for directing treatment. MRI has been demonstrated to be an accurate method for evaluation of articular cartilage injuries. For this purpose, high-resolution cartilage-sensitive pulse sequences should be used in routine MRI of the knee. Generally, normal cartilage should be intermediate in signal intensity and of rather uniform thickness. With high-resolution cartilage-sensitive sequences, however, a normal gray scale stratification of the cartilage may be seen, which corresponds to normal cartilage zonal anatomy (31).

■ MRI accuracy for diagnosis of internal derangement of the knee is excellent, with high sensitivity and specificity (9,16). It is the most commonly evaluated joint by MRI (29). In a study of 200 patients who had MRI of the knee and subsequent arthroscopy, Vincken et al. (34) demonstrated high sensitivity and specificity of MRI for diagnosis of both medial and lateral meniscal tears, concluding that MRI is effective as a test for directing clinical treatment.

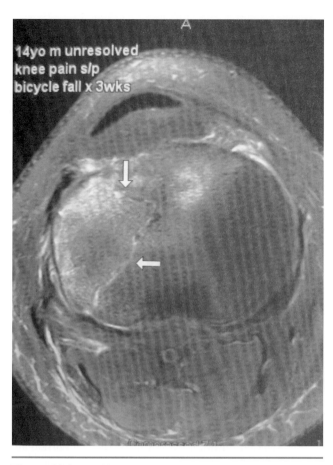

Figure 58.3: Axial fat suppression intermediate-weighted MRI demonstrating a subacute nondisplaced occult tibial plateau fracture (*arrows*), which was not suspected clinically.

■ MRI has a high sensitivity for diagnosing bone marrow edema, the causes of which are varied and include trauma, AVN, subchondral stress reaction or insufficiency fractures due to altered biomechanics, or arthritic changes (Fig. 58.3).

■ Many injury patterns are encountered in sports injuries to the knee, and certain bone marrow contusion patterns seen at MRI correlate with particular mechanisms of injury. Sanders et al. (29) described 5 such patterns that have a high correlation with specific soft tissue injuries of the knee. One particularly common contusion pattern is the "pivot shift injury," in which the classic bone marrow edema pattern involves the posterolateral tibial plateau and the midportion of the lateral femoral condyle. The anterior cruciate ligament (ACL) is invariably torn with this mechanism of injury. Other soft tissue injuries to the knee that can be seen in this pattern include medial collateral ligament sprains, longitudinal tears through the peripheral aspect of the posterior menisci, and posterior capsular injuries (29).

■ The normal ligamentous and tendinous structures of the knee have uniformly low signal intensity on all MRI sequences. The cruciate ligaments are best seen on sagittal sequences, and the collateral ligaments are best seen on coronal sequences. However, correlation with orthogonal imaging planes is often

valuable in corroborating pathology because, occasionally, volume averaging of signal with adjacent soft tissue structures may falsely suggest pathology (27).

■ The ACL is commonly injured in athletes. On MRI, the ACL is a thick dark band-like structure that parallels the roof of the intercondylar notch. Direct MR signs of ACL disruption include focal discontinuity of ligament fibers, abnormal slope of the ACL, and avulsion of the anterior tibial spine (Fig. 58.4).

■ Additional indirect MR signs of ACL disruption that can increase confidence of an ACL tear include a deep sulcus sign, a Segond fracture (capsular avulsion fracture of lateral tibial plateau), anterior translation of the tibia relative to the femur, hyperextension bone contusion injuries involving the anterior tibia and femur, and buckling of the posterior cruciate ligament (PCL) (28).

■ Full-thickness ACL tears are diagnosed by observation of complete discontinuity of the ligament fibers, as described previously. Partial-thickness ACL tears can be difficult to diagnose because there is only partial ligament fiber discontinuity. Confirmation of the diagnosis of partial ACL tear not only in the sagittal but also in the axial plane may be necessary (27). In the athletic population, ACL tears are typically repaired, because an unrepaired torn ACL may subsequently lead to chronic ACL deficiency. This condition is associated with a higher risk of medial meniscal degenerative tearing.

■ The ACL can be evaluated postoperatively with MRI and should parallel the roof of the intercondylar notch, without buckling, as seen in the sagittal plane. Tears of ACL grafts are diagnosed by observing focal discontinuity of graft fibers, not unlike that seen in a native ACL tear. Postoperatively, fast spin echo and inversion recovery sequences should be used rather than frequency selective fat suppression as the

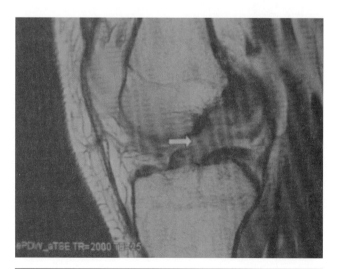

Figure 58.4: Sagittal intermediate-weighted MRI demonstrating abnormal signal and fiber discontinuity of the anterior cruciate ligament (ACL) consistent with a full-thickness tear (*arrow*).

water-sensitive sequence, because the latter is more susceptible to metallic particle-associated magnetic field inhomogeneities resulting in susceptibility artifact.

■ A post-ACL reconstruction complication that can be accurately evaluated with MRI includes a focal form of arthrofibrosis ("cyclops lesion") seen in the anterior intercondylar region, which may impede full joint extension (6).

■ Tears of the PCL are much less common than ACL tears and can be seen in association with significant trauma resulting in posterior translation of the tibia in relation to the femur, such as seen in significant falls or "dashboard" injuries to the tibia. Direct signs of PCL disruption include focal discontinuity of ligament fibers with high signal traversing fibers of the PCL on fluid sensitive images (28).

■ Ligamentous sprains of the medial and lateral collateral ligaments of the knee are common injuries in the athletic population and can be seen in isolation or in conjunction with other injuries to the knee. Ligamentous sprains are graded depending on the continuity or disruption of the fibers of the ligament on MRI as follows: grade 1: high signal within the ligament with intact fibers; grade 2: partial ligamentous tearing; and grade 3: complete ligamentous tear with discontinuity of fibers (Fig. 58.5).

■ The normal menisci are composed of fibrocartilage and therefore dark on all MRI pulse sequences. As evaluated in the sagittal plane, the normal meniscus appears as a triangular low signal intensity structure. The lateral meniscus is smaller and more circular in shape than the medial meniscus, with the anterior and posterior horns nearly equal in size. Conversely, the normal posterior horn of the medial meniscus is 1 and one-half to 2 times the size of the anterior horn, as viewed sagittally.

■ Short echo time sequences, T1 or intermediate weighted, are the most sensitive for identifying meniscal tears. Meniscal tears are diagnosed on MRI by abnormal morphology, displaced or missing meniscal tissue, and/or abnormal hyperintense linear signal extending to an articular margin of the meniscus (grade 3) (Fig. 58.6). Increased intrasubstance signal within a meniscus (grade 1 or 2) that does not extend to a meniscal articular margin, does not represent a meniscal tear, but rather intrasubstance degeneration within an adult meniscus, and likely normal vascularity in an adolescent. Various normal anatomic structures closely apposed to the meniscus can mimic tears on MRI, and therefore, understanding of normal anatomy and variants is necessary for accurate diagnosis.

■ On MRI, meniscal tears are categorized as horizontal, longitudinal, radial, or parrot beak in configuration. Description of the location of the tear with respect to the periphery of the meniscus is important in determining reparability of the tear. Typically, meniscal tears in the peripheral portion are repaired in the young athletic population because there is a greater likelihood of viability due to greater vascular supply to the peripheral meniscus.

■ Longitudinal meniscal tears deserve special note because they may become displaced within the joint and form a "bucket handle tear," wherein the cleaved displaced inner meniscal fragment may be displaced into the intercondylar

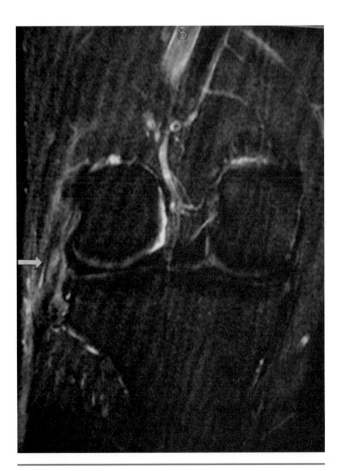

Figure 58.5: Coronal fat suppression intermediate-weighted MRI of the knee demonstrating abnormal signal and partial fiber discontinuity of a moderate acute sprain of the lateral collateral ligament (*arrow*).

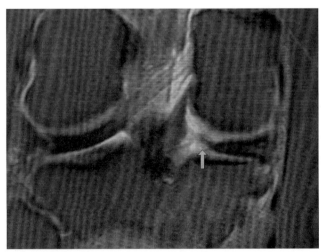

Figure 58.6: Coronal fat suppression intermediate-weighted MRI demonstrating a posterior medial meniscal root tear (*arrow*). Notice the fluid-filled gap in the posterior horn of the meniscus.

notch, anteriorly, posteriorly, or laterally. A bucket handle tear of the medial meniscus may be displaced into the intercondylar notch adjacent and inferior to the PCL, a configuration termed the "double PCL sign." Bucket handle tears of the lateral meniscus are hindered from displacement into the intercondylar notch to the level of the PCL due to be presence of the ACL and, therefore, typically displace anteriorly, forming the so-called "double anterior horn sign" (26,35).

- In the postoperative meniscus, a retear of the meniscus on MRI can be diagnosed if any of the following criteria are met: grade 3 signal of the meniscus that is as bright as fluid on T2-weighted sequences, a displaced meniscal fragment, or grade 3 signal in a new location when compared to preoperative findings. Grade 3 signal seen only on short echo time sequences is indeterminate for retear and can be further assessed with MR arthrography (28).

- With use of appropriate high-resolution cartilage-sensitive sequences, a high degree of accuracy in evaluation of articular cartilage abnormalities with MRI can be obtained (7,31).

- Subchondral stress fractures and osteochondral injuries typically occur on weight-bearing articular surfaces. Classic osteochondritis dissecans, however, is seen on the lateral non–weight-bearing aspect of the medial femoral condyle. MRI is important in determining size, location, and stability characteristics of osteochondral lesions. Signs of an unstable lesion include size > 5 mm, fluid equivalent signal surrounding the fragment, or cystic changes undermining the lesion (10).

- MRI is well suited for assessment of articular cartilage injuries of the knee. As previously discussed, normal cartilage demonstrates intermediate signal intensity on MRI. Chondral injuries, including focal abnormal signal, fibrillation and fissuring, partial- and full-thickness chondral defects, and chondral shear injuries, can be evaluated with appropriate cartilage-sensitive sequences (Figs. 58.7 and 58.8) (1).

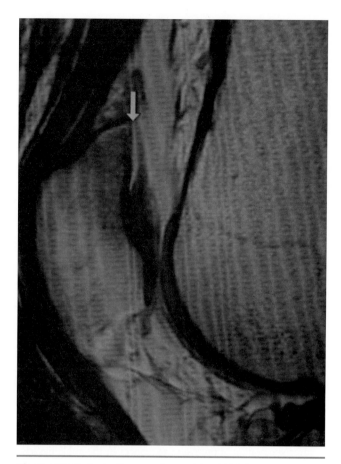

Figure 58.8: Sagittal intermediate-weighted MRI demonstrating a patellar chondral delamination injury (*arrow*).

- Various surgical repair techniques of articular cartilage defects are used, including subchondral microfracture, autologous chondrocyte implantation, cadaver allografts, and mosaicplasty, all of which can be successfully imaged with MRI postoperatively (13).

- Lateral patellar dislocation is common in the young athletic population and associated with anterolateral femoral condylar and inferomedial patellar bone contusions and osteochondral injuries (Fig. 58.9). Associated medial patellofemoral ligament injury is common.

- Proximal patellar tendinosis, as diagnosed on MRI, demonstrates localized hyperintensity and thickening of the proximal patellar tendon near the origin at the inferior pole of the patella. Reactive marrow edema in the inferior pole of the patella can also be seen. Complete tears of the patellar tendon or quadriceps tendon are diagnosed as focal tendinous discontinuity.

FOOT AND ANKLE

- Triplanar MRI of the foot and ankle is recommended for adequate evaluation of the ligaments and tendons, osseous and articular structures, and adjacent soft tissues. Although foot

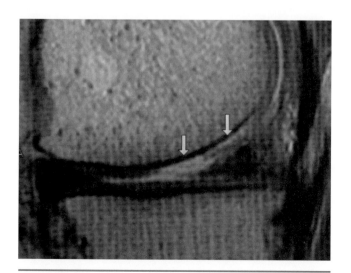

Figure 58.7: Sagittal intermediate-weighted MRI demonstrating a full-thickness chondral defect (*left arrow*) with an associated chondral flap tear (*right arrow*).

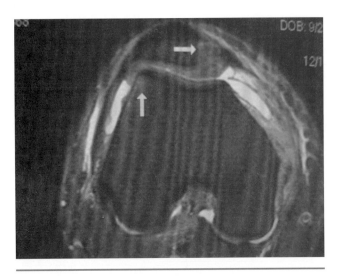

Figure 58.9: Axial fat suppression intermediate-weighted MRI of the knee demonstrating the sequela of recent lateral transient patellar dislocation with an anterolateral condylar bone contusion (*vertical arrow*) and inferomedial patellar osteochondral injury (*horizontal arrow*).

and ankle MRI protocols vary, it is important to include a T2-weighted sequence without fat saturation, a STIR sequence, a short TE sequence in the axial plane, and a T1-weighted sequence in particular for bone marrow evaluation. Typically, STIR sequences are preferred as a fluid-sensitive sequence over spectral fat suppression sequences in the ankle because the latter is more susceptible to regional field inhomogeneities, resulting in areas of failed fat suppression (2).

■ The ankle is one of the most frequently injured joints in the athletic population. The use of MRI in foot and ankle injuries in athletes has become common, allowing simultaneous evaluation of both osseous and soft tissue structures. Although less indicated in the acutely injured ankle, MRI evaluation of chronic ankle pain is useful for determining causes of pain or instability that are not readily apparent on clinical exam, including occult fractures or bone contusions, osseous stress injuries, osteochondral injuries, and tendinous or ligamentous injuries.

■ Stress and insufficiency fractures of the ankle and foot are common in athletes who typically have undergone a change in their training routines, wherein normal bone is exposed to repeated excessive stress. In a report of 320 cases of stress fractures in athletes, the most commonly injured bones included the tibia followed by the tarsals, metatarsals, fibula, and sesamoids (17). Stress fractures with high risk for potential nonunion or AVN include the tarsal navicular and sesamoid bones. Exercise- and sports-related stress fractures (and their common associated activity) include those of the metatarsals and calcaneus (military recruits), tarsal navicular (runners), sesamoids (ballet dancers/runners, sprinters), and the fibula (ballet dancers/runners) (4,15,21). Initial radiographs of stress fractures are often negative, and because of its high sensitivity and specificity, even exceeding that of bone scintigraphy, MRI is considered the modality of choice for confirmation of stress fractures in cases in which

radiographs are normal or equivocal (19). MRI findings of stress fractures typically demonstrate marrow edema with a low signal intensity fracture line (Fig. 58.10) (32).

■ Occult nondisplaced fractures can be missed on conventional radiographs, such as calcaneal and talar fractures. MRI can help detect radiographically occult fractures of the ankle and foot by demonstrating a low signal intensity fracture line associated with cortical disruption and marrow hyperintensity.

■ Osteochondral lesions of the talus (OLTs) are articular surface impaction injuries that typically affect the talar dome because of ankle inversion injuries. OLTs, especially lower stage lesions, may not be well detected with conventional radiographs but are well depicted with MRI, and MRI allows accurate staging of OLTs into stable and unstable groups (Fig. 58.11) (19).

■ On MRI, ligaments are seen as smooth, low-signal bands or thin strands on all sequences, with continuity from bone to bone. Sprains of the ankle ligaments are common and predominantly involve the lateral collateral ligamentous complex (Fig. 58.12) and less often the distal syndesmotic ligaments and the medial deltoid ligament complex. Direct signs of acute ligament tears on MRI include abnormal morphology and increased signal abnormality within the ligament. Ligament discontinuity implies a complete tear. Chronic tears may demonstrate ligamentous thickening or thinning (22).

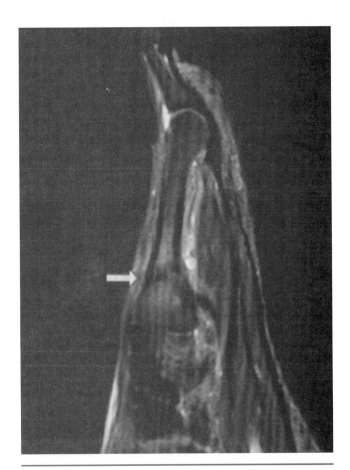

Figure 58.10: Sagittal fat suppression intermediate-weighted MRI demonstrating a subacute nondisplaced metatarsal stress fracture.

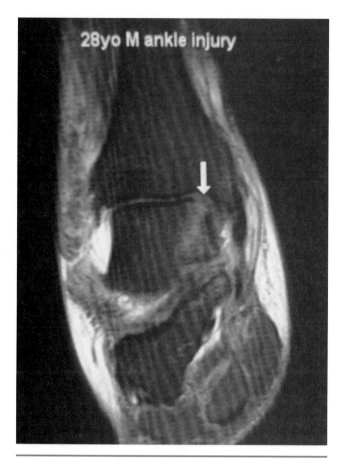

Figure 58.11: Coronal fat suppression intermediate-weighted MRI demonstrating a medial talar dome osteochondral lesion.

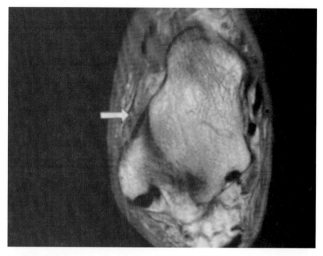

Figure 58.12: Axial T1 MRI of the ankle demonstrating an acute mild sprain of the anterior talofibular ligament (*arrow*). The ligament remains intact with periligamentous edema.

- An advantage of MRI includes depiction of other lesions associated with ligamentous injury. Sinus tarsi syndrome (STS) is a clinical condition characterized by pain along the lateral aspect of the foot with associated hindfoot instability. STS may develop after an inversion injury and can be suggested on MRI when low-signal intensity fibrous scarring or inflammatory tissue replaces the normal fat signal intensity within the tarsal sinus and/or when there is disruption of the sinus tarsi ligaments.

- There are four main functional tendon groups about the ankle, which can be evaluated on MRI. Normal tendons about the ankle are uniformly low-signal intensity structures that are best evaluated in axial imaging or perpendicular to the long axis of the tendon. Tendon tears are diagnosed by observing fluid signal intensity within the tendon or tendon fiber discontinuity. Tendinosis is characterized by variable tendinous thickening and increased signal intensity on short TE sequences (T1 and Intermediate weighted sequences). Tenosynovitis is inflammation of the tendon sheath characterized on MRI by excessive fluid distention of the tendon sheath. Tendons commonly injured among athletes include the peroneus brevis and tibialis posterior tendons (TPT).

- TPT tears, which generally occur in older athletes, are categorized as either partial tears (hypertrophic or atrophic types) or complete tears with tendon discontinuity. Injury of the TPT is important to recognize because insufficiency of the TPT can contribute to and is associated with abnormalities of the sinus tarsi and plantar fascia and can lead to loss of the longitudinal arch of the foot (flatfoot deformity) (Fig. 58.13) (11).

- Longitudinal split tears of the peroneal tendons, especially the peroneus brevis tendon, are increasingly recognized and are well depicted with MRI. Additionally, lateral dislocation of the peroneus brevis tendon from the retromalleolar groove can occur with disruption of the superior peroneal retinaculum, and therefore, tendon location should be evaluated.

- As the largest tendon in the body, the Achilles tendon is normally seen as a thick low-signal intensity band inserting into the calcaneus. Tendinosis of the Achilles tendon is manifest on MR imaging by thickening and abnormally increased signal on short TE sequences, findings common to tendinosis of most tendons. Achilles tendon injuries may be divided by location into insertional and noninsertional. Most sports-related Achilles tendon injuries consist of tendinosis and peritendinitis near the insertional region. Most Achilles tendon tears occur approximately 2–6 cm proximal to the calcaneal enthesis. MRI is useful to differentiate between partial and complete ruptures and demonstrates tendinous thickening and increased signal on T1- and T2-weighted sequences in the former and complete disruption of tendon fibers in the latter. Dystrophic calcifications and ossification within the tendon can be seen in cases of chronic tendinosis (30).

- Various ankle impingement syndromes can be evaluated with MRI. In anterior impingement, marginal osteophytes at the anterior margin of the tibiotalar joint may be seen in association with perifocal marrow edema. Posterior ankle impingement (PAI) refers to a group of pathologic entities resulting from repetitive forced plantarflexion of the foot (classically in ballet dancers) with the most common causes implicated including an os trigonum, elongated lateral tubercle (Stieda process), or prominent posterior process of the calcaneus. MRI findings of

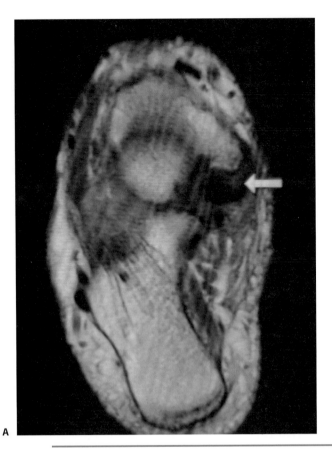
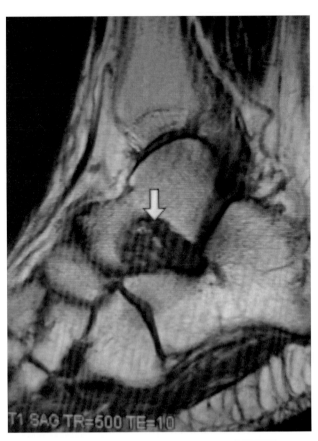

Figure 58.13: **A:** Axial T1 MRI demonstrating evidence of tibialis posterior tendon (TPT) insufficiency with hypertrophic partial-thickness tearing of TPT (*arrow*). **B:** Sagittal T1 MRI of the same ankle demonstrating scarring within the sinus tarsi (*arrow*), a finding suggestive of associated sinus tarsi syndrome (STS) in this patient with TPT insufficiency.

PAI typically show marrow edema within these osseous structures with adjacent periostitis (33). Anterolateral impingement may be implicated with a history of chronic anterolateral ankle pain and manifests on MRI as abnormal soft tissue mass or fibrous band in the anterolateral gutter (20).

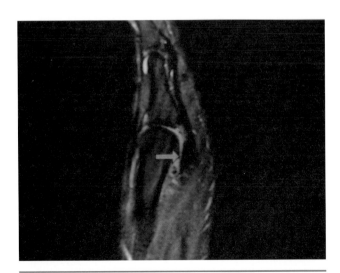

Figure 58.14: Sagittal fat suppression intermediate-weighted MRI demonstrating a plantar plate avulsion from the great toe proximal phalanx (turf toe).

- Plantar fasciitis is a common overuse injury seen in athletes involved in running and jumping sports. Although essentially a clinical diagnosis, MRI may be helpful in clinically equivocal or refractory cases. Imaging findings include focal fascial thickening with intrafascial hyperintensity and perifascial edema, most commonly near the calcaneal insertion. Partial and complete fascial tears can also be diagnosed.

- The term "turf toe" refers to a sprain of the plantar capsuloligamentous complex of the metatarsophalangeal joint of the great toe, which is due to severe dorsiflexion at the joint. With high-resolution MRI sequences, the osseous and capsuloligamentous structures can be evaluated (Fig. 58.14) to help direct treatment and avoid further morbidity such as hallux rigidus and osteoarthrosis of the joint (8).

REFERENCES

1. Alatakis S, Naidoo P. MR imaging of meniscal and cartilage injuries of the knee. *Magn Reson Imaging Clin N Am.* 2009;17(4):741–56, vii.

2. Ali M, Chen TS, Crues JV III. MRI of the ankle. *Appl Radiol.* 2006; 35(8):27.

3. Anderson MW, Kaplan PA, Dussault RG. Adductor insertion avulsion syndrome (thigh splints): spectrum of MR imaging features. *AJR Am J Roentgenol.* 2001;177(3):673–5.

4. Bergman A, Fredericson M. MR imaging of stress reactions, muscle injuries, and other overuse injuries in runners. *Magn Reson Imaging Clin N Am.* 1999;7(1):151–74, ix.

5. Boutin R, Newman JS. MR imaging of sports-related hip disorders. *Magn Reson Imaging Clin N Am.* 2003;11(2):255–81.

6. Bradley DM, Bergman AG, Dillingham MF. MR imaging of cyclops lesions. *AJR Am J Roentgenol.* 2000;174(3):719–26.

7. Bredella MA, Tirman PF, Peterfy CG, et al. Accuracy of T2- weighted fast spin-echo MR-imaging with fat saturation in detecting cartilage defects in the knee: comparison with arthroscopy in 130 patients. *AJR Am J Roentgenol.* 1999;172(4):1073–80.

8. Crain JM, Phancao JP, Stidham K. MR imaging of turf toe. *Magn Reson Imaging Clin N Am.* 2008;16(1):93–103, vi.

9. Crues JV III, Mink J, Levy TL, Lotysch M, Stoller DW. Meniscal tears of the knee: accuracy of MR imaging. *Radiology.* 1987;164(2):445–8.

10. De Smet AA, Ilahi OA, Graf BK. Reassessment of the MR criteria for stability of osteochondritis dissecans in the knee and ankle. *Skeletal Radiol.* 1996;25(2):159–63.

11. Geideman WM, Johnson JE. Posterior tibial tendon dysfunction. *J Orthop Sports Phys Ther.* 2000;30(2):68–77.

12. Guanche CA. Clinical update: MR imaging of the hip. *Sports Med Arthrosc.* 2009;17(1):49–55.

13. Hangody L, Kish G, Kárpáti Z, Szerb I, Udvarhelyi I. Arthroscopic autogenous osteochondral mosaicplasty for the treatment of femoral condylar articular defects. A preliminary report. *Knee Surg Sports Traumatol Arthrosc.* 1997;5(4):262–7.

14. James SL, Ali K, Malara F, Young D, O'Donnell J, Connell DA. MRI findings of femoroacetabular impingement. *AJR Am J Roentgenol.* 2006; 187(6):1412–9.

15. Khan K, Brown J, Way S, et al. Overuse injuries in classical ballet. *Sports Med.* 1995;19:341–57.

16. Mackenzie R, Palmer CR, Lomas DJ, Dixon AK. Magnetic resonance imaging of the knee: diagnostic performance statistics. *Clin Radiol.* 1996; 51(4):251–7.

17. Matheson GO, Clement D, McKenzie DC, Tauton JE, Llyod-Smith DR, MacIntyre JG. Stress fractures in athletes. A study of 320 cases. *Am J Sports Med.* 1987;15(1):46–58.

18. Mintz D, Hooper T, Connell D, Buly R, Padgett DE, Potter HG. Magnetic resonance imaging of the hip: detection of labral and chondral abnormalities using non-contrast imaging. *Arthroscopy.* 2005;21(4):385–93.

19. Narváez JA, Cerezal L, Narváez J. MRI of sports-related injuries of the foot and ankle: part 1. *Curr Probl Diagn Radiol.* 2003;32(4):139–55.

20. Narváez JA, Cerezal L, Narváez J. MRI of sports-related injuries of the foot and ankle: part 2. *Curr Probl Diagn Radiol.* 2003;32(5):177–93.

21. Niva MH, Sormaala MJ, Kiuru MJ, Haataja R, Ahovuo J, Pihlajamaki H. Bone stress injuries of the ankle and foot: an 86-month magnetic resonance imaging-based study of physically active young adults. *Am J Sports Med.* 2007;35(4):643–9.

22. Perrich KD, Goodwin DW, Hecht PJ, Cheung Y. Ankle ligaments on MRI: appearance of normal and injured ligaments. *AJR Am J Roentgenol.* 2009;193(3):687–95.

23. Pfirrmann CW, Mengiardi B, Dora C, Kalberer F, Zanetti M, Hodler J. Cam and pincer femoroacetabular impingement: characteristic MR arthrographic findings in 50 patients. *Radiology.* 2006;240(3):778–85.

24. Potter HG, Black BR, Chong le R. New techniques in articular cartilage imaging. *Clin Sports Med.* 2009;28(1):77–94.

25. Potter HG, Schachar J. High resolution noncontrast MRI of the hip. *J Magn Reson Imaging.* 2010;31(2):268–78.

26. Rosas HG, De Smet AA. Magnetic resonance imaging of the meniscus. *Top Magn Reson Imaging.* 2009;20(3):151–73.

27. Roychowdhury S, Fitzgerald SW, Sonin AH, Peduto AJ, Miller FH, Hoff FL. Using MR imaging to diagnose partial tears of the anterior cruciate ligament: value of axial images. *AJR Am J Roentgenol.* 1997;168(6):1487–91.

28. Sanders T, Miller M. A systematic approach to magnetic resonance imaging interpretation of sports medicine injuries of the knee. *Am J Sports Med.* 2005;33(1):131–48.

29. Sanders TG, Medynski MA, Feller JF, Lawhorn KW. Bone contusion patterns of the knee at MR imaging: footprint of the mechanism of injury. *Radiographics.* 2000;20(Spec No):S135–51.

30. Schweitzer ME, Karasick D. MR imaging of disorders of the Achilles tendon. *AJR Am J Roentgenol.* 2000;175(3):613–25.

31. Shindle M, Foo L, Kelly B, et al. Magnetic resonance imaging of cartilage in the athlete: current techniques and spectrum of disease. *J Bone Joint Surg Am.* 2006;88(suppl 4):27–46.

32. Sofka CM. Imaging of stress fractures. *Clin Sports Med.* 2006;25(1): 53–62, viii.

33. Sofka CM. Posterior ankle impingement: clarification and confirmation of the pathoanatomy. *HSS J.* 2010;6(1):99–101.

34. Vincken PW, ter Braak BP, van Erkell AR, et al. Effectiveness of MR imaging in selection of patients for arthroscopy of the knee. *Radiology.* 2002;223(3):739–46.

35. Wright DH, De Smet AA, Norris M. Bucket-handle tears of the medial and lateral menisci of the knee: value of MR imaging in detecting displaced fragments. *AJR Am J Roentgenol.* 1995;165(3):621–5.

36. Zoga AC, Kavanagh EC, Omar IM, et al. Athletic pubalgia and the "sports hernia": MR imaging findings. *Radiology.* 2008;247(3):797–807.

59 Pelvis, Hip, and Thigh Injuries

Matthew Diltz

AVULSION FRACTURES AND APOPHYSEAL INJURIES

History/Findings

- Avulsion fractures about the hip and pelvis are the result of failure of the bone at the tendinous insertion rather than the tendon itself. These injuries are more common in skeletally immature athletes with open apophyses that are more susceptible to failure than the tendinous insertion. These are usually the result of a sudden, forceful concentric or eccentric contracture or rapid, excessive passive lengthening.

- Common sites of these avulsions about the pelvis are the insertion of the sartorius into the anterior-superior iliac spine, the rectus femoris superior head insertion into the anterior-inferior iliac spine, and the insertion of the hamstrings into the ischial tuberosity. These injuries are also seen in the proximal femur with the insertion of the hip abductors into the greater trochanter and the insertion of the iliopsoas into the lesser trochanter.

- Radiographs may show avulsions that involve the bone. Magnetic resonance imaging (MRI) is a more sensitive test and can demonstrate the extent of injury to the muscle.

Treatment

- Nonsurgical management has been the mainstay of treatment in most series with good to excellent results reported.

- Indications for surgery include complete ruptures of the origin of the hamstring with retraction in active patient with functional disability, chronic ruptures associated with sciatic nerve compression, and large bone avulsion fragment that results in discomfort with sitting (8); however, most authorities do not recommend surgery for these injuries.

- Metzmaker and Pappas (12) defined a rehabilitation treatment protocol for these injuries including (a) rest, using proper positioning to unload the injured apophysis and ice/analgesics; (b) initiation of gentle active and passive range of motion (ROM) exercises; (c) progressive resistance beginning when 75% of motion is achieved and ending when 50% of strength is returned; (d) integration of stretching and strengthening exercises with functional activity; and (e) return to competitive sport at 8–10 weeks. Skeletally immature patients are also susceptible to chronic traction injuries at these apophyses, and this is referred to as apophysitis.

Apophysitis is treated conservatively with rest followed by functional rehabilitation of the involved muscle group.

STRESS FRACTURES

Pelvis

- Pelvic stress fractures should be suspected in athletes such as long-distance runners and military recruits. The most common site is the junction between the ischium and inferior pubic ramus. Tenderness to palpation directly over the fractured bone can be helpful in locating the lesion. A positive standing sign has been described in which a patient develops discomfort in the groin while standing unsupported on the ipsilateral leg.

- Plain radiographic signs, such as periosteal reaction or fracture line, can lag behind the clinical presentation by as long as 3 weeks. MRI and bone scan can provide an earlier diagnosis. Tumors should at least be considered in the differential diagnosis.

- Treatment consists of rest with emphasis on protected weight-bearing, flexibility, and aerobic nonimpact exercises such as swimming or cycling. Return to sport can be delayed up to 6 months.

Femoral Neck

- Although femoral neck stress fractures are not as common as pelvic stress fractures, if treated incorrectly, the results can be disastrous. Similar to pelvic stress fractures, these present with groin pain and an antalgic gait. Pain will be worsened by flexion and internal rotation of the hip. Again, radiographic evidence may lag behind by 3–4 weeks. MRI and bone scan may be helpful in earlier diagnosis.

- Two types of femoral neck stress fractures exist. The first type is a compression-side femoral neck stress fracture. This occurs in the inferior medial aspect of the neck and usually respond to restriction to non–weight-bearing status until radiographic evidence of healing has occurred. The more worrisome type is the tension-side femoral neck stress fracture. This is a transverse fracture along the superior margin of the neck. Internal fixation is recommended for nondisplaced fractures. Immediate closed or open reduction and internal fixation is recommended for displaced fractures. Fracture displacement can lead to avascular necrosis of the femoral head (3).

SOFT TISSUE INJURIES

Muscle Strains

- Soft tissue injuries to the periarticular structures surrounding the hip and pelvis are the most common injuries seen in athletes. In general, the great majority of soft tissue injuries about the hip and pelvis are musculotendinous strains.

- The type of injury sustained is highly dependent on (a) skeletal age of the athlete, (b) physical condition, and (c) biomechanical forces involved in both the sport and nature of the trauma. The degree of injury can range from repetitive microinjury associated with each performance to a more significant single macroinjury caused by an abnormal biomechanical force. A certain degree of microtrauma occurs with every major exertional performance immediately manifested by swelling, sensitivity, and a recovery interval. If additional moderate or severe microinjury or macroinjury occurs, there may not be a normal healing response, which may lead to more significant changes in tissue structure and a negative effect on future athletic performance (4).

- A strain is an injury to a musculotendinous structure caused by an indirectly applied force. The most common mechanism of injury is a result of eccentric contraction or stretching of an activated muscle. The site of injury is influenced by the rate of loading, mechanism of injury, and local anatomic factors. Low rates of loading will result in a failure at the tendon–bone junction by bone avulsion or disruption at its insertion. High rates of loading result in intratendinous or myotendinous juncture injuries.

- These injuries can be graded on a 3-scale clinical grading system. Grade 1 injuries involve a simple stretching of soft tissue fibers. Grade 2 strains involve partial tearing of the musculotendinous unit; and grade 3, which are unusual, are secondary to extreme violent forces causing complete disruptions.

Contusions

- Among the most frequently experienced hip and pelvic injuries sustained by athletes are soft tissue contusions. Contusions usually result from direct blows to a specific soft tissue area usually overlying a bony prominence. Contusions are most common in contact sports, especially football, but are also seen in other sports as well. In contact sports, the blow is usually caused by contact with another athlete. In noncontact sports, athletes usually sustain blows from contact with equipment (gymnastics), contact with high-velocity projectiles (lacrosse ball), or contact from the playing surface.

- Contusions are often found over areas of bony prominences of the pelvis including the iliac crest (hip pointer), greater trochanter, ischial tuberosity, and pubic rami. Because of the varied anatomy of the pelvis, contusions can be superficial, especially when they overlie a relatively subcutaneous bone or lie deep within a large muscle mass. It is important to determine possible presence and extent of muscular hemorrhage because an increase in muscular hemorrhage often results in more severe symptoms and longer time before returning to sport (4).

HIP POINTER

- Pain and hemorrhage over the iliac crest have been referred to as a hip pointer. These injuries include contusions, avulsion of the iliac apophysis, periostitis, or avulsion of the muscles that insert onto the iliac crest. On physical examination, the patient will have superficial or muscular hemorrhage, which will be painful on palpation. It is important to note by touch a defect, which would indicate an avulsion injury. Patients will have difficulty with rotation and side bending of the trunk.

- Anterior-posterior and oblique x-rays of the pelvis will rule out an avulsion fracture, periostitis, or an acute fracture of the iliac wing.

HAMSTRING SYNDROME

- Hamstring syndrome, described in track athletes, involves severe pain in and around the ischial tuberosity that radiates down the posterior aspect of the thigh to the popliteal area. Any activity that puts the hamstring in stretch can create this radiating pain. Sprinting, hurdling, and even sitting for long periods will cause pain.

- Physical examination elicits exquisite tenderness at the ischial tuberosity and, at times, reproduction of sciatic pain with percussion of the nerve at the ischial tuberosity. Resisted leg extension will reproduce the pain. The sciatic nerve is thought to be entrapped between the semitendinosus and the biceps femoris by a fibrous band that constricts the 2 muscles (4).

THIGH CONTUSIONS/QUADRICEPS INJURY

- Thigh contusions are common athletic injuries, most often encountered in football from direct trauma. These injuries can involve significant muscular damage, hematoma formation, and swelling. Therefore, the athlete can be extremely uncomfortable.

- Initial treatment is rest, ice, and compression to minimize hematoma formation. Immobilization in flexion and initiation of early flexion exercises have been recommended to decrease myositis ossificans formation and improve functional outcome (16).

SPECIFIC CONDITIONS

Athletic Pubalgia

History/Findings

- The term athletic pubalgia is often used interchangeably with sports hernia. It is a condition of chronic groin pain. The condition is common in soccer and ice hockey athletes. Typically, the patient reports activity-related pain that resolves with rest.

Most patients describe a hyperextension injury in association with hyperabduction of the thigh. Usually, the abdominal pain involves the inguinal canal near the insertion of the rectus abdominis muscle at the pubis.

■ Maneuvers that increase intra-abdominal pressure, such as a resisted sit-up, can reproduce the symptoms. A gross hernia is not detected. On imaging studies, 12% of patients have derangement of the insertion of the rectus on MRI. Adductor longus inflammation can also be present. Dynamic ultrasound can detect posterior wall defects.

Pathophysiology

■ The rectus insertion on the pubis with or without the origin of the adductor longus tendon appears to be the primary site of pathology.

■ The proposed mechanism of injury involves repetitive hyperextension of the trunk in association with hyperabduction of the thigh pivoting on the anterior pelvis and pubic symphysis. Only a small percentage of patients are found to have occult hernia at the time of surgery.

Treatment

■ The initial treatment of athletic pubalgia consists of rest, ice, compression, and elevation. There are medical grade compression shorts that can help alleviate symptoms. After the symptoms resolve, an overseen slow transition back to sport is employed.

■ Often athletes present for evaluation after exhaustion of nonoperative management. These patients are on the verge of cessation of sport. In this case, surgical options are discussed. Many approaches have been tried in the treatment of sports hernia. Options include tissue repair, laparoscopic repairs, anterior repairs, and mesh repairs. The goal of surgery is repair or reinforcement of the anterior abdominal wall.

Outcomes

■ With appropriate indications and surgical techniques, return to previous level of performance without pain has been reported at 80%–97% (14).

Osteitis Pubis

■ Osteitis pubis is a painful inflammation of the pubis bone, symphysis, and surrounding structures. The pelvic pain can be sharp or aching. It originates over the symphysis and can radiate to the medial thigh along the adductor musculature.

■ Physical exam findings include the presence of a positive lateral compression test. With the patient in a lateral decubitus position, force is applied to the iliac crest. This should reproduce the symptoms at the pubis. MRI and computed tomography (CT) findings consist of bone resorption, widening of the symphysis pubis, and periarticular sclerosis.

Pathophysiology

■ The condition can be associated with a primary infection or secondary to repetitive microtrauma from the pull of the rectus muscle or gracilis.

Treatment

■ Nonoperative management is typically successful. A period of rest, ice, and compression is followed with a rehabilitation protocol. Core strengthening and stretch of the hamstrings is employed. If there is an infectious component, antibiotics are added.

■ After failure of nonoperative management, surgical alternatives include debridement of the joint with curette, arthrodesis, and an either partial or complete resection of the joint.

Outcomes

■ Surgical outcomes of osteitis pubis are variable (7).

Trochanteric Pain Syndrome

History/Findings

■ Trochanteric pain syndrome refers to pain at the lateral and posterior aspect of the hip. There are two related conditions that contribute to the symptoms. Trochanteric bursitis is an inflammation of the bursa overlying the trochanter. Patients are typically found to have a tight iliotibial (IT) band. This can be tested with the Ober test; taking the hip from extension and abduction into an adducted position demonstrates tightness and an inability to reach the neutral position.

■ Gluteus medius syndrome is recognized as a common cause of posterolateral hip pain. It is an overuse syndrome that can lead to tendinosis and partial and complete tears of the tendon. Single-leg squat or simulated stair step can reproduce the symptoms. Resisted abduction and external rotation from an internally rotated position also produce symptoms.

Pathophysiology

■ Bursitis can be secondary to direct injury, overuse of the adjacent musculotendinous structures, or degenerative changes in those structures. The bursa is lined with synovial tissue. Systemic conditions that lead to synovitis can affect the bursa as well.

■ Gluteus medius syndrome is an overuse injury to the tendon. It is common in women who participate in running or step aerobics.

Treatment

■ In both conditions, the first line of treatment is activity modification, ice, massage, and stretch of the involved muscle. Local anesthetic and steroid injection can be a useful clinical and therapeutic tool. Recalcitrant cases may require surgery to alleviate the symptoms. The posterior aspect of the IT band can be lengthened or released for bursitis. The gluteus medius tendon may be debrided or repaired depending on the type of injury.

Piriformis Syndrome

History/Findings

■ Piriformis syndrome involves compression of the sciatic nerve as it exits deep to the piriformis muscle. Patients complain of pain in the sciatic nerve distribution. A history of an acute injury to the buttock is common.

- On physical exam, the low back should be examined to rule out more proximal nerve root impingement. In the case of piriformis syndrome, typically the area of maximal tenderness is over the piriformis muscle in the gluteal area. Provocative tests include Pace sign — pain and weakness on resisted abduction and external rotation of the thigh. Forced internal rotation on an extended thigh can also reproduce the symptoms.

- An MRI can demonstrate sciatic nerve inflammation in the area of the piriformis tendon. Depending on the cause of the syndrome, myopathic and neuropathic changes can be present on electromyographic studies including a prolonged H-reflex.

Pathophysiology

- Piriformis syndrome can be caused by a traumatic injury to the piriformis muscle that leads to hypertrophy and impingement of the sciatic nerve. There can also be anatomic variations that contribute to the development of the syndrome.

- Examination of the relationship between the muscle and nerve in 240 cadavers revealed that, in 90% of cases, the sciatic nerve emerges from below the piriformis muscle; in 7%, the piriformis and the sciatic nerve are divided, with one branch of the sciatic nerve passing through the split and the other branch passing distal to the muscle; in 2%, only the sciatic nerve is divided; and in 1%, the piriformis is divided by the sciatic nerve (1).

Treatment

- Treatment of piriformis syndrome with a history of trauma is directed toward soothing the muscle. Anti-inflammatory medications and muscle relaxants can provide relief. Directed massage, heat, and ultrasound can help to break up scar tissue. Physical therapy can assist with these modalities as well as muscle stretch and activity modification. Often muscle imbalance is a contributing factor. Injections of anesthetic and cortisone can help with diagnosis and provide therapeutic benefit.

- If these treatments fail to provide relief, surgery can evaluate the relationship between the piriformis muscle and the sciatic nerve. The nerve can be decompressed, and the muscle can be released to provide relief.

Outcomes

- Benson and Schutzer (2) reported the results of 15 cases of traumatic piriformis syndrome. They had 11 excellent and 4 good results with clinical follow-up at 2 years.

Internal/External Snapping Hip

History/Findings

- A snapping hip, or coxa saltans, refers to the catching of a muscle as it crosses the hip joint. The two most common muscles that can get caught are the IT band as it crosses the greater trochanter and the iliopsoas as it crosses over the anterior hip joint.

- The posterior aspect of the IT band catches at the greater trochanter at the outside of the hip joint and is referred to as an external snapping hip. The patient is often able to make the

hip snap. Visually, it can appear dramatic and be confused with a subluxing hip. Over time, the catching can lead to irritation at the trochanteric bursa.

- The internal snapping hip involves the iliopsoas getting caught as it crosses the iliopectineal eminence. The internal snapping hip is often associated with an audible "pop." The bursa around the muscle can be irritated over time and lead to pain. The snap is reproduced when taking the hip from flexion, abduction, and external rotation to a neutral extended position. MRI is useful to rule out other conditions and can demonstrate associated bursitis.

Pathophysiology

- Both snapping hip conditions are associated with tight muscles. In adolescents, a growth spurt can precede the development of the muscle tightness. Typically, the snapping muscle does not cause pain, but over time, the compression and shear across the bursa can lead to the development of irritation and bursitis, which is painful.

- In each condition, it is important to rule out additional pathology. The external snapping hip can be associated with tears of the gluteus medius. Both the gluteus medius and the IT band assist in abduction of the hip. If surgical intervention is considered, a tear must be ruled out first.

- The internal snapping hip is common in cases of intra-articular pathology. The iliopsoas or hip flexor crosses directly over the anterior superior labrum. An intra-articular hip derangement can lead to an effusion that exacerbates the symptoms. Conditions such as loose bodies, labral tears, and impingement should be ruled out in a persistent symptomatic internal snapping hip.

Treatment

- Initial management focuses on treatment of the muscle tightness. Physical therapy is an essential adjuvant to selectively stretch the responsible muscle and tendon. Deep massage and ultrasound can assist in alleviating symptoms. An elastic spica wrap or medical grade compression shorts help to control symptoms while stretching the muscles. IT band syndrome and external snapping hip are associated with hill training. Activity modification and cross-training assist in reducing symptoms. When the condition has become painful, steroid injections can decrease the inflammation of the bursa.

- With failed nonoperative management, there are a number of surgical interventions that can lengthen the muscle and address the bursa. More recently, these procedures have been performed endoscopically with encouraging results.

Outcomes

- Ilizaliturri and Camacho-Galindo (9) reviewed their results of both endoscopic IT band releases and iliopsoas releases. With at least 2 years of follow-up, 10 patients with endoscopic release of the IT band had resolution of pain. One patient had a painless snapping hip (10). For the hip flexor release, 6 patients were followed for at least 2 years. All patients had complete relief of symptoms. There was no residual flexion weakness (11).

Femoroacetabular Impingement

History/Findings

■ Femoroacetabular impingement is an abnormal contact between femur and acetabulum, specifically the anterosuperior femoral head/neck and acetabulum rim. This abnormal contact can lead to damage to the labrum and chondral surface over time.

■ Patients typically present in young to middle age with decreased ROM and progressive groin pain exacerbated with physical activity. The abnormal contour of the hip is not by definition painful, but the lesions to the cartilage and labrum result in symptoms.

■ On physical exam, pain in the groin and catching with flexion, adduction, and internal rotation are associated with chondral damage and labral injury at the anterolateral rim of the acetabulum. Often patients describe the discomfort as deep within the hip by cupping their hand; this is referred to as the "C" sign. Decreased ROM with flexion, abduction, and external rotation is also indicative of impingement.

■ Plain films can demonstrate an abnormal orientation of the acetabulum and contour of the femoral head–neck junction. CT scans with three-dimensional reconstructions are useful to evaluate the relationship between the acetabulum and femoral head–neck junction for abnormal cases of impingement. An MRI arthrogram is necessary to evaluate soft tissue damage to the labrum and articular surface of the acetabulum.

Pathophysiology

■ The two components of femoroacetabular impingement are impingement from the acetabulum, or "pincer," and impingement from the femoral head neck junction, or "cam."

■ Pincer impingement is the result of a deep acetabulum (coxa profunda) or abnormal orientation of the acetabulum resulting in anterior overcoverage (acetabular retroversion).

■ Cam impingement is typically an aspherical contour of the anterolateral head–neck junction. This can be visualized on the frog leg lateral view of the femur and the axial images of a CT scan or MRI.

■ Most patients present with a mixture of cam and pincer impingement. The abnormal anatomy can be congenital or acquired (18).

Treatment

■ Treatment is dependent on the degree of abnormal anatomy and the patient goals. The use of an anti-inflammatory medication to calm down the soft tissue irritation followed by physical therapy to strengthen the surrounding musculature and adjust pelvic tilt to avoid the abnormal contact is the first line of treatment.

■ Often, these patients present after months or years of pain and limitation. In these cases, the nonoperative modalities can exacerbate the symptoms and necessitate surgery. In the past, the impingement was treated with open surgical dislocation of the hip and osteoplasty of the femur and acetabulum. Within the last 15 years, many of the procedures to address the abnormal anatomy and soft tissue injuries have been performed arthroscopically (17).

Outcomes

■ The midterm results of both open and arthroscopic procedures are directly related to the degree of osteoarthritis at the time of surgery. Patients with minimal arthritis treated arthroscopically have demonstrated good and excellent results after 3 years of follow-up with significant improvement in pain and function (15).

Acetabular Labral Tear

History/Findings

■ The labrum is the fibrocartilaginous rim around the articular surface of the acetabulum. Biomechanic studies have shown that it has little function in distribution of forces or in stability. The labrum does have significant function as a hydraulic seal.

■ The clinical findings depend on the location of the labral tear and can be variable. Groin pain and mechanical symptoms with flexion, adduction, and internal rotation are indicative of an anterior-superior lesion.

■ An MRI arthrogram with radial reconstructions is the study of choice to evaluate the labrum. Fluid can be seen tracking under the injured labrum.

Pathophysiology

■ Labral tears can be the result of abnormal morphology such as femoroacetabular impingement or normal anatomy that is placed in supraphysiologic positions. Isolated labral tears are common in elite athletes and dancers who present with groin pain. These injuries can also be seen in acute trauma, such as a hip dislocation or subluxation. Isolated labral tears are rare in patients who present with an insidious onset of pain. In these cases, it is important to rule out associated conditions such as femoroacetabular impingement. Degenerative tears of the labrum occur with the progression of osteoarthritis.

Treatment

■ Initial management of labral tears consists of rest, anti-inflammatory medications, and physical therapy followed by a slow transition back to sport.

■ If the symptoms fail to resolve with rest or recur with advancing activity, surgical management is a consideration. The majority of the treatments to address the labrum can now be performed arthroscopically. The choice of a removal of the irritated portion of the labrum versus repair is dependent on a number of factors including the location of the tear, age of the patient, chronicity of the injury, and associated findings.

Outcomes

■ A recent study with 10-year follow-up demonstrated 82% continued successful outcomes in patients treated with labral debridement in the absence of osteoarthritis (5). Long-term results of arthroscopic repair have not been reported to date. Conceptually, it would make sense that restoration of the anatomy and maintenance of the fluid seal would be beneficial. Regardless of the whether the labrum is repaired or removed, it is essential that additional pathology be diagnosed and addressed at the time of surgery.

Loose Bodies

History/Findings

- Loose bodies are common after acute trauma to the hip including subluxations and dislocations. In the setting of dislocation, the incidence has been reported at 92% (13). The patient typically reports mechanical symptoms, including locking, catching, or clicking.
- Plain films, CT, and MRI can demonstrate the presence of loose bodies.

Pathophysiology

- The overall stability of the hip joint is related to the bony congruency. With a traumatic dislocation, the force at the edge of the acetabulum can lead to a fracture or commonly a shear injury to the cartilage at the edge of the acetabulum. With reduction of the dislocation, those fragments can be caught within the joint. Even without radiographic evidence of loose bodies, arthroscopic evaluation can demonstrate fragments in the joint.
- Other atraumatic conditions that are associated with loose bodies include synovial chondromatosis, dislodged osteophytes, and foreign bodies.

Treatment

- Mechanical symptoms in the presence of a corresponding clinical history are an indication for arthroscopic evaluation.

Ruptured Ligamentum Teres

History/Findings

- The ligamentum teres is the connection between the cotyloid fossa of the acetabulum and the fovea capitis of the femoral head. It provides blood supply to the developing hip. After adolescence, the function of the structure is not fully known. It is postulated that it provides additional stability and resists dislocation forces at the hip. Injury to the ligamentum teres results in catching, popping, locking, and giving way. These findings are common in intra-articular pathology.
- There is no a physical exam test that is pathognomonic for ligamentum teres injury. Imaging findings can be variable as well. In a study by Byrd and Jones (6), the diagnosis was made preoperatively in 2 of 23 patients.

Pathophysiology

- Disruption of the ligamentum teres is common after trauma and hip dislocation, but it can occur without dislocation as well. The structure is tight in adduction, flexion, and external rotation. Acute disruptions are believed to occur with exaggerated adduction and external rotation.

Treatment

- The symptoms associated with an injury to the ligamentum teres are believed to be secondary to hyperplasia of the surrounding tissue and soft tissue impingement. Initial management should consist of modalities to rest the hip and control inflammation.

- Arthroscopic management consists of debridement of the torn fibers of the ligamentum teres.

Outcomes

- Byrd and Jones (6) published the results of their experience in 23 cases of traumatic tears. The results demonstrated a significant improvement in pain and function.

REFERENCES

1. Beaton LE, Anson BJ. The sciatic nerve and the piriformis muscle: their interrelation a possible cause of coccygodynia. *J Bone Joint Surg Am.* 1938;20(3):686–8.
2. Benson ER, Schutzer SF. Posttraumatic piriformis syndrome: diagnosis and results of operative treatment. *J Bone Joint Surg Am.* 1999;81(7):941–9.
3. Boden BP, Osbahr DC. High-risk stress fractures: evaluation and treatment. *J Am Acad Orthop Surg.* 2000;8(6):344–53.
4. Busconi BD, Wixted JJ, Owens BD. Differential diagnosis of the painful hip. In: McCarthy JC, editor. *Early Hip Disease: Advances in Detection and Minimally Invasive Treatment.* New York: Springer-Verlag; 2003. p. 97–103.
5. Byrd JW, Jones KS. Prospective analysis of hip arthroscopy with 10-year followup. *Clin Orthop Relat Res.* 2010;468(3):741–6.
6. Byrd JW, Jones KS. Traumatic rupture of the ligamentum teres as a source of hip pain. *Arthroscopy.* 2004;20(4):385–91.
7. Choi H, McCartney M, Best TM. Treatment of osteitis pubis and osteomyelitis of the pubic symphysis in athletes: a systematic review. *Br J Sports Med.* 2011;45(1):57–64.
8. Cohen S, Bradley J. Acute proximal hamstring rupture. *J Am Acad Orthop Surg.* 2007;15(6):350–5.
9. Ilizaliturri VM Jr, Camacho-Galindo J. Endoscopic treatment of snapping hips, iliotibial band, and iliopsoas tendon. *Sports Med Arthrosc.* 2010;18(2):120–7.
10. Ilizaliturri VM Jr, Martinez-Escalante FA, Chaidez PA, Camacho-Galindo J. Endoscopic iliotibial band release for external snapping hip syndrome. *Arthroscopy.* 2006;22(5):505–10.
11. Ilizaliturri VM Jr, Villalobos FE Jr, Chaidez PA, Valero FS, Aguilera JM. Internal snapping hip syndrome: treatment by endoscopic release of the iliopsoas tendon. *Arthroscopy.* 2005;21(11):1375–80.
12. Metzmaker JN, Pappas AM. Avulsion fractures of the pelvis. *Am J Sports Med.* 1985;13(5):349–58.
13. Mullis BH, Dahners LE. Hip arthroscopy to remove loose bodies after traumatic dislocation. *J Orthop Trauma.* 2006;20(1):22–6.
14. Paajanen H, Brinck T, Hermunen H, Airo I. Laparoscopic surgery for chronic groin pain in athletes is more effective than nonoperative treatment: a randomized clinical trial with magnetic resonance imaging of 60 patients with sportsman's hernia (athletic pubalgia). *Surgery.* 2011;150(1):99–107.
15. Philippon MJ, Briggs KK, Yen YM, Kuppersmith DA. Outcomes following hip arthroscopy for femoroacetabular impingement with associated chondrolabral dysfunction: minimum two-year follow-up. *J Bone Joint Surg Br.* 2009;91(1):16–23.
16. Ryan JB, Wheeler JH, Hopkinson WJ, Arciero RA, Kolakowski KR. Quadriceps contusions. West Point update. *Am J Sports Med.* 1991;19(3):299–304.
17. Safran MR. Hip arthroscopy: the basics. In: Wiesel SW, editor. *Operative Techniques in Orthopaedic Surgery.* Philadelphia: Lippincott Williams & Wilkins; 2010. p. 191–202.
18. Safran MR. Hip joint injuries. In: Kibler WB, editor. *Orthopaedic Knowledge Update.* Rosemont: American Academy of Orthopaedic Surgeons; 2009. p. 91–100.

60 Knee Meniscal Injuries

John P. Goldblatt, John C. Richmond, Dipak B. Ramkumar, and Anthony S. Albert

INTRODUCTION

- The meniscus plays an important role in weight distribution, reduction in joint contact stresses, joint stabilization, and energy absorption (2,9,11,20,26). Injury to the meniscus can result in marked physical impairment.
- Once thought to be a vestigial organ, it is now recognized that meniscectomy often leads to a recognizable pattern of joint deterioration including joint space narrowing, osteophyte formation, and squaring of the femoral condyles (9).
- Meniscal preservation is the goal of new surgical procedures.
- Arthroscopy facilitates optimal treatment of meniscal tears with minimally invasive techniques.

ANATOMY AND BASIC SCIENCE

- Each of the medial and lateral compartments of a knee has an intervening meniscus located between the femur and tibia.
- The menisci are peripherally thick and convex and centrally taper to a thin free margin (2).
- The meniscal surfaces conform to the femoral and tibial contours.
- Each meniscus has anterior and posterior bony attachment sites.

Medial Meniscus

- The medial meniscus is semicircular, crescent-shaped, and measures approximately 3.5 cm in length.
- The medial meniscus covers 50%–60% of the medial tibial plateau. The posterior horn is wider than the anterior horn in the anteroposterior (AP) dimension (20,26).
- The attachment site for the anterior horn is variable, in the area of the intercondylar fossa in front of the anterior cruciate ligament (ACL), often to the anterior surface of the tibial plateau.
- The posterior fibers of the anterior horn merge with the transverse fibers of the intermeniscal ligament, which connects the anterior horns of the medial and lateral menisci. The intermeniscal ligament is located approximately 8 mm anterior to the ACL (2).

- The posterior horn is firmly attached to the posterior intercondylar fossa of the tibia, anterior and medial to the posterior cruciate ligament attachment site (2).
- The periphery is attached to the capsule throughout its length, and the tibial portion of this attachment is called the coronary ligament. In addition, at its midpoint, the medial meniscus is firmly attached to the femur and tibia through a condensation of the joint capsule known as the deep medial collateral ligament (26).

Lateral Meniscus

- The lateral meniscus is almost circular in gross morphology and covers 70%–80% of the lateral tibial plateau (2,26).
- The lateral meniscus is nearly uniform in width from front to back.
- The bony attachments of the lateral meniscus are much closer to each other than those of the medial meniscus. The anterior horn inserts adjacent to the ACL, and the posterior horn inserts just posterior to the ACL, anterior to the posterior horn of the medial meniscus.
- There is a loose peripheral attachment of the lateral meniscus to the joint capsule that allows greater translation of the lateral meniscus, when compared to the medial meniscus (11.2 vs. 5.2 mm) (2).
- The area of the lateral meniscus with no coronary ligament attachment, anterior to the popliteus tendon, is called the bare area of the lateral meniscus, or popliteal hiatus.

Lateral Meniscus Attachments

- Motion of the lateral meniscus is guided by the capsular attachments, as well as additional ligamentous attachments. These ligaments include the meniscofemoral ligaments (MFLs) and the anterior inferior and posterior superior popliteomeniscal fascicles from the popliteus muscle.
- The posterior horn has variably present attachments to the medial femoral condyle through the MFLs. The MFLs originate from the posterior horn of the lateral meniscus.
- The anterior MFL (of Humphrey) passes anterior to the posterior cruciate ligament (PCL) to insert on the femur between the distal margin of the femoral attachment of the PCL and the edge of the condylar articular cartilage.

- The posterior MFL (of Wrisberg) passes posterior to the PCL to insert at the proximal margin of the femoral attachment of the PCL.
- The overall incidence of at least one MFL is 91%. In the knees demonstrating at least one structure, the incidence of an anterior MFL is 48.2%, and the incidence of posterior MFL is 70.4%. The incidence of both ligaments coexisting in one knee is 31.8% (13).

Meniscal Variants

- Discoid variants occur with an estimated incidence of 3.5%–5.0%, most commonly the incomplete type (11).
- Discoid meniscus is almost universally located in the lateral compartment.
- Three types exist — incomplete, complete, and Wrisberg.
- Both the incomplete and complete types have firm posterior tibial attachments and are considered stable.
- The Wrisberg variant occurs when the posterior horn bony attachment is absent, and the posterior MFL of Wrisberg is the only stabilizing structure (11).

Microscopic Anatomy

- The menisci are fibrocartilaginous tissue comprised of cells interspersed in a matrix largely composed of collagen bundles, along with noncollagenous proteins including elastin and proteoglycans.
- Two cell types are present — a more fusiform, fibroblastic cell, and a more rounded, chondrocytic cell.
- Water constitutes 72% of the extracellular matrix, and collagen makes up 75% of the dry weight (20).
- Elastin is estimated to be less than 0.6%, and noncollagenous proteins 8%–13%, of the meniscus dry weight in humans (20).
- Type I collagen represents 90% of collagen present, and types II, III, V, and VI are present in varying quantities depending on location and age (20).
- The principle orientation of collagen fiber bundles is circumferential, with few radially directed "tie" fibers. Tie fibers provide structural rigidity to help resist forces that would split the circumferential fibers with compressive loading (2,20).
- Fiber orientation changes with depth from the surface. Surface fibers are arranged as a network of irregularly oriented bundles. The deeper fibers are primarily circumferential (20).

Neurovascular Anatomy

- Both medial and lateral menisci demonstrate an extensive microvascular network, arising from the respective superior and inferior geniculate arteries (16,26).
- The perimeniscal capillary plexus is oriented circumferentially and branches extensively into smaller vessels to supply the peripheral border of the meniscus through its attachment to the capsule.

- The branches terminate after supplying the peripheral 10%–30% of the meniscus, leaving the remainder avascular (16,20).
- Free nerve endings and specialized end-receptors are present within the menisci. The most densely innervated regions are the anterior and posterior horns of both menisci (20).
- Nerve fibers originate in the perimeniscal tissues and radiate into the peripheral 30% of the meniscus.
- Three receptor types have been identified — Ruffini endings, Golgi tendon organs, and Pacinian corpuscles.
- It is hypothesized that the nerves play a proprioceptive role in normal joint function. Meniscal-derived signals generated during deformation and loading may be important to joint position sense and for protective neuromuscular reflex control of joint motion and loading (20).

Nutrition of the Menisci

- The bulk of meniscus nutrition is supplied by the synovial fluid, most notably to the avascular regions.
- Nutrients reach the tissue via passive diffusion and mechanical pumping with intermittent compression during loading (20).

BIOMECHANICS AND MENISCAL FUNCTION

- The menisci serve in load transmission, shock absorption, lubrication, prevention of synovial impingement, synovial fluid distribution, stability, and improved gliding motion (26).
- Long-term follow-up demonstrates that virtually all knees after total meniscectomy develop degenerative changes, and this is less frequent after partial meniscectomy (1,9).

Meniscus Motion

- With knee flexion from 0–120 degrees, the menisci move posteriorly. In the midcondylar, parasagittal plane, the medial meniscus moves approximately 5.1 mm, and the lateral meniscus moves 11.2 mm (2).
- The medial meniscus lacks the controlled mobility of the lateral meniscus.
- Posterior motion of the medial meniscus is guided by the deep medial collateral ligament and semimembranosus, whereas anterior translation is caused by the push of the anterior femoral condyle (33).
- The posterior oblique fibers of the deep medial collateral ligament limit motion in rotation, and therefore, the medial meniscus is at increased risk of tear (2,16).
- The lateral meniscus is stabilized, and motion guided, by the popliteus tendon, popliteomeniscal ligaments, popliteofibular ligament, MFLs, and lateral capsule.
- Meniscal motion allows continued load distribution during changes of position of the joint, during which the radius of curvature of the femoral condyles changes (33).

Knee Stability

- The medial meniscus provides greater restraint to anterior translation than the lateral meniscus by acting as a buttress (17,18).

- ACL-deficient knees demonstrate increased anterior translation when subjected to an anteriorly directed force, and this translation increases significantly with combined meniscectomy at all angles of flexion. This confirms the role of the ACL as a primary restraint to anterior translation and demonstrates that the medial meniscus acts as a secondary stabilizer to resist anterior translation (18).

- With sufficient anterior translation (in the ACL-deficient knee), the posterior horn of the medial meniscus is wedged between the tibial plateau and the femoral condyle and is the mechanism suggested for the resistance provided by the meniscus.

- In contrast, the soft tissue attachments of the lateral meniscus do not affix the lateral meniscus as firmly to the tibia. Combined lateral meniscectomy and ACL sectioning does not increase anterior translation significantly over ACL sectioning alone. This implies that the greater mobility of the lateral meniscus prevents it from contributing as efficiently as a posterior wedge to resist anterior translation of the tibia on the femur (17).

Additional Functional Roles of the Menisci

- The menisci serve additional functional roles, including load bearing and shock absorption (26). The menisci transmit large loads across the joint, and their contact areas change with different degrees of knee flexion and rotation.

- Up to 50%–70% of compressive load is transmitted through the menisci in extension, and 85% at 90 degrees of flexion (2,11,16,26).

- Removal of a portion of the meniscus results in a decreased contact area between the femur and tibia. Medial meniscectomy decreases the contact area by up to 70%.

- Resection of as little as 15%–34% of the meniscus results in increased contact pressure by up to 350% (33).

EPIDEMIOLOGY

- The annual incidence of meniscal injury is 60–70 per 100,000 persons (11).

- Meniscus injury is more common in males, with a male-to-female ratio between 2.5:1 and 4:1 (11).

- Approximately one-third of all tears are associated with ACL injury, and approximately 80% of repairable meniscal tears occur during ACL injury (16).

- Meniscal tears are also commonly associated with tibia plateau fractures and femoral shaft fractures.

- Degenerative tears peak in the fourth through sixth decade in men and remain relatively constant after the second decade in women (11).

- Medial meniscus tears are more common than lateral tears, and tears are most frequently located in the midportion and posterior horns of the meniscus.

- Medial meniscal tears are more commonly longitudinal type, whereas laterally, a radial component is more frequent (16).

DIAGNOSIS OF MENISCAL INJURY

History

- Meniscal injury during sport occurs most frequently during noncontact cutting, deceleration, hyperflexion, or landing from a jump.

- Degenerative meniscal injury with aging (> 40 years) often occurs after trivial insult. The tear may not be noticed at the time of injury. The mechanical symptoms that follow often trigger the patient to seek attention.

- Mechanical symptoms of popping, catching, locking, or buckling, along with joint line pain, are suggestive of meniscal tear. These are nonspecific symptoms and may be secondary to chondral injury or patellofemoral chondrosis (11).

- Mild synovitis often results from the injury, with swelling present for several days after the event. The synovitis may be recurrent and activity related.

- An audible pop at the time of injury is more characteristic of an ACL tear; however, a meniscus tear is commonly present in this scenario.

- Immediate swelling suggests bleeding and is frequently not present after isolated meniscus tear; however, it may be present with a more peripherally based tear.

- A delayed effusion is more characteristic of meniscus injury, with the production of reactive joint fluid.

- The reporting of loss of motion with a sensation of a mechanical block to extension is suggestive of a displaced meniscus tear (11).

- A history of a snapping or popping knee may suggest a discoid variant. Mechanical symptoms present in childhood or adolescence, without a history of trauma, should raise the suspicion of the presence of a discoid meniscus (26).

- The complete history should include assessment of the patient's lifestyle, activity level, occupation, and medical history. Younger, more active individuals often require more aggressive management.

Physical Examination

- Examination begins with evaluation of gait. A limp is common after meniscus tear, and pain after an acute injury may result in the inability to bear weight.

- Inspection of the knee includes evaluation for an effusion, as well as thigh asymmetry in the setting of a chronic tear.

- Range of motion is assessed in comparison to the opposite extremity. A displaced tear may block the knee from achieving full extension, as well as impair flexion. A mechanical block to motion is termed the locked knee.

- Palpation of the joint lines is performed in an effort to elicit tenderness and may be the best clinical sign of a tear, with 74% sensitivity and 50% positive predictive value (11).

- Pain at terminal flexion or extension may be present, depending on the location of the tear.

- The McMurray test is performed with the patient supine. The hip and knee are flexed, and the foot is alternately internally and externally rotated during application of a circumduction maneuver to the knee. Concurrently, the examiner palpates the posterolateral and posteromedial joint lines.

- Medial meniscal injury is tested by extending the knee with the foot externally rotated. Lateral meniscal injury is assessed with the foot internally rotated.

- A palpable and audible clunk is considered a positive McMurray test. A true positive test is uncommon, even in the presence of a tear, but is nearly 100% specific. The sensitivity of the test is as low as 15% (11). More commonly, the test elicits pain (27).

- Cysts at or below the joint line may be palpable and are highly correlated with meniscal tears, most commonly lateral (11).

- No clinical examination finding is consistently predictive of meniscus tear; however, the combination of several positive tests from the following list is highly predictive of meniscus tear: joint line tenderness, pain on forced flexion, positive McMurray test, and a block to extension.

- Sensitivity of thorough examination reaches 95% and specificity 72% (11).

- Confounding diagnoses include fibrotic plica, fat pad impingement, chondral lesions, and synovitis (11).

Imaging

- Diagnostic studies should begin with plain radiography. Radiographs are assessed for associated skeletal injury, loose bodies, and presence of degenerative changes.

- Radiographs should include a 45-degree flexed knee posteroanterior weight-bearing view for individuals who may have knee arthrosis. Flexion weight-bearing views allow evaluation of the posterior tibiofemoral contact region, which is most frequently involved in early degenerative arthritis. Identification of arthrosis may have significant influence on treatment planning.

- Arthrograms are generally reserved for individuals for whom magnetic resonance imaging (MRI) is not possible. This includes individuals with metal implants (pacemaker, aneurysm clips, foreign body, and the like), individuals too large for the MRI equipment, or individuals with severe claustrophobia.

- MRI is the diagnostic modality of choice to evaluate the menisci.

- Accuracy of modern MRI scans in detection of meniscus tears approaches 95% (11).

- MRI studies have shown that the meniscal substance is not always homogeneous.

- Abnormal signal has been found in up to 30% of asymptomatic patients without any history of knee injury (26).

- Normal anatomic structures adjacent to the meniscus, such as the intermeniscal ligament and hiatus for the popliteus tendon, can be a source of confusion in interpretation of MRI scans (11).

- False-positive results occur more frequently than false-negative results, which emphasize the need for clinical correlation.

- Routine preoperative MRI scan does not significantly improve diagnostic accuracy over clinical examination alone (22). Each has accuracy in competitive athletes of approximately 90% (23).

- MRI does provide information regarding the extent of the tear and identification of occult chondral and osseous injuries.

- Judicious use of MRI is recommended, particularly in patients in whom arthroscopic surgery is anticipated.

MRI Interpretation

- Meniscal signals as shown by MRI have been classified into 4 grades.
  - Grade 0 signal: Uniformly low signal intensity (normal meniscus).
  - Grade I signal: Irregular increases in intrameniscal signal.
  - Grade II signal: Linear increases in intrameniscal signal, not communicating with the superior or inferior meniscal surface.
  - Grade III signal: Abnormal increased signal extends to one meniscal surface.

- Grades I and II have no surgical significance. Grade III signal is visible arthroscopically and represents a meniscus tear.

MENISCUS TEAR PATTERNS

- Meniscus injuries are commonly classified by the description of the pattern of tear.

- Patterns of tear include vertical longitudinal, oblique (flap, parrot beak), horizontal, radial (transverse), and complex.

- Vertical and oblique patterns constitute approximately 80% of tears (11).

- Complex, degenerative tears increase in frequency with age (> 4 years).

- A complete, displaced vertical tear is termed a bucket handle tear and is the pattern often associated with mechanical block to motion.

- Radial tears disrupt the circumferential fibers of the meniscus and, when they extend to the periphery, result in loss of the load-bearing function of the meniscus.

TREATMENT

- Treatment of meniscal injury is influenced by patient factors, as well as the nature of the meniscal pathology. Patient factors include the chronicity of symptoms, tolerance for activity modification following repair versus resection, tolerance for risk of failure, expectations, age, and underlying condition of the joint (16).

- The determinants of successful healing of a torn meniscus include tear location and configuration.

- No more than the peripheral one-third of the meniscus has a vascular supply. Therefore, the central 70%–80% demonstrates inferior conditions for healing.

- It is important to classify the location of the tear relative to the blood supply of the meniscus in order to predict repair potential.

- Tear classification based on location is as follows: red–red tear, located at the meniscal periphery within the vascular zone; red–white, no blood supply from the inner surface of the lesion; and white–white, located in the avascular zone.

- Red–red tears have the greatest potential for healing, and white–white tears the least (16).

Nonoperative Management

- Surgical treatment is recommended for most meniscal tears, except those causing minor symptoms in less active patients.

- If nonoperative management is selected, treatment is directed at minimizing symptoms of pain and swelling.

- A trial of activity modification, rehabilitation, and nonsteroidal anti-inflammatory medications is warranted until symptoms abate. This may be successful; however, symptoms may recur.

Operative Management

- Arthroscopic treatment of meniscal injuries has become one of the most common orthopedic surgical procedures in the United States (11).

- Operative treatment of meniscus tears is warranted in patients with high physical demands associated with work or sport, because the activity modification required to reduce symptoms often is not acceptable.

- Surgical indications include symptoms that affect activities of daily living, work, or sport; failure to respond to nonsurgical management; and absence of other causes of knee pain identified by radiographs or other imaging.

- Results of early treatment of peripheral tears (suspected with development of an effusion over the first 48 hours) are improved with surgical repair performed within the first 4 months from the time of injury (ideally < 10 weeks) (12).

- Additional predictors of favorable outcome from repair include peripheral location (within 3 mm of the meniscosynovial junction), patient age less than 30 years, tear length less than 2.5 cm, tear of the lateral meniscus, and simultaneous ACL reconstruction (secondary to intra-articular bleeding and fibrin clot formation) (6,12).

- The goal of meniscal surgery is to maximize meniscal preservation. Tears with the potential to heal should be repaired.

- Tears most likely to heal without treatment include tears less than 10 mm in length, tears with less than 3 mm of displacement on arthroscopic probing, partial-thickness tears (< 50% meniscal depth), and radial tears less than 3 mm in length (16).

- Arthroscopic rasping of the tear and synovium, or trephination, of these tears to encourage neovascularization may encourage healing and may be successful in as many as 90% of cases (12,16).

- Displaced tears that result in a block to motion should be treated expeditiously.

Meniscus Repair

- Repair techniques include open, arthroscopically assisted, and all arthroscopic repair.

- Traditional techniques for repair use suture fixation, passed using a variety of devices that are tied through a posterior counterincision.

- Meniscus repair implants continue to evolve since their introduction in the mid-1990s. Current-generation implants incorporate a suture-based repair and allow for an all arthroscopic technique (34).

- Criteria for meniscus repair include complete vertical longitudinal tear > 10 mm in length, location within the peripheral 10%–30% of the meniscus (or within 3–4 mm of the meniscosynovial junction), displaceable more than 3–5 mm on arthroscopic probing, no significant secondary joint degeneration or deformity, and a stable knee (12,16).

- Situations not meeting the above criteria must be individualized. It may be appropriate to extend the indications in younger individuals or in cases where resection would lead to nonfunctional remaining tissue (16).

- Suture repairs should be performed with vertical mattress stitches when possible, because these demonstrate superior repair strength compared to the horizontal pattern (12). This is predominately due to the histologic arrangement of the circumferential fiber bundles within the meniscus (34).

Partial Meniscectomy

- Meniscal injury leads to partial meniscectomy in the majority of cases, as a result of the anatomy of the tear, underlying degeneration of the substance of the meniscus, or distance from the blood supply (16).

- Meniscal tears that do not fall into the category of stable (with possible spontaneous healing), or repairable, should be treated with partial meniscectomy to remove unstable fragments, eliminate mechanical symptoms, and reduce pain and associated swelling (11).

■ Indications for partial meniscectomy include complete oblique, radial, horizontal, degenerative, or complex tears and tears located in the white–white zone (16).

■ The goal during meniscectomy is to remove nonfunctioning tissue, maximize meniscus preservation, maintain hoop stresses, and create a stable configuration of the remaining tissue.

OUTCOMES

■ As previously outlined, the meniscus serves a chondroprotective function in the knee.

■ Precocious arthropathy may result from partial or total meniscectomy. This is thought to be secondary to the increased contact stresses on the articular surfaces.

■ Total meniscectomy in previously normal knees results in significant arthrosis in two-thirds of patients by 15 years from surgery (1).

■ Better outcome is noted after successful repair compared to resection, with lower incidence of degenerative change after 5 years (16).

■ More rapid degeneration is noted after lateral meniscectomy compared to medial meniscectomy (15,16,28).

■ The factor with the greatest impact on long-term outcome is whether articular damage is present at the time of partial meniscectomy (12).

■ Other factors that influence risk of future arthritis include amount of resection (more resection, higher risk), type of resection (radial resection destroys the meniscus ability to convert compression forces to hoop stresses), associated instability, overall weight-bearing alignment, body habitus, age, and activity level (16).

■ A recent systematic review (30) has concluded that the preoperative and intraoperative predictors of poor clinical and/or radiographic outcomes include the following: total meniscectomy (7), removal of the peripheral meniscal rim (14), lateral meniscectomy (4), degenerative meniscal tears (8), presence of chondral damage (32), genetic predisposition as correlated with the presence of hand osteoarthritis (8), and increased body mass index (5).

■ Variables that had poor predictive values of clinical and/or radiographic outcomes include meniscal tear pattern, age, mechanical alignment, patient gender, activity level, and meniscal tears associated with ACL reconstruction (30).

■ Results of partial meniscectomy remain good or excellent in over 90% of patients not demonstrating articular cartilage damage at the time of meniscectomy, and this declines to approximately 60% if damage is present (12). In general, 80%–90% of patients have documented good to excellent results within the first 5 years after partial meniscectomy (16).

■ Functional results do not always correlate with radiographic findings. Up to 50% of patients at 8 years after partial meniscectomy, versus 25% of patients with untreated knees, will demonstrate radiographic changes (11,15,16).

■ Meniscus repair is successful in approximately 80% of cases. Healing rates increase to approximately 95% in the setting of concomitant ACL reconstruction (12).

COMPLICATIONS

■ Complications specific to meniscus repair include neurovascular injuries.

■ The peroneal nerve is at greatest risk with lateral meniscus repair. The popliteal artery, popliteal vein, and tibial nerve are also at risk.

■ The saphenous nerve, particularly the infrapatellar branch, is at greatest risk with medial repair.

■ Failure of repair resulting in the need for repeat arthroscopy is possible, and the risk increases as indications for repair are extended.

■ Meniscus repair done concurrently with ACL reconstruction increases the risk of motion loss; however, the appropriateness of staged repair remains controversial.

MENISCAL SUBSTITUTES

■ Substitutes for meniscus tissue injury, or loss, are in development.

■ Current replacements include meniscal allograft transplantation and collagen meniscal implants (CMI).

Meniscal Allograft Transplantation

■ Meniscal allograft transplantation has been used in humans for over 20 years.

■ The general indication has been disabling pain after loss of a meniscus in a skeletally mature individual (10).

■ A patient with symptoms referable to a meniscus-deficient tibiofemoral compartment is the most common indication for meniscal transplant (25).

■ A patient who has undergone prior meniscectomy should be carefully examined for early onset of joint degeneration, with the physical exam focusing on the presence of effusion, joint-line tenderness, crepitus, stability, and axial alignment (25).

■ The allograft tissue is most commonly fresh-frozen or cryopreserved. Fresh allografts have also been used; however, logistical difficulties in the routine use of fresh grafts make them impractical for widespread use (12).

■ Four types of meniscus allografts are currently available, including fresh, cryopreserved, fresh-frozen, and lyophilized. Fresh and cryopreserved allografts contain viable cells, whereas fresh-frozen and lyophilized allografts are acellular (25).

- Fresh grafts have the theoretical advantage of harboring viable cells, but the proportion of cells that survive and the duration of cell survival following transplantation are not known (25).

- Immune response against the transplant has been shown; however, frank rejection does not appear to occur (28).

- The technique of allograft transplantation has proved to be reproducible in terms of healing and control of postmeniscectomy pain and swelling. The exact indications for allograft transplantation, however, continue to be developed (28). When properly indicated, transplantation leads to predictable good results in over 90% of patients (16).

- Meniscal allograft transplantation may be considered for patients with symptoms referable to a meniscus-deficient tibiofemoral compartment. These symptoms include pain and swelling, more commonly than mechanical symptoms (16,28).

- It is not possible, at this time, to identify patients who will develop symptomatic arthrosis after meniscectomy, and therefore, prophylactic transplantation in the asymptomatic patient after meniscectomy has not been justified (16).

- Ideally, an objective marker of early pathologic changes to articular surfaces will be identified to allow identification of appropriate patients for early meniscus replacement. Such markers may be found through advanced imaging techniques or synovial fluid analysis for cartilage degradation products.

- Transplantation results are poor in cases of advanced joint degeneration and therefore should only be considered when no more than fibrillation and fissuring of the articular surfaces is present.

- Full-thickness articular cartilage lesions on the flexion weight-bearing zone of the femoral condyle or tibia greater than 10–15 mm in diameter are a contraindication to transplantation (12,28).

- Additionally, in order to be a candidate for transplantation, the knee must be stable, without malalignment. An unstable knee must be stabilized, and malalignment requires correction to avoid direct weight-bearing through the involved compartment receiving the meniscus transplant (16,28).

Meniscus Scaffolds

- Several biologics and materials such as autologous tendons, submucosa, collagen matrices, and carbon fiber prostheses were developed, but only CMIs, made from bovine Achilles tendons, have been used clinically with varying success rates (31).

- Bovine collagen meniscal scaffolds, termed CMIs, have been approved for human implantation in Europe, Australia, and Chile. The scaffold is gradually replaced by meniscus-like tissue as fibrochondrocytes proliferate within the scaffold. This device was briefly approved for implantation by the Food and Drug Administration (FDA) in the United States in 2009–2010, but that approval was withdrawn in 2010 when it became apparent that political intervention had influenced the initial approval process.

- Linke et al. (19) have demonstrated that the clinical outcome after implantation of a CMI combined with high-tibial osteotomy was not different compared with the control group with high-tibial osteotomy alone after 2 years.

- Recently, Rodkey et al. (29) published a multicentric randomized clinical trial comparing the clinical results of the CMI with partial meniscectomy at 5 years of follow-up. These authors concluded that CMI has the utility to be used to replace irreparable or lost meniscal tissue in patients who had had 1, 2, or 3 prior meniscal surgical procedures. The CMI did not provide any apparent benefit for patients with an acute injury when compared to a control group treated with meniscectomy at 5 years of follow-up.

- Porcine small intestine submucosa, which contains collagen and multiple growth factors, is an alternative scaffold under consideration and currently used in animal trials (35).

FUTURE DIRECTIONS

- Future treatments in both meniscus repair and replacement continue to evolve.

- Several growth factors and cytokines are under investigation as potential adjuncts to potentiate healing.

- Meniscal fibrochondrocytes respond with migration and proliferation to growth factors, including platelet-derived growth factor (PDGF), hepatocyte growth factor (HGF), bone morphogenic protein-2 (BMP-2), insulinlike growth factor-1 (IGF-1), and transforming growth factor-beta (TGF-β) (3,24).

- Suggested delivery systems for growth factors include impregnated absorbable scaffolds, impregnated fixation devices, or even virus vectors for gene therapy (21).

- Tissue engineering may be the next step in development of a durable meniscal replacement. This technique combines the technology of cell culture, polymer chemistry, and biology to create tissues that are appropriate for tissue replacement or reconstruction. The implant would incorporate fibrochondrocytes that have been multiplied in cell culture, in appropriate-shaped polymer scaffolds.

REFERENCES

1. Andersson-Molina H, Karlsson H, Rockborn P. Arthroscopic partial and total meniscectomy: a long-term follow-up study with matched controls. *Arthroscopy.* 2002;18(2):183–9.

2. Arnoczky SP, McDevitt CA. The meniscus: structure, function, repair, and replacement. In: Buckwalter JA, editor. *Orthopaedic Basic Science: Biology and Biomechanics of the Musculoskeletal System.* 2nd ed. Rosemont: American Academy of Orthopedic Surgeons; 2000. p. 531–45.

3. Bhargava MM, Attia ET, Murrell GA, Dolan MM, Warren RF, Hannafin JA. The effect of cytokines on the proliferation and migration of bovine meniscal cells. *Am J Sports Med.* 1999;27(5):636–43.

4. Chatain F, Adeleine P, Chambat P, Neyret P; Société Française d'Arthroscopie. A comparative study of medial versus lateral arthroscopic partial meniscectomy on stable knees: 10-year minimum follow-up. *Arthroscopy.* 2003;19(8):842–9.

5. Cicuttini FM, Baker JR, Spector TD. The association of obesity with osteoarthritis of the hand and knee in women: a twin study. *J Rheumatol.* 1996;23(7):1221–6.

6. Eggli S, Wegmüller H, Kosina J, Huckell C, Jakob RP. Long-term results of arthroscopic meniscal repair. An analysis of isolated tears. *Am J Sports Med.* 1995;23(6):715–20.

7. Englund M, Lohmander LS. Risk factors for symptomatic knee osteoarthritis fifteen to twenty-two years after meniscectomy. *Arthritis Rheum.* 2004;50(9):2811–9.

8. Englund M, Paradowski PT, Lohamnder LS. Association of radiographic hand osteoarthritis with radiographic knee osteoarthritis after meniscectomy. *Arthritis Rheum.* 2004;50(2):469–75.

9. Fairbank TJ. Knee joint changes after meniscectomy. *J Bone Joint Surg Br.* 1948;30B(4):664–70.

10. Goble EM, Kohn D, Verdonk R, Kane SM. Meniscal substitutes — human experience. *Scand J Med Sci Sports.* 1999;9(3):146–57.

11. Greis PE, Bardana DD, Holmstrom MC, Burks RT. Meniscal injury: I. Basic science and evaluation. *J Am Acad Orthop Surg.* 2002;10(3):168–76.

12. Greis PE, Holmstrom MC, Bardana DD, Burks RT. Meniscal injury: II. Management. *J Am Acad Orthop Surg.* 2002;10(3):177–87.

13. Gupte CM, Bull AM, Thomas RD, Amis AA. A review of the function and biomechanics of the meniscofemoral ligaments. *Arthroscopy.* 2003;19(2):161–71.

14. Higuchi H, Kimura M, Shirakura K, Terauchi M, Takagishi K. Factors affecting long-term results after arthroscopic partial meniscectomy. *Clin Orthop Relat Res.* 2000;377:161–8.

15. Jaureguito JW, Elliot JS, Lietner T, Dixon LB, Reider B. The effects of arthroscopic partial lateral meniscectomy in an otherwise normal knee: a retrospective review of functional, clinical, and radiographic results. *Arthroscopy.* 1995;11(1):29–36.

16. Klimkiewicz JJ, Shaffer B. Meniscal surgery. 2002 Update: indications and techniques for resection, repair, regeneration, and replacement. *Arthroscopy.* 2002;18(9)(suppl 2):14–25.

17. Levy IM, Torzilli PA, Gould JD, Warren RF. The effect of lateral meniscectomy on motion of the knee. *J Bone Joint Surg Am.* 1989;71(3):401–6.

18. Levy IM, Torzilli PA, Warren RF. The effect of medial meniscectomy on anterior-posterior motion of the knee. *J Bone Joint Surg Am.* 1982;64(6):883–8.

19. Linke RD, Ulmer M, Imhoff AB. Replacement of the meniscus with a collagen implant (CMI). *Oper Orthop Traumatol.* 2006;18(5–6):453–62.

20. Lo IKY, Thornton G, Miniaci A, et al. Structure and function of diarthrodial joints. In: McGinty JB, editor. *Operative Arthroscopy.* 3rd ed. Philadelphia: Lippincott Williams & Wilkins; 2003. p. 41–126.

21. Martinek V, Usas A, Pelinkovic D, Robbins P, Fu FH, Huard J. Genetic engineering of meniscal allografts. *Tissue Eng.* 2002;8(1):107–17.

22. Miller GK. A prospective study comparing the accuracy of the clinical diagnosis of meniscus tear with magnetic resonance imaging and its effect on clinical outcome. *Arthroscopy.* 1996;12(4):406–13.

23. Muellner T, Weinstabl R, Schabus R, Vécsei V, Kainberger F. The diagnosis of meniscal tears in athletes. A comparison of clinical and magnetic resonance imaging investigations. *Am J Sports Med.* 1997;25(1):7–12.

24. Ochi M, Uchio Y, Okuda K, Shu N, Yamaguchi H, Sakai Y. Expression of cytokines after meniscal rasping to promote meniscal healing. *Arthroscopy.* 2001;17(7):724–31.

25. Packer JD, Rodeo SA. Meniscal allograft transplantation. *Clin Sports Med.* 2009;28(2):259–83, viii.

26. Rath E, Richmond JC. The menisci: basic science and advances in treatment. *Br J Sports Med.* 2000;34(4):252–7.

27. Richmond JC. The knee. In: Richmond JC, Shahady EJ, editors. *Sports Medicine for Primary Care.* Oxford: Blackwell Science; 1996. p. 387–444.

28. Rodeo SA. Meniscal allografts — where do we stand? *Am J Sports Med.* 2001;29(2):246–61.

29. Rodkey WG, DeHaven KE, Montgomery WH III, et al. Comparison of the collagen meniscus implant with partial meniscectomy. A prospective randomized trial. *J Bone Joint Surg Am.* 2008;90(7):1413–26.

30. Salata MJ, Gibbs AE, Sekiya JK. A systematic review of clinical outcomes in patients undergoing meniscectomy. *Am J Sports Med.* 2010;38(9):1907–16.

31. Sandmann GH, Eichorn S, Vogt S, et al. Generation and characterization of a human acellular meniscus scaffold for tissue engineering. *J Biomed Mater Res.* 2009;91(2):567–74.

32. Shelbourne KD, Gray T. Results of anterior cruciate ligament reconstruction based on meniscus and articular cartilage status at the time of surgery. Five- to fifteen-year evaluations. *Am J Sports Med.* 2000;28(4):446–52.

33. Simon SR, Alaranta H, An KN, et al. Kinesiology. In: Buckwalter JA, editor. *Orthopaedic Basic Science: Biology and Biomechanics of the Musculoskeletal System.* 2nd ed. Rosemont: American Academy of Orthopedic Surgeons; 2000. p. 730–827.

34. Stärke C, Kopf S, Petersen W, Becker R. Meniscal repair. *Arthroscopy.* 2009;25(9):1033–44.

35. Welch JA, Montgomery RD, Lenz SD, Plouhar P, Shelton WR. Evaluation of small-intestinal submucosa implants for repair of meniscal defects in dogs. *Am J Vet Res.* 2002;63(3):427–31.

61 Knee Instability

Matthew C. Bessette, Frank Winston Gwathmey, Jr, and Mark Miller

INTRODUCTION

- The knee is an encapsulated compound joint consisting of two condyloid joints at the medial and lateral articulations of the tibia and femur and one saddle joint between the patella and femur. Lacking intrinsic bony stability, most of its overall stability is derived from the major ligaments and smaller supporting structures in and around the knee. Disruption of one or more of these ligaments, commonly from injury in athletics or major trauma, results in instability. Injuries to the anterior cruciate ligament (ACL) and medial collateral ligament (MCL) make up the vast majority of ligamentous knee injuries.

ANATOMY

Anterior Cruciate Ligament

- The ACL is one of two major intra-articular ligaments of the knee. Its femoral origin is on the posteromedial aspect of the lateral femoral condyle. It inserts on the tibial plateau, just anterior to the area between the intercondylar eminences.

- The ACL is compromised of two distinct bundles, each identified by their relative insertion on the tibia. The anteromedial bundle tightens in flexion, while the posterolateral bundle tightens in full extension. The overall tension on the ACL is greatest when the knee is in 30 degrees of flexion (59).

- The blood supply to the ACL is from the middle geniculate artery, a branch of the popliteal artery. Innervation from branches of the tibial nerve aids proprioception.

- The primary role of the ACL is to prevent excessive anterior tibial translation in relation to the femur, providing 90% of total anterior translational stability. The anteromedial bundle serves this function, while the posterolateral bundle adds protection against internal rotation (15). The ACL also stabilizes the knee against varus and valgus stress when the knee is in full extension. It contributes to the "screw home" mechanism, by which the femur is internally rotated over the tibia in full extension to "lock" the knee while standing (44).

Posterior Cruciate Ligament

- The intra-articular posterior cruciate ligament (PCL) originates on the anterolateral aspect of the medial femoral condyle and inserts in a depression approximately 1–1.5 cm distal to the articular surface in a fovea between the posterior aspects of the medial and lateral tibial plateaus.

- Like the ACL, the PCL is composed of two bundles, a larger anterolateral bundle that tightens in flexion and a posteromedial bundle that tightens in extension. Overall, the ligament bears the most tension in 90 degrees of knee flexion. These bundles are less distinct than those of the ACL and are described by some as a continuum of one ligament.

- The PCL shares its neurovascular supply with the nearby ACL. Present in 90% of the population, the meniscofemoral ligaments of Humphry and Wrisberg originate on the posterior horn of the lateral meniscus and straddle the PCL anteriorly and posteriorly before inserting on the medial femoral condyle (27).

- The primary role of the PCL is to resist posterior tibial translation, providing up to 100% of posterior stability at 90 degrees of flexion (3). It also protects against varus and valgus stress in full extension. With the ACL, it contributes to the "screw-home" mechanism (5).

Medial Collateral Ligament

- The MCL is an extraarticular ligament composed of superficial and deep components. The superficial MCL is 10–12 cm long and originates just proximal and posterior to the medial epicondyle. It courses distally deep to the pes anserinus tendons and inserts on the medial tibial metaphysis approximately 5 cm distal to the joint line. The shorter deep MCL is deep and adherent to the superficial MCL. It is connected to the medial meniscus by its meniscofemoral and meniscotibial components.

- Once thought to be a posterior portion of the superficial MCL, the posterior oblique ligament (POL) is a distinct, fan-like ligament spanning from a femoral origin posterior and superior to that of the superficial MCL distally to the joint capsule and distal semimembranosus tendon (33).

- The superficial MCL is the primary restraint to valgus instability of the knee and aids in rotational stability. The POL acts synergistically with the MCL to stabilize the knee against internal tibial rotation and valgus deformity with the knee in extension (26).

- The medial structures of the knee are described in three layers.
  - Sartorius and fascia
  - Superficial MCL, POL, semimembranosus
  - Deep MCL, capsule

Posterolateral Corner and Lateral Collateral Ligament

- Multiple static and dynamic stabilizers form a complex, interrelated network to secure the lateral knee against varus deformity, external tibial rotation, and posterior tibial translation. Collectively, these are known as the posterolateral corner (PLC). The lateral collateral ligament (LCL), popliteus muscle, and popliteofibular ligaments are the most important stabilizing structures of the region (32).

- The LCL originates just proximal and posterior to the lateral epicondyle and travels 7 cm distally to insert on the lateral portion of the fibular head. It is the primary restraint to varus instability of the knee and also aids in rotational stability in the extended knee.

- From its origin on the posteromedial proximal tibia, the popliteus muscle arcs laterally and proximally. Its tendon becomes intra-articular, coursing through the popliteal hiatus before inserting on the femur deep, distal, and anterior to the LCL. It has interconnections to the fibula, tibia, and meniscus that form the popliteus complex, giving it both static and dynamic stabilizing properties.

- The popliteofibular (arcuate) ligament is a "Y" shaped structure connecting the popliteus to the fibular head. The popliteus and popliteofibular ligament provide the primary restraint against external tibial rotation (34).

- Other structures involved with the PLC include the fabellofibular ligament, iliotibial band, biceps femoris tendon, lateral head of the gastrocnemius, and the lateral joint capsule. The PLC works in concert with the PCL to prevent excessive posterior tibial translation, contributing more in extension (54).

- The lateral structures of the knee can be considered in three layers.
  - Fascia, iliotibial band, and biceps femoris tendon
  - Patellar retinaculum and patellofemoral ligament
  - Popliteofibular ligament, popliteus, fabellofibular ligament, LCL, and capsule

ANTERIOR CRUCIATE LIGAMENT

Mechanism of Injury

- It is estimated that more than 100,000 ACL injuries occur in the United States each year, many of them during athletic activity. Seventy percent of injuries to the ACL occur by noncontact mechanisms (11). Tension is created primarily by forces in the sagittal plane that cause large anterior tibial sheer forces. A combination of small knee flexion angles, large posterior ground reaction forces, and substantial quadriceps contractions all contribute to anterior sheer stress. This is augmented but not duplicated by rotational and valgus forces acting upon the knee. The posterior sheer forces on the tibia exerted by the hamstrings are protective from ACL injury.

- Common mechanisms of injury include pivoting during acceleration or deceleration and forcefully landing on the heel with a small knee flexion angle (1). Contact-induced injury often involves valgus loading of the fixed and straightened knee (11).

- While males and females sustain an approximately equal number of total ACL injuries, women who participate in athletics are three to eight times more likely than their male counterparts to sustain injury (23). Reasons for this discrepancy include smaller ligaments relative to body size, increased joint laxity, higher levels of estrogen, and smaller intercondylar notch dimensions. Females have also been shown to have different neuromuscular mechanics that predispose them to ACL injury. They tend to land from jumps with less knee flexion, have more valgus loading of the knee, and have greater activation of their quadriceps relative to their hamstrings.

- Other risk factors for ACL injury include game situations in comparison to practice, an increased coefficient of friction of footwear, and prior ACL injury with or without reconstruction of the ipsilateral or contralateral knee (13).

Evaluation

- A thorough history and physical exam is the most important aspect of the evaluation of a possible ACL injury. Patients often report pain and instability occurring after landing or cutting in a noncontact situation. An audible "pop" is common. Swelling within the joint occurs rapidly, and athletes are typically unable to return to play. It is not uncommon to see ACL, MCL, and lateral meniscal injury from the same event (5).

- The Lachman test is the most important physical exam for ACL injuries, having a high sensitivity and specificity (85% and 94%, respectively). With the patient supine and the quadriceps relaxed, the knee is placed in 30 degrees of flexion. The patient's thigh is stabilized, and the examiner grasps the patient's proximal tibia and applies anterior force, noting the amount of anterior translation and the endpoint. Anterior translation of greater than 3 mm compared to the contralateral knee and a "soft" endpoint signifies ACL injury.

- The pivot shift test is an important indicator of rotational instability. With the leg fully extended, the ankle is internally rotated while a valgus force is applied to the proximal tibia. In the ACL-deficient knee, this causes anterior subluxation of the lateral tibial plateau beneath the lateral femoral condyle. As the knee is slowly flexed past 30 degrees, the iliotibial band induces a sudden reduction of the subluxed lateral tibia, interpreted as a positive pivot shift. Although the test is not very sensitive (24%), it is extremely specific (98%). It is much more sensitive (74%) and comfortable for the patient when preformed under anesthesia (7).

- Although not as sensitive or specific as the Lachman test, the anterior drawer test is useful in the evaluation of chronic ACL injury. With a supine patient's knee in 90 degrees of flexion and foot resting on the table, anterior force is applied to the tibia. The difference in anterior translation between the two knees is evaluated (7). All tests have been shown to be highly examiner dependent and are most effectively preformed by trained orthopedists (23). Mechanical devices such as the KT-1000 or KT-2000 arthrometers (MEDmetric, San Diego, CA) can evaluate the anterior translation of the tibia in a more standardized fashion but are typically used for research purposes only (44).

- Although radiographs typically do not diagnose ligamentous injury, they are helpful to evaluate for other injuries. Avulsion of the tibial spine and Segond fractures (lateral tibial capsular avulsion fractures) can be seen with ACL injuries, the latter of which is pathognomonic. A magnetic resonance imaging (MRI) is usually not necessary to make the diagnosis of an ACL rupture, but it is useful to visualize the ligament and to evaluate for other pathology (5).

Natural History

- Injury to the ACL rarely occurs in isolation. Characteristic bone bruise on the central lateral femoral condyle and posterior lateral tibial plateau can be found in nearly all patients on MRI (24), although the clinical significance is unknown at this point (20). Approximately half will have meniscal tears, commonly located in the posterior horn of the lateral meniscus in acute injury (6). Chronic instability stresses the posterior horn of the medial meniscus, resulting in tears in this region. When meniscal repair is performed concomitantly with ACL reconstruction, there is a greater chance of healing of the meniscus in comparison to delayed treatment. Meniscal repairs in the chronically unstable knee typically have poor outcomes (6).

- There is a 50% incidence of clinical and radiographic evidence of osteoarthritis in patients between 10 and 20 years after ACL injury regardless of their treatment. This increased risk of osteoarthritis is especially evident in those who sustain injury to the menisci (39).

Management

- Indications for surgical reconstruction include athletes, patients with associated repairable meniscal injury, patients with complete tears to any of the three other major knee ligaments, and patients experiencing instability that interferes with activities of daily living (22).

- Conservative (nonoperative) treatment focuses on regaining normal knee range of motion and strengthening the secondary stabilizers of the knee, in particular the hamstrings. Rotation and lateral movement should be avoided for 6–12 weeks, and competitive situations should be avoided for at least 3 months (20). Bracing may be used for patient comfort but is not necessary. It is important to counsel the patient about episodes of instability and behavioral modifications to protect the joint (30). These patients are typically self-reported to be satisfied with their condition, but suffer from instability issues and a reduction in activity levels (47).

- If surgical treatment is elected, it should be performed after acute hemarthrosis and accompanying synovitis have resolved and knee range of motion has returned to normal, usually 3–4 weeks after injury. Early reconstruction may result in arthrofibrosis, whereas late repair may be associated with additional injury to the joint (30). Restoring range of motion, weight bearing, and closed-chain exercises are key aspects of both preoperative and postoperative management.

- Primary repair does not result in adequate healing due to the intra-articular environment, and thus, reconstruction is necessary. This involves drilling tunnels through the tibia and femur and placing a graft through the tunnels to serve as scaffolding for new ligament growth. Surgeons commonly use the central third of the patient's patellar tendon with bone plugs from the patella and tibial tubercle (bone-tendon-bone [BTB]), the patient's own semitendinosus and gracilis tendons (hamstring), or cadaveric (allograft) grafts.

- BTB autografts incorporate into the bone tunnels more rapidly and have been shown by some to have lower failure rates than hamstring grafts, making them ideal for more active, younger patients. They are associated with increased radiographic osteoarthritis changes as well as anterior knee pain (29).

- Hamstring tendon grafts have lower donor-site morbidity and have a greater tensile strength when quadrupled, but are slower to incorporate in the tunnels at the bone–tendon interface (21).

- Allografts are associated with no donor-site morbidity and decreased operative time. Disease transmission and graft preservation are less of a concern with modern harvesting techniques, but allografts have an increased cost and delayed graft incorporation. Younger, more active patients have been shown to have significantly higher rates of failure with allografts (12).

- New methods of double-bundle repair using two separate grafts to mimic the natural ACL's distinct bundles and two tibial tunnels have been gaining popularity in recent years. They have been shown to have superior results in terms of postoperative measurements of anterior translation and rotation, but studies have yet to show a difference in terms of clinical outcome (55).

Pediatrics

- ACL injuries in skeletally immature patients are increasingly common and now make up 3.3% of all ACL injuries. Children typically suffer from poor outcomes with conservative treatment, but reconstruction is complicated by the proximity of the physeal growth plates to the joint, as the distal tibial and proximal femur contribute to 65% of the growth of the lower extremity. Several different surgical techniques have been shown to be successful in reconstructing the ligament while respecting the physis and thus maintaining normal bone growth (55).

POSTERIOR CRUCIATE LIGAMENT

Mechanism of Injury

- PCL injuries make up approximately 3% of all ligamentous knee injuries, but up to 38% in trauma situations. There are associated injuries in approximately half of all PCL injuries, most notably to the PLC. This proportion rises to 95% in the setting of severe trauma (3,40).

- A "dashboard injury" occurs when contact of the tibia with the dashboard during collision exerts a large posterior sheer force on the tibia, often resulting in multiligament damage. In athletics, damage to the PCL is more often isolated and can occur when falling onto a flexed knee with a plantar-flexed foot or from a direct blow to the anterior tibia. Severe hyperextension and hyperflexion are other mechanisms of injury (42).

- Unless associated with obvious trauma, the presentation of a PCL injury is subtle, especially if isolated. There is usually no "popping" reported, and athletes are often able to continue competition after injury or may not be able to recall the event at all. Reported symptoms include stiffness, mild swelling, moderate posterior knee pain, and pain with deep knee flexion (42).

Evaluation

- Acute hemarthrosis due to PCL injury will be mild. Observation of gait may reveal a slight varus deformity in the setting of chronic instability.

- The posterior drawer test is the most important physical examination for evaluation of the PCL, having a sensitivity and specificity of 90% and 99%, respectively (26). With the patient supine, the knees are flexed to 90 degrees and the hips to 45 degrees while the feet rest on the table. It is important to detect a posterior "sag." Normally, the tibial plateau should be more than 1 cm anterior to the medial femoral condyle. Otherwise, there is likely PCL injury and the tibia must be anteriorly reduced to an anatomically neutral position before testing. A posterior force is directed upon the anterior proximal tibia, and the magnitude of displacement and characteristics of the endpoint are observed.

- Displacement of 3–5 mm indicates a grade I posterior drawer with the medial tibial plateau remaining anterior to the medial femoral condyle. In grade II displacement, there is 6–10 mm of displacement and the tibial plateau is flush with the femoral condyle. More than 10 mm of displacement, pushing the plateau posterior to the condyle, is a grade III injury (41). In grade III injury, there is likely a concurrent injury to the PCL (56).

- The posterior sag test is done with the patient supine and the hip and knee flexed to 90 degrees. The examiner holds the patient's ankles and observes the knee for a step-off between the tibial plateau and femoral condyles. For the quadriceps active test, the supine patient's feet are set flush on the table and the patient is asked to advance the feet away from the body. Anterior shift of the tibial plateau greater than 2 mm is indicative of PCL pathology (42).

- Plain radiographs may show bony avulsions in the acute setting or degenerative changes in the medial and patellofemoral compartments in chronic cases. Stress radiographs are useful to quantify the degree of posterior instability, with greater than 10 mm of displacement compared to the contralateral side indicating injury to the PCL and PLC. MRI is excellent for assessment of the PCL and other structures of the knee in acute settings, but lacks adequate sensitivity for detection of chronic PCL injury (42).

Natural History

- Injuries to the PCL can be subtle and have a varied course. At the time of injury, it is difficult to predict future consequences from instability. One study found that 2% of highly functioning college football players had asymptomatic PCL deficiencies (49), whereas another study evaluated symptomatic patients 5 years after injury and found articular cartilage damage in almost 80% of medial femoral condyles and nearly 50% of patellae via arthroscopy (57).

- Knee kinematics are altered such that there is persistent anterior subluxation of the medial femoral condyle, leading to increased rates of osteoarthritis in the medial and patellofemoral compartments and higher rates of meniscal tears (38). MRI studies have shown partial healing ability of the ligament (1). Although some do well with conservative treatment, others suffer from continued instability and osteoarthritic changes.

Management

- Patients with both acute and chronic isolated grade I or II injuries should undergo nonoperative treatment, because surgical reconstruction has not been shown to be helpful for either. Protected weight bearing in an extension brace is followed by quadriceps rehabilitation and range-of-motion exercises. Return to sports is usually possible within 2–6 weeks.

- Surgical intervention is recommended for patients with associated injuries to the ACL, MCL, and PLC (grade III PCL injury), preferably within 1–2 weeks. In the case of chronic injury, a tibial osteotomy may be necessary to correct for varus deformity (3).

- There is no clear superior surgical technique for PCL reconstruction, and results of such procedures are inferior to ACL reconstruction. Grafts may be single- (anterolateral) or double-bundled.

- Traditionally, the graft is fixed to the tibia through a trans-tibial tunnel. It is forced to make a sharp "killer turn" superiorly over the posterior edge of the tunnel, resulting in loosening of the graft over time. Berg (8) described the tibial inlay technique, using a bony fragment to fix the graft directly to the fovea at the origin of the native PCL, resulting in decreased laxity (9,10). As with ACL reconstruction, exercises are gradually introduced, and full recovery generally takes 9 months.

MEDIAL COLLATERAL LIGAMENT

Mechanism of Injury

- The annual incidence of MCL injuries is 0.24 per 1,000 and is twice as common in men (17). They typically occur in isolation and during athletics.

- The mechanism of injury often involves a valgus force on the partially flexed knee, opening the medial compartment of the knee and stressing the medial support structures. Patients often report localized pain and swelling along the medial aspect of the knee. Instability is not a common symptom, but when it does occur, it is described as affecting side-to-side motion.

Examination

- Physical examination begins with inspection, which may reveal localized swelling or ecchymosis at the site of injury, most often near the femoral origin of the superficial MCL. Areas of tenderness are usually discrete and identifiable.

- Valgus stress testing is done with the knee in 30 degrees of flexion and the patient relaxed. Stabilizing the femur, a valgus load is applied to the tibia. Injury is characterized as grade I for pain and no joint laxity compared to the contralateral knee, grade II for some laxity with a solid endpoint, and grade III for laxity and a soft or no endpoint. Grade I and II injuries usually correlate with partial sprains, whereas grade III injuries involve a complete tear. In the case of a grade III tear, careful evaluation should be done for other ligamentous injuries. At 0 degrees of flexion, both the cruciate ligaments and the POL stabilize the knee against valgus deformity; instability in this position should prompt further exam for injury to additional structures.

- Radiographic examination can assess for avulsion and for growth plate injury in skeletally immature patients.

Valgus stress views are useful to quantify medial compartment opening. A Pellegrini-Stieda lesion, calcification of the MCL at its femoral origin, may be seen with chronic injuries. Ultrasound is also a useful tool for diagnosis but is highly user dependent (37). MRI is a very sensitive tool for diagnosis and detects bone bruises in almost half of all isolated injuries, mostly in the lateral compartment (45).

Natural History

- Although most MCL injuries are isolated, it is important to evaluate for other lesions. Meniscal tears may occur in 5% of presentations. Grade III injuries severe enough to require surgery are associated with POL and ACL injury in 99% and 78% of patients, respectively.

- Because of its rich vascular supply, the MCL exhibits excellent healing characteristics. When chronic injury does occur, it exposes other medial knee structures to altered loads that increase the risk of further injury (4).

Treatment

- Most MCL injuries are amenable to nonoperative treatment. For simple grade I and II injuries, a short course of rest, ice, compression, elevation, and possibly bracing may be all that is necessary. Weight-bearing and range-of-motion exercises are initiated as soon as tolerable. Adequate strength and flexibility along with control of pain are the primary goals of treatment.

- Nonoperative treatment of grade III injuries and proper rehabilitation have been shown to be just as effective as surgery when the injury is isolated (52). A hinged knee brace is used for 6 weeks after pain and swelling are controlled, and as with lower grade injuries, strength, range of motion, and early weight bearing are key.

- Longer use of bracing is commonly used for comfort in nonoperative patients with grade II or III injuries. Studies of prophylactic bracing by athletes such as football linemen have been shown to be protective of the MCL as well as other knee structures (2).

- Operative treatment is reserved for chronic injuries with instability despite appropriate rehabilitation or MCL injury in combination with other surgically amenable injuries, especially involving the ACL or menisci. Primary repair, imbrications, advancement of insertions, tendon transfers, and reconstruction are all possible techniques, and none has been adequately proven to be superior. Chronic injuries usually require reconstruction of the superficial MCL and POL.

- Postoperatively, early range of motion is necessary to prevent adhesions. Closed-chain exercises are started around 6 weeks after surgery, and full weight bearing is permitted shortly thereafter. Wearing a brace throughout rehabilitation will increase the patient's sense of stability and comfort but will not accelerate healing (50,58).

POSTEROLATERAL CORNER AND LATERAL COLLATERAL LIGAMENT

Mechanism of Injury

- Accounting for approximately 16% of knee ligament injuries, damage to the PLC is becoming an increasingly recognized source of instability in the knee. Eighty-seven percent of new presentations have multiple ligament injuries, most often involving the ACL. O'Brien et al. (48) found that chronic PLC deficiency was the most frequently identifiable reason for ACL reconstruction failure. With a ruptured PCL, there is a high likelihood of concomitant PLC injury (36).

- The most common mechanism of PLC injury occurs with a blow to the anteromedial tibia. Hyperextension and excessive varus loading can also precipitate injury (50).

Evaluation

- Patients with PLC injury typically report pain along the posterolateral aspect of the knee. Because isolated injury is rare, careful examination of other knee structures is necessary. Peroneal nerve palsy is found in approximately 15% of presentations, and evaluation of foot dorsiflexion, eversion, and sensation is vital (35).

- A patient's gait may be altered, revealing varus thrust, internal rotation with swing, and knee hyperextension in stance. Evaluation of the LCL is completed and graded in the same manner as MCL injury, but with varus stress.

- The external rotation recurvatum test is done by lifting the feet of a supine patient off the table by the greater toes. Hyperextension of the knee, external tibial rotation, and varus deformity are all signs of a PLC lesion. The posterolateral drawer test is a modification of the posterior drawer test done with the foot externally rotated. Excessive translation indicates PLC injury.

- The dial test can be done with the patient prone or supine. The patient's feet are externally rotated, and the orientation of the medial sole is compared to that of the femoral shaft. A difference of greater than 10 or 15 degrees with the knee flexed at 30 degrees indicates a PLC injury, and a difference at 90 degrees of knee flexion indicates a combined PLC and PCL injury.

- Plain films may show avulsions of the fibular head in acute presentations or lateral compartment degenerative changes with chronic instability. Varus stress films will show lateral laxity. Although MRI is helpful to identify additional pathology, it may overdiagnose PLC injury due to extensive edema visualized in posterolateral structures. It should be used in combination with physical examination and stress radiographs (14).

Natural History

- Prognosis typically depends on the extent of injury and associated findings. Patients with low-grade injuries typically do quite well in the long run with nonoperative treatment. Complete tears, however, are associated with increased laxity, damage to the ACL, muscle weakness, and osteoarthritis (31).

Treatment

- Isolated incomplete injuries are treated nonoperatively. Two to 3 weeks of knee immobilization in extension are followed by gradual increases in strength and movement, emphasizing range of motion throughout. A return to full activity is generally seen within 12–14 weeks.

- Grade III injuries are treated operatively, ideally between 2 and 3 weeks of an acute injury to avoid excessive scar tissue formation and to allow primary repair. Augmentation of a primary repair with tendon reconstruction is frequently used. Chronic injuries are not amenable to primary repair and require reconstruction. Anatomic and nonanatomic methods have been described (16).

- Injuries to other ligaments in the knee should be addressed at the same time or in a staged fashion, because the structures are reliant on one another for stability and proper healing.

KNEE DISLOCATION

Mechanism of Injury

- When an injury leads to disruption of multiple ligaments, there exists the possibility that a femoral–tibial knee dislocation has occurred. In contrast to patellar dislocations, which are common, dislocations between the femur and tibia are much less common and carry a high risk of limb-threatening consequences. Physicians must maintain a high index of suspicion for dislocation because spontaneous reduction may occur prior to examination.

- Dislocations are classified by the direction of tibial displacement in reference to the femur, but because of spontaneous reduction, any injury with three or more damaged ligaments should be considered a dislocation. In most cases, both cruciate ligaments are ruptured, and approximately three-quarters are either anterior or posterior dislocations. Tethering of the popliteal artery above and below the joint predisposes it to injury in 32%–45% of presentations, with an increased incidence in posterior displacement (25). Nerve damage occurs in 16%–40% of patients, more often to the common peroneal nerve, where it is constrained in its path around the proximal fibula (53).

- The mechanism of injury typically involves high-energy impact from motor vehicle accidents, although low-energy injuries do occur in athletes and in the morbidly obese.

Evaluation

- After the patient is stabilized, the first step in evaluation is to obtain a brief history, if possible, regarding the mechanism of injury. Reduction is undertaken if the knee is grossly displaced.

- Physical examination starts with palpation for pulses. The ankle–brachial index (ABI) has been shown to be highly sensitive and specific as a screening tool for vascular injury. Any patient with an ABI < 0.9 should undergo further workup and likely has a lesion requiring surgery, whereas the rest can be monitored with serial physical examination (46). Although arteriography has been the gold standard in further evaluation, CT angiography has been shown to be an effective and less invasive alternative (51).

- Sensory and motor exams for tibial or peroneal nerve injury can be difficult in the multitrauma patient, but are important. Anteroposterior and lateral films should be taken before and after manipulation to evaluate for malalignment and for fractures, found in up to 60% of injuries in high-energy trauma (43). Careful evaluation of all ligamentous structures is necessary for proper characterization of the injury (19).

Management

- Emergent surgery is indicated for patients with vascular injury. Other surgical emergencies include compartment syndrome, open injury, and irreducible dislocations (53). Posterolateral dislocations are more likely to be irreducible because of medial femoral condyle entrapment in the medial capsule. Vascular compromise for more than 8 hours has a high association with above-knee amputation (25). Significant instability after reduction may require spanning external fixation.

- In the absence of surgical emergencies and gross instability, the knee should be splinted in extension. Serial vascular examinations are done during a period of observation over the next 24–48 hours. Early surgical intervention within 2–3 weeks is recommended to facilitate primary repair of medial and lateral structures before excessive scar tissue formation. Cruciate reconstruction is concomitant or staged. Nonoperative treatment leads to unacceptable outcomes in terms of stiffness and instability, and thus, surgical treatment is recommended for nearly all knee dislocations.

- While most patients are able to return to work after recovery is complete (28), few are able to return to competitive sports (18).

REFERENCES

1. Akisue T, Kurosaka M, Yoshiya S, Kuroda R, Mizuno K. Evaluation of healing of the injured posterior cruciate ligament: analysis of instability and magnetic resonance imaging. *Arthroscopy*. 2001;17(3):264–9.
2. Albright JP, Powell JW, Smith W, et al. Medial collateral ligament knee sprains in college football. Effectiveness of preventive braces. *Am J Sports Med*. 1994;22(1):12–8.
3. Allen CR, Kaplan LD, Fluhme DJ, Harner CD. Posterior cruciate ligament injuries. *Curr Opin Rheumatol*. 2002;14(2):142–9.
4. Battaglia MJ 2nd, Lenhoff MW, Ehteshami JR, et al. Medial collateral ligament injuries and subsequent load on the anterior cruciate ligament: a biomechanical evaluation in a cadaveric model. *Am J Sports Med*. 2009;37(2):305–11.
5. Baumfeld JA, Hart JA, Miller MD. Sports medicine. In: Miller MD, editor. *Review of Orthopaedics*. 5th ed. Philadelphia: Saunders; 2008. p. 245–305.
6. Bellabarba C, Bush-Joseph CA, Bach BR Jr. Patterns of meniscal injury in the anterior cruciate-deficient knee: a review of the literature. *Am J Orthop (Belle Med NJ)*. 1997;26(1):18–23.
7. Benjaminse A, Gokeler A, van der Schans CP. Clinical diagnosis of an anterior cruciate ligament rupture: a meta-analysis. *J Orthop Sports Phys Ther*. 2006;36(5):267–88.
8. Berg EE. Posterior cruciate ligament tibial inlay reconstruction. *Arthroscopy*. 1995;11(1):69–76.
9. Bergfeld JA, Graham SM, Parker RD, Valdevit ADC, Kambic HE. A biomechanical comparison of posterior cruciate ligament reconstructions using single- and double-bundle tibial inlay techniques. *Am J Sports Med*. 2005;33(7):976–81.
10. Bergfeld JA, McAllister DR, Parker RD, Valdevit AD, Kambic HE. A biomechanical comparison of posterior cruciate ligament reconstruction techniques. *Am J Sports Med*. 2001;29(2):129–36.
11. Boden BP, Dean GS, Feagin JA Jr, Garrett WE Jr. Mechanisms of anterior cruciate ligament injury. *Orthopedics*. 2000;23(6):573–8.
12. Borchers JR, Pedroza A, Kaedig C. Activity level and graft type as risk factors for anterior cruciate ligament graft failure: a case-control study. *Am J Sports Med*. 2009;37(12):2362–7.
13. Brophy RH, Silvers HJ, Mandelbaum BR. Anterior cruciate ligament injuries: etiology and prevention. *Sports Med Arthrosc*. 2010;18(1):2–11.
14. Chen FS, Rokito AS, Pitman MI. Acute and chronic posterolateral rotatory instability of the knee. *J Am Acad Orthop Surg*. 2000;8(2):97–110.
15. Chhabra A, Starman JS, Ferretti M, Vidal AF, Zantop T, Fu FH. Anatomic, radiographic, biomechanical, and kenematic evaluation of the anterior cruciate ligament and its two functional bundles. *J Bone Joint Surg Am*. 2006;88(Suppl 4):2–10.
16. Cooper JM, McAndrews PT, LaPrade RF. Posterolateral corner injuries of the knee: anatomy, diagnosis, and treatment. *Sports Med Arthrosc*. 2006;14(4):213–20.
17. Daniel DM, Pedowitz RA, O'Connor JJ, Akeson WH. *Daniel's Knee Injuries: Ligament and Cartilage Structure, Function, Injury, and Repair*. 2nd ed. Philadelphia (PA): Lippincott Williams & Wilkins; 2003.
18. Eranki V, Begg C, Wallace B. Outcomes of operatively treated acute knee dislocations. *Open Orthop J*. 2010;4:22–30.
19. Fanelli GC, Orcutt DR, Edson CJ. The multiple-ligament injured knee: evaluation, treatment, and results. *Arthroscopy*. 2005;21(4):471–86.
20. Fithian DC, Paxton EW, Stone ML, et al. Prospective trial of a treatment algorithm for the management of the anterior cruciate ligament-injured knee. *Am J Sports Med*. 2005;33(3):335–46.
21. Foster TE, Wolfe BL, Ryan S, Silvestri L, Kaye EK. Does the graft source really matter in the outcome of patients undergoing anterior cruciate ligament reconstruction? An evaluation of autograft versus allograft reconstruction results: a systematic review. *Am J Sports Med*. 2010;38(1):189–99.
22. Fu FH, Schulte KR. Anterior cruciate ligament surgery 1996: state of the art? *Clin Orthop Relat Res*. 1996;(325):19–24.
23. Goldstein J, Bosco JA 3rd. The ACL-deficient knee: natural history and treatment options. *Bull Hosp Jt Dis*. 2001–2002;60(3–4):173–8.
24. Graf BK, Cook DA, De Smet AA, Keene JS. "Bone bruises" on magnetic resonance imaging evaluation of anterior cruciate ligament injuries. *Am J Sports Med*. 1993;21(2):220–3.
25. Green NE, Allen BL. Vascular injuries associated with dislocations of the knee. *J Bone Joint Surg Am*. 1977;59(2):236–9.
26. Griffith CJ, Wijdicks CA, LaPrade RF, Armitage BM, Johansen S, Engebretsen L. Force measurements on the POL and superficial medial collateral ligament proximal and distal divisions to applied loads. *Am J Sports Med*. 2009;37(1):140–8.

27. Gupte CM, Smith A, McDermott ID, Bull AM, Thomas RD, Amis AA. Mensicofemoral ligaments revisited. Anatomical study, age correlation and clinical implications. *J Bone Joint Surg Br*. 2002;84(6):846–51.

28. Hirschmann MT, Zimmermann N, Rychen T, et al. Clinical and radiological outcomes after management of traumatic knee dislocation by open single stage complete reconstruction/repair. *BMC Musculoskelet Disord*. 2010;11:102.

29. Hospodor SJ, Miller MD. Controversies in ACL reconstruction: bone-patellar tendon-bone anterior cruciate ligament reconstruction remains the gold standard. *Sports Med Arthrosc*. 2009;17(4):242–6.

30. Johnson RJ, Beynnon BD, Nichols CE, Renstrom PA. The treatment of injuries of the anterior cruciate ligament. *J Bone Joint Surg Am*. 1992; 74(1):140–51.

31. Kannus P. Nonoperative treatment of grade II and III sprains of the lateral ligament compartment of the knee. *Am J Sports Med*. 1989;17(1):83–8.

32. LaPrade RF, Bollom TS, Wentorf FA, Wills NJ, Meister K. Mechanical properties of the posterolateral structures of the knee. *Am J Sports Med*. 2005;33(9):1386–91.

33. LaPrade RF, Engebretsen AH, Ly TV, Johansen S, Wentorf FA, Engebretsen L. The anatomy of the medial part of the knee. *J Bone Joint Surg Am*. 2007;89(9):2000–10.

34. LaPrade RF, Ly TV, Wentorf FA, Engebretsen L. The posterolateral attachments of the knee: a qualitative and quantitative morphologic analysis of the fibular collateral ligament, popliteus tendon, popliteofibular ligament, and lateral gastrocnemius tendon. *Am J Sports Med*. 2003; 31(6):854–60.

35. LaPrade RF, Terry GC. Injuries to the posterolateral aspect of the knee: association of anatomic injury patterns with clinical instability. *Am J Sports Med*. 1997;25(4):433–8.

36. LaPrade RF, Wentorf FA, Fritts H, Gundry C, Hightower CD. A propective magnetic resonance imaging study of the incidence of posterolateral and multiple ligament injuries in actue knee injuries presenting with hemarthrosis. *Arthroscopy*. 2007;23(12):1341–7.

37. Lee JI, Song IS, Jung YB, et al. Medial collateral ligament injuries of the knee: ultrasonographic findings. *J Ultrasound Med*. 1996;15(9):621–5.

38. Logan M, Williams A, Lavelle J, Gedroyc W, Freeman M. The effect of posterior cruciate ligament deficiency on knee kinematics. *Am J Sports Med*. 2004;32(8):1915–22.

39. Lohmander LS, Englund PM, Dahl LL, Roos EM. The long-term consequences of anterior cruciate ligament and meniscus injuries: osteoarthritis. *Am J Sports Med*. 2007;35(10):1756–69.

40. Margheritini F, Rihn J, Musahl V, Mariani PP, Harner C. Posterior cruciate ligament injuries in the athlete: an anatomical, biomechanical and clinical review. *Sports Med*. 2002;32(6):393–408.

41. Matava MJ, Ellis E, Gruber B. Surgical treatment of posterior cruciate ligament tears: an evolving technique. *J Am Acad Orthop Surg*. 2009; 17(7):435–46.

42. McAllister DR Petrigliano FA. Diagnosis and treatment of posterior cruciate ligament injuries. *Curr Sports Med Rep*. 2007;6(5):293–9.

43. Meyers MH, Moore TM, Harvey JP Jr. Traumatic dislocation of the knee joint. *J Bone Joint Surg Am*. 1975;57(3):430–3.

44. Miller MD. The knee and lower leg. In: Miller MD, Hart JA, MacKnight JM, editors. *Essential Orthopaedics*. 1st ed. Philadelphia: Saunders; 2010.

45. Miller MD, Osborne JR, Gordon WT, Hinkin DT, Brinker MR. The natural history of bone bruises. A prospective study of magnetic resonance imaging-detected trabecular microfractures in patients with isolated medial collateral ligament injuries. *Am J Sports Med*. 1998;26(1): 15–9.

46. Mills WJ, Barei DP, McNair P. The value of the ankle-brachial index for diagnosing arterial injury after knee dislocation: a prospective study. *J Trauma*. 2004;56(6):1261–5.

47. Muaidi QI, Nicholson LL, Refshuge KM, Herbert RD, Maher CG. Prognosis of conservatively managed anterior cruciate ligament injury: a systematic review. *Sports Med*. 2007;37(8):703–16.

48. O'Brien SJ, Warren RF, Pavlov H, Panariello R, Wickiewicz TL. Reconstruction of the chronically insufficient anterior cruciate ligament with the central third of the patellar ligament. *J Bone Joint Surg Am*. 1991;73(2):278–86.

49. Parolie JM, Bergfeld JA. Long-term results of nonoperative treatment of isolated posterior cruciate ligament injuries in the athlete. *Am J Sports Med*. 1986;14(1):35–8.

50. Quarles JD, Hosey RG. Medial and lateral collateral injuries: prognosis and treatment. *Prim Care*. 2004;31(4):957–75, ix.

51. Redmond JM, Levy BA, Dajani KA, Cass JR, Cole PA. Detecting vascular injury in lower-extremity orthopedic trauma: the role of CT angiography. *Orthopedics*. 2008;31(8):761–7.

52. Reider B, Sathy MR, Talkington J, Blyznak N, Kollias S. Treatment of isolated medial collateral ligament injuries in athletes with early functional rehabilitation. A five-year follow-up study. *Am J Sports Med*. 1994;22(4):470–7.

53. Rihn JA, Cha PS, Groff YJ, Harner CD. The acutely dislocated knee: evaluation and management. *J Am Acad Orthop Surg*. 2004;12(5): 334–46.

54. Sanchez AR 2nd, Sugalski MT, LaPrade RF. Anatomy and biomechanics of the lateral side of the knee. *Sports Med Arthrosc*. 2006;14(1):2–11.

55. Schreiber VM, van Eck CF, Fu FH. Anatomic double-bundle ACL reconstruction. *Sports Med Arthroc*. 2010;18(1):27–32.

56. Sekiya JK, Whiddon DR, Zehms CT, Miller MD. A clinically relevant assessment of posterior cruciate ligmanet and posterolateral corner injuries. Evaluation of isolated and combined deficiency. *J Bone Joint Surg Am*. 2008;90(8):1621–7.

57. Strobel MJ, Weiler A, Schulz MS, Russe K, Eichhorn HJ. Arthroscopic evaluation of articular cartilage lesions in posterior-cruciate-ligament-deficient knees. *Arthroscopy*. 2003;19(3):262–8.

58. Wijdicks CA, Griffith CJ, Johansen S, Engebretsen L, LaPrade RF. Injuries to the medial collateral ligament and associated medial structures of the knee. *J Bone Joint Surg Am*. 2010;92(5):1266–80.

59. Yu B, Garrett WE. Mechanisms of non-contact ACL injuries. *Br J Sports Med*. 2007;41:i47–51.

62 The Patellofemoral Joint

Robert J. Nascimento and Anthony A. Schepsis

ANATOMY

- The patella is the largest sesamoid bone in the body. Its blood supply arises mainly from the peripatellar plexus. The patella articulates with the femoral sulcus, otherwise known as the trochlea. It is asymmetrically oval in shape with the apex distal. It is enveloped by fibers of the quadriceps tendon and blends with the patellar tendon distally. The patella serves as a fulcrum for the quadriceps muscles. The main biomechanical function of the patella is to increase the moment arm of the quadriceps mechanism.

- The patellar surface is divided into two large facets — medial and lateral, which are separated by a central ridge. The facets are covered by the thickest hyaline cartilage in the body that may measure up to 6.5 mm. The superior three-fourths of the patella are articular, and the inferior one-fourth is non-articular. The contact area between the patella and femur varies with knee position. At 10–20 degrees of knee flexion, the distal pole of the patella contacts the femoral trochlea. As flexion increases, the contact of the patella moves proximally and medially with the most extensive contact being made at approximately 45 degrees (2,6,12,23). Contact stresses on the patellofemoral joint are higher than any other major weight-bearing joint in the body. The contact area and load across the joint increase with knee flexion. Compressive forces on the patella can range from 3.3 times body weight with stair climbing up to 7.6 times body weight with squatting (20).

- The patellar medial facet varies anatomically. It may be divided into a medial facet proper and a small odd facet. The odd facet may develop as a response to functional loads and does not contact the medial femoral condyle except in extreme flexion.

- Several ossification centers contribute to the patella. Failure of fusion can lead to bipartite patella that can be classified into three types: type I — inferior; type II — lateral; and type III — superolateral (most common). Bipartite patella is most often discovered accidentally during radiographic examination of the knee for another disorder. The rate of bipartite patellae is approximately 1%, and of these cases, more than 55% are unilateral. A bipartite patella may mimic a patellar sleeve fracture in children or an osteochondral fracture after trauma on plain radiographs.

- Within the medial retinaculum is the medial patellofemoral ligament and the medial patellotibial ligament. The medial patellofemoral ligament originates from the adductor tubercle and inserts on the medial border of the patella. This ligament plays a major role in preventing lateral displacement of the patella (4) and is the most commonly injured structure in acute patellar dislocations. The lateral retinaculum is composed of a superficial and deep layer and runs from lateral margin of the patella and patellar tendon to the anterior aspect of the iliotibial band.

- The patellar tendon varies in length from 4.0–6.9 cm (average, 4.6 cm) (18,24,27,32). It connects the apex of the patella to the tibial tuberosity and is slightly wider proximally than distally. The patella is commonly associated with either alta or baja, meaning it is high or low, respectively, in reference to standardized controls. Patients with patella alta may have instability (32), whereas patients with patella baja may display limited range of motion; this is commonly a consequence of surgery or trauma. The thickness of the patellar tendon is 4–7 cm, with the mean being 5.5 cm, proximally and 5–7 cm, with a mean of 5.4 cm, in its midsubstance (18,24,27).

PATELLAR PAIN

- The single most common cause of knee pain involves pathology related to the patella (9,29,35). Patellar pain or discomfort may be the result of direct trauma, repetitive direct pressure, constant repetitive movements with the knee in a flexed position, instability, malalignment, or a combination of these factors. It can arise from bony, soft tissue structures or even can be referred pain from the hip or spine.

- Symptoms of patellar pain that begin during relatively normal activities/sports should alert the physician that the knee may not have been normal in the first place or that there is a chronic overuse entity. If the knee swells significantly within the first 12–24 hours after traumatic knee injury, this signifies that there is blood or a hemarthrosis within the joint. The most common cause of an acute hemarthrosis after a sports-related knee injury is a tear of the anterior cruciate ligament, with the second most common cause being a traumatic patellar dislocation/subluxation with bleeding as a result of either soft tissue tearing, osteochondral fracture, or both.

PHYSICAL EXAMINATION (12)

- The physical examination should begin with general inspection for skin abrasions, contusions, lacerations, and prior surgical incisions.

- It is important to document the overall alignment of the leg while the patient is standing, seated, and supine. Start with the patient in the standing position and observe the amount of standing varus or valgus alignment. Patellofemoral crepitus is best elicited by having the patient stand and then squat down with the examiner's hands over the patella noting at what arc of motion the crepitus occurs. Retropatellar crepitus that is painful and occurs in either early flexion or terminal extension indicates disease on the distal part of the patella. A painful arc with crepitus in greater degrees of flexion indicates disease on the more proximal portion of the patella. Also observe for excessive pes planus or other abnormal foot alignments while standing. This is usually best accomplished by standing behind the patient.

- With the patient in the seated position, observe patellofemoral tracking with the patient seated over the edge of the table while slowly flexing and extending the knee from 0–90 degrees. Observe for high or lateral patellar positioning (grasshopper eyes), small patella, patella alta (the patella faces the ceiling rather than straight ahead), and vastus medialis oblique (VMO) dysplasia. Also, the examiner should observe for signs of J tracking (the patella deviates laterally in terminal extension as the patient extends the knee from a flexed position, thus mimicking a J). Thigh circumference should be measured at a consistent level above the knee to assess for quadriceps atrophy. Palpate for crepitation, suggesting possible chondral injury, noting at what degree of knee flexion that crepitus is present to delineate between proximal and distal lesions.

- With the patient supine, patellar alignment and Q angle (angle between anterior superior iliac spine, patella, and tibial tubercle) are measured. A Q angle of less than 15 degrees is generally considered normal. The Q angle should be assessed with the knee flexed at 30 degrees when the patella should be centered in the trochlear groove. An angle greater than 25 degrees with this method is indicative of an abnormally lateralized patellar vector. If the patella is subluxated, the Q angle can yield a falsely low measurement (21). One-finger palpation is important to localize tenderness, whether it is in the retinaculum or the medial and lateral patellar facets. These are best palpated by placing one finger under the respective facet and pushing the patella over to that side with the other hand. The quadriceps tendon and patellar tendon are also best palpated in a resting position with the knee extended. Point tenderness at the inferior pole of the patella at the attachment of the patellar tendon is typically consistent with patellar tendonitis (24) or jumper's knee. The tenderness is more pronounced with the patellar tendon relaxed with the knee in the extended position. Usually, this area is less tender with the knee in the flexed position. Lateral displacement may cause apprehension in patients with patellar instability; this is called the "apprehension sign." When assessing for instability, measure patellar mobility (patellar glide). This is based on the maximum amount of passive displacement of the patella (using quadrant system with the patella divided into four vertical quadrants) both medially and laterally with the knee at 0 and 30 degrees of flexion. This test evaluates the integrity and tightness of the medial and lateral restraints. The sage sign tests the amount of medial translation of the patella in 20–30 degrees of flexion with respect to the same quadrant system. Any translation greater than two quadrants or a side-to-side difference is considered abnormal. The passive patellar tilt test determines the tension of the lateral restraints. With the knee fully extended, the patella is manually elevated. A passive tilt of less than 0 degrees (neutral or below the horizontal plane) may imply lateral retinacular tightness, increased patellar tilt, and a diagnosis of excessive lateral pressure syndrome (ELPS). Documentation of the full range of motion should be done in the supine position as well. Femoral anteversion and tibial torsion should be examined with the patient in the prone position.

RADIOGRAPHS

- Patients who present with patellofemoral complaints should undergo standard knee radiographs in order to rule out associated pathology. These radiographs include bilateral weight-bearing anteroposterior (AP), bilateral weight-bearing flexion posteroanterior (PA), a true lateral radiograph at 30 degrees of flexion, and bilateral axial views at 30, 60, and 90 degrees. The standard patellar radiograph is the axial view or sunrise view. It is generally performed with the patient supine with the knee flexed 45 degrees to evaluate for articular cartilage loss, tilt, and subluxation (30). The Laurin view (20-degree sunrise view) may be more sensitive for delineating subluxation or tilt (26). The flexion lateral view at 30 degrees is important to evaluate for patella alta and infera, as well as trochlear dysplasia (8).

- A computed tomography (CT) scan from 0–60 degrees of knee flexion may be useful to evaluate for tilt and subluxation (14). The axial images will allow measurement of the tibial tubercle to trochlear groove (TT-TG) distance — a radiographic Q angle. This important measurement gives an accurate quantitative assessment of subluxation.

- Magnetic resonance imaging (MRI) can also help delineate patellofemoral pathology. There have been many studies examining the role of MRI for evaluation of the articular surfaces of the patellofemoral joint. Most of these note an underestimation of damage in early stages of cartilage damage. MRI was more useful in moderate to advanced patellar cartilage damage (17,31). MRI is also useful in detecting intra-articular pathology such as meniscal tears, cruciate or collateral ligament injuries, and osteochondral defects.

GENERAL TREATMENT OF PATELLOFEMORAL PAIN

■ Nonoperative treatment is the mainstay for patellofemoral pain (2,3,5,6,11–15,19,22,28,34). Nonsteroidal anti-inflammatory drugs (NSAIDs) may be beneficial if there is an inflammatory component to the patellar dysfunction. Simple bracing with a patellar cutout or patellar stabilizing braces may be beneficial to many patients. Differing types of braces act either to help recreate proper tracking or via a lateral buttress effect. Taping techniques, such as those described by McConnell (28) to stabilize subluxation or tilt, may also be beneficial to patients. Simple stretching and exercises can be easily learned by patients and are very useful. Prone quadriceps stretching, retinacular stretching, and short arc isotonic closed- or open-chain quadriceps strengthening can all be useful in diminishing pain from patellofemoral dysfunction. Isokinetic, eccentric, and high-torque exercises can cause high articular surface pressures and should be avoided.

SYNOVIAL PLICA

■ A synovial plica is a redundant fold in the synovial lining of the knee. This is a normal finding, but it may rarely become symptomatic when it becomes inflamed or fibrotic. A symptomatic plica is most commonly located on the medial side with a localized tender thickening along the medial border of the patella or condyle on palpation (knee at 45 degrees of flexion). An audible snap with flexion may sometimes be elicited with a plica. Nonoperative management of a synovial plica includes relative rest, flexibility exercises especially of the hamstrings, quadriceps strengthening, and anti-inflammatory medication. If the synovial plica is significantly scarred or fibrotic and cannot be rehabilitated, arthroscopic excision is indicated.

EXCESSIVE LATERAL PRESSURE SYNDROME

■ Excessive lateral patellar compression syndrome, or ELPS or lateral facet syndrome, represents a loss of equilibrium of the patella in the trochlea associated with tilt (11,13). This results in increased pressure on the lateral patellar facet. This is usually secondary to a tight lateral retinaculum. The patient with ELPS usually has a spontaneous or posttraumatic onset with patellofemoral arthralgia (dull aching in the center of the knee), and occasionally, swelling and giving way may be present. These patients are commonly tender over the lateral patellar facet. Radiographs or CT of patients with ELPS will usually show lateral patellar tilt on the axial views. Early treatment consists of nonoperative measures including lateral retinacular stretching, taping, and strengthening (11,13,34).

Operative management may include lateral release alone or with lateral patellar facetectomy (33) after conservative treatment fails to provide relief.

PATELLAR MALALIGNMENT AND INSTABILITY

■ Patellar malalignment and instability are two separate issues:
  ■ Malalignment indicates maltracking of the patella based on physical examination and imaging studies such as x-rays or CT. As discussed earlier, the TT-TG distance can give a quantitative measure of trochlear groove to tibial tubercle offset, which along with history and physical examination can suggest distal malalignment. A TT-TG distance of 12–15 mm is considered normal, whereas greater than 20 mm is abnormal (1,7,25).
  ■ Instability is a functional symptom with the patella transiently displacing (usually lateral) either partially (subluxation) or completely (dislocation). The main soft tissue restraint to lateral subluxation of the patella is the medial patellofemoral ligament (4). This is usually injured in an acute traumatic patellar dislocation. Initial treatment for instability is nonoperative with stretching, strengthening, McConnell taping, and bracing (15). Surgical correction is indicated when there is failure of nonoperative management or evidence of progressive articular cartilage damage as a result of the instability. Patellar realignment for recurrent instability is categorized as either proximal realignment (tightening, repairing, or reconstructing the medial soft tissue patellar restraints) or distal realignment (transposing the tibial tubercle medially or anteromedially (10) to correct tubercle malalignment, as documented by an abnormal Q angle or TT-TG distance. Moving the tibial tubercle (distal realignment) cannot be performed before skeletal maturity. Medial patellar instability is uncommon but can occur following previous lateral retinacular release (16).
  ■ Traumatic versus atraumatic instability is treated differently in regard to referral and surgical planning. Both entities should have all radiographic views upon presentation (weight-bearing AP, flexion PA, lateral at 30 degrees of flexion, and axial images). It is imperative to obtain the axial radiograph in the emergency department for an acute traumatic patellar dislocation/subluxation. Immediate referral should be obtained for acute traumatic subluxation/dislocation. Acute patellar dislocations are treated surgically if there are displaced osteochondral defects or for failure of reduction (which can only be assessed on the axial view) (11).

OSTEOCHONDRAL INJURY

■ Osteochondral injuries are frequently encountered following acute traumatic subluxation/dislocation. The patient will commonly give a history of a traumatic event with possible continued instability. They also may have symptoms of a loose body within the knee joint. These injuries are best evaluated with plain x-rays (all four radiographic views), CT scan, and MRI in order to determine the size and location of the fragment. Osteochondral fractures should be evaluated acutely with arthroscopy. Large articular fragments can and should be fixed acutely, whereas nondisplaced stable fractures can be managed nonsurgically.

FRACTURES

■ Fractures of the patella are most commonly from direct trauma to the anterior knee. Patella fractures can also occur via indirect mechanisms such as jumping or rapid flexion of the knee with maximal quadriceps contraction. Patellar fractures are most commonly transverse in orientation and are seen best on a lateral x-ray. Vertical fractures are rare and best seen on the sunrise view. Fracture types include undisplaced, transverse, lower or upper pole, comminuted, vertical, and stellate. Undisplaced fractures with an intact articular surface and preserved extensor mechanism are treated nonoperatively with 6 weeks of bracing/casting in extension followed by progressive range-of-motion exercises. Displaced fractures are those with at least 3 mm of cortical disruption or 2 mm of articular step-off on radiographs. These are treated with open reduction internal fixation (ORIF). Fractures that occur with patellar dislocation most commonly involve the lateral condyle or medial patellar facet. With a traumatic avulsion of the VMO in a previously normal knee, surgical repair and early motion are advocated.

REFERENCES

1. Beaconsfield T, Pintore E, Mafulli N, Petri GJ. Radiological measurements in patellofemoral disorders. A review. *Clin Orthop Relat Res.* 1994;(308):18–28.

2. Bentley G, Dowd G. Current concepts of etiology and treatment of chondromalacia patellae. *Clin Orthop Relat Res.* 1984;(189):209–28.

3. Boden BP, Pearsall AW, Garrett WE Jr, Feagin JA Jr. Patellofemoral instability: evaluation and management. *J Am Acad Orthop Surg.* 1997; 5(1):47–57.

4. Conlan T, Garth WP Jr, Lemons JE. Evaluation of the medial soft-tissue restraints of the extensor mechanism of the knee. *J Bone Joint Surg Am.* 1993;75(5):682–93.

5. Crossley K, Bennell K, Green S, Cowan S, McConnell J. Physical therapy for patellofemoral pain: a randomized, double-blinded, placebo-controlled trial. *Am J Sports Med.* 2002;30(6):857–65.

6. Dehaven KE, Dolan WA, Mayer PJ. Chondromalacia patella in athletes. Clinical preservation and conservative management. *Am J Sports Med.* 1979;7(1):5–11.

7. Dejour D, Le Coultre B. Osteotomies in patello-femoral instabilities. *Sports Med Arthrosc.* 2007;15(1):39–46.

8. Dejour H, Walch G, Neyret P, Adeleine P. La dysplasie de la trochlée femorale. *Rev Chir Orthop Reparatrice Appar Mot.* 1990;76(1):45–54.

9. Dye SF, Boll DA. Radionuclide imaging of the patellofemoral joint in young adults with anterior knee pain. *Orthop Clin North Am.* 1986;17(2):249–62.

10. Fulkerson JP. Anteromedialization of the tibial tuberosity for patellofemoral malalignment. *Clin Orthop Relat Res.* 1983;(177):176–81.

11. Fulkerson JP. Diagnosis and treatment of patients with patellofemoral pain. *Am J Sports Med.* 2002;30(3):447–56.

12. Fulkerson JP. *Disorders of the Patellofemoral Joint.* 4th ed. New York (NY): Lippincott Williams & Wilkins; 2004. 314 p.

13. Fulkerson JP. Patellofemoral pain disorders: evaluation and management. *J Am Acad Orthop Surg.* 1994;2(2):124–32.

14. Fulkerson JP, Schutzer SF, Ramsby GR, Bernstein RA. Computerized tomography of the patellofemoral joint before and after lateral release or realignment. *Arthroscopy.* 1987;3(1):19–24.

15. Fulkerson JP, Shea KP. Current concepts review disorders of patellofemoral alignment. *J Bone Joint Surg.* 1990;72–A(9):1424–9.

16. Gambardella RA. Technical pitfalls of patellofemoral surgery. *Clin Sports Med.* 1999;18(4):897–903.

17. Ghelman B, Hodge JC. Imaging of the patellofemoral joint. *Orthop Clin North Am.* 1992;23(4):523–43.

18. Griffiths GP, Selesnick FH. Operative treatment and arthroscopic findings in chronic patellar tendinitis. *Arthroscopy.* 1998;14(8):836–9.

19. Henry JH. Conservative treatment of patellofemoral subluxation. *Clin Sports Med.* 1989;8(2):261–78.

20. Huberti HH, Hayes WC. Contact pressures in chondromalacia patellae and the effects of capsular reconstructive procedures. *J Orthop Res.* 1988;6(4):499–508.

21. Hughston JC. Subluxation of the patella. *J Bone Joint Surg Am.* 1968; 50(5):1003–26.

22. Hungerford DS, Lennox DW. Rehabilitation of the knee in disorders of the patellofemoral joint: relevant biomechanics. *Orthop Clin North Am.* 1983;14(2):397–402.

23. Insall J. "Chondromalacia patellae": patellar malalignment syndrome. *Orthop Clin North Am.* 1979;10(1):117–27.

24. Johnson DP, Wakeley CJ, Watt I. Magnetic resonance imaging of patellar tendonitis. *J Bone Joint Surg Br.* 1996;78(3):452–7.

25. Jones R, Barlett EC, Vainright JR, Carroll RG. CT determination of tibial tubercle lateralization in patients presenting with anterior knee pain. *Skeletal Radiol.* 1995;24(7):505–9.

26. Laurin CA, Lévesque HP, Dussault R, Labelle H, Peides JP. The abnormal lateral patellofemoral angle. A diagnostic roentgenographic sign of recurrent patellar subluxation. *J Bone Joint Surg Am.* 1978;60(1):55–60.

27. Matava MJ. Patellar Tendon Ruptures. *J Am Acad Orthop Surg.* 1996; 4(6):287–96.

28. McConnell J. The management of chondromalacia patellae: a long-term solution. *Aust J Physiotherapy.* 1986;32(4):215–23.

29. Merchant AC. Classification of patellofemoral disorders. *Arthroscopy.* 1988;4(4):235–40.

30. Merchant AC, Mercer RL, Jacobsen RH, Cool CR. Roentgenographic analysis of patellofemoral congruence. *J Bone Joint Surg.* 1974;56(7):1391–6.

31. Nakanishi K, Inoue M, Harada K, et al. Subluxation of the patella: evaluation of patellar articular cartilage with MR imaging. *Br J Radiol.* 1992;65(776):662–7.

32. Neyret P, Robinson AH, Le Coultre B, Lapra C, Chambat P. Patellar tendon length — the factor in patellar instability. *Knee.* 2002;9(1):3–6.

33. Paulos LE, O'Connor DL, Karistinos A. Partial lateral patellar facetectomy for treatment of arthritis due to lateral patellar compression syndrome. *Arthroscopy.* 2008;24(5):547–53.

34. Radin EL. A rational approach to the treatment of patellofemoral pain. *Clin Orthop Relat Res.* 1979;144:107–9.

35. Wiles Philip, Andrews PS, Devas MB. Chondromalacia of the patella. *J Bone Joint Surg Br.* 1956;38–B(1):95–113.

63 Soft Tissue Knee Injuries (Tendon and Bursae)

Bryan J. Whitfield and John J. Klimkiewicz

BIOMECHANICS OF TENDON RUPTURES

Extensor mechanism force ratio

$$= \frac{\text{Patellar tendon force}}{\text{Quadriceps tendon force}}$$

- Position of knee flexion directly affects this ratio. At knee flexion angles < 45 degrees, this ratio is > 1, whereas at knee flexion angles > 45 degrees, this ratio is < 1 (16).
- At > 45 degrees, the patellar tendon has a mechanical advantage and is less susceptible to injury through tensile failure, whereas at positions < 45 degrees, the quadriceps tendon has a mechanical advantage and is less vulnerable to injury.
- Tendon strain in response to tensile load is up to three times greater at the insertion sites than at the tendon midsubstance. Additionally, collagen fiber stiffness is less at the insertion sites. These biomechanical properties contribute to tendon rupture commonly occurring at their insertion sites rather than at their midsubstance (50,51).
- Failure usually occurs during rapid eccentric muscular contraction when markedly higher forces can be generated as compared to concentric muscular contraction (12).
- This most often occurs with trauma causing forced extension of a flexed joint.
- Several metabolic diseases or direct steroid injection can predispose to tendon rupture. These conditions include hyperparathyroidism, calcium pyrophosphate deposition disease (CPPD), diabetes mellitus, chronic renal disease, gout, systemic lupus erythematosus, and rheumatoid arthritis (11,50).
- Fluoroquinolone antibiotics and isotretinoin treatment have been associated with pathologic tendon alteration and increased incidence of tendon rupture (47,49).

PATELLAR TENDON RUPTURES

- The patellar tendon receives its blood supply from the vessels within the infrapatellar fat pad and retinacular structures (2,45).
- The origin and insertion of the patellar tendon are relatively avascular.

- Ruptures of the patella tendon most typically occur in patients less than 40 years of age and are frequently associated with sporting activities including football, basketball, and soccer (33).
- Ruptures are most common through the tendon–bone junction at the distal pole of the patella.
- Histologic examination of rupture tendon often demonstrates an area of degeneration thought to predispose these patients to injury.
- Previous surgeries, including total knee arthroplasty, anterior cruciate ligament (ACL) reconstruction using autograft patellar tendon, and tibial intramedullary nailing, have been associated with postoperative patellar tendon ruptures (4,6,24).

Clinical Presentation

- At time of injury, a pop is often heard with an acute onset of pain and swelling. Patient is usually unable to actively extend knee or maintain it in an extended position against gravity. Chronic cases present with an extensor lag (33).
- A palpable defect is commonly present just below the distal pole of the patella.
- Concomitant ACL injuries are not uncommon and should be clinically ruled out.
- Plain radiographs often demonstrate a patella alta in comparison to the opposite knee using the Insall-Salvati Index (> 1.2) (1).

$$\text{Insall} - \text{Salvati Index} = \frac{\text{Length of patellar tendon}}{\text{Length of patella}}$$

(Normal value 0.8–1.2)

- An osseous fragment is present at times at the distal pole of the patella when an avulsion is part of the injury.
- Magnetic resonance imaging (MRI) is useful in cases where partial injury is suspected.

Treatment

- Partial tendon injuries can be treated conservatively by cylinder cast or brace with the leg placed in full extension for 4–6 weeks followed by progressive range of motion and strengthening.

- Complete ruptures should be directly repaired on an acute basis through transosseous drill holes through the patella. Once secured, the knee should have at least 90 degrees of flexion to avoid overconstraint. Primary repairs are often augmented with wire, mersilene tape, suture, or autologous hamstring tendon or iliotibial band (27).

- Chronic ruptures can involve proximal patellar migration and can often require quadriceps mobilization or V-Y advancement in order to restore patellar height.

- Semitendinosus/gracilis augmentation is recommended in the chronic scenario. Achilles tendon or patellar tendon allograft has often been found useful to replace/reinforce the reconstruction in chronic situations (17).

Complications

- After surgery, complications include knee stiffness and weakness. Rerupture is rare. Restoration of normal patellofemoral tracking and height at the time of surgery is essential to achieve optimal results. Residual weakness of extensor mechanism is more common in delayed repairs.

QUADRICEPS TENDON RUPTURES

- The quadriceps tendon is a coalescence of tendinous portions of the rectus femoris, vastus lateralis, vastus intermedius, and vastus medialis muscles.

- The quadriceps tendon receives its vascular supply from an anastomotic network including the lateral circumflex femoral artery, descending geniculate artery, and medial/lateral geniculate arteries (40).

- There is an avascular region of the deep part of the quadriceps tendon measuring 1.5×3.0 cm.

- Ruptures of the quadriceps tendon most typically occur in patients over 40 years of age and are three times more frequent than patella tendon ruptures. Unilateral injuries are up to 20 times more frequent than bilateral injury (18).

- The site of rupture usually occurs through a degenerative area within the tendon and seldom occurs in younger individuals. Systemic disease can lead to tendon degeneration and predispose to infrequent bilateral tendon ruptures (29).

Clinical Presentation

- Pain is often present before rupture. At time of injury, a pop is often heard with an acute onset of pain and swelling.

- In cases of partial injury or complete injuries that do not extend to include the retinacular tissue, the patient may be able to extend and resist gravity with an associated extensor lag, but in complete injuries, this is not possible.

- A palpable defect at the site of rupture is usually felt just superior to the proximal pole of the patella.

- Plain radiographs often demonstrate patellar baja, an avulsion of the superior pole of the patella, spurring of the superior patellar region, or calcification within the quadriceps tendon. Insall-Salvati Index is less than 0.8 (1).

- MRI is a useful adjunct study because it can demonstrate partial ruptures or preexisting disease within the quadriceps tendon.

Treatment

- Partial tears are often responsive to conservative treatment when the patient presents primarily with pain and has little loss of strength, retaining the ability to actively extend the knee against gravity.

- Conservative treatment consists of a long leg cylinder cast in full extension for 4–6 weeks, with progressive range of motion and strengthening thereafter for partial injuries.

- Complete ruptures respond best to immediate surgical repair in a direct end-to-end fashion after tendon debridement of necrotic tissue or with transosseous tunnels through the patella (42).

- Chronic rupture involving more significant tendon retraction often require quadriceps tendon advancement through a tendon Z-plasty or V-Y tendon lengthening and advancement technique. Interpositional autograft/allograft tendon has been used with success in this scenario (46).

- Success of repair is directly related to the length of time between injury and the time of surgery, with more chronic repairs producing less favorable outcomes. Age is also a factor, with better results in younger patients (26).

- The most common complications after surgery or conservative treatment include decreased quadriceps strength/function with an associated extensor lag and lack of knee flexion.

GASTROCNEMIUS RUPTURE

- Often referred to as *tennis leg*.

- Traumatic injury to middle-aged athlete presenting as sudden pain in posterior proximal calf region. Significant pain, swelling, and ecchymosis usually occur with 24 hours.

- Involves tearing of the medial head of the gastrocnemius muscle typically at its musculotendinous junction (35).

- Mechanism of injury combines ankle dorsiflexion in combination with knee hyperextension.

Differential Diagnoses

- Differential diagnoses involve plantaris rupture, thrombophlebitis, and an acute compartment syndrome (48).

- MRI remains the imaging modality of choice. Ultrasound can be employed to rule out thrombophlebitis.

- Can be associated with an acute compartment syndrome secondary to swelling.

Treatment

■ Treatment of isolated ruptures of the medial gastrocnemius involves compressive wrapping, activity modification including crutches if necessary, ankle range of motion, ice, and anti-inflammatory medications (13).

PATELLAR TENDINITIS

■ Caused by activities involving repeated extension of the knee.

■ Termed *jumper's knee*, because it is most common in sporting activities such as basketball, volleyball, and soccer. Seen most commonly in younger individuals from their adolescent years to 40 years of age (10).

■ Predisposing factors include abnormal patellofemoral tracking, patellar alta, chondromalacia, Osgood-Schlatter disease, and leg length discrepancy.

■ Can be confused with Sindig-Larsen-Johansson disease, which is a traction apophysitis of the distal pole of the patella that presents with similar complaints in a younger age group (usually under 20 years old).

■ Involves the most proximal part of the patellar tendon and its attachment to the distal pole of the patella. This area of tendon is thought to impinge under the patella during knee flexion, causing injury to the tendon (25).

■ The affected area of tendon resembles tendinosis in the form of tendon degeneration and not inflammation. Histologically, this tissue is characterized as undergoing *angiofibroblastic hyperplasia* with fibroblast proliferation, new blood vessel formation, chondromucoid deposition, and collagen fragmentation (23).

Clinical Presentation

■ Pain occurs with palpation in the area of tendon involvement just distal to its insertion on the inferior pole of the patella.

■ Pain is increased with activity requiring knee extension against resistance.

■ Tendon may acquire bogginess; however, there is no associated joint effusion.

■ Blazina et al. (3) have classified this condition based on the patients' symptoms: (a) Pain only after activity. (b) Pain is present before activity, and then disappears, only to return near the end of activity with muscular fatigue. (c) Pain is constant with both rest and activity. (d) Patellar tendon rupture.

Radiographic Evaluation

■ Mainly a clinical diagnosis, but plain x-rays, although usually normal, can at times demonstrate an osteopenia at the distal pole of the patella, a traction osteophyte in the area of involvement, and calcification of the tendon.

■ MRI is the study of choice in the chronic setting because it can clearly identify the area of tendon involvement. This area usually involves the posterior aspect of the tendon in its proximal third (20).

Treatment

■ Conservative treatment is usually successful and includes rest, ice, and anti-inflammatory medication. Therapeutic modalities including ultrasound, iontophoresis, and phonophoresis are helpful in pain relief (31,39).

■ Once the pain has subsided, physiotherapy in the form of quadriceps strengthening and hamstring stretching is begun with gradual return to activity.

■ An elastic knee sleeve or counterforce brace (Cho-Pat–type brace) has also proved beneficial.

■ More chronic cases with pathology demonstrable on MRI scan require surgical debridement and excision of the diseased tendon and adjacent bone through either an open or arthroscopic approach (5,14,44).

QUADRICEPS TENDINITIS

■ Not as common as patellar tendonitis but has similar risk factors.

■ Repetitive microtrauma through overuse can lead to localized degeneration of the quadriceps tendon at its insertion into the superior pole of the patella.

■ Chronic symptoms in this area appear to be a risk factor for future tendon rupture.

Clinical Presentation

■ Pain with exertion and tenderness over affected area of quadriceps insertion. This most commonly is the lateral aspect of the tendon.

■ Radiographs often demonstrate calcification of the tendon at its insertion to the patella or a traction osteophyte at the osseous margin.

Treatment

■ Treatment is similar to that of patellar tendonitis. Results of conservative treatment are excellent, although more chronic cases can require open surgical debridement (19).

POPLITEUS TENDINITIS

■ Popliteus tendon travels from its origin on the lateral femoral condyle posterolaterally through the popliteal hiatus to insert on the posterior aspect of the proximal tibia (30).

■ Injuries to this area are a cause of posterolateral knee pain and can occur both acutely (*i.e.*, ACL rupture or posterolateral corner injuries) or more chronically as an overuse phenomenon. Chronic injuries most often occur with excessive downhill running or walking (*i.e.*, backpacking) (34,37).

Clinical Presentation

- Pain to palpation posterolaterally over the popliteus tendon. This is best appreciated clinically by placing the leg in a figure-of-four position and palpating at the origin of the popliteus just anterior to the lateral femoral epicondyle.
- Differential diagnosis includes iliotibial band syndrome, lateral meniscal tear, and biceps femoris tendonitis. LCL and posterolateral corner ligamentous injuries usually occur with acute trauma as opposed to a chronic injury.

Treatment

- Includes rest and activity modification in the form of eliminating downhill activity. Anti-inflammatory medication and physiotherapeutic modalities are also helpful (34). A generalized knee-strengthening program is instituted following resolution of symptoms.

ILIOTIBIAL BAND SYNDROME

- Most common cause of lateral-sided knee pain in long-distance runners. Also seen in cyclists, weightlifters, and football, soccer, and tennis players. Often precipitated by downhill running (38).
- Caused by excessive friction between iliotibial band and lateral epicondyle. Knee flexion angle of 30 degrees maximizes friction between these two structures, causing an ensuing bursitis.
- Anatomic factors predisposing to this condition include genu varum, tibial varum, varus hindfoot, and compensatory foot hyperpronation.

Clinical Presentation

- Lateral-sided knee pain that usually is present after initial warm-up that often causes cessation of activity. Pain not present at rest.
- Point of maximal tenderness is approximately 3 cm proximal to lateral joint line over lateral epicondylar region.
- *Ober's* and *Noble's* tests are positive and can confirm diagnosis.
- Ober's test: Patient is placed in lateral decubitus position with the affected extremity upwards. The unaffected knee and hip are flexed. The involved knee is flexed and hip hyperextended and adducted. Tightness or pain along the iliotibial tract will prevent the affected extremity from adducting below the horizontal created by the patient's torso (43).
- Noble's test: Patient is in supine position with the knee flexed 90 degrees. Pain is elicited in lateral epicondylar region when the patient's knee is extended between 30 and 40 degrees.

- Radiographs are negative in this condition. MRI can confirm more chronic cases unresponsive to conservative treatment.

Treatment

- Conservative treatment focusing on iliotibial tract, hamstring, and hip external rotator stretching combined with strengthening of the hip abductors is usually successful when combined with activity modification and anti-inflammatory treatment. Foot orthotics can also be a useful adjunct in conservative treatment.
- Surgical excision of the posterior aspect of the iliotibial tract overlying the lateral epicondyle at 30–40 degrees of knee flexion is effective in chronic cases not responding to conservative treatment (32).

PREPATELLAR BURSITIS

- Prepatellar bursa is a potential space of synovial tissue that functions to decrease the friction between the overlying subcutaneous tissue and patella.
- A bursitis can result from an acute injury, infection, systemic disease (*i.e.*, gout), or chronic activity or overuse (8).
- Commonly seen in the sport of wrestling (36).

Clinical Presentation

- Patients typically present with swelling superficial to the patella. Knee range of motion may be limited at the extremes of flexion pending the size of the collection but is painless. There is no associated effusion. Crepitation and thickening of the tissue involving the bursal tissue are often present in more chronic cases.
- Warmth, erythema, and pain to palpation may signify a septic process, but aspiration is necessary to confirm this because not all infected bursae are clinically demonstrable.
- Most common infecting organisms include *Staphylococcus aureus* and streptococcal species.
- On synovial fluid analysis, greater than 75% polymorphonuclear cell differential is most accurate in confirming a septic process. Total white blood cell count and glucose levels are less predictable (15).
- Radiographs are usually negative aside from radiolucency in the area of the bursitis. In cases involving gouty deposits, calcific stippling can be seen.

Treatment

- Treatment for aseptic bursitis in this region is activity modification, compressive wrapping, and anti-inflammatory medications. In more chronic situations, aspiration in combination with immobilization in extension can be useful.

- Septic or more chronic aseptic processes are best treated with surgical excision via open or arthroscopic techniques. Cases of septic bursitis should be treated with postoperative antibiotics sensitive to the infecting organism (22).

PES ANSERINE BURSITIS

- Pes anserine bursa is the synovial tissue overlying the attachment of the sartorius, gracilis, and semitendinosus tendons.
- Patients present with pain over this bursal region with often some swelling in this region.
- Differential diagnoses include medial collateral ligament injury, medial meniscal tear, medial compartmental arthritis, patellofemoral syndrome, saphenous neuritis, and stress fracture or avascular necrosis of the medial tibial plateau (28).

Treatment

- Treatment comprises activity modification, anti-inflammatory medications, hamstring stretching, and physiotherapy modalities. Recalcitrant cases often respond to a corticosteroid injection.

SYNOVIAL PLICAE SYNDROME

- Plicae are defined as synovial folds of tissue within the knee. They are described as suprapatellar, infrapatellar, medial, or lateral based on their position within the knee (7).
- Ninety percent of cadavers studied on anatomic dissection have the presence of at least one of the synovial plicae described.
- Not all plicae are symptomatic. Differential diagnoses include patellofemoral syndrome and meniscal/chondral pathology. Medial plicae are most commonly associated with symptoms. Its presence noted at the time of arthroscopy in all patients ranges from 19% to 70% (21,41).
- Patients often describe pain over the affected plicae in combination with intermittent snapping or giving way.
- Clinically, this snapping can often be elicited with manipulation of the plicae at varying degrees of flexion between 45 and 60 degrees.
- Radiographic studies, including x-rays and MRI, are usually negative. The latter is often obtained to rule out other intra-articular pathology.

Treatment

- Treatment is usually conservative with nonsteroidal anti-inflammatory drugs and activity modification. Steroid injections, either into the plica or placed into the intra-articular space, have proven to be effective in more unresponsive cases.

- Arthroscopic resection is limited to patients not responding to conservative treatment and has mixed results. Associated chondral injuries and concurrent patellofemoral maltracking have been implicated in arthroscopic failures, which have been reported to be as high as 30% (9).

REFERENCES

1. Aglietti P, Buzzi R, Insall J. Disorders of the patellofemoral joint. In: Insall JN, Scott WN, editors. *Surgery of the Knee.* 3rd ed. New York: Churchill Livingstone; 2001. p. 930–1.
2. Arnoczky SP. Blood supply to the anterior cruciate ligament and supporting structures. *Orthop Clin North Am.* 1985;16(1):15–28.
3. Blazina ME, Kerlan RK, Jobe FW, Carter VS, Carlson GJ. Jumper's knee. *Orthop Clin North Am.* 1973;4(3):665–78.
4. Bonamo JJ, Krinick RM, Sporn AA. Rupture of the patellar ligament after use of its central third for anterior cruciate reconstruction. A report of two cases. *J Bone Joint Surg Am.* 1984;66(8):1294–7.
5. Coleman BD, Khan KM, Kiss ZS, Bartlett J, Young DA, Wark JD. Open and arthroscopic patellar tenotomy for chronic patellar tendinopathy. A retrospective outcome study. Victorian Institute of Sport Tendon Study Group. *Am J Sports Med.* 2000;28(2):183–90.
6. Crossett LS, Sinha RK, Sechriest VF, Rubash, HE. Reconstruction of a ruptured patellar tendon with Achilles tendon allograft following total knee arthroplasty. *J Bone Joint Surg Am.* 2002;84-A:1354–61.
7. Dandy DJ. Anatomy of the medial suprapatellar plicae and medial synovial shelf. *Arthroscopy.* 1990;6(2):79–85.
8. Dawn B, Williams JK, Walter SE. Prepatellar bursitis. A unique presentation in tophaceous gout in an normouricemic patient. *J Rheumatol.* 1997;24(5):976–8.
9. Dupont JY. Synovial plicae of the knee. Controversies and review. *Clin Sports Med.* 1997;16(1):87–122.
10. Ferretti A, Puddu G, Mariani PP, Neri M. The natural history of jumper's knee. Patellar or quadriceps tendonitis. *Int Orthop.* 1985;8(4):239–42.
11. Ford LT, DeBender J. Tendon rupture after local steroid injection. *South Med J.* 1979;72(7):827–30.
12. Garrett WE Jr. Injuries to muscle-tendon unit. *Instr Course Lect.* 1988;37:275–82.
13. Gecha S, Torg E. Knee injuries in tennis. *Clin Sports Med.* 1988;7(2):435–52.
14. Griffiths GP, Selesnick FH. Operative treatment and arthroscopic findings in chronic patellar tendinitis. *Arthroscopy.* 1998;14(8):836–9.
15. Ho G Jr, Tice AC. Comparison of nonseptic and septic bursitis. Further observations on the treatment of septic bursitis. *Arch Intern Med.* 1979;139(11):1269–73.
16. Huberti HH, Hayes WC, Stone JL, Shybut GT. Force ratios in the quadriceps tendon and ligamentum patellae. *J Orthop Res.* 1984;2(1):49–54.
17. Hyman J, Rodeo SA, Wickiewicz T. Patellofemoral tendinopathy. In: Drez D Jr, DeLee JC, Miller M, editors. *DeLee & Drez's Orthopaedic Sports Medicine: Principles and Practice.* 2nd ed. Philadelphia: Saunders; 2003. p. 1849–54.
18. Ilan DI, Tejwani N, Keschner M, Leibman M. Quadriceps tendon rupture. J Am Acad Orthop Surg. 2003;11(3):192–200.
19. James SL. Running injuries to the knee. *J Am Acad Orthop Surg.* 1995;3(6):309–18.
20. Johnson DP, Wakely CJ, Watt I. Magnetic resonance imaging of patellar tendonitis. *J Bone Joint Surg Br.* 1996;78(3):452–7.
21. Joyce JJ, Harty M. Surgery of the synovial fold. In: Cassells W, editor. *Arthroscopy: Diagnosis in Surgical Practice.* Philadelphia: Lea & Febiger; 1984. p. 201–9.

22. Kaalund S, Breddam M, Kristensen G,. Endoscopic resection of the septic prepatellar bursa. *Arthroscopy*. 1998;14(7):757–8.

23. Kannus P, Józsa L. Histopathologic changes preceding spontaneous rupture of a tendon. A controlled study of 891 patients. *J Bone Joint Surg Am*. 1991;73(10):1507–25.

24. Keating JF, Orfaly R, O'Brien PJ. Knee pain after tibial nailing. *J Orthop Trauma*. 1997;11(1):10–3.

25. King JB, Perry DJ, Mourad K, Kumar SJ. Lesions of the patellar ligament. *J Bone Joint Surg Br*. 1990;72(1):46–8.

26. Konrath GA, Chen D, Lock T, et al. Outcomes following repairs of quadriceps tendon ruptures. *J Orthop Trauma*. 1998;12(4):273–9.

27. Larson E, Lund PN. Ruptures of the extensor mechanism of the knee joint. Clinical results and patellofemoral articulation. *Clin Orthop Relat Res*. 1986;(213):150–3.

28. Larsson LG, Baum J. The syndrome of anserine bursitis: an overlooked diagnosis. *Arthritis Rheum*. 1985;28(9):1062–5.

29. Lauerman WC, Smith BG, Kenmore PI. Spontaneous bilateral rupture of the extensor mechanism of the knee in two patients on chronic ambulatory peritoneal dialysis. *Orthopedics*. 1987;10(4):589–91.

30. Mann RA, Hagy JL. The popliteus muscle. *J Bone Joint Surg Am*. 1977;59(7):924–7.

31. Martens M, Libbrecht P, Burssens A. Surgical treatment of iliotibial band friction syndrome. *Am J Sports Med*. 1989;17(5):651–4.

32. Martens M, Wouters P, Burssens A, Mulier JC. Patellar tendinitis: pathology and results of treatment. *ACTA Orthop Scand*. 1982;53(3):445–50.

33. Matava MJ. Patella tendon ruptures. *J Am Acad Orthop Surg*. 1996;4(6):287–96.

34. Mayfield GW. Popliteus tendon tenosynovitis. *Am J Sports Med*. 1977;5(1):31–6.

35. Miller WA. Rupture of the musculotendinous juncture of the medial head of the gastrocnemius muscle. *Am J Sports Med*. 1977;5(5):191–3.

36. Mysnyk MC, Wroble RR, Foster DT, Albright JP. Prepatellar bursitis in wrestlers. *Am J Sports Med*. 1986;14(1):46–54.

37. Naver L, Aalberg JR. Avulsion of the popliteus tendon. A rare cause of chondral fracture and hemarthrosis. *Am J Sports Med*. 1985;13(6):423–4.

38. Orava S. Iliotibial friction syndrome in athletes — an uncommon exertion syndrome on the lateral side of the knee. *Br J Sports Med*. 1978;12(2):69–73.

39. Panni AS, Tartarone M, Maffulli N. Patellar tendinopathy in athletes. Outcome of nonoperative and operative management. *Am J Sports Med*. 2000;28(3):392–7.

40. Petersen W, Stein V, Tillmann B. Blood supply of the quadriceps tendon. *Unfallchirurg*. 1999;102(7):543–7.

41. Pipkin G. Knee injuries: the role of the suprapatellar plica and suprapatellar bursa in simulating internal derangements. *Clin Orthop Relat Res*. 1971;74:161–76.

42. Rasul AT Jr, Fischer DA. Primary repair of quadriceps tendon ruptures. Results of treatment. *Clin Orthop Relat Res*. 1993;289:205–7.

43. Renne JW. The iliotibial band friction syndrome. *J Bone Joint Surg Am*. 1975;57(8):1110–1.

44. Romeo AA, Larson RV. Arthroscopic treatment of infrapatellar tendonitis. *Arthroscopy*. 1999;15(3):341–5.

45. Scapinelli R. Studies on the vasculature of the human knee joint. *Acta Anat (Basel)*. 1968;70(3):305–31.

46. Scuderi C. Rupture of the quadriceps tendon; study of twenty tendon ruptures. *Am J Surg*. 1958;95(4):626–34.

47. Scuderi AJ, Datz FL, Valdivia S, Morton KA. Enesthopathy of the patellar tendon insertion associated with isotretinoin therapy. *J Nucl Med*. 1993;34(3):455–7.

48. Severence HW Jr, Bassett FH 3rd. Rupture of the plantaris — does it exist? *J Bone Joint Surg Am*. 1982;64(9):1387–8.

49. Williams RJ 3rd, Attia E, Wickiewicz TL, Hannafin JA. The effect of ciprofloxacin on tendon, paratenon, and capsular fibroblast metabolism. *Am J Sports Med*. 2000;28(3):364–9.

50. Woo SLY, Maynard J, Butler D, et al. Ligament, tendon and joint capsule insertions into bone. In: Woo S, Buckwalter JJA, editors. *Injury and Repair of the Musculoskeletal Soft Tissues*. Park Ridge: American Academy of Orthopedic Surgeons; 1988. p. 133–66.

51. Zernicke RF, Garhammer J, Jobe FW. Human patellar tendon rupture. *J Bone Joint Surg*. 1977;59(2):179–83.

64 Ankle Instability

R. Todd Hockenbury

DEFINITION OF ANKLE SPRAIN

- An ankle sprain is a tear of the ligaments supporting the ankle joint.
- Ankle sprains are common. They constitute 25% of all sports-related injuries (33).
- Ankle sprains make up 21%–53% of basketball injuries and 17%–29% of all soccer injuries (13,19).
- An age of 10–19 years old is associated with higher rates of ankle sprain. Nearly half of all ankle sprains occur during athletic activity, with basketball (41.1%), football (9.3%), and soccer (7.9%) being associated with the highest percentage of ankle sprains during sports (61).

ANATOMY AND PATHOPHYSIOLOGY

Anatomy

- The ankle, or talocrural, joint consists of the talus, tibial plafond, medial malleolus, and lateral malleolus. The distal tibia and lateral malleolus form a mortise, in which the talus sits.
- The talus is wider anteriorly than posterior, thus resulting in a tighter fit and more stable articulation between the talus and mortise during ankle dorsiflexion.
- Ankle joint stability depends on joint congruency and the supporting ligamentous structures.
- The lateral ankle ligaments are the anterior talofibular ligament (ATFL), calcaneofibular ligament (CFL), and posterior talofibular ligament (PTFL). The medial ankle ligaments are the deep and superficial portions of the deltoid ligament.
- The relative strengths of the ankle ligaments from weakest to strongest are ATFL, CFL, PTFL, and deltoid (4).
- The syndesmotic ligaments connect and stabilize the distal fibula to the distal tibia. The syndesmotic ligaments are the anterior tibiofibular ligament, posterior tibiofibular ligament, transverse tibiofibular ligament, interosseous ligament, and interosseous membrane.
- The subtalar (talocalcaneal) joint lies inferior to the ankle joint and is responsible for hindfoot inversion and eversion. Up to 50% of clinical ankle inversion occurs at the subtalar joint (51).

Joint Mechanics

- The ankle is a hinge joint that permits flexion, extension, and rotation. The talus externally rotates with ankle dorsiflexion and internally rotates during plantarflexion (46).
- The distal fibula externally rotates during ankle dorsiflexion and moves distally during weight bearing, thus deepening and stabilizing the ankle mortise (60).
- The ankle mortise widens with ankle dorsiflexion and with weight bearing.
- The ATFL and CFL act synergistically to resist ankle inversion forces. The ATFL resists ankle inversion in plantarflexion, and the CFL resists ankle inversion during ankle dorsiflexion.
- The CFL spans both the lateral ankle joint and lateral subtalar joint, thus contributing to both ankle and subtalar joint stability (51).
- The PTFL limits posterior talar displacement and external rotation (48).
- The deltoid ligament resists ankle eversion, external rotation, and plantarflexion. In cases of distal fibular fracture and mortise instability, it restrains lateral talar translation (23).

Injury Mechanisms

- The most commonly sprained ankle ligament is the ATFL, followed by the CFL and then the PTFL. An isolated CFL or PTFL tear is rare. A tear of the ATFL almost always precedes a CFL tear. The ATFL is almost always torn, the CFL and PTFL are torn 50%–75% of the time, and the PTFL is torn in < 10% of ankle sprains (16).
- Lateral ankle sprains occur as a result of landing on a plantar flexed and inverted foot. These injuries occur while running on uneven terrain, stepping in a hole, stepping on another athlete's foot during play, or landing from a jump in an unbalanced position.
- A syndesmotic ankle sprain, or "high ankle sprain," occurs as a result of forced external rotation of a dorsiflexed foot or during internal rotation of the tibia on a fixed planted foot. A common mechanism is a direct blow to the back of the ankle while the patient is lying prone with the foot externally rotated (64).
- Isolated deltoid ligament sprains are rare and are usually accompanied by a lateral malleolar fracture and/or a syndesmotic injury. The deltoid ligament is injured through a mechanism of external rotation or eversion.

Injury Prevention

■ A balance training program has been shown to reduce the rate of ankle sprains in high school soccer and basketball players by one-third to one-half (14,34).

■ Studies are mixed regarding the efficacy of prophylactic bracing of athletes. A retrospective study of female college volleyball players who wore bilateral double-upright padded ankle braces showed a 93% reduction in ankle sprain incidence compared to the overall ankle injury rate in the National Collegiate Athletic Association (NCAA) (38). A prospective study of high school volleyball players found that ankle bracing did not overall decrease the incidence of sprains, except in those players who had not had a previous sprain. Players with a previous history of ankle sprain did not benefit from prophylactic bracing to prevent additional sprains. Players who had never had a sprain did show a lower incidence of initial ankle sprains with bracing (18).

Ligament Pathophysiology

■ Ligamentous injuries undergo a series of phases during the healing process: hemorrhage and inflammation, fibroblastic proliferation, collagen protein formation, and collagen maturation (1,9).

■ Early mobilization of joints following ligamentous injury actually stimulates collagen bundle orientation and promotes healing, although full ligamentous strength is not reestablished for several months (36,56,58).

■ Early treatment focuses on limiting soft tissue effusion, which speeds the healing process by lessening the amount of extracellular fluid and hematoma to be reabsorbed (24,43,55).

PHYSICAL EXAMINATION

■ Lateral ankle swelling and ecchymosis are present and are proportional to the degree of ligament damage.

■ Careful one-finger palpation is essential to define areas of tenderness and avoid misdiagnosis of associated fractures or tendon ruptures.

■ Common fractures that mimic ankle sprains are fractures of the lateral malleolus and medial malleolus, fifth metatarsal base, anterior process of the calcaneus, lateral process of the talus, posterior talar process, talar dome, and navicular.

■ Commonly missed tendon injuries are Achilles ruptures, peroneal tendon tears, peroneal tendon subluxation/dislocation, posterior tibial tendon injuries, anterior tibial tendon tears, and flexor hallucis longus tendon ruptures.

■ A careful neurologic examination is essential to rule out loss of sensation or motor weakness, because peroneal nerve and tibial nerve injuries are sometimes seen with severe lateral ankle sprains (35).

DIAGNOSTIC TESTS

Anterior Drawer Test

■ Tests the integrity of the ATFL.

■ Performed by stabilizing the anterior tibia just above the ankle with one hand while grasping the posterior heel with the other hand and applying an anteriorly directed force, and therefore attempting to translate the talus anteriorly.

■ The test should be performed on a relaxed leg with the knee bent and the ankle held in slight plantarflexion.

■ Normal anterior talar translation is less than 5 mm. The contralateral asymptomatic ankle should also be tested as a baseline.

Inversion Stress Test or Talar Tilt Test

■ Tests the integrity of the ATFL and CFL.

■ Performed by grasping the heel and inverting the ankle. A clunk may be heard or palpated in unstable ankles, as the medial talar dome impacts the distal tibial medial articular surface, indicating injury to one or both ligaments.

■ This test should be performed with the ankle in both dorsiflexion (to test the CFL) and plantarflexion (to test the ATFL).

Suction Sign

■ Tests the integrity of the ATFL.

■ During performance of the anterior drawer test, an unstable ankle will produce a dimple in the anterolateral ankle as the talus reaches it full anterior excursion. The dimple is formed by negative pressure within the ankle joint (26).

Squeeze Test

■ Tests the integrity of the syndesmotic ligaments.

■ The squeeze test is performed by placing the fingers over the proximal half of the fibula and thumb around the tibia and squeezing the two bones together. Pain in the distal ankle may indicate a syndesmotic injury (28,42).

External Rotation Stress Test

■ Tests the integrity of the syndesmotic ligaments.

■ The external rotation stress test is performed on the seated patient by externally rotating the foot while stabilizing the tibia with the other hand. Medial ankle pain or lateral talar motion indicates that a syndesmotic injury may be present.

■ Confirmatory anteroposterior and lateral external rotation stress radiographs will document widening of the syndesmosis and lateral talar subluxation (12,65).

IMAGING

Ottawa Ankle Rules (52)

- Every sprained ankle does not require screening radiographs.
- Anteroposterior, lateral, and oblique radiographs should be obtained if any of the below criteria are present:
  - Lateral or medial malleolar bone tenderness is present.
  - Patient is unable to bear weight for four steps both immediately after injury and in the emergency department.
- The Ottawa ankle rules do NOT apply in the following settings:
  - Age less than 18 years
  - Multiple painful injuries
  - Pregnancy
  - Diminished sensation due to neurologic deficit
- These criteria have been found to be 100% sensitive for detecting fracture while decreasing the incidence of unneeded radiographs (52).

Radiographs

- If radiographs are warranted, they should be examined closely for the following fractures that mimic ankle sprains:
  - Medial or lateral malleolus
  - Talar dome
  - Posterior malleolus (posterior distal tibia)
  - Posterior talar process
  - Lateral talar process
  - Anterior calcaneal process
  - "Flake fracture" off the posterior distal fibular rim, indicating a tear of the superior peroneal retinaculum and peroneal tendon dislocation
  - Navicular fracture
  - Widening of the medial clear space between the medial talar facet and medial malleolus, produced by lateral talar subluxation indicative of a tear of the deltoid ligament and probable syndesmotic ligament instability

Stress Radiographs

- Not required to make a diagnosis of an acute ankle sprain.
- Used primarily to document mechanical instability as a cause of chronic lateral ankle instability symptoms.
- Can be performed with or without the injection of local anesthetic into the lateral ankle. An injection of 5 cc of 1% Xylocaine (lidocaine) into the anterolateral ankle may yield a more reliable test due to patient comfort.
- Talar tilt test
  - The talar tilt test is performed by taking an anteroposterior or mortise view of the ankle while performing an inversion stress on the slightly plantarflexed ankle.
  - The talar tilt angle is obtained by measuring the angle subtended by a line parallel to the distal tibial articular surface and a line drawn along the superior articular surface of the talus.
  - Most authors agree that a difference of 5–15 degrees in talar tilt between the injured and uninjured side is diagnostic of mechanical ankle instability (44).
- Anterior drawer test
  - Anterior drawer stress radiographs are performed by taking a lateral radiograph of the ankle while attempting to translate the talus anteriorly within the mortise, as in the clinical anterior drawer test.
  - The anterior drawer is measured as the shortest distance between a point on the posterior aspect of the distal tibial articular surface and a point on the posterior aspect of the talar dome.
  - An anterior drawer difference of greater than 3 mm between injured and uninjured ankles is thought to be diagnostic of ATFL laxity (2).
- Stress radiographs for syndesmotic instability
  - A mortise stress radiograph of the ankle syndesmosis can be obtained by placing an external rotation force on the ankle while stabilizing the proximal tibia with the knee flexed 90 degrees.
  - Abnormal widening of the mortise and lateral talar shift indicates distal syndesmotic instability.

Magnetic Resonance Imaging

- Magnetic resonance imaging (MRI) is not needed for diagnosis in the acute setting unless occult fractures or tendon injury is suspected.
- MRI is most useful in diagnosing causes of the "chronically sprained" ankle, and MRI can diagnose talar dome injuries, peroneal tendon tears, bone bruises, or other occult fractures.

Computed Tomography Scan

- Not needed in the acute setting unless an occult fracture is suspected.
- More valuable than MRI in delineating bone or joint pathology (*i.e.*, talar dome fractures, lateral talar process fractures, tarsal coalition, subtalar arthritis, and loose bodies).

GRADING

- Grading of ankle sprains helps to guide treatment, rehabilitation, and prognosis. The grade is based on the number of ligaments injured, degree of ligament tearing (partial vs. complete tear), and amount of swelling and ecchymosis.
- The West Point ankle grading system is a useful tool for grading ankle sprains (Table 64.1) (21).

Table 64.1	West Point Ankle Sprain Grading System		
	Stage 1	**Stage 2**	**Stage 3**
Edema/ecchymosis	Localized/slight	Localized/moderate	Diffuse/significant
Weight-bearing ability	Full or partial without significant pain	Difficult without crutches	Impossible
Ligament pathology	Ligament stretch	Partial tear	Complete tear
Instability testing	None	None or slight	Definite
Time to return to sporting activities	11 days	2–6 weeks	4–26 weeks

INITIAL TREATMENT

PRICE — Protection, Rest, Ice, Compression, Elevation (44)

- Protection — Accomplished with the use of taping, a lace-up splint, a thermoplastic ankle stirrup splint, a functional walking orthosis, or a short leg cast. Early protected range of motion in a flexible or semirigid orthosis is superior to rigid cast immobilization in terms of patient satisfaction, return of motion and strength, and earlier return to function (3,30,31,41). Protected weight bearing in an orthosis is allowed with weight bearing to tolerance as soon as possible following injury. Crutches are used until pain-free weight bearing is achieved.

- Rest — Interruption of training in running or jumping sports is essential in limiting swelling and preventing early reinjury. Length of time to return to sports depends on injury grade (see Table 64.1).

- Ice — Cryotherapy is the application of cold to the ankle in the form of ice bags, a cold whirlpool, or a commercially available compressive cuff filled with circulating coolant. Early use of cryotherapy has been shown to enable patients to return to full activity more quickly (27).

- Compression — Compression can be applied to the ankle by means of an elastic bandage, felt doughnut, neoprene or elastic orthosis, or pneumatic device.

- Elevation — This initial treatment attempts to limit the amount of hematoma and extracellular fluid accumulation edema around the ankle in order to speed ligamentous healing.

Rehabilitation: 5 Phases (44)

- Acute — PRICE: Goal is to limit effusion, reduce pain, and protect from further injury.

- Subacute — Focus is on eliminating pain, increasing pain-free range of motion, continued protection against reinjury with bracing, limiting loss of strength with isometric exercises, and continued modalities to decrease pain and effusion.

- Rehabilitative — Emphasizes regaining full pain-free motion with joint mobilization and stretching, increasing strength with isotonic and isokinetic exercises, and proprioceptive training.

- Functional — Focuses on sports-specific exercises with a goal to return the patient to sports participation.

- Prophylactic — Seeks to prevent recurrence of injury through preventative strengthening, functional proprioceptive drills, and prophylactic support as needed. An 8-week proprioceptive training program has been shown to reduce the recurrence of ankle sprains and to be cost effective (29).

Treatment of Syndesmotic Ligament Injury, or "High Ankle Sprain"

- PRICE

- If the mortise is not widened or fractured, protection is in the form of a short leg cast or brace for 4 weeks, followed by physical therapy.

- In the presence of diastasis between the distal fibula and tibia on x-ray, operative stabilization of the syndesmotic ligament is required with a syndesmotic screw placed through the distal fibula and tibia parallel to the ankle joint.

- The patient should be warned that these injuries result in longer periods of disability than do injuries to the lateral collateral ligaments. In one study, only 44% of 16 patients had an acceptable outcome at 6 months (21).

- Heterotopic ossification of the distal syndesmosis has been reported in up to 25% of patients, although no correlation to ossification with functional outcome has been found (54).

Nonsurgical Treatment Results

- Primary ligamentous repair has not been supported by studies comparing early surgery to functional treatment of ankle sprains (50,62,66). MRI has documented satisfactory healing of lateral ankle ligaments with the use of a functional ankle brace (11).

- A prospective study of 146 patients with grade 3 ankle sprains who were randomized into operative and nonoperative groups found that the group treated with an ankle orthosis returned to work faster. No difference in joint laxity was found on stress radiographs 2 years after injury (40).

- A second controlled prospective study of 51 patients with grade III sprains randomized into operative and nonoperative groups followed for a mean of 14 years showed no difference in mean ankle score, ankle stability on stress radiographs, and return to preinjury functional level. Surprisingly, osteoarthritis was more common in the operative group (39).

CHRONIC ANKLE PAIN AND INSTABILITY

Pain versus Instability

■ For residual symptoms following an ankle sprain, initial work-up should center on whether the patient's chief complaint is pain or instability. This determination dictates further workup on the different sides of the diagnostic algorithm (Fig. 64.1).

Chronic Ankle Pain

■ In a retrospective study of 457 patients treated with immobilization or bracing, 72.6% reported residual symptoms at 6–18 months (6). A study of 96 ankle sprains in West Point cadets found residual symptoms in 40% of ankles at 6 months after injury (21).

■ Common causes of chronic ankle pain are occult fractures, tendon tears, nerve injury, or ankle soft tissue impingement.

■ An MRI or bone scan (technetium-labeled nuclear medicine study) is an excellent screening test to rule out occult fractures and to guide further treatment. If either test reveals an abnormality, then a spot radiograph or computed tomography scan is useful in further identifying the exact location of fracture.

■ Occult or associated injuries to the tendons of the foot and ankle should also be considered. The physical exam is crucial in testing for tendon integrity, strength, or tendon sheath swelling. MRI is the most useful exam to identify and confirm tendon injuries.

■ Injury to the lateral ankle ligaments may produce scarring of the ATFL and joint capsule, leading to the formation of "meniscoid tissue" in the anterolateral ankle. This inflamed tissue is pinched between the talus, fibula, and tibia, leading to a condition called anterolateral impingement (63).

■ MRI has been shown to have a 78.9% accuracy, 83.3% sensitivity, and 78.6% specificity in the diagnosis of anterolateral soft tissue impingement (15).

■ The distal fascicle of the anteroinferior tibiofibular ligament may abrade the anterolateral surface of the talus during ankle dorsiflexion during abnormal anterior translation of the talus (5).

■ An anomalous or accessory peroneal tendon may also cause chronic posterolateral ankle pain (57). Its presence is confirmed by MRI.

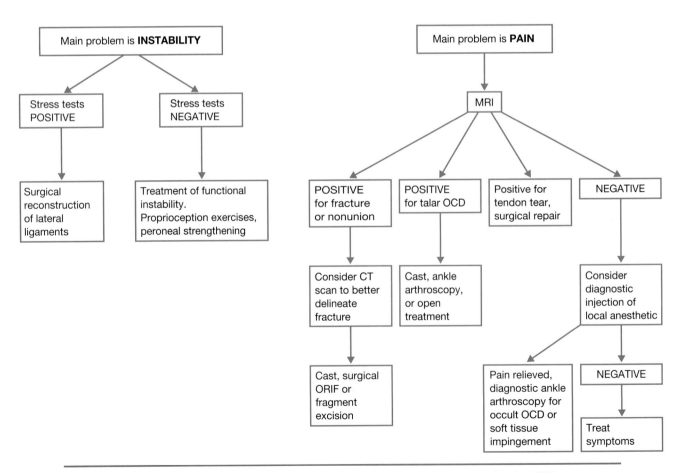

Figure 64.1: Chronic ankle pain algorithm. CT, computed tomography; MRI, magnetic resonance imaging; ORIF, open reduction internal fixation.

■ Nerve injury may result due to traction on the nerve during an inversion sprain. Electromyography performed 2 weeks after lateral ankle sprains in 36 patients with grade III injuries showed an 86% incidence of peroneal nerve injury and 83% incidence of tibial nerve injury (35). A cadaver study of a simulated ankle sprain has shown that traction on the superficial peroneal nerve causes nerve strain of enough magnitude to result in nerve injury (37).

Chronic Ankle Instability

■ If the primary problem is ankle instability, the patient will experience feelings of "giving way" of the ankle on uneven ground, inability to play cutting or jumping sports, loss of confidence in ankle support, and reliance on braces, and give a history of multiple ankle sprains.

■ The ankle should be evaluated with stress radiographs. If the stress radiographs are positive for mechanical lateral ligamentous laxity, then surgery is indicated to reconstruct the deficient ligaments.

■ If stress radiographs disprove mechanical laxity of the lateral ankle ligaments, then the patient may have functional ankle instability rather than true mechanical ankle instability. Functional instability is due to deficient neuromuscular control of the ankle, impaired proprioception, and peroneal weakness (17,20). Treatment in this case should be directed toward restoring peroneal tendon strength, restoring ankle motion, and improving ankle proprioception with physical therapy.

■ Chronic recurrent lateral ankle instability is associated with chondral damage. Ankle arthroscopy in 93 patients with chronic ankle instability showed moderate to severe cartilage damage in 41 patients (44%) (53). A retrospective study of 247 patients with ankle arthritis identified 33 patients with ligamentous end-stage ankle osteoarthritis. Eighty-five percent of patents had injured the lateral ligaments, and 15% of patients had injured both medial and lateral ankle ligaments. Mean time from injury to osteoarthritis was 34.3 years (59).

■ Other causes for ankle instability not demonstrated by stress radiographs include rotational instability of the talus, subtalar instability, distal syndesmotic (tibiofibular) instability, and hindfoot varus malalignment (25).

SURGICAL TREATMENT

Indications for Surgery

■ Multiple episodes of mechanical instability, *i.e.,* difficulty walking on uneven ground, inability to play cutting sports, lack of confidence in ankle stability

■ Demonstration of mechanical instability on stress radiographs

■ Failure of a full course of physical therapy emphasizing peroneal strengthening and proprioceptive training

■ Failure of a course of bracing

Surgical Procedures

■ Most procedures are designed to tighten or reconstruct the ATFL and CFL.

■ Ankle reconstructive procedures are described either as anatomic or nonanatomic procedures. Anatomic reconstructions attempt to tighten lateral ligaments or transfer tendons into the exact anatomic locations of the ATFL and CFL. Nonanatomic reconstructions use tendon transfers to act as a tenodesis on the lateral side of the ankle, although they do not attempt to place the transferred tendons to the exact anatomic origins of the ATFL or CFL. Most surgeons agree that anatomic reconstructions are preferable. A retrospective study comparing anatomic to nonanatomic ankle ligament reconstruction in 77 patients showed superior results in the anatomic reconstruction group (32).

■ The Brostrom procedure is an anatomic reconstruction in which the ATFL and CFL are divided and imbricated (7). Some authors advance the shortened ligaments into the distal fibula. This procedure is sometimes modified by advancing the extensor retinaculum proximally (the Gould modification) to further tighten the lateral aspects of the ankle and subtalar joints (22).

■ Tendon transfers most commonly use one-half of the peroneus brevis tendon, which is divided proximally about 15 cm proximal to its insertion in the base of the fifth metatarsal. The transferred peroneus brevis tendon is then passed through holes in the talar neck, distal fibula, and lateral calcaneus in order to reconstruct the lateral ligamentous structures. In lieu of drill holes, the transferred tendon may be sutured directly to bone using suture anchors. Due to concern of potentially weakening ankle eversion strength following harvest, Coughlin et al. (10) have successfully used gracilis autograft. Tendon allograft may also be used in lieu of autograft (8). A detailed discussion of all these procedures is beyond the scope of this chapter (45,47,49).

Postoperative Care

■ Following lateral ankle ligamentous reconstructive procedures, most postoperative regimens immobilize the ankle in a cast for 4 weeks followed by an orthosis for 4 additional weeks.

■ Physical therapy is instituted at 6–8 weeks after surgery with an emphasis on peroneal strengthening and proprioceptive training.

■ Return to sports occurs at about 3 months after surgery.

REFERENCES

1. Akeson WH, Woo SLY, Amiel D, et al. The chemical basis for tissue repair. In: Hunter LH, Funk FJ, editors. *Rehabilitation of the Injured Knee.* St. Louis: CV Mosby; 1984. p. 93.
2. Anderson KJ, Lecocq JF. Operative treatment of injury to the fibular collateral ligament of the ankle. *J Bone Joint Surg Am.* 1954;36-A(4):825–32.

3. Ardèvol J, Bolíbar I, Belda V, Argilaga S. Treatment of complete rupture of the lateral ligaments of the ankle: a randomized clinical trial comparing cast immobilization with functional treatment. *Knee Surg Sports Traumatol Arthrosc.* 2002;10(6):371–7.

4. Attarian DE, McCrackin HJ, DeVito DP, McElhaney JH, Garrett WE Jr. Biomechanical characteristics of human ankle ligaments. *Foot Ankle.* 1985;6(2):54–8.

5. Bassett FH 3rd, Gates HS 3rd, Billys JB, Morris HB, Nikolaou PK. Talar impingement by the anteroinferior tibiofibular ligament. A cause of chronic pain in the ankle after inversion sprain. *J Bone Joint Surg Am.* 1990;72(1):55–9.

6. Braun BL. Effects of ankle sprain in a general clinic population 6 to 18 months after medical evaluation. *Arch Fam Med.* 1999;8(2):143–8.

7. Broström L. Sprained ankles. VI. Surgical treatment of "chronic" ligament ruptures. *Acta Chir Scand.* 1966;132(5):551–65.

8. Caprio A, Oliva F, Treia F, Maffuli N. Reconstruction of the lateral ankle ligaments with allograft in patients with chronic ankle instability. *Foot Ankle Clin.* 2006;11(3):597–605.

9. Chvapil M. *Physiology of Connective Tissue.* London (UK): Butterworth's Scientific Publications; 1967. p. 246–86.

10. Coughlin MJ, Schenck RC Jr, Grebing BR, Treme G. Comprehensive reconstruction of the lateral ankle for chronic ankle instability using a free gracilis graft. *Foot Ankle Int.* 2004;25(4):231–41.

11. De Simoni C, Wetz HH, Zanetti M, Hodler J, Jacob H, Zollinger H. Clinical examination and magnetic resonance imaging in the assessment of ankle sprains treated with an orthosis. *Foot Ankle Int.* 1996;17(3):177–82.

12. Edwards GS Jr, DeLee JC. Ankle diastasis without fracture. *Foot Ankle.* 1984;4(6):305–12.

13. Ekstrand J, Tropp H. The incidence of ankle sprains in soccer. *Foot Ankle.* 1990;11(1):41–4.

14. Emery CA, Meeuwisse WH. The effectiveness of a neuromuscular prevention strategy to reduce injuries in youth soccer: a cluster-randomised controlled trial. *Br J Sports Med.* 2010;44(8):555–62.

15. Ferkel RD, Tyorkin M, Applegate GR, Heinen GT. MRI evaluation of anterolateral soft tissue impingement of the ankle. *Foot Ankle Int.* 2010;31(8):655–61.

16. Ferran NA, Maffulli N. Epidemiology of sprains of the lateral ankle ligament complex. *Foot Ankle Clin.* 2006;11(3):659–62.

17. Freeman MA, Dean MR, Hanham IW. The etiology and prevention of functional instability of the foot. *J Bone Joint Surg Br.* 1965;47(4):678–85.

18. Frey C, Feder KS, Sleight J. Prophylactic ankle brace in high school volleyball players: a prospective study. *Foot Ankle Int.* 2010;31(4):296–300.

19. Garrick JG, Requa RK. The epidemiology of foot and ankle injuries in sports. *Clin Sports Med.* 1988;7(1):29–36.

20. Gauffin H, Tropp H, Odenrick P. Effect of ankle disk training on postural control in patients with functional instability of the ankle joint. *Int J Sports Med.* 1988;9(2):141–4.

21. Gerber JP, Williams GN, Scoville CR, Arciero RA, Taylor DC. Persistent disability associated with ankle sprains: a prospective examination of an athletic population. *Foot Ankle Int.* 1998;19(10):653–60.

22. Gould N, Seligson D, Gassman J. Early and late repair of lateral ligament of the ankle. *Foot Ankle.* 1980;1(2):84–9.

23. Harper MC. Deltoid ligament: an anatomical evaluation of function. *Foot Ankle.* 1987;8(1):19–22.

24. Hettinga DL. Inflammatory response of synovial joint structures. In: Gould JA, Davies GJ, editors. *Orthopaedic and Sports Physical Therapy.* St. Louis: CV Mosby; 1985. p. 87.

25. Hintermann B. Biomechanics of the unstable ankle joint and clinical implications. *Med Sci Sports Exerc.* 1999;31(7 Suppl):S459–69.

26. Hockenbury RT, Sammarco GJ. Evaluation and treatment of ankle sprains: clinical recommendations for a positive outcome. *Phy Sportsmed.* 2001;29(2):57–64.

27. Hocutt JE Jr, Jaffee R, Rylander CR, Beebe JK. Cryotherapy in ankle sprains. *Am J Sports Med.* 1982;10(5):316–9.

28. Hopkinson WJ, St Pierre P, Ryan JB, Wheeler JH. Syndesmosis sprains of the ankle. *Foot Ankle.* 1990;10(6):325–30.

29. Hupperets MD, Verhagen EA, Heymans MW, Bosmans JE, van Tulder MW, van Mechelen W. Potential savings of a program to prevent ankle sprains recurrence: economic evaluation of a randomized controlled trial. *Am J Sports Med.* 2010;38(11):2194–200.

30. Kerkhoffs GM, Rowe BH, Assendelft WJ, Kelly K, Struijs PA, van Dijk CN. Immobilisation and functional treatment for acute lateral ankle ligament injuries in adults. *Cochrane Database Syst Rev.* 2002;3:CD003762.

31. Klein J, Höher J, Tiling T. Comparative study of therapies for fibular ligament rupture of the lateral ankle joint in competitive basketball players. *Foot Ankle.* 1993;14(6):320–4.

32. Krips R, van Dijk CN, Lehtonen H, Halasi T, Moyen B, Karlsson J. Sports activity level after surgical treatment for chronic anterolateral ankle instability. A multicenter study. *Am J Sports Med.* 2002;301(1):13–9.

33. Mack RP. Ankle injuries in athletes. *Clin Sports Med.* 1982;1(1):71–84.

34. McGuine TA, Keene JS. The effect of a balance training program on the risk of ankle sprains in high school athletes. *Am J Sports Med.* 2006;34(7):1103–11.

35. Nitz AJ, Dobner JJ, Kersey D. Nerve injury and grades II and III ankle sprains. *Am J Sports Med.* 1994;13(3):177–82.

36. Noyes FR, Torvik PJ, Hyde WB, DeLucas JL. Biomechanics of ligament failure: II. An analysis of immobilization, exercise, and reconditioning effects in primates. *J Bone Joint Surg Am.* 1974;56(7):1406–18.

37. O'Neill PJ, Parks BG, Walsh R, Simmons LM, Miller SD. Excursion and strain of the superficial peroneal nerve during inversion ankle sprain. *J Bone Joint Surg Am.* 2007;89(5):979–86.

38. Pedowitz DI, Reddy S, Parekh SG, Huffman GR, Sennett BJ. Prophylactic bracing decreases ankle injuries in collegiate female volleyball players. *Am J Sports Med.* 2008;36(2):324–7.

39. Pihlajamäki H, Hietaniemi K, Paavola M, Visuri T, Mattila VM. Surgical versus functional treatment for acute ruptures of the lateral ligament complex of the ankle in young men: a randomized controlled trial. *J Bone Joint Surg Am.* 2010;92(14):2367–74.

40. Povacz P, Unger SF, Miller WK, Tockner R, Resch H. A randomized, prospective study of operative and non-operative treatment of injuries of the fibular collateral ligaments of the ankle. *J Bone Joint Surg Am.* 1998;80(3):345–51.

41. Regis D, Montanari M, Magnan B, Spagnol S, Bragantini A. Dynamic orthopedic brace in the treatment of ankle sprains. *Foot Ankle Int.* 1995;16(7):422–6.

42. Ryan JB, Hopkinson WJ, Wheeler JH, Arciero RA, Swain JH. Office management of the acute ankle sprain. *Clin Sports Med.* 1989;8(3):477–95.

43. Safran MR, Benedetti RS, Bartolozzi AR 3rd, Mandelbaum BR. Lateral ankle sprains: a comprehensive review. Part 1: etiology, pathoanatomy, histopathogenesis, and diagnosis. *Med Sci Sports Exerc.* 1999;31 (7 Suppl):S429–37.

44. Safran MR, Zachazewski JE, Benedetti RS Bartolozzi AR 3rd, Mandelbaum BR. Lateral ankle sprains: a comprehensive review. Part 2: treatment and rehabilitation with an emphasis on the athlete. *Med Sci Sports Exerc.* 1999;31(7 Suppl):S438–47.

45. Sammarco GJ, DiRaimondo CV. Surgical treatment of lateral ankle instability syndrome. *Am J Sports Med.* 1988;16(5):501–11.

46. Sammarco GJ, Hockenbury RT. Biomechanics of the foot and ankle. In: Nordin M, Frankel VH, editors. *Basic Biomechanics of the Musculoskeletal System.* 3rd ed. Baltimore: Lippincott Williams & Wilkins; 2001. p. 242.

47. Sammarco GJ, Idusuyi OB. Reconstruction of the lateral ankle ligaments using a split peroneus brevis tendon graft. *Foot Ankle Int.* 1999; 20(2):97–103.

48. Sarrafian SK. *Anatomy of the Foot and Ankle*. 2nd ed. Philadelphia (PA): JB Lippincott; 1993. p. 159–87, 474–551.

49. Snook GA, Chrisman OD, Wilson TC. Long-term results of the Chrisman-Snook operation for reconstruction of the lateral ligaments of the ankle. *J Bone Joint Surg Am*. 1985;67(1):1–7.

50. Sommer HM, Arza D. Functional treatment of recent ruptures of the fibular ligament of the ankle. *Int Orthop*. 1989;13(2):157–60.

51. Stephens MM, Sammarco GJ. The stabilizing role of the lateral ligament complex around the ankle and subtalar joints. *Foot Ankle*. 1992;13(3):130–6.

52. Stiell IG, Greenberg GH, McKnight RD, et al. Decision rules for the use of radiography in acute ankle injuries: refinement and prospective validation. *JAMA* 1993;269(9):1127–32.

53. Sugiomoto K, Takakura Y, Okahashi K, Samoto N, Kawate K, Iwai M. Chondral injuries of the ankle with recurrent lateral instability: an arthroscopic study. J Bone Joint Surg Am. 2009;91(1):99–106.

54. Taylor DC, Englehardt DL, Basset FH III. Syndesmosis sprains of the ankle: the influence of heterotopic ossification. *Am J Sports Med*. 1992; 20(2):146–50.

55. Thorndike A. *Athletic Injuries: Prevention, Diagnosis, and Treatment*. Philadelphia (PA): Lea & Febinger; 1962. 59 p.

56. Tipton CM, James SL, Mergner W, Tcheng TK. Influence of exercise in strength of medial collateral ligaments in dogs. *Am J Physiol*. 1970; 218(3):894–902.

57. Trono M, Tueche S, Quintart C, Libotte M, Baillon J. Peroneus quartus muscle: a case report and review of the literature. *Foot Ankle Int*. 1999;20(10):659–62.

58. Vailas AC, Tipton CM, Mathes RD, Gart M. Physical activity and its influence on the repair process of medial collateral ligaments. *Connect Tissue Res*. 1981;9(1):25–31.

59. Valderrabano V, Hintermann B, Horisberger M, Fung TS. Ligamentous posttraumatic ankle osteoarthritis. *Am J Sports Med*. 2006;34(4): 612–20.

60. Wang Q, Whittle M, Cunningham J, Kenwright J. Fibula and its ligaments in load transmission and ankle joint stability. *Clin Orthop Relat Res*. 1996;(330):261–70.

61. Waterman BR, Owens BD, Davey S, Zacchilli MA, Belmont PJ Jr. The epidemiology of ankle sprains in the United States. *J Bone Joint Surg*. 2010;92(13):2279–84.

62. Weise K, Rupf G, Weinelt J. Die laterale bandverletzung des OSG beim sport. *Aktuelle Traumatol*. 1988;1(18 Supp l):54–66.

63. Wolin I, Glassman F, Sideman S, Levinthal DH. Internal derangement of the talofibular component of the ankle. *Surg Gynechol Obstet*. 1950;91(2):193–200.

64. Wuest TK. Injuries to the distal lower extremity syndesmosis. *J Am Acad Orthop Surg*. 1997;5(3):172–181.

65. Xenos, JS, Hopkinson WJ, Mulligan ME, Olson EJ, Popovic NA. The tibiofibular syndesmosis: evaluation of the ligamentous structures, methods of fixation, and radiographic assessment. *J Bone Joint Surg*. 1995;77(6):847–56.

66. Zwipp H, Hoffmann R, Wippermann B, Thermann H, Gottschalk F. Fibulare bandruptur am oberen Sprunggelenk. *Orthopäde* 1989;18(4): 336–40.

65 Soft Tissue Injuries of the Leg, Ankle, and Foot

Keith Lynn Jackson, II and Brian E. Abell

■ As the number of participants in both recreational and competitive activities increases, soft tissue injuries to the lower extremity are encountered more frequently by the primary care provider. If left untreated, these injuries could jeopardize participation and quality of life for those affected. The purpose of this chapter is to outline the characteristics and treatment of the more frequently encountered soft tissue pathologies by region.

SOFT TISSUE INJURIES OF THE LEG

■ The leg extends from the knee to the ankle. Some of the soft tissue injuries affecting this portion of the extremity include exertional compartment syndrome, posterior tibial tendon injury, and peroneal tendon injury.

Exertional Compartment Syndrome

■ Exertional compartment syndrome is activity-related pain caused by an increased intermuscular pressure within an anatomic compartment. In the leg, there are four compartments that contain muscle, blood vessels, and nerves. The compartments are enclosed by fascia, which limit muscular expansion during activity and can cause compression of the contents of the compartment. As pressure within the compartment approaches the mean arterial pressure, the blood flow through the microvasculature is diminished and ischemia ensues.

■ Knowledge of the anatomy of the lower leg is vital to the diagnosis of exertional compartment syndrome (Fig. 65.1). The anterior compartment contains the extensor hallucis longus, extensor digitorum longus, peroneus tertius, and tibialis anterior as well as the deep peroneal nerve. The lateral compartment contains the peroneus longus and brevis as well as the superficial peroneal nerve. The superficial posterior compartment contains the gastrocnemius and soleus muscles and the sural nerve. The deep posterior compartment contains the flexor hallucis longus, flexor digitorum longus, and posterior tibialis muscle as well as the posterior tibial nerve.

■ The patient is usually asymptomatic upon initiating exercise. The pain will begin at a predictable time during the workout. The pain is described as aching or cramping associated with feelings of swelling, fullness, or tightness. Dysesthesias often accompany the pain along the nerve within the affected compartment. Patients may also complain of altered running style. For example, a runner may state that the foot seems to be slapping the ground when the pain comes on.

Physical Examination

■ The physical examination at rest is often normal. In advanced cases, there may be tenderness to deep palpation along the affected compartment or a palpable fascial defect with hernia within the affected compartment.

■ Examination immediately after exercise reveals a firm, tender compartment with increased pain on passive stretch of the muscles within the compartment. Fascial defects with resultant herniations are more identifiable at this time.

■ Several techniques have been described for measuring compartment pressures: These include needle manometry, wick catheter, and slit catheter. Our preferred method of measuring compartment pressure is with a battery-operated, hand-held, digital, fluid pressure monitor. The Stryker Intracompartmental Pressure Monitor (Stryker Corporation, Kalamazoo, MI) is a convenient and easy-to-use measuring device.

■ Compartment pressures should be taken before exercise, 1 minute after exercise, and if necessary, 5 minutes after exercise. One or more of the following pressure criteria must be met in addition to a history and physical that is consistent with the diagnosis of exertional compartment syndrome. Preexercise pressure > 15 mm Hg, 1-minute postexercise pressure > 30 mm Hg, or 5-minute postexercise pressure > 20 mm Hg (16).

Treatment

■ Nonoperative care generally consists of activity modification to levels below symptomatic threshold, ice, nonsteroidal anti-inflammatory medications, and massage. The patient should be counseled that return to previous level of activity is likely to cause recurrence of symptoms.

■ A fasciotomy is the surgical treatment of an exertional compartment syndrome. In this procedure, the fascia is divided longitudinally over the entire length of the involved compartment. Indications for this procedure include an appropriate history for chronic exertional compartment syndrome,

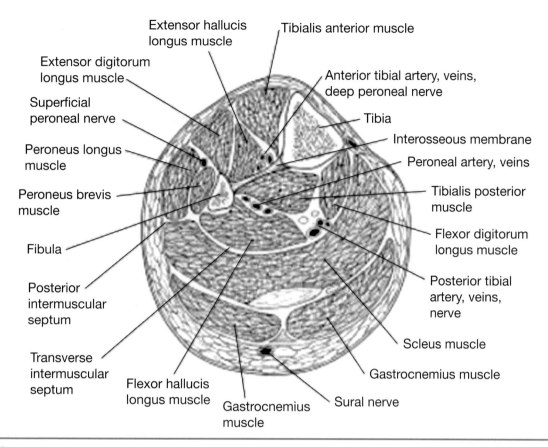

Extensor hallucis longus muscle

Tibialis anterior muscle

Extensor digitorum longus muscle

Anterior tibial artery, veins, deep peroneal nerve

Superficial peroneal nerve

Tibia

Peroneus longus muscle

Interosseous membrane

Peroneal artery, veins

Peroneus brevis muscle

Tibialis posterior muscle

Fibula

Flexor digitorum longus muscle

Posterior intermuscular septum

Posterior tibial artery, veins, nerve

Transverse intermuscular septum

Scleus muscle

Flexor hallucis longus muscle

Gastrocnemius muscle

Gastrocnemius muscle

Sural nerve

Figure 65.1: Cross-sectional anatomy of the compartments of the leg. © 2003 American Academy of Orthopaedic Surgeons. Reprinted from the *Journal of the American Academy of Orthopaedic Surgeons*, Volume 11(4), p. 268–276, with permission.

a 1-minute postexercise compartment pressure greater than 30 mm Hg, or the presence of a fascial defect.

Posterior Tibial Tendon Injury

■ Injury to the posterior tibial tendon may occur acutely or as a component of chronic overuse syndrome. The posterior tibial tendon helps invert and plantarflex the foot and has an important role in maintaining the longitudinal arch.

■ Patients with posterior tibial tendon injury often report pain along the medial aspect of the leg posterior to the medial malleolus. The onset of symptoms is usually gradual with increases in such activities as walking, running, or jumping.

Physical Examination

■ There may be loss of the longitudinal arch and a clinical planovalgus deformity. When observing the patient from behind, the affected side will reveal more toes lateral to the heel than the unaffected side.

■ With an attempted single leg heel raise, there is loss of foot supination and heel inversion. In the later stages of posterior tibial dysfunction, patients cannot perform a single leg heel rise. In earlier stages of dysfunction, patients will perform the single leg heel rise in a slow deliberated fashion with associated pain.

■ There is tenderness and fullness along the course of the tendon.

■ Pain and weakness are present with resisted inversion.

Radiographic Examination

■ The x-ray evaluation should include standing anteroposterior and lateral views. The anteroposterior (AP) x-ray may show medial talar displacement in relation to the navicular. This is best seen with uncovering of the talar head. The lateral x-ray may reveal decreased height of the longitudinal arch and increased overlap of the metatarsals (20).

■ Magnetic resonance imaging (MRI) is the test of choice to evaluate the posterior tibial tendon (20). Significant findings on MRI include heterogenous signal along the course of the tendon and possible increase in size.

Treatment

■ The initial treatment for posterior tibial tendon deficiency is generally nonoperative and begins with a period of immobilization with the use of a short leg walking boot or short leg walking cast. Once immobilization is complete, an orthotic should be used to support the arch and relieve stress on the tendon by posting the heel in a neutral position.

■ Corticosteroid injections are not recommended because of the risk of tendon rupture.

- Surgery should be considered in those who do not respond to nonoperative management after 3–6 months, patients with loss of the arch, or patients with midfoot arthritis (13). Surgical options include synovectomy/debridement, flexor digitorum longus transfer, or calcaneal osteotomy.

Peroneal Tendon Injury

- Peroneal tendon pathology is a commonly missed source of chronic lateral-sided ankle pain. The spectrum of peroneal tendon injury includes tenosynovitis, tendon tear, and peroneal tendon instability.

- The peroneus longus originates from the proximal aspect of the lateral fibula. Its tendinous portion runs posterior to the lateral malleolus before inserting primarily onto the plantar proximal surface of the first metatarsal. Its function is primarily eversion and plantarflexion of the foot. The peroneus brevis originates from the lateral fibula. Its tendinous portion courses anterior and medial to the peroneus longus tendon at the level of the ankle and inserts onto the base of the fifth metatarsal. Its primary function is to evert the foot.

- The patient will often complain of lateral ankle pain that localizes posterior to the lateral malleolus. The patient may also relay a history of pain, "popping," and transient swelling in this area usually after an inversion injury.

Physical Examination

- Pain and swelling over the course of the tendons posterior to the lateral malleolus will be present on examination. The patient may also report pain with resisted eversion of the ankle, passive inversion of the ankle, or resisted plantarflexion of the first metatarsal. In cases of peroneal instability, tendon subluxation or dislocation may be elicited with resisted eversion and dorsiflexion of the ankle.

Radiographic Examination

- Standard radiographic review should include weight-bearing AP, mortise, and lateral x-rays.

- Ultrasonography may show areas of heterogeneity within the tendons as well as subluxation.

- MRI may show increased or heterogenous signal within the substance of the tendon. Circumferential fluid within the tendon sheath measuring greater than 3 mm suggests tenosynovitis (11,17).

Treatment

- The initial treatment of peroneal tendon tenosynovitis begins with rest, ice, and nonsteroidal anti-inflammatory medications. An ankle brace or lateral heel wedge may also help alleviate symptoms. For more severe cases of tenosynovitis, the patient may be placed in a short leg cast or walking boot for a period of 2–4 weeks. In cases of peroneal tendon instability, nonoperative treatment is associated with a high rate of failure.

- Corticosteroid injections are not recommended because of the risk of tendon rupture.

- Operative intervention is indicated if symptoms persist after a trial on nonoperative care. Surgical treatment includes exploration, synovectomy, primary tendon repair, tenodesis, or retinacular repair.

SOFT TISSUE INJURIES OF THE HINDFOOT AND MIDFOOT

- The hindfoot consists of the talus and calcaneus and their articulations, whereas the midfoot consists of the navicular, cuboid, and three cuneiform bones and their related articulations. Foot function hinges on the stability provided by the osseous anatomy and overlying soft tissue structures. Some of the more frequently encountered soft tissue pathologies affecting this region include os trigonum, jogger's foot, tarsal tunnel syndrome, plantar heel pain, and posterior heel pain.

Painful Os Trigonum

- The os trigonum is an ossicle present in 7%–11% of the population as a continuation of the posterior talar process. Painful os trigonum syndrome is one cause of posteromedial ankle pain. This syndrome is most prevalent in athletes who perform frequent or forced plantarflexion. The condition may be misdiagnosed as other conditions such as Achilles tendonitis (14).

- Presentation is commonly with pain in the posterior medial ankle that may be worsened with plantarflexion activities (en pointe position in ballet).

Physical Examination

- On examination, there may be tenderness to palpation over the os or the posteromedial ankle. Passive dorsiflexion/plantarflexion of the great toe may also illicit pain due to the close anatomic relationship of the flexor hallucis longus tendon and the trigonal process.

Radiographic Examination

- Standard radiographs should include weight-bearing AP and oblique and lateral views of the foot. The os trigonum may be appreciated on the lateral view.

- MRI will demonstrate fluid between the os trigonum and the lateral talar process (8). MRI may also demonstrate associated flexor hallucis longus tenosynovitis.

Treatment

- The initial treatment for symptomatic os trigonum is nonoperative and generally begins with a brief (4–6 weeks) period of immobilization in a short leg cast or controlled ankle movement (CAM) boot. Nonsteroidal anti-inflammatory drugs (NSAIDs) and activity modification may help alleviate symptoms.

- Surgical excision may be required with failure of nonoperative management (3).

Compression Neuropathy (Jogger's Foot)

- Entrapment of the medial plantar nerve distal to the tarsal tunnel can cause a neuropathy known as *jogger's foot*. The medial plantar nerve courses plantarward after it exits the tarsal tunnel, where it may be compressed by osteophytes from the talonavicular joint or a fibrotic master knot of Henry.

- Patients often complain of pain or numbness of the medial sole of the foot and medial toes that increases with physical activity.

Physical Examination

- There may be tenderness to palpation along the medial aspect of the longitudinal arch. Numbness and tingling may also be recreated with a Tinel test over this area.

Treatment

- The initial treatment of this condition is generally nonoperative and should consist of rest, nonsteroidal anti-inflammatories, or soft orthoses. Patients with a planovalgus or flatfoot may benefit from a University of California Biomechanics Laboratory (UCBL) orthosis.

- Injection of corticosteroid with local anesthetic can be diagnostic as well as therapeutic.

- Surgical release of the medial plantar nerve may be indicated for cases that fail trials of nonoperative care.

Tarsal Tunnel Syndrome

- Tarsal tunnel syndrome is the most common compression neuropathy of the foot and ankle. The etiology is entrapment of the posterior tibial nerve in the tarsal tunnel or one of its terminal branches after leaving the tarsal tunnel. Tarsal tunnel syndrome may be posttraumatic, idiopathic or the result of a space occupying lesion or accessory muscle (12,18).

- The tarsal tunnel is a fibro-osseous tunnel. The osseous boundaries are the medial surface of the talus, the medial surface of the os calcis, the sustentaculum tali, and inferomedial navicular. The fibrous portion of the canal consists of the flexor retinaculum as the roof and the abductor hallucis with its investing fascia.

- Patients often complain of burning, tingling, or numbness on plantar aspect of foot and may have night pain or discomfort with even light bedcovers.

Physical Examination

- Examination may demonstrate a positive Tinel's sign at the tarsal tunnel or reproduction of symptoms with compression for 60 seconds.

- Other causes of peripheral neuropathy should be considered such as diabetes, hypothyroidism, and alcoholism.

- Electrodiagnostic studies are helpful in differentiating tarsal tunnel syndrome from peripheral neuropathy or lumbosacral radiculopathy.

Treatment

- Conservative treatment consists of avoidance of aggravating activities and control of generalized edema, if present, with medications or compressive stockings as indicated. Arch supports or medial heel wedges may help alleviate symptoms. A NSAID or injection of corticosteroid into the tarsal tunnel is often of benefit to patients with tenosynovitis.

- Surgical management consists of complete release of the tibial nerve and all its branches and has been shown to result in improved outcome measures after failure of conservative management (2).

Plantar Fasciitis

- Insertional plantar fasciitis is the most common cause of plantar heel pain. Repetitive or acute trauma leads to microtears at the calcaneal insertion of the plantar fascia. The patient often describes the pain as worse with the "first step in the morning."

- A variation of insertional plantar fasciitis is a posterior fourchette (PF) tear. In this condition, the plantar fascia is acutely torn.

- An infrequent but unique cause of plantar heel pain that can be confused with plantar fasciitis is fat pad insufficiency. This condition is often seen in older athletes or in patients after multiple corticosteroid injections to the heel. Other causes of heel pain should be excluded prior to making the diagnosis of fat pad atrophy. Treatment consists of a viscoelastic heel cup and well-cushioned shoes (2,10).

Physical Examination

- Patients with insertional plantar fasciitis typically presents with pain localized to the plantar medial heel. The pain is often worse with the first few steps in the morning or after rest.

- In a PF tear, a palpable defect in the plantar fascia may be appreciated. A loss of arch height may be appreciated in cases of complete tear.

Radiographic Examination

- Standing AP, lateral, and oblique radiographs show a plantar heel spur in 50% of patients with insertional plantar fasciitis and 15% of asymptomatic patients.

- A bone scan can help differentiate plantar fasciitis from calcaneal stress fracture.

Treatment

- The primary treatment of plantar fasciitis is nonoperative, consisting of Achilles stretching and activity modification. Hand massage, ice massage, or anti-inflammatories may also be helpful. Cushioned heel cups are often prescribed.

- Injection of corticosteroids with local anesthetic may be considered after failure of other methods. Repeat steroid injections may cause atrophy of the heel fat pad and should be avoided.

- Ninety-five percent of patients with plantar fasciitis will have resolution of their symptoms within 12–18 months.

- For the 5% of patients who fail conservative treatment, surgical release of the plantar fascia may be considered.
- Although surgery generally results in improvement in symptoms, patients should be counseled that recovery can be prolonged and that exercises to maintain Achilles length must be continued.

Insertional Achilles Tendinitis

- The most common site of posterior heel pain is in the area of the insertion of the Achilles tendon. Factors that predispose this area to pathology include the hypovascular nature of the distal Achilles tendon, the repetitive forces seen at the bone tendon interface, and the prominence of the area becoming irritated with shoe wear.
- Insertional Achilles tendinitis is a common condition in jumping athletes but may also be precipitated by a direct blow or poorly fitting shoes.
- Patients with this condition may complain of pain at the distal portion of the Achilles tendon and note weakness in plantarflexion.

Physical Examination

- On examination, there is tenderness to palpation directly over the insertion of the Achilles. The patient with this condition may also experience pain with resisted plantar flexion.

Treatment

- Initial treatment is conservative with NSAIDs, Achilles stretching, and activity modification. Felt or Silipos pads placed over the posterior heel may also be beneficial.
- Corticosteroid injections have been associated with tendon rupture and are discouraged.
- Operative intervention may be indicated in select cases after a 6-month trial on nonoperative care. Surgical options include Achilles tendon debridement and flexor hallucis longus tendon transfer.

Retrocalcaneal Bursitis

- The retrocalcaneal bursa is a synovial-lined bursa between the posterior calcaneus and the Achilles tendon.
- Patients with this condition frequently present with posterior heel pain and direct tenderness to palpation of the posterior heel.
- Frequently, patients with retrocalcaneal bursitis have an associated pathologic prominence of the posterior superior aspect of the calcaneal tuberosity. This prominence is commonly referred to as a Haglund deformity and is often associated with rigid shoe wear.

Physical Examination

- On examination, there is generally tenderness to palpation just proximal to the insertion of the Achilles tendon. The patient may also demonstrate weakness with plantarflexion of the ankle.

- Patients with an associated Haglund deformity may have a visible prominence at the insertion of the Achilles tendon.

Radiographic Examination

- Standard weight-bearing AP, oblique, and lateral x-rays should be obtained in the initial evaluation. In cases with an associated Haglund deformity, a prominence of the posterior superior portion of the calcaneal tuberosity will be seen on the lateral view.

Treatment

- The initial treatment generally consists of rest, ice, heel cord stretches, and shoe modification.
- In cases that have failed a trial of nonoperative treatment, a bursectomy or surgical excision of the Haglund deformity may be required (19).

SOFT TISSUE INJURIES OF THE FOREFOOT

- The forefoot consists of the metatarsals and phalanges and their corresponding articulations. Injury in this region of the lower extremity is common in both the recreational and competitive athlete.
- During ambulation, the contact forces are equally distributed among the second through fifth metatarsal heads and two sesamoids.
- Because of the higher loads distributed across the first metatarsal phalangeal joint in weight-bearing activities, the great toe is commonly injured.

Hallux Rigidus

- Hallux rigidus is a common disorder, seen in about 1 in 45 individuals over the age of 50. It is characterized by limitation of motion of the first metatarsophalangeal (MTP) joint, particularly in dorsiflexion.
- Patients present complaining of limitation of motion and pain at the MTP joint with ambulation or athletic activity.
- Hallux rigidus has been attributed to many causes, including trauma, inflammatory or metabolic conditions, and congenital disorders.

Physical Examination

- Patients with hallux rigidus will demonstrate pain with both active and passive motion of the first MTP joint. Occasionally, a palpable dorsal exostosis may also be present over the dorsal aspect of the joint.
- Cases with a large exostosis may demonstrate irritation of the overlying skin from improperly fitting shoe wear.

Radiographic Examination

- Weight-bearing AP, oblique, and lateral x-rays obtained during the initial evaluation of hallux rigidus may demonstrate narrowing of the first MTP joint as well as a dorsal osteophyte.

Treatment

- Initial treatment is nonoperative, consisting of NSAIDs and avoidance of high-impact activities.
- A steel or fiberglass shank in the sole of the shoe can relieve symptoms by limiting dorsiflexion. Rocker bottom shoes and custom insoles may have a similar effect.
- Failure of nonoperative treatment is an indication for surgery. Surgical treatment can consist of cheilectomy, arthrodesis, or Keller arthroplasty.

Hallux Valgus

- Hallux valgus, or bunion deformity, is common in the general population and occurs in athletes as well. Hallux valgus in athletes demands different considerations and treatment than in the general population.
- Hallux valgus occurs with lateral deviation of the great toe and progressive subluxation of the first MTP joint. The medial eminence of the first MTP joint becomes prominent. The overlying soft tissue becomes irritated, swollen, and inflamed, creating the bunion (from the Greek for turnip).
- Several intrinsic and extrinsic factors may contribute to hallux valgus. The most important extrinsic factor is constricting footwear. Shoes with heels and a narrow toe box have been associated with bunions. Athletic activities that increase the lateral stress on the first MTP joint can be another extrinsic cause. Intrinsic factors include a pronated foot, contracted heel cord, hypermobility of the first metatarsocuneiform joint, and metatarsus primus varus. Injury to the first MTP joint, such as turf toe or first MTP dislocation, may weaken the joint capsule and collateral ligament, predisposing to hallux valgus.
- Patients typically present complaining of pain over the medial eminence and irritation with shoe wear. The skin and bursa over the medial eminence may be irritated.

Physical Examination

- The patient's feet should be examined sitting and standing. Standing may accentuate the deformity.
- Range of motion at the first MTP should be noted, as well as any hypermobility at the metatarsocuneiform joint. The foot should be examined for pes planus and pronation.

Radiographic Examination

- Radiographic evaluation consists of AP, lateral, and sesamoid views with the patient standing.
- The angle formed by the proximal phalanx and first metatarsal, or hallux valgus angle, is measured. A normal hallux valgus angle is less than 15 degrees. An angle between 15 and 20 degrees is considered mild hallux valgus. Moderate deformity is characterized by a hallux valgus angle between 20 and 40 degrees, with an angle greater than 40 degrees being severe deformity.
- Other radiographic angles measured include the intermetatarsal angle between the shafts of the first and second metatarsal and the distal metatarsal articular angle, a measurement of joint congruity.

Treatment

- The initial treatment of hallux valgus is nonoperative and consists of shoe wear modification. Irritation of the medial eminence may be relieved with a wider toe box, shoe stretching, or pads around the bunion. Patients with pes planus may benefit from an orthosis.
- Contracture of the Achilles, if present, should be treated appropriately.
- Persistent pain after exhausting nonoperative treatment options is an indication for surgery.
- Surgery can result in postoperative restriction of MTP motion, which should be considered by athletes requiring a great range of MTP motion, such as dancers and sprinters (1,5).

Turf Toe

- Injury to the first MTP joint has ranked third in collegiate athletes after knee and ankle injuries.
- Turf toe represents an acute injury to the plantar MTP capsuloligamentous structures of the great toe.
- The most common mechanism of injury is when an axial load is delivered to the heel with the ankle plantarflexed and the great toe in dorsiflexion.
- Turf toe is classified into three grades. In grade I, the plantar tissues remain intact, and symptoms are minimal. There may be minor swelling but no ecchymosis. Grade II injuries represent a partial tear of the capsule. Symptoms are pain, swelling, ecchymosis, and restricted motion. The patient will be unable to perform at his or her usual level of sport. Grade III injuries are complete capsuloligamentous tears. There may have been an occult MTP dislocation that spontaneously reduced.

Physical Examination

- On physical examination, there may be swelling or ecchymosis about the MTP joint on inspection. The patient may also demonstrate pain with passive motion and tenderness to palpation. In more severe injuries, there may be instability of the MTP joint.

Radiographic Examination

- X-rays of the affected foot may reveal proximal migration of the sesamoids on the AP view or a lag in sesamoid tracking on the lateral view.
- X-rays of the uninjured foot may be helpful for comparative purposes.
- MRI may reveal increased uptake or frank disruption of the plantar capsuloligamentous structures.

Treatment

- Treatment is generally conservative, consisting of rest, ice, elevation, and possibly anti-inflammatory drugs. Buddy taping or rigid orthoses to limit MTP motion may also provide symptomatic relief.
- Operative treatment may be indicated in patients with symptoms refractory to conservative management.

- Turf toe injuries may predispose toward osteoarthritis of the first MTP joint and hallux rigidus (4,7).

Metatarsalgia

- Metatarsalgia is a descriptive term for pain beneath the metatarsal heads that may have a number of etiologies including stress fracture, synovitis, or neuroma. Forefoot pain has been associated with tightness of the gastrocnemius–soleus complex. Patients presenting with forefoot or midfoot symptoms have less dorsiflexion on average than asymptomatic controls (6).

- Synovitis of the MTP joint most commonly affects the second metatarsal. It occurs most frequently in middle-aged athletes. Symptoms typically include pain in the forefoot exacerbated by running, walking, or forced dorsiflexion of the MTP joint.

- Interdigital neuroma, or Morton neuroma, is a common cause of forefoot pain that classically presents as neurogenic pain in the ball of the foot between the third and fourth toes. It is thought to be caused by irritation of the interdigital nerve as it passes beneath the deep transverse metatarsal ligament. It occurs in all populations but is most frequently reported in runners and dancers.

Physical Examination

- On examination, there may be swelling dorsally or tenderness to palpation of the MTP joint in cases of MTP synovitis.

- In cases of interdigital neuroma, palpation of the interspace while compressing the forefoot by pressing on the first and fifth metatarsal heads may reproduce the pain.

Radiographic Examination

- Weight-bearing radiographs of the foot should be obtained to rule out joint degeneration and metatarsal stress fracture.

- Cases of MTP joint synovitis may demonstrate joint space widening.

Treatment

- Treatment is initially conservative, including activity modification, shock-absorbing insoles, and NSAIDs. Additionally, in cases of interdigital neuroma, avoiding heels or shoes with narrow toe boxes may decrease extrinsic compression on the nerve. In cases where shoe modification has failed, injection of corticosteroid with local anesthetic may give lasting or permanent relief.

- In cases of MTP synovitis, surgical management may be necessary with failure of conservative treatment and development of deformity (15).

- Excision of the neuroma has demonstrated good pain relief in 80% of patients (9).

REFERENCES

1. Baxter DE. Treatment of bunion deformity in the athlete. *Orthop Clin North Am.* 1994;25(1):33–9.
2. Baxter DE, Pfeffer GB, Thigpen M. Chronic heel pain. Treatment rationale. *Orthop Clin North Am.* 1989;20(4):563–9.
3. Blake RL, Lallas PJ, Ferguson H. The os trigonum syndrome. A literature review. *J Foot Surg.* 1989;28(4):312–8.
4. Clanton TO, Ford JJ. Turf toe injury. *Clin Sports Med.* 1994;13(4):731–41.
5. Coughlin M. Hallux valgus. *Instr Course Lect.* 1997;46:357–91.
6. Digiovani CW, Kuo R, Tejwani N, et al. Isolated gastrocnemius tightness. *J Bone Joint Surg Am.* 2002;84-A(6):962–70.
7. Fleming LL. Turf toe injuries and related conditions. In: Garrett WE, Speer KP, Kirkendall DT, editors. *Principles and Practice of Orthopedic Sports Medicine.* Philadelphia: Lippincott Williams & Wilkins; 2000. p. 965–7.
8. Karasick D, Schweitzer ME. The os trigonum syndrome: imaging features. *AJR Am J Roentgenol.* 1996;166(1):125–9.
9. Karr SD. Subcalcaneal heel pain. *Orthop Clin North Am.* 1994;25(1):161–75.
10. Kay D, Bennett GL. Morton's neuroma. *Foot Ankle Clin.* 2003;8(1):49–59.
11. Kijowski R, De Smet A, Mukharjee R. Magnetic resonance imaging findings in patients with peroneal tendinopathy and peroneal tenosynovitis. *Skeletal Radiol* 2007;36(2):105–14.
12. Lau JTC, Daniels TR. Tarsal tunnel syndrome. *Foot Ankle Int.* 1999;19(11):770–7.
13. Mann RA. Flatfoot in adults. In Mann RA, Coughlin MJ, editors. *Surgery of the Foot and Ankle.* 6th ed. St. Louis (MO): Mosby; 1993. p. 757.
14. Martin BF. Posterior triangle pain: the os trigonum. *Foot Ankle Int.* 2000;21(8):669–72.
15. Mizel MS, Yodlowski ML. Disorders of the lesser metatarsophalangeal joints. *J Am Acad Orthop Surg.* 1995;3(3):166–73.
16. Pedowitz RA, Hargens AR, Mubarak SJ, Gershuni DH. Modified criteria for the objective diagnosis of chronic compartment syndrome of the leg. *Am J Sports Med.* 1990;18(1):35–40.
17. Philbin TM, Landis GS, Smtih, B. Peroneal tendon injuries. *J Am Acad Orthop Surg.* 2009;17(5):306–17.
18. Schon LC. Nerve entrapment, neuropathy and nerve dysfunction in athletes. *Orthop Clin North Am.* 1994;25(1):47–59.
19. Stephens MM. Haglund's deformity and retrocalcaneal bursistis. *Orthop Clin North Am.* 1994;25(1):41–6.
20. Trevino S, Baumhauer JF. Tendon injuries of the foot and ankle. *Clin Sports Med.* 1992;11:727–39.

Foot and Ankle Fractures

66

Brian E. Abell and J. Richard Lee Evanson

ANKLE FRACTURES

- The true incidence of ankle fractures in the general population is unknown, as it changes with increased participation in athletics and trends in fashion footwear. There is also a great deal of interobserver reliability when it comes to classifying these fractures.

- A great deal of research has been conducted to determine the incidence of age-related fractures, particularly in the elderly population. Barrett et al. (1) analyzed Medicare data in 1999 and found that ankle fractures were the fourth most common fracture in the elderly population (65–90 years of age). The study also demonstrated that elderly blacks were less likely than whites to fracture the ankle.

- The most current data suggest that 8.3 per 1,000 Medicare patients will sustain an ankle fracture (11). Among Finnish patients older than 70 years of age, the number of ankle fractures has increased threefold from 1970 to 2000, with a larger number of fractures classified as unstable (19).

Physical Examination

- The examination of the ankle should begin with a thorough visual inspection noting abnormal swelling, redness, or deformities. The physician should also palpate the ankle to determine the extent of any swelling, identify any abnormal bony prominences or incongruities, determine specific areas of point tenderness or extreme pain, and evaluate the neurovascular status of the patient.

- The neurovascular examination should include an assessment of the dorsalis pedis and posterior tibial pulses. Additionally, the physician should evaluate the capillary refill, light touch, and two-point discrimination distal to the ankle.

- Gross deformity of the ankle is a likely indicator of dislocation, which should be reduced and splinted prior to radiographic examination or further evaluation.

- The physician will then evaluate the range of motion of the ankle. The normal range of ankle motion is 30 degrees of dorsiflexion and 45 degrees of plantarflexion. The range of motion necessary for ankle functionality or ambulation is 10 degrees of dorsiflexion and 20 degrees of plantarflexion (21).

- It is important to evaluate the stability of the ankle when suspecting a fracture. The squeeze test is performed to rule out disruption of the tibiofibular syndesmosis. The squeeze test is performed by squeezing the leg, approximating the tibia and fibula, at or slightly above the level of the belly of the gastrocnemius. An indicator of syndesmotic disruption is pain at the distal tibiofibular articulation when the squeeze test is performed (18). The physician should also perform an anterior drawer test to evaluate the laxity of the complex ligamentous support network of the ankle. Pain with dorsiflexion and external rotation should also be noted because this may represent posterior bony injury or tendinous disruption.

Radiographic Examination

- The *Ottawa ankle rules* are a valuable guideline in determining the need for radiographic examination in a patient suspected to have an ankle fracture. Radiographic examination is required if the patient is unable to bear weight, if the patient has pain with palpation within 6 cm proximal or distal to the talar articulation, or if the patient has bony tenderness at the posterior edge or tip of either malleolus (34).

- The ankle is best examined radiographically with an anteroposterior (AP), lateral, and mortise view. Three-view radiographs demonstrate greater reliability when compared to various combinations of two-view radiographs (4). Abnormal radiographic findings are greater than 2 mm of talar tilt (difference in lateral and medial joint spaces in AP view), misalignment of the talar dome under the tibia in AP or lateral views, and a demonstrated tibiofibular overlap of less than 10 mm in the AP view or the mortise view (25). Stress radiographs may be valuable but are difficult to standardize. Patients are most tolerant of the gravity stress test whereby a mortise view of the ankle is obtained with the patient lying on their injured side and their distal tibia and injured ankle off of the table unsupported (32). Although normative data are not adequately reported in the literature, the Telos stress device is being used to standardize the amount of stress about the ankle during routine radiographic stress examinations.

- Magnetic resonance imaging (MRI) is best suited for the examination of the integrity of the ankle ligaments, and a bone scan is often helpful to rule out osteochondral lesions in patients with chronic ankle injuries.

Classification

- There are three primary classification systems used to define ankle fractures. The Danis-Weber classification is based solely on the fibula and the location of the fracture in relation to the ankle mortise (10). The Lauge-Hansen classification describes the ankle fracture according to foot position and movement of the foot in relation to the leg (supination-adduction, supination-external rotation, pronation-abduction, pronation-eversion, and pronation-dorsiflexion). The most common mechanism of ankle fracture is of the supination-external rotation variety (22). Lastly, the AO classification is based on the level of the fibula fracture, medial malleolar involvement, and syndesmotic disruption (16). A summary of the aforementioned classifications can be found in Table 66.1.

Treatment

- The goal of treatment of ankle fractures is to restore the anatomic congruity of the ankle joint, promote pain-free restoration of range of motion, and restore and maintain fibular length.
- Nondisplaced, stable ankle fractures and stable, reduced ankle fractures can be managed nonoperatively with great success. Once swelling is reduced, long leg casting is indicated with transition to short leg cast or fracture bracing after 4–6 weeks (25). Diabetics are a special subgroup of patients who may need more time in the long leg cast before adequate bone growth is evident and are less likely candidates for operative intervention. Recent studies suggest that diabetics have higher postoperative complication rates when compared to nondiabetics. Blotter et al. (3) reported a 43% complication rate in diabetics as compared to a 15% complication rate in nondiabetics. Diabetics also demonstrate a higher postoperative infection rate after ankle surgery as reported by Flynn et al. (14) in 2000 and Leyes et al. (23) in 2003.

- Displaced, unstable, open, or unreducible ankle fractures must be treated operatively with reduction and internal or external fixation (8,35).

- Open fractures require emergent orthopedic consult, and it is very likely that these patients will be taken to the operating room urgently. Studies have shown that most open ankle fractures are associated with wounds less than 1 cm long and that infection rates after operative treatment of these fractures are comparable to infection rates seen in the treatment of closed fractures. Chapman and Mahoney (7) demonstrated in their series of open ankle fractures in which immediate fixation was achieved, that the rate of infection in open fracture wounds less than 1 cm was 2% and the rate of infection in open fracture wounds with extensive soft tissue damage and wounds greater than 1 cm was 29%.

Table 66.1	**Classification Systems of Ankle Fractures**		
Fracture Classification	**Type**	**Location of Fracture**	**Associated Injuries**
Danis-Weber	A	Below ankle mortise and tibiofibular articulation	Syndesmosis likely intact
	B	At level of mortise and tibiofibular articulation	Syndesmosis likely intact
	C	Above level of mortise and tibiofibular articulation	Likely disruption of syndesmosis with positive squeeze test
Lauge-Hansen	Supination-adduction	Transverse fracture of lateral malleolus	Stage 1: Tear of lateral ligaments Stage 2: Fracture of medial malleolus
	Supination-external rotation	Avulsion fracture of lateral malleolus	Stage 1: Rupture of anterior tibiofibular ligament Stage 2: Spiral or oblique fracture of lateral malleolus Stage 3: Posterior tibial fracture Stage 4: Fracture of medial malleolus or torn deltoid ligament
	Pronation-abduction	Medial malleolus	Stage 1: Torn deltoid ligament Stage 2: Syndesmotic disruption and posterior tibial fracture Stage 3: Oblique fracture of fibula above mortise
	Pronation-external rotation	Medial malleolus	Stage 1: Torn deltoid ligament Stage 2: Syndesmotic disruption Stage 3: Spiral fracture of fibula above mortise Stage 4: Posterior tibial fracture
AO	A	Fibula at or below plafond	Intact or possible avulsions medial and posterior
	B	Fibula at plafond extending proximally	Tibiofibular ligaments torn; possible avulsions medially and posteriorly
	C	Fibula above plafond	Syndesmosis always torn; deltoid ligament torn

- The most important aspects of ankle fracture management are to immediately reduce dislocated ankles prior to radiographic study, clean and dress open wounds in a proper sterile fashion, document and evaluate neurovascular status, and apply a posterior splint with a U-shaped component at the ankle when transporting the patient or preparing them for further workup by an orthopedic surgeon.

FOOT FRACTURES

- The foot comprises a total of 26 bones. The hindfoot consists of the talus and calcaneus, whereas the midfoot includes the navicular, cuboid, and cuneiforms, and their articulations with the proximal metatarsals. The metatarsals and phalanges make up the forefoot.

- Most foot injuries involve innocuous sprains; however, a small percentage of them involve significant injuries with subtle radiographic findings. The rarity of these injuries limits physician familiarity and accounts for frequent misdiagnosis (36). Foot injuries involving the talus are the most often misdiagnosed (20).

FRACTURES OF THE TALUS

- Fractures of the talus are the second most common tarsal bone injury, with an incidence ranging from 0.1% to 0.85% of all fractures (30).

- The talus has five articulating surfaces as 60% of the talus is covered with articular cartilage. There are no muscle or tendinous attachments. Blood supply to the talus is tenuous, and fractures can easily disrupt the blood supply, resulting in osteonecrosis (15).

- Talus fractures can occur at the talar head, neck, body, or lateral or posterior processes. An os trigonum remains a separate ossicle in 14% of normal feet and can sometimes be mistaken for an acute fracture posterior to the lateral tubercle of the talus (2).

Physical Examination

- Patients with fractures of the talus may present with swelling and ecchymosis of the hindfoot or midfoot. Pain with palpation or with motion of the hindfoot should raise suspicion for the presence of a fracture.

Radiographic Examination

- Physicians evaluating talus fractures should obtain three-view radiographs of both the foot and ankle. The Canale view can provide an optimal view of the talar neck (6). This is performed with the foot placed flat on the cassette and the ankle in equinus and pronated 15 degrees with the beam directed 15 degrees cephalad from the vertical (Fig. 66.1).

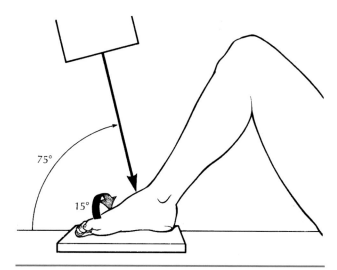

Figure 66.1: The correct position of the foot for x-ray evaluation of the talar neck is shown. From Bucholz RW, MD and Heckman JD, MD. Rockwood & Green's Fractures in Adults, 5th ed. Philadelphia (PA): Lippincott Williams & Wilkins; 2001.

- Computed tomography (CT) is indicated when displacement cannot be ruled out with plain radiographs. A CT will assist with characterization of fracture patterns, displacement, and articular involvement. The role of bone scans or MRI is limited to the evaluation of occult fractures or cartilage lesions.

Talar Neck Fractures

- Most fractures of the talar neck occur from a forced dorsiflexion injury against the anterior margin of the tibia that usually occurs from a motor vehicle accident or fall.

- The Hawkins fracture classification system may be used to guide treatment decisions and predict the risk of osteonecrosis (17). Fracture classification is based on displacement and articular surface involvement (Fig. 66.2). Displaced fractures may injure arteries of the tarsal canal or tarsal sinus, placing the talar body at risk for osteonecrosis.

- Nonsurgical treatment is reserved for type I nondisplaced fractures without comminution or articular step-off. Treatment consists of a short leg cast and non–weight bearing.

- Operative intervention is indicated for all displaced fractures of the talar neck. Urgent surgical treatment is required when subluxation or dislocation leads to soft tissue compromise.

Talar Body Fractures

- Talar body fractures are less common than fractures of the talar neck and are usually the result of high-energy injuries (9).

- Radiographs may underestimate the amount of articular involvement, indicating the need to obtain a CT to identify the fracture pattern and amount of comminution. These fractures can be classified according to their anatomic location.

- Open reduction internal fixation (ORIF) is indicated when the articular surfaces are displaced more than 2 mm (15).

Figure 66.2: Diagrammatic representation of Hawkins' classification of talar neck fractures. I, nondisplaced; II, displaced with associated subtalar joint subluxation; III, talar body dislocated from the ankle mortise; IV, talonavicular joint subluxated also. From Hansen ST, Swiontkowski MF. Orthopaedic trauma protocols. New York: Raven, 1993:340, with permission.

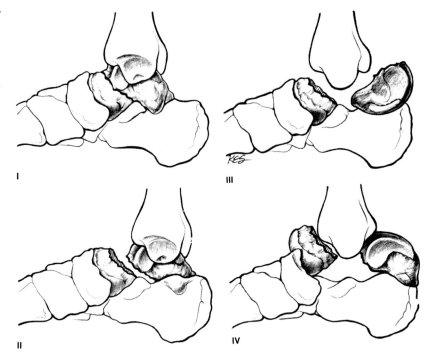

Talar Head Fractures

■ Talar head fractures are the least common subtype of talus fractures. These fractures typically result from plantarflexion and compression along the longitudinal axis of the forefoot.

■ Radiographic examination should include a careful evaluation of the talonavicular joint for associated navicular injuries or talonavicular joint disruption.

■ Nonsurgical treatment consisting of immobilization and non–weight bearing is indicated for nondisplaced fractures. For displaced fractures, the talonavicular joint should be reduced and the fracture fragments stabilized.

Lateral Process Fractures of the Talus

■ Lateral process fractures occur with dorsiflexion and external rotation and most commonly occur during snowboarding. These fractures may be seen on the AP view of the ankle; however, they typically require a CT scan. Physicians should have a high index of suspicion for this injury in patients who have anterolateral ankle pain and normal plain radiographs following an ankle injury while snowboarding.

■ Nondisplaced lateral process fractures are commonly treated with a period of cast immobilization and non–weight bearing. ORIF is indicated for fractures displaced more than 2 mm. Comminuted fractures not amenable to ORIF can be treated with casting or excision.

Posterior Process Fractures of the Talus

■ The posterior process includes the posteromedial and posterolateral tubercles, which are separated by a groove for the flexor hallucis longus tendon. A CT scan is recommended for fractures through this area because they are difficult to visualize on plain radiographs (2).

■ Posteromedial tubercle fractures typically occur from an avulsion of the posterior talotibial ligament or posterior deltoid ligament. Small avulsion fractures are treated with casting and non–weight bearing. Large displaced fragments are treated with ORIF.

■ The posterolateral tubercle fractures are usually an avulsion of the posterior talofibular ligament. Clinically, the patient may exhibit pain with flexion and extension of the great toe caused by the flexor hallucis longus rubbing along the fracture fragment.

■ Posterolateral tubercle fractures with no subtalar involvement are best treated with nonsurgical management. If there is subtalar involvement, then ORIF is warranted.

FRACTURES OF THE CALCANEUS

■ The calcaneus is the most frequently fractured tarsal bone and accounts for 2% of fractures overall. Between 60% and 75% are displaced intra-articular fractures, with open injuries occurring between 7% and 15% of the time. The primary mechanism of injury is an axial load as a result of a fall from a height or motor vehicle accident (21).

■ The calcaneus has three facets along its superior articular surface with the talus. These include the anterior, middle, and posterior facets. The middle facet lies over the sustentaculum tali and is separated from the posterior facet by the sinus tarsi and its corresponding artery. The posterior facet is the largest of the three facets and is the primary weight-bearing surface (15).

Physical Examination

■ Patients with calcaneus fractures typically present with significant swelling and severe heel pain. Ecchymosis around the heel and foot arch is highly suggestive of a fracture of the calcaneus. Fracture blisters are common. To minimize soft tissue compromise, the foot should be elevated and immediately splinted with the ankle in a neutral position (24).

■ Physicians evaluating these injuries should carefully evaluate patients for any neurovascular injury, compartment syndrome, or skin disruption. Wounds associated with open calcaneus fractures typically occur medially (5). Compartment syndrome develops in up to 10% of patients and could lead to a hammer toe deformity (24).

■ Associated injuries occur nearly 50% of the time in patients with calcaneus fractures. A thorough exam should be performed on all joints above and below the injury, along with an exam of the lower back. Ten percent of patients with calcaneus fractures also have fractures of the lumbar spine, and 25% have concomitant injuries in the lower extremities (21).

Radiographic Examination

■ For patients with a suspected fracture of the calcaneus, appropriate radiographs should include AP, lateral, and oblique views of the foot and ankle, in addition to a Harris axial view. The Harris view helps visualize widening, shortening, or varus position of a tuberosity fragment. This view is obtained with the heel against the plate and the ankle in dorsiflexion. The x-ray beam is aimed approximately 30 degrees cephalad toward the heel of the foot.

■ A CT scan is the most complete and reliable means of visualizing and classifying calcaneal fractures. Coronal views are best for evaluating the articular surfaces as well as the position of the peroneal and flexor hallucis tendons. Axial and sagittal views will help evaluate the congruency of the calcaneocuboid joint as well as the posterior facet and calcaneal tuberosity (21,29).

■ Other important fracture characteristics include the degree of shortening, widening, and lateral wall displacement, which may cause injury to the peroneal tendons.

Extraarticular Fractures of the Calcaneus

■ Extraarticular fractures include the anterior process, tuberosity, medial process, sustentacular, and body fractures. These injuries often occur in patients with osteopenic bone, making secure fixation difficult.

■ Early reduction is important because displaced fractures can cause pressure necrosis of the overlying skin. Small fragments can be excised, but fractures with larger fragments may require ORIF.

■ Tuberosity fractures result from a strong contraction of the gastrocnemius–soleus complex with avulsion at its insertion.

■ Anterior process fractures occur with inversion and plantarflexion and result from avulsion of the bifurcate ligament.

Small extraarticular fragments can be treated with casting. Fragments larger than 1 cm may involve the calcaneocuboid joint and require ORIF if joint displacement is present (24).

Intra-Articular Fractures of the Calcaneus

■ The Sanders classification for calcaneal fractures uses a 30-degree semicoronal CT to visualize the subtalar joint at its widest point in the coronal plane (Fig. 66.3). Types are based on the number of articular fragments, which may guide treatment options and help predict treatment outcomes (28,29).

■ Nonsurgical treatment is reserved for type I nondisplaced fractures. Patients should not bear weight for 10–12 weeks, and range-of-motion exercises are initiated once soft tissue swelling allows.

■ Surgical indications include the following: displaced intra-articular fractures of the posterior facet, fragments with greater than 25% of calcaneocuboid articulation involvement, displaced fractures of the tuberosity, fracture dislocations, and selected open fractures. ORIF generally is delayed for 2–3 weeks to allow for resolution of soft tissue swelling (24).

■ Negative prognostic factors include severity, advanced age, male sex, obesity, bilateral fractures, multiple trauma, or worker's compensation (27).

■ A complication rate of up to 40% has been reported. Factors that predict an increased risk of complications include a fall from a height, early surgery, and smoking. Outcomes correlate with the accuracy of the reduction and the number of articular fragments. Type II fractures have better outcomes than type III fractures, whereas type IV fractures have the worst outcomes. Wound-related complications are the most common. Other potential complications include malunion, subtalar arthritis, and lateral impingement with peroneal tendon pathology.

MIDFOOT FRACTURES

■ Fractures of the midfoot are relatively uncommon. The bones of the midfoot include the navicular, cuboid, cuneiforms, and bases of the metatarsals. The midfoot has osseous stability due to the recessed articulation of the base of the second metatarsal. The trapezoidal shape of the first three metatarsal bases contributes to stability, as do the plantar ligaments. The calcaneocuboid and talonavicular joints make up the midtarsal joint, whereas the Lisfranc joint complex is between the tarsi and the first two metatarsals (31).

■ Most midfoot fractures are a result of high-energy trauma from a motor vehicle collision or the lower energy combination of an axial load and twisting of the foot during an athletic event.

Physical Examination

■ When examining a patient with a potential midfoot injury, it is important to recognize there is a wide range of injury severity and patient presentation. Injuries may involve anything from

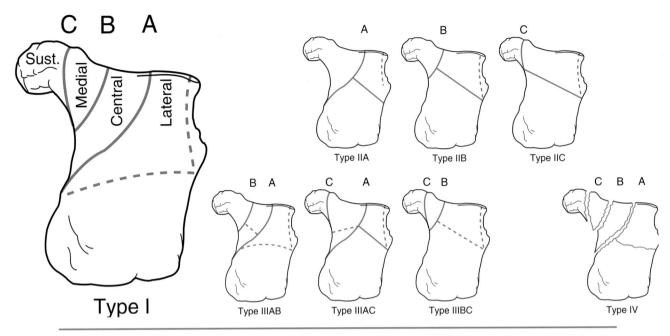

Figure 66.3: Schematic depiction of Sanders classification of intraarticular fractures of the calcaneus. Fracture lines A, B, and C describe the position of the primary fracture line in relation to the posterior facet and the subtalar joint. Types II and III have two or three fragments. Type IV represents severe comminution. From Bucholz RW, MD and Heckman JD, MD. Rockwood & Green's Fractures in Adults, 5th ed. Philadelphia (PA): Lippincott Williams & Wilkins; 2001.

a simple sprain to an injury with potential to cause significant chronic disability such as a Lisfranc injury (31).

- Physicians should perform and document a careful neurovascular exam. Serial examinations may be warranted to rule out an impending foot compartment syndrome anytime a patient presents with extreme pain and swelling.

Radiographic Examination

- Three-view radiographs should be obtained including an AP, lateral, and oblique view of the foot as well as an AP, lateral, and mortise view of the ankle. If tolerated, then stress views or weight-bearing films can assist with defining subtle injuries.

- Obtaining a CT can help distinguish any articular incongruities or comminution and can help characterize the fracture pattern. MRI is more beneficial for evaluating a potential ligamentous injury or for detection of stress fractures.

Navicular Fractures

- The navicular articulates with the cuneiforms, cuboid, calcaneus, and talus. The talonavicular articulation is critical to maintaining inversion and eversion range of motion. The blood supply is limited in the central portion of the navicular, making this area susceptible to fractures.

- Avulsion fractures of the navicular are primarily caused by a plantarflexion injury. Acute treatment consists of immobilization with delayed excision of painful fragments. ORIF is required for fractures involving more than 25% of the articular surface (21).

- Tuberosity fractures commonly result from forced eversion and posterior tibial tendon contraction. An oblique radiograph at 45 degrees of internal rotation can be obtained to appreciate the injury. Most tuberosity avulsions can be managed with cast immobilization. Acute ORIF is indicated with more than 5 mm of diastasis or with large intra-articular fragments (26).

- Fractures of the navicular body are usually caused by axial loading. The Sangeorzan fracture classification is based on the plane of the fracture and degree of comminution. Minimally displaced type I and II fractures are treated nonsurgically, whereas ORIF is used for displaced fractures, disruption of the talonavicular joint, comminution, or type III fractures (26).

Lisfranc Joint Injuries

- Lisfranc injuries can lead to chronic disability if they are not appropriately recognized and treated. The Lisfranc ligament runs from the base of the second metatarsal to the medial cuneiform (Fig. 66.4). This injury can be caused directly from a dorsal force or from an indirect injury by axial loading and twisting on a loaded, plantarflexed foot. Patients may report a history of a fixed foot with rotation of the body around the midfoot (33).

- Physicians evaluating for disruption of the Lisfranc ligament should look for diastasis or a small avulsed fragment of bone between the base of the first and second metatarsals on an AP radiograph. Anatomic alignment should be maintained on the oblique view, and there should be no dorsal subluxation of the metatarsal bases on the lateral. Weight-bearing or stress radiographs will accentuate the deformity and can be

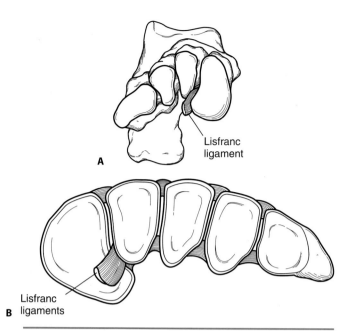

A

Lisfranc ligament

B Lisfranc ligaments

Figure 66.4: The anatomy of the tarsometatarsal joints of the foot. A: Proximal view of the cuneiform and cuboid articular surfaces. B: Distal view of the corresponding articular surfaces of the metatarsals. From Bucholz RW, MD and Heckman JD, MD. Rockwood & Green's Fractures in Adults, 5th ed. Philadelphia (PA): Lippincott Williams & Wilkins; 2001.

ordered when the results of physical examination and plain radiographs are equivocal.

- Treatment consists of ORIF for displaced midfoot fractures and dislocations. Reduction and screw fixation are indicated to stabilize any intercuneiform instability (31).

- Late posttraumatic osteoarthritis is common, occurring in up to 58% of patients. Anatomic reduction, the presence of an open injury, and comminution will affect long-term outcomes.

Cuboid Fractures

- Compression fractures of the cuboid can occur as part of a Lisfranc injury, whereas isolated cuboid fractures are uncommon. Cuboid fractures with significant compression can result in collapse of the lateral column requiring the use of an external fixator to restore length and disimpact fragments. Avulsion fractures are treated symptomatically (26).

Cuneiform Fractures

- Isolated cuneiform fractures are uncommon. Discovering the mechanism of injury is vital for understanding the severity of the injury since the radiographic appearance does not always demonstrate the inciting displacement.

- Avulsion fractures are treated symptomatically. Displaced fractures and intercuneiform instability can occur as part of a Lisfranc fracture-dislocation and should be treated as such. Displacement should be reduced and stabilized during operative fixation of the tarsometatarsal injuries (26).

METATARSAL AND PHALANGEAL FRACTURES

- Metatarsal and phalangeal fractures are common injuries treated by a variety of physicians. The fifth followed by the first toes are the most frequently injured digits due to their vulnerable positions along the medial and lateral borders of the foot (13).

- Metatarsal fractures can result in a disruption of the major weight-bearing complex of the forefoot leading to other problems such as metatarsalgia or transfer lesions. Injuries to this region should not be overlooked and require a thorough workup and appropriate treatment and referral to avoid further complications and disability. With a careful physical exam, a good history, and appropriate radiographs, the diagnosis of most forefoot injuries is straightforward (31).

Physical Examination

- The physician must always evaluate and document the neurovascular status of the patient with a suspected metatarsal or phalangeal fracture. It is most important to evaluate and document the capillary refill and sensation to each toe.

Radiographic Examination

- Radiographs of a suspected forefoot injury should include AP, oblique, and lateral radiographic views of the foot and ipsilateral ankle.

- CT may aid in determining the precise location, depth, and articular involvement; however, these are not a part of the initial radiologic evaluation for these fractures. MRI may be used to investigate stress fractures, but a bone scan is the radiographic study of choice (13).

- When describing fractures of the metatarsal or phalanx, the reporting physician should include the following: open versus closed, incongruent joints, proximal versus distal, comminution, transverse/spiral/oblique pattern, angulation and displacement, and shortening or overlap.

Metatarsal Shaft Fractures

- The plantar flexors are the deforming force involved with fractures of the metatarsal shaft. Mechanisms of injury include a direct blow, avulsion, twisting, inversion, or repetitive stress.

- Nonsurgical treatment is appropriate for fractures of the second, third, and fourth metatarsal shafts when there is < 3 mm of displacement or < 10 degrees of angulation. A prominent plantar fragment can result in callus formation, whereas a dorsiflexion malunion can result in transfer metatarsalgia.

- Indications for surgical treatment include displaced fractures of the first metatarsal. Patients do not tolerate these fractures well because the first ray bears more weight than the lesser metatarsals. Fractures of the second through fourth metatarsals should also undergo operative fixation with > 3 mm of displacement, > 10 degrees of sagittal displacement, or when there are multiple metatarsal fractures (31).

Metatarsal Neck and Head Fractures

■ Metatarsal head and neck fractures are rare and usually occur from a direct blow to the foot involving multiple metatarsals. Failure to recognize and appropriately treat these injuries can disrupt the normal weight-bearing function of the forefoot, causing transfer metatarsalgia (13).

■ Most metatarsal head and neck fractures can be treated nonoperatively. Fractures with severe angulation or prominence may require reduction and fixation if closed reduction is unsuccessful (31).

Fifth Metatarsal Base Fractures

■ Fifth metatarsal fractures usually result from direct trauma and are generally separated into proximal base and distal spiral fractures. Proximal fractures are further divided into three anatomic fracture zones, which help distinguish treatment options. From proximal to distal, zone 1 includes the tuberosity, zone 2 is from the tuberosity to the metaphyseal–diaphyseal junction, and zone 3 includes the proximal diaphysis (Fig. 66.5).

■ Zone 1 fractures are caused by avulsion of the long plantar ligament or the lateral band of the plantar fascia. Treatment consists of weight bearing as tolerated in a stiff-soled shoe. Surgery may be indicated for fractures with large, displaced, intra-articular fragments.

■ Zone 2 fractures represent an area of circulatory watershed, resulting in limited blood supply, and are commonly called Jones fractures. Because of the compromised blood supply in this area, the fracture is at risk of nonunion. Therefore, patients should not bear weight for 6–8 weeks. Acute ORIF using screws is often used in athletes to minimize the possibility of nonunion and prolonged restriction from activity.

■ Zone 3 fractures are typically diaphyseal stress fractures. Nonsurgical treatment consisting of non–weight bearing in

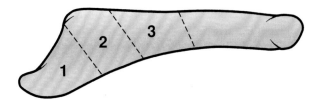

Figure 66.5: Three zones of proximal fifth metatarsal fracture. Zone 1: avulsion fracture. Zone 2: fracture at the metaphyseal-diaphyseal junction. Zone 3: proximal shaft stress fracture. From Bucholz RW, Heckman JD, Court-Brown C, et al., eds. Rockwood and Green's Fractures in Adults, 6th ed. Philadelphia (PA): Lippincott Williams & Wilkins; 2006.

a short leg cast is the appropriate treatment for fractures in this zone in the absence of prodromal symptoms (12).

Phalangeal Fractures

■ The mechanism of injury is a crush injury or axial loading. Painful subungual hematomas should be evacuated through a hole in the nail.

■ Distal phalanx fractures of the hallux are treated nonsurgically, as are lesser toe injuries. Nonsurgical treatment should consist of closed reduction and buddy taping for 4 weeks.

■ Surgical treatment is indicated for displaced articular injuries or angulated proximal phalanx fractures of the hallux if closed reduction and percutaneous pinning fail (13).

Sesamoid Fractures

■ Sesamoid injuries can occur by either a direct impact with compression, hyperdorsiflexion causing a transverse fracture, or repetitive trauma.

■ Plain radiographs can include a sesamoid view to evaluate the articulation of the sesamoid with the plantar aspect of the metatarsal head. MRI is useful in determining the presence of stress reaction or stress fracture; however, a CT is usually not indicated.

■ Acute fractures or stress fractures are treated with padding and immobilization in a hard-soled shoe for 4–8 weeks, and patients can be followed up as outpatients. Excision of the sesamoid is used for chronic symptomatic nonunions and not typically for acute fractures (13).

REFERENCES

1. Barrett JA, Baron JA, Karagas MR, Beach ML. Fracture risk in the U.S. Medicare population. *J Clin Epidemiol.* 1999;52(3):243–9.
2. Berkowitz MJ, Kim DH. Process and tubercle fractures of the hindfoot. J Am *Acad Orthop Surg.* 2005;13(8):492–502.
3. Blotter RH, Connolly E, Wasan A, Chapman MW. Acute complications in the operative treatment of isolated ankle fractures in patients with diabetes mellitus. *Foot Ankle Int.* 1999;20:687–94.
4. Brandser EA, Berbaum KS, Dorfman DD, et al. Contribution of individual projections alone and in combination for radiographic detection of ankle fractures. *AJR Am J Roentgenol.* 2000;174(6):1691–7.
5. Buckley RE, Tough S. Displaced Intra-articular calcaneal fractures. *J Am Acad Orthop Surg.* 2004;12(3):172–8.
6. Canale ST, Kelly FB Jr. Fractures of the neck of the talus: long-term evaluation of seventy-one cases. *J Bone Joint Surg Am.* 1978;60(2):143–56.
7. Chapman MW, Mahoney M. The place of immediate internal fixation in the management of open fracture. *Abbott Soc Bull.* 1976;8:85.
8. Court-Brown CM. Fractures of the tibia and fibula. In: Rockwood CA, Green DB, Bucholz RW, et al., editors. *Fractures in Adults.* 5th ed. Philadelphia: Lippincott Williams & Wilkins; 2001. p. 1939–2000.
9. Daniels TR, Smith JW, Ross TI. Varus malalignment of the talar neck: its effect on the position of the foot and on subtalar motion. *J Bone Joint Surg Am.* 1996;78(10):1559–67.

10. Danis R. Les fractures malleolaires. In: Danis R, editor. *Theories et Pratique de l'Osteosynthese.* 1949. p. 133–65.

11. Davidovitch RI, Egol KE. Ankle fractures. In: Rockwood CA, Green DB, Bucholz RW, et al., editors. *Fractures in Adults.* 7th ed. Philadelphia (PA): Lippincott Williams & Wilkins; 2010. p. 1975–2021.

12. Den Hartog BD. Fracture of the proximal fifth metatarsal. *J Am Acad Orthop Surg.* 2009;17(7):458–64.

13. Early JS. Fractures and dislocations of the midfoot and forefoot. In: Rockwood CA, Green DB, Bucholz RW, et al., editors. *Fractures in Adults.* 6th ed. Philadelphia (PA): Lippincott Williams & Wilkins; 2006. p. 2337–99.

14. Flynn JM, Rodriguez-del Rio F, Pizá PA. Closed ankle fractures in the diabetic patient. *Foot Ankle Int.* 2000;21(4):311–9.

15. Fortin PT, Balazsy JE. Talus fractures: evaluation and treatment. *J Am Acad Orthop Surg.* 2001;9(2):114–27.

16. Fracture and dislocation compendium. Orthopedic Trauma Association Committee for Coding and Classification. *J Orthop Trauma* 1996; 10(Suppl 1):v–ix, 1–154.

17. Hawkins LG. Fractures of the neck of the talus. *J Bone Joint Surg Am.* 1970;52(5):991–1002.

18. Hopkinson WJ, St Pierre P, Ryan JB, Wheeler JH. Syndesmosis sprains of the ankle. *Foot Ankle.* 1990;10(6):325–30.

19. Kannus P, Palvanen M, Niemi S, Parkarri J, Järvinen M. Increasing number and incidence of low trauma ankle fractures in elderly people: Finnish statistics 1970–2000 and projections for the future. *Bone.* 2002;31(3):430–3.

20. Kou JX, Fortin PT. Commonly missed peritalar injuries. *J Am Acad Orthop Surg.* 2009;17(12):775–86.

21. Koval KJ, Zuckerman JD. *Handbook of Fractures.* 4th ed. Philadelphia: Lippincott Williams & Wilkins; 2010. p. 645–59.

22. Lauge-Hansen N. Fractures of the ankle. II. Combined experimental-surgical and experimental roentgenologic investigations. *Arch Surg.* 1950;60(5):957–85.

23. Leyes M, Torres R, Guillén P. Complications of open reduction and internal fixation of ankle fractures. *Foot Ankle Clin.* 2003;8: 131–47, ix.

24. Macey LR, Benirschke SK, Sangeorzan BJ, Hansen ST. Acute calcaneal fractures: treatment options and results. *J Am Acad Orthop Surg.* 1994;2(1):36–43.

25. Marsh JL, Saltzman C. Ankle fractures. In: Rockwood CA, Green DB, Bucholz RW, et al., editors. *Fractures in Adults.* 5th ed. Philadelphia: Lippincott Williams & Wilkins; 2001. p. 2001–89.

26. Miller CM, Winter WG, Bucknell AL, Jonassen EA. Injuries to the midtarsal joint and lesser tarsal bones. *J Am Acad Orthop Surg.* 1998;6(4):249–58.

27. Potter MQ, Nunley JA. Long-term functional outcomes after operative treatment for intra-articular fractures of the calcaneus. *J Bone Joint Surg Am.* 2009;91(8):1854–60.

28. Sanders R. Intra-articular fractures of the calcaneus: present state of the art. *J Orthop Trauma.* 1992;6(2):252–65.

29. Sanders R, Fortin P, Pasquale T, Walling A. Operative treatment in 120 displaced intra-articular calcaneal fractures. Results using a prognostic computed tomography scan classification. *Clin Orthop Relat Res.* 1993;(290):87–95.

30. Santavirta S, Seitsalo S, Kiviluoto O, Myllynen P. Fractures of the talus. *J Trauma* 1984;24(11):986–9.

31. Schenck RC Jr, Heckman JD. Fractures and dislocations of the forefoot: operative and nonoperative treatment. *J Am Acad Orthop Surg.* 1995;3(2):70–8.

32. Schock HJ, Pinzur M, Manion L, Stover M. The use of gravity or manual-stress radiographs in the assessment of supination external rotation fractures of the ankle. *J Bone Joint Surg Br.* 2007;89(8):1055–9.

33. Solan MC, Moorman CT III, Miyamoto RG, Jasper LE, Belkoff SM. Ligamentous restraints of the second tarsometatarsal joint: a biomechanical evaluation. *Foot Ankle Int.* 2001;22:637–41.

34. Stiell IG, Greenberg GH, McKnight RD, et al. Decision rules for the use of radiography in acute ankle injuries. Refinement and prospective validation. *JAMA.* 1993;269(9):1127–32.

35. Vrahas M, Fu F, Veenis B. Intraarticular contact stresses with simulated ankle malunions. *J Orthop Trauma.* 1994;8(2):159–66.

36. Wei CJ, Tsai WC, Tiu CM, Wu HT, Chiou HJ, Chang CY. Systematic analysis of missed extremity fractures in emergency radiology. *Acta Radiol.* 2006;47(7):710–7.

67 Lower Extremity Stress Fractures

Michael Fredericson and Julia Arroyo

INCIDENCE

- Stress fractures account for 0.5%–21% of all injuries in recreational or competitive athletes presenting to sports medicine clinics (53). The highest incidence of stress fractures occurs among track and field athletes (6%–20% of total injuries), compared with athletes in other sports such as football, basketball, soccer, or rowing (1,29,53).

- The site of injury varies from sport to sport. For example, among track athletes, stress fractures of the navicular, tibia, and metatarsals are the most common, whereas in distance runners, the most common locations are the tibia and fibula, and in dancers, the metatarsals (19,53).

ETIOLOGY

- A stress fracture may best be described as an accelerated bony remodeling in response to repetitive submaximal stress. Histologic studies (37,54) have shown that repetitive response to stress leads to osteoclastic activity that surpasses the rate of osteoblastic new bone formation, resulting in temporary weakening of bone.

- It has been debated whether stress fractures occur due to the increased load after fatigue of supporting structures or to contractile muscular forces acting across and on the bone (12,54); in principle, both factors contribute.

- If the activity continues, trabecular microfractures result, which are believed to explain the early bone marrow edema seen on magnetic resonance imaging (MRI) scanning (16). The bone responds by forming new periosteal bone for reinforcement. Eventually, if the osteoclastic activity continues to exceed the rate of osteoblastic new bone formation, a full cortical break occurs. It is important to recognize this process as a continuum accumulation of damage that results clinically in a spectrum of injuries, from the early stages called stress reactions, to stress fractures, and ultimately complete bone fractures (19,58).

RISK FACTORS

- Alteration in the training program is considered one of the most important factors related to the occurrence of stress fractures. Any rapid change in mileage, pace, intensity, or some other factor inserted into the program without adequate time for physiologic adaptation may predispose to stress fractures (27,39).

- Failure to follow intensive training days with easy ones also can contribute to injury. Hard or cambered training surfaces and training in older shoes are also important precursors to lower extremity overuse injuries (16,25).

- Anatomic variables such as narrow width of the tibia, smaller calf girth, and less muscle mass in the lower limb have been associated with stress fractures. In a study (11) comparing 23 running athletes with a history of tibial stress fractures and 23 healthy runners, the stress fracture group had a significantly smaller tibial cross-sectional area. Bony geometry plays a role in stress fracture development. In runners, repetitive loading in a single plane leads to asymmetric cross-sectional geometry of the tibia in contrast to soccer players who load in multiple directions and are found to have a more robust and symmetric bone geometry (8).

- Statistics suggest that women are at greater risk for sustaining stress fractures than men (53). The female athlete triad (menstrual irregularity, disordered eating, and osteopenia) emphasizes this susceptibility in this group of athletes. Other studies have failed to show a significant gender difference (28).

HISTORY

- The typical history of a stress fracture is that of localized pain that is not present at the start but occurs after or toward the end of physical activity. This pattern is opposite to that of many soft tissue injuries that cause pain first thing in the morning and with day-to-day activities but reduced pain during physical activity.

- Untreated stress reactions display pain that occurs earlier during the physical activity and lingers longer; with continued training, pain will be present throughout the training and persist into daily ambulation.

- A careful history often reveals some change in the training regimen during the preceding 2–6 weeks, and it is critical that the physician ask detailed questions to identify training changes as a cause.

PHYSICAL EXAMINATION

- The physical examination typically reveals local tenderness over the involved bone (12). Other tests for the clinical detection of stress fracture such as the fulcrum test (femur), hop test (tibia), and spinal extension test (pars interarticularis) are helpful but not as reliable as direct palpation (29).

- The fulcrum test is performed by gradually applying a force across the distal femur in the seated position using the edge of the examination table as a fulcrum while fixing the proximal femur (15). In the hop test, patients are asked to repeat single-legged hops over the affected leg. The spinal extension test is performed with the patient standing, balancing on one leg to increase the load over the ipsilateral pars interarticularis. Pain provocation with these maneuvers is a positive finding.

- Assessment of biomechanical factors such as varus alignment of the lower extremity, true leg length discrepancies, femoral neck anteversion, muscle weakness, excessive Q angles, excessive subtalar pronation, or a pes cavus style is recommended, because these may contribute to the mechanical load imparted to the affected site (41).

IMAGING

- Radiographic findings are insensitive in the detection of early-stage stress injuries, and their usefulness is limited to the late phase. The time from onset of pain to positive radiographic evidence of a stress fracture can vary from 2–12 weeks (45). Early radiographic findings of a stress fracture in the long bones may include the visualization of a faint fracture radiolucency in the cortical bone (46). As the bone remodels, the endosteum can become ill defined, thickened, and sclerotic. As the fracture heals and remodels, periosteal reaction follows both on the cortical and endosteal surfaces. Stress fractures present differently in trabecular and cortical bone. The former is characterized by a predictable pattern manifested by a line of sclerosis perpendicular to the trabeculae, whereas the latter demonstrates periosteal reaction or a cortical fracture line.

- Radionuclide scanning is a more sensitive but less specific method for imaging bony stress injuries (36,45). Radionuclide technetium-99 diphosphonate triple-phase scanning can provide the diagnosis as early as 2–8 days after the onset of symptoms (16). In acute stress fractures, all three phases of the bone scan are positive. One must be aware of the possibility of increased uptake in nonpainful sites, indicating subclinical accelerated remodeling (5).

- MRI is considered as the gold standard for the evaluation of stress injuries (5,35,45). Fat suppression technique allows for early detection of injuries improving sensitivity and accuracy. A four-stage grading system has been developed:

A grade 1 injury simply shows periosteal edema on the fat suppressed or short tau inversion recovery (STIR) images. In grade 2 injuries, abnormal increased signal intensity is also seen within the marrow cavity or along the endosteal surface on fat-suppressed T2-weighted images. In grade 3 injuries, signal abnormalities are also present on T1-weighted images. Grade 4 injuries involve an actual fracture line often seen on both T1- and T2-weighted images (16). One study (2) showed that grade 3 and 4 injuries took longer to heal than grade 1 and 2 injuries and demonstrated that the grade of injury has prognostic implications regarding the time of healing. Reported false-negative MRI findings have been because of reader errors, suboptimal choice of imaging planes and sequences, inhomogeneities in fat suppression, and partial volume effects (19).

- Before making therapeutic decisions, it is important to correlate MRI findings with clinical symptoms. Bergman and Fredericson (5) studied 21 asymptomatic runners with MRI of the tibia. Nine (43%) of them showed abnormalities indicating stress injuries. After 12 months, none of the asymptomatic runners developed a bone stress injury. Stress response to exercise may cause bone marrow edema, and interpretation should always be made in conjunction with the patient's clinical history (45).

GENERAL PRINCIPLES OF TREATMENT

- It is important to distinguish stress fractures at higher risk for delayed union, nonunion, displacement, or intra-articular component. These fractures require early diagnosis, aggressive treatment, and occasionally internal fixation. High-risk stress fractures include fractures of the femoral neck, patella, tibial diaphysis, fifth metatarsal diaphysis (Jones fracture), tarsal navicular, body of the talus, base of second metatarsal, sesamoids, and pars interarticularis.

- Less critical or not-at-risk fractures can be treated with a two-phase protocol. Phase 1 includes pain control with analgesics and physical therapy modalities. Weight bearing is allowed for normal activities within the tolerance of pain.

- A modified activity program such as elliptical, rowing, or cycling can be used to maintain strength and fitness but to reduce impact loading to the skeleton. A program of deep water training or pool running can be indicated. In our experience, we have found it useful to include an antigravity treadmill device as part of the cross-training recovery protocol. This device allows controlled, progressive weight bearing while permitting unrestricted mobility and natural mechanics and enables the athlete to preserve aerobic condition.

- Phase 2, graduated return to sport, generally begins once the athlete has been pain free for 10–14 days. The athlete can return to running only every other day for the first 2 weeks. Then, over a 3- to 6-week period, a gradual increase in distance and frequency is permitted (17).

- Functional foot orthoses may play a role in treatment and prevention of stress fractures (15). Orthoses are useful either for reducing abnormal pronation in patients with a markedly everted rear foot or providing better shock absorption in athletes with a rigid, inverted rear foot (10).

- If there is a positive history of irregular menses or amenorrhea, then consideration should be given to obtaining a bone mineral density test and endocrine workup. Hormonal replacement therapy indication should be cautiously considered only if the athlete is unable to resume normal menses through weight gain and is not indicated as a long-term solution. Calcium and vitamin D supplementation and additional nutritional deficiencies should be assessed and corrected (20).

- The role of calcium and vitamin D supplementation in the prevention of stress fractures is still to be determined. Recent evidence shows that a daily calcium dietary intake of 1,500 mg in female adolescent athletes reduced incidence of stress fractures and increased bone mineral density (55).

- There is still not conclusive evidence to prove any beneficial effect of bisphosphonates for the treatment of stress fractures in humans (51,52). Adverse effects should be considered, especially in adolescents with open physis and women of childbearing age. In these patients, the safety of bisphosphonate use has not yet been established (51).

- Electrical stimulation has proven to be effective in enhancing regular fracture healing, but limited experience exists on its benefits for stress fractures (22,44). Electric fields can be useful to accelerate stress fracture healing, but treatment protocol requires compliance with the use of the device for 15 hours per day in combination with rest and limited weight bearing. Electrical stimulation may be particularly indicated in the more severe cases or in the elite athlete with higher motivation for superior compliance (3).

SPECIFIC SITES OF STRESS FRACTURE

Pelvis

Sacrum

- Stress fractures in the sacrum are most common in women distance runners with low bone density, but can be seen in those with normal bone mineralization. These stress fractures tend to involve the anteroinferior aspect of the sacral wing unilaterally, mimicking a sacroiliitis (21).

- MRI is recommended for diagnosis, with intermediate signal intensity on T1-weighted images and high-signal intensity on T2-weighted images in the anterior aspect of the sacral ala (19).

Pubic Rami

- More commonly, a bony stress reaction may develop in runners at the symphysis pubis (osteitis pubis) or at the inferior pubic ramus adjacent to the symphysis and is believed to be related to overuse of the adductor muscles for pelvis stabilization.

- Treatment for both of the above pelvic stress fractures requires a period of rest and temporary use of crutches if there is any pain during ambulation. Symptoms usually resolve within several weeks, and a gradual return to athletic activity can typically be safely advised between 10 and 12 weeks.

Ischium

- An ischial ramus stress reaction is not considered a true stress fracture, because it is seen in association with proximal hamstring tendinopathy or hamstring bursitis, secondary to chronic traction of the muscle origin (17).

Femoral Neck

- Stress fractures of the femoral neck are high-risk fractures and should be considered in any athlete, especially a distance runner, who presents with hip, thigh, or groin pain. Pain and symptoms are worse with weight bearing, and there is often reduced range of movement in the hip, particularly internal rotation.

- Early detection of femoral neck stress fractures is crucial, because continued stress may lead to a displaced fracture, with associated risk of avascular necrosis and irreversible damages to the joint (38).

- Compression fractures are more common in younger athletic patients and are located at the cortex of the lower medial margin of the femoral neck. The early radiographic appearance of these fractures is subtle endosteal lysis or sclerosis along the inferior cortex of the femoral neck, followed by progressive sclerosis and appearance of a fracture line. If radiographic findings are negative, MRI should be indicated to detect bone marrow edema and the presence or absence of a low signal intensity line that indicates a fracture.

- If there is no fracture line present, treatment is conservative, with a period of non–weight bearing to allow healing (19,57). Athletes are allowed to continue conditioning exercises such as swimming or cycling during the period of rest. The return-to-play criteria are based on asymptomatic full weight bearing, no pain with passive range of motion of the hip, and follow-up imaging studies with signs of a healed fracture. As a rule, 2–3 months are required for complete healing of stress fractures of this type (19).

- Surgical management of this injury is considered under the following circumstances: failure of nonoperative management, prophylactic stabilization of a fracture at high risk for displacement, any displaced femoral stress fracture, and malunion or nonunion (19).

Femoral Diaphysis

- Stress fractures of the femoral diaphysis are relatively common but often misdiagnosed as muscle or tendon injuries. The most common site of injury is the posteromedial cortex of the proximal femur (18).

- Athletes typically complain of an insidious onset of vague poorly localized thigh pain that is activity related. Physical examination may reveal local tenderness, with normal hip range of motion. Hopping on the affected side will typically reproduce pain in the involved bone. The fulcrum test can be helpful in localizing the anatomic site of involvement (29).

- MRI shows periosteal and bone marrow edema involving the medial aspect of the femur approximately at the junction of the proximal and middle thirds of the femoral diaphysis (4).

- If there is no evidence of cortical break or displacement, conservative treatment is indicated. Once the athlete can ambulate without pain, a cross-training program is appropriate and return to athletic activities can be initiated after 8–12 weeks.

Patella

- Stress fracture of the patella is a rare injury that occurs typically in young athletes and jumping sports (13,14).

- The clinical findings are localized tenderness over the patella. Most patellar stress fractures are of the transverse type. These may be confused radiographically with bipartite patella; however, a patella fracture line tends to be more oblique than the bipartite patella.

Tibia

Posterior-Medial Tibial Shaft

- Many athletes, particularly runners, commonly experience pain along the medial border of the tibia related to training. Pain in this location from medial tibial stress syndrome (tibial periostitis) and tibial stress fractures accounts for up to 75% of injuries presenting to a sports medicine clinic (47).

- Pain is located along the posteromedial border of the tibia, usually in the middle or distal thirds. It is often difficult to clinically distinguish the more severe tibial stress reaction or fracture from the more common medial tibial stress or shin splint syndrome. It has been suggested that the periostitis (seen as periosteal edema on MRI) may be the initial injury on a spectrum that, if allowed to progress, may evolve into a more serious bone injury (16).

- The physical examination findings such as localized tibial tenderness and pain with direct or indirect (at a distance from the site of tenderness) percussion over the involved bone help distinguish it from the more common medial tibial stress syndrome.

- The pain is occasionally aggravated by testing muscle strength actively, particularly in those muscles that have origins on the posterior medial tibial border including the soleus (best tested by repetitive toe raises), posterior tibialis, and flexor digitorum longus.

- It is also important to evaluate the lower extremity alignment as well as mechanical gait. Athletes with increased subtalar pronation have shown a tendency toward developing tibial stress injuries (43). It has been found that both the degree of pronation and also the timing of pronation during gait are important discriminators between athletes at higher risk (56).

- The temporary cessation of running is essential to allow for bony remodeling and repair. This can range from a few days to 3 weeks for a minor injury to 12 weeks for a severe injury with frank cortical fracture. If there is pain with daily activities, a pneumatic tibial brace can be used to immobilize distal and midtibial injuries (16).

Anterior Tibial Diaphysis

- Stress fractures of the anterior cortex of the midtibia require a different approach and treatment. They occur most commonly in athletes performing jumping or leaping activities. Located in the tension side of the bone, they are prone to delayed union, nonunion, or even complete fracture (48).

- Radiographs show a radiolucent cortical defect surrounded by sclerosis, known as the dreaded black line for its propensity for nonunion or even progression to complete fracture that may displace (48).

- These patients require treatment in a non–weight bearing brace for 6–8 weeks. Surgical excision and bone grafting or placement of an intramedullary rod is indicated after 3–6 months of failed closed management (32).

Proximal Tibial Metaphysis

- The proximal tibial metaphysis is a less common site of stress fracture. Tenderness is located along the medial aspect of the proximal tibia just below the medial joint line and is often misdiagnosed as pes anserinus tendinitis or bursitis (24).

- Radiographs may show a linear transverse region of sclerosis 2–3 mm wide in the medial plateau close to the level of the epiphyseal scar.

- An MRI examination may demonstrate bone marrow edema of the proximal tibial and medial tibial plateau before radiographic signs appear, with periosteal edema and sometimes a fracture line (4).

Fibula

- Fibular stress fractures are relatively common, accounting for up to 21% of all stress fractures in athletes (25). Although fibular stress fractures can occur more proximally, the majority occur in the lower third of the fibula, just proximal to the tibiofibular ligament attachment.

- The subcutaneous location of the fibula makes it easy to recreate symptoms with direct palpation over the involved bone. These athletes are often found to have a cavus-type foot.

- Radiographs may not be diagnostic at early stages, whereas MRI examination allows for early diagnosis showing periosteal as well as bone marrow edema and often a fracture line (4).

- Fibular stress fractures are noncritical injuries, and a gradual return to running can typically resume when local tenderness resolves.

Medial Malleolus

- The repetitive stress of running and jumping can create a vertical stress fracture starting at the junction of the medial malleolus and the tibial plafond and continuing proximally and slightly medially.

- It is hypothesized that chronic anteromedial impingement of the talus on the medial malleolus during ankle dorsiflexion may result in a medial malleolar stress fracture (31).

- Stress reactions without frank cortical fracture can be treated with temporary immobilization. Unlimited ambulation in a brace is permitted and a gradual return to sport is allowed as symptoms resolve.

- The presence of a radiographically detectable fracture line or displaced fragment, particularly in a high-level or in-season athlete, is considered an indication for surgical intervention (50).

Calcaneus

- Calcaneal stress fractures usually present as heel pain with localized tenderness over the bone, usually in the body of the calcaneus posterior to the talus (23). Initially, these injuries may present similar to plantar fasciitis. A less common stress injury involves the anterior process of the calcaneus (6).

- Pain elicited by squeezing the calcaneus from both sides simultaneously can usually differentiate this condition from retrocalcaneal bursitis, Achilles tendinitis, plantar nerve entrapment, subtalar arthritis, and radiculopathy (17).

- Radiographs generally become positive within the first month after pain presentation and show callus formation perpendicular to the trabecular axis of the calcaneus, usually located between the calcaneal tuberosity and the posterior facet of the subtalar joint.

- This is a noncritical stress fracture with rapid healing, and return to activity is usually possible within 6 weeks following restriction of activity and partial weight bearing.

Navicular Bone

- Tarsal navicular stress fractures are especially important, as they are particularly difficult to diagnose in their early stages and have a high risk of nonunion.

- Patients report an insidious onset of vague foot pain that is worse with certain activities, such as explosive sprinting, rapid changes in direction, jumping, and push-off (40). Tenderness is often located over the dorsal border of the navicular near the talonavicular joint (34).

- Investigation usually requires bone scan or MRI. Computed tomography (CT) is often needed to detect early separation of bone fragments or more clearly define the degree of fracture (4).

- The most common site of stress fracture within the navicular is the central third, which is an area of relative avascularity.

- Treatment of an uncomplicated partial stress fracture should include at least 6 weeks of non–weight-bearing cast immobilization until the navicular is no longer tender. This is followed by a further 6-week program of rehabilitation (17).

- Athletes who have sustained a navicular stress fracture are at high risk of developing a recurrent stress fracture at the same site if they return to their preinjury level of activity. A surgical option should be considered in the athlete to minimize time out of competition and additional risks (40). One study (49) used the CT fracture pattern to classify the lesion and determine the best treatment. Type I shows a cortical break, type II fractures propagate into the navicular body, and type III fractures propagate into the opposite cortex. Early operative intervention was recommended for type II and III injuries, with return to activity of approximately 4 months for all groups.

Talus, Cuboid, and Cuneiform

- Stress fractures of the talus, cuboid, and cuneiform bones are uncommon. In general, joint involvement, displacement, and nonunion do not occur, and treatment can be the same as that for other noncritical stress fracture (34).

- Stress fractures of the talus may have poorer long-term outcomes, and patients may suffer from persistent pain (6). In particular, fractures of the body of the talus can extend into the subtalar joint, which places them into the critical-at-risk category and requires at least 4–6 weeks of immobilization and occasionally open reduction and internal fixation (7,34).

Metatarsals

- Stress fractures of the metatarsal bones were first described in military recruits and referred to as a march fracture. This fracture typically occurs in the neck or distal shaft, with the second and third metatarsals most commonly affected (26,41).

- The stress fracture at the base of the second metatarsals is known as the dancer's fracture. Pain is noted to be greatest when in the full en pointe position. During this maneuver, the foot is maximally plantarflexed, and weight is borne on the plantar aspect and tip of the first and second distal phalanges (42). These injuries can be difficult to differentiate from synovitis of the Lisfranc joint (23). MRI is often necessary for diagnosis. The injury involves the volar and medial aspect of the Lisfranc joint and should be recognized early and treated with at least 4 weeks of non–weight-bearing immobilization (33,42).

- Stress fractures of the proximal fifth metatarsal diaphysis that occur more than approximately 1.5 cm distal to the tuberosity are known as Jones fractures (30). It is important to differentiate this fracture from the acute avulsion fracture of the tuberosity of the fifth metatarsal (7). The avulsion injury is noncritical and is treated with relative rest and then gradual progression. The Jones fracture is notorious for poor healing and requires prolonged immobilization (6–12 weeks) followed by a functional splint for another 4–8 weeks. In the athletic population, open reduction and screw fixation are recommended (33).

Sesamoids

- Stress fracture of a sesamoid of the great toe can be particularly disabling and can result in delayed union or nonunion. Passive distal push of the sesamoid, direct tenderness, and sesamoid area pain with stretch of the flexor hallucis suggest the diagnosis.

- Radiographic changes may be difficult to detect in sesamoid stress fracture, but occasionally, axial views or magnification views can assist in the diagnosis. Separation of the sesamoid fragments and irregular edges suggest a stress fracture rather than a bipartite sesamoid. MRI is often indicated to confirm the diagnosis (4).

- Rest from the offending activity is clearly advised. For non-operative treatment, it is essential to include a non–weight-bearing 6-week immobilization period with the use of an orthotic designed to off-load the sesamoids and specifically prevent dorsiflexion. Surgical excision is advocated if conservative treatment fails (9).

REFERENCES

1. Arendt E, Agel J, Heikes C, Griffiths H. Stress injuries to bone in college athletes: a retrospective review of experience at a single institution. *Am J Sports Med.* 2003;31(6):959–68.

2. Arendt EA, Griffiths HJ. The use of MR imaging in the assessment and clinical management of stress reactions of bone in high-performance athletes. *Clin Sports Med.* 1997;16(2):291–306.

3. Beck BR, Matheson GO, Bergman G, et al. Do capacitively coupled electric fields accelerate tibial stress fracture healing? A randomized controlled trial. *Am J Sports Med.* 2008;36(3):545–53.

4. Bergman AG, Fredericson M. MR imaging of stress reactions, muscle injuries, and other overuse injuries in runners. *Magn Reson Imaging Clin N Am.* 1999;7(1):151–74, ix.

5. Bergman AG, Fredericson M, Ho C, Matheson GO. Asymptomatic tibial stress reactions: MRI detection and clinical follow-up in distance runners. *AJR Am J Roentgenol.* 2004;183(3):635–8.

6. Brockwell J, Yeung Y, Griffith JF. Stress fractures of the foot and ankle. *Sports Med Arthrosc.* 2009;17(3):149–59.

7. Chuckpaiwong B, Queen RM, Easley ME, Nunley JA. Distinguishing Jones and proximal diaphyseal fractures of the fifth metatarsal. *Clin Orthop Relat Res.* 2008;466(8):1966–70.

8. Cleek TM, Whalen RT. Effect of activity and age on long bones using a new densitometric technique. *Med Sci Sports Exerc.* 2005;37(10):1806–13.

9. Cohen BE. Hallux sesamoid disorders. *Foot Ankle Clin.* 2009;14(1):91–104.

10. Craig DI. Medial tibial stress syndrome: evidence-based prevention. *J Athl Train.* 2008;43(3):316–8.

11. Crossley K, Bennel KL, Wrigley T, Oakes BW. Ground reaction forces, bone characteristics, and tibial stress fracture in male runners. *Med Sci Sports Exerc.* 1999;31(8):1088–93.

12. Daffner RH, Pavlov H. Stress fractures: current concepts. *AJR Am J Roentgenol.* 1992;159(2):245–52.

13. Devas MB. Stress fractures of the patella. *J Bone Joint Surg Br.* 1960;42-B:71–4.

14. Drabicki RR, Greer WJ, DeMeo PJ. Stress fractures around the knee. *Clin Sports Med.* 2006;25(1):105–15, ix.

15. Dugan SA, Weber KM. Stress fractures and rehabilitation. *Phys Med Rehabil Clin N Am.* 2007;18(3):401–16, viii.

16. Fredericson M, Bergman AG, Hoffman KL, Dillingham MS. Tibial stress reaction in runners: correlation of clinical symptoms and scintigraphy with a new magnetic imaging grading system. *Am J Sports Med.* 1995;23(4):472–81.

17. Fredericson M, Bergman AG, Matheson GO. Stress fractures in athletes. *Orthopade.* 1997;26(11):961–71.

18. Fredericson M, Jang KU, Bergman G, Gold G. Femoral diaphyseal stress fractures: results of a systematic bone scan and magnetic resonance imaging evaluation in 25 runners. *Phys Ther Sport.* 2004;5:188–93.

19. Fredericson M, Jennings F, Beaulieu C, Matheson GO. Stress fractures in athletes. *Top Magn Reson Imaging.* 2006;17(5):309–25.

20. Fredericson M, Kent K. Normalization of bone density in a previously amenorrheic runner with osteoporosis. *Med Sci Sports Exerc.* 2005;37(9):1481–6.

21. Fredericson M, Salamancha L, Beaulieu C. Sacral stress fractures: tracking down nonspecific pain in distance runners. *Phys Sportsmed.* 2003;31(2):31–42.

22. Goldstein C, Sprague S, Petrisor BA. Electrical stimulation for fracture healing: current evidence. *J Orthop Trauma.* 2010;24(Suppl 1):S62–5.

23. Goulart M, O'Malley MJ, Hodgkins CW, Charlton TP. Foot and ankle fractures in dancers. *Clin Sports Med.* 2008;27(2):295–304.

24. Harolds JA. Fatigue fractures of the medial tibial plateau. *South Med J.* 1981;74(5):578–81.

25. Harrast MA, Colonno D. Stress fractures in runners. *Clin Sports Med.* 2010;29(3):399–416.

26. Heaslet MW, Kanda-Mehtani SL. Return-to-activity levels in 96 athletes with stress fractures of the foot, ankle, and leg: a retrospective analysis. *J Am Podiatr Med Assoc.* 2007;97(1):81–4.

27. Hubbard TJ, Carpenter EM, Cordova ML. Contributing factors to medial tibial stress syndrome: a prospective investigation. *Med Sci Sports Exerc.* 2009;41(3):490–6.

28. Iwamoto J, Takeda T. Stress fractures in athletes: review of 196 cases. *J Orthop Sci.* 2003;8(3):273–8.

29. Johnson AW, Weiss CB Jr, Wheeler DL. Stress fractures of the femoral shaft in athletes—more common than expected: a new clinical test. *Am J Sports Med.* 1994;22(2):248–56.

30. Jones R. I. Fracture of the base of the fifth metatarsal bone by indirect violence. *Ann Surg.* 1902;35(6):697–700.

31. Jowett AJ, Birks CL, Blackney MC. Medial malleolar stress fracture secondary to chronic ankle impingement. *Foot Ankle Int.* 2008;29(7):716–21.

32. Kaeding CC, Yu JR, Wright R, Amendola A, Spindler KP. Management and return to play of stress fractures. *Clin J Sport Med.* 2005;15(6):442–7.

33. Khan K, Brown J, Way S, et al. Overuse injuries in classical ballet. *Sports Med.* 1995;19(5):341–57.

34. Khan KM, Brukner PD, Kearney C, Fuller PJ, Bradshaw CJ, Kiss ZS. Tarsal navicular stress fracture in athletes. *Sport Med.* 1994;17:65–76.

35. Kiuru MJ, Pihlajamaki HK, Hietanen HJ, Ahovuo JA. MR imaging, bone scintigraphy, and radiography in bone stress injuries of the pelvis and the lower extremity. *Acta Radiol.* 2008;43(2):207–12.

36. Leffers D, Collins L. An overview of the use of bone scintigraphy in sports medicine. *Sports Med Arthrosc.* 2009;17(1):21–4.

37. Li GP, Zhang SD, Chen G, Chen H, Wang AM. Radiologic and histologic analysis of stress fracture in rabbit tibias. *Am J Sports Med.* 1985;13(5): 285–94.

38. Lombardo SJ, Benson DW. Stress fractures of the femur in runners. *Am J Sports Med.* 1982;10(4):219–27.

39. Macera CA. Lower extremity injuries in runners. Advances in prediction. *Sports Med.* 1992;13(1):50–7.

40. Mann JA, Pedowitz DI. Evaluation and treatment of navicular stress fractures, including nonunions, revision surgery, and persistent pain after treatment. *Foot Ankle Clin.* 2009;14(2):187–204.

41. Matheson GO, Clement DB, Mckenzie DC, Tauton JE, Llyod-Smith DR, MacIntyre JG. Stress fractures in athletes. A study of 320 cases. *Am J Sports Med.* 1987;15(1):46–58.

42. Micheli LJ, Sohn RS, Soloman R. Stress fractures of the second metatarsal involving Lisfranc's joint in ballet dancer: a new overuse injury of the foot. *J Bone Joint Surg.* 1985;67(9):1372–5.

43. Moen MH, Tol JL, Weir A, Steunebrink M, De Winter TC. Medial tibial stress syndrome: a critical review. *Sports Med.* 2009;39(7): 523–46.

44. Mollon B, da Silva V, Busse JW, Einhorn TA, Bhandari M. Electrical stimulation for long-bone fracture-healing: a meta-analysis of randomized controlled trials. *J Bone Joint Surg Am.* 2008;90(11): 2322–30.

45. Moran DS, Evans RK, Hadad E. Imaging of lower extremity stress fracture injuries. *Sports Med.* 2008;38(4):345–56.

46. Mulligan ME. The "gray cortex": an early sign of stress fracture. *Skeletal Radiol.* 1995;24(3):201–3.

47. Orava S, Puranen J. Athlete's leg pains. *Br J Sports Med.* 1979;13:92–7.

48. Orava S, Hulkko A. Stress fracture of the mid-tibial shaft. *Acta Orthop Scand.* 1984;55(1):35–7.

49. Saxena A, Fullem B. Navicular stress fractures: a prospective study on athletes. *Foot Ankle Int.* 2006;27(11):917–21.

50. Sherbondy PS, Sebastianelli WJ. Stress fractures of the medial malleolus and distal fibula. *Clin Sports Med.* 2006;25:129–37, x.

51. Shima Y, Engebretsen L, Iwasa J, Kitaoka K, Tomita K. Use of bisphosphonates for the treatment of stress fractures in athletes. *Knee Surg Sports Traumatol Arthrosc.* 2009;17(5):542–50.

52. Sloan AV, Martin JR, Li S, Li J. Parathyroid hormone and bisphosphonate have opposite effects on stress fracture repair. *Bone.* 2010;47(2):235–40.

53. Snyder RA, Koester MC, Dunn WR. Epidemiology of stress fractures. *Clin Sports Med.* 2006;25(1):37–52, viii.

54. Stanitski CL, McMaster JH, Scranton PE. On the nature of stress fractures. *Am J Sports Med.* 1978;6(6):391–6.

55. Tenforde AS, Sayres LC, Sainani KL, Fredericson M. Evaluating the relationship of calcium and vitamin D in the prevention of stress fracture injuries in the young athlete: a review of the literature. *PMR.* 2010; 2(10):945–9.

56. Tweed JL, Campbell JA, Avil SJ. Biomechanical risk factors in the development of medial tibial stress syndrome in distance runners. *J Am Podiatr Med Assoc.* 2008;98(6):436–44.

57. Volpin G, Hoerer D, Groisman G, Zaltzman S, Stein H. Stress fractures of the femoral neck following strenuous activity. *J Orthop Trauma.* 1990;4(4):394–8.

58. Warden SJ, Creaby MW, Bryant AL, Crossley KM. Stress fracture risk factors in female football players and their clinical implications. *Br J Sports Med.* 2007;41(Suppl 1):i38–43.

Lower Extremity Nerve Entrapments

Evan Peck and Jay Smith

68

INTRODUCTION

- Neurologic conditions account for 10–15% of all exercise-induced leg pain among runners (15,79,82,88). Causes include contusion, compression, stretching, and iatrogenic injury (3,5,6,78–80). The interdigital (interdigital or Morton neuroma), lateral plantar (LPN), medial plantar (MPN), tibial (TN), peroneal (common [CPN], deep [DPN], and/or superficial [SPN]), sural (SN), or saphenous nerves may be affected (79).

- Figures 68.1 through 68.7 show the relevant neuroanatomy, including as it pertains to entrapment sites.

- Table 68.1 outlines the anatomic relationship among the lower limb nerves.

COMMON NERVE ENTRAPMENT SYNDROMES

Interdigital Neuroma (Morton Neuroma)

Definition

- Most commonly affects the third web space; rarely the first or fourth web spaces (Figs. 68.1 and 68.2) (82).

- Typically affects ages 20 or older; more common in women (5,78,79,98).

Anatomy, Pathophysiology, and Risk Factors

- During push-off, forceful toe dorsiflexion compresses and stretches the interdigital nerve across the dorsal intermetatarsal ligament, resulting in demyelination, scarring, and hypertrophy (5).

- Others suggest that Morton neuromas result from the pressure of the metatarsal heads and metatarsophalangeal (MTP) joints (41).

- Risk factors: prolonged running, squatting, high-heeled or narrow toe-boxed shoes, or demi-pointe in ballet (98).

- Hyperpronation dorsiflexes the third metatarsal relative to the fourth, exposing the nerve to injury during push-off (79).

- Idiopathic MTP synovitis may cause local edema and interdigital nerve compression (78).

Symptoms and Signs

- Tenderness in affected intermetatarsal space; neuropathic pain, typically between the third and fourth toes, increased with running, standing, walking, toe dorsiflexion, and squatting.

- Provocative testing: pressure over plantar aspect of the web space between the metatarsal heads, or squeezing metatarsals together during palpation. The squeeze test may also result in a click ("Mulder click") as the neuroma subluxates from between the metatarsals in a plantar direction (79).

Differential Diagnosis and Evaluation

- Differential diagnosis includes proximal and systemic neurologic conditions, stress fractures, MTP joint synovitis or arthritis, and flexor tenosynovitis.

- Diagnostic interdigital nerve block is confirmatory.

- Diagnostic ultrasound (US) can be used for diagnosis or to guide therapeutic injection (34,36,70,83).

- Magnetic resonance imaging (MRI) and US have comparable detection rates for evaluation of Morton neuroma (45).

Treatment

- Activity modification, nonsteroidal anti-inflammatory drugs (NSAIDs), footwear modifications, physical therapy, and biomechanical interventions to reduce toe dorsiflexion, control hyperpronation, and maintain greater metatarsal separation.

- Corticosteroids have been used with good results in some cases (52).

- Sonographically guided alcohol ablation of the neuroma may be used (36). One study reported resolution of pain in 80.3% of cases at a mean follow-up of 36 months (50).

- Surgery is generally indicated when diagnosis is firm and symptoms refractory. One study noted that 76% of cases were asymptomatic at a minimum of 2 years postoperatively after surgical resection (22). Minimally invasive techniques have also been described, with similarly favorable outcomes reported in one small study (100).

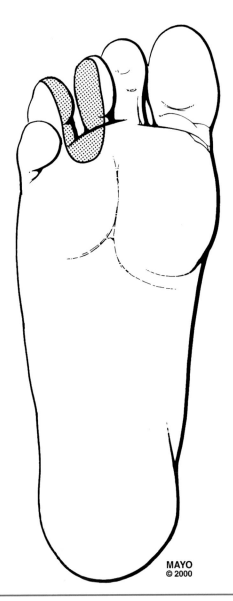

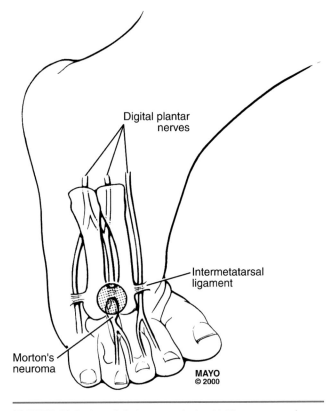

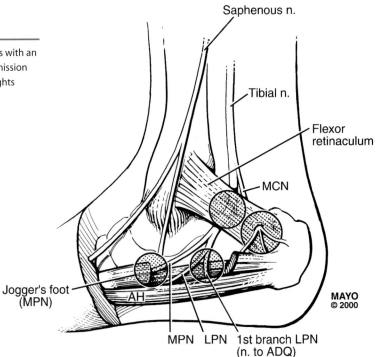

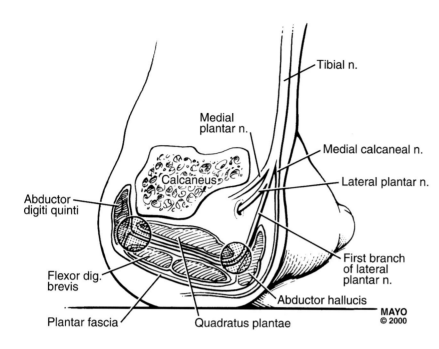

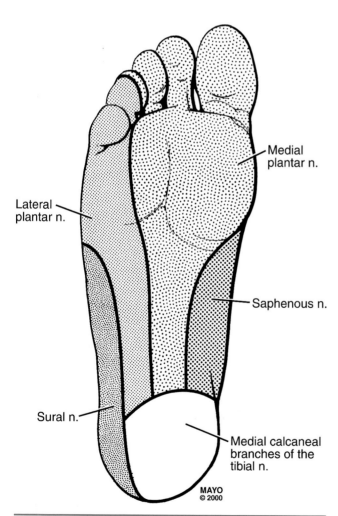

FIGURE 68.5: Cutaneous innervation of the plantar surface of the foot. By permission of Mayo Foundation for Medical Education and Research. All rights reserved.

Tibial Nerve (TN): Tarsal Tunnel Syndrome (TTS)

Definition

- TN entrapment most commonly occurs at the level of the tarsal tunnel (Fig. 68.3) (82). There is a slight (56%) female predilection (43). TN entrapment may also occur at the level of the medial gastrocnemius (high TTS), under the fibromuscular arch of the soleus, or as a result of popliteus muscle tear (5,6,19,24,67,78,79).

Anatomy, Pathophysiology, and Risk Factors

- The TN originates from the L4 to S3 spinal segments and is the larger terminal branch of the sciatic nerve (52). The tarsal tunnel is a fibro-osseous space formed by the flexor retinaculum, medial calcaneus, posterior talus, distal tibia, and medial malleolus, and extends from the distal tibia to the navicular bone. Over 90% of the time, the TN will divide into the MPN and LPN within the tarsal tunnel (43). Within 1–2 cm below the medial malleolar-calcaneal line, the MPN and LPN enter separate fibro-osseous canals at the origin of the abductor hallucis muscle (AHM) (62,79). At this point, the LPN may be particularly vulnerable to injury (43).

- Etiologies include trauma, compression by space-occupying lesions (*e.g.*, venous varicosities, ganglion, neurilemmoma, tenosynovitis, os trigonum, bone fragments, tumors, or accessory muscles), systemic disease, and biomechanical factors (38,55,58,59,62,64,65,69,77,87,99). Hyperpronation increases AHM tension and may entrap the TN or plantar nerves (43). Eversion and inversion of the foot and ankle have been shown to decrease tarsal tunnel compartment volume (9). A specific cause is identified in only 60%–80% of cases (43).

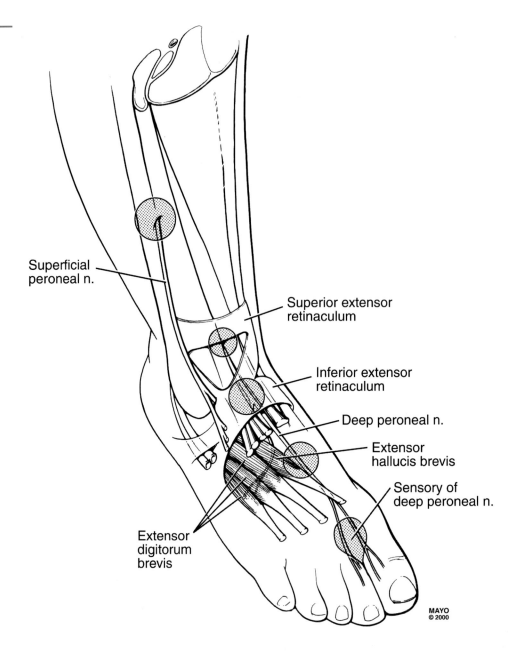

Symptoms and Signs

- Symptoms include cramping, burning, and tingling at the medial ankle, medial foot, and/or plantar foot. The medial heel is usually spared because of the proximal origin of the MCN (43). Symptoms increase with activity. Running on a banked surface promotes hyperpronation and may aggravate symptoms (52). Resting and night pain may occur in provocative positions, and shaking the foot or walking may provide relief, similar to carpal tunnel syndrome (78,79).

- Examination includes inspection for malalignment, deformity, or muscular atrophy causing or resulting from TTS, such as forefoot pronation, claw toe, talipes calcaneus, or calcaneovalgus. Percussion testing is completed over the TN and all its terminal branches; a Valleix phenomenon (proximal radiation from the site of entrapment) may be elicited (21).

Provocative maneuvers include sustained passive eversion or great toe dorsiflexion, and postexercise examination.

- In severe cases, weakness of toe plantarflexion manifests by reduced push-off on the affected side (52).

Differential Diagnosis and Evaluation

- Differential diagnosis includes polyneuropathy, proximal or distal neuropathy, deep posterior compartment syndrome, popliteal artery entrapment, vascular claudication, venous disease, tenosynovitis, ganglia, plantar fasciitis, tibiotalar or subtalar synovitis, accessory muscles, and osseous compression (76,93).

- TN injury just distal to the SN contribution spares lateral calcaneal and foot sensation and gastrocnemius-soleus function. Injury distal to the midportion of the leg affects plantar

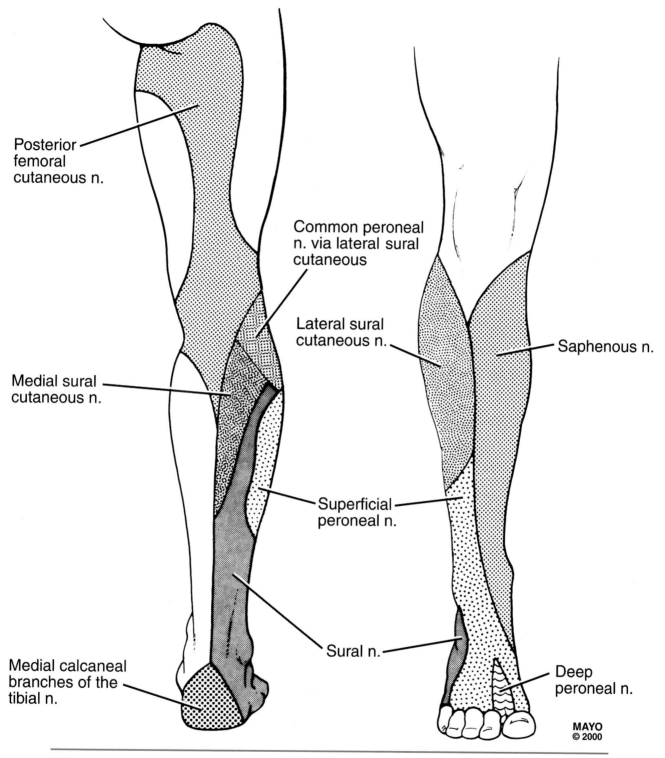

FIGURE 68.7: Cutaneous innervation of the thigh, leg, and dorsal surface of the foot. By permission of Mayo Foundation for Medical Education and Research. All rights reserved.

Table 68.1 | Neuroanatomy of the Lower Limb

Sciatic nerve (L4–S3 spinal segments)	Tibial nerve (TN)	Medial sural cutaneous nerve (MSCN)	
		Medial calcaneal nerve (MCN)[1]	
		Medial plantar nerve (MPN)	Contribution to third interdigital nerve
			Medial hallucal nerve
		Lateral plantar nerve (LPN)	First branch of LPN (FB-LPN)[2]
			Contribution to third interdigital nerve
	Common peroneal nerve (CPN)	Lateral sural cutaneous nerve (LSCN)	
		Superficial peroneal nerve (SPN)	
		Deep peroneal nerve (DPN)	
Femoral nerve (FN; L2–4 spinal segments)			Saphenous nerve
Lateral femoral cutaneous nerve (LFCN; L2–3 spinal segments)			
Obturator nerve (ON; L2–4 spinal segments)			

[1] May arise from the LPN or from the bifurcation of the LPN and MPN.
[2] May arise directly from the TN.

sensation and results in claw toe deformity caused by imbalance between the affected foot intrinsic muscles and the unaffected flexor digitorum longus (FDL) and extensor digitorum brevis (EDB) muscles (52).

■ Night pain, proximal radiation, and lack of pain during the first steps in the morning help differentiate TTS from plantar fasciitis (39).

■ MRI is effective for examining the tarsal tunnel and reveals an inflammatory lesion or mass in up to 88% of patients with a firm clinical diagnosis of TTS (27). Diagnostic US can also effectively visualize structures within the tarsal tunnel and accurately identify compressive mass lesions and/or focal changes in TN cross-sectional area (2,59,94).

■ Electrodiagnostic (EDX) studies may be positive in up to 90% of patients with tarsal tunnel syndrome; whether EDX findings correlate with surgical outcome is controversial (28,32). Of note, increased spontaneous activity can be seen in normal subjects in the AHM (8).

Treatment

■ Treatment includes activity modification, NSAIDs, neuromodulatory medications (tricyclic and antiepileptic medications), physical therapy, and biomechanical interventions including pronation control (43). A change in running habits to reduce TN tension may be useful (71).

■ Corticosteroid injection may be useful; a period of postinjection protected weight bearing is recommended (43). Injections around the TN are more accurate with US guidance (72).

■ Surgery may be indicated when diagnosis is firm and symptoms are refractory (43). Up to 65% of patients required surgical treatment in one study (12).

■ Postoperatively, neuropathic symptoms generally improve after 6 weeks, but maximal recovery may take 6 months or more (78). Although traditionally good or excellent results were reported in 79–95% of cases, a more methodologically stringent study indicated only 44% of patients significantly

benefited at a minimum 24-month follow-up (43,68). Another investigation found that 54% of patients obtained satisfactory benefit following surgical decompression of TTS (91). Endoscopic techniques exist, but adequacy of decompression has been questioned (62).

First Branch of the Lateral Plantar Nerve (FB-LPN)

Definition

■ FB-LPN entrapment is reported to be the most common neurologic cause of heel pain (6,82). Up to 15% of athletes with chronic, recalcitrant heel pain may have FB-LPN entrapment (79). The average age of runners in the largest series to date was 38 years, and 88% were men (6).

Anatomy, Pathophysiology, and Risk Factors

■ The FB-LPN usually arises from the LPN in the tarsal tunnel, but in 46% of cases, it may originate directly from the TN (Fig. 68.3) (62). After penetrating the AHM and its fascia, the FB-LPN courses inferiorly, passing between the deep fascia of the AHM medially and the medial-caudal margin of the medial head of the quadratus plantae muscle laterally (6). The nerve then courses between the flexor digitorum brevis and quadratus plantae muscles (Fig. 68.4). The FB-LPN ramifies into three terminal branches supplying the flexor digitorum brevis, the medial calcaneal periosteum, and the abductor digiti quinti. The branch to the calcaneal periosteum often supplies branches to the long plantar ligament as well as an inconsistent branch to the quadratus plantae muscle (79).

■ FB-LPN entrapment may occur at the site of direction change from an inferior to lateral course deep to the AHM (most likely), between the calcaneus and flexor digitorum brevis muscle, or at the plantar aspect of the long plantar ligament (6,40). FB-LPN entrapment has been reported secondary to AHM or quadratus plantae hypertrophy, accessory muscles, abnormal bursae, venous varicosities, calcaneal spurs, and scar tissue from adjacent repetitive injury (5,6,26,40,63).

- FB-LPN irritation is believed to occur in up to 15%–20% of cases of chronic plantar fasciitis (5,6,40,52,78). Those with proximal edema of the flexor digitorum brevis or microtears in the plantar fascia may be more susceptible (52). The FB-LPN may be injured by a large calcaneal spur (80).

Symptoms and Signs

- Chronic, neuropathic, medial heel pain is seen. Symptoms are precipitated by sports in 50% of cases (6). Up to 25% of patients have severe pain in the morning secondary to venous engorgement, but night pain is rare (80).

- A suggested pathognomonic sign of FB-LPN entrapment is maximal pain over the medial heel, superior to the plantar fascia origin, along a line drawn parallel to the posterior tibia. In one study, 100% of patients exhibited maximal pain over this site, although 42% also had mild tenderness of the plantar fascia origin (6).

Differential Diagnosis and Evaluation

- Heel pain syndrome, plantar fasciitis, and fat pad disorders are suggested by finding maximal tenderness in the plantar calcaneal region, anterior medial calcaneus, or mid-medial edge of the plantar fascia, respectively (6). Sensory loss on the medial heel suggests another disorder.

- In 27 patients with 38 symptomatic heels from surgically documented FB-LPN entrapment, only 44% had involvement of the LPN on EDX testing (80).

Treatment

- Most cases of FB-LPN entrapment respond to nonoperative measures (40). Recommended interventions include activity modification, NSAIDs, neuromodulatory medications, physical therapy, biomechanical management for pronation control, and corticosteroid injections (40). One author recommends no more than three injections at 2- to 4-week intervals be attempted (52).

- Most clinicians advocate at least 6–12 months of nonoperative care before considering surgery. Postoperative recovery typically takes 3–6 months, but may be longer if small toe abduction is weak preoperatively (78). With careful patient selection and firm diagnosis, good or excellent results may be seen in approximately 85% of patients (6). A retrospective analysis of outcomes after FB-LPN surgical release found 50% of cases to be asymptomatic and 50% to be mildly symptomatic with activity, at a mean follow-up of 32.8 months (31). Endoscopic techniques have been described (49).

Medial Plantar Nerve (MPN): Jogger's Foot

Definition

- Syndrome of neuropathic pain radiating along the medial heel and longitudinal arch resulting from local entrapment of the MPN (71,82).

Anatomy, Pathophysiology, and Risk Factors

- The MPN enters the sole of the foot, passes superficial to the traversing FDL tendon at the master knot of Henry, and continues distally along the flexor hallucis longus tendon to divide into terminal medial and lateral branches at the level of the base of the first metatarsal (79). These branches ramify and terminate as three common plantar digital nerves within the medial three web spaces. The MPN is a mixed sensorimotor nerve providing sensation to the medial sole and plantar aspect of the first to third and medial fourth toes, as well as motor innervation to the AHM, flexor hallucis brevis, flexor digitorum brevis, and first lumbrical muscles (Figs. 68.3 and 68.5).

- MPN entrapment typically occurs at the AHM fibro-osseous canal or master knot of Henry (5). The MPN may be compressed by AHM hypertrophy, functional hyperpronation, high-arched orthoses, or in association with hallux rigidus or tibial artery schwannoma (5,71,79,84).

Symptoms and Signs

- Exercise-induced neuropathic pain is reported, radiating along the medial arch toward the plantar aspect of the first and second toes. The most useful palpatory finding is maximal tenderness at the superior aspect of the AHM at the navicular tuberosity, with distally radiating pain (52,71). Provocative testing includes forceful passive heel eversion, standing on the forefoot, or percussion over the nerve. Examination may be normal unless the athlete is examined after running (5).

Differential Diagnosis and Evaluation

- MPN entrapment typically presents with burning medial heel pain, longitudinal arch aching, and medial sole paresthesias (71). Differential diagnosis parallels that of TTS, with the exception of additional local pathologic processes. Resisted great toe plantarflexion or passive dorsiflexion induces pain with flexor hallucis longus tendinopathy, but not typically with nerve entrapment (52).

- EDX studies should be interpreted with caution; asymptomatic runners have been found to have abnormal nerve conduction velocities in the MPN and sural nerve (14).

Treatment

- Rigid orthoses should be removed to avoid MPN compression. Functional hyperpronation may be addressed by medial arch strengthening, kinetic chain rehabilitation, modifying running mechanics (less valgus) or terrain, or altering footwear (71).

- Surgical release has been successful in refractory cases and is generally a distal extension of TTS surgery.

Common Peroneal Nerve (CPN)

Definition

- CPN entrapment typically occurs at the fibular head, proximal to the bifurcation into the SPN and DPN, and produces dorsiflexion weakness and neuropathic pain over the anterolateral leg and foot dorsum (82). It is the most prevalent peroneal nerve injury seen in runners (44,52,57).

Anatomy, Pathophysiology, and Risk Factors

- The CPN contains sensory and motor fibers from the L4–S2 segments and is the smaller terminal branch of the sciatic nerve (Figs. 68.5 through 68.7). The CPN separates from the sciatic nerve at the apex of the popliteal fossa, where it supplies innervation to the short head of the biceps femoris muscle and divides into the SPN, DPN, and lateral sural cutaneous nerve at the level of the fibular head.

- The SPN innervates lateral compartment leg muscles and emerges from the lateral compartment by penetrating the crural fascia 10.5–12.5 cm proximal to the tip of the lateral malleolus. It supplies sensation to the anterolateral leg and divides into terminal medial and intermediate cutaneous branches about 6 cm above the lateral malleolus (Figs. 68.6 and 68.7). These branches enter the dorsal foot superficial to the inferior extensor retinaculum and supply sensation to the dorsal foot, with the exception of the first web space.

- The DPN innervates anterior compartment leg muscles, divides into medial and lateral branches 1–2 cm proximal to the ankle, and enters the foot deep to the inferior extensor retinaculum. The medial branch supplies sensation to the first web space; the lateral branch innervates the EDB and local joints. Up to 20% of individuals may have accessory innervation of the EDB from the SPN (52).

- The CPN is vulnerable to compression at the fibular head. Causes include external compression, aneurysms, tumors, tibiofibular joint ganglia, tibiofibular or knee dislocation or instability, Baker cyst, generalized ligamentous laxity, genu varum, genu recurvatum, compartment syndrome, stress fracture, fabella syndrome, fascial compression by the edge of the peroneus longus muscle, direct ice injury, ischemia, and complication of an ankle sprain or after knee surgery (1,7,17,20,44,54,56,57,60,66,85).

Symptoms and Signs

- The DPN is often more severely affected than the SPN. Neuropathic symptoms may affect the anterior or anterolateral leg, extending into the dorsal foot and toe web spaces. The most common complaint is weakness, most often with ankle dorsiflexion (52).

- Postexercise percussion sensitivity or weakness was detected in all seven patients with CPN injury who had normal baseline examinations in one study (44).

Differential Diagnosis and Evaluation

- A focal CPN injury would not involve the TN sensorimotor functions or the cutaneous distribution of the saphenous nerve. Sciatic neuropathy, lumbosacral plexopathy, and L5 radiculopathy may also produce foot drop, but typically produce weakness in nonperoneal innervated muscles, nonperoneal territory sensory loss, and nonperoneal reflex loss. Multiple sclerosis may present as relatively painless, exercise-induced foot drop (Uhthoff phenomenon).

- Diagnostic US can detect intraneural ganglia and other CPN abnormalities (95). EDX abnormalities may only occur postexercise (44).

Treatment

- Treatment may include nerve protection, neuromodulatory medications, transcutaneous electrical nerve stimulation (TENS), biomechanical interventions, dorsiflexion support, knee stabilization, or change in running technique.

- If the clinical diagnosis is firm, operative decompression usually provides satisfactory results. In one small study, 86% of runners returned to normal activities within 6 weeks of surgical treatment (44).

Superficial Peroneal Nerve (SPN)

Definition

- Typically occurs as the nerve penetrates the crural fascia above the ankle, resulting in neuropathic pain in the SPN distribution (Figs. 68.6 and 68.7). Among athletes, the mean age is 28 years, and men and women are equally affected (79).

Anatomy, Pathophysiology, and Risk Factors

- May result from sharp fascial edges, chronic ankle sprains, muscular herniation, direct contusive trauma, fibular fracture, edema, varicose veins, wearing tight ski boots or roller blades, biomechanical factors, space-occupying lesions (such as nerve sheath tumors, lipomas, and ganglia), ankle fractures, or a complication of ankle surgery (74,86,92). Up to 10% of affected individuals may have lateral chronic exertional compartment syndrome (90).

Symptoms and Signs

- Diffuse ache over the sinus tarsi or dorsolateral foot. One-third of patients report numbness or tingling (89). Sensation may be an achy distal anterolateral leg discomfort, and proximal radiation has been reported (48).

- Examination may reveal percussion tenderness, a fascial defect (60% of patients), or muscular herniation at the exit site approximately 10.5–12.5 cm above the ankle.

- Provocative testing before and after exercise is the most useful clinical indicator of SPN entrapment and includes: (a) pressure over the exit site during resisted ankle dorsiflexion-eversion, (b) pressure over the same area during passive plantarflexion combined with inversion, and (c) percussion over the SPN course while passive plantarflexion and inversion are maintained. Pain or paresthesias indicate a positive test, and the presence of two positive tests strongly supports the diagnosis (89,90). Sensation may be diminished, but this is uncommon (79).

Differential Diagnosis and Evaluation

- Postexercise nerve conduction testing has been advocated when necessary (90). Diagnostic US can trace the course of the SPN to assess for abnormalities (11).

Treatment

- Parallels that for CPN entrapment, but may also include corticosteroid injection, ankle instability rehabilitation, myofascial release, or lateral heel wedges.

- In refractory confirmed cases, surgery typically consists of isolated release at the fascial exit site, reduction of muscular herniation, fat nodule resection, and fasciotomy if compartment syndrome is documented. One study reported that up to 75% of patients who underwent surgical decompression remained improved at 18-month follow-up; however, only 4 of 17 patients had unlimited activity levels, whereas 10 of 17 patients categorized their activity as improved but still limited (89,90).

Deep Peroneal Nerve (DPN): Anterior Tarsal Tunnel Syndrome (ATTS)

Definition

- DPN irritation in the vicinity of the extensor retinaculum, resulting in neuropathic pain extending into the dorsomedial foot and first web space (Figs. 68.6 and 68.7) (82).

Anatomy, Pathophysiology, and Risk Factors

- The DPN traverses deep to the extensor retinaculum and between the extensor hallucis longus and extensor digitorum longus tendons, approximately 3–5 cm above the ankle joint. At the level of the oblique superior band of the inferior extensor retinaculum, about 1 cm above the ankle joint, the DPN forms its terminal lateral and medial branches. The lateral branch innervates the EDB muscle. The medial branch courses distally with the dorsalis pedis artery, passing deep to the oblique inferior medial band of the inferior extensor retinaculum, where it may be entrapped by processes affecting the talonavicular joint (79).

- DPN entrapment may occur at the inferior aspect of the superior extensor retinaculum where the extensor hallucis longus crosses over the DPN, the inferior extensor retinaculum (most common), or where the EDB crosses the DPN in the first intermetatarsal space. In the latter two cases, an isolated sensory neuropathy of the medial branch occurs. Entrapment may occur due to trauma, shoe contact pressure ("boot top" neuropathy), osteophytic compression, edema, or synovitis or ganglia (16,18,29,46).

Symptoms and Signs

- Symptoms include dorsal midfoot pain and neuropathic symptoms extending into the first web space. Symptoms are worse with activity, prolonged standing, and wearing tight-fitting or high-top shoes, and relieved by rest. Night pain can occur from pressure or prolonged plantarflexion positioning (62). Depending on entrapment site, symptom provocation may occur with either plantarflexion or dorsiflexion of the ankle (5,62).

Differential Diagnosis and Evaluation

- Parallels that for CPN and SPN entrapments but also includes anterior compartment syndrome. Because CPN entrapments often preferentially affect the DPN fascicles, CPN injury presenting as DPN injury should be excluded (52). Involvement of the EDB localizes injury above the extensor retinaculum.

- Radiographs may reveal dorsal midfoot osteophytes or accessory ossicles that may irritate terminal branches of the DPN (58).

Treatment

- Treatment includes footwear changes to avoid direct pressure, neuromodulatory and anti-inflammatory medications, TENS, edema control, ankle stability rehabilitation, and local corticosteroid injections. Surgery involves partial sectioning of the extensor retinaculum and osteophyte removal. Recovery may take 6–8 weeks.

MISCELLANEOUS NERVE ENTRAPMENT SYNDROMES

Medial Calcaneal Nerve (MCN)

- MCN entrapment produces neuropathic pain at the medial heel secondary to entrapment in the tarsal tunnel region (82). The purely sensory MCN usually arises from the TN, but may arise from the LPN or at the MPN-LPN bifurcation; thus, the MCN many originate proximal to or within the tarsal tunnel. The MCN pierces the flexor retinaculum to provide cutaneous innervation to the posterior, medial, and plantar surfaces of the heel (Figs. 68.3, 68.5, and 68.7). Entrapment usually occurs as the MCN pierces the flexor retinaculum.

- Contributing factors may include excessive pronation, direct compression, or repetitive heel impact on hard surfaces. Neuropathic pain is limited to the medial heel, and there is no motor or reflex deficit. Symptoms increase with activity. Percussion tenderness may be present, or paresthesia may occur when palpating the MCN as it pierces the retinaculum posterior to the TN (Fig. 68.3). Examination will less commonly reveal proximal radiation, or a "lamp cord sign," a hypersensitive, tender thickening of the MCN along its oblique-posterior course (13).

- Differential diagnosis is similar to TTS, but medial heel involvement suggests MCN entrapment.

- Nonoperative management follows general principles previously discussed, including measures to improve pronation control, corticosteroid injections, and cut-out pads and footwear alterations to reduce direct pressure on the MCN. A small study showed promising results with extracorporeal shockwave treatment (4). The "lamp cord" sign is often a poor prognostic factor, and surgery is often recommended to remove this "pseudoneuroma" (13).

Sural Nerve (SN)

- The SN is formed by branches of the TN and CPN in the posterior calf, 11–20 cm proximal to the lateral malleolus (82). Two centimeters proximal to the lateral malleolus, the SN provides a sensory branch to the lateral heel, and then courses subcutaneously inferior to the peroneal tendons to the base of the fifth metatarsal, where it ramifies into distal sensory branches (Figs. 68.5 and 68.7). Causes include recurrent ankle sprains, calcaneal or fifth metatarsal fractures, Achilles tendinopathy, space-occupying lesions such as ganglia, direct contusion, footwear-induced pressure, or iatrogenic (33,61).

- Symptoms consist of achy, posterolateral calf pain, with neuropathic pain in the SN distribution. Examination includes percussion testing along the nerve and provocative testing by passive dorsiflexion and inversion.

- Sural nerve conduction studies in asymptomatic runners may be abnormal (14).

- Treatment emphasizes pressure reduction from footwear, Achilles stretching, neuropathic pain treatment, edema control, and ankle stability rehabilitation. When SN block is indicated, US guidance has been shown to improve clinical outcome (73). A retrospective study found good to excellent results in 17 of 18 sural nerve entrapment cases undergoing surgical neurolysis (23).

Saphenous Nerve

- The saphenous nerve is the largest cutaneous branch of the femoral nerve. This purely sensory nerve arises from the femoral nerve in the femoral triangle and courses with the femoral artery to the medial knee, where its infrapatellar branch supplies cutaneous sensation to the medial knee (82). It then courses inferiorly with the saphenous vein to supply cutaneous sensation to the medial calf to the level of the ankle (78). At the ankle, a branch passes anterior to the medial malleolus to innervate the medial foot (Figs. 68.3 and 68.5). The saphenous nerve is most vulnerable at the medial knee, where it pierces the fascia and emerges from the distal subsartorial canal (Hunter adductor canal).

- Causes of saphenous neuropathy include entrapment at the adductor canal, pes anserine bursitis, contusion, patellar dislocation, and iatrogenic injury from knee surgery or injection (25,30,35,37,47,97).

- Athletes report neuropathic pain and numbness in the area of the medial knee and/or calf, depending on whether there is isolated infrapatellar branch or complete saphenous nerve involvement. Saphenous neuropathy related to pes anserine bursitis may clinically resemble tibial stress fracture (35).

- Examination includes percussion testing along the nerve starting at the adductor canal.

- Differential diagnosis includes all proximal femoral nerve, plexus, and root lesions, as well as musculoskeletal disorders about the knee. Diagnosis and treatment principles resemble those for SN entrapment but focus on different anatomic areas. Surgical release or excision of a neuroma may be necessary.

Obturator Nerve (ON)

- ON entrapment is a potential source of groin pain in some athletes (53). The ON arises from the L2–4 spinal segments, exits the pelvis via a fibro-osseous tunnel (obturator canal),

and divides into terminal anterior and posterior branches (53). These branches provide the predominant motor innervation to the thigh adductor group and sensory innervations to the distal one-half to two-thirds of the medial thigh (82). ON entrapment most commonly occurs at the exit of the obturator canal due to compressive fibrous bands located in this area (10,53). Rarely, ON entrapment may occur secondary to the local inflammatory changes of osteitis pubis or from an obturator hernia (42,53).

- The athlete will typically complain of activity-related groin pain of a deep, burning, achy quality. Pain radiation, numbness, tingling, and weakness are rare. Examination is largely unremarkable, but assists in excluding more common causes of hip and groin pain among athletes.

- EDX studies may reveal fibrillation potentials in the adductor muscles in some cases but are not uniformly helpful (10,53). Local anesthetic and corticosteroid injections may assist in making the diagnosis and have successfully treated some cases when combined with rehabilitation. Surgical treatment may be necessary (10). A laparoscopic method has been described (75).

Lateral Femoral Cutaneous Nerve (LFCN): Meralgia Paresthetica

- LFCN injury has been reported in athletes (51). The purely sensory LFCN arises from the L2–3 spinal segments and typically exits the pelvis by passing underneath or through the lateral aspect of the ilioinguinal ligament, just medial to the anterior superior iliac spine (ASIS) (53). The LFCN then splits into two terminal branches, supplying cutaneous innervation to the anterolateral thigh (82). LFCN injury usually occurs at the level of the ilioinguinal ligament, where repetitive hip flexion-extension can injure the nerve, and the nerve is susceptible to local contusive trauma due to its superficial location.

- Etiologies include rapid weight change, compression from tight clothing or belts, and systemic disease affecting nerves such as thyroid disease and diabetes.

- Athletes report burning, aching discomfort over the anterolateral thigh, with or without clear inciting factors. Examination is often normal but may reveal percussion tenderness or a percussion sign approximately 1 cm anterior and inferior to the ASIS, or a sensory deficit in the cutaneous distribution.

- Differential diagnosis includes focal musculoskeletal pathologies or lesions affecting the lumbosacral plexus or L2–3 nerve roots. Local anesthetic and corticosteroid injections may be diagnostic and therapeutic. Treatment involves removal of inciting factor, treatment of neuropathic pain, and injections. Up to 90% of cases resolve with nonoperative management (96). Surgical release is sometimes necessary (53). One series reported complete symptom resolution in 73% of cases following surgical decompression at a mean follow-up of 4.1 years (81).

Medial Hallucal Nerve

- The medial hallucal nerve is a distal terminal branch of the MPN, providing sensation to the medial aspect of the great toe (82). This nerve may be rarely entrapped as it exits the distal end of the AHM, producing medial first MTP joint pain and neuropathic pain extending along the medial great toe. Etiologies include pressure from hallux valgus, prominent tibial sesamoid, abductor hallucis tendinopathy, and poorly fitting footwear.

- Percussion tenderness or a percussion sign over the nerve may be useful on examination. Differential diagnosis includes medial tibial sesamoid disorders, MTP joint disorders, and polyneuropathy. Treatment includes removal of inciting factors and treatment of neuropathic pain as previously described.

REFERENCES

1. Al-Kashmiri A, Delaney JS. Case report: fatigue fracture of the proximal fibula with secondary common peroneal nerve injury. *Clin Orthop Relat Res.* 2007;463:225–8.

2. Alshami AM, Cairns CW, Wylie BK, Souvlis T, Coppieters MW. Reliability and size of the measurement error when determining cross-sectional area of the tibial nerve at the tarsal tunnel with ultrasonography. *Ultrasound Med Biol.* 2009;35(7):1098–102.

3. Babcock JL. Cervical spine injuries. Diagnosis and classification. *Arch Surg.* 1976;111(6):646–51.

4. Barrett SL, Reese MM, Tassone J, Buitrago M. The use of low-energy radial shockwave in the treatment of entrapment neuropathy of the medial calcaneal nerve: a pilot study. *Foot Ankle Spec.* 2008;1(4):231–42.

5. Baxter DE. Functional nerve disorders in the athlete's foot, ankle and leg. *Instr Course Lect.* 1993;42:185–94.

6. Baxter DE, Pfeffer GB. Treatment of chronic heel pain by surgical release of the first branch of the lateral plantar nerve. *Clin Orthop Relat Res.* 1992;(279):229–36.

7. Bonnevialle P, Dubrana F, Galau B, et al. Common peroneal nerve palsy complicating knee dislocation and bicruciate ligaments tears. *Orthop Traumatol Surg Res.* 2010;96(1):64–9.

8. Boon AJ, Harper CM. Needle EMG of abductor hallucis and peroneus tertius in normal subjects. *Muscle Nerve.* 2003;27(6):752–6.

9. Bracilovic A, Nihal A, Houston VL, Beattie AC, Rosenberg ZS, Trepman E. Effect of foot and ankle position on tarsal tunnel compartment volume. *Foot Ankle Int.* 2006;27(6):431–7.

10. Bradshaw C, McCrory P, Bell S, Brukner P. Obturator nerve entrapment. A cause of groin pain in athletes. *Am J Sports Med.* 1997;25(3):402–8.

11. Canella C, Demondion X, Guillin R, Boutry N, Peltier J, Cotten A. Anatomic study of the superficial peroneal nerve using sonography. *AJR Am J Roentgenol.* 2009;193(1):174–9.

12. Cimino WR. Tarsal tunnel syndrome: review of the literature. *Foot Ankle.* 1990;11(1):47–52.

13. Cohen S. Another consideration in the diagnosis of heel pain: neuroma of the medial calcaneal nerve. *J Foot Ankle Surg.* 1974;13:128.

14. Colak T, Bamaç B, Gönener A, Ozbek A, Budak F. Comparison of nerve conduction velocities of lower extremities between runners and controls. *J Sci Med Sport.* 2005;8(4):403–10.

15. Coughlin MJ, Mann RA, Saltzman CL. *Surgery of the Foot and Ankle.* 8th ed. St. Louis (MO): Mosby; 2006. 1511 p.

16. Dallari D, Pellacani A, Marinelli A, Verni E, Giunti A. Deep peroneal nerve paresis in a runner caused by ganglion at capitulum peronei. Case report and review of the literature. *J Sports Med Phys Fitness.* 2004;44(4):436–40.

17. Dawson DM, Hallett M, Wilbourn AJ, editors. *Entrapment Neuropathies.* 3rd ed. Philadelphia: Lippincott-Raven; 1999. p. 273–8.

18. Dellon A. Deep peroneal nerve entrapment on the dorsum of the foot. *Foot Ankle.* 1990;11(2):73–80.

19. de Ruiter GC, Torchia ME, Amrami KK, Spinner RJ. Neurovascular compression following isolated popliteus muscle rupture: a case report. *J Surg Orthop Adv.* 2005;14(3):129–32.

20. DiRisio D, Lazaro R, Popp AJ. Nerve entrapment and calf atrophy caused by a Baker's cyst: case report. *Neurosurgery.* 1994;35(2):333–4.

21. Dumitru D, Amato AA, Zwarts MJ, editors. *Electrodiagnostic Medicine.* 2nd ed. Philadelphia (PA): Hanley & Belfus; 2001. 1103 p.

22. Espinosa N, Schmitt JW, Saupe N, et al. Morton neuroma: MR imaging after resection — postoperative MR and histologic findings in asymptomatic and symptomatic intermetatarsal spaces. *Radiology.* 2010; 255(3):850–6.

23. Fabre T, Montero C, Gaujard E, Gervais-Dellion F, Durandeau A. Chronic calf pain in athletes due to sural nerve entrapment. A report of 18 cases. *Am J Sports Med.* 2000;28(5):679–82.

24. Feinberg JH, Spielholz NI, editors. *Peripheral Nerve Injuries in the Athlete.* Champaign: Human Kinetics; 2003. p. 106–41.

25. Ferkel RD, Heath DD, Guhl JF. Neurological complications of ankle arthroscopy. *Arthroscopy.* 1996;12(2):200–8.

26. Fredericson M, Standage S, Chou L, Matheson G. Lateral plantar nerve entrapment in a competitive gymnast. *Clin J Sport Med.* 2001;11(2):111–4.

27. Frey C, Kerr R. Magnetic resonance imaging and the evaluation of tarsal tunnel syndrome. *Foot Ankle.* 1993;14(3):159–64.

28. Galardi G, Amadio S, Maderna L, et al. Electrophysiologic studies in tarsal tunnel syndrome. Diagnostic reliability of motor distal latency, mixed nerve and sensory nerve conduction studies. *Am J Phys Med Rehabil.* 1994;73(3):193–8.

29. Gessini L, Jandolo B, Pietrangeli A. The anterior tarsal syndrome. Report of four cases. *J Bone Joint Surg Am.* 1984;66(5):786–7.

30. Gleeson AP, Kerr JG. Patella dislocation neurapraxia — a report of two cases. *Injury.* 1996;27(7):519–20.

31. Goecker RM, Banks AS. Analysis of release of the first branch of the lateral plantar nerve. *J Am Podiatr Med Assoc.* 2000;90(6):281–6.

32. Gondring WH, Trepman E, Shields B. Tarsal tunnel syndrome: assessment of treatment outcome with an anatomic pain intensity scale. *Foot Ankle Surg.* 2009;15(3):133–8.

33. Gould N, Trevino S. Sural nerve entrapment by avulsion fracture of the base of the fifth metatarsal bone. *Foot Ankle.* 1981;2(3):153–5.

34. Gregg J, Marks P. Metatarsalgia: an ultrasound perspective. *Australas Radiol.* 2007;51(6):493–9.

35. Hemler DE, Ward WK, Karstetter KW, Bryant PM. Saphenous nerve entrapment caused by pes anserine bursitis mimicking stress fracture of the tibia. *Arch Phys Med Rehabil.* 1991;72(5):336–7.

36. Hughes RJ, Ali K, Jones H, Kendall S, Connell DA. Treatment of Morton's neuroma with alcohol injection under sonographic guidance: follow-up of 101 cases. *AJR Am J Roentgenol.* 2007;188(6):1535–9.

37. Iizuka M, Yao R, Wainapel S. Saphenous nerve injury following medial knee joint injection: a case report. *Arch Phys Med Rehabil.* 2005; 86(10):2062–5.

38. Jackson DL, Haglund B. Tarsal tunnel syndrome in athletes. Case reports and literature review. *Am J Sports Med.* 1991;19(1):61–5.

39. Jackson DL, Haglund BL. Tarsal tunnel syndrome in runners. *Sports Med.* 1992;13(2):146–9.

40. Johnson MR. Nerve entrapment causing heel pain. *Clin Podiatr Med Surg.* 1994;11(4):617–24.

41. Kim JY, Choi JH, Park J, Wang J, Lee I. An anatomical study of Morton's interdigital neuroma: the relationship between the occurring site and the deep transverse metatarsal ligament (DTML). *Foot Ankle Int.* 2007;28(9):1007–10.

42. Kopell H, Thompson W. Peripheral nerve entrapments of the lower extremity. *New Engl J Med.* 1962;266:216–9.

43. Lau JT, Daniels TR. Tarsal tunnel syndrome: a review of the literature. *Foot Ankle Int.* 1999;20(3):201–9.

44. Leach RE, Purnell MB, Saito A. Peroneal nerve entrapment in runners. *Am J Sports Med.* 1989;17(2):287–91.

45. Lee MJ, Kim S, Huh YM, et al. Morton neuroma: evaluated with ultrasonography and MR imaging. *Korean J Radiol.* 2007;8(2):148–55.

46. Lindenbaum BL. Ski boot compression syndrome. *Clin Orthop Relat Res.* 1979;140:109–10.

47. Logue EJ 3rd, Drez D Jr. Dermatitis complicating saphenous nerve injury after arthroscopic debridement of a medial meniscal cyst. *Arthroscopy.* 1996;12(2):228–31.

48. Lowdon IM. Superficial peroneal nerve entrapment. A case report. *J Bone Joint Surg Br.* 1985;67(1):58–9.

49. Lui TH. Endoscopic decompression of the first branch of the lateral plantar nerve. *Arch Orthop Trauma Surg.* 2007;127(9):859–61.

50. Magnan B, Marangon A, Frigo A, Bartolozzi P. Local phenol injection in the treatment of interdigital neuritis of the foot (Morton's neuroma). *Chir Organi Mov.* 2005;90(4):371–7.

51. Massey EW, Pleet AB. Neuropathy in joggers. *Am J Sports Med.* 1978;6(4):209–11.

52. McCluskey LF, Webb LB. Compression and entrapment neuropathies of the lower extremity. *Clin Podiatr Med Surg.* 1999;16(1):96–125, vii.

53. McCrory P, Bell S. Nerve entrapment syndromes as a cause of pain in the hip, groin, and buttock. *Sports Med.* 1999;27(4):261–74.

54. Meals RA. Peroneal-nerve palsy complicating ankle sprain. Report of two cases and review of the literature. *J Bone Joint Surg Am.* 1977;59(7):966–8.

55. Miranpuri S, Snook E, Vang D, Yong RM, Chagares WE. Neurilemoma of the posterior tibial nerve and tarsal tunnel syndrome. *J Am Podiatr Med Assoc.* 2007;97(2):148–50.

56. Moeller JL, Monroe J, McKeag DB. Cryotherapy-induced common peroneal nerve palsy. *Clin J Sport Med.* 1997;7(3):212–6.

57. Møller B, Kadin S. Entrapment of the common peroneal nerve. *Am J Sports Med.* 1987;15(1):90–1.

58. Murphy PC, Baxter DE. Nerve entrapment of the foot and ankle in runners. *Clin Sports Med.* 1985;4(4):753–63.

59. Nagaoka M, Matsuzaki H. Ultrasonography in tarsal tunnel syndrome. *J Ultrasound Med.* 2005;24(8):1035–40.

60. Nagel A, Greenebaum E, Singson RD, Rosenwasser MP, McCann PD. Foot drop in a long-distance runner. An unusual presentation of neurofibromatosis. *Orthop Rev.* 1994;23(6):526–30.

61. Nakano KK. Entrapment neuropathy from Baker's cyst. *JAMA.* 1978;239(2):135.

62. Park TA, Del Toro DR. Electrodiagnostic evaluation of the foot. *Phys Med Rehabil Clin N Am.* 1998;9(4):871–96, vii–viii.

63. Park TA, Del Toro DR. Isolated inferior calcaneal neuropathy. *Muscle Nerve.* 1996;19(1):106–8.

64. Park TA, Del Toro DR. The medial calcaneal nerve: anatomy and nerve conduction technique. *Muscle Nerve.* 1995;18(1):32–8.

65. Pasku DS, Karampekios SK, Kontakis GM, Katonis PG. Varicosities as an etiology of tarsal tunnel syndrome and the significance of Tinel's sign: report of two cases in young men and a review of the literature. *J Am Podiatr Med Assoc.* 2009;99(2):144–7.

66. Peicha G, Pascher A, Schwarzl F, Pierer G, Fellinger M, Passler JM. Transsection of the peroneal nerve complicating knee arthroscopy: case report and cadaver study. *Arthroscopy.* 1998;14(2):221–3.

67. Peri G. The "critical zones" of entrapment of the nerves of the lower limb. *Surg Radiol Anat.* 1991;13(2):139–43.

68. Pfeiffer WH, Cracchiolo A 3rd. Clinical results after tarsal tunnel decompression. *J Bone Joint Surg Am.* 1994;76(8):1222–30.

69. Pla ME, Dillingham TR, Spellman NT, Colon E, Jabbari B. Painful legs and moving toes associates with tarsal tunnel syndrome and accessory soleus muscle. *Mov Disord.* 1996;11(1):82–6.

70. Quinn TJ, Jacobson JA, Craig JG, van Holsbeeck MT. Sonography of Morton's neuromas. *Am J Roentgenol.* 2000;174(6):1723–8.

71. Rask MR. Medial plantar neurapraxia (jogger's foot): report of 3 cases. *Clin Orthop Relat Res.* 1978;(134):193–95.

72. Redborg KE, Antonakakis JG, Beach ML, Chinn CD, Sites BD. Ultrasound improves the success rate of a tibial nerve block at the ankle. *Reg Anesth Pain Med.* 2009;34(3):256–60.

73. Redborg KE, Sites BD, Chinn CD, et al. Ultrasound improves the success rate of a sural nerve block at the ankle. *Reg Anesth Pain Med.* 2009;34(1):24–8.

74. Redfern DJ, Sauvé PS, Sakellariou A. Investigation of incidence of superficial peroneal nerve injury following ankle fracture. *Foot Ankle Int.* 2003;24(10):771–4.

75. Rigaud J, Labat JJ, Riant T, Bouchot O, Robert R. Obturator nerve entrapment: diagnosis and laparoscopic treatment: technical case report. *Neurosurgery.* 2007;61(1):E175.

76. Sammarco GJ, Chalk DE, Feibel JH. Tarsal tunnel syndrome and additional nerve lesions in the same limb. *Foot Ankle.* 1993;14(2):71–7.

77. Sammarco GJ, Stephens MM. Tarsal tunnel syndrome caused by the flexor digitorum accessorius longus. A case report. *J Bone Joint Surg Am.* 1990;72(3):453–4.

78. Schon LC. Nerve entrapment, neuropathy, and nerve dysfunction in the athlete. *Orthop Clin North Am.* 1994;25(1):47–59.

79. Schon LC, Baxter DE. Neuropathies of the foot and ankle in athletes. *Clin Sports Med.* 1990;9(2):489–509.

80. Schon LC, Glennon TP, Baxter DE. Heel pain syndrome: electrodiagnostic support for nerve entrapment. *Foot Ankle.* 1993;14(3):129–35.

81. Siu TL, Chandran KN. Neurolysis for meralgia paresthetica: an operative series of 45 cases. *Surg Neurol.* 2005;63(1):19–23.

82. Smith J, Dahm DL. Nerve entrapments. In: O'Connor FG, Wilder R, Nirschl R, editors. *The Textbook of Running Medicine.* New York: McGraw-Hill; 2001. p. 257–72.

83. Sofka CM, Adler RS. Ultrasound guided interventions in the foot and ankle. *Semin Musculoskelet Radiol.* 2002;6(2):163–8.

84. Spinner RJ, Scheithauer BW, Amrami KK. Medial plantar nerve compression by a tibial artery schwannoma. Case report. *J Neurosurg.* 2007;106(5):921–3.

85. Sprowson AP, Rankin K, Shand JE, Ferrier G. Common peroneal and posterior tibial ischemic nerve damage, a rare cause. *Foot Ankle Surg.* 2010;16(2):e16–7.

86. Stamatis ED, Manidakis NE, Patouras PP. Intraneural ganglion of the superficial peroneal nerve: a case report. *J Foot Ankle Surg.* 2010;49(4):400.

87. Stefko RM, Lauerman WC, Heckman JD. Tarsal tunnel syndrome caused by an unrecognized fracture of the posterior process of the talus (Cedell fracture). A case report. *J Bone Joint Surg Am.* 1994;76(1):116–8.

88. Styf J. Chronic exercise induced pain in the anterior aspect of the lower leg. An overview of diagnosis. *Sports Med.* 1989;7(5):331–9.

89. Styf J. Entrapment of the superficial peroneal nerve. Diagnosis and results of decompression. *J Bone Joint Surg Br.* 1989;71(1):131–5.

90. Styf J, Morberg P. The superficial peroneal tunnel syndrome. Results of treatment by decompression. *J Bone Joint Surg Br.* 1997;79(5):801–3.

91. Sung KS, Park SJ. Short-term operative outcome of tarsal tunnel syndrome due to benign space-occupying lesions. *Foot Ankle Int.* 2009; 30(8):741–5.

92. Takao M, Ochi M, Shu N, et al. A case of superficial peroneal nerve injury during ankle arthroscopy. *Arthroscopy.* 2001;17(4):403–4.

93. Turnipseed W, Pozniak M. Popliteal entrapment as a result of neurovascular compression by the soleus and plantaris muscles. *J Vasc Surg.* 1992;15(2):285–92.

94. Vijayan J, Therimadasamy AK, Teoh HL, Chan YC, Wilder-Smith EP. Sonography as an aid to neurophysiological studies in diagnosing tarsal tunnel syndrome. *Am J Phys Med Rehabil.* 2009;88(6):500–1.

95. Visser LH. High resolution sonography of the common peroneal nerve: detection of intraneural ganglia. *Neurology.* 2006;67(8):1473–5.

96. Williams PH, Trzil KP. Management of meralgia paresthetica. *J Neurosurg.* 1991;74(1):76–80.

97. Worth RM, Kettelkamp DB, Defalque RJ, Duane KU. Saphenous nerve entrapment. A cause of medial knee pain. *Am J Sports Med.* 1984;12(1):80–1.

98. Wu KK. Morton's interdigital neuroma: a clinical review of its etiology, treatment, and results. *J Foot Ankle Surg.* 1996;35(2):112–9.

99. Yamamoto S, Tominaga Y, Yura S, Tada H. Tarsal tunnel syndrome with double causes (ganglion, tarsal coalition) evoked by ski boots. Case report. *J Sports Med Phys Fitness.* 1995;35(2):143–5.

100. Zelent ME, Kane RM, Neese DJ, Lockner WB. Minimally invasive Morton's intermetatarsal neuroma decompression. *Foot Ankle Int.* 2007; 28(2):263–5.

69 Physical Modalities in Sports Medicine

Sarah A. Eby and Alan P. Alfano

- The physical modalities use physical forces to speed healing and return an athlete to as full a level of function as possible.
- These agents should not be used in isolation: They are more effective when used as a part of a comprehensive treatment approach including medical and/or surgical intervention as well as exercise and education (5).

THERAPEUTIC HEAT

- Energy transfer by physical modalities typically occurs by one of three processes: *conduction, convection,* or *conversion.*
- **Conduction:** Heat energy is transferred by contact from the object of highest energy to the object of lowest energy.
- **Convection:** The process of heat energy transfer between a solid object and a moving gas or liquid.
- **Conversion:** The process of energy transfer that involves converting one form of energy to a different form. Use of high-frequency sound waves or electromagnetic (EM) waves to heat tissue will be discussed.
- Heating modalities are divided into *superficial* and *deep.*

PHYSIOLOGY OF SUPERFICIAL HEAT

- Predominant mode of heating is conduction; however, some superficial applications use convection or conversion.
- Superficial heat effects include vasodilatation, pain relief, reduction of muscle tone and spasticity, increased cellular metabolic activity, decreased joint stiffness, increased soft tissue extensibility, and promotion of hyperemia. Elevation of tissue temperature does not generally exceed 40°C and is usually short lived.
- Causes superficial vasodilatation preferentially.
- May be associated with consensual vasodilatation of areas distant to the area being heated; for example, the contralateral limb.
- Changes of 13–15°C in the finger joint may change joint viscosity by about 20% (93).

- There is moderate evidence that heat wrap therapy provides short-term pain reduction and disability in patients with acute and subacute low back pain. There is further pain reduction and functional improvement with the addition of exercise (30).

General Indications

- Pain
- Muscle spasm
- Contracture
- Tension myalgia
- Hematoma resolution
- Bursitis
- Tenosynovitis
- Fibromyalgia
- Superficial thrombophlebitis
- Acceleration of metabolic process

General Contraindications and Precautions

- Acute inflammation, trauma, or hemorrhage
- Bleeding dyscrasia
- Ischemia
- Insensitivity
- Atrophic skin
- Scar tissue
- Inability to communicate
- Poor thermal regulation (systemic applications)
- Malignancy
- Edema

Application Methods

Hot Packs (Hydrocollator)

- Transfer of heat energy by conduction
- **Application:** Silicate gel in a canvas cover
- When not in use, these packs are kept in thermostatically controlled water baths at 70–80°C.

- Used in terry cloth insulating covers or used with towels placed between the pack and the patient for periods of 20–30 minutes.
- **Advantages:** Low cost, easy use, long life, and patient acceptance
- **Disadvantages:** Difficult to apply to curved surfaces
- **Safety:** One should never lie on top on the pack, as it is more likely to cause burns. Towels should be applied between the skin and hydrocollator pack.

Heat Lamps

- Heat primarily by the conversion of radiant energy to heat, *i.e.,* the direct application of photons to living tissue leading to heat production.
- **Application:** Simple to use but require some attention to avoid injuries or burns.
- In practice, therapeutic temperatures are usually obtained when the heat sources are about 50 cm from the skin.
- The intensity of heating of point heat sources, such as incandescent bulbs, drops off in accordance with the inverse squared $(1/r^2)$ law; the heating effectiveness of linear sources, such as some quartz lamps, may follow a more slowly decreasing $1/r$ relationship.
- **Safety:** These agents produce erythema (known as *erythema ab igne* and *erythema calor*).
- Chronic use may produce a permanent brownish discoloration.

Hydrotherapy

- Heat transfer is primarily by convection.
  - Uses a fluid medium (usually water) to apply heat and cold.
  - Immersion of large portion of the body in water at neutral temperatures between 36.5°C and 40°C for 20 minutes.
  - Water temperatures are limited to about 39°C if a significant fraction of the body is immersed.
  - Hydrotherapy medium may be stationary or in motion.

Specific Modes

- Whirlpool baths and Hubbard tanks
  - Tanks range in size/construction from small portable units to treat a portion of a limb to fixed Hubbard tanks for the entire body.
  - Hydrotherapy is expensive in terms of labor and resources.

Advantages/Specific Uses

- **Wounds and burns:** Hydrotherapy may lessen pain and speed healing of open wounds (20,48).
- Used for wounds and treatments when gentle mechanical debridement, heat, and solvent actions are desired.
- For larger wounds, a 0.9% NaCl solution improves comfort and lessens the risks of hemolysis and electrolyte imbalance.
- **Musculoskeletal/pain applications:** Hydrotherapy is often used as an adjunct to joint mobilization after cast removal or prolonged immobilization.

- Sitz baths (small warm water bath) for perineal and anal pain.
- Used to treat musculoskeletal pain, spasms, and tension myalgia.
- In clinical institutions where disinfecting procedures are followed and areas of stagnant water are avoided, infection appears to be rare.

Disadvantages

- Should not be used with edematous limbs.
- Treatment systems and infection control are time consuming.

Contrast Baths

Application

- Contrast baths consist of two baths: a warm bath at 38–44°C and a cool reservoir at about 10–18°C.
- Treatment begins by soaking the involved limb in the warm reservoir for about 10 minutes and then progressing to about four cycles of 1- to 4-minute cold and 4- to 6-minute warm soaks (92).

Advantages/Disadvantages

- Most commonly used to produce reflex hyperemia and desensitization in patients with complex regional pain syndrome.
- Athletes may find the cold baths uncomfortable.
- May increase superficial blood flow and skin temperature; however, no effect on functional outcome (17).

Spa Therapy (Balneotherapy)

- Little research has addressed these issues for athletes.
- In addition, a comparison of the effects of spa therapy, underwater traction, and water jets on low-back pain found no specific benefits attributable to balneotherapy (58).

Fluidotherapy

Application

- **Heats by convection:** Fine particles fluidized by turbulent, high-velocity hot air, frequently used in hand therapy.
- Despite widespread use, benefits of this high temperature remain poorly established (3,16).
- May be used for analgesia or desensitization.

Paraffin Baths

Application

- **Heats primarily by conduction:** Liquid mixture of paraffin wax and mineral oil.
- Helpful in the treatment of scars and hand contractures. Temperatures (52–54°C) are higher than those of hydrotherapy (< 40–45°C) but are well tolerated due to the low heat capacity of the paraffin–mineral oil mixture and a lack of convection.
- Can be used in combination with exercise for patients with rheumatoid arthritis of the hands with beneficial short-term effects including improved range of motion and function and decreased swelling and pain (76).
- **Treatment:** Dipping, immersion, occasionally brushed onto the area of treatment.

- **Safety:** Burns are the main safety concern with paraffin treatment.
- **Visual inspection is important:** Paraffin bath should have a thin film of white paraffin on its surface or an edging around the reservoir.

DIATHERMY (DEEP HEATING)

- The following differences set diathermy apart from superficial heating:
  - Produces higher temperatures
  - Heats tissue faster and heat dissipates more slowly
  - Predominantly uses sound waves or EM energy

Deep Heating Modalities

Ultrasound

- *Ultrasound* is defined as sound waves at a frequency above the threshold of human hearing (frequencies higher than 20 kHz).

Heats by Conversion

- Ultrasound uses sound waves to heat tissues. A wide range of frequencies are potentially useful, but in the United States, most machines operate between 0.8 and 1 MHz.
- Uses piezoelectric transducers to convert electrical energy into sound.

Physiology

- The most vigorous and deeply penetrating heating agent can elevate intramuscular temperatures by about 3.5–4.0°C (25).
- Penetration is not uniform and depends markedly on tissue properties. Ultrasound beam will selectively heat tissue with high water content.
- The ability of ultrasound to heat tissue by the conversion of sound energy into heat is its best-understood capability.
- Nonthermal processes such as *cavitation, shock waves, streaming,* and *mechanical deformation* have been identified.
- Cavitation occurs when small gaseous bubbles are formed in the presence of a high-intensity ultrasound beam and either oscillate stably or grow rapidly in size and collapse (28).
- No irreversible harmful effects of cavitation have been demonstrated in animal tissue (31).
- Streaming is described as movements in water-rich tissues and standing waves. Streaming may damage tissue or possibly speed healing.
- Typical intensity for application is 0.8–1.5 W/cm^2.
- Low-intensity ultrasound (15–400 mW/cm^2) may also stimulate cell proliferation, protein synthesis, and cytokine production. Although these findings are limited to the laboratory, they furnish some support for the clinical interest in low-intensity ultrasound in wound healing.

Indications

- Tendonitis and bursitis
- Muscle pain and overuse
- Contractures
- Inflammation and trauma
- Scars and keloids
- The evidence is mixed. In most cases, ultrasound comparisons have been performed against placebo controls; therefore, the relative effectiveness of this agent over that of other conventional approaches is unknown. There is, however, promising evidence of effectiveness in lateral epicondylitis (85).
- **Fractures:** Low-intensity ultrasound (*e.g.*, 30 mW/cm^2) accelerates bone healing and is approved by the Food and Drug Administration (FDA) for the treatment of some fractures (36).
- Low-intensity pulse ultrasound (LIPUS) has been shown in vivo to enhance collagen synthesis after tendon injury during the granulation phase (2 weeks after injury) but to slow repair during the remodeling phase (4 weeks after injury) (32).

Precautions

- Ultrasound is typically avoided in the acute stages of an injury due to concerns that it may aggravate bleeding, tissue damage, and swelling.
- The subacute situation may be different, because many feel that ultrasound may speed healing and the resolution of symptoms in the later stages of injury.

Phonophoresis

- Ultrasound may be used to deliver medication into tissues. The active substance is mixed into a coupling medium, and ultrasound is used to drive the material through the skin.
- Phonophoresis with corticosteroids is frequently used in sports medicine.
- Clinical studies are conflicting.
- In a comparison of phonophoresis of 0.05% fluocinonide with ultrasound alone at 1.5 W/cm^2, both treatments were found to be beneficial but were indistinguishable in their effects on superficial musculoskeletal conditions (55).
- Another study did not find lidocaine and corticosteroid phonophoresis to be more effective than the same treatment with an inert coupling agent (68).

Contraindications

- Fluid-filled areas (*i.e.*, eye and the pregnant uterus)
- Growth plates, immature or inflamed joints (27,87,88)
- Acute hemorrhages, ischemic tissue, tumors, laminectomy sites, infections, and implanted devices such as pacemakers and pumps
- **Caution:** Relatively contraindicated near metal plates or cemented artificial joints because the effects of localized heating (19,34,79) or mechanical forces on prosthetic–cement interfaces are not well known.

Shortwave Diathermy

Heats by Conversion

- *Shortwave diathermy* (SWD) uses EM energy to interact with tissue and produce heat.
- Both thermal and nonthermal effects are possible.
- Tissue warming is produced by two processes:
  - Resistive heating
  - Degradation of molecular oscillatory motions that EM waves induce when they interact with tissue
- SWD is the dominant EM diathermy in sports medicine, although it is relatively rarely used in comparison to other heating modalities.
- Most devices operate at 27.12 MHz. The U.S. Federal Communications Commission also approves frequencies of 13.56 and 40.68 MHz for use.

Mechanism

- An SWD machine is a signal generator that uses either inductive or capacitive electrodes to deliver energy to the body.
- Inductive electrodes act as an antenna, and the body absorbs energy from an EM field produced by the shortwave machine.
- With capacitive electrodes, the portion of the body being treated is placed in series between the electrodes and serves as the dielectric (resistance) between two plates of a capacitor.
- Inductive applicators induce currents that preferentially flow in water-rich tissues such as muscles that are highly conductive.
- Capacitive applicators, on the other hand, heat poorly conductive substances, such as fat preferentially (52).
- SWD can increase subcutaneous fat temperatures by 15°C and intramuscular temperatures at depths of 4–5 cm by 4–6°C (26,61,62).

Technique

- Two common inductive applicators are typically used (pads or drums).
- Pad applicators are moderately flexible mats that contain a coil.
- Drum applicators are characterized by fixed coils and hinges.

Indications

- Heating in tissues that are either too deep or too extensive to be treated by other modalities, *e.g.*, the low back, the knee.

Precautions and Contraindications/Safety

- Jewelry is removed.
- Treatment is performed on nonconductive tables.
- Contraindications include metal implants or electrical devices (*e.g.*, joints, pacemakers, pumps, and metallic intrauterine devices), contact lenses, and the menstruating or pregnant uterus.
- Treating the immature skeleton is generally not recommended and has not been well studied.

Low-Power and Pulsed Electromagnetic Field

Heats by Conversion

- Nonthermal effects can be obtained and tissue heating avoided altogether by using low-power fields delivered in either continuous or pulsed modes.
- Research offers little to support the specificity or certainty of benefits.

THERAPEUTIC COLD

- The cooling agents are often used for their analgesic, metabolic, and perfusion-limiting effects.
- Cooling therapies are restricted to conductive and convective means.

General Indications

- Acute musculoskeletal trauma
- Pain
- Arthrogenic muscle inhibition
- Muscle spasm: spasticity
- Reduction of metabolic activity

General Contraindication and Precautions

- Ischemia
- Insensitivity
- Cold intolerance
- Raynaud phenomenon and disease
- Severe cold pressor responses
- Cold allergy

Physiology of Cryotherapy

- Superficial cold produces analgesia (37), reduces metabolic activity, slows and may block nerve conduction (24), decreases muscle tone and spasticity (56–58,67), increases gastrointestinal motility (14), reduces conduction velocity, inhibits the release of histamine, and slows chemical reactions.
- Relative hyperemia after cold application stimulates tissue repair and healing.
- Ice is the most common cryotherapy agent.
- Skin temperatures initially fall rapidly following the application of ice and then decrease more slowly toward an equilibrium value of 12–13°C. The target temperature reduction is 10–15°C (64).
- Recent systematic review showed that ice is most effective when applied in repeated applications of 10 minutes, which helps sustain lower muscle temperatures without compromising overlying skin (64).

Technique

- Ice packs and compression wraps are most common.
- Ice massage is a vigorous approach suitable for limited portions of the body. A piece of ice is rubbed over the painful area for 7–10 minutes.
- Iced whirlpools cool large areas vigorously.
- Vapocoolant and liquid nitrogen sprays produce large (as much as 20°C), rapid drops in skin temperature and are used at times to produces superficial analgesia as well as in *spray and stretch* treatments (74,82).
- Chemical ice packs are also common.
- A mixture of ice water and alcohol was shown to lower skin temperatures significantly more than gels packs or frozen peas (51).
- Postexercise ice water immersion is often used as a method of recovery after intense workouts. It is postulated that ice water immersion will constrict blood vessels, flush waste products and lactic acid out of the affected tissues, slow tissue metabolism, reduce swelling, and prevent further tissue damage (60). Results of several studies on the efficacy of this method in reducing muscle soreness or improving performance and recovery are mixed (47,60,78,90).
- Whole-body cryotherapy (WBC) consists of several-minute exposure to very cold air (−110 to −140°C) in special temperature-controlled cryochambers or cryosaunas. WBC is used to relieve pain and inflammatory symptoms primarily in Europe and is becoming more popular in the United States because of its use in elite athletes. Research is limited; however, recent studies have shown that it does not cause deleterious effects in athletes (7) and provides short-term relief of pain and inflammatory symptoms in rheumatologic patients (41,66).
- Reflex activity and motor function are impaired for up to 30 minutes after cold application (64).

Trauma Indications

- Cooling applied soon after trauma may decrease edema, lessen metabolic activity, reduce blood flow, lower compartmental pressures, diminish tissue damage, and accelerate healing (11,13,40,42,70,77,80).
- *Rest, ice, compression, and elevation* (RICE) are the mainstay of treatment.
- Opinions regarding usefulness of cryotherapy for injuries more than 24–48 hours old are divergent.
- Cryotherapy may hasten return to play after ankle sprains (43,45,80).

Precautions and Contraindications

- When sensation is compromised, circulation is impaired, or tissues are compressed (9).

- Rare but possible problems include pressor responses aggravating cardiovascular disease, Raynaud phenomenon, cold hypersensitivity, urticaria, and cold allergy/cryoprecipitation.
- Because reflex activity and motor function are impaired for up to 30 minutes after ice application, return to play should not be immediate in order to prevent further injury (64).

ELECTROTHERAPY

General Indications

- Today, high-intensity electrical stimulation is used to strengthen muscles and to move paralyzed limbs.
- Less intense stimulation produces analgesia and delivers medications percutaneously.
- Stimulation at still lower intensities has gained FDA approval for fracture healing.
- Soft tissue wounds, osteoporosis, and musculoskeletal pain represent additional potentially important, but still investigational, applications (8,91).

Specific Applications

Transcutaneous Electrical Nerve Stimulators

- It is clear that transcutaneous electrical nerve stimulators (TENS) produce localized analgesia, and research suggests that stimulation at 110 Hz (as well as H-wave therapy at 2 and 60 Hz) results in a hypoalgesia that persists for up to 5 minutes after stimulation is stopped (65).
- Dorsal horn cell activity is reduced following stimulation (33).
- High-frequency, low-intensity TENS (barely or not perceptible, 10–100+ Hz) may work more according to the gate theory than higher intensity, low-frequency (1–4 Hz) stimulation, which may be more dependent on endorphins.
- Electrodes are usually placed over the painful region, but other locations are common.
- TENS units are expensive (often as much as $800) and annoying to put on. Benefits may appear to wane with time; purchase is not warranted unless its improvements persist for several months.
- There are inconsistent outcomes and insufficient data in the literature regarding TENS and clinical improvement of low back pain (86).

Indications
- Pain reduction

Precautions and Contraindications
- Skin irritation and contact dermatitis (53).
- Cardiac pacemakers may be relatively resistant to TENS signals, but there is at least one report that an intracardiac defibrillator was triggered by a TENS unit (22).
- The pregnant uterus should not be treated.

Functional Electric Stimulation

Neuromuscular Electrical Stimulation/Muscle Stimulation

- In summary, electrical muscle stimulation is more effective in maintaining muscle mass after an injury than it is in reversing atrophy once it is established (6).
- Review of the literature shows that use of neuromuscular electrical stimulation after anterior cruciate ligament repair is associated with increased quadriceps strength compared with exercise alone; however, the effect on functional outcome is inconsistent (54). This effect was not seen after total knee arthroplasty (69).

Iontophoresis

- Iontophoresis uses electrical fields to force charged or polarized substances into tissue (21,39,73).
- Iontophoretic devices consist basically of a direct-current (possibly pulsed) power source and two electrodes. A dilute solution of the active substance (which must exist in an ionized or polar form) is placed under the electrode of the same polarity, and the device is turned on.
- Medication is not always required as the electric current alone may have therapeutic benefits.
- Iontophoresis with dexamethasone has been shown to be effective in the treatment of bicipital tendonitis, epicondylitis, plantar fasciitis, and tendon sheath inflammation (23,35,38,71,81).
- Direct comparison of iontophoresis with oral medication, transdermal patches, or alternative physical therapy approaches is rare.
- **Safety:** Allergies to the materials (pads, electrodes, and medication) used are always possible, and the passage of electrical current into the skin can cause erythema, rashes, and, if the current intensity is high, pain (12).

Interferential and Kilohertz Frequency Currents

- Skin impedance falls as frequency increases. As a result, stimuli that are painful at the low < 70-Hz frequencies of TENS and many muscle simulators are well tolerated at a few thousand hertz.
- There are at least two ways to take advantage of this fact. One of these arranges two sets of electrodes so that two sine waves in the low-kilohertz range differing by 20–100 Hz cross. The waves thus interfere with each other and produce beneath the skin barrier a *difference* frequency comparable to that of TENS units and muscle stimulators.
- **Safety:** There is no conclusive and consistent evidence that EM field exposure causes a significant increase in the risk of cancer or neurobehavioral or reproductive dysfunction (49,50).

COMPLEMENTARY AND ALTERNATIVE THERAPIES

- Athletes and the general population are intrigued by the potential use of complementary and alternative medicine.

Low-Intensity Laser Therapy

- Low-power lasers are widely used to treat musculoskeletal injuries, speed healing, and lessen pain.
- Lasers have been shown to decrease pain and inflammation in tendinopathies and Achilles tendonitis (15,83); however, there is no evidence to support use in osteoarthritis (18).
- Unfortunately, demonstration of clinical benefits has been difficult, and these devices have yet to gain FDA approval for clinical use (10).

Static Magnetic Fields (Magnetic Devices)

- Magnetic discs, pads, bandages, and blankets are promoted in sports, veterinary, and general circulation magazines as a cure for a variety of musculoskeletal injuries.
- Various magnetic products have been studied with field strengths generally in the 300–3,950 Gs range (4,84).
- Results are generally mixed. In one study, efficacy was demonstrated in patients with painful diabetic neuropathy (89); another study comparing magnet pad versus control groups suffering from fibromyalgia showed statistical significance for pain relief, but no clear functional improvement in the magnet user group (4).
- Many animal studies have shown significant cellular physiologic changes with static magnetic fields, but functional and long-term consequences remain unknown.
- Observed physiologic effects have included increased nerve excitability (44) and circulatory stimulation (72).

Acupuncture

- Treatment consists of using acupuncture needles to pierce the skin to differing depths at designated acupuncture points to bring about pain relief or physiologic change.
- Needles are commonly stimulated by hand, electricity, or heat.
- Research is scarce regarding treatment of athletic injuries; in 1997, the National Institutes of Health sponsored a consensus panel that concluded: "promising results have emerged, for example, showing efficacy of acupuncture in adult postoperative and chemotherapy associated nausea and vomiting and in postoperative dental pain. There are other situations such as addiction, stroke rehabilitation, headache, menstrual cramps, tennis elbow, fibromyalgia, myofascial pain, osteoarthritis, low back pain, carpal tunnel syndrome, and asthma, in which acupuncture may be useful" (1).

- Dry needling in elite volleyball players during competition provided short-term pain relief and improved function in shoulder injuries (75).

- Acupuncture, in combination with traditional Chinese medicine including massage and herbs, was effective in reducing pain, decreasing edema, and restoring ankle function in acute ankle ligamentous sprains in sports (29).

- Studies have shown increased muscle strength and power, improved performance, and improved hemodynamic parameters in endurance activities after acupuncture. There is also associated decrease in acute muscle soreness with acupuncture (2).

- Single acupuncture treatment improved isometric quadriceps strength in recreational athletes (46).

- Male basketball players treated with acupuncture had decreased maximum heart rate, $\dot{V}O_{2max}$, and blood lactate levels after 30 minutes of exercise compared to controls (63).

REFERENCES

1. Acupuncture. *NIH Consens Statement.* 1997;15(5):1–34.
2. Ahmedov S. Ergogenic effect of acupuncture in sport and exercise: a brief review. *J Strength Cond Res.* 2010;24(5):1421–7.
3. Alcorn R, Bowser B, Henley EJ, Holloway V. Fluidotherapy and exercise in the management of sickle cell anemia. A clinical report. *Phys Ther.* 1984;64(10):1520–2.
4. Alfano AP, Taylor AG, Foresman PA, et al. Static magnetic fields for the treatment of fibromyalgia: a randomized controlled trial. *J Altern Complement Med.* 2001;7(1):53–64.
5. Allen RJ. Physical agents used in the management of chronic pain by physical therapists. *Phys Med Rehabil Clin N Am.* 2006;17(2):315–45.
6. Baldi JC, Jackson RD, Moraille R, Mysiw WJ. Muscle atrophy is prevented in patients with acute spinal cord injury using functional electrical stimulation. *Spinal Cord.* 1998;36(7):463–9.
7. Banfi G, Lombardi G, Colombini A, Melegati G. Whole-body cryotherapy in athletes. *Sports Med.* 2010;40(6):509–17.
8. Banon JJ, Jacobson WE, Tidd G. Treatment of decubitus ulcers. A new approach. *Minn Med.* 1985;68(2):103–6.
9. Barlas D, Homan CS, Thode HC Jr. In vivo tissue temperature comparison of cyrotherapy with and without external compression. *Ann Emerg Med.* 1996;28(4):436–9.
10. Basford JR. Low intensity laser therapy: still not an established clinical tool. *Lasers Surg Med.* 1995;16(4):331–42.
11. Basur RL, Shephard E, Mouzas GL. A cooling method in the treatment of ankle sprains. *Practitioner.* 1976;216(1296):708–11.
12. Berliner MN. Reduced skin hyperemia during tap water iontophoresis after intake of acetylsalicylic acid. *Am J Phys Med Rehabil.* 1997;76(6):482–7.
13. Bert JM, Stark JG, Maschka K, Chock C. The effect of cold therapy on morbidity subsequent to arthroscopic lateral retinacular release. *Orthop Rev.* 1991;20(9):755–8.
14. Bisgard JD, Nye D. The influence of hot and cold application upon gastric and intestinal motor activity. *Surg Gynecol Obstet.* 1940;71:172–80.
15. Bjordal JM, Lopes-Martins RA, Iversen VV. A randomized, placebo controlled trial of low level laser therapy for activated Achilles tendinitis with microdialysis measurement of peritendinous prostaglandin E2 concentrations. *Br J Sports Med.* 2006;40(1):76–80.
16. Borrell RM, Parker R, Henley EJ, Masley D, Repinecz M. Comparison of in vivo temperatures produced by hydrotherapy, paraffin wax treatment, and fluidotherapy. *Phys Ther.* 1980;60(10):1273–6.
17. Breger Stanton DE, Lazaro R, Macdermid JC. A systematic review of the effectiveness of contrast baths. ;22(1):57–69.
18. Brosseau L, Welch V, Wells G, et al. Low level laser therapy (Classes I, II and III) for treating osteoarthritis. *Cochrane Database Syst Rev.* 2004;3:CD002046.
19. Brunner GD, Lehmann JF, McMillan JA, Lane KE, Bell JW. Can ultrasound be used in the presence of surgical metal implants: an experimental approach. *Phys Ther Rev.* 1958;38(12):823–4.
20. Burke DT, Ho CH, Saucier MA, Stewart G. Effects of hydrotherapy on pressure ulcer healing. *Am J Phys Med Rehabil.* 1998;77(5):394–8.
21. Chantraine A, Ludy JP, Berger D. Is cortisone iontophoresis possible? *Arch Phys Med Rehabil.* 1986;67(1):38–40.
22. Curwin JH, Coyne RF, Winters SL. Inappropriate defibrillator (ICD) shocks caused by transcutaneous electronic nerve stimulation (TENS) units [letter, comment]. *Pacing Clin Electrophysiol.* 1999;22(4 Pt 1):692–3.
23. Demirtaş RN, Oner C. The treatment of lateral epicondylitis by iontophoresis of sodium salicylate and sodium diclofenac. *Clin Rehabil.* 1998;12(1):23–9.
24. Denys EH. AAEM minimonograph # 14: the influence of temperature in clinical neurophysiology. *Muscle Nerve.* 1991;14(9):795–811.
25. Draper DO, Harris ST, Schulthies S, Durrant, E, Knight KL, Ricard M. Hot-pack and 1-MHz ultrasound treatments have an additive effect on muscle temperature increase. *J Athl Train.* 1998;33(1):21–4.
26. Draper DO, Knight K, Fujiwara T, Castel JC. Temperature change in human muscle during and after pulsed shortwave diathermy. *J Orthop Sports Phys Ther.* 1999;29(1):13–8.
27. Dussick KT, Fritch DJ, Kyriazidou M, Sear RS. Measurement of articular tissues with ultrasound. *Am J Phys Med.* 1958;37(3):160–5.
28. Flint EB, Suslick KS. The temperature of cavitation. *Science.* 1991;253(5026):1397–9.
29. Fong DT, Chan YY, Mok KM, Yung PSh, Chan KM. Understanding acute ankle ligamentous sprain injury in sports. *Sports Med Arthrosc Rehabil Ther Technol.* 2009;1:14.
30. French SD, Cameron M, Walker BF, Reggars JW, Esterman AJ. A Cochrane review of superficial heat or cold for low back pain. *Spine (Phila Pa 1976).* 2006;31(9):998–1006.
31. Frizzell LA, Dunn F. Biophysics of ultrasound. In: Lehman J, editor. *Therapeutic Heat and Cold.* 4th ed. Baltimore (MD): Williams & Wilkins; 1990. p. 404–5.
32. Fu SC, Hung LK, Shum WT, et al. In vivo low-intensity pulsed ultrasound (LIPUS) following tendon injury promotes repair during granulation but suppresses decorin and biglycan expression during remodeling. *J Orthop Sports Phys Ther.* 2010;40(7):422–9.
33. Garrison DW, Foreman RD. Effects of transcutaneous electrical nerve stimulation (TENS) on spontaneous and noxiously evoked dorsal horn cell activity in cats with transected spinal cords. *Neurosci Lett.* 1996;216(2):125–8.
34. Gersten JW. Effects of metallic objects on temperature rises produced in tissue by ultrasound. *Am J Phys Med.* 1958;37(2):75–82.
35. Gudeman SD, Eisele SA, Heidt RS Jr, Colosimo AJ, Stroupe AL. Treatment of plantar fasciitis by iontophoresis of 0.4% dexamethasone. A randomized, double-blind, placebo controlled study. *Am J Sports Med.* 1997;25(3):312–6.
36. Hadjiargyrou M, McLeod K, Ryaby JP, Rubin C. Enhancement of fracture healing by low intensity ultrasound. *Clin Orthop Relat Res.* 1998;355(Suppl):S216–29.
37. Hartviksen K. Ice therapy in spasticity. *Acta Neurol Scand.* 1962;38(Suppl 3):79–84.

38. Hendricks HJM, Verbeek ALM, van de Putte LBA, Vermeulen RA. Effect of dexamethason-iontophoresis on patients with muscle tendinopathy. *Dutch J Phys Ther.* 1992;102:198–207.

39. Hill AC, Baker GF, Jansen GT. Mechanism of action of iontophoresis in the treatment of palmar hyperhidrosis. *Cutis.* 1981;28(1):69–70,72.

40. Hirasé Y. Postoperative cooling enhances composite graft survival in nasal-alar and fingertip reconstruction. *Br J Plast Surg.* 1993;46(8):707–11.

41. Hirvonen HE, Mikkelsson MK, Kautiainen H, Pohjolainen TH, Leirisalo-Repo M. Effectiveness of different cryotherapies on pain and disease activity in active rheumatoid arthritis. A randomised single blinded controlled trial. *Clin Exp Rheumatol.* 2006;24(3):295–301.

42. Ho SS, Illgen RL, Meyer RW, Torok PJ, Cooper MD, Reider B. Comparison of various icing times in decreasing bone metabolism and blood flow in the know. *Am J Sports Med.* 1995;23(1):74–6.

43. Hocutt JE Jr, Jaffe R, Rylander CR, Beebe JK. Cryotherapy in ankle sprains. *Am J Sports Med.* 1982;10(5):316–9.

44. Hong CZ. Static magnetic field influence on human nerve function. *Arch Phys Med Rehabil.* 1987;68(3):162–4.

45. Hubbard TJ, Aronson SL, Denegar CR. Does cryotherapy hasten return to participation? A systematic review. *J Athl Train.* 2004;39(1):88–94.

46. Hübscher M, Vogt L, Ziebart T, Banzer W. Immediate effects of acupuncture on strength performance: a randomized, controlled crossover trial. *Eur J Appl Physiol.* 2010;110(2):353–8.

47. Ingram J, Dawson B, Goodman C, Wallman K, Beilby J. Effect of water immersion methods on post-exercise recovery from simulated team sport exercise. *J Sci Med Sport.* 2009;12(3):417–21.

48. Juvé Meeker B. Whirlpool therapy on postoperative pain and surgical wound healing: an exploration. *Patient Educ Couns.* 1998;33(1):39–48.

49. Kaiser J. NIH panel revives EMF-cancer link. *Science.* 1998;281(5373):21–2.

50. Kaiser J. Panel finds EMFs pose no threat. *Science.* 1996;274(5289):910.

51. Kanlayanaphotporn R, Janwantanakul P. Comparison of skin surface temperature during the application of various cryotherapy modalities. *Arch Phys Med Rehabil.* 2005;86(7):1411–5.

52. Kantor G. Evaluation and survey of microwave and radiofrequency applicators. *J Microw Power.* 1981;16(2):135–50.

53. Khadilkar A, Odebiyi DO, Brosseau L, Wells GA. Transcutaneous electrical nerve stimulation (TENS) versus placebo for chronic low-back pain. *Cochrane Database Syst Rev.* 2008;4:CD003008.

54. Kim KM, Croy T, Hertel J, Saliba S. Effects of neuromuscular electrical stimulation after anterior cruciate ligament reconstruction on quadriceps strength, function, and patient-oriented outcomes: a systematic review. *J Orthop Sports Phys Ther.* 2010;40(7):383–91.

55. Klaiman MD, Shrader JA, Danoff JV, Hicks JE, Pesce WJ, Ferland J. Phonophoresis versus ultrasound in the treatment of common musculoskeletal conditions. *Med Sci Sports Exerc.* 1998;30(9):1349–55.

56. Knight KL. *Cryotherapy: Theory, Technique and Physiology.* 1st ed. Chattanooga (TN): Chattanooga; 1985. p. 15.

57. Knight KL. *Cryotherapy: Theory, Technique and Physiology.* 1st ed. Chattanooga (TN): Chattanooga; 1985. p. 83.

58. Knutsson E, Mattsson E. Effects of local cooling on monosynaptic reflexes in man. *Scand J Rehabil Med.* 1969;1(3):126–32.

59. Konrad K, Tatrai T, Hunka A, Vereckei E, Korondi I. Controlled trial of balneotherapy in treatment of low back pain. *Ann Rheum Dis.* 1992;51(6):820–2.

60. Lateef F. Post exercise water immersion: is it a form of active recovery? *J Emerg Trauma Shock.* 2010;3(3):302.

61. Lehmann JF, de Lateur BJ. Diathermy and superficial heat and cold therapy. In: Kottke FJ, Stilllwell GK, Lehmann JF, editors. *Krusen's Handbook of Physical Medicine and Rehabilitation.* 3rd ed. Philadelphia (PA): Saunders. 1982. p. 275.

62. Lehmann JF, DeLateur BJ, Stonebridge JB. Selective muscle heating by shortwave diathermy with a helical coil. *Arch Phys Med Rehabil.* 1969;50(3):117–23.

63. Lin ZP, Lan LW, He TY, et al. Effects of acupuncture stimulation on recovery ability of male elite basketball athletes. *Am J Chin Med.* 2009;37(3):471–81.

64. MacAuley DC. Ice therapy: how good is the evidence? *Int J Sports Med.* 2001;22(5):379–84.

65. McDowell BC, McCormack K, Walsh DM, Baxter DG, Allen JM. Comparative analgesic effects of H-wave therapy and transcutaneous electrical nerve stimulation on pain threshold in humans. *Arch Phys Med Rehabil.* 1999;80(9):1001–4.

66. Metzger D, Zwingmann C, Protz W, Jäckel WH. Whole-body cryotherapy in rehabilitation of patients with rheumatoid diseases — pilot study. *Rehabilitation (Stuttg).* 2000;39(2):93–100.

67. Miglietta O. Action of cold on spasticity. *Am J Phys Med.* 1973;52(4):198–205.

68. Moll MJ. A new approach to pain: lidocaine and decadron with ultrasound. *USAF Med Service Dig.* 1979;30:8–11.

69. Monaghan B, Caulfield B, O'Mathúna DP. Surface neuromuscular electrical stimulation for quadriceps strengthening pre and post total knee replacement. *Cochrane Database Syst Rev.* 2010;1:CD007177.

70. Moore CD, Cardea JA. Vascular changes in leg trauma. *South Med J.* 1977;70(11):1285–6.

71. Nirschl RP, Rodin DM, Ochiai DH, Maartmann-Moe C; DEX-AHE-01-99 Study Group. Iontophoretic administration of dexamethason sodium phosphate for acute epicondylitis. A randomized, double-blinded, placebo-controlled study. *Am J Sports Med.* 2003;31(2):189–95.

72. Ohkubo C, Xu S. Acute effects of static magnetic fields on cutaneous circulation in rabbits. *In Vivo.* 1997;11(3):221–5.

73. O'Malley EP, Oester YT. Influence of some physical chemical factors on iontophoresis using radioisotopes. *Arch Phys Med Rehabil.* 1955;36(5):310–6.

74. Oosterveld FG, Rasker JJ. Effects of local heat and cold treatment on surface and articular temperature of arthritic knees. *Arthritis Rheum.* 1994;37(11):1578–82.

75. Osborne NJ, Gatt IT. Management of shoulder injuries using dry needling in elite volleyball players. *Acupunct Med.* 2010;28(1):42–5.

76. Robinson V, Brosseau L, Casimiro L, et al. Thermotherapy for treating rheumatoid arthritis. *Cochrane Database Syst Rev.* 2002;2:CD002826.

77. Schaubel HJ. The local use of ice after orthopedic procedures. *Am J Surg.* 1946;72(5):711–4.

78. Sellwood KL, Brukner P, Williams D, Nicol A, Hinman R. Ice-water immersion and delayed-onset muscle soreness: a randomised controlled trial. *Br J Sports Med.* 2007;41(6):392–7.

79. Skoubo-Kristensen E, Sommer J. Ultrasound influence on internal fixation with a rigid plate in dogs. *Arch Phys Med Rehabil.* 1982;63(8):371–3.

80. Sloan JP, Hain R, Pownall R. Clinical benefits of early cold therapy in accident and emergency following ankle sprain. *Arch Emerg Med.* 1989;6(1):1–6.

81. Taskaynatan MA, Ozgul A, Ozdemir A, Tan AK, Kalyon TA. Effects of steroid iontophoresis and electrotherapy on bicipital tendonitis. *J Musculoskeletal Pain.* 2007;15(4):47–54.

82. Travell J. Ethyl chloride spray for painful muscle spasm. *Arch Phys Med Rehabil.* 1952;33(5):291–8.

83. Tumilty S, Munn J, McDonough S, Hurley DA, Basford JR, Baxter GD. Low level laser treatment of tendinopathy: a systematic review with meta-analysis. *Photomed Laser Surg.* 2010;28(1):3–16.

84. Vallbona C, Hazelwood CF, Jurida G. Response of pain to static magnetic fields in post-polio patients: a double blind pilot study. *Arch Phys Med Rehabil.* 1997;78(11):1200–3.

85. van der Windt DA, van der Heijden GJ, van den Berg SG, ter Riet G, de Winter AF, Bouter LM. Ultrasound therapy for musculoskeletal disorders: a systematic review. *Pain*. 1999;81(3):257–71.

86. van Middelkoop M, Rubinstein SM, Kuijpers T, et al. A systematic review on the effectiveness of physical and rehabilitation interventions for chronic non-specific low back pain. *Eur Spine J*. 2010;20(1):19–39.

87. Weinberger A, Fadilah R, Lev A, Levi A, Pinkhas J. Deep heat in the treatment of inflammatory joint disease. *Med Hypotheses*. 1988;25(4):231–3.

88. Weinberger A, Fadilah R, Lev A, Shohami E, Pinkhas J. Treatment of articular effusions with local deep microwave hyperthermia. *Clin Rheumatol*. 1989;8(4):461–6.

89. Weintraub MI, Wolfe GI, Barohn RA, et al. Static magnetic field therapy for symptomatic diabetic neuropathy: a randomized, double-blind, placebo-controlled trial. *Arch Phys Med Rehabil*. 2003;84(5):736–46.

90. Wilcock IM, Cronin JB, Hing WA. Physiologic response to water immersion: a method for sport recovery? *Sports Med*. 2006;36(9):747–65.

91. Wood JM, Evans PE 3rd, Schallreuter KU, et al. A multicenter study on the use of pulsed low-intensity direct current for healing chronic stage II and stage III decubitus ulcers. *Arch Dermatol*. 1993;129(8):999–1009.

92. Woodmansey A, Collins DH, Ernst MM. Vascular reactions to the contrast bath in health and in rheumatoid arthritis. *Lancet*. 1938; 2:1350–4.

93. Wright V, Johns RJ. Quantitative and qualitative analysis of joint stiffness in normal subjects and in patients with connective tissue disease. *Ann Rheum Dis*. 1961;20:36–46.

Core Strengthening

Joel Press

70

OVERVIEW

- Core rehabilitation allows the multisegmented spinal column to maintain its center of gravity through multiple ranges of motion, counteracting gravity, and applied forces to decrease torsion and shear on the spinal structures (ligaments, disc, nerve).
- Definition of core
    - The core is the lumbopelvic hip complex.
    - The core is where the center of gravity is located and where all movement begins (6).
    - An efficient core allows for maintenance of the normal length–tension relationship of functional agonists and antagonists, which allows for the maintenance of normal force–couple relationships in the lumbopelvic hip complex (6).
- Why is the core important?
    - When a limb is moved, reactive forces are imposed on the spine acting in parallel and opposing those forces producing the movement (3).
    - The spine is particularly prone to the effect of these reactive forces due to its multisegmental nature and the requirement for muscle contractions to provide stability of the spine (22).
    - Without muscular support and contraction, buckling of the spine occurs with compressive forces of as little as 2 kg (19).
    - Significant microtrauma of the lumbar spine will occur with rotation of as little as 2 degrees (12).
    - The musculature of the spine has been shown repeatedly to be most important in maintaining spinal stability during movements (10,25).
    - Function of core muscles: oppose the movements of limbs, hold spine together, and decrease lumbar shearing.
    - Muscle dysfunction in low back pain is a problem with motor control in the deep muscles related to segmental joint stabilization (23).
    - Back pain can occur as a consequence of deficits in control of the spinal segment when abnormally large segmental motions cause abnormal deformation of ligaments and pain-sensitive structures (22).
        - Loss of joint stiffness
        - Increase in mobility and abnormal spinal motion
        - Changes in the ratios of segmental rotations and translations

WHAT ARE CORE MUSCLES? ANATOMY/ BIOMECHANICS OF THE "CORE"

- Local paravertebral-multifidi
    - Stabilizing role: Protecting articular structures, discs, and ligaments from excessive bending, strains, and injury.
    - Multisegmental column is unstable and will buckle under compression at individual joints unless locally stabilized.
    - Short muscles provide local support for longer muscles to work (2).
    - Neutral zone control
        - The neutral zone is a region of intervertebral motion around the neutral posture where little resistance is offered by the passive spinal column (bones and ligaments).
        - Sensitive region for stabilization of joints (22)
        - Multifidi contribute to control of the neutral zone (21,26,27) and contribute more than two-thirds of stiffness increase at L4–L5 (27).
- Polysegmental: Erector spinae
    - Important for posture: Contract intermittently during the swaying movements that take place from an upright position.
    - Contraction of the erector spinae extends the trunk, a movement controlled largely by opposing activity of the rectus abdominis.
    - In slow trunk flexion movements, the erector spinae lowers the trunk into flexion (eccentrically contract) against the action of gravity during slow movements (20).
    - Role: Balance external loads and minimize forces on the spine (2).
    - Only a very small increase in activation of the multifidi and abdominal muscles is required to stiffen the spinal segments — 5% maximal voluntary contraction (MVC) for activities of daily living and 10% MVC for rigorous activity (5).
    - Endurance of muscles to maintain spinal stability during prolonged activities, not absolute strength, is most important (18).

- Abdominals: transversus abdominis (TrA), internal and external obliques, and rectus abdominis
  - Contraction of abdominals (especially TrA), pelvic floor, and diaphragm correlates closely with increased abdominal pressure in a variety of postural tasks (7,15,16).
  - TrA: Critical in stabilization of lumbar spine (7).
  - Contracting TrA increases intra-abdominal pressure and tensions the thoracolumbar fascia.
  - Helps create rigid cylinder, enhancing stiffness of lumbar spine (18).
  - Rectus abdominis and oblique abdominals are activated in direction-specific patterns with respect to limb movements, thus providing postural support *before* limb movements (1,16).
  - Contraction increasing intra-abdominal pressure occurs *before* initiation of large segment movement of the upper limbs (9,15,16).
- Quadratus lumborum
  - Fibers cross-link the vertebrae.
  - From transverse process to rib cage to iliac crests, can buttress shearing of spine in all planes
  - Active during flexion, extension, and lateral bending — not just a frontal plane muscle
- Diaphragm
  - To minimize the displacement of the abdominal contents within the abdomen and pelvis, it is necessary to elevate the intra-abdominal pressure by simultaneously contracting the diaphragm, the pelvic floor, and the abdominal muscles (5,8).
  - Diaphragm increases intra-abdominal pressure and segmental unloading of the spine, and thus increases trunk stability.
- Pelvic floor
  - Coactivation of the TrA, abdominals, multifidi, and pelvic floor muscles contributes to spine stability (24).
- Lower extremity muscles — gluteus maximus, hamstrings
  - Hip and pelvic muscles: base of support for lumbar spine and upper limbs
  - Thoracolumbar fascia
    - Covers the deep muscles of the back and trunk (including multifidi)
    - Connects the lower limbs to the upper via the latissimus dorsi
    - Internal obliques, TrA, latissimus dorsi, gluteus maximus
    - Enhances stiffness of the lumbar spine
  - Multifidi blend with superior medial aspect of gluteus maximus.
  - Multifidi attach to sacrotuberous ligaments and are mechanically linked to gluteus maximus.

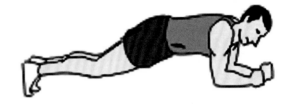

Figure 70.1: Plank core-strengthening exercise.

HOW DO WE STRENGTHEN CORE MUSCLES?

- Balance: Control center of gravity (COG) as it moves through various planes of motion and then shift the COG through various planes.
- Goals of core-strengthening exercise:
  - Improve multifidus activity and endurance
  - Restore the control of deep abdominal muscles
  - Restore coordination and position sense
  - Restore mobility, especially in rotational and lateral flexion directions
  - Restore normal gluteal muscle activity and lumbopelvic rhythm
  - Train motor and postural control and balance
  - Make exercises functional

PRACTICAL APPLICATIONS OF CORE STRENGTHENING

- Turn on the light.
  - Abdominal bracing: Tightening the abdominal muscles isometrically like you are going to be punched in the stomach.
  - May require cueing and instruction.
    - Need core stability for global mobility.
    - Abdominal bracing is more effective and puts less stress on the spine than hollowing (which is sucking in the abdominal muscles and then holding them tight) (13).

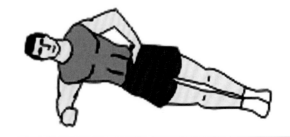

Figure 70.2: Side plank core-strengthening exercise.

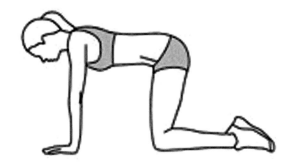

Figure 70.3: "Bird dog" core-strengthening exercise.

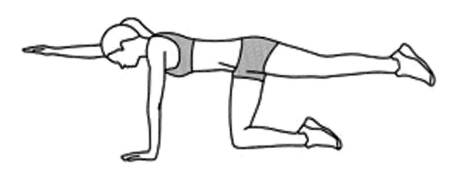

- Reeducation of stabilization muscles — pelvic clocks.
    - Learn how to turn on pelvic and hip muscles.
- Get the engines going.
    - Abdominal bracing in supine > prone, side lying > quadruped
    - Progress to kneeling > sitting > standing
    - Three basic core exercises that put the least load on the spine: plank (Fig. 70.1), side plank (Fig. 70.2), and "bird dog" (Fig. 70.3) (17)
- Make it functional and fun to do.
    - Start in pain-free ranges
    - Progress to multiple planes of motions
        - Frontal plane core
        - Sagittal plane core
        - Transverse plane core
    - Dynamic challenges — easy to hard
    - Include balance/proprioception
    - Need to make it subconscious

IS THERE EVIDENCE FOR CORE STABILIZATION EXERCISES AS TREATMENT FOR LOW BACK PAIN?

- No effect: No difference compared to other exercise treatments or manual therapy for randomized patients with chronic low back pain (4,11).

- Positive effect: Prediction rules indicate that patients most likely to benefit are those in specific subgroups with negative straight leg raise, positive prone instability test, aberrant motion, lumbar hypermobility, or low fear of avoidance (14).
- Conclusion: If patients are first subgrouped into those responding to specific maneuvers, there is a greater chance of predicting benefit from core exercises. Core exercises for everyone with nonspecific back pain may not provide any better results than other nonspecific exercises as part of an activating program.

REFERENCES

1. Aruin AS, Latash ML. Directional specificity of postural muscles in a feed-forward postural reaction during fast voluntary arm movements. *Exp Brain Res.* 1995;103(2):323–32.
2. Bergmark A. Stability of the lumbar spine. A study in mechanical engineering. *Acta Orthop Scand Suppl.* 1989;230:1–54.
3. Bouisset S, Zattara M. Biomechanical study of the programming and anticipatory postural adjustments associated with voluntary movement. *J Biomech.* 1987;20(8):735–42.
4. Cairns MC, Foster NE, Wright C. Randomized controlled trial of specific spinal stabilization exercises and conventional physiotherapy for recurrent low back pain. *Spine (Phila Pa 1976).* 2006;31(19):E670–81.
5. Cholewicki J, Juluru K, McGill SM. Intra-abdominal pressure for stabilizing the lumbar spine. *J Biomech.* 1999;32(1):13–7.
6. Clark MA, Fater D, Reuteman P. Core (trunk) stabilization and its importance for closed kinetic chain rehabilitation. *Orthop Phys Ther Clin North Am.* 2000;9(2):119–32.
7. Cresswell AG, Oddsson L, Thorstensson A. The influence of sudden perturbations on trunk muscle activity and intraabdominal pressure while standing. *Exp Brain Res.* 1994;98(2):336–41.

8. Daggfeldt K, Thorstensson A. The role of intra-abdominal pressure in spinal unloading. *J Biomech.* 1997;30(11–12):1149–55.

9. Ferreira ML, Ferreira PH, Hodges PW. Changes in postural activity of the trunk muscles following spinal manipulative therapy. *Man Ther.* 2007;12(3):240–8.

10. Gardner-Morse M, Stokes IA, Laible JP. Role of the muscles in lumbar spine stability in maximum extension efforts. *J Orthop Res.* 1995;13(5):802–8.

11. Goldby LJ, Moore AP, Doust J, Trew ME. A randomized controlled trial investigating the efficiency of musculoskeletal physiotherapy on chronic low back disorder. *Spine (Phila Pa 1976).* 2006;31(10):1083–93.

12. Gracovetsky S, Farfan H, Helleur C. The abdominal mechanism. *Spine (Phila Pa 1976).* 1985;10(4):317–24.

13. Grenier SG, McGill SM. Quantification of lumbar stability by using 2 different abdominal activation strategies. *Arch Phys Med Rehabil.* 2007; 88(1):54–62.

14. Hicks GE, Fritz JM, Delitto A, McGill SM. Preliminary development of a clinical prediction rule for determining which patients with low back pain will respond to a stabilization exercise program. *Arch Phys Med Rehabil.* 2005;86(9):1753–62.

15. Hodges PW, Butler JE, McKenzie DK, Gandevia SC. Contraction of the human diaphragm during rapid postural adjustments. *J Physiol.* 1997;505(Pt 2):539–48.

16. Hodges PW, Richardson CA. Feedforward contraction of transverses abdominis is not influenced by the direction of the arm movement. *Exp Brain Res.* 1997;114(2):362–70.

17. McGill SM. *Corrective and Therapeutic Exercise for the Painful Lumbar Spine: Technique Matters.* Rochester (MN): American Academy of Neuromuscular and Electrodiagnostic Medicine; 2009.

18. McGill SM, Norman RW. Reassessment of the role of intra-abdominal pressure in spinal compression. *Ergonomics.* 1987;30(11): 1565–88.

19. Morris JM, Lucas DM, Bresler B. Role of the trunk in the stability of the spine. *J Bone Joint Surg Am.* 1961;43:327–51.

20. Oddsson LI. Control of voluntary trunk movements in man: mechanisms for postural equilibrium in standing. *Acta Physiol Scan Suppl.* 1990;595:1–60.

21. Panjabi MM. The stabilizing system of the spine. Part 1. Function, dysfunction, adaptation, and enhancement. *J Spinal Disord.* 1991;5(4): 383–9.

22. Panjabi MM. The stabilizing system of the spine. Part II. Neutral zone and stability hypothesis. *J Spinal Disord.* 1992;5(4):390–6.

23. Richardson C, Jull G, Hodges PW, Hides JA. *Therapeutic Exercise for Spinal Segmental Stabilization in Low Back Pain: Scientific Basis and Clinical Approach.* Edinburgh (UK): Churchill Livingstone; 1999. 192 p.

24. Sapsford RR, Hodges PW, Richardson CA, Cooper DH, Makwell SJ, Jull GA. Co-activation of the abdominal and pelvic floor muscles during voluntary exercise. *Neurourol Urodyn.* 2001;20(1):31–42.

25. Solomonow M, Zhou BH, Harris M, Lu Y, Baratta RV. The ligamento-muscular stabilizing system of the spine. *Spine (Phila Pa 1976).* 1998; 23(23):2552–62.

26. Steffen R, Nolte LP, Pingel TH. Importance of back muscles in rehabilitation of postoperative lumber instability; a biomechanical analysis. *Rehabilitation (Stuttg).* 1994;33(3):164–70.

27. Wilke HJ, Wolf S, Claes LE, Arand M, Wiesend A. Stability increase of the lumbar spine with different muscle groups. A biomechanical in vitro study. *Spine (Phila Pa 1976).* 1995;20(2):192–8.

Medications and Ergogenic Aids

71

Scott Flinn and Andrew J. McMarlin

OVERVIEW

■ Many athletes self-medicate using various pharmacologic or nutritional substances in an effort to improve performance and speed recovery from injury. For example, over-the-counter anti-inflammatory medications are often used to limit pain and inflammation in an effort to reduce swelling, limit inflammation, and presumably speed healing from injury.

■ Other substances, some of which may be illegal, are used specifically in an effort to improve workload and performance.

DEFINITION

■ Ergogenic aids are defined as items designed to increase work or improve performance above that of regular training and diet.

■ Ergogenic aids are usually classified into five groups: mechanical aids such as running shoes, psychological aids, physiologic aids such as fluids and blood, pharmacologic aids that generally are thought of as requiring a prescription, and nutritional aids.

HISTORY

■ In 1994, Congress passed the Dietary Supplement Health and Education Act (DSHEA), which substantially changed the regulation and marketing of dietary supplements (23). Essentially, substances can be sold without U.S. Food and Drug Administration (FDA) approval as long as the products are labeled and sold as dietary supplements and the label makes no claim as a drug.

■ These supplements are not held to the same quality control standards as FDA-approved drugs; the content and purity of these products are not regulated, and they may contain too much of the product to none at all (13). Furthermore, these substances do not require evaluation for safety or efficacy.

■ Despite all this, ergogenic aids are commonly used, sometimes with cataclysmic consequences, often with no effect, and occasionally with good effect.

EVALUATING ERGOGENIC AIDS

■ Objective evaluations of ergogenic aids are often difficult to perform. Additionally, the scientific literature usually differs significantly from the advertising on many products (13).

■ There is no burden of proof on the manufacturer to prove efficacy or product content like there is for drugs (23).

■ Products may contain lower amounts of the product than those listed on the label, with some products having zero amount of the supposedly ergogenic substance, whereas others may be contaminated by the previous drug manufactured in the equipment (55).

■ Furthermore, the placebo effect can have a huge impact on the perceived benefits derived by the user.

EFFICACY OF ERGOGENIC AIDS

■ Ergogenic aids can affect various aspects of physical fitness to improve performance. Six components of fitness that may be affected include aerobic fitness, anaerobic fitness, strength, body composition, psychological factors, and healing of injuries.

■ Aerobic metabolism uses oxygen, whereas anaerobic metabolism does not.

■ Aerobic fitness is the ability to produce work using aerobic metabolism, generally lasting longer than 1 minute and often lasting for hours, and is important especially in endurance events. It comprises two parts: maximal aerobic power and aerobic capacity.

■ Anaerobic fitness is important in activities generally lasting less than 1 minute and is fueled primarily through anaerobic metabolism.

■ Maximum strength, usually measured by the one-repetition maximum, refers to the amount of power that can be generated in a brief burst and is fueled by anaerobic metabolism.

■ Body composition can affect performance by increasing lean muscle mass. More muscle can perform more work, whereas decreasing body fat decreases the inert weight that has to be carried through space to the finish line.

■ Psychological factors may affect performance through various mind–body mechanisms including decreased perceptions of fatigue and pain.

■ Enhancing the healing of injuries and soreness promotes a more rapid return to training and maintenance of fitness.

SAFETY CONSIDERATIONS

■ Ergogenic aids can have side effects like any other substance.
■ Heart attacks, seizures, strokes, coma, and death have been attributed to the use of ergogenic products (13).
■ Injectable products carry the risk of disease transmission if needles are shared.

ETHICAL AND LEGAL CONSIDERATIONS

■ The athletic ideal is winning through natural training, which maximizes native ability and performance. However, this is often not the reality. Athletes are constantly caught in the dilemma of trying to keep up with what their competitors may be trying to do. Many athletes will try ergogenic aids even though the product has not been shown to work, has serious side effects, or is banned by the sport's governing body ruling over the sport in which the athlete is competing.
■ In an attempt to keep the playing field level, various amateur and professional organizations have instituted drug policies. These policies are targeted toward substances that may be dangerous, illegal, and/or give an unfair competitive advantage. For example, the use of anabolic steroids had become so widespread by the 1964 Olympics that drug testing began at the 1968 Olympic Games in Mexico City, with the National Collegiate Athletic Association (NCAA) following in 1986.
■ The American College of Sports Medicine® (ACSM) and other organizations have taken a position on anabolic steroids stating that they are unethical, they have dangerous side effects, and their use should be deplored (2).

■ The Anabolic Steroids Control Act of 1991 made anabolic steroids a Schedule III controlled substance.
■ Anabolic steroids are not the only substances banned by sports governing bodies such as the International Olympic Committee (IOC), the World Anti-Doping Agency (WADA), and the NCAA. The IOC developed their list in 1967.
■ Because of many doping scandals, the U.S. Anti-Doping Agency (USADA) was formed in 2000 as an independent antidoping organization for Olympic sports in the United States. The list of substances banned by the IOC can be viewed on the WADA Web site at http://www.wada-ama.org/en/World-Anti-Doping-Program/ (72).
■ The NCAA has their list at http://www.ncaa.org/wps/wcm/connect/public/NCAA/Student-Athlete+Experience/NCAA+banned+drugs+list (48).
■ Because the lists are continually changing, physicians caring for athletes in these or other organizations should always consult them prior to writing a prescription or suggesting over-the-counter remedies.
■ Testing is usually done by analyzing urine samples through a number of methods, with most confirmatory tests done using gas chromatography/mass spectrometry. In the future, blood or hair samples may be used to detect banned substances. See Chapter 25, Drug Testing.
■ Further discussion of ethical considerations related to supplements, medications, and ergogenic aids can be found in Chapter 2, Ethical Considerations in Sports Medicine.

SPECIFIC ERGOGENIC AIDS

■ Specific ergogenic aids will be reviewed here regarding their efficacy, safety, and use in Olympic and NCAA competition. Table 71.1 gives an overview of many ergogenic aids, their effects on the six fitness components, and their safety.

Table 71.1	**Ergogenic Aids, Their Effect on Fitness Components, and Dangerous Side Effects**						
Product	**Aerobic**	**Anaerobic**	**Strength**	**Body Composition**	**Psychological**	**Healing**	**Danger**
Anabolic steroids	—	—	+	+	+	?	+
Androstenedione/DHEA	—	—	+	+	+	?	+
β_2-agonist (clenbuterol)	?	—	—	?	?	—	?
Blood doping	+	—	—	—	—	—	++
Caffeine	+	+	—	—	?	—	—
Corticosteroids	—	—	—	—	—	?	?
Creatine	—	+	?	+	—	?	—
Ephedrine/amphetamines	+	+	+	+	+		++
Gene therapy	?	?	?	?	?	?	?
Growth hormone	—	—	—	+	—	—	?
NSAIDs	—	—	—	—	—	?	+

DHEA, dehydroepiandrosterone; NSAIDs, nonsteroidal anti-inflammatory drugs.

Anabolic-Androgenic Steroids and Selective Androgen Receptor Modulators

Efficacy

- Anabolic steroids have both anabolic (tissue-building) and androgenic side effects. Anabolic steroids have been shown to increase lean muscle mass and strength when used with an adequate diet and with progressive weight training. Supraphysiologic doses seem to increase these effects (2,7).

- There does not appear to be a direct effect on aerobic power or capacity, although decreased healing time may allow for increased training volume.

- Surveys of anabolic steroid users show increases in the incidence of mood disorders and in aggression.

- Researchers are developing selective androgen receptor modulators in attempts to achieve anabolic effects in specific tissues without the systemic side effects of older androgenic agents (16).

- The concordant use of human chorionic gonadotropin along with estrogen blockers may increase athletes' testosterone levels, maintain normal (3:1) testosterone-to-epitestosterone levels, and minimize androgenic side effects (29).

Safety

- Anabolic steroids are Schedule III drugs. Legal indications to prescribe and common contraindications to steroids are listed in Table 71.2.

- Anabolic steroids have a long list of reported side effects, some of which may have been exaggerated in the medical literature.

- A concerning increase in low-density lipoprotein and decrease in high-density lipoprotein (HDL) by an average of 50% in both male and female users, combined with hypertension, have been shown with no direct link yet to increased cardiovascular mortality (2).

- Adverse effects have been noted in the liver including jaundice, benign tumors, and, rarely, peliosis hepatis (blood-filled cysts in the liver), which has caused a few fatalities when the cysts ruptured. Causation of malignant liver tumors has not been proven (10).

- Other side effects include acne, female masculinization (alopecia, hirsutism, clitoromegaly, deepening of the voice) and enhancement of aggression.

- Physiologic doses of testosterone hasten closure of epiphyses (growth plates). Surveys suggest that 6% of high school football players (and 4% of all high school students) have taken anabolic steroids and that half of them started taking them before age 14 (19).

- Long-term side effects have been harder to establish a causal relationship.

Legality

- Steroids are Schedule III controlled substances.

- Banned by IOC and NCAA (WADA 2011, NCAA 2011), although athletes having certain medical conditions (*i.e.*, bilateral orchiectomy for testicular cancer treatment) may apply for a therapeutic use exemption (TUE).

- Users attempt to avoid detection by tapering in advance of announced tests, staying within the WADA cutoff of 4:1 urinary testosterone-to-epitestosterone ratio, or using masking agents such as diuretics. Recent development of a hair test may change the way testing is done in the future.

Androstenedione and Dehydroepiandrosterone

Efficacy

- Androstenedione, a testosterone precursor, is one of the few oral "supplements" that is converted into testosterone when ingested. Despite a serum increase in testosterone and estradiol after high doses of androstenedione, double-blinded studies have failed to demonstrate any significant change in lean body mass or strength (68).

- Dehydroepiandrosterone (DHEA) is a hormone secreted by the adrenal gland that is a precursor to both androgens and estrogens. DHEA levels peak at puberty and young adulthood and gradually fade as aging progresses. Although the FDA banned the manufacture of DHEA as a drug due to insufficient evidence of efficacy and safety, it continues to be available as a nutritional supplement.

- Studies showed that physiologic doses (50 mg d^{-1}) and supraphysiologic doses (1,600 mg d^{-1}) of DHEA increased circulating androgen levels in older women but not in older men. DHEA increased androstenedione levels but not testosterone levels and had a small, not statistically significant increase in lean body mass when given at supraphysiologic doses to five young males (61).

- DHEA did not appear to affect energy or protein metabolism in young males (70). In summary, DHEA does not appear to increase testosterone in young healthy males, and it does not appear to have an ergogenic effect.

Table 71.2 | Indications and Contraindications for Anabolic Steroids

Indications	Contraindications
Primary hypogonadism	Known or suspected prostate cancer
Hypogonadotropic hypogonadism	Breast cancer in females with high Ca^{2+}
Hereditary angioedema	Breast cancer in males
Antithrombin III deficiency	Nephritis
Anemia from renal disease	Pregnancy or nursing
Catabolic disease such as AIDS	
Delayed-onset puberty	

AIDS, acquired immunodeficiency syndrome.

Safety

- Side effects of androstenedione are likely to be similar to anabolic steroids.

- Short-term use of DHEA has been associated with few side effects, but risks of long-term use are unknown. There is a theoretical risk of prostate and endometrial cancer as well as gynecomastia. DHEA effects on lipids are unknown.

Legality

- Androstenedione, although banned, currently is not frequently specifically tested (10).

- DHEA is currently banned by both the NCAA and IOC and is available only as a nutritional supplement in the United States (48,72).

β₂-Adrenergic Receptor Agonists

Efficacy

- β₂-adrenergic agonists, such as albuterol and salmeterol, are sympathomimetics and are used widely as bronchodilators for the treatment of many types of asthma, including exercise-induced asthma. Clenbuterol, available by prescription in some countries, is a longer acting β₂-agonist that may increase aerobic capacity and decrease body fat.

- There are no human studies to support athletes' use of clenbuterol for their potential anabolic effects, either as an anabolic steroid substitute or to prevent some of the muscle loss after cessation of anabolic steroids. Animal studies have shown that clenbuterol in high doses increases lean body mass and decreases adipose tissue (50).

- However, a study on a relative drug, salbutamol, showed increased quadriceps and hamstring strength, while another showed that 6 weeks of oral albuterol may augment strength gains in isokinetic strength training of the knee (14,42).

- Taken together, these studies imply that there may be an ergogenic effect of prolonged oral β₂-agonists on strength, but no ergogenic effect of short-term administration of inhaled medicines. Confirmatory studies on humans remain to be done regarding their potential anabolic effects.

Safety

- Side effects of β₂-agonists are common and similar to other sympathomimetics and include tachycardia, tremor, palpitations, anxiety, headache, anorexia, and insomnia. Serious side effects include dysrhythmias, cardiac muscle hypertrophy, myocardial infarction, or stroke (11,50).

Legality

- Because of its potential ergogenic effect, clenbuterol in all its forms and all oral β₂-agonists are banned by the IOC and NCAA. Inhaled salbutamol and salmeterol are allowed when used in accordance with manufacturer's recommendations. Salbutamol may not exceed a urinary concentration of $1,000 \ \text{ng} \cdot \text{mL}^{-1}$, which would correlate to over 1,600 μg in 24 hours (48,72).

- Advances in testing may eventually enable detection of these drugs through hair analysis.

- Clenbuterol is not FDA approved.

- It is interesting to note there was an increase in the percentage of U.S. Olympic athletes with exercise-induced asthma from 10% in the 1984 Summer Olympics to over 20% in the 1996 Summer Olympics, thus greatly increasing the number of athletes who can "legally" use these products (69).

Blood Doping, Recombinant Erythropoietin, and Continuous Erythropoietin Receptor Activators

Efficacy

- Blood doping refers to the process of artificially increasing red blood cell (RBC) mass to improve exercise performance. Increasing RBC mass can be accomplished through infusion of RBCs or through the use of the recombinant erythropoietin (rEPO) to stimulate RBC production (54).

- By increasing the RBC mass, oxygen-carrying capacity is increased with resultant increase in both maximal aerobic power and aerobic capacity. The increased $\dot{V}O_{2max}$ and time to exhaustion enable improvements in race performance, especially in distance runners and cyclists (21,54).

- Blood doping also seems to help performance in the heat, especially in acclimatized individuals (54).

- Effects of synthetic erythropoietin last up to six times longer than human erythropoietin, whereas the newer continuous erythropoietin receptor activators (CERAs) last up to 20 times longer, allowing for monthly dosing.

Safety

- Although rare, the major risk from blood transfusions is transfusion reactions. Other complications include infection from the blood or procedure.

- Hyperviscosity can occur with hemoglobin levels over 55%, which may increase the risk of thrombosis causing strokes or myocardial infarction in athletes using rEPO or blood transfusions. It has been postulated that numerous deaths among cyclists have been caused by rEPO-induced hyperviscosity, causing vascular sludging and myocardial artery occlusion (20,54).

- Blood pressure may also be increased by rEPO and is contraindicated in uncontrolled hypertension (21).

Legality

- Banned by the IOC and NCAA (48,72).

- Blood transfusions can be detected if homologous blood is used, but autologous blood is harder to detect (54). Erythropoietin isoforms can be measured directly from blood testing and in the urine, but because rEPO currently can only be detected for a few days after administration but has effects that last for weeks, reliable testing is difficult. At this time, it is unclear for how long the newer, longer acting CERAs can be detected in the blood, and there is no current urine test available (36).

Caffeine

Efficacy

- Caffeine enhances performance during both prolonged activity and shorter intense activity lasting from 1–60 minutes (*e.g.*, rowing, swimming, middle distance races) and during stop-and-go sports such as team and racquet sports (12).

- In events involving strength and power, such as lifts, throws, and sprints, caffeine's effects are unclear.

- Caffeine has been hypothesized to work for runners by increasing free fatty acid production (which would spare muscle glycogen), elevating cyclic adenosine 3′,5′-monophosphate (cAMP) levels in cells, altering the movement of calcium by the sarcoplasmic reticulum, increasing levels of catecholamines, increasing neuromuscular transmissions, and decreasing perceived effort and fatigue (3).

- The effectiveness of caffeine may not be as great in habitual users or in hot humid environments.

Safety

- In normal doses (3–8 mg · kg^{-1}) caffeine appears safe and produces a few side effects such as diarrhea, insomnia, restlessness, and anxiety.

- Caffeine does not appear to increase risk for heatstroke or compromise cardiovascular activity in endurance performance (49).

- Very high doses, over 10 mg · kg^{-1}, may cause seizures, and overdosing may lead to death.

Legality

- Caffeine, although ergogenic at 5–10 mg · kg^{-1}, is not completely banned by the IOC and NCAA. Habitual users may consume their usual caffeine in small amounts. Ingestion of around 7 mg · kg^{-1}, roughly two cups of coffee, produces urinary levels close to the limit of 12 μg · mL^{-1} for the IOC. The NCAA levels are slightly more liberal at 15 μg · mL^{-1} (48,72).

Corticosteroids

Efficacy

- Corticosteroids are a class of medications acting on a number of body systems, including inflammation. Glucocorticoids downregulate the expression of inflammatory genes in cells, thus decreasing inflammatory cytokines, enzymes, and adhesion molecules, while upregulating the production of anti-inflammatory proteins such as interleukin-1 receptor antagonist and interleukin-10.

- Although commonly used for a variety of acute and chronic injuries, most of the literature evaluating steroids for treating sports medicine injuries is retrospective in nature, involves case series, or is anecdotal.

- Steroids may be given by numerous routes, but when used to treat musculoskeletal injuries, they are usually given orally, as a topical agent, or via injection.

- There are no prospective studies that evaluate the effectiveness of steroids in treating acute injuries. Anecdotally, some clinicians use short courses of oral steroids for 3 to 5 days on acute injuries including radicular back pain, but this has not been evaluated prospectively. Because of the potential side effects from steroid use, treatment with corticosteroids for acute injuries in the sports setting should be of short duration and left up to the individual clinician to develop any treatment protocol until better information becomes available.

- For overuse injuries, many chronic tendon injuries seem to be a tendinosis of a degenerative nature and do not involve classic chronic inflammatory cells. However, clinicians frequently use corticosteroids for these conditions, which often provide the patient with temporary pain control (1).

- In patients with lateral epicondylitis (tennis elbow), a review of randomized controlled trials showed that pain improved faster in patients with new-onset epicondylitis with steroid injection as compared to nonsteroidal anti-inflammatory drugs (NSAIDs) and simple analgesics, but pain relief was similar at 1 year (30). Another review showed better short-term relief with corticosteroid injection (4).

- Trigger finger has been shown to be well treated in two small double-blind, randomized, placebo-controlled trials (34,47).

- Subacromial injections for rotator cuff tendinopathy have been shown to improve range of motion in two randomized placebo-controlled trials but were no better than lidocaine injection alone in another (25,67).

- There is no evidenced-based guideline or consensus on the number, interval, type, or dose of steroid that should be used at a particular site. Suggestions include mixing anesthetic with the corticosteroid to provide some immediate pain relief, not injecting tendons, using extra caution when performing peritendinous injections or injecting structures that communicate with a joint, resting the injected area for 2–6 weeks, and limiting injections to no closer than 6 weeks apart and no more than three injections in one site (39).

Safety

- Steroid injection has a complication rate of 1%–5.8% (60).

- Infection, hypopigmentation, postinjection flare, and fat pad atrophy are the most common adverse effects.

- Steroid injection directly into a tendon weakens it and may cause tendon rupture (24).

- Long-term therapy or extremely high dosages of steroids may cause avascular necrosis, adrenal suppression, gastrointestinal ulcer, diabetes, cataracts, and hypertension.

Legality

- WADA prohibits all glucocorticosteroids when administered by oral, intravenous, intramuscular, or rectal routes, but they are not banned by the NCAA (48,72).

Creatine

Efficacy

- Creatine is a naturally occurring organic acid made by the kidneys, liver, and pancreas and is stored in skeletal muscle.

Studies have shown an increase in available intracellular adenosine triphosphate with supplementation of creatine monohydrate (26).

- Numerous studies have shown that supplementation may improve maximal weight lifted and performance in very short-cycling sprints (< 10 seconds) as well as increase fat-free body mass by 1–7 kg (18,66).
- Studies that have used double-blinded protocols have not been able to demonstrate performance improvement in endurance efforts or sprints at the end of endurance efforts (31).
- Enhancement of performance is most likely in sports or positions where increased mass (*i.e.*, American football linemen or Sumo wrestlers) or a single pushing, lifting, or striking effort is required (*i.e.*, baseball or softball hitter, non–weight-class powerlifting).
- To transfer these research data to creatine's usefulness within individual sports, the potential enhancement from a very short-lived power increase needs to be balanced with the increased body mass for the entire activity.

Safety

- Concerns that increased uptake of water by muscle may hinder heat tolerance and hydration status or that metabolism of creatine by the kidneys may result in kidney damage have not been supported by controlled trials (38). Long-term studies of the safety of this supplement are ongoing.

Legality

- Use of creatine by athletes is allowed by the IOC and the NCAA. The latter organization did ban the purchase and dispersal of this supplement to athletes by its affiliated universities and university employees (*i.e.*, coaches and athletic trainers) (48,72).

Ephedra, Pseudoephedrine, and Amphetamines

Efficacy

- Ephedra and its derivatives pseudoephedrine and amphetamine, and other related compounds, are sympathomimetic amines and are used as stimulants, appetite suppressants, and decongestants. Some derivatives are used to treat obesity and attention-deficit hyperactivity disorder.
- Ephedrine is a sympathomimetic drug that is the active ingredient in the Chinese herbal medicine ma huang.
- Ephedrine acts physiologically to increase heart rate and blood pressure. When used with caffeine, ephedrine has been shown to improve time to exhaustion during exercise tests. When used with caffeine, it also seems to be effective in producing weight loss. Low-dose (24 mg) ephedrine did not show an improvement in performance (57).
- Pseudoephedrine has not been shown to improve aerobic performance in controlled trials (63).
- Acutely, this class probably improves strength, muscular power (endurance), and time to exhaustion, possibly due to the masking of fatigue (59). Studies have not shown improvement in aerobic power ($\dot{V}O_{2max}$) or running speed.
- Ephedrine has been shown to maintain vigilance, reaction time, and cognitive function during sleep deprivation (15).
- Amphetamines also act as appetite suppressants.

Safety

- The side effects often depend on dose. Deaths have been associated with use of these drugs due to myocardial infarctions, arrhythmias, cerebrovascular accidents, and heat stroke (15,28,59).
- Other problems include hypertension, restlessness, vomiting, arrhythmias, and seizures.
- Side effects are potentiated when used with certain antidepressants including selective serotonin reuptake inhibitors, bupropion, and monoamine oxidase inhibitors.
- Amphetamine and its derivatives are Schedule II drugs and are considered potentially addicting, with particular dependency risk with chronic use.

Legality

- Amphetamines are banned by both the IOC and NCAA (48,72).
- Ephedrine is illegal as a food supplement in the United States (65). It is banned by the NCAA and WADA.
- Pseudoephedrine is allowed in Olympic competition when the urine concentration is less than 150 $\mu g \cdot mL^{-1}$. It is not banned by the NCAA. Because of their potential to be used in the manufacture of methamphetamine, the drugs were regulated in the United States by the Combat Methamphetamine Epidemic Act of 2005 (CMEA) and have limits on daily sales, 30-day purchases, and other restrictions regarding their sale (17).

Gene Therapy

Efficacy

- The newest modalities for increasing muscle size and strength are currently undergoing in vivo studies in animals and are primarily designed to inhibit the myostatin gene. Myostatin is a member of the transforming growth factor-β family that regulates, and limits, the number and growth of myocytes (37). Proteins that block the myostatin receptor, called myostatin inhibitors or antagonists, have been identified and encoded into viral DNA. In studies in several different animal models, a single injection into hind limb skeletal muscle results in significantly increased size and strength of hind limb and fore limb skeletal muscles, which persists for more than 2 years. These results held true for both young and middle-aged animals (27). The most tested myostatin inhibitors thus far include follistatin, follistatin-related gene (FLRG), and growth and differentiation factor-associated protein-1 (GASP-1).
- The cumulative results are very promising for the future treatment of skeletal muscle disorders, but there will almost

inevitably be attempts to use these for performance enhancement if and when they reach the human trial phase.

Safety

- Changes to tissues outside of skeletal muscle have not been detected in these studies. Researchers have specifically looked for changes in cardiac muscle size or function and for changes in test animals' reproductive capacity, and positive findings of any change are currently absent from the literature.

Legality

- All of these investigational myostatin inhibitors fall under the Nonapproved Substances (S0 Subsection) of the WADA 2011 Prohibited List as substances that have no current governmental approval for therapeutic use in humans (72).

Growth Hormone and Insulin-Like Growth Factor

Efficacy

- Growth hormone (GH) is secreted by the hypothalamus and is important in the growth and development of normal bones and muscle.
- GH seems to be intricately related to, and its effects are primarily mediated by, insulin-like growth factor-1 (IGF-1) and the regulation of insulin (40).
- GH and IGF-1 appear to provide an anabolic effect and increases bone mass and lean body mass while decreasing adipose tissue (6,46).
- Administration of GH in GH-deficient individuals has been shown to increase height, decrease body fat, and improve respiratory muscle function, strength, and agility.
- Results of supplementation with GH in normal individuals have been varied in regard to whether it improves athletic performance (44) or not (5,20,53).
- Although there are myocardial receptors for GH, administration of recombinant human growth hormone (rhGH) did not affect cardiovascular performance as measured by left ventricular ejection fraction, heart rate, or blood pressure in seven normal male volunteers (9).
- GH levels can be increased by exercise, and the level of release is related directly to exercise intensity, but the duration of the secretion and effects of long-term training are not known (51).
- In summary, GH and IGF-1 appear to increase lean body mass and decrease body fat, but it is still unclear whether they have any effect on athletic performance.

Safety

- Long-term human GH doping will probably result in the symptoms of acromegaly: fluid retention, increased risk of developing diabetes mellitus, and hypertension. Other risks include cardiomyopathy, decreased HDL, osteoporosis, menstrual irregularities, and impotence.

- As with any drug that is injected, users have increased risks for cross infection with human immunodeficiency virus (HIV) and hepatitis.
- Although cadaveric GH may not be used as commonly as in the past, its use increases risk for prion disease (Creutzfeldt-Jakob disease), which is characterized by progressive dementia. (53).

Legality

- Current testing for GH is limited to blood testing for elevated levels of IGF-1 and measuring changes in GH isoforms, which requires having had a previous blood test evaluating baseline GH isoforms (8).
- GH and the proteins in the GH signaling pathway are banned by the NCAA and the IOC, although it is possible an athlete with a genetic deficiency of GH may obtain a TUE from the IOC (48,72).

Nonsteroidal Anti-Inflammatory Drugs

Efficacy

- NSAIDs are commonly used medications to treat both acute and chronic injuries. Over 50 million people in the United States take daily prescription NSAIDs, with over 100 million Americans using prescription NSAIDs during a year (58). They are widely available over the counter.
- The major pharmacologic effect of NSAIDs is to inhibit the enzyme cyclooxygenase (COX), thus decreasing prostaglandin production. The decreased prostaglandins produce decreased inflammation and promote analgesia in the injured tissue. There are at least two forms of the COX enzyme, COX-1 and COX-2.
- COX-1 is important in the production of prostaglandins involved in the homeostasis of various tissues including renal parenchyma, gastric mucosa, and platelets.
- COX-2 produces prostaglandins involved in pain and inflammation. Most NSAIDs inhibit both COX-1 and COX-2 at various levels, with newer agents developed to be more COX-2 selective. Theoretically, this enhances the desired effects while limiting the side effects.
- NSAIDs have been shown to decrease pain, increase functional ability, and allow for a more rapid return to training in ankle sprains (43).
- NSAIDs may provide benefit in treating delayed-onset muscle soreness by decreasing pain and improving short-term muscle recovery (71), but given their potential to impair healing, they should only be used for 3–7 days after injury.

Safety

- Because of the risks associated with NSAIDs, consideration should be given to avoidance of these NSAIDs and using acetaminophen and exercise therapy as alternatives (62).
- Acetaminophen may be as effective as NSAIDs in acute pain reduction (70).
- NSAIDs should be used for as short a duration as possible.

- Which NSAID to recommend may be a complex risk–benefit decision, with gastrointestinal (GI) bleeding risk, cardiovascular risk, and aspirin use variables to consider. Based on the available data, in a patient with limited GI bleed risk (defined as no history of bleeding ulcers or concomitant corticosteroid use) and limited cardiovascular risk (defined as those without a history of ischemic heart, cerebrovascular, or peripheral arterial disease, and whose Framingham 10-year risk is < 10%), nonselective NSAIDs are appropriate for a short duration.

- Cardiovascular side effects from NSAIDs, namely an increased risk in acute myocardial infarctions, were thought to be linked to the COX-2–specific NSAIDs, but recent studies suggest that there may also be an increased risk with the nonselective NSAIDs (32,52,64).

- Naproxen appears to have the lowest cardiovascular risk and, until more data become available, should be considered one of the safer choices.

- NSAIDs can potentially damage the GI tract, principally through systemic effects including disruption of the mucous layer, decreased bicarbonate secretion, vasoconstriction, and a direct topical effect causing epithelial necrosis (56). GI bleeds can occur with both chronic and acute use, sometimes within days of starting the medication. Although much more common in the elderly, GI bleeds can occur in younger individuals. Those that appear to be at increased risk include patients with concurrent *Helicobacter pylori* infections and those on medications such as anticoagulants, including aspirin and corticosteroids (22,35).

- COX-2–selective NSAIDs were introduced in the 1990s to decrease the GI bleed risk, but some had a higher risk of cardiovascular side effects including myocardial infarction and had to be withdrawn from the market (45).

- Other methods that have been attempted to reduce the risk of GI bleed include using proton pump inhibitors, misoprostol, H_2-receptor antagonists, and *H. pylori* eradication. These methods have variable outcomes and side effects. Overall, the addition of a proton pump inhibitor and/or switching to a COX-2–selective NSAID seems to be the best options to reduce GI bleed risk (33).

- For patients with both high risk of GI bleed and cardiac complications, use of a COX-2 NSAID plus a proton pump inhibitor may be prudent because the risk of a fatal bleed may be higher than a cardiovascular event.

- If the patient will be on NSAIDs for a long duration, consideration should be given to *H. pylori* eradication (41).

Legality

- NSAIDs are allowed by WADA and the NCAA.

REFERENCES

1. Almekinders LC, Temple JD. Etiology, diagnosis and treatment of tendonitis: an analysis of the literature. *Med Sci Sports Exerc.* 1998;30(8):1183–90.

2. American College of Sports Medicine position stand on the use of anabolic-androgenic steroids in sports. *Med Sci Sports Exerc.* 1987;19(5):534–9.

3. Applegate E. Effective nutritional ergogenic aids. *Int J Sport Nutr.* 1999;9(2):229–39.

4. Assendelft WJ, Hay EM, Adshead R, Bouter LM. Corticosteroid injections for lateral epicondylitis: a systematic overview. *Br J Gen Pract.* 1996;46(405):209–16.

5. Berggren A, Ehrnborg C, Rosén T, Ellegård L, Bengtsson BA, Caidahl K. Short-term administration of supraphysiological recombinant human growth hormone (GH) does not increase maximum endurance exercise capacity in healthy, active young men and women with normal GH-insulin-like growth factor I axes. *J Clin Endocrinol Metab.* 2005;90(6):3268–73.

6. Berneis K, Keller U. Metabolic actions of growth hormone: direct and indirect. *Baillieres Clin Endocrinol Metab.* 1996;10(3):337–52.

7. Bhasin S, Storer TW, Berman N, et al. The effects of supraphysiologic doses of testosterone on muscle size and strength in normal men. *N Engl J Med.* 1996;335(1):1–7.

8. Bidlingmaier M, Strasburger CJ, Technology insight: detecting growth hormone abuse in athletes. *Nat Clin Pract Endocrinol Metab.* 2007;3(11):769–77.

9. Bisi G, Podio V, Valetto MR, et al. Acute cardiovascular and hormonal effects of GH and hexarelin, a synthetic GH-releasing peptide, in humans. *J Endocrinol Invest.* 1999;22(4):266–72.

10. Blue JG, Lombardo JA. Steroids and steroid–like compounds. *Clin Sports Med.* 1999;18(3):667–89, ix.

11. Botré F, Pavan A. Enhancement drugs and the athlete. *Neurol Clin.* 2008;26(1):149–67, ix.

12. Burke LM. Caffeine and sports performance. *Appl Physiol Nutr Metab.* 2008;33(6):1319–34.

13. Butterfield G. Ergogenic aids: evaluating sport nutrition products. *Int J Sport Nutr.* 1996;6(2):191–7.

14. Caruso JF, Signorile JF, Perry AC, et al. The effects of albuterol and isokinetic exercise on the quadriceps muscle group. *Med Sci Sports Exerc.* 1995;27(11):1471–6.

15. Chandler JV, Blair SN. The effect of amphetamines on selected physiological components related to athletic success. *Med Sci Sports Exerc.* 1980;12(1):65–9.

16. Chen J, Kim J, Dalton JT. Discovery and therapeutic promise of selective androgen receptor modulators. *Mol Interv.* 2005;5(3):173–88.

17. Combat Methamphetamine Epidemic Act of 2005 (CMEA) [Internet]. United States Department of Justice; [cited 2011 Jan 8]. Available from: http://www.deadiversion.usdoj.gov/meth/index.html.

18. Dempsey RL, Mazzone MF, Meurer LN. Does oral creatine supplementation improve strength? A meta-analysis. *J Fam Pract.* 2002;51(11):945–51.

19. Eaton DK, Kann L, Kinchen S, et al. Youth risk behavior surveillance—United States 2005. *MMWR Surveill Summ.* 2006;55(5):1–108.

20. Eichner ER. Sports anemia, iron supplements, and blood doping. *Med Sci Sports Exerc.* 1992;24(9 Suppl):S315–8.

21. Ekblom B. Blood doping and erythropoietin. The effects of variation in hemoglobin concentration and other related factors on physical performance. *Am J Sports Med.* 1996;24(6 Suppl):S40–2.

22. Gabriel SE, Jaakkimainen L, Bombardier C. Risk for serious gastrointestinal complications related to the use of nonsteroidal anti-inflammatory drugs. A meta-analysis. *Ann Intern Med.* 1991;115(10):787–96.

23. Glade MJ. The Dietary Supplement Health and Education Act of 1994—focus on labeling issues. *Nutrition.* 1997;13(11–12):999–1001.

24. Gottlieb NL, Riskin WG. Complications of local corticosteroid injections. *JAMA.* 1980;243(15):1547–8.

25. Green S, Buchbinder R, Glazier R, Forbes A. Interventions for shoulder pain. *Cochrane Database Syst Rev.* 2000;2:CD001156.

26. Greenhaff PL, Bodin K, Soderlund K, Hultman E. Effect of oral creatine supplementation on skeletal muscle phosphocreatine resynthesis. *Am J Physiol.* 1994;266(5 Pt 1):E725–30.

27. Haidet AM, Rizo L, Handy C, et al. Long-term enhancement of skeletal muscle mass and strength by single gene administration of myostatin inhibitors. *Proc Natl Acad Sci USA.* 2008;18:105(11):4318–22.

28. Haller CA, Benowitz NL. Adverse cardiovascular and central nervous system events associated with dietary supplements containing ephedra alkaloids. *N Engl J Med.* 2000;343(25):1833–8.

29. Handelsman DJ. Clinical review: the rationale for banning human chorionic gonadotropin and estrogen blockers in sport. *J Clin Endocrinol Metab.* 2006;91(5):1646–53.

30. Hay EM, Paterson SM, Lewis M, Hosie G, Croft P. Pragmatic randomized controlled trial of local corticosteroid injection and naproxen for treatment of lateral epicondylitis of elbow in primary care. *BMJ.* 1999;319(7215):964–8.

31. Hickner RC, Dyck DJ, Sklar J, Hatley H, Byrd P. Effect of 28 days of creatine ingestion on muscle metabolism and performance of a simulated cycling road race. *J Int Soc Sports Nutr.* 2010;7:26.

32. Hippisley-Cox J, Coupland C, Logan R. Risk of adverse gastrointestinal outcomes in patients taking cyclo-oxygenase-2 inhibitors or conventional non-steroidal anti-inflammatory drugs: population based nested case-control analysis. *BMJ.* 2005;331(7528):1310–6.

33. Jones R, Rubin G, Berenbaum F, Scheiman J. Gastrointestinal and cardiovascular risks of nonsteroidal anti-inflammatory drugs. *Am J Med.* 2008;121(6):464–74.

34. Lambert MA, Morton RJ, Sloan JP. Controlled study of the use of local steroid injection in the treatment of trigger finger and thumb. *J Hand Surg.* 1992;17(1):69–70.

35. Lanza LL, Walker AM, Bortnichak EA, Dreyer NA. Peptic ulcer and gastrointestinal hemorrhage associated with nonsteroidal anti-inflammatory drug use in patients younger than 65 years. A large health maintenance organization cohort study. *Arch Intern Med.* 1995;155(13):1371–7.

36. Lasne F, Martin L, Martin JA, de Ceaurriz J. Detection of continuous erythropoietin receptor activator in blood and urine in anti-doping control. *Haematologica.* 2009;94(6):888–90.

37. Lee SJ. Regulation of muscle mass by myostatin. *Annu Rev Cell Dev Biol.* 2004;20:61–86.

38. Lopez RM, Casa DJ, McDermott BP, Ganio MS, Armstrong LE, Maresh CM. Does creatine supplementation hinder exercise heat tolerance or hydration status? A systematic review with meta-analyses. *J Athl Train.* 2009;44(2):215–23.

39. Louis LJ. Musculoskeletal ultrasound intervention: principles and advances. *Radiol Clin North Am.* 2008;46(3): 515–33, vi.

40. Maki RG. Small is beautiful: insulin-like growth factors and their role in growth, development, and cancer. *J Clin Oncol.* 2010;28(33):4985–95.

41. Malfertheiner P, Mégraud F, O'Morain C, et al. Current concepts in the management of Helicobacter pylori infection—the Maastricht 2–2000 Consensus Report. *Aliment Pharmacol Ther.* 2002;16(2):167–80.

42. Martineau L, Horan MA, Rothwell NJ, Little RA. Salbutamol a beta 2-adrenoceptor agonist, increases skeletal muscle strength in young men. *Clin Sci (Lond).* 1992;83(5):615–21.

43. Mehallo CJ, Drezner JA, Bytomski JR. Practical management: nonsteroidal anti-inflammatory drug (NSAID) use in athletic injuries. *Clin J Sport Med.* 2006;16(2):170–4.

44. Meinhardt U, Nelson AE, Hansen JL, et al. The effects on growth hormone on body composition and physical performance in recreational athletes: a randomized trial. *Ann Intern Med.* 2010;152(9):568–77.

45. Micklewright R, Lane S, Linley W, McQuade C, Thompson F, Maskrey N. Review article: NSAIDs, gastroprotection and cyclo-oxygenase II selective inhibitors. *Aliment Pharmacol Ther.* 2003;17(3):321–32.

46. Møller N, Jørgensen J. Effects of growth hormone on glucose, lipid, and protein metabolism in human subjects. *Endocr Rev.* 2009;30(2):152–77.

47. Murphy D, Failla JM, Koniuch MP. Steroid versus placebo injection for trigger finger. *J Hand Surg Am.* 1995;20(4):628–31.

48. NCAA Web site [Internet]. NCAA Banned Drug List. [cited 2011 Mar 10]. Available from: http://www.ncaa.org/wps/wcm/connect/public/NCAA/Student-Athlete+Experience/NCAA+banned+drugs+list.

49. Pasman WJ, van Baak MA, Jeukendrup AE, de Haan A. The effect of different dosages of caffeine on endurance performance time. *Int J Sports Med.* 1995;16(4):225–30.

50. Prather ID, Brown DE, North P, Wilson JR. Clenbuterol: a substitute for anabolic steroids? *Med Sci Sports Exerc.* 1995;27(8):1118–21.

51. Pritzlaff CJ, Wideman L, Weltman JY, et al. Impact of acute exercise intensity on pulsatile growth hormone release in men. *J Appl Physiol.* 1999;87(2):498–504.

52. Salpeter SR, Gregor P, Ormiston TM, et al. Meta-analysis: cardiovascular events associated with nonsteroidal anti-inflammatory drugs. *Am J Med.* 2006;119(7):552–9.

53. Saugy M, Robinson N, Saudan C, Baume N, Avois L, Mangin P. Human growth hormone doping in sport. *Br J Sports Med.* 2006;40(Suppl 1):i35–9.

54. Sawka MN, Joyner MJ, Miles DS, Robertson RJ, Spriet LL, Young AJ. American College of Sports Medicine position stand. The use of blood doping as an ergogenic aid. *Med Sci Sports Exerc.* 1996;28(6):i–viii.

55. Schardt D. Relieving arthritis, can supplements help? *Nutr Action.* 1998;Jan/Feb:3–6.

56. Schoen RT, Vender RJ. Mechanisms of nonsteroidal anti-inflammatory drug-induced gastric damage. *Am J Med.* 1989;86(4):449–58.

57. Sidney KH, Lefcoe NM. The effects of ephedrine on the physiological and psychological responses to submaximal and maximal exercise in man. *Med Sci Sports.* 1977;9(2):95–9.

58. Simon LS, Smith TJ. *NSAID mechanism of action, efficacy, and relative safety. Managing Arthritis: A Postgraduate Medicine Special Report.* 1998 March 17–22.

59. Smith GM, Beecher HK. Amphetamine sulfate and athletic performance. *J Am Med Assoc.* 1959;170(5):524–57.

60. Speed CA. Fortnightly review: corticosteroid injections in tendon lesions. *BMJ.* 2001;323(7309):382–6.

61. Stricker PR. Other ergogenic agents. *Clin Sports Med.* 1998;17(2):283–97.

62. Superuio-Cabuslay E, Ward MM, Lorig KR. Patient education interventions in osteoarthritis and rheumatoid arthritis: a meta-analytic comparison with nonsteroidal anti-inflammatory drug treatment. *Arthritis Care Res.* 1996;9(4):292–301.

63. Swain RA, Harsha DM, Baenziger J, Saywell RM Jr. Do pseudoephedrine or phenylpropanolamine improve maximum oxygen uptake and time to exhaustion? *Clin J Sports Med.* 1997;7(3):168–73.

64. Trelle S, Reichenbach S, Wandel S, et al. Cardiovascular safety of nonsteroidal anti-inflammatory drugs: network meta-analysis. *BMJ.* 2011;342:c7086.

65. U.S. Food and Drug Administration Web site [Internet]. FDA announces rule prohibiting sale of dietary supplements containing ephedrine alkaloids effective April 12, 2004. Department of Health and Human Services, FDA Statement. [cited 2011 Apr 24]. Available from: http://www.fda.gov/bbs/topics/news/2004/NEW01050.html.

66. Vandebeurie F, Vanden Eynde B, Vandenberghe K, Hespel P. Effect of creatine loading on endurance capacity and sprint power in cyclists. *Int J Sports Med.* 1998;19(7):490–5.

67. Vecchio PC, Hazleman BL, King RH. A double blind trial comparing subacromial methylprednisolone and lignocaine in acute rotator cuff tendinitis. *Br J Rheumatol.* 1993;32(8):743–5.

68. Wallace MB, Lim J, Cutler A, Bucci L. Effects of dehydroepiandrosterone vs. androstenedione supplementation in men. *Med Sci Sports Exerc.* 1999;31(2):1788–92.

69. Weiler JM, Layton T, Hunt M. Asthma in United States Olympic athletes who participated in the 1996 Summer Games. *J Allergy Clin Immunol.* 1998;102(5):722–6.

70. Welle S, Jozefowicz R, Statt M. Failure of dehydroepiandrosterone to influence energy and protein metabolism in humans. *J Clin Endocrinol Metab.* 1990;71(5):1259–64.

71. Woo WW, Man SY, Lam PK, Rainer TH. Randomized double-blind trial comparing oral paracetamol and oral nonsteroidal anti-inflammatory drugs for treating pain after musculoskeletal injury. *Ann Emerg Med.* 2005;46(4):352–61.

72. World Anti-Doping Agency [Internet]. World Anti-Doping Agency Prohibited List 2011 [cited 2011 Mar 10]. Available from: http://www.wada-ama.org/en/World-Anti-Doping-Program/Sports-and-Anti-Doping-Organizations/International-Standards/Prohibited-List/

Prolotherapy

Keith A. Scorza and Manik Singh

72

INTRODUCTION

- Overuse injuries remain a constant challenge for the sports medicine physician. Injuries such as chronic tendinopathies are traditionally treated with corticosteroids or nonsteroidal anti-inflammatory drugs (NSAIDs), although it has been decades since Puddu et al. (22) demonstrated that tendinosis is not an inflammatory condition. Most investigations demonstrate that such treatments provide at best a short-term decrease in pain. With growing concern of complications associated with corticosteroids and NSAIDs, the search for other treatment modalities continues (14).

- Proinflammatory therapies ("prolotherapy") are a subject of growing interest and research. Although not a new concept, prolotherapy is new to the rigors of evidence-based medicine. As such, research is subject to skepticism, and providers are reluctant to adopt these techniques.

- Prolotherapy is an injection technique that uses the body's own inflammation and repair system for treatment of chronic musculoskeletal pain. It is a unique alternative to standard care that can be performed quickly in an outpatient setting. The theoretic basis and state of current evidence regarding prolotherapy are discussed in this chapter.

DEFINITIONS

- Injection of a solution that will stimulate the production of new cells (11,12).

- Injection of growth factors or growth factor stimulants that cause growth of normal cells or tissues (24,25).

COMMON USES

- Commonly used for chronic musculoskeletal pain; most frequently used for chronic tendinopathies, chronic ligament pain, and chronic back pain.

- Growing interest in use for osteoarthritis; may contribute to correcting instabilities that contribute to osteoarthritis.

- Case reports additionally claim success in treatment of neck pain, groin pain, and traumatic migraines.

HISTORICAL PERSPECTIVES

- Hippocratic treatises suggested the utilization of scar tissue to add stability to joints, advising the use of a "hot poker" as treatment for recurrent dislocating shoulders.

- During the 1800s, sclerosing agents were used for treatment of varicose veins, hemorrhoids, and nonsurgical hernias.

- Prolotherapy was first described in modern literature by Dr. Louis Schultz (30).
  - Injected sodium psylliate into painful temporomandibular joints and reported effectiveness for treatment of chronic pain.
  - Performed animal studies revealing soft tissue fibrosis within 4–6 days after injections, suggesting that agents might stabilize joints by tightening ligaments.

- The term "prolotherapy" was popularized by Dr. George S. Hackett (11,12).
  - Theorized that chronic musculoskeletal pain was secondary to chronic laxity of ligaments and bone–tendon junctions.
  - Used the term "prolotherapy" to simplify phrases such as fibroproliferative therapy, proliferant therapy, sclerotherapy, and regenerative injection therapy.
  - Term derived from "prolo" meaning offspring and "proliferative" meaning to produce new cells in rapid succession. Dr. Hackett considered prolotherapy the "rehabilitation of an incompetent structure by the generation of new cellular tissue."
  - Published works in 1953 describing use of prolotherapy for treatment of chronic sacroiliac pain on 253 patients over a 14-year period (11).

- The current prevalence of physicians practicing prolotherapy is uncertain.
  - A 2003 survey of osteopathic physicians identified 95 practitioners in the United States with treatment of approximately 450,000 patients. Only 27% of the surveys were returned; therefore, the prevalence was likely much greater (7).
  - A 2006 investigation of prolotherapy side effects identified 314 members of the American Academy of Orthopaedic Medicine listed as performing prolotherapy in the member directory (6).

■ A survey of 908 primary care patients using narcotic therapies for chronic musculoskeletal pain revealed that 8.3% of the patients had received prolotherapy treatments in the past, with 5.9% receiving treatment during the previous 12 months (8).

PROLOTHERAPY AGENTS

Traditional Agents

■ Irritants
  ■ Examples: phenol, guaiacol, tannic acid
  ■ Irritants contain a phenol hydroxyl group that is oxidized to quinine derivatives. Such agents are thought to alkylate surface proteins of cells, either damaging the cell wall or making the cell antigenic. The end result is an initiation of an inflammatory cascade.
■ Osmotics
  ■ Examples: dextrose, glycerin
  ■ Osmotics are thought to increase extracellular osmotic pressure and, therefore, dehydrate cells at the injection site. This may lead to cell lysis with the release of cell fragments, attraction of granulocytes and macrophages, and a resultant inflammatory cascade.
■ Chemotactics
  ■ Examples: sodium morrhuate, polidocanol
  ■ Chemotactics are thought to be direct precursors of and may undergo conversion into inflammatory mediators (*e.g.*, prostaglandins, leukotrienes, thromboxanes).
■ Particulates
  ■ Example: pumice flour
  ■ Particulates are thought to attract macrophages to the injection site, initiating an inflammatory cascade.

Modern Agents (see Chapter 73, Platelet-Rich Plasma Therapy and Autologous Blood)

■ Specific growth factors, whole blood, platelet-rich plasma
  ■ Modern agents use specific growth factors or carriers of growth factors (*e.g.*, platelets) to initiate an inflammatory cascade (2,9,28).

MECHANISM OF ACTION

■ The mechanism of action of prolotherapy is not fully understood.
■ Prolotherapy agents are proposed to either attract inflammatory mediators or induce the release of growth factors to induce an inflammatory reaction. Such reaction is the first stage of the healing process and theoretically promotes repair of degenerated structures. See "Prolotherapy Agents" section for individual mechanisms of action.
■ Other mechanisms not involving inflammatory responses have been suggested.
  ■ Macrophages responding to particulate agents may secrete a polypeptide promoting fibroplasia.
  ■ Irritant agents may cause neurolysis/denervation of nociceptive fibers.
  ■ Injections with significant volume may result in lysis of connective tissue adhesions.

THEORETIC BASIS OF PROLOTHERAPY

■ It is well known that growth factors play a critical role in the healing process (28).
  ■ Numerous in vitro studies demonstrate increased gene expression when cells are exposed to growth factors (1,16).
  ■ Numerous animal studies demonstrate increases in growth factors after induced musculoskeletal injuries (20).
■ In vitro studies have demonstrated that cells bathed in traditional agents show increased expression of genes for inflammation and growth factors (15).
  ■ Clarkson et al. (1) observed that human renal mesangial cells exposed to 5–30 mM of dextrose demonstrated increased expression of 200 genes, many encoding for cytoskeleton P-proteins and growth factors (1).
  ■ Lam et al. (16) observed that renal fibroblasts exposed to dextrose demonstrated increased expression of connective tissue growth factor and insulin-like growth factor gene expression (16).
■ Animal studies with traditional agents demonstrate soft tissue fibrosis, increases in tendon diameters, and ligament hypertrophy with increased tensile strength (15).
  ■ Schultz (30) noted soft tissue fibrosis 4–6 days after injections of sodium psylliate.
  ■ Hackett injected synasol (sodium salt fatty acid) into gastrocnemius and superficial flexor tendons and noted an increase in bone formation at tendon junctions at 1–3 months. At 9–12 months, a 40% increase in tendon diameter and 30% increase in thickness of tendon–osseous junctions was noted. Tensile strengths were not tested (12).
  ■ Liu et al. (18) injected 5% sodium morrhuate in the medial collateral ligaments of rabbits and reported a 27% increase in ligament–bone junction strength and 56% increase in collagen diameter.
  ■ Maynard et al. (19) injected 5% sodium morrhuate into the patellar and Achilles tendons of rabbits and noted increased tendon diameters as well as increased collagen content of fibrils, water, glucosamine, and fibroblasts. Such

effects were not noted with a single injection, but required three to five iterations. They did not test tensile strength.

- Human case reports utilizing medical imaging have suggested evidence of tissue repair following prolotherapy (10).

PROLOTHERAPY TECHNIQUE

- There are no formal practice guidelines.
  - The procedure is not currently regulated, and certification is not required.
  - Techniques are typically taught through workshops, continuing medical education activities, and provider-to-provider education.
- Choice of best agent for injection, volume of agent, or concentration of agent is not clear.
  - No clinical trials have compared efficacy of different agents, concentrations of agents, or the volume of solutions injected.
  - Most clinicians report use of single-agent injections.
  - The most common combined agent is a combination of phenol, glycerin, and dextrose (referred to as P2G, commonly with concentrations of 1% phenol, 12.5% glycerin, and 12.5% dextrose).
  - Common concentrations of dextrose range from 10% to 25% dextrose in either saline or an anesthetic agent.
  - Common concentration of sodium morrhuate is 5% solution.
  - Common concentration of polidocanol is $5-10 \, \text{mg} \cdot \text{mL}^{-1}$ (0.5%–1% solution).
  - Total volume injected varies according to target area. Techniques studied for lower back pain have ranged from 10–30 mL of solution. Joint injections and injections near or in ligaments and tendons are often performed with 0.5–1 mL at each injection site, with total volume ranging from 1–10 mL.
- Therapeutic injections are often performed at the site of greatest tenderness or along the path of a painful ligament or tendon. For large areas of pain, injections are performed at small intervals (*e.g.*, 1 cm) with an injection of 0.5–1 mL of agent at each site.
- Current technology allows use of musculoskeletal ultrasound to guide injections into ligaments, degenerated regions of tendons, neovessels within tendons, and joint spaces.
- Injections are commonly performed at intervals ranging from every 1–6 weeks. Procedure is often repeated one to two times prior to determining whether intervention is successful. Total duration of therapy is guided by clinical results, typically continuing therapy until beneficial changes plateau.
- Postinjection pain is anticipated for 72 hours and typically resolves by 5–7 days. Acetaminophen or narcotic medications are often used for pain control during this period.

Anti-inflammatory medications are generally avoided because they theoretically offset the proposed desired inflammatory action for prolotherapy techniques.

CURRENT EVIDENCE

- Evidence is limited but growing in volume. The majority of literature involves case reports. Most studies are small or lacking a control group. There are very few randomized controlled trials.

The Knee

- Hoksrud et al. (13) used polidocanol to sclerose neovessels in patellar tendinopathies. He recruited 33 patients, with 17 in the intervention group and 16 in a control group that crossed over at 4 months. The initial treatment group demonstrated improvements in pain compared to the control group. Upon crossover, the remaining 16 patients demonstrated pain improvement.
- Ryan et al. (27) used dextrose injections under ultrasound guidance for patellar tendinopathies that failed conservative treatment. They recruited 47 patients who received a mean of 4 ($\pm$ 3) injections. They reported improvements in visual analog pain scales (at rest, with activities of daily living, and with sporting activities) at a mean of 45 weeks and noted improvements in appearance of the tendons under ultrasound evaluation. There was no control group.

The Elbow

- Zeisig et al. (32) used polidocanol and sclerosed neovessels under ultrasound guidance in 11 of 13 elbows with lateral epicondylitis for an average duration of 23 months with 8 months of follow-up. They noted good results in 11 of 13 elbows, with visual analog scale pain scores decreasing from 75 to 34 and grip strength increasing from 29 to 40 kg. This was a small study, and there was no control group (32).
- Scarpone et al. (29) compared injections of sodium morrhuate with dextrose to a saline placebo at 0, 4, and 8 weeks. The intervention group improved in pain at all points with significance reached over placebo by 16 weeks and maintained at 52 weeks. This study had a control group, but had overall limited size (24 patients).

The Achilles Tendon

- Ohberg et al. (21) used polidocanol to sclerose neovessels in 11 subjects with a mean duration of 23 months of insertional Achilles tendon pain. At 8-month follow-up, 8 of 11 patients noted improvement of pain with a decrease in the visual analog scale pain rating from an average of 82 to 14 during tendon-loading activities. This was a small pilot study, and there was no control group.

■ Lind et al. (17) used polidocanol and sclerosed neovessels in 42 patient tendons with mean duration of 32 months of midportion Achilles pain. Initially, 37 of 42 subject tendons demonstrated satisfaction with treatment. At 2-year follow-up, 38 patients noted satisfaction with treatment and reported a reduction in the visual analog pain scale rating from 75 to 7. Researchers reported improved appearance of tendons under ultrasound evaluation. There was no control group (17).

■ Yelland et al. (31) performed a single-blinded randomized study involving 43 patients with Achilles tendinopathy. Subjects were randomized into three groups: prolotherapy only, eccentric exercises only, and combination of prolotherapy and eccentric exercises. The combined group had superior results, whereas the prolotherapy and the eccentric exercise groups were equivalent. Of note, the prolotherapy group achieved maximum improvement more rapidly than the eccentric exercise group.

Plantar Fascia

■ Ryan et al. (26) used hypertonic dextrose (25% solution) in 20 subjects with chronic plantar fasciitis that had failed conservative treatment. Injections were performed at 6-week intervals with an average number of three injections. Telephone follow-up at a mean of 11.8 months after treatment reported improvements in 16 of 20 patients with visual analog scale pain scores decreasing from 36.8 to 10.3 at rest, from 74.7 to 25 for activities of daily living, and from 91.6 to 38.7 during or after physical activity. This was a small pilot study, and there was no control group (26).

Lower Back Pain

■ There are numerous studies of the use of traditional prolotherapy for lower back and sacroiliac pain. Such studies are confounded by lack of consistency in formulating a specific diagnosis prior to therapy and location of injection sites. Of the studies that are prospective and randomized with control groups, the results are mixed (3,4,5).

Osteoarthritis

■ Reeves and Hassanein (25) studied the use of 10% dextrose solution for osteoarthritis of the fingers. This study included individuals with at least a 6-month history of pain at the metacarpophalangeal, proximal interphalangeal, or distal interphalangeal joints. Thirteen patients were randomized to the intervention group and 14 to the control group, and injections were performed to the medial and lateral joint lines. Evaluation was performed at 0, 2, and 4 months. The intervention group was noted to have significant improvement in pain with motion and improved flexion range of motion. There was no change in rest pain or grip strength.

■ Reeves and Hassanein (24) studied the use of 10% dextrose solution for osteoarthritis of the knee in a randomized double-blinded study. The intervention group had improvement compared with the control group in knee buckling; however, both groups improved in pain, range of motion, and sense of swelling.

Other Conditions

■ Case reports have claimed use of prolotherapy for treatment of neck pain, groin pain, and traumatic migraine pain. No organized studies are available.

CONTRAINDICATIONS AND ADVERSE REACTIONS

■ There are no well-defined contraindications to prolotherapy. Suggested contraindications include standard contraindications to any needle technique, as well as reasonable precautions for the induction of inflammation.

■ Suggested contraindications include acute illness, infection at proposed injection site, anatomic defects precluding injection, metastatic cancer, systemic inflammation, gouty arthritis, bleeding disorders, inability to perform postprocedure range-of-motion exercises, nonmusculoskeletal pain, whole-body pain, and low pain tolerance.

■ There are very limited data regarding adverse effects of prolotherapy. Data suggest similar adverse effect profiles to other similar needling techniques.

■ Common adverse effects include needle trauma (*e.g.*, pain, bruising, bleeding, fullness, or numbness at injection site), light headedness, local infection, and local nerve damage. For procedures to the spine and neck, risks include pneumothorax, spinal headache, disc injury, and potential spinal nerve/cord injury, although injury rates are similar to other commonly performed back procedures.

■ Prolotherapy agents are considered relatively safe. Dextrose has been used safely as an intravenous treatment for hypoglycemia for over 50 years. Sodium morrhuate is used in gastrointestinal procedures, and reports of allergic reactions are rare. P2G has not been reported in clinical trials to have significant side effects or adverse reactions (23).

REFERENCES

1. Clarkson M, Murphy M, Gupta S, et al. High glucose-altered gene expression in mesangial cells. Actin-regulatory protein gene expression is triggered by oxidative stress and cytoskeletal disassembly. *J Biol Chem.* 2002;277(12):9707–12.

2. Creaney L, Hamilton B. Growth factor delivery methods in the management of sports injuries: the state of play. *Br J Sports Med.* 2008; 42(5):314–20.

3. Cusi M, Saunders J, Hungerford B, Wisbey-Roth T, Lucas P, Wilson S. The use of prolotherapy in the sacroiliac joint. *Br J Sports Med.* 2010; 44(2):100–4.

4. Dagenais S, Mayer J, Haldeman S, Borg-Stein J. Evidence-informed management of chronic low back pain with prolotherapy. *Spine J.* 2008;8(1):203–12.

5. Dagenais S, Haldeman S, Wooley JR. Intraligamentous injection of sclerosing solutions (prolotherapy) for spinal pain: a critical review of the literature. *Spine J.* 2005;5(3):310–28.

6. Dagenais S, Ogunseitan O, Haldeman S, Wooley JR, Newcomb RL. Side effects and adverse events related to intraligamentous injection of sclerosing solutions (prolotherapy) for back and neck pain: a survey of practitioners. *Arch Phys Med Rehabil.* 2006;87(7):909–13.

7. Dorman TA. Prolotherapy: a survey. *J Orthopaed Med.* 1993;15(2):49–50.

8. Fleming S, Rabago DP, Mundt MP, Fleming MF. CAM therapies among primary care patients using opioid therapy for chronic pain. *BMC Complement Altern Med.* 2007;7:15.

9. Foster TE, Puskas BL, Mandelbaum BR, Gerhardt MB, Rodeo SA. Platelet-rich plasma: from basic science to clinical applications. *Am J Sports Med.* 2009;37(11):2259–72.

10. Fullerton BD. High-resolution ultrasound and magnetic resonance imaging to document tissue repair after prolotherapy: a report of three cases. *Arch Phys Med Rehabil.* 2008;89(2):377–85.

11. Hackett GS. Joint stabilization through induced ligament sclerosis. *Ohio Med.* 1953;49(10):877–84.

12. Hackett GS, Henderson DG. Joint stabilization: an experimental histologic study with comments on the clinical application in ligament proliferation. *Am J Surg.* 1955;89(5):968–73.

13. Hoksrud A, Ohberg L, Alfredson H, Bahr R. Ultrasound-guided sclerosis of neovessels in painful chronic patellar tendinopathy: a randomized controlled trial. *Am J Sports Med.* 2006;34(11):1738–46.

14. Kaeding C, Best TM. Tendinosis: pathophysiology and nonoperative treatment. *Sports Health: A Multidisciplinary Approach.* 2009;1(4):284–92.

15. Kim SR, Stitik TP, Foye PM, Greenwald BD, Campagnolo DI. Critical review of prolotherapy for osteoarthritis, low back pain, and other musculoskeletal conditions: a physiatric perspective. *Am J Phys Med Rehabil.* 2004;83(5):379–89.

16. Lam S, van der Geest RN, Verhagen NA, et al. Connective tissue growth factor and IGF-I are produced by human renal fibroblasts and cooperate in the induction of collagen production by high glucose. *Diabetes.* 2003;52(12):2975–83.

17. Lind B, Ohberg L, Alfredson H. Sclerosing polidocanol injections in mid-portion Achilles tendinosis: remaining good clinical results and decreased tendon thickness at 2-year follow-up. *Knee Surg Sports Traumatol Arthrosc.* 2006;14(12):1327–32.

18. Liu YK, Tipton CM, Matthes RD, Bedford TG, Maynard JA, Walmer HC. An in situ study of the influence of a sclerosing solution in rabbit medial collateral ligaments and its junction strength. *Connect Tissue Res.* 1983;11(2–3):95–102.

19. Maynard JA, Pedrini VA, Pedrini-Mille A, Romanus B, Ohlerking F. Morphological and biochemical effects of sodium morrhuate on tendons. *J Orthop Res.* 1985;3(2):236–48.

20. Molloy T, Wang Y, Murrell G. The roles of growth factors in tendon and ligament healing. *Sports Med.* 2003;33(5):381–94.

21. Ohberg L, Alfredson H. Sclerosing therapy in Achilles tendon insertional pain: results of a pilot study. *Knee Surg Sports Traumatol Arthrosc.* 2003;11(5):339–43.

22. Puddu G, Ippolito E, Postacchini F. A classification of Achilles tendon disease. *Am J Sports Med.* 1976;4(4):145–50.

23. Rabago D, Slattengren A, Zgierska A. Prolotherapy in primary care practice. *Prim Care.* 2010;37(1):65–80.

24. Reeves KD, Hassanein K. Randomized prospective double-blind placebo controlled study of dextrose therapy for knee osteoarthritis with or without ACL laxity. *Altern Ther Health Med.* 2000;6(2):68–74, 77–80.

25. Reeves KD, Hassanein K. Randomized, prospective, placebo-controlled double-blind study of dextrose prolotherapy for osteoarthritic thumb and finger (DIP, PIP, and trapeziometacarpal) joints: evidence of clinical efficacy. *J Altern Complement Med.* 2000;6(4):311–20.

26. Ryan MB, Wong AD, Gillies JH, Wong J, Taunton JE. Sonographically guided intratendinous injections of hyperosmolar dextrose/lidocaine: a pilot study for the treatment of chronic plantar fasciitis. *Br J Sports Med.* 2009;43(4):303–6.

27. Ryan M, Wong A, Rabago D, Lee K, Taunton J. Ultrasound-guided injections of hyperosmolar dextrose for overuse patellar tendinopathy: a pilot study. *Br J Sports Med.* 2011;45(12):972–7.

28. Sampson S, Gerhardt M, Mandelbaum B. Platelet rich plasma injection grafts for musculoskeletal injuries: a review. *Curr Rev Musculoskelet Med.* 2008;1(3–4):165–74.

29. Scarpone M, Rabago D, Zgierska, Arbogest J, Snell E. The efficacy of prolotherapy for lateral epicondylitis: a pilot study. *Clin J Sport Med.* 2008;18(3):248–54.

30. Schultz L. A treatment for subluxation of the temporomandibular joint. *JAMA.* 1937;190:1032–5.

31. Yelland MJ, Sweeting KR, Lyftogt JA, Ng SK, Scuffham PA, Evans KA. Prolotherapy injections and eccentric loading exercises for painful Achilles tendinosis: a randomized trial. *Br J Sports Med.* 2011;45(5):421–8.

32. Zeisig E, Ohberg L, Alfredson H. Sclerosing polidocanol injections in chronic painful tennis elbow-promising results in a pilot study. *Knee Surg Sports Traumatol Arthrosc.* 2006;14(11):1218–24.

73

Platelet-Rich Plasma Therapy and Autologous Blood

Kimberly G. Harmon and Jonathan A. Drezner

INTRODUCTION

■ Soft tissue injuries including tendon, muscle, and ligament injuries account for a large proportion of injuries to recreational and elite athletes. Enhancing the healing of these injuries beyond ice, rest, activity modification, and the tincture of time has been the goal of sports medicine physicians.

■ It is now known that nonsteroidal anti-inflammatory drugs (NSAIDs), commonly prescribed for soft tissue injury, do not enhance healing, but alleviate pain. The advent of autologous growth factor therapies holds the potential to use the body's own healing ability to speed up and improve tissue repair. A number of different options have been investigated.

■ This chapter will explore the pathophysiology of autologous blood and platelet-rich plasma, examine the human literature to date, and offer conclusions based on the best available data.

AUTOLOGOUS GROWTH FACTOR THERAPIES

Concept

■ Growth factors mediate the biologic process of repair; individual growth factors have been shown to enhance injury repair in animal models.

■ By increasing the amount of growth factors to the injury, healing may be accelerated or enhanced in terms of outcome (repaired tissue more closely approximates original tissue).

■ Platelets are one of the first cells to arrive at injury and are filled with growth factors; growth factors in platelets are in a physiologic balance.
  ■ Contain multiple growth factors in α-granules:
    ❑ Platelet-derived growth factor (PDGF)
    ❑ Transforming growth factor-β (TGF-β)
    ❑ Insulin-like growth factor (IGF)
    ❑ Epidermal growth factor (EGF)
    ❑ Vascular endothelial growth factor (VEGF)
    ❑ Fibroblast growth factor (FGF)
  ■ Also contain other factors that modulate healing:
    ❑ Serotonin
    ❑ Adenosine diphosphate (ADP)
    ❑ Stromal cell-derived factor-1α (SDF-1α)
      ▪ Recruits circulating stem cells to site of injury
      ▪ Stimulates bone marrow to release additional stem cells

Variables to Consider

■ The use of ultrasound (US) guidance:
  ■ 24%–71% failure rate with palpation-guided injections to subacromial bursa, glenohumeral, knee, and ankle joints (12,13,21,22)
  ■ Approximately a 5% failure rate with US-guided injections (26,41,45)

■ Amount of injectate: typically 2–5 cc is used depending on location and type of tissue being treated. There is a volume effect from the injection of any fluid as well as an effect from the substance itself.

■ Amount of and location of local anesthetic used:
  ■ Lidocaine has been shown to be toxic to platelets in vitro (4,25,28).
  ■ Anesthetics may also be toxic to tenocytes (44).
  ■ No in vivo studies.
  ■ Procedures with tenotomy are painful without anesthetic.
  ■ Negative effect of intratendinous anesthetic should be considered.

■ Whether or not a fenestration is performed:
  ■ Fenestration is the repetitive passing of a needle in a tissue.
  ■ Called tenotomy when done in a tendon.
  ■ There are retrospective studies that show that tenotomy alone is 60% effective in treatment of tendinosis (24,36,37).

■ Immobilization and/or rehabilitation after the injury.

AUTOLOGOUS BLOOD

History

- Percutaneous release of extensor tendons of elbow shown to be effective treatment of lateral epicondylitis (1).
- Theorized by Edwards and Calandruccio (10) that the benefits of this treatment were secondary to beneficial effect of bleeding in the area, which started an inflammatory reaction that led to a cascade of healing.

Definition

- Injection of a small amount (2–3 cc) of the patient's own blood back into a damaged or injured area.

Studies

- Edwards and Calandruccio, 2003 (10):
  - Design was case series.
  - Twenty-eight patients with mean age of 46 with lateral epicondylitis for at least 3 months.
  - Injected 2 mL of autologous blood plus 1 mL bupivacaine blindly.
  - Thirty-two percent got second injection at 6 weeks if pain not completely relieved.
  - Visual analog pain scale (VAS) decreased from 7.8 to 2.3 mm.
  - Seventy-nine percent of patients had complete relief of pain.
  - One patient (4%) failed treatment.
- Connell et al., 2006 (6):
  - Design was case series.
  - Thirty-five patients with lateral epicondylitis with a mean duration of symptoms of 13.8 months; average age was 40.9.
  - Injected 2 mL of autologous blood under US guidance after dry needling for 1 minute.
  - Seventy-five percent had second injection at 4 weeks.
  - VAS decreased from 9 to 6 at 4 weeks and to 0 at 6 months.
  - Two patients (6%) failed treatment.
- Suresh et al., 2006 (47):
  - Design was case series.
  - Twenty patients (average age, 48.5) with medial epicondylitis with a mean duration of symptoms for 12 months.
  - Injected 2 mL of autologous blood under US guidance after dry needling.
  - Second injection done at 4 weeks (100%).
  - VAS decreased from 8 to 5.65 in 4 weeks and to 2.15 at 10 months.
  - Three patients (15%) failed.

- James et al., 2007 (27):
  - Design was case series.
  - Forty-seven patients (average age, 34.5) with patellar tendinosis for a mean duration of 12.9 months.
  - Injected 3 mL of autologous blood under US guidance after dry needling for 1 minute.
  - Second injection done at 4 weeks per protocol.
  - Victorian Institute of Sport Assessment Scale – Patellar (VISA-P) is a validated outcome measure for pain and functional activity in individuals with patellar tendinosis ranging from 0–100, with 100 being normal. VISA-P increased from 39.8 to 74.3.
  - Three treatment failures (6%).

Conclusion

- Level III evidence (case series) that autologous blood injection is an effective treatment for tendinosis.
- Techniques, protocols, and rehabilitation varied between studies.

PLATELET-RICH PLASMA

History

- First use reported in maxillofacial surgery to enhance healing of bone grafts (35).
- The use spread to cardiac, plastic surgery, and orthopedic procedures.
- First use in tendons documented in 2006 by Mishra and Pavelko (38).

Definition

- A volume of autologous plasma that has a platelet concentration above baseline (35).
- The plasma allows platelets to clot.
- Clot is composed of fibrin, fibronectin, and vitronectin, which are cell adhesion molecules required to promote tissue healing (35).

Terminology

- Platelet rich in growth factors (PRGF)
  - Another term for platelet-rich plasma (PRP)
- Platelet-rich fibrin matrix
  - Typically used to refer to PRP that has been clotted
  - The clot provides substance and is usually used in surgical techniques.
- Platelet concentrate
  - A solid composition of platelets without plasma
  - Will not clot without plasma (no fibrin)

- Platelet releasate
  - The product created from activated platelets, *i.e.*, the released growth factors from the platelets
  - Typically created by creating a pellet of platelets in plasma and then adding thrombin to activate platelets
- Fibrin glue
  - First described in 1970s
  - Polymerized fibrin induced by thrombin and calcium
  - Used as a tissue adhesive and to achieve hemostasis
- Autologous conditioned serum
  - Initially described by Wright-Carpenter et al. (50,51)
  - Whole blood (without anticoagulant) is incubated with glass beads for 24 hours.
  - Blood clots and glass beads serve as slow activators of platelets with release of growth factors.
  - Serum is removed.
  - Has increased growth factors compared to serum not incubated with glass beads (FGF and TGF-β)
  - Should not be confused with Autologous Conditioned Plasma, a proprietary product

Variables to Consider in PRP Product

- Platelet concentration
  - There may be an optimum concentration of platelets above which the concentration may be inhibitory.
  - Graziani et al., 2006 (18) demonstrated that 2.5× baseline was optimal concentration in vitro
  - Han et al. (19) demonstrated that PRP with 50 ng · mL^{-1} TGF-β was more stimulatory then 200 ng · mL^{-1}.
  - Other studies have shown that proliferation is dependent on platelet concentration, with higher concentrations being more effective (33)
  - Marx (34) suggested that the minimum effective amount of platelets was a concentration of 1,000,000/μL in 6 mL of PRP. Many modern platelet concentrating systems do not achieve this concentration.
- Presence or absence of leukocytes
  - There is debate regarding whether white blood cells (WBCs) enhance or are a detriment to healing.
  - There are three subtypes of WBCs.
    - Neutrophils
      - Contain hydrolytic enzymes
      - Release proteases and free radicals
      - In muscle injury, neutrophils promote secondary damage after the initial injury (3,48).
    - Monocytes
      - Primary role is removal of debris.
      - Balance anti-inflammatory and proinflammatory aspects of healing (11)

- Lymphocytes
  - Initiate cell-to-cell interactions
  - Play an important role in vessel formation by supporting the proliferation and differentiation of stem cells
- Viability of platelets
  - Once platelets are activated (by thrombin, calcium chloride, or collagen), they release 95% of their growth factors in the first hour (34).
  - Platelets can be damaged during the collection process (mechanical trauma).
- Anticoagulation
  - Anticoagulant citrate dextrose-A (ACD-A)
    - Reversible
    - Citrate binds to calcium to inhibit initiation of the clotting cascade.
    - Dextrose and other buffers support the viability of the platelet (32).
  - Citrate phosphate dextrose (CPD) also binds calcium but is 10% less effective at supporting platelet viability (32).
  - Once anticoagulated, PRP will remain stable and sterile for 8 hours (34).
  - ACD-A is acidic and thus will lower pH.
    - This makes it more painful to inject.
    - Some PRP protocols use bicarbonate to buffer back acidity.
    - There is some evidence that release of PDGF-α (and early healing) is enhanced by acidic environment (31).
- How and when PRP is activated
  - Can be activated by:
    - Thrombin
    - Calcium chloride activates clotting cascade by allowing polymerization of fibrin fibers required for clotting.
    - Collagen is an endogenous activator of PRP.
  - Exogenous activation
    - When activated, a fibrin clot is formed and the PRP increases in density, forming a globule or membrane.
      - For surgical use, this can allow the product to be incorporated into repairs with suture.
      - For use with injections, the product will gel and be difficult or impossible to inject.
      - Growth factor release begins as soon as PRP is activated, so product should be used relatively quickly. This will occur with products that use no anticoagulation.
    - Some techniques use double-barrelled syringes to inject the PRP and thrombin simultaneously so the activation occurs at the time of injection.
- Amount of fibrinogen
  - Fibrinogen forms a matrix that enmeshes platelets and supports cell migration.

- Depending on how PRP is activated, different molecular structures can be formed.
  - Drastic activation from high thrombin concentrations may form a less stable tetramolecule or bilateral junctions, which leads to fibrin monomers that are not favorable for cytokine enmeshment or cell migration (9).
  - Slower activation encourages more stable trivalent or equilateral junctions, which leads to a multifiber assembly that supports cytokine enmeshment and cell migration (9).
  - A recent study showed that both leukocyte-rich and leukocyte-poor PRP had similar amounts of fibrinogen present (5).
- pH of product
  - Growth factor function is dependent on pH.
  - Some protocols suggest buffering back PRP to physiologic pH by the addition of bicarbonate to the PRP.
  - Liu et al. (31) demonstrated that PRP was more effective in an acidic environment.

Categories

- Buffy coat product
  - PRP that is made up by isolating the buffy coat.
  - The buffy coat is composed of platelets and leukocytes.
  - To obtain the buffy coat, some red blood cells are included in the product.
  - Mesenchymal stem cells also reside in this layer.
- Plasma-based products
  - Have a lower concentration of leukocytes
  - Also have lower platelet concentrations

PRP in Tendons

- Pathogenesis of tendon injury
  - Tendon pain that lasts more than 3–6 weeks is not inflammatory.
  - Tendinosis or tendinopathy is degenerative on biopsies with an absence of inflammatory cells.
- Theory
  - PRP can stimulate healing by starting an inflammatory reaction.
  - Inflammation is the first stage of healing.
- Case series studies
  - Mishra and Pavelko, 2006 (38)
    - Lateral epicondylosis
    - Fifteen patients with a mean age of 48 who had had an average duration of symptoms for 15 months.
    - Had one injection of 2 mL of leukocyte-rich PRP (Biomet) with five needle penetrations. No US guidance.

- VAS score decreased from an average of 80.3 at baseline to 5.7 at 6 months; 93% of patients were completely satisfied with their treatment.
  - One treatment failure
- Volpi et al., 2007 (49)
  - Patellar tendinosis
  - Ten patients with mean age of 27
  - One injection with leukocyte-rich PRP (Biomet) with five to eight needle penetrations under US guidance.
  - Average VISA increased 36 points, and magnetic resonance imaging appearance improved.
  - One treatment failure went to surgery.
- Filardo et al., 2009 (15)
  - Patellar tendon
  - Case control
  - Fifteen patients treated and 16 controls, with average duration of symptoms for 3 months
  - Three injections 15 days apart with 6× baseline platelet concentration. PRP was leukocyte rich, and 10% CaCl was added prior to injection.
  - Eleven patients in PRP group showed complete or marked recovery, and two had no improvement.
  - Eight patients in control group showed complete or marked recovery, and three had no improvement.
  - Difference was not statistically significant.
- Kon et al., 2009 (30)
  - Patellar tendon
  - Twenty patients with a mean age of 25.5 with an average duration of symptoms of 20.7 months
  - Three injections 15 days apart with 6× baseline platelet concentration. PRP was leukocyte rich, and 10% CaCl was added prior to injection using a 22-g needle with four to six needle penetrations.
  - Fourteen patients had marked improvement, and four had no improvement.
- Gaweda et al., 2010 (16)
  - Achilles tendon
  - Fifteen patients with a mean age of 40 and symptoms for at least 6 months
  - One injection of 3 mL of leukocyte-rich PRP (Curasan) with US guidance
  - Achilles VISA increased from 24 to 96
  - On American Orthopedic Foot and Ankle Society (AOFAS) scale, two patients continued to have pain with activity.
- Hechtman et al., 2011 (20)
  - Lateral epicondylosis
  - Thirty-one patients with average age of 47 with elbow pain > 6 months

- ❏ One injection of leukocyte-poor PRP (Cascade) using 18-g needle with nine needle penetrations without US guidance
- ❏ VAS score decreased > 25% in 96% of patients at 12 months.
- ❏ Two patients had surgery, and one had no improvement.
- ■ Double-blind, randomized studies
  - ▦ de Vos et al., 2010 (8)
    - ❏ Achilles tendinosis
    - ❏ Fifty-four patients total (27 in each group), with an average age of 49 and at least 3 months of pain
    - ❏ Could not have performed eccentric exercises prior to study
    - ❏ Control group received saline injection with 15 needle penetrations.
    - ❏ PRP group received leukocyte-rich PRP (Biomet) with 15 needle penetrations.
    - ❏ Outcome
      - ▦ VISA-Achilles (VISA-A) score increased an average of 22 points in both groups.
      - ▦ PRP with tenotomy was effective, but no more effective than saline with tenotomy.
    - ❏ Study flaws
      - ▦ Eccentric exercises alone will increase VISA-A scores in similar demographic by 27 points (40).
      - ▦ Tenotomy (15 needle penetrations) improved tendinosis approximately 60% of the time (24,36,37).
    - ❏ PRP should be used after other treatments have failed.
  - ▦ Peerbooms et al., 2010 (39), and Gosens et al., 2011 (17)
    - ❏ Lateral epicondylosis
    - ❏ One hundred patients (49 in control group, 51 in PRP group) with at least 6 months of elbow pain failing other treatments
    - ❏ Control group received corticosteroid (*i.e.*, "standard of care").
    - ❏ PRP group received leukocyte-rich PRP (Biomet) with 22-g needle and five needle penetrations without US guidance.
    - ❏ Outcome
      - ▦ VAS and Disabilities of the Arm, Shoulder and Hand (DASH) scores were followed.
      - ▦ Corticosteroid group initially improved but returned to near baseline after 9 weeks.
      - ▦ PRP group had significant improvement of VAS and DASH scores, which continued to improve up to 2 years.
      - ▦ Level I evidence that PRP is effective treatment for lateral epicondylosis.
- ■ There is ample evidence and sound theory that PRP is effective for chronic tendinopathy that is unresponsive to other treatments.

PRP in Muscle Injuries

- ■ Pathogenesis of muscle injury (3,48)
  - ■ Muscle injury (strain or contusion) leads to a three-phase healing reaction.
  - ■ Days 1–3 represent the degeneration and inflammation phase.
    - ❏ A clot forms and neutrophils begin to invade at 1–2 hours.
    - ❏ Peak muscle damage does not occur at the time of injury but corresponds to time of peak neutrophil count.
    - ❏ Peak injury is attenuated if neutrophils are blocked.
    - ❏ Sometimes, this is referred to as "secondary injury" or the "respiratory burst."
  - ■ Day 2 to 2 weeks is the regenerative phase.
    - ❏ Satellite cells are quiescent muscle cells that become activated at the time of injury. Growth factors play a critical role in influencing the fate of satellite cells, which can become either myofibroblasts (scar-producing) or myoblasts (muscle fiber–producing).
    - ❏ Myoblasts fuse with other myoblasts to create multinucleated myofibers.
    - ❏ TGF-β and IGF-1 are key growth factors.
    - ❏ NSAIDs increase TGF-β and decrease prostaglandin E_2, which enhances satellite cell differentiation (2).
  - ■ From 2 weeks and on is the remodeling phase.
    - ❏ Maturation of regenerated fibers
    - ❏ Remodeling of scar
    - ❏ Fibrosis is key inhibitor of complete healing.
- ■ Theory
  - ▦ Platelets in initial clot are "spent" after 3–7 days.
  - ■ Initial clot has high density of red blood cells due to vascularity of muscle and significant bleeding with injury.
  - ■ PRP can increase the density of platelets in the clot, and the fibrin can form a scaffold for repair and cell migration.
  - ■ PRP may speed healing or may just increase the quality of the repair by influencing the satellite cells to become myoblasts and thus increase the amount of new muscle formed versus fibrous scar tissue, which is prone to reinjury.
  - ■ PRP may not enhance this already acutely inflammatory healing process.
  - ■ PRP with increased neutrophil density (leukocyte-rich PRP) may increase secondary injury (43).
  - ■ PRP with increased plasma component has increased levels of IGF-1.
    - ❏ IGF-1 is also referred to as mechanogrowth factor.
    - ❏ There is very little IGF-1 in platelets; 99% is in plasma (7).

❑ IGF-1 increases satellite cell differentiation to myoblasts (over myofibroblasts), which theoretically may produce a better repair.

■ Studies

  ■ Very limited human studies

    ❑ Muscle injuries are heterogeneous, and it is difficult to predict how long a muscle injury will take to heal.

    ❑ Muscle injuries are self-limited, and the vast majority will heal if given enough time without other intervention.

  ■ Sánchez et al., 2009 (43)

    ❑ Case series

    ❑ Twenty professional athletes with 22 muscle injuries were injected with leukocyte-poor PRP under US guidance.

    ❑ Healing was reported to be half of the expected time, and there were no incidences of recurrence.

    ❑ Flaws

      ▪ No control

      ▪ No quantification of injury

      ▪ Difficult to accurately predict expected time loss

  ■ Wright-Carpenter et al., 2004 (50)

    ❑ Eighteen professional athletes were treated with 2 mL of autologous conditioned serum (ACS). ACS is whole blood that is allowed to clot and is incubated with glass beads to release growth factors into supernatant. There is no fibrin in ACS. Up to five injections were done 2 days apart.

    ❑ Control group was 11 professional athletes treated with a combination of Actovegin and Traumeel (naturopathic anti-inflammatories). Up to five injections were done 2 days apart.

    ❑ The group treated with ACS returned to play at 16 days versus 22 days for the "control" group.

    ❑ Flaws

      ▪ No true control group

      ▪ No quantification of injury

  ■ Wright-Carpenter et al., 2004 (51)

    ❑ One hundred eight mice had experimental muscle contusion model induced.

    ❑ Fifty-four were treated with ACS injections at 2, 24, and 48 hours.

    ❑ Fifty-four were treated with normal saline at 2, 24, and 48 hours.

    ❑ Results showed that ACS-treated mice had increased satellite cell activation at 30 and 48 hours after injury, and the diameter of regenerating myofibrils was increased compared to controls within the first week after injury.

■ Conclusion

  ■ There is little evidence that PRP improves time to return to play in muscle injuries, although limited, low-quality evidence and anecdotal reports suggest it may decrease healing time by about one-third.

  ■ PRP may improve outcome of natural repair process by increasing myoblast differentiation.

PRP in Ligament Injuries

■ Theory

  ■ PRP will speed or improve outcome of healing.

■ Studies

  ■ No human studies.

  ■ Increased matrix synthesis in ligaments in vitro (46)

  ■ PRP enhances ligament cell adhesion, proliferation, and differentiation in vitro (19).

  ■ PRP-treated rabbit medial collateral ligaments had increased load to failure (23).

■ Conclusion

  ■ Additional human and animal studies are needed before recommendations can be made.

PRP in Arthritis

■ Theory

  ■ PRP may be able to stimulate chondral anabolism and inhibit the catabolic process.

  ■ PRP may reduce synovial membrane hyperplasia and modulate cytokine level.

■ Studies

  ■ Kon et al., 2010 (29) (1-year follow-up), and Filardo et al., 2011 (14) (2-year follow-up)

    ❑ One hundred fifteen knees had leukocyte-rich PRP injected intra-articularly for a total of three injections 3 weeks apart.

    ❑ Both International Knee Documentation Committee objective and subjective score as well as EuroQol VAS increased at 2 months, and although they decreased slightly by 12 months, they were still significantly higher than baseline.

    ❑ Ninety-one patients were available for follow-up at 2 years. There was a further decrease in scores at 2 years, but scores were still above baseline (14).

    ❑ Patients who were younger and had less severe arthritis did better.

  ■ Sampson et al., 2010 (42)

    ❑ Fourteen patients with a median age of 51.8 years had leukocyte-rich PRP (Biomet) injected for a total of three injections approximately 4 weeks apart.

    ❑ VAS and Knee Injury and Osteoarthritis Outcome Score improved in most patients.

■ Conclusion

  ■ There may be a modest, beneficial effect of PRP in osteoarthritis that declines over time. Further study is needed.

Conclusions Regarding PRP

■ Most human research has been done in tendinopathy.

    ■ Level III evidence suggests PRP is effective in the treatment of chronic tendinopathy (15,16,20,30,38,49).

    ■ Level I evidence suggests PRP is effective in the treatment of chronic tendinopathy (8,17,39).

■ There have been no adverse effects reported in the literature.

■ More study is needed in acute muscle and ligament injuries and osteoarthritis.

REFERENCES

1. Baumgard SH, Schwartz DR. Percutaneous release of the epicondylar muscles for humeral epicondylitis. *Am J Sports Med.* 1982;10(4):233–6.

2. Bedair HS, Karthikeyan T, Quintero A, Li Y, Huard J. Angiotensin II receptor blockade administered after injury improves muscle regeneration and decreases fibrosis in normal skeletal muscle. *Am J Sports Med.* 2008;36(8):1548–54.

3. Best TM, Hunter KD. Muscle injury and repair. *Phys Med Rehabil Clin N Am.* 2000;11(2):251–66.

4. Borg T, Modig J. Potential anti-thrombotic effects of local anaesthetics due to their inhibition of platelet aggregation. *Acta Anaesthesiol Scand.* 1985;29(7):739–42.

5. Castillo TN, Pouliot MA, Kim HJ, Dragoo JL. Comparison of growth factor and platelet concentration from commercial platelet-rich plasma separation systems. *Am J Sports Med.* 2011;39(2):266–71.

6. Connell DA, Ali KE, Ahmad M, Lambert S, Corbett S, Curtis M. Ultrasound-guided autologous blood injection for tennis elbow. *Skeletal Radiol.* 2006;35(6):371–7.

7. Creaney L, Hamilton B. Growth factor delivery methods in the management of sports injuries: the state of play. *Br J Sports Med.* 2008;42(5):314–20.

8. de Vos RJ, Weir A, van Schie HT, et al. Platelet-rich plasma injection for chronic Achilles tendinopathy: a randomized controlled trial. *JAMA.* 2010;303(2):144–9.

9. Dohan Ehrenfest DM, Rasmusson L, Albrektsson T. Classification of platelet concentrates: from pure platelet-rich plasma (P-PRP) to leucocyte- and platelet-rich fibrin (L-PRF). *Trends Biotechnol.* 2009; 27(3):158–67.

10. Edwards SG, Calandruccio JH. Autologous blood injections for refractory lateral epicondylitis. *J Hand Surg Am.* 2003;28(2):272–8.

11. El-Sharkawy H, Kantarci A, Deady J, et al. Platelet-rich plasma: growth factors and pro- and anti-inflammatory properties. *J Periodontol.* 2007; 78(4):661–9.

12. Esenyel C, Demirhan M, Esenyel M, et al. Comparison of four different intra-articular injection sites in the knee: a cadaver study. *Knee Surg Sports Traumatol Arthrosc.* 2007;15(5):573–7.

13. Eustace JA, Brophy DP, Gibney RP, Bresnihan B, FitzGerald O. Comparison of the accuracy of steroid placement with clinical outcome in patients with shoulder symptoms. *Ann Rheum Dis.* 1997;56(1):59–63.

14. Filardo G, Kon E, Buda R, et al. Platelet-rich plasma intra-articular knee injections for the treatment of degenerative cartilage lesions and osteoarthritis. *Knee Surg Sports Traumatol Arthrosc.* 2011;19(4):528–35.

15. Filardo G, Kon E, Della Villa S, Vincentelli F, Fornasari PM, Marcacci M. Use of platelet-rich plasma for the treatment of refractory jumper's knee. *Int Orthop.* 2010;34(6):909–15.

16. Gaweda K, Tarczynska M, Krzyzanowski W. Treatment of Achilles tendinopathy with platelet-rich plasma. *Int J Sports Med.* 2010;31(8):577–83.

17. Gosens T, Peerbooms JC, van Laar W, den Oudsten BL. Ongoing positive effect of platelet-rich plasma versus corticosteroid injection in lateral epicondylitis: a double-blind randomized controlled trial with 2-year follow-up. *Am J Sports Med.* 2011;39(6):1200–8.

18. Graziani F, Ivanovski S, Cei S, Ducci F, Tonetti M, Gabriele M. The in vitro effect of different PRP concentrations on osteoblasts and fibroblasts. *Clin Oral Implants Res.* 2006;17(2):212–9.

19. Han J, Meng HX, Tang JM, Li SL, Tang Y, Chen ZB. The effect of different platelet-rich plasma concentrations on proliferation and differentiation of human periodontal ligament cells in vitro. *Cell Prolif.* 2007; 40(2):241–52.

20. Hechtman KS, Uribe JW, Botto-vanDemden A, Kiebzak GM. Platelet-rich plasma injection reduces pain in patients with recalcitrant epicondylitis. *Orthopedics.* 2011;34(2):92.

20. Heidari N, Pichler W, Grechenig S, Grechenig W, Weinberg AM. Does the anteromedial or anterolateral approach alter the rate of joint puncture in injection of the ankle? A cadaver study. *J Bone Joint Surg Br.* 2010;92(1):176–8.

22. Henkus HE, Cobben LP, Coerkamp EG, Nelissen RG, van Arkel ER. The accuracy of subacromial injections: a prospective randomized magnetic resonance imaging study. *Arthroscopy.* 2006;22(3):277–82.

23. Hildebrand KA, Woo SL, Smith DW, et al. The effects of platelet-derived growth factor-BB on healing of the rabbit medial collateral ligament. An in vivo study. *Am J Sports Med.* 1998;26(4):549–54.

24. Housner JA, Jacobson JA, Misko R. Sonographically guided percutaneous needle tenotomy for the treatment of chronic tendinosis. *J Ultrasound Med.* 2009;28(9):1187–92.

25. Huang GS, Lin TC, Wang JY, Ku CH, Ho ST, Li CY. Lidocaine priming reduces ADP-induced P-selectin expression and platelet-leukocyte aggregation. *Acta Anaesthesiol Taiwan.* 2009;47(2):56–61.

26. Im SH, Lee SC, Park YB, Cho SR, Kim JC. Feasibility of sonography for intra-articular injections in the knee through a medial patellar portal. *J Ultrasound Med.* 2009;28(11):1465–70.

27. James SL, Ali K, Pocock C, et al. Ultrasound guided dry needling and autologous blood injection for patellar tendinosis. *Br J Sports Med.* 2007;41(8):518–21; discussion 22.

28. Kangasaho M. Effects of lidocaine, codeine and vadocaine hydrochloride on platelet aggregation in human platelet-rich plasma. *Arzneimittelforschung.* 1988;38(4A):613–6.

29. Kon E, Buda R, Filardo G, et al. Platelet-rich plasma: intra-articular knee injections produced favorable results on degenerative cartilage lesions. *Knee Surg Sports Traumatol Arthrosc.* 2010;18(4):472–9.

30. Kon E, Filardo G, Delcogliano M, et al. Platelet-rich plasma: new clinical application: a pilot study for treatment of jumper's knee. *Injury.* 2009;40(6):598–603.

31. Liu Y, Kalén A, Risto O, Wahlström O. Fibroblast proliferation due to exposure to a platelet concentrate in vitro is pH dependent. *Wound Repair Regen.* 2002;10(5):336–40.

32. Lucarelli E, Beccheroni A, Donati D, et al. Platelet-derived growth factors enhance proliferation of human stromal stem cells. *Biomaterials.* 2003;24(18):3095–100.

33. Marx RE. Platelet-rich plasma: evidence to support its use. *J Oral Maxillofac Surg.* 2004;62(4):489–96.

34. Marx RE. Platelet-rich plasma (PRP): what is PRP and what is not PRP? *Implant Dent.* 2001;10(4):225–8.

35. Marx RE, Carlson ER, Eichstaedt RM, Schimmele SR, Strauss JE, Georgeff KR. Platelet-rich plasma: growth factor enhancement for bone grafts. *Oral Surg Oral Med Oral Pathol Oral Radiol Endod.* 1998;85(6):638–46.

36. McShane JM, Nazarian LN, Harwood MI. Sonographically guided percutaneous needle tenotomy for treatment of common extensor tendinosis in the elbow. *J Ultrasound Med*. 2006;25(10):1281–9.

37. McShane JM, Shah VN, Nazarian LN. Sonographically guided percutaneous needle tenotomy for treatment of common extensor tendinosis in the elbow: is a corticosteroid necessary? *J Ultrasound Med*. 2008;27(8):1137–44.

38. Mishra A, Pavelko T. Treatment of chronic elbow tendinosis with buffered platelet-rich plasma. *Am J Sports Med*. 2006;34(11):1774–8.

39. Peerbooms JC, Sluimer J, Bruijn DJ, Gosens T. Positive effect of an autologous platelet concentrate in lateral epicondylitis in a double-blind randomized controlled trial: platelet-rich plasma versus corticosteroid injection with a 1-year follow-up. *Am J Sports Med*. 2010;38(2):255–62.

40. Rompe JD, Nafe B, Furia JP, Maffulli N. Eccentric loading, shock-wave treatment, or a wait-and-see policy for tendinopathy of the main body of tendo Achillis: a randomized controlled trial. *Am J Sports Med*. 2007;35(3):374–83.

41. Rutten MJ, Maresch BJ, Jager GJ, de Waal Malefijt MC. Injection of the subacromial-subdeltoid bursa: blind or ultrasound-guided? *Acta Orthop*. 2007;78(2):254–7.

42. Sampson S, Reed M, Silvers H, Meng M, Mandelbaum B. Injection of platelet-rich plasma in patients with primary and secondary knee osteoarthritis: a pilot study. *Am J Phys Med Rehabil*. 2010;89(12):961–9.

43. Sánchez M, Anitua E, Orive G, Mujika I, Andia I. Platelet-rich therapies in the treatment of orthopaedic sport injuries. *Sports Med*. 2009;39(5):345–54.

44. Scherb MB, Han SH, Courneya JP, Guyton GP, Schon LC. Effect of bupivacaine on cultured tenocytes. *Orthopedics*. 2009;32(1):26.

45. Smith J, Hurdle MF, Weingarten TN. Accuracy of sonographically guided intra-articular injections in the native adult hip. *J Ultrasound Med*. 2009;28(3):329–35.

46. Smith JJ, Ross, MW, Smith RK. Anabolic effects of acellular bone marrow, platelet rich plasma, and serum on equine suspensory ligament fibroblasts in vitro. *Vet Comp Orthop Traumatol*. 2006;19(1):43–7.

47. Suresh SP, Ali KE, Jones H, Connell DA. Medial epicondylitis: is ultrasound guided autologous blood injection an effective treatment? *Br J Sports Med*. 2006;40(11):935–9; discussion 9.

48. Tidball JG. Inflammatory processes in muscle injury and repair. *Am J Physiol Regul Integr Comp Physiol*. 2005;288(2):R345–53.

49. Volpi P, Marinoni L, Bait C, De Girolamo, Schoenhuber H. Treatment of chronic patellar tendinitis with buffered platelet rich plasma: a preliminary study. *Med Sport*. 2007;60:595–603.

50. Wright-Carpenter T, Klein P, Schäferhoff P, Appell HJ, Mir LM, Wehling P. Treatment of muscle injuries by local administration of autologous conditioned serum: a pilot study on sportsmen with muscle strains. *Int J Sports Med*. 2004;25(8):588–93.

51. Wright-Carpenter T, Opolon P, Appell HJ, Meijer H, Wehling P, Mir LM. Treatment of muscle injuries by local administration of autologous conditioned serum: animal experiments using a muscle contusion model. *Int J Sports Med*. 2004;25(8):582–7.

74 Common Injections in Sports Medicine: General Principles and Specific Techniques

Christopher J. Lutrzykowski, Francis G. O'Connor, and Thad Barkdull

INTRODUCTION

- Injections are a common intervention provided by sports clinicians. Injections can be both diagnostic and therapeutic. If delivered properly and with sound indications, injections can be very rewarding for both the patient and the provider.

- This chapter details the indications, benefits, risks, and technique for administering common injections in sports medicine. These injections, while in most cases simple to administer, should be done only after proper training and appropriate supervision. Most injections are simple to learn (see one, do one, teach one); judgment on their use, however, takes time and effort to acquire.

INDICATIONS

- Injections/aspirations are indicated for both diagnosis and therapy.
  - Diagnosis:
    - ❑ Synovial fluid analysis to rule out infection, traumatic, rheumatic, or crystal-induced etiology (Table 74.1)
    - ❑ To perform a therapeutic trial to differentiate various etiologies
    - ❑ Imaging studies
    - ❑ Synovial biopsy
  - Therapy:
    - ❑ To remove tense effusions to relieve pain and improve function
    - ❑ To remove blood or pus from a joint
    - ❑ For injection of steroids and other intra-articular therapies
    - ❑ For therapeutic lavage of joints

Risks/Complications (58) (Table 74.2)

- **Infection (9,37,60):** The risk of postinjection infection is extremely rare, on the order of one infection per 3,000–50,000 injections when sterile technique is used. *Staphylococcus aureus* is the most common organism involved, with recent reports also implicating methicillin-resistant *S. aureus* (MRSA).

- **Tendon rupture (29):** Collagen atrophy and tendon rupture are rare but have been described in the literature. Injections into tendons should be avoided. In addition, corticosteroid injections into the synovial sheath or peritendinous region of major weight-bearing tendons (Achilles, patellar, and plantar fascia) should be done with extreme caution, and the athlete should be protected from weight-bearing exercise for a period of 2–4 weeks.

- **Postinjection flare:** This entity is seen in 2%–10% of patients. In this setting, the patient develops a flare of pain in the immediate 6- to 12-hour period after an injection. The etiology for this reaction is thought to be secondary to a local reaction to the microcrystalline steroid suspension and is generally self-limited. The postinjection flare has also been attributed to the preservative that accompanies the anesthetic. This complication may be treated with ice, activity modification, and a short course of a nonsteroidal anti-inflammatory drug (NSAID). Patients with pain beyond 36 hours should be evaluated for a septic joint.

- **Skin atrophy/depigmentation/hyperpigmentation:** When local steroid is applied too close to the surface of the skin, local atrophy and depigmentation/hyperpigmentation can occur. These changes may be irreversible.

- **Hyperglycemia:** In some diabetics, there may be short-term difficulties with glycemic control secondary to the local absorption of corticosteroid. This effect has been rarely reported and may be overstated (53).

- **Cartilage degeneration:** Traditional teaching limits injections into a weight-bearing joint to no more than three injections per year, because there is some concern about weakening articular cartilage or frank chondrotoxicity from

Table 74.1 | **Classification of Synovial Fluid**

Classification	Appearance	WBC	PMNs (%)	Crystals	Culture
Normal	Clear to straw colored	< 150	< 25	None	Negative
Noninflammatory	Yellow	< 3,000	< 30	None	Negative
Inflammatory	Yellow or cloudy	3,000–75,000	> 50	None	Negative
Infectious	Yellow or purulent	50,000–200,000	> 90	None	Positive
Crystal-induced	Cloudy, turbid	500–200,00	< 90	Yes	Negative
Hemorrhagic	Red-brown	50–10,000	< 50	None	Negative

PMNs, polymorphonuclear leukocytes; WBC, white blood cell.
SOURCE: O'Connell TX. Interpreting tests from joint aspirates. In: Phenninger JL, editor. *The Clinics Atlas of Office Procedures — Joint Injection Techniques.* Vol. 5 (no. 4). Philadelphia (PA): WB Saunders Company; 2002.

studies on postoperative bupivacaine continuous drips (18,44,58). Recent studies indicate that more frequent injections are well tolerated, particularly when used in a disease-specific manner (54). Please see later section on use of anesthetics.

- **Intravascular injection**
- **Traumatic injection:** Possible to cause a pneumothorax and damage articular cartilage, local nerves, or soft tissue structures
- **Vasovagal reactions**
- **Facial flushing (10):** Up to 15% and described mostly in women
- **Intramuscular injection**

CONTRAINDICATIONS (54)

- Cellulitis or broken skin over the needle entry site would increase the risk for infection.

Table 74.2 | **Common Adverse Outcomes**

Complication	Estimated Incidence (%)
Postinjection flare	2–10
Steroid arthropathy	0.8
Tendon rupture	< 1
Facial flushing	< 1
Skin atrophy, depigmentation	< 1
Iatrogenic infectious arthritis	< 0.001–0.072
Transient paresis of injected extremity	Rare
Hypersensitivity reaction	Rare
Asymptomatic pericapsular calcification	43
Acceleration of cartilage attrition	Unknown

SOURCE: Gray RG, Gottlieb NL. Intra-articular corticosteroids. An updated assessment. *Clin Orthop Relat Res.* 1983;(177):253–63.

- Unstable coagulopathy
- Intra-articular fractures are a contraindication to a corticosteroid injection.
- Septic effusion of a bursa or a periarticular structure
- Lack of response to prior injections
- More than three prior injections in the last year to a weight-bearing joint
- Inaccessible joints, *e.g.,* hip, spine, sternoclavicular (62), and sacroiliac joints
- Joint prostheses — relative contraindication
- Known hypersensitivity to any component of the injection

GENERAL PRINCIPLES (38,63)

- **Consent:** Because there are inherent risks and complications associated with corticosteroid injections, informed consent should be obtained, witnessed, and documented.
- **Equipment:** Most injections are performed using an alcohol, chlorhexidine, or povidone-iodine wipe; some authors recommend a sterile scrub before injecting into a large joint (9,54). Sterile versus nonsterile gloves are another area of controversy; as a rule, the authors teach that sterile gloves are used for joints and nonsterile gloves may be used for soft tissue structures. Some advocate sterile gloves for all injections, whereas others prefer using the one sterile glove technique. In this technique, the physician wears the sterile glove on the noninjecting hand to ensure proper positioning after the local preparation. Finally, the "sterile no touch" technique may be employed as well, with only the needle touching the patient after preparation. Other equipment includes the following:
  - Povidone-iodine wipes and/or alcohol wipes
  - Sterile or nonsterile gloves
  - Sterile drapes: optional
  - 21- to 27-gauge 1.5-inches needles for injection
  - 18- to 20-gauge needles for aspirations

■ 1- to 10-cc syringes for injections

■ 3- to 50-cc syringes for aspirations

■ Ethyl chloride surface coolant

■ 1% lidocaine

■ 0.5% bupivacaine

■ 2 × 2 gauze sponges

■ Small dressings such as Band-Aids

■ Access to equipment to treat severe allergic reactions: oxygen; epinephrine 1:1,000; Benadryl 25–50 mg intramural (IM); advanced cardiac life support (ACLS) equipment

■ **Anesthesia:** The three main uses of anesthesia include diminishing pain, aiding in diagnosis, and providing a volume for corticosteroid injections. Although there are many local anesthetics, the two most commonly used are the amide compounds lidocaine and bupivacaine.

■ Recent studies have indicated evidence of chondrolysis in postoperative patients treated with continuous intra-articular bupivacaine (3,47). Because no minimum volume has been described, cautious use of intra-articular anesthetic is recommended until this risk has been clearly defined.

■ Lidocaine (Xylocaine) is available commercially as a 0.5%–2% concentration. The most commonly used concentration is 1%; 2% may be used in small areas where a small volume is required. Time from injection to onset of effect is 1–2 minutes, with duration of action of approximately 1–2 hours. The upper limit of dosing is 10 mL for 2% and 20 mL for 1%; above these levels, side effects can be expected.

■ Bupivacaine (Marcaine) is available commercially in 0.25%–0.5% concentrations. Time from injection to onset of effect is 5–30 minutes, with duration of action of approximately 8 hours. The upper limit of dosing is 30 mL for 0.5% and 60 mL for 0.25%; above these levels, side effects can be expected.

■ Side effects including anaphylaxis can occur; resuscitation equipment should be available.

■ An alternative to a local anesthetic injection is topical ethyl chloride. When used, however, spray lightly to avoid cold injury and secondary skin changes.

■ It is recommended to draw the anesthetic prior to the corticosteroid with multiuse vials to limit anesthetic contamination by the steroid ("clear to cloudy").

■ **Corticosteroids (54):** Corticosteroids are commonly used in musculoskeletal medicine. The corticosteroid treats the local inflammatory response and not the clinical problem. Steroids have both mineralocorticoid and glucocorticoid effects. The mineralocorticoid effects modify salt and water balance, while the glucocorticoid effect suppresses the inflammatory response. The ideal choice is to use a medication that maximizes the anti-inflammatory effect. Steroids also differ in their solubilities, potencies, and duration of action (Table 74.3). The duration of the effect is thought to vary inversely with the drug's solubility. Shorter acting agents tend to have a lower incidence of postinjection flare. In general, higher solubility agents (*e.g.,* betamethasone [Celestone], dexamethasone, and methylprednisolone) tend to be better for soft tissues, whereas lower solubility agents (*e.g.,* triamcinolone hexacetonide) tend to favor joint injections. Selected dosing is found in Table 74.4.

■ Alternative injections such as platelet-rich plasma, autologous blood, and prolotherapy are discussed elsewhere in this text.

■ **Technique**

■ Patient: The patient should be in a comfortable position, preferably sitting or lying down. The most important

Table 74.3 | **Relative Potencies and Solubilities of Corticosteroids**

Corticosteroid	Relative Anti-Inflammatory Potency	Equivalent Dose (mg)	Solubility	Concentration (mg · mL⁻¹)
Short-acting				
Cortisone	0.8	25	NA	25, 50
Hydrocortisone	1	20	0.002	25
Intermediate-acting				
Triamcinolone Hexacetonide	5	4	0.0002	20
Methylprednisolone	5	4	0.001	20, 40, 80
Long-acting				
Dexamethasone Sodium phosphate	25	0.6	0.01	4,8
Betamethasone	25	0.6	NA	6

NA, not applicable.

SOURCE: Genovese MC. Joint and soft tissue injection: a useful adjuvant to systemic and local treatment. *Postgrad Med.* 1998;103(2):125–34.

Table 74.4	Recommended Corticosteroid and Lidocaine Dosages for Injections		
Site of Injection	Dose of 1% Lidocaine (mL)	Dose of Triamcinolone (mg)	Dose of Betamethasone (mg)
de Quervain	1–2	40	6
Carpal tunnel	0.5–1	40	6
Trigger finger	1	20	3
Tennis elbow	0.5–1	40	6
Subacromial space	6–8	40	6
Glenohumeral	6–8	40–60	6–9
Acromioclavicular	1–2	40	6
Plantar fascia	1–2	40	6
Anserine bursa	2–3	40	6
Trochanteric bursa	4–5	40–60	6–9
Intra-articular knee	4–6	40–60	6–9
Morton neuroma	1–2	20–40	3–6
Myofascial	1–2	NA	NA
Iliotibial band	1–2	20–40	3–6
Ankle	2–3	40	6

NA, not applicable.
SOURCE: Stankus SJ. Inflammation and the role of anti-inflammatory medications. In: Lillegard WA, Butcher JD, Rucker KS, editors. *Handbook of Sports Medicine*. 2nd ed. Boston (MA): Butterworth-Heinemann; 1999.

aspect of the patient's position, however, is that the physician injecting is comfortable and can easily identify anatomic landmarks and administer the injection.

■ Be prepared: Have all your equipment ready so that you can move quickly. Have your combination of steroid and anesthetic already drawn up and ready to go. Remember to use separate needles for drawing up different agents.

■ Identify structure: Put the skin under traction and identify anatomic landmarks. If needed, the skin can be marked with a fingernail, a retracted end of a ballpoint pen, or ink.

■ Aseptic technique: The area may be cleansed with alcohol, povidone, or betadine using nonsterile gloves. When entering a joint, a sterile prep may be used, but swabbing with betadine or other suitable antimicrobial prep is common practice.

■ Local anesthesia: The practice of using a preinjection anesthetic varies among practitioners. Some authors will only use local anesthesia when using needles larger than 22 gauge. Prior to a joint preparation and injection, some providers will cleanse only with alcohol swabs and use lidocaine to raise a wheal and anesthetize the tract they are planning to inject. In those cases where no joint will be entered, the use of an assistant to give a quick spray of surface coolant prior to the introduction of the injection needle can provide pain relief. When using smaller gauge needles (22 gauge and higher), no subcutaneous anesthetic is also an acceptable choice because the same bore needle is often used when anesthetizing skin as for the actual injection.

■ When performing diagnostic arthrocentesis, it is recommended to use local anesthetic to minimize the pain experienced by the entrance of a larger bore needle through the skin and synovium (often 18 gauge).

■ Needle insertion: The needle should be an extension of the finger and inserted quickly and preferably perpendicular to the skin. When introducing the agent, aspirate first to ensure you are not in the artery or vein. Aspirated contents should be sent for appropriate analysis. The patient should not complain of neurologic symptoms such as paresthesias; reposition needle if this occurs.

■ Delivering the steroid: The bolus technique may be used when entering a joint; there should be a free flow with no resistance. When injecting near a ligament or tendon, some authors recommend a peppering technique. When injecting in a tendon sheath, the ideal injection demonstrates a free flow of fluid that fills the sheath. Prior to injection, the patient can be asked to move the affected tendon, or an assistant can passively move the finger; if the needle moves, this suggests that the clinician is in the tendon, and the needle should be withdrawn slightly and repositioned.

■ **Postprocedure care:** Any postinjection pain can be relieved with ice or a short course of a nonsteroidal anti-inflammatory medication. The patient should be informed that the anti-inflammatory effect of the corticosteroid may not kick in for 48–72 hours and that the anesthetic will quickly wear off. It is recommended that strenuous activity be avoided for a period of 10 days to 2 weeks following an injection. Rehabilitative exercise, however, may be commenced within 2–3 days.

■ **Evidence-based medicine evaluation of steroid injections (9,40,54):** There are currently conflicting or insufficient quality data to provide a definitive answer on the efficacy of steroid injections. With some injection locations, corticosteroid may provide lasting relief, but with others, short-term or no relief has also been found. Available data regarding efficacy of corticosteroid injection are listed below for each injection site. The addition of image-guided injection may help improve efficacy as accuracy of injection improves. Where available, evidence regarding accuracy of palpation-guided injection is also included.

SPECIFIC INJECTIONS (2,10,31,44,49,50,55)

Subacromial Space

■ **Indications:** For the relief of pain in subacromial impingement syndrome

■ **Clinical anatomy/landmarks:** Useful landmarks include the acromioclavicular (AC) joint, the posterior glenohumeral joint, and the posterolateral corner of the acromion.

■ **Technique:** This injection is most easily accomplished with the patient in a seated position. The arm should be in a relaxed, dependent position; the other arm may be used to provide traction on the shoulder to be injected. The posterior edge of the acromion is palpated, with a recess identified inferior to this edge providing the portal for the injection. The needle is inserted bevel-up in a slightly cephalad angulation, pointed to the AC joint. If bony resistance is felt, the needle is most probably in the acromion, and the needle should be redirected inferiorly. Insertion depth is approximately 1 inch. Alternate approaches such as the lateral, anterior, and AC joint approach can also be used. In the lateral approach, the lateral border of the acromion is palpated and the needle inserted at a 30- to 45-degree angle just below the acromion. Depth is variable given the habitus of the patient. Anterior and AC access to the subacromial space will not be discussed, but see later discussion regarding accuracy.

■ **Needle size and dosage:** One milliliter of corticosteroid in combination with 6–10 mL of long- and short-acting anesthetics. A 22-gauge long 1.5-inch needle is recommended when injecting a large volume.

■ **Accuracy (23,36,39,65):** 70%–80% accurate in unguided injections. There is conflicting evidence regarding location of injection, with some favoring posterolateral approach (23,35) and others indicating no difference between techniques (39). Additionally, other structures are infiltrated such as rotator cuff tendons, deltoid, and ligamentous structures.

■ **Efficacy:** Short-term (2 weeks–2 months) improvement in pain symptoms and function has been reported (7,20). Conflicting evidence is present regarding efficacy with improved accuracy (12,16,17).

Glenohumeral Joint

■ **Indications:** Inflammatory or degenerative arthritis, adhesive capsulitis

■ **Clinical anatomy/landmarks:** Posterior approach: coracoid process, humeral head, and the acromion process of the scapula. Anterior approach: coracoid process, humeral head, acromion.

■ **Technique:** Posterior approach: The seated position is most comfortable for this injection. The coracoid process is identified inferomedial to the AC joint, with the anterior glenohumeral joint inferior to the coracoid and appreciated by internally and externally rotating the shoulder. At the same time, the posterior glenohumeral joint can be appreciated. The technique is the same as the subacromial injection; however, the needle is now aimed to the coracoid process. The depth of penetration is approximately 1 inch. Anterior approach (54): Patient placement is the same as the posterior approach. Landmarks are identified, and the needle is placed medial to the head of the humerus and just lateral to the coracoid process. The needle is directed slightly superiorly and laterally. If bone is encountered, needle is redirected. Depth is variable depending on body habitus.

■ **Needle size and dosage:** A 22- to 25-gauge 1.5-inch needle is recommended; 1–2 mL of corticosteroid can be combined with 5–10 mL of anesthetic.

■ **Accuracy:** Variable success with palpation-guided injections. Accuracy ranges from 24% to 99% anteriorly (46,52) and 50% posteriorly (59,28,52).

■ **Efficacy:** Improvement is seen in adhesive capsulitis patients with corticosteroid injection, but limited data exist for degenerative disease in palpation-guided injections (7,8,17,33). Some authors have found that improved accuracy may improve pain relief (19).

Acromioclavicular Joint

■ **Indications:** AC degenerative disease

■ **Clinical anatomy/landmarks:** Important landmarks are the clavicle and acromion. The AC joint can be conveniently located by abducting the shoulder.

■ **Technique:** The injection is conveniently administered by having the patient in a seated position. The injection is most easily accomplished by coming from above with the needle directed inferiorly. An insertion depth of 3/8–1/2 inch is required. A preinjection radiograph of the angle of the AC joint can be useful.

■ **Needle size and dosage:** 0.5- to 1-inch 25-gauge needle is appropriate; 0.5 mL each of anesthetic and corticosteroid are adequate.

■ **Accuracy:** Small studies indicate surprisingly low degrees of accuracy with palpation-guided injection (6,45).

■ **Efficacy:** Limited small studies advocate use of intra-articular corticosteroid for AC degenerative changes (25).

Lateral Epicondylitis

- **Indications:** Lateral tennis elbow that fails to improve with conservative therapy.
- **Clinical anatomy/landmarks:** Key landmarks include the radial head, appreciated by pronation and supination of the elbow, and the humeral lateral epicondyle. The most common location of tennis elbow is at the extensor *carpi radialis brevis* origin, which is one fingerbreadth inferior and medial to the lateral epicondyle.
- **Technique:** The injection can be administered in a supine or seated position. If seated, the elbow should be comfortably resting at 90 degrees with the forearm supinated. The area of maximal tenderness is identified, and the needle is inserted at an oblique angle to infiltrate the soft tissues over the extensor aponeurosis. There should be little resistance to the injection; if encountered, the needle should be withdrawn until there is little resistance to flow. Some authors advocate for a "peppering" technique (1,13).
- **Needle size and dosage:** A 1-inch 25-gauge needle is recommended; 0.5 mL of corticosteroid should be mixed with 1–2 mL of anesthetic.
- **Efficacy:** Short-term limited benefit noted (4,17) with corticosteroid.

De Quervain Tenosynovitis

- **Indications:** This disorder is caused by an inflammation and swelling of the tendons of the abductor pollicis longus and the extensor pollicis brevis at the level of the radial styloid process. Patients who fail to improve with NSAIDs and wrist support may be candidates for an injection.
- **Clinical anatomy/landmarks:** The anatomic snuffbox is the anatomic landmark. The anterior border is the first dorsal compartment of the wrist (abductor pollicis longus and extensor pollicis brevis), and the posterior border is the extensor pollicis longus tendon.
- **Technique:** This injection can be done in the seated or supine position, with the wrist in a vertical position, resting over a folded towel, with the thumb flexed. The point of maximal tenderness is identified, which is generally over the radial styloid. The needle is inserted bevel-up, directed in an oblique, cephalad angle, nearly parallel to the tendons. If the gap between the two tendons can be appreciated, the needle should be placed in this gap. When the needle is approximately 1/4 inch, an attempt should be made to aspirate, and then gently push the plunger. If there is resistance, the needle should be withdrawn slightly and the process repeated.
- **Needle size and dosage:** 0.5- to 1-inch, 25- to 27-gauge needle; 0.5 mL of anesthetic and 0.5 mL of corticosteroid
- **Efficacy:** Limited studies but considered effective treatment (41,54).

Carpal Tunnel Syndrome

- **Indications:** Carpal tunnel syndrome
- **Clinical anatomy/landmarks:** Key landmarks include the palmaris longus and flexor carpi radialis tendons, the distal wrist crease, and the median nerve. The median nerve lies deep to and between the tendons of the palmaris longus and the flexor carpi radialis at the wrist.
- **Technique:** The injection can be given in the supine position or the seated position. The dorsum of the hand should rest on a folded towel. The needle is inserted just proximal to the distal wrist crease at a 45-degree angle just ulnar to the palmaris longus and angled toward the index finger. The needle may be felt to pop through the dense transverse carpal ligament. If pain or paresthesias are reported in the palm or fingertips during needle placement, the needle should be withdrawn and reangled prior to reinsertion. Free flow of solute is required to ensure that a tendon is not injected inadvertently. Depth of penetration should be approximately one-half inch.
- **Needle size and dosage:** A 25- to 27-gauge needle may be used, with 0.5 mL of steroid and a similar dose volume of anesthetic.
- **Efficacy:** Found to be effective in short term but limited studies (26,34,43).

Trigger Finger

- **Indications:** Trigger finger/stenosing tenosynovitis
- **Clinical anatomy/landmarks:** The key landmark is the first annular pulley. This condition is secondary to an inflammation and swelling of the flexor tendon of the flexor digitorum superficialis. Repetitive irritation leads to a nodule in this tendon, which becomes obstructed as the nodule passes beneath the pulley, which is proximal to the metacarpophalangeal (MP) joint.
- **Technique:** The patient may be administered the injection in the seated or supine position. The site for the injection is the distal palmar crease, just proximal to the MP joint. The needle is inserted bevel-up, directed at an oblique angle parallel with the tendon, toward the fingertips. When an increase in resistance is felt, at approximately 1/4-inch depth, the plunger should be gently pushed. If there is resistance, the needle may be in the tendon, and the needle should be slightly withdrawn, aspirated, and reinjected.
- **Needle size and dosage:** A 25- to 27-gauge needle may be used; a preparation of 0.5 mL of corticosteroid with 0.5 mL of anesthetic can be mixed, with half to all of this suspension injected.
- **Efficacy:** Recent Cochrane review found efficacy in adults (42).

Trochanteric Bursitis

- **Indications:** Recalcitrant trochanteric bursitis
- **Clinical anatomy/landmarks:** The key landmark is the greater trochanteric prominence; most bursitis is posterosuperior to this prominence. This prominence is best appreciated with the patient in a lateral decubitus position.

- **Technique:** The point of maximal tenderness is palpated. The needle should be inserted perpendicular to the skin and slowly advanced to the greater trochanter; depth of penetration may vary from 0.5–1.5 inches (up to 4–5 inches if there is significant adipose tissue). If paresthesias are appreciated, the needle should be withdrawn and reinserted laterally. Once bone is appreciated, the needle should be slightly withdrawn, aspiration should be performed, and then gentle *peppering* of the bursa is performed.
- **Needle size and dosage:** A 21- to 23-gauge needle, 1.5 inches long, should be used; 1 mL of corticosteroid with 3–5 mL of local anesthetic should be used.
- **Efficacy:** Small trials of palpation-guided corticosteroid injection indicate it is a safe and effective treatment (48,54).

Knee Joint

- **Indications:** Inflammatory or degenerative arthritis, aspiration of joint fluid
- **Clinical anatomy/landmarks:** Patellar tendon and medial and lateral joint lines
- **Technique:** Injections are most easily administered through the lateral joint line recess just lateral to the patellar tendon. This injection can be accomplished in the seated position or in the supine position with the knee flexed to approximately 90 degrees. The portal for injection should be identified as lateral and inferior to the patellar tendon border at the level of the joint line. The needle is directed toward the center of the knee, medially, posteriorly, and slightly cephalad. Depth of insertion is approximately 1 inch. One should be careful to ensure needle clearance of the fat pad and avoid injecting the anterior cruciate ligament; there should be a free flow to the injection, with any resistance prompting needle repositioning. An alternative injection but common technique is to inject the patient in the supine position in the suprapatellar space. This space is most commonly reached by identifying a portal one fingerbreadth superior and one fingerbreadth lateral to the superolateral aspect of the patella. Multiple other locations have been proposed and studied (see accuracy below).
- **Needle size and dosage:** A 22- to 25-gauge, 1.5-inch needle is recommended; 1 mL of corticosteroid should be mixed with 2–3 mL of anesthetic.
- **Accuracy:** Several small studies have shown variable outcomes. Lateral mid-patella is favored over anteromedial or anterolateral lateral with accuracy of 93% (27), with another recent study (15) showing similar results (56% with medial mid-patella, 85% with all others).
- **Efficacy:** Short-term benefit reported in multiple studies/reviews for corticosteroid injection for osteoarthritis of the knee (5,24).

Iliotibial Band Syndrome

- **Indications:** Recalcitrant iliotibial band friction syndrome at the knee

- **Clinical anatomy/landmarks:** The key landmark is the lateral femoral epicondyle, which is the site of repetitive irritation. The bursa lies deep to the iliotibial band just above the lateral condyle of the femur.
- **Technique:** The injection may be performed in a seated position or in a lateral decubitus position. The knee should be flexed to 90 degrees, and the maximal point of tenderness identified; the intent is to inject between the epicondyle and the iliotibial band. The skin is entered to the point of maximal tenderness and angled posteriorly and slightly medially. The needle is inserted to a depth of 1/4–3/8 inch just above the periosteum. If bone is contacted, withdraw the needle very slightly, aspirate, and then inject. Additionally, it is important not to inject the iliotibial band itself; if resistance is felt with injection, withdraw, redirect the needle, aspirate, and inject.
- **Needle size and dosage:** A 25- to 27-gauge, 1-inch needle is recommended, with 0.5 mL of corticosteroid with 0.5–1 mL of anesthetic.
- **Efficacy:** There are limited data indicating improvement at 2 weeks with corticosteroid injection (14,21).

Pes Anserine Bursitis

- **Indications:** Pes anserine bursitis
- **Clinical anatomy/landmarks:** Medial aspect of the proximal tibia, where the sartorius, gracilis, and semitendinosus insert. The pes is identified by making the patient strongly flex the knee against resistance. The bursa is found as an area of tenderness deep to the insertion.
- **Technique:** This injection can be administered in the supine or seated position; the authors prefer the seated position. The objective of the injection is to slip the needle between the tibia and the pes tendons. The skin should be entered just lateral to the point of maximal tenderness, with the needle angled posteriorly and medially. Depth of insertion is approximately 1/4 inch. If resistance is felt with the injection, withdraw, redirect the needle, aspirate, and inject.
- **Needle size and dosage:** A 25-gauge needle, 1 inch long, is recommended, with 0.5 mL of corticosteroid and 0.5–1 mL of anesthetic.
- **Efficacy:** Limited studies. May need accurate diagnosis by ultrasound for improved efficacy as referred pain from medial compartment arthritis also presents at pes anserinus (66).

Ankle Joint

- **Indications:** Diagnostic injection for synovitis; chronic capsulitis. Can be used to treat soft tissue impingement.
- **Clinical anatomy/landmarks:** There is a readily identifiable hollow between the medial malleolus and the articulation between the tibia and the talus. This area is readily located just medial to the anterior tibial tendon.
- **Technique:** The patient may be seated or lying supine with a towel beneath the knee. Distraction of the ankle can be

accomplished by an assistant. The skin is entered just medial to the anterior tibial tendon in the anteromedial recess; depth of insertion is approximately 0.5–1 inch.

- **Needle size and dosage:** A 25-gauge needle, 1–1.5 inches long, may be used; 0.5 mL of corticosteroid may be injected with 3–5 mL of anesthetic.
- **Accuracy:** 77%–100% using either anteromedial or anterolateral approach (22,30,64).
- **Efficacy:** Improvement is short term as with other intra-articular injections. Pain relief at 2 months may predict long-term benefit (61).

Plantar Fascia

- **Indications:** Recalcitrant plantar fasciitis
- **Clinical anatomy/landmarks:** Key landmarks include the medial calcaneal tubercle and the junction between the skin of the sole of foot and the skin of the lower extremity.
- **Technique:** This examination is best administered with the patient in the supine position. The needle is inserted medial to lateral toward the point of maximal tenderness, which is generally at the plantar insertion into the medial calcaneal tubercle. Avoid injecting through the plantar fat pad because this may induce fat pad atrophy. If pain is felt radiating across the heel or into the arch or there is excessive resistance, withdraw, change the angle slightly, and reinsert.
- **Needle size and dosage:** A 25- to 27-gauge needle, 1–1.5 inches long, may be used; 1 mL of corticosteroid may be injected with 1–2 mL of anesthetic.
- **Efficacy:** Effective in short term, but outcome long term may be improved with ultrasound guidance (11,57). Harms may outweigh benefits of corticosteroid injection (32).

Morton Neuroma

- **Indications:** Morton neuroma is thought to be the result of perineural fibrosis of an interdigital nerve.
- **Clinical anatomy/landmarks:** Key landmarks are the metatarsal heads.
- **Technique:** The point of maximal discomfort should be identified between the metatarsal heads; the neuroma is typically between and slightly plantar to the metatarsal heads. The patient should be placed in the supine position with a pillow under the knee so that the foot can be slightly plantarflexed. The nerve is approached from a dorsal approach, with the needle entering between the metatarsal heads, advanced perpendicular through the transverse tarsal ligament. The depth of insertion is approximately 0.5 inch. A giving way can be felt as the needle passes through the ligament.
- **Needle size and dosage:** A 25-gauge 1-inch needle is appropriate; 0.5 mL of corticosteroid is mixed with 1–2 mL of local anesthetic.
- **Efficacy:** A recent small study indicated short-term improvement with ultrasound-guided corticosteroid injection (34).

Myofascial Trigger Points

- **Indications:** Diagnosis and treatment of myofascial trigger points
- **Clinical anatomy/landmarks:** Dependent on location of trigger points; knowledge of local anatomy is recommended, as well as knowledge of common trigger point sites and their referral patterns.
- **Technique:** Trigger points are often palpable as fusiform firm nodules running parallel to the fibers in a muscle. The nodule should be identified and trapped with the fingers of the nondominant hand. After a sterile preparation, the skin is penetrated in a perpendicular fashion with the needle into the center of the trigger point. Occasionally, a local twitch response may be noted where the muscle twitches as the center of the trigger point is entered.
- **Needle size and dosage:** A 25- to 27-gauge needle, 1–1.5 inches long, is used; 1–5 mL of anesthetic is used for injection.
- **Efficacy:** Unclear (51,56)

REFERENCES

1. Altay T, Günal I, Oztürk H. Local injection treatment for lateral epicondylitis. *Clin Orthop Relat Res.* 2002;(398):127–30.
2. Anderson BC. *Office Orthopedics for Primary Care: Diagnosis and Treatment.* 2nd ed. Philadelphia (PA): WB Saunders; 1999. 342 p.
3. Bailie DS, Ellenbecker TS. Severe chondrolysis after shoulder arthroscopy: a case series. *J Shoulder Elbow Surg.* 2009;18(5):742–7.
4. Barr S, Cerisola FL, Blanchard V. Effectiveness of corticosteroid injections compared with physiotherapeutic interventions for lateral epicondylitis: a systematic review. *Physiotherapy.* 2009;95(4):251–65.
5. Bellamy N, Campbell J, Robinson V, Gee T, Bourne R, Wells G. Intraarticular corticosteroid for treatment of osteoarthritis of the knee. *Cochrane Database Syst Rev.* 2006;19(2):CD005328.
6. Bisbinas I, Belthur M, Said HG, Green M, Learmonth DJ. Accuracy of needle placement in ACJ injections. *Knee Surg Sports Traumatol Arthrosc.* 2006;14(8):762–5.
7. Buchbinder R, Green S, Youd JM. Corticosteroid injections for shoulder pain. *Cochrane Database Syst Rev.* 2003;(1):CD004016.
8. Carette S, Moffet H, Tardif J, et al. Intraarticular corticosteroids, supervised physiotherapy, or a combination of the two in the treatment of adhesive capsulitis of the shoulder: a placebo-controlled trial. *Arthritis Rheum.* 2003;48(3):829–38.
9. Charalambous CP, Tryfonidis M, Sadiq S, Hirst P, Paul A. Septic arthritis following intra-articular steroid injection of the knee — a survey of current practice regarding antiseptic technique used during intra-articular steroid injection of the knee. *Clin Rheumatol.* 2003;22(6):386–90.
10. Cole BJ, Schumacher HR Jr. Injectable corticosteroids in modern practice. *J Am Acad Orthop Surg.* 2005;13(1):37–46.
11. Crawford F, Atkins D, Young P, Edwards J. Steroid injection for heel pain: evidence of short-term effectiveness. A randomized controlled trial. *Rheumatology (Oxford).* 1999;38(10):974–7.
12. Cunnington J, Marshall N, Hide G, et al. A randomized, double-blind, controlled study of ultrasound-guided corticosteroid injection into the joint of patients with inflammatory arthritis. *Arthritis Rheum.* 2010;62(7):1862–9.

13. Dogramaci Y, Kalici A, Savaş N, Duman G, Yanat AN. Treatment of lateral epicondylitis using three different local injection modalities: a randomized prospective clinical trial. *Arch Orthop Trauma Surg.* 2009;129(10):1409–14.

14. Ellis R, Hing W, Reid D. Iliotibial band friction syndrome — a systematic review. *Man Ther.* 2007;12(3):200–8.

15. Esenyel C, Demirhan M, Esenyel M, et al. Comparison of four different intra-articular injection sites in the knee: a cadaver study. *Knee Surg Sports Traumatol Arthrosc.* 2007;15(5):573–7.

16. Eustace JA, Brophy DP, Gibney RP, Bresnihan B, FitzGerald O. Comparison of the accuracy of steroid placement with clinical outcome in patients with shoulder symptoms. *Ann Rheum Dis.* 1997;56(1):59–63.

17. Gaujoux-Viala C, Dougados M, Gossec L. Efficacy and safety of steroid injections for shoulder and elbow tendonitis: a meta-analysis of randomised controlled trials. *Ann Rheum Dis.* 2009;68(12):1843–9.

18. Genovese MC. Joint and soft-tissue injection. A useful adjuvant to systemic and local treatment. *Postgrad Med.* 1998;103(2):125–134.

19. Goh GJ, Over KE, Daroszewska A, Whitehouse GH, Bucknall RC. The value of arthrography in steroid injection of the shoulder joint. *Br J Rheumatol.* 1997;36(6):709–10.

20. Gruson KI, Ruchelsman DE, Zuckerman JD. Subacromial corticosteroid injections. *J Shoulder Elbow Surg.* 2008;17(1 Suppl):118S–30S.

21. Gunter P, Schwellnus MP. Local corticosteroid injection in iliotibial band friction syndrome in runners: a randomised controlled trial. *Br J Sports Med.* 2004;38(3):269–72.

22. Heidari N, Pichler W, Grechenig S, Grechenig W, Weinberg AM. Does the anteromedial or anterolateral approach alter the rate of joint puncture in injection of the ankle? A cadaver study. *J Bone Joint Surg Br.* 2010;92(1):176–8.

23. Henkus HE, Cobben LP, Coerkamp EG, Nelissen RG, van Arkel ER. The accuracy of subacromial injections: a prospective randomized magnetic resonance imaging study. *Arthroscopy.* 2006;22(3):277–82.

24. Hepper CT, Halvorson JJ, Duncan ST, Gregory AJ, Dunn WR, Spindler KP. The efficacy and duration of intra-articular corticosteroid injection for knee osteoarthritis: a systematic review of level I studies. *J Am Acad Orthop Surg.* 2009;17(10):638–46.

25. Hossain S, Jacobs LG, Hashmi R. The long-term effectiveness of steroid injections in primary acromioclavicular joint arthritis: a five-year prospective study. *J Shoulder Elbow Surg.* 2008;17(4):535–8.

26. Huisstede BM, Hoogvliet P, Randsdorp MS, Glerum S, van Middelkoop M, Koes BW. Carpal tunnel syndrome. Part I: effectiveness of nonsurgical treatments — a systematic review. *Arch Phys Med Rehabil.* 2010;91(7):981–1004.

27. Jackson DW, Evans NA, Thomas BM. Accuracy of needle placement into the intra-articular space of the knee. *J Bone Joint Surg Am.* 2002;84-A(9):1522–7.

28. Jones A, Regan M, Ledingham J, Pattrick M, Manhire A, Doherty M. Importance of placement of intra-articular steroid injections. *BMJ.* 1993;307(6915):1329–30.

29. Kennedy JC, Willis RB. The effects of local steroids on tendons: a biomechanical and microscopic correlative study. *Am J Sports Med.* 1976;4(1):11–21.

30. Khosla S, Thiele R, Baumhauer JF. Ultrasound guidance for intra-articular injections of the foot and ankle. *Foot Ankle Int.* 2009;30(9):886–90.

31. Klippel JH, Dieppe PA. *Practical Rheumatology.* Baltimore (MD): Mosby; 1997.

32. Landorf KB, Menz HB. Plantar heel pain and fasciitis. *Clin Evid.* 2008;1111.

33. Lorbach O, Anagnostakos K, Scherf C, Seil R, Kohn D, Pape D. Nonoperative management of adhesive capsulitis of the shoulder: oral cortisone application versus intra-articular cortisone injections. *J Shoulder Elbow Surg.* 2010;19(2):172–9.

34. Marcovic M, Crichton K, Read JW, Lam P, Slater HK. Effectiveness of ultrasound-guided corticosteroid injection in the treatment of Morton's neuroma. *Foot Ankle Int.* 2008;29(5):483–7.

35. Marshall S, Tardif G, Ashworth N. Local corticosteroid injection for carpal tunnel syndrome. *Cochrane Database Syst Rev.* 2007;2:CD001554.

36. Mathews PV, Glousman RE. Accuracy of subacromial injection: anterolateral versus posterior approach. *J Shoulder Elbow Surg.* 2005;14(2):145–8.

37. Murray RJ, Pearson JC, Coombs GW, et al. Outbreak of invasive methicillin-resistant Staphylococcus aureus infection associated with acupuncture and joint injection. *Infect Control Hosp Epidemiol.* 2008;29(9):859–65.

38. Paluska AS. Indications, contraindications, and overview for aspirating or injecting a joint or related structure. In: Pfenninger JL, editor. *The Clinics Atlas of Office Procedures: Joint Injection Techniques.* Vol. 5 (4). Philadelphia: WB Saunders; 2002.

39. Partington PF, Broome GH. Diagnostic injection around the shoulder: hit or miss? A cadaveric study of injection accuracy. *J Shoulder Elbow Surg.* 1998;7(2):147–50.

40. Peterson C, Hodler J. Evidence-based radiology (part 2): is there sufficient research to support the use of therapeutic injections into the peripheral joints? *Skeletal Radiol.* 2010;39(1):11–8.

41. Peters-Veluthamaningal C, van der Windt DA, Winters JC, Meyboom-de Jong B. Corticosteroid injection for de Quervain's tenosynovitis. *Cochrane Database Syst Rev.* 2009;3:CD005616.

42. Peters-Veluthamaningal C, van der Windt DA, Winters JC, Meyboom-de Jong B. Corticosteroid injection for trigger finger in adults. *Cochrane Database Syst Rev.* 2009;1:CD005617.

43. Peters-Veluthamaningal C, Winters JC, Groenier KH, Meyboom-de Jong B. Randomised controlled trial of local corticosteroid injections for carpal tunnel syndrome in general practice. *BMC Fam Pract.* 2010;11:54.

44. Pfenninger JL. Joint and soft tissue aspiration and injection. In: Pfenninger JL, Fowler GC, editors. *Procedures for Primary Care Physicians.* St. Louis: Mosby; 1994.

45. Pichler W, Weinberg AM, Grechenig S, Tesch NP, Heidari N, Grechenig W. Intra-articular injection of the acromioclavicular joint. *J Bone Joint Surg Br.* 2009;91(12):1638–40.

46. Porat S, Leupold JA, Burnett KR, Nottage WM. Reliability of non-imaging-guided glenohumeral joint injection through rotator interval approach in patients undergoing diagnostic MR arthrography. *AJR Am J Roentgenol.* 2008;191(3):W96–9.

47. Rapley JH, Beavis RC, Barber FA. Glenohumeral chondrolysis after shoulder arthroscopy with continuous bupivacaine infusion. *Arthroscopy.* 2010;26(4):439–40.

48. Rowand M, Chambliss ML, Mackler L. Clinical inquiries. How should you treat trochanteric bursitis? *J Fam Pract.* 2009;58(9):494–500.

49. Safran MR. Injections. In: Safran MR, McKeag DB, Van Camp SP, editors. *Manual of Sports Medicine.* Philadelphia: Lippincott-Raven Publishers; 1998.

50. Saunders S, Cameron G. *Injection Techniques in Orthopedic and Sports Medicine.* Philadelphia (PA): WB Saunders; 1997. 160 p.

51. Scott NA, Guo B, Barton PM, Gerwin RD. Trigger point injections for chronic non-malignant musculoskeletal pain: a systematic review. *Pain Med.* 2009;10(1):54–69.

52. Sethi PM, Kingston S, Elattrache N. Accuracy of anterior intra-articular injection of the glenohumeral joint. *Anthroscopy.* 2005;21(1):77–80.

53. Slotkoff A, Clauw D, Nashel D. Effect of soft tissue corticosteroid injection on glucose control in diabetics. *Arthritis Rheum.* 1994;37 (Suppl 9):s347.

54. Stephens MB, Beutler AI, O'Connor FG. Musculoskeletal injections: a review of the evidence. *Am Fam Physician*. 2008;78(8):971–6.

55. Tallia AF, Cardone DA. Diagnostic and therapeutic injection of the shoulder region. *Am Fam Physician*. 2003;67(6):1271–8.

56. Tough EA, White AR, Cummings M, Richards SH, Campbell JL. Acupuncture and dry needling in the management of myofascial trigger point pain: a systematic review and meta-analysis of randomised controlled trials. *Eur J Pain*. 2009;13(1):3–10.

57. Tsai WC, Hsu CC, Chen CP, Chen MJ, Yu TY, Chen YJ. Plantar fasciitis treated with local steroid injection: comparison between sonographic and palpation guidance. *J Clin Ultrasound*. 2006;34(1):12–6.

58. Turner JL, McKeag DB. Complications of joint aspirations and injections. In: Phenninger JL, editor. *The Clinics Atlas of Office Procedures: Joint Injection Techniques*. Philadelphia: WB Saunders Company; 2002. p. 433–43.

59. van der Heijden GJ, van der Windt DA, Kleijnen J, Koes BW, Bouter LM. Steroid injections for shoulder disorders: a systematic review of randomized clinical trials. *Br J Gen Pract*. 1996;46(406):309–16.

60. von Essen R, Savolainen HA. Bacterial infection following intra-articular injection. A brief review. *Scand J Rheumatol*. 1989;18(1):7–12.

61. Ward ST, Williams PL, Purkayastha S. Intra-articular corticosteroid injections in the foot and ankle: a prospective 1-year follow-up investigation. *J Foot Ankle Surg*. 2008;47(2):138–44.

62. Weinberg AM, Pichler W, Grechenig S, Tesch NP, Heidari N, Grechenig W. Frequency of successful intra-articular puncture of the sternoclavicular joint: a cadaver study. *Scand J Rheumatol*. 2008;38(5):396–8.

63. White RD. Supplies and equipment needed for joint injection. In: Pfenninger JL, editor. *The Clinics Atlas of Office Procedures: Joint Injection Techniques*. Vol 5(4). Philadelphia: WB Saunders; 2002. p. 403–12.

64. Wisniewski SJ, Smith J, Patterson DG, Carmichael SW, Pawlina W. Ultrasound-guided versus nonguided tibiotalar joint and sinus tarsi injections: a cadaveric study. *MR*. 2010;2(4):277–81.

65. Yamakado K. The targeting accuracy of subacromial injection to the shoulder: an arthrographic evaluation. *Arthroscopy*. 2002;18(8):887–91.

66. Yoon HS, Kim SE, Suh YR, Seo Y, Kim HA. Correlation between ultrasonographic findings and the response to corticosteroid injection in pes anserinus tendinobursitis syndrome in knee osteoarthritis patients. *J Korean Med Sci*. 2005;20(1):109–12.

75 Footwear and Orthotics

Jay Dicharry and Eric M. Magrum

FOOTWEAR

- The goal of this chapter is to educate clinicians on current footwear design, to enable them to select beneficial aspects of footwear as part of a patient's comprehensive rehabilitation plan. Most of what is known and prescribed with regard to footwear recommendations is based on "running lore" and the rapidly changing footwear model revisions driven by industry. There has been very little independent research done to prove or disprove footwear claims, and the lack of prospective footwear studies limits our knowledge base. At the time of this writing, there is a revolution in footwear design by most manufacturers due to elevated interest in this field as well as the recent focus on barefoot and minimal shoe design. Clinicians will have better results recommending types of shoes based on construction and features over specific model designations.

- The basis of overuse injury risk lies within the balance of intrinsic and extrinsic factors. Running shoes are a modifiable extrinsic factor. To assess proper footwear selection, the athlete's intrinsic factors (alignment, stability, flexibility, and imbalances) must be assessed to determine the best functional outcome (60).

- Despite the lack of conclusive data on how to best match the runner to shoe type, shoe design clearly has an effect. Running mechanics can be influenced by shoe midsole stiffness/geometry as demonstrated in studies where subjects ran in shoes with varied specific stiffness/geometry (30,51,57,58,72,77).

- Incorrect footwear choices can exacerbate or cause lower extremity dysfunction, while ideal footwear can help in prevention or even speed healing due to decreased tissue stress on impaired structures (4,33,57,70,81,89).

- The goal of any shoe/foot interface is to allow shock attenuation and functional stability about the foot's three-dimensional motions of pronation and supination throughout the stance phase of gait and provide a proper support for the propulsion phase of the gait cycle (4).

Shoe Construction and Anatomy

- Upper — Usually made of highly breathable fabric to minimize heat buildup. May be reinforced by Gore-Tex or similar fabric for water resistance. Typically includes a heel counter — plastic molding wraps around the heel that are thought to control pronation at the rear foot. Achilles tab cutouts in the rear can be used to decrease friction on the Achilles complex.

- Lacing — Various lacing techniques are available to minimize pressure or increase stability and tension on the foot.

- Midsole — Functional part of the shoe. The midsole is usually made up of a mixture of ethyl vinyl acetate (EVA) and polyurethane. EVA has the advantage of being light in weight and available in multiple densities so that the manufacturer can manipulate the amount of support for a given shoe type. Polyurethane is heavier but longer lasting. Most shoes use a combination of the two to achieve the desired balance between weight and cushioning. Most shoe companies have developed a trademark insert such as Air, Gel, Grid, Hydro Flow, Torsion, Roller Bar, Wave, or Adeprene. Their goal is to provide cushioning, dissipate stress, and increase durability, while keeping weight low. Increased density materials are commonly used on the medial aspect of the stability and motion control midsoles in an attempt to control pronation.

- Lastings — The lasting sits on top of the midsole and is glued or stitched depending on the stability requirements. The following are types of lastings: board — increases torsional rigidity; slip or California — favors cushion and flexibility; combination — board last rear, slip last in the forefoot.

- Insole or sock liner — Thin layer of cushion material, mostly to smooth the surface of the foot. The insole does not provide any functional stability to the shoe and usually breaks down in its cushioning properties with 1 week. This is removed if the individual uses orthotics or over-the-counter inserts.

- Outsole — Most current shoe models are a mixture of carbon rubber for firm support and durability and blown rubber, which is softer and provides increased cushioning. Flex grooves in the outsole influence how the midsole deforms during loading (more flex grooves yield a more compressible midsole).

- Last or shape — This is different from the lasting and is not a separate component of the shoe, but the design shape on which the shoe is built. A straight last will provide more contact for a flatter foot and may increase torsional rigidity of the shoe, whereas a curved last will better fit the shape of a higher arched foot while decreasing torsional rigidity. A semi-curved last is a popular shape for the top-selling stability category of shoes and has elements of both.

- Geometry — The angle of the posterolateral aspect of the shoe (heel bevel angle) is typically beveled (reduced) or even increased to vary the lever arm of the shoe. The toe spring refers to the flex placement of the forefoot.

Common Descriptors of the Five Shoe Types (25)

- Motion control: Board lasting, dense midsole, straight last, rear and forefoot postings, for overpronators and heavy runners
- Stability: Combination last, semi-curved shape, dense midsole, usually only rearfoot posting, usually forefoot cushion, for mild pronators and light runners
- Cushion: Slip lasting, soft midsole, curved shape last, cushion in the heel and forefoot, mostly for supinators
- Trail: Usually a stability shoe for increased support on uneven surface; carbon rubber for additional durability
- Racing flats: Light thin midsole with little to no posting

Shoe Selection

- Shoe selection for an individual athlete is an art, because the literature is limited in its ability to assist providers. In light of the lack of evidence-based information to assign shoe type to a runner, clinicians have traditionally used foot type to guide shoe prescriptions. Although the efficacy of this approach in either reducing or mitigating injury has not been demonstrated, this technique remains one of the most commonly used strategies in the United States.
- Traditional beliefs about shoe selection use three different shoe categories (cushioned, stability, and motion control) for each respective foot type (cavus, neutral, and planus foot type). This hierarchy is widespread among shoe manufacturers, media, stores, and clinicians.
- This type of shoe prescription can be done using objective tests such as navicular drop or arch index, or more subjectively using the wet foot test, during which the athlete, with a wet foot, steps across an absorbent surface to observe the high or low arch alignment of the foot.
- Foot structure plays a significant role in the quantity of force transmitted to bone and soft tissues (4). The rigid arch of a cavus foot, while stable, passes on a significant amount of stress up the kinetic chain (4). Thus, traditionally, cavus foot types are shod with a curved shaped last with slip lasting, a soft midsole, and no medial posting (25,73) with a goal to increase shock absorption. Conversely, the flexible or planus foot dissipates considerable vertical force loads inside the foot structure and is commonly thought to benefit from additional stability control from the shoe (4). Planus feet are traditionally shod with a straight last, board lasting, firm heel counter, multidensity midsole, and medial heel posting (25,73).
- In this traditional approach, the athlete's foot type should guide your recommendation toward the ideal last configuration with the goal of increasing shock absorption

of the cavus (high) hypomobile arch, increasing stability of the planus (low) arch, or promoting the mechanics of the neutral foot.

- Despite their wide use, these current conventions for assigning stability categories are likely simplistic and are not successful in preventing pain and injury in runners (74,87).
- A critical look at the literature reveals that the clinical efficacy of typical running shoe construction (elevated heel height with pronation control systems) is not as commonly accepted. Their effect on running injury rates, enjoyment, performance, osteoarthritis risk, physical activity levels, and overall athlete health and well-being remain unknown, and they may in fact have potential to cause harm. The prescription of shoe categories to runners is not evidence based (67).
- Peak pronation in the running gait cycle occurs after heel off (20). Thus, at the time of maximum foot deformation, pronation control systems used in typical running shoe designs are not in contact with the ground to limit foot pronation.
- In light of the lack of evidence-based information to assign shoe type to a runner, the clinician is encouraged to combine clinical evaluation of a runner's structural alignment, flexibility, and intrinsic muscular stability with dynamic walking and running assessments to identify the runner's unique needs regarding footwear. Once the runner's individual needs have been identified, the clinician can recommend footwear that contains specific design aspects for that runner's needs.
- The experience of the runner with their current footwear is valuable. If they have had success with a given shoe, continue its use, or suggest other brands/models within a specific category to improve comfort. Different models feature subtle differences in construction/shape that may fit the individual's foot contour better. A subjective impression of improved comfort yields improved function with the individual's foot.

What to Look for When Buying Shoes

- Athlete structural alignment, flexibility, and muscle control
- Weight: Typical running shoes are made for a 160-lb male and a 125-lb female. Runner weight significantly above or under this range may impact selection or longevity.
- Lightweight shoes: It is speculated that there is energy savings from lighter shoes.
- Previous pathology and wear patterns
- Try on shoes in early evening due to the foot swelling during the day.
- One-half inch between longest toe and the shoe
- Check to ensure that the flex point of the toe spring is underneath the metatarsal heads.
- Adequate width (most shoes are a size D). A wide toe box allows the forefoot to spread out during contact. Narrow shoes limit this normal motion of the foot and may alter foot shape.
- If using orthotics for stability purposes, use board or California lasting to provide a stable base for the orthotic.

■ Arch cookies should not be used to make up for poor fit because the arch is not a weight-bearing part of the foot. It should be allowed to move as needed.

Barefoot Running and Minimal Footwear Design

■ Recent work has highlighted the differences between barefoot running and shoes. Barefoot running typically results in a more plantarflexed ankle at contact and reduction/elimination of the impact peak component of the ground reaction force (GRF) and a decreased loading rate (39,46,80).

■ Barefoot running results in a shorter stride length and increased cadence compared to shod running (39,80). These temporal spatial changes in stride length act to lower joint torques across the board, but they do not alone explain the significant decrease in hip rotation, knee varus, and sagittal plane knee torques (39).

■ The previously discussed studies do not clearly state that barefoot is "better" than shod running, but that shoes allow the runner to adopt a gait style that is different from barefoot and potentially shift stresses to the body in the wrong direction (19).

■ There is an emerging category of "natural running" shoes that feature minimal heel–toe drops (typically ~0–4 mm) to achieve a contact style more similar to barefoot running (forefoot/midfoot) than the heel contact style observed in traditional elevated heel shoes (18,80).

■ New "natural running" shoes feature firmer midsoles to improve proprioceptive feedback to maximize the elastic recoil of the body's connective tissues.

■ Traditional running shoes are built with a 2:1 ratio, where the rearfoot is twice as high as the forefoot. This impacts contact style and muscle activation. Heel elevation during stance places the ankle joint in a position where proprioception is inherently poor (76). Further, this translates loading toward the forefoot, which creates a quadriceps-dominant firing pattern above the gluteus maximus, which results in postural changes in the runner (75).

■ Supporters of existing footwear design argue that reducing the heel heights of existing shoes would spark a number of lower leg (specifically Achilles) injuries. However, several studies have shown no decrease in stress to the Achilles with elevated heel shoes, with one study finding an increase in injuries with elevated heels (21,37,66).

Special Considerations

■ Midsole characteristics are the primary determinant of the rate of loading imposed during initial ground contact (50). Midsole stiffness has a marked effect on proprioception, illustrating that peripheral sensory information is a variable in performance (42).

■ Too much cushioning causes the runner to land with increased limb stiffness and can lead to instability due to less proprioceptive feedback for stability (4,8).

■ Shoes with a softer durometer midsole allowed significantly increased pronation and total rearfoot movement when compared to medium or hard midsoles (12).

■ Functional stability of the foot requires effective muscle contraction, coordination, and firing patterns. Fatigued muscle firing patterns cause increased peak strain on the lower extremity, thus leading to injury. Patellofemoral pain syndrome, osteoarthritis, iliotibial band syndrome, and tibial stress syndrome have been linked to abnormal muscle firing patterns (1,4,35,38,78).

■ Proper footwear has been shown to increase internal stability and decrease onset time to achieve stabilization in the low back via postural changes (61).

■ Race flats and spikes: GRFs have been found to increase in race flats and spikes as compared to traditional running shoes. Thus, runners should adopt a gradual transition into race footwear prior to competition season to allow the body to acclimate to the increased stress (47).

■ Durability: Expect 300–500 miles or 3–6 months out of a pair of shoes prior to midsole break down. Midsoles lose 40% of their cushioning ability after 400–500 miles (65). Look to purchase new shoes when the midsole shows signs of compression, the outer sole shows signs of wear, or injury rate increases.

■ Shoe wear adaptations: Running in worn shoes caused increased stance time and kinematic adaptations but did not change force variables, suggesting that as shoe cushioning decreases, runners modify their patterns to maintain constant external loads (41).

■ Footwear cost: Low- and medium-cost running shoes in three brands tested provided the same (if not better) cushioning of plantar pressure as high-cost running shoes (13).

■ Despite claims, no manufacturer has successfully achieved energy return to the runner. Shoemakers have made functional gains in minimizing energy lost through lightweight alterations in materials (82).

■ Results of the majority of footwear studies apply to runners using a heel contact style. However, between 25% and 53% of runners do not use a heel contact style. High intrasubject variability in running pattern warrants further investigation (41).

■ Increases in ankle stability due to structural support and high collars have not been supported. However, a firm midsole will provide benefits in tactile sensitivity and proprioception, which increase foot position awareness and decrease time to initiation of intrinsic muscles (5,69)

■ The market continues to drive shoe trends. Current research does not indicate definitive benefits to specific shoe construction in those with a specific foot type or injury diagnosis. Changes in shoe construction induce alterations in gait pattern that vary from a barefoot running gait (42,57,89). This net effect makes it tough to discern whether the benefits are attributed to proprioceptive feedback to the runner or true shifts in biomechanical force as applied through the shoe. Prospective research into the effects of specific footwear components is needed to examine footwear's true effect on injury and performance in the running athlete.

ORTHOTICS

- Prescription custom foot orthoses are frequently used as part of a management strategy for the treatment of various lower quarter injuries in the athlete (79,86,90).
- Significant success treating many common lower quarter injuries with orthotic intervention has been demonstrated with multiple frequently referenced classic studies. James et al. (36) reported that 78% of runners were able to return to prior level of running following a knee injury with orthotic management. Donatelli et al. (22) reported that 96% of patients with knee pain, ankle pain, shin splints, or chondromalacia experienced pain relief and 70% were able to return to prior level of activity. Gross et al. (27) reported that 76% of long-distance runners had complete recovery or substantial improvement in a variety of lower quarter injuries with orthotic management. More recently, both Nigg et al. (56) and Nawoczenski et al. (54) agree that at least 70% of runners with lower extremity symptoms will show symptom reduction with orthotic use.

Goals of Orthotic Management

- The classic balanced foot orthosis is aimed to allow the subtalar joint to function near and around its neutral position by maintaining the angular anatomic relationships of the forefoot to the rearfoot and the rearfoot to the ground and to control functional pathomechanics in the lower quarter.
- An orthotic device should alter foot function with the expectation that it will control excessive movement of the foot through the stance phase of gait, through stimulation of the somatosensory system, to promote overall biomechanical efficiency and reduce abnormal tissue stress (14,48).

Indications/Effects

- Numerous clinicians and authors have proposed various indications for the rationale to prescribe custom biomechanical foot orthoses.
- Support and correction of rearfoot and forefoot intrinsic deformities
- Reduce the frequency of lower quarter injuries, by altering applied tissue stresses (22,27,36)
- Support or control range of motion (43,48,54,64)
- Treatment of postural dysfunction caused by foot abnormalities (7)
- Improve sensory feedback and proprioception (7,48,53,56)
- Dissipate pathologic GRFs and improve shock absorption (43,56)

- Improve neuromuscular responses (43,55,56)
- Redistribute plantar weight-bearing forces (23,48)
- Improve lower extremity biomechanics/kinematics:
  - Decrease amount of pronation, reduce maximal velocity of pronation, reduce time to maximal pronation, and decrease total rearfoot motion (40,48,59)
  - Significant orthotic effects shown for rotation from heel contact to peak tibial internal rotation and in the coupling relationship between tibial transverse rotation and calcaneal inversion/eversion (54,85)
- **Electromyography changes:** A recent systematic review concluded that foot orthoses increase activation of the tibialis anterior and peroneus longus and may alter lower back muscle activation. However, there were substantial limitations in the data presented in the majority of studies reviewed (52,53).
- **Prevention:** A recent systematic review concluded that a few studies showed moderate or large beneficial effects of orthotics in preventing injuries. Customized semirigid orthotics have moderate to large beneficial effects in treating and preventing plantar fasciitis and posterior tibial stress fractures and small to moderate effects in treating patellofemoral pain syndrome (34).
- **Kinematic/kinetic changes:** A recent study by MacLean et al. (49) concluded that, in a group of runners, custom foot orthoses influenced several variables during the loading phase. The study revealed significant decreases in vertical loading rate, maximum rearfoot eversion velocity, and ankle inversion angular impulse during the loading phase with custom foot orthosis intervention. All of these variables occur in the initial 50% of the stance phase and have been associated with running injuries (49). Kinematic studies have reported small changes in foot and lower extremity rotation patterns that may initially seem inconsequential, but when considered over time and repetition, even these small changes may have a positive impact.

Clinical Conditions

- **Patellofemoral pain syndrome:** A recent systematic review summarized the evidence for the benefits of orthoses in patellofemoral pain syndrome. Limited evidence exists for greater improvements, with short-term improvements and patient perceived success with prefabricated orthotics. Limited evidence also exists that combining physical therapy and orthotics improves short- and long-term functional outcomes (6).
- **Plantar fasciitis:** A recent meta-analysis concluded that orthotic intervention provides short-, intermediate-, and long-term improvements in pain and foot function (45). A recent Cochrane review concluded that there is silver-level evidence for the use of orthotics for treatment of plantar fasciitis (31).
- **Posterior tibial tendon dysfunction:** Orthotic management has been described for all four stages based on progressive deformity and loss of forefoot/rearfoot flexibility (3,62).

A recent review concluded that there appears to be a general consensus in the literature to employ orthotic therapy in the treatment of posterior tibial tendon dysfunction (9).

■ **Lower quarter stress fracture:** Conflicting evidence exists for the use of orthotics in the prevention and management of stress fractures. However, studies using various orthotic devices have been shown to decreased incidence of metatarsal, tibial, and femoral stress fractures, with shock-absorbing materials as a primary component of the device (22,24,27,31,45). A recent Cochrane review concluded that shock-absorbing inserts reduce the incidence of stress fractures (71).

■ **Medial tibial stress syndrome:** A recent review of the literature concluded that there is some evidence for effective prevention of shin splints involves the use of shock-absorbing insoles. Previous reports have demonstrated significant clinical success treating shin splints with various orthotic devices. The American College of Foot & Ankle Orthopedics & Medicine's position statement is that custom foot orthoses can be used to treat the symptoms of shin splints and stabilize the etiology that causes the condition (9,22,27,36,62,84).

■ **Pes cavus:** Two recent Cochrane reviews investigated orthotic management in the cavus foot type. One study concluded that custom-made foot orthoses were significantly more beneficial than sham orthoses for treating chronic musculoskeletal foot pain associated with pes cavus in a variety of clinical populations. They also concluded that there is no evidence for any other type of intervention for the treatment or prevention of foot pain in people with a cavus foot type (10). The second Cochrane systematic review concluded that there is gold-level evidence for painful pes cavus (31).

■ **Flexible flatfoot:** The symptomatic adult hyperpronated foot has been shown to be effectively treated with various orthotic interventions regarding alleviating pain and deformity (3,10,62,68).

■ **Hallux valgus/hallux rigidus:** Custom orthoses have been clinically shown to redistribute weight, prevent excessive dorsiflexion forces, and improve gait transition with pathology of the great toe (11,17,28,53,62,83). A recent Cochrane review concluded that there is silver-level evidence for the use of custom orthotics with painful hallux valgus (31).

■ **Ankle sprain:** A recent review concluded that foot orthoses have been shown to have a positive influence on subjects who have recently experienced an ankle sprain and on subjects with chronic ankle instability. There is evidence that foot orthoses can influence multiple levels of neuromuscular control of the ankle. Improvements in somatosensory feedback and reduced muscular load seem to be the most viable mechanisms by which foot orthoses may positively affect patients with chronic ankle instability (29,68).

■ **Low back pain:** There is limited evidence for the use of orthotics with low back pain. One study reported that pain has been shown to be effectively treated with custom-fabricated foot orthoses following a comprehensive gait evaluation to address the pathomechanical process to decrease the degree of pain and rate of reoccurrence (16,26).

Types of Orthotics

■ **Accommodative:** A device designed with a primary goal of conforming to the individual's foot, allowing plantar-grade floor contact that permits forces to be distributed evenly to the foot. An accommodative device allows the foot to compensate and yields to abnormal foot forces. It is primarily prescribed to improve foot function and improve shock absorption for patients who are poor candidates for biomechanical devices secondary to congenital malformations, restrictions of foot or lower quarter motion, neuromuscular dysfunction, insensitive feet, or physiologic old age. Most devices are full length and total contact and made of materials such as Plastazote, PPT, Spenco, Pelite, Sorbathane, EVA, and Neoprene foam rubber.

■ **Biomechanical:** A custom prescription device fabricated specifically to address pathomechanical components of a lower quarter condition by controlling and resisting abnormal compensatory foot forces (62). The prescription aspect of the device involves clinical decision making for type of materials to be used for rigidity, length of the device (full, metatarsal, or sulcus), degree of correction/posting, and depth of heel seat. Decision making should be based on a comprehensive evaluation of active/passive foot and ankle range of motion, including joint mobility; neurovascular integrity; lower quarter biomechanics; and walking/running gait assessment.

■ **Temporary:** A device fabricated in the clinic primarily for the purpose of assessing the need/benefit for permanent device, unloading tissues for healing, or controlling hyperpronation. Common materials are Aquaplast, or orthopedic felt medial buttress, and navicular-sustentaculum tali support (88). The majority of studies have shown minimal differences regarding comfort and rearfoot kinematic differences between over-the-counter prefabricated inserts and custom biomechanical orthotics (28).

Selection

■ Specific aspects of subjective and objective examination guide clinical decision making for choosing the proper components of a prescription custom-fabricated orthosis.

■ Chief complaint/diagnosis, including stage, intensity, severity, and nature of the disorder

■ Control versus bias of subtalar motion

■ Mobility of the rearfoot, forefoot, midfoot, first ray: hypermobile → normal → hypomobile

■ Primary use of the orthosis: Type of street, sport, or dress shoe to be worn in helps to determine material selection and thickness. Specific sport and competition level also guide choice of components.

■ Physiologic, not chronologic, age: Older patients tolerate semirigid devices better, and younger patients tolerate more rigid management.

■ Need for shock absorption to dissipate GRFs

■ Weight of patient determines durometer (rigidity) of the orthotic.

- Neurologic or anatomic abnormality helps to determine the need for accommodation with cutouts, pressure distribution modifications, and material selection.

Casting

- Numerous techniques have been used to capture the foot for fabrication of a custom orthosis (2). Plaster casting may be preferable when capturing rearfoot to forefoot relationship is of prime importance for fabrication of a functional device (44). Weight-bearing measures of a loaded foot to determine forefoot posting have proven to be reliable, and further investigation into clinical application needs to be evaluated for orthotic prescription and fabrication (15). Neutral suspension casting with the foot positioned by holding the sulcus of the fourth and fifth toes obtained in prone or supine is the preferred method for a functional prescription foot orthoses (62).

- Plaster cast: The goal is to capture the relationship of the forefoot to rearfoot and reproduce the ideal position of the foot in midstance just prior to heel off.

- Compressive foam box: Partial weight-bearing technique most appropriate for accommodative devices, with the benefits of simplicity of use/clean up, but typically provides an inconsistent representation of forefoot relationship (62). A recent study quantified the differences between custom-made foot orthoses made from foam impressions and plaster impressions regarding contact area, plantar pressures, gait lines, and walking convenience. Foam box casting is preferable for the construction of accommodative and functional orthoses because it is easier to use, quicker, cleaner, and less expensive and because it leads to better walking convenience (28).

- Computer imaging/scanning: Another technique to capture the contour and shape of the foot for orthotic fabrication where the device is milled from an image or a positive model of the foot is created. The benefits of an imaging system are exactness of forefoot to rearfoot relationship for posting, image created in partial or non–weight bearing, and simplicity of use; the drawback is expense (62).

Requirements

- Requirements for successful orthotic intervention are based on patient- and condition-specific goals developed after a comprehensive subjective and objective evaluation as stated previously. The device must have certain components to increase treatment success and compliance.
- Conform precisely to all contours of foot, especially heel, calcaneal, and forefoot inclinations
- Rigid enough to maintain shape, contour, and angular relationships
- Control abnormal motion, allow normal motion, and provide proper sequencing/timing of motion
- Improve muscle function
- Able to withstand stress and wear

- Comfortable to assure compliance
- Adjustable
- End proximal to metatarsal heads
- Narrow enough to fit in shoes and allow first and fifth ray function

Specific Orthotic Components

- Specific components can be added to the device based on clinical goals for management of the lower quarter pathology, problem-solving information from the biomechanical evaluation, and assessment of the patient using the device.
- Heel lift to accommodate a leg length inequality or to unload the Achilles tendon
- Metatarsal head cut out to accommodate a rigid plantarflexed first ray
- Heel cushioning for increased shock absorption
- Metatarsal pads to redistribute weight from second to fourth metatarsal heads to first and fifth
- Morton's extension to redistribute weight from second to first metatarsal
- Rigid forefoot extension to limit mobility of great toe
- Toe crests can be added to prevent the toes from sliding back over the insole of the shoe and prevent clawing.
- Lateral rearfoot posting to unload medial knee compartment (degenerative joint disease/osteoarthritis)
- Highly inverted (Blake) orthotic when decreasing inversion moment and work at the rearfoot and increasing knee adduction and abduction moment are the treatment goals (90).

CONTROVERSIES, CONCLUSIONS, AND FURTHER RESEARCH

- In a review of the literature, Pratt (63) judged 40 orthotic-related articles using Sackett's "levels of evidence" criteria for scientific merit and concluded that the literature is rather weak, with only one study achieving a level of 2 and none achieving a level 1 qualification.
- There are several different classification systems of evaluating foot type that have shown poor interrater reliability and measurement accuracy, questioning the practical usefulness and validity (2,31,59,62).
- There is significant debate about whether functional kinematics and pathomechanics of the foot can be based principally on morphology. Mechanisms causing lower quarter injuries are poorly understood with very few adequate randomized controlled studies relating specific foot type or pathomechanics with injury incidence (2,59,62).
- Recent research has debated the assumptions that the rearfoot achieves subtalar joint neutral position near midstance in gait and the functional significance of rearfoot neutral (2,3,48,59).

- Studies have shown that static measurements in a classic biomechanical exam are poor predictors of dynamic foot motion (3,32,48,62).

- Research evaluating orthotic effectiveness in gait has substantial inadequacies including: various biomechanical assessment tools for gait analysis; nonstandardized orthotic device or footwear; modifications to shoe counter; motion analysis markers on shoe or skin; differences in calibration of equipment; and anecdotal descriptions of gait changes (3,23,48,62).

- The literature demonstrates a lack of controlled studies with consistently poor methodology, including variable orthotic prescription, patient presentation, fabrication of the orthoses, and outcome measurement tools (23,62).

- Overall, throughout the orthotic literature, there is a significant amount of inconclusive or conflicting data (2,3,23).

- The review of the literature highlights the fact that the current research can be greatly improved upon with further randomized controlled trials for specific measurable clinical outcomes to more effectively prescribe a custom orthotic device for treatment and prevention of lower quarter injuries in patients and athletes.

- A recent trend in the research proposes orthotic intervention to influence lower quarter dynamic function by increased afferent feedback from cutaneous receptors in the foot and minimizing muscle activity with the concept combining biomechanical control and proprioceptive feedback with custom-fabricated biomechanical orthotics to reduce tissue stress. As with previous work, more randomized controlled research must be completed to justify these hypotheses (7,54,56,59).

REFERENCES

1. Arroll B, Ellis-Pegler E, Edwards A, Sutcliffe G. Patellofemoral pain syndrome. A critical review of the clinical trials on nonoperative therapy. *Am J Sports Med.* 1997;25(2):207–12.

2. Ball KA, Afheldt MJ. Evolution of foot orthotics — part 1: coherent theory or coherent practice? *J Manipulative Physiol Ther.* 2002;25(2):116–24.

3. Ball KA, Afheldt MJ. Evolution of foot orthotics — part 2: research reshapes long-standing theory. *J Manipulative Physiol Ther.* 2002; 25(2):125–34.

4. Barnes RA, Smith PD. The role of footwear in minimizing lower limb injury. *J Sports Sci.* 1994;12(4):341–53.

5. Barrett JR, Tanji JL, Drake C, Fuller D, Kawasaki RI, Fenton RM. High- versus low-top shoes for the prevention of ankle sprains in basketball players. A prospective randomized study. *Am J Sports Med.* 1993;21(4):582–5.

6. Barton CJ, Munteanu SE, Menz HB, Crossley KM. The efficacy of foot orthoses in the treatment of individuals with patellofemoral pain syndrome: a systematic review. *Sports Med.* 2010;40(5):377–95.

7. Benard M, Goldsmith H, Gurnick K, et al. Prescription custom foot orthoses practice guidelines. *The American College of Foot and Ankle Orthopedics and Medicine.* 2002;32.

8. Bishop M, Fiolkowski P, Conrad B, Brunt D, Horodyski M. Athletic footwear, leg stiffness, and running kinematics. *J Athl Train.* 2006; 41(4):387–92.

9. Bowring B, Chockalingam N. Conservative treatment of tibialis posterior tendon dysfunction — a review. *Foot (Edinb).* 2010;20(1):18–26.

10. Burns J, Landorf KB, Ryan MM, Crosbie J, Ouvrier RA. Interventions for the prevention and treatment of pes cavus. *Cochrane Database Syst Rev.* 2007;4:CD006154.

11. Churchill RS, Donley BG. Managing injuries of the great toe. *Phys Sportsmed.* 1998;26(9):29–39.

12. Clarke TE, Frederick EC, Hamill CL. The effects of shoe design parameters on rearfoot control in running. *Med Sci Sports Exerc.* 1983;15(5): 376–81.

13. Clinghan R, Arnold GP, Drew TS, Cochrane LA, Abboud RJ. Do you get value for money when you buy an expensive pair of running shoes? *Br J Sports Med.* 2008;42(3):189–93.

14. Cornwall M, McPoil T. The foot and ankle: current concepts in mechanics, examination, and orthotic intervention. In: *Proceedings of Annual Conference & Exposition of the American Physical Therapy Association.* Washington (DC); 2003.

15. Cummings GS, Higbie EJ. A weight bearing method for determining forefoot posting for orthotic fabrication. *Physiother Res Int.* 1997; 2(1):42–50.

16. Dananberg HJ, Guiliano M. Chronic low-back pain and its response to custom-made foot orthoses. *J Am Podiatr Med Assoc.* 1999;89(3): 109–17.

17. Davis IS, Zifchock RA, Deleo AT. A comparison of rear foot motion control and comfort between custom and semicustom foot orthotic devices. *J Am Podiatr Med Assoc.* 2008;98(5):394–403.

18. De Wit B, De Clercq D, Aerts P. Biomechanical analysis of the stance phase during barefoot and shod running. *J Biomech.* 2000;33(3): 269–78.

19. Dicharry JM. Barefoot running: is barefoot better? In: *UVA Running Medicine Conference.* Charlottesville (VA); 2010.

20. Dicharry JM, Franz JR, Della Croce U, Wilder RP, Riley PO, Kerrigan DC. Differences in static and dynamic measures in evaluation of talonavicular mobility in gait. *J Orthop Sports Phys Ther.* 2009;39(8):628–34.

21. Dixon SJ, Kerwin DG. The influence of heel lift manipulation on sagittal plane kinematics in running. *J Appl Biomech.* 1999;15:139–51.

22. Donatelli RA, Hurlburt C, Conaway D, St Pierre R. Biomechanical foot orthotics: a retrospective study. *J Ortho Sports Phys Ther.* 1988; 10(6):205–12.

23. Ekenman I, Milgrom C, Finestone A, et al. The role of biomechanical shoe orthoses in tibial stress fracture prevention. *Am J Sports Med.* 2002;30(6):866–70.

24. Finestone A, Giladi M, Elad H, et al. Prevention of stress fractures using custom biomechanical shoe orthoses. *Clin Orthop Relat Res.* 1999; 360:182–90.

25. Foot and ankle update. In: *Proceedings of Healthsouth Educational Program.* Charlottesville (VA); 2002.

26. Genova JM, Gross MT. Effect of foot orthotics on calcaneal eversion during standing and treadmill walking for subjects with abnormal pronation. *J Orthop Sports Phys Ther.* 2000;30(11):664–75.

27. Gross ML, Davlin LB, Evanski PM. Effectiveness of orthotic shoe inserts in the long-distance runner. *Am J Sports Med.* 1991;19(4):409–12.

28. Guldemond NA, Leffers P, Sanders AP, Emmen H, Schaper NC, Walenkamp GH. Casting methods and plantar pressure: effects of custom-made foot orthoses on dynamic plantar pressure distribution. *J Am Podiatr Med Assoc.* 2006;96(1):9–18.

29. Handoll HH, Rowe BH, Quinn KM, de Bie R. Intervention for preventing ankle ligament injuries. *Cochrane Database Syst Rev.* 2001;3:CD000018.

30. Hardin EC, van den Bogert AJ, Hamill J. Kinematic adaptations during running: effects of footwear, surface, and duration. *Med Sci Sports Exerc.* 2004;36(5):838–44.

31. Hawke F, Burns J, Radford JA, du Toit V. Custom-made foot orthoses for the treatment of foot pain. *Cochrane Database Syst Rev*. 2008; 16(3):CD006801.

32. Heiderscheit B, Hamill J, Tiberio D. A biomechanical perspective: do foot orthoses work? *Br J Sports Med*. 2001;35(1):4–5.

33. Hennig EM, Milani TL. Pressure distribution measurements for evaluation of running shoe properties. *Sportverletz Sportschaden*. 2000; 14(3):90–7.

34. Hume P, Hopkins W, Rome K, Maulder P, Coyle G, Nigg B. Effectiveness of foot orthoses for treatment and prevention of lower limb injuries: a review. *Sports Med*. 2008;38(9):759–79.

35. Hurley MV. The role of muscle weakness in the pathogenesis of osteoarthritis. *Rheum Dis Clin North Am*. 1999;25(2):283–98, vi.

36. James S, Bates B, Osternig LR. Injuries to runners. *Am J Sports Med*. 1978;6:40–50.

37. Järvinen TA, Kannus P, Maffulli N, Khan KM. Achilles tendon disorders: etiology and epidemiology. *Foot Ankle Clin*. 2005;10(2):255–66.

38. Kannus P, Niittymäki S. Which factors predict outcome in the nonoperative treatment of patellofemoral pain syndrome? A prospective follow-up study. *Med Sci Sports Exerc*. 1994;26(3):289–96.

39. Kerrigan DC, Franz JR, Keenan GS, Dicharry J, Della Croce U, Wilder RP. The effect of running shoes on lower extremity joint torques. *PMR*. 2009;1(12):1058–63.

40. Kitaoka HB, Luo ZP, Kura H, An KN. Effect of foot orthoses on 3-dimensional kinematics of flatfoot: a cadaveric study. *Arch Phys Med Rehabil*. 2002;83(6):876–9.

41. Kong PW, Candelaria NG, Smith DR. Running in new and worn shoes: a comparison of three types of cushioning footwear. *Br J Sports Med*. 2009;43(10):745–9.

42. Kurz MJ, Stergiou N. The spanning set indicates that variability during the stance period of running is affected by footwear. *Gait Posture*. 2003;17(2):132–5.

43. Landorf KB, Keenan AM. Efficacy of foot orthoses. What does the literature tell us? *J Am Podiatr Med Assoc*. 2000;90(3):149–58.

44. Laughton C, McClay Davis I, Williams DS. A comparison of four methods of obtaining a negative impression of the foot. *J Am Podiatr Med Assoc*.2002;92(5):261–8.

45. Lee SY, McKeon P, Hertel J. Does the use of orthoses improve self-reported pain and function measures in patients with plantar fasciitis? A meta-analysis. *Phys Ther Sport*. 2009;10(1):12–8.

46. Lieberman DE, Venkadesan M, Werbel WA, et al. Foot strike patterns and collision forces in habitually barefoot versus shod runners. *Nature*. 2010;463(7280):531–5.

47. Logan S, Hunter I, Hopkins JT, et al. Ground reaction force differences between running shoes, racing flats, and distance spikes in runners. *J Sports Sci Med*. 2010;9:147–53.

48. MacLean CL. Custom foot orthoses for running. *Clin Podiatr Med Surg*. 2001;18(2):217–24.

49. MacLean CL, Davis IS, Hamill J. Short- and long-term influences of a custom foot orthotic intervention on lower extremity dynamics. *Clin J Sport Med*. 2008;18(4):338–43.

50. McCaw ST, Heil ME, Hamill J. The effect of comments about shoe construction on impact forces during walking. *Med Sci Sports Exerc*. 2000;32(7):1258–64.

51. Milgrom C, Finestone A, Ekenman I, Simkin A, Nyska M. The effect of shoe sole composition on in vivo tibial strains during walking. *Foot Ankle Int*. 2001;22(7):598–602.

52. Murley GS, Landorf KB, Menz HB, Bird AR. Effect of foot posture, foot orthoses and footwear on lower limb muscle activity during walking and running: a systematic review. *Gait Posture*. 2009;29(2): 172–87.

53. Nawoczenski DA. Nonoperative and operative intervention for hallux rigidus. *J Orthop Sports Phys Ther*. 1999;29(12):727–35.

54. Nawoczenski DA, Cook TM, Saltzman CL. The effect of foot orthotics on three-dimensional kinematics of the leg and rearfoot during running. *J Orthop Sports Phys Ther*. 1995;21(6):317–27.

55. Nigg BM. The role of impact forces and foot pronation: a new paradigm. *Clin J Sports Med*. 2001;11(1):2–9.

56. Nigg BM, Nurse MA, Stefanyshyn CJ. Shoe inserts and orthotics for sport and physical activities. *Med Sci Sports Exerc*. 1999;31(7 Suppl):S421–8.

57. Nigg BM, Stefanyshyn D, Cole G, Stergiou P, Miller J. The effect of material characteristics of shoe soles on muscle activation and energy aspects during running. *J Biomech*. 2003;36(4):569–75.

58. Nigg BM, Stergiou P, Cole G, Stefanyshyn D, Mündermann A, Humble N. Effect of shoe inserts on kinematics, center of pressure, and leg joint moments during running. *Med Sci Sports Exerc*. 2003;35(2):314–9.

59. Noll KH. The use of orthotic devices in adult acquired flatfoot deformity. *Foot Ankle Clin*. 2001;6(1):25–36.

60. O'Connor FG, Wilder RP, Nirschl R, editors. *Textbook of Running Medicine. Running Medicine*. New York (NY): McGraw-Hill, Medical Pub. Division; 2001.

61. Ogon M, Aleksiev AR, Spratt KF, Pope MH, Saltzman CL. Footwear affects the behavior of low back muscles when jogging. *Int J Sports Med*. 2001;22(6):414–9.

62. Payne C, Chuter V. The clash between theory and science on the kinematic effectiveness of foot orthoses. *Clin Podiatr Med Surg*. 2001; 18(4):705–13, vi.

63. Pratt DJ. A critical review of the literature on foot orthoses. *J Am Podiatr Med Assoc*. 2000;90(7):339–41.

64. Razeghi M, Batt ME. Biomechanical analysis of the effect of orthotic shoe inserts: a review of the literature. *Sports Med*. 2000;29(6):425–38.

65. Reinschmidt C, Nigg BM. Current issues in the design of running and court shoes. *Sportverletz Sportschaden*. 2000;14(3):71–81.

66. Reinschmidt C, Nigg BM. Influence of heel height on ankle joint moments in running. *Med Sci Sports Exerc*. 1995;27(3):410–6.

67. Richards CE, Magin PJ, Callister R. Is your prescription of distance running shoes evidence-based? *Br J Sports Med*. 2009;43(3):159–62.

68. Richie DH Jr. Effects of foot orthoses on patients with chronic ankle instability. *J Am Podiatr Med Assoc*. 2007;97(1):19–30.

69. Robbins S, Waked E. Factors associated with ankle injuries. Preventive measures. *Sports Med*. 1998;25(1):63–72.

70. Roberts ME, Gordon CE. Orthopedic footwear. Custom-made and commercially manufactured footwear. *Foot Ankle Clin*. 2001;6(2): 243–7.

71. Rome K, Handoll HH, Ashford R. Interventions for preventing and treating stress fractures and stress reactions of bone of the lower limbs in young adults. *Cochrane Database Syst Rev*. 2005;18(2):CD000450.

72. Roy JP, Stefanyshyn DJ. Shoe midsole longitudinal bending stiffness and running economy, joint energy, and EMG. *Med Sci Sports Exerc*. 2006;38(3):562–9.

73. Running course. In: *Proceedings of Healthsouth Educational Program*. Charlottesville (VA); 2002.

74. Ryan MB, Valiant GA, McDonald K, Taunton JE. The effect of three different levels of footwear stability on pain outcomes in women runners: a randomised control trial. *Br J Sports Med*. 2011;45(9):715–21.

75. Sahrmann S. *Diagnosis and Treatment of Movement Impairment Syndromes*. St. Louis (MO): Mosby; 2002.

76. Sekizawa K, Sandrey MA, Ingersoll CD, Cordova ML. Effects of shoe sole thickness on joint position sense. *Gait Posture*. 2001;13(3):221–8.

77. Sharkey NA, Ferris L, Smith TS, Matthews DK. Strain and loading of the second metatarsal during heel-lift. *J Bone Joint Surg Am*. 1995; 77(7):1050–7.

78. Slemenda C, Brandt KD, Heilman DK, et al. Quadriceps weakness and osteoarthritis of the knee. *Ann Intern Med.* 1997;127(2):97–104.

79. Sobel E, Levitz SJ, Caselli MA. Orthoses in the treatment of rear foot problems. *J Am Podiatr Med Assoc.* 1999;89(5):220–33.

80. Squadrone R, Gallozzi C. Biomechanical and physiological comparison of barefoot and two shod conditions in experienced barefoot runners. *J Sports Med Phys Fitness.* 2009;49(1):6–13.

81. Stacoff A, Kälin X, Stüssi E. The effects of shoes on the torsion and rearfoot motion in running. *Med Sci Sports Exerc.* 1991;23(4): 482–90.

82. Stefanyshyn DJ, Nigg BM. Energy aspects associated with sport shoes. *Sportverletz Sportschaden.* 2000;14(3):82–9.

83. Tang SF, Chen CP, Pan JL, Chen JL, Leong CP, Chu NK. The effects of a new foot-toe orthosis in treating painful hallux valgus. *Arch Phys Med Rehabil.* 2002;83(12):1792–5.

84. Thacker SB, Gilchrist J, Stroup DF, Kimsey CD. The prevention of shin splints in sports: a systematic review of literature. *Med Sci Sports Exerc.* 2002;34(1):32–40.

85. Tillman MD, Chiumento AB, Trimble MH, et al. Tibiofemoral rotation in landing: the influence of medially and laterally posted orthotics. *Physical Ther Sport.* 2003;4:34–9.

86. Valmassy R. Orthoses. In: Subotnick S, editor. *Sports Medicine of the Lower Extremity.* New York (NY): Churchill Livingstone; 1989.

87. van Gent RN, Siem D, van Middelkoop M, van Os AG, Bierma-Zeinstra SM, Koes BW. Incidence and determinants of lower extremity running injuries in long distance runners: a systematic review. *Br J Sports Med.* 2007;41(8):469–80.

88. Vicenzino B, Griffiths S, Griffiths LA, Hadley A. Effect of antipronation tape and temporary orthotic on vertical navicular height before and after exercise. *J Orthop Sports Phys Ther.* 2000;30(6):333–9.

89. Wakeling JM, Pascual SA, Nigg BM. Altering muscle activity in the lower extremities by running with different shoes. *Med Sci Sports Exerc.* 2002;34(9):1529–32.

90. Williams DS 3rd, McClay Davis I, Baitch SP. Effect of inverted orthoses on lower-extremity mechanics in runners. *Med Sci Sports Exerc.* 2003;35(12):2060–8.

Taping in Sports Medicine

76

Jessica M. Poole, Casey Hulsey, and RM Barney Poole

INTRODUCTION

- Taping in sports medicine has been a long-standing rehabilitative adjunct to assist sports medicine providers in preventing injury and facilitating a safe return to play (18).

- The most basic way to restrict motion is by applying simple athletic taping methods to the affected area. Tape can aid in the support and compression of a soft tissue injury and can additionally unload the amount of force placed on damaged ligaments during the healing process. Taping a joint to reduce the risk of injury or increase patient confidence in the integrity of a joint may be the most common reason for athletic taping (3,13).

- Restricting motion of certain joints has been demonstrated to effectively protect, prevent, and limit further injury (16).

- This chapter reviews the role of athletic taping in sports medicine, specifically addressing indications, current methods, recommended materials, principles of application, site-specific techniques and the current evidence for efficacy.

INDICATIONS

- There are two principal indications for taping: prevention and rehabilitation.

- Prevention: Taping normal or injured tissue for practice and games to help keep a recreational or occupational athlete safe from injury or to protect from potential or further injury with early return to activity.

- Rehabilitation: Tape may be applied to speed the process of return to activity and protect the area during early return; tape may also be applied to modify the activity of a joint to allow for joint retraining during rehabilitation.

CURRENT METHODS

- As the manufacture of tape becomes more sophisticated, its uses become ever more varied. There are many forms of taping presently used in sports medicine, but the principal techniques involve: classic nonstretch athletic taping, McConnell taping and Kinesio taping.

- Classic athletic taping
  - Classic nonstretch linen high–thread count athletic tape has been used for years to support and protect athletes' joints for practice and games.
  - Traditional nonstretch athletic tapes are generally applied to form an inflexible bandage with the goal of supporting, and usually immobilizing, a joint or muscle.
- McConnell taping
  - McConnell taping was originally developed by Jenny McConnell, PT, to be used in the treatment of patellofemoral pain syndrome (15).
  - This method uses a good exam of the affected joint and a high–thread count nonstretch tape to potentially correct tracking and alignment issues in the patella, support the patella, and retrain muscles to correct the issue. The tape required consists of elastic underwrap and the nonstretch adhesive tape. Leukotape is a brand often used for McConnell taping.
- Kinesio taping
  - Kinesio taping is a relatively new technique that has recently come into wide use throughout the world to facilitate healing and provide stability and support without restricting motion. Kinesio tape may be used for days at a time (5).
  - Kinesio tape has the properties of being both strong and flexible. Kinesio taping additionally uses a proprietary taping method complete with certification classes and seminars for practitioners. The tape is applied in a specific pattern and is either stretched or not stretched, depending on the injury and rehabilitative goals. Kinesio tape is thought to work by not only supporting injured muscles and joints, but also helping to relieve pain by lifting the skin and allowing blood to flow more freely to the injured area (20,21).

RECOMMENDED MATERIALS

- Prior to applying tape to a joint for protection, prevention, or prophylactic means, there are several concepts that need to be addressed. First, proper materials are needed. There is a wide variety of taping materials on the market for the provider to choose from.

539

- The principal types of tape matter the most; there is no evidence to suggest one brand is superior to another. Be sure to find the best type of tape that accommodates budgets while providing the best result for the patient. A good supply of the following types and sizes of tape is recommended:
  - 1-, 1.5-, and 2-inch linen athletic tape
  - 1.5-, 2-, and 3-inch light elastic Lightplast
  - 2- and 3-inch heavy elastic tape such as Elastikon
  - Adhesive covering such as CoverRoll
  - Leukotape for McConnell taping
  - Kinesio tape: rolls or prefabricated for a particular joint; both are available
- Other supplies necessary for the application of tape are tape adherent (such as Tuff Skin or QDA), heel and lace pads to prevent friction in areas of concern, skin lube for application of friction pads, prewrap foam to prevent skin irritation, bandage scissors or any blunt nose scissors, and tape cutters (2).

PRINCIPLES OF APPLICATION

- When applying tape to a joint, there are several basic rules that need to be followed in order to ensure comfort, correct joint mechanics and function, and limit further injury to the joint or cutaneous tissue. The following rules apply:
  - Rule out any factors that could pose harm (*e.g.*, an injury in close proximity, open wounds such as cuts or blisters).
  - Shave the area if applying tape directly to the skin.
  - Always place joint in position to be stabilized.
  - Apply tape adhesive to area for maximum adhesion.
  - Cover area to be taped with a prewrap or a pretape product.
  - Always begin with anchor strips and end with close strips.
  - Keep tape roll in same hand at all times.
  - Always overlap tape by half the width to prevent gaps that may cause friction blisters and/or cuts.
  - Do not apply tape to anesthetized skin or after a heat or cold modality application or to areas of poor circulation (2,16,18).

SITE PREPARATION

- Clean the area to be taped.
- Shave if tape is to be applied directly to the skin.
- Use a tape-adherent spray to maximize adhesion.
- Cover broken skin, cuts, skin moles tags, etc., prior to taping (2).
- Use lubricated pads over bony prominence for comfort.
- Apply pretape or prewrap to the skin to protect it; a single layer is usually all that is needed.
- Avoid wrinkles in the tape to prevent blisters beneath the tape.

REMOVAL

- Tape is removed using scissors or tape cutters.
- A liquid tape adhesive remover may be used to remove tape residue.

SITE-SPECIFIC TECHNIQUES

- The most common areas of the body to tape are as follows: toes, ankle, arch, Achilles tendon, patella, acromioclavicular joint, elbow, wrist, and fingers. The knee and hip benefit most from bracing, which will be discussed in a subsequent chapter. A complete review of taping is beyond the scope of this text, and the interested reader is referred to the following excellent resources at end of chapter (2,15,16,18). This section will, however, discuss and review standard application procedures for the ankle joint and the plantar fascia and introduce the McConnell taping technique used for patellofemoral pain.

Plantar Fascia Taping

- Arch (weave technique): Relieves pain in foot, anterior compartment, or knee due to plantar fasciitis, medial tibial stress syndrome, patellar tendonitis, and iliotibial band syndrome all caused by overpronation or due to a falling high arch (8,9). If application relieves pain; orthoses or foot orthotic devices may be the next best course of action for continuous arch support in a variety of shoes and decrease the reliance on tape. Procedure is as follows:
  - Apply tape adherent to foot.
  - Place ankle joint in neutral position.
  - Place anchor strip around forefoot at metatarsal heads.
  - Using 1-inch tape, begin at fifth metatarsal head and tape and loop around the lateral heel and back to the fifth toe.
  - Beginning at base of hallux, apply tape and loop around the medial heel and back to the base of the hallux.
  - Repeat steps 4 and 5 three more times, overlapping by half tape width (Fig. 76.1).
  - Apply 1-inch linen tape in circular anchors over the arch for added support (Fig. 76.2).

Ankle Sprain Taping

- Closed basket weave for inversion ankle sprain: Prevents an inversion ankle sprain by improving mechanical stability of the subtalar joint reference. Taping will limit inversion or eversion stresses depending on application. Applying stirrups medial to lateral provides support and prevention of lateral ankle sprains, while pulling stirrups from the bottom of the heel proximally will limit motion due to an eversion sprain. Taping will support the subtalar and talocrural joints from excessive movement due to force. Proprioceptive qualities of the ankle joint may also be improved. It is important to remember that taping will help prevent recurrent ankle sprains, but there is no substitute for

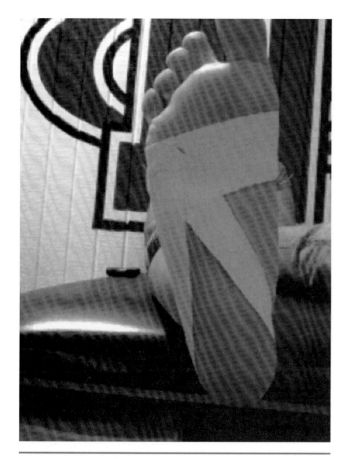

Figure 76.1: Completed arch weave.

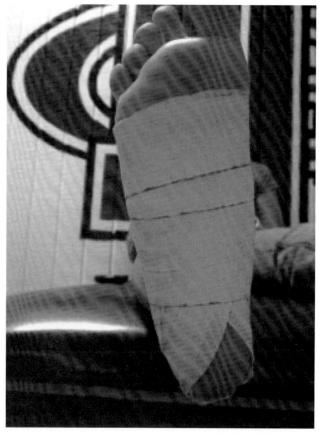

Figure 76.2: One-inch linen tape anchors to provide added support over arch weave.

appropriate rehabilitation focusing on strength and proprioception improvement. The procedure is as follows:

■ Apply tape adherent.

■ Apply heel pad over the distal Achilles tendon and lace pad over the anterior ankle joint to prevent friction injuries. Apply prewrap material.

■ Using 1.5-inch linen tape, apply a circular anchor at the musculotendinous junction of the gastrocnemius/soleus complex (Fig. 76.3).

■ Apply another anchor around the forefoot directly covering the fifth styloid.

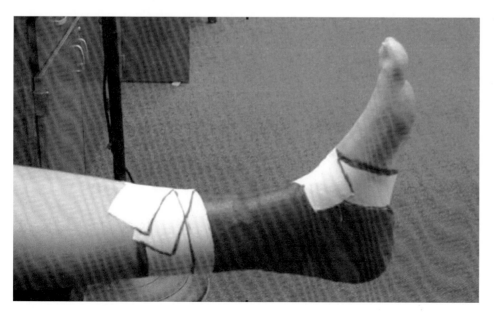

Figure 76.3: Proximal and distal anchors for closed basket weave inversion ankle sprain taping.

Figure 76.4: Medial stirrups and alternating C-strips (Gibney strips) for closed basket weave inversion ankle sprain taping.

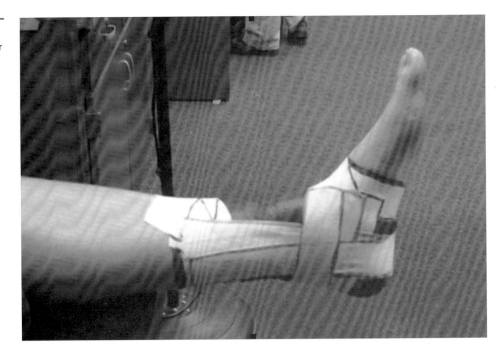

- Apply three stirrups and alternate with C-Strips (Gibney strips). Place first stirrup at top anchor just posterior to the medial malleolus. With adequate tension, pull medially to laterally underneath the heel and up the fibula. Begin C-strip on medial side of the foot anchor and wrap around posterior heel and finish on lateral aspect of foot anchor. Apply next stirrup, using same method as before and overlapping by half. Apply the next C-strip, overlapping by half moving proximally. Repeat with final stirrup and final C-strip (Fig.76.4).

- Next, apply four alternating heel locks. Begin high on the instep and pull under the arch and toward the lateral heel, hooking the heel, and then come around the opposite side and back to the starting point. Repeat on the opposite side and then apply two more overlapping by half (Figs. 76.5 and 76.6).

- Complete the taping by applying close strips to secure all the loose tape ends. Check for circulation and warmth (Fig. 76.7) (9).

Figure 76.5: Heel lock for closed basket weave inversion ankle sprain taping.

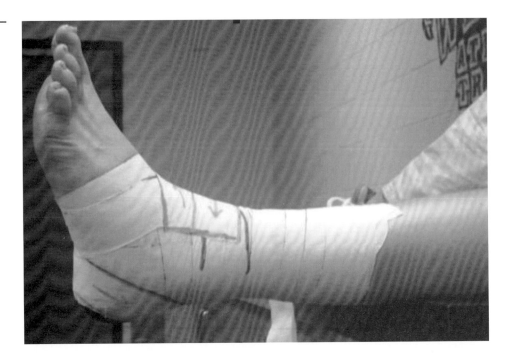

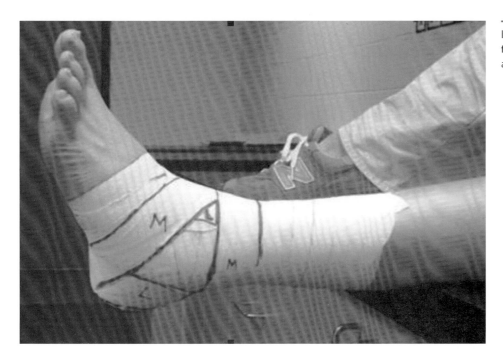

Figure 76.6: Alternating heel lock for closed basket weave inversion ankle sprain taping.

- Variations: One may increase the integrity by increasing the strength of the tape. Using a heavy-duty elastic tape for the stirrups and heel locks will make for a more restrictive tape application. To decrease the restrictive qualities, use a lightweight elastic tape. Other variations are the Spartan, where stirrups are applied with heavy elastic tape and as the stirrup comes across the lateral malleolus, the tape is split, forming two tails that can be wrapped around the fibula and tibia for added strength and support. A continuous elastic tape technique will give less restriction and is a faster application.

McConnell Taping

- The only recommended tape application for the knee is McConnell taping for poor patellar tracking or patellar displacement (4,15). Taping for medial collateral ligament (MCL) or lateral collateral ligament (LCL) sprains or rotary

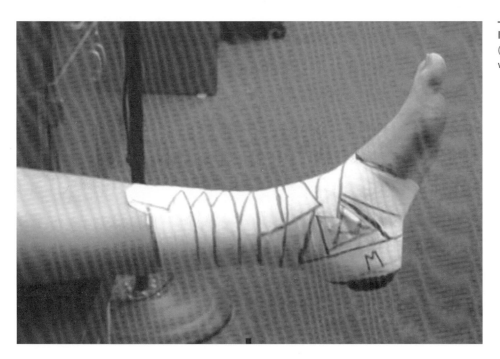

Figure 76.7: Close strips (completed tape job) for closed basket weave inversion ankle sprain taping.

Figure 76.8: Squat to assess patellar tracking and pain.

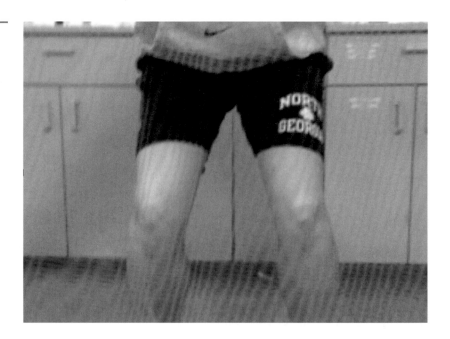

instability is not as effective as bracing, due to the dynamics of the knee. Bracing affords the patient more continuous support and dissipation of forces.

■ McConnell taping for patellar tracking or poor patellar alignment: We recommend that a through history and assessment be completed prior to taping the patella. One must realize that although this tape application may ease the patient's symptoms, it should only be used as a temporary solution to allow completion of activities of daily living or sports competition in comfort. It is essential for the clinician to address why the patella is sitting high, low, medially, laterally, or poorly tracking (15). These issues should be addressed with a rehabilitation program to correct the underlying causes, specifically a weak vastus medialis oblique and hip musculature (17). The procedure is as follows:

■ Assess the patella and decide how to locate the patella to limit pain. In the following figures, the patient's left patella tracked from the superior lateral side to the inferior medial side of the femur; therefore, the goal of the taping will be to pull the left patella superiorly and laterally using Leukotape to try and relieve pain associated with poor tracking due to a weak vastus medialis oblique muscle and overpronation. The patient wears corrective orthoses regularly (Fig 76.8).

■ Apply tape adherent to a shaved knee area.

■ Apply a tape base, such as CoverRoll, over the patella, but not all the way around the knee (Fig 76.9).

■ Cut three strips of Leukotape. Leukotape is a heavy non-elastic tape with very little yield. It will securely hold the patella in the desired positioning to relieve pain.

■ Place the patella in the position to be stabilized and secure with the Leukotape, securing the patella superior and medially (Fig. 76.10A and B).

■ Apply two more strips to adequately secure the patella in the proper position (18).

■ Reassess your patient to determine if the taping adequately decreases the symptoms. If not, you may need to readjust the patella. We use a squat to determine tracking and to assess pain level before and after application (Fig. 76.11).

CURRENT EVIDENCE

■ The ankle is the most commonly taped joint in sport (10).

■ The scientific evidence favoring the efficacy of taping for ankle sprains and other injuries is mixed; however, the clinical use of taping and anecdotal evidence of its efficacy are widespread (14).

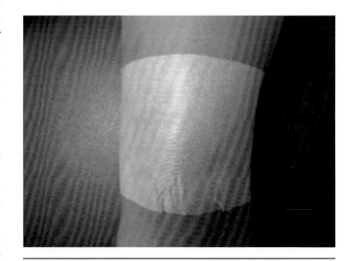

Figure 76.9: Application of CoverRoll for McConnell taping.

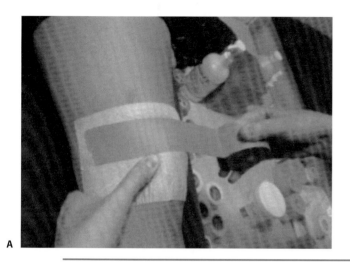

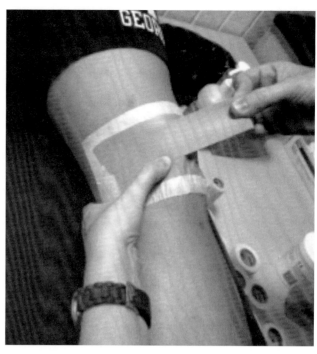

A   B

Figure 76.10: **A:** Using Leukotape to stabilize the patella laterally. **B:** Using Leukotape to stabilize the patella superiorly.

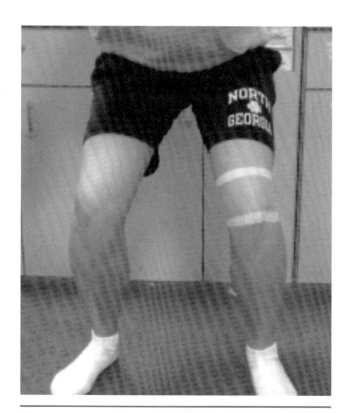

Figure 76.11: Patient in a squat position to reassess for corrected tracking and reduction of pain.

- A randomized controlled study by Garrick and Requa (7) examined the effectiveness of taping on the incidence of ankle sprains in basketball players; subjects who were taped had 14.7 sprains per 1,000 games, and those who were not taped had 32.8 sprains per 1,000 games (7).

- The Garrick and Requa (7) study in 1973 is also credited with demonstrating that tape loosens just 10 minutes after application and provides little mechanical support after 30 minutes.

- Other studies proposed that the benefit of taping comes through increased proprioceptive input, allowing muscles to react faster in potential injury situations (6,11).

- The current evidence on taping versus bracing is inconclusive regarding efficacy and efficiency.

- In a retrospective study comparing taping to bracing, athletes with tape had 4.9 ankle sprains per 1,000 games, and those who wore ankle braces had 2.6 sprains per 1,000 games (19).

- No evidence has been found to support McConnell taping for the knee; one randomized controlled study found no evidence to support that McConnell taping enhanced a regular physical therapy treatment program when compared to a control group (1,2,12).

REFERENCES

1. Aminaka N, Gribble PA. A systematic review of the effects of therapeutic taping on patellofemoral pain syndrome. *J Athl Train*. 2005;40(4):341–51.

2. Beam JW. *Orthopedic Taping, Wrapping, Bracing, & Padding*. Philadelphia (PA): F.A. Davis; 2006. 512 p.

3. Callaghan MJ. Role of ankle taping and bracing in the athlete. *Br J Sports Med*. 1997;31(2):102–8.

4. Derasari A, Brindle TJ, Alter KE, Sheehan FT. McConnell taping shifts the patella inferiorly in patients with patellofemoral pain: a dynamic magnetic resonance imaging study. *Phys Ther.* 2010;90(3):411–9.

5. Fu TC, Wong AM, Pei YC, Wu KP, Chou SW, Lin YC. Effect of Kinesio taping on muscle strength in athletes-a pilot study. *J Sci Med Sport.* 2008;11(2):198–201.

6. Garn SN, Newton RA. Kinesthetic awareness in subjects with multiple ankle sprains. *Phys Ther.* 1998;68(11):1667–71.

7. Garrick JG, Requa RK. Role of external support in the prevention of ankle sprains. *Med Sci Sports.*1973;5(3):200–3.

8. Hatch RL, Hacking S. Evaluation and management of toe fractures. *Am Fam Physician.* 2003;68(12):2413–8.

9. Jamali B, Walker M, Hoke B, Echternach J. Windlass taping technique for symptomatic relief of plantar fasciitis. *J Sport Rehabil.* 2004;13(3);228–43.

10. Junge A, Rösch D, Peterson L, Graf-Baumann T, Dvorak J. Prevention of soccer injuries: a prospective intervention study in youth amateur players. *Am J Sports Med.* 2002;30(5):652–9.

11. Karlsson J, Andreasson GO. The effect of external ankle support in chronic lateral ankle joint instability. An electromyographic study. *Am J Sports Med.* 1992;20(3):257–61.

12. Kowall MG, Kolk G, Nuber GW, Cassisi JE, Stern SH. Patellar taping in the treatment of patellofemoral pain. A prospective randomized study. *Am J Sports Med.* 1996;24(1):61–6.

13. Lohkamp M, Craven S, Walker-Johnson C, Greig M. The influence of ankle taping on changes in postural stability during soccer-specific activity. *J Sport Rehabil.* 2009;18(4):482–92.

14. Macdonald R, editor. *Taping Techniques: Principles and Practice.* Oxford (UK): Butterworth-Heinemann; 1994.

15. McConnell JS. The management of chondromalacia patellae: a long term solution. *Aust J Physiotherapy.* 1986;32:215–23.

16. Mitchell L. Brace Yourself Taping Essentials [Internet]. Available from: http://www.sportex.net.

17. Ng GY, Cheng JM. The effects of patellar taping on pain and neuromuscular performance in subjects with patellofemoral pain syndrome. *Clin Rehabil.* 2002;16(8):821–7.

18. Prentice WE. Bandaging and taping. In: *Principles of Athletic Training.* 14th ed. New York: McGraw-Hill; 2011. p. 176–205.

19. Rovere GD, Clarke TJ, Yates CS, Burley K. Retrospective comparison of taping and ankle stabilizers in preventing ankle injuries. *Am J Sports Med.* 1988;16(3):228–33.

20. Thelen MD, Dauber JA, Stoneman PD. The clinical efficacy of Kinesio tape for shoulder pain: a randomized, double-blinded, clinical trial. *J Orthop Sports Phys Ther.* 2008;38(7):389–95.

21. Yoshida A, Kahanov L. The effect of Kinesio taping on lower trunk range of motions. *Res Sports Med.* 2007;15(2):103–12.

Bracing in Sports Medicine

77

Jessica M. Poole, Casey Hulsey, and RM Barney Poole

INTRODUCTION

- Bernhart and Anderson (1) state that, "In an attempt to reduce sport injuries, many athletes are turning to pro-phylactic and functional braces for protection, support, compression, restriction of movement, immobilization, and proprioceptive enhancement."
- There are two principal types of braces used in sports medi-cine: rehabilitative and prophylactic.
- In rehabilitative bracing, the prime focus is to allow a protected range of motion after surgery for the injured joint.
- Prophylactic braces are designed to stop or lessen the severity of injuries, so their focus is prevention.
- Custom-made braces, which non-restrictive are principally rehabilitative, provide security for unstable joints and are fabricated from measurements and/or cast molds to fit the athlete for a specific purpose (11).

INDICATIONS

- There are two principal indications for bracing: support of injured tissue and prevention of injury (10).
- Prevention of injury may also include support for safe and early return to activity.
- When choosing a brace, consider the type of injury to be prevented and the area that needs to be supported.

SELECTING A BRACE

- Braces may be purchased in a variety of shapes, sizes, and colors and range in price from the relatively inexpensive off-the-shelf variety found in large-box athletic stores and some grocery store pharmacy areas to custom-fabricated braces fitted and personalized for the athlete.
- Braces are made to fit a wide variety of joint types and come in various sizes. When choosing a brace, the most important factor is the purpose for which the brace is in-tended. For example, an ankle brace for a basketball athlete may not be the same as one chosen for an airline baggage handler.

- When choosing a brace, consider the type of injury to be prevented and the area that needs to be supported.
- Braces should increase the stability of joints and limit pathomechanical stress to adjacent joints.
- Braces should not interfere with normal joint function.
- Bracing worn in contact sports should not endanger others.
- Bracing should be adaptable to all somatotypes.
- Braces should be chosen that are cost effective.
- Selected bracing should have evidence to support its use (5).

SITE-SPECIFIC INDICATIONS

Ankle

- Ankle sprains are one of the most common traumatic injuries in sports; the most common mechanism of injury for the ankle is an inversion ankle sprain.
- Two types of braces can be worn to help reduce ankle injuries: lace-up braces and rigid support braces. Both types of braces derive some of their support of the ankle from the shoe in which they are worn.
- Lace-up ankle braces fit comfortably in a shoe and may have extra lateral support from figure-eight straps that provide assistance to support the ankle in cutting situations that may stress the lateral structures.
- Rigid support ankle braces fit in a shoe or boot and may be better for supporting injured workers who may not be exposed to running or cutting forces or athletes needing firmer support.
- Size shoe and heel width properly; apply over sock.
- Ankle range of motion should be within normal limits for dorsiflexion/plantarflexion; inversion and eversion should be limited.
- Inspect for friction areas.
- Demonstrate donning and doffing technique, making correc-tions as needed.

Knee

- Bracing for the knee is determined by the area of the knee where support is needed and the reason the athlete is using the brace (support of injury, prophylaxis, or rehabilitation).

- Measure for correct sizing; circumferentially 6 inches above patella and at the joint line are the most common measures.
- Center patella between hinges; hinges are centered at joint.
- Check for movement up and down and rotationally.
- Check for normal range of motion of the knee.
- Set range of motion restrictions if applicable.
- Demonstrate donning and doffing technique and make changes as indicated.

Hip

- There are no known braces for the hip joint; however, Coreshorts™ by Under Armour can help reduce reoccurring injuries in the hip.
- Coreshorts™ are expandable compression shorts that not only compress, but also add resistance to increased range of motion (1).

Back

- Mechanical low back pain is a major health care problem; some evidence is available to support the use of bracing as an adjunct to standard treatment plans (6).
- Select the proper lumbar support and size by measuring circumferentially at the waist.
- Fit the brace to support the low back and maintain comfortable positional lumbar lordosis.
- Demonstrate donning and doffing technique and make changes as indicated.

CURRENT EVIDENCE

- Current evidence regarding the prophylactic use of ankle bracing in sports indicates that use of ankle bracing significantly reduces injury (4).
- One study using female volleyball players indicated an injury rate of 0.07 per 1,000 exposures as opposed to a rate of 0.98 per 1,000 exposures in a comparison group (8).
- Two studies, each looking at the effects of ankle brace usage on knee and ankle kinematics and ground force reaction, concluded that although there may be a slight increase on the knee axial rotation with some activities (14), overall ankle and knee kinematics and ankle ground reaction forces remained the same over time (3).
- Knee bracing was also found to have beneficial effects in prevention of medial collateral and anterior cruciate ligament injuries (11,13). However, a recent systematic review noted that there remains a lack of evidence to support the routine use of prophylactic knee bracing in uninjured

knees (12). More research is needed in this area to reach a definitive conclusion.

- A Cochrane review found that knee bracing in osteoarthritis increases the distance one is able to walk; the brace, however, may not lead to any difference in pain, knee function, or quality of life (2).
- Some recent studies have shown that lumbar bracing and other elements of a plan of care have a beneficial effect on maintaining proper lumbar lordosis when sitting and standing, thus helping to decrease low back pain (7,9).

REFERENCES

1. Bernhardt T, Anderson GS. Influence of moderate prophylactic compression on sport performance. *J Strength Cond Res.* 2005;19(2):292–7.
2. Brouwer RW, Jakma TSC, Verhagen AP, Verhaar JAN, Bierma-Zeinstra SMA. Braces and orthoses for treating osteoarthritis of the knee. *Cochrane Database Syst Rev.* 2005;25(1):CD004020.
3. DiStefano LJ, Padua DA, Brown CN, Guskiewicz KM. Lower extremity kinematics and ground reaction forces after prophylactic lace-up ankle bracing. *J Athl Train.* 2008;43(3):234–41.
4. Hume PA, Gerrard DF. Effectiveness of external ankle support. Bracing and taping in rugby union. *Sports Med.* 1998;25(5):285–312.
5. Jepson KK. The use of orthoses for athletes. In: Birrer RB, editor. *Sports Medicine for the Primary Care Physician.* 2nd ed. New York: Informa Healthcare; 1994. p. 285–95.
6. Mathias M, Rougier PR. In healthy subjects, the sitting position can be used to validate the postural effects induced by wearing a lumbar lordosis brace. *Ann Phys Rehabil Med.* 2010;53(8):511–9.
7. Munoz F, Salmochi JF, Faouën P, Rougier P. Low back pain sufferers: is standing postural balance facilitated by a lordotic lumbar brace? *Orthop Traumatol Surg Res.* 2010;96(4):362–6.
8. Pedowitz DI, Reddy S, Parekh SG, Huffman RG, Sennett BJ. Prophylactic bracing decreases ankle injuries in collegiate female volleyball players. *Am J Sports Med.* 2008;36(2):324–7.
9. Phaner V, Fayolle-Minon I, Lequang B, Valayer-Chaleat E, Calmels P. Are there indications (other than scoliosis) for rigid orthopedic brace treatment of chronic, mechanical low back pain? *Ann Phys Rehabil Med.* 2009;52(5):382–93.
10. Prentice WE. *Arnheim's Principles of Athletic Training: A Competency-Based Approach.* New York (NY): McGraw-Hill; 2009. p. 225–6.
11. Rishiraj N, Taunton JE, Lloyd-Smith R, Woollard R, Regan W, Clement DB. The potential role of prophylactic/functional knee bracing in preventing knee ligament injury. *Sports Med.* 2009;39(11):937–60.
12. Salata MJ, Gibbs AE, Sekiya JK. The effectiveness of prophylactic knee bracing in American football: a systematic review. *Sports Health.* 2010;2(5):375–9.
13. Sanders MS, Cates RA, Baker MD, Barber-Westin SD, Gladin WM, Levy MS. Knee injuries and the use of prophylactic knee bracing in off-road motorcycling: results of a large-scale epidemiological study. *Am J Sports Med.* 2011;39(7):1395–400.
14. Santos MJ, McIntire K, Foecking J, Liu W. The effects of ankle bracing on motion of the knee and the hip joint during trunk rotation tasks. *Clin Biomech (Bristol, Avon).* 2004;19(9):964–71.

Casting and Splinting

Jennifer M. Garrison and Chad A. Asplund

78

PRINCIPLES OF CASTING AND SPLINTING

- The initial approach to casting and splinting involves a thorough assessment of the injury for proper diagnosis to include an exam above and below the injured area.
- The purpose of splinting and casting is to immobilize, protect, aid in healing, and decrease pain.
- Immobilization offers three benefits: prevention of loss of position, protection of adjacent structures, and pain relief.
- Conditions that benefit from immobilization include fractures, sprains, severe soft tissue injuries, reduced joint dislocations, inflammatory conditions, deep lacerations across joints, and tendon lacerations.
- Complications can occur regardless of how long the device is used (13).

SPLINTING VERSUS CASTING

- Consideration for casting versus splinting requires assessment of the stage and severity of the injury, the potential for instability, the risk of complications, and the patient's functional requirements.
- Splinting is more commonly used in the primary care setting (6).
- If an injury is associated with significant swelling or more swelling is anticipated, initial splinting followed by casting for definitive treatment is recommended.
- Maximal immobilization cannot be obtained unless the joints above and below the fracture are immobilized, which is required for most unstable or potentially unstable fractures.

SPLINTING

- Splinting offers many advantages over casting, including easier application and removal and decreased pressure-related complications because they are noncircumferential.
- Disadvantages include decreased patient compliance and increased motion at the injury site.

- Splints may be used in the acute setting and later replaced by a cast for definitive treatment of unstable of potentially unstable fractures (6).

CASTING

- Casting is the mainstay of treatment for most fractures (6).
- Casts provide superior immobilization and are reserved for complex and/or definitive fracture management (13).
- They require more skill and time for application.

SPLINTING/CASTING MATERIALS

- Plaster is traditionally preferred for splints because it is pliable and has a longer setting time than fiberglass and produces less heat, which avoids burns and patient discomfort (15).
- Fiberglass is less messy and lighter than plaster and is typically used for nondisplaced fractures and severe soft tissue injuries.
- Casts set slower in colder water than warm water (3).
- Regardless of material used, water temperature is the most important variable. Heat is inversely proportional to the setting time and directly proportional to the number of layers of casting material used (4,5).
- Plaster is cheaper and has a longer shelf life, while fiberglass is more durable and lighter.
- Fiberglass is generally preferred for casting by providers who have more experience casting and who treat larger numbers of fractures.
- Other materials and equipment include: adhesive tape for splints, bandage scissors, casting gloves for fiberglass, elastic bandage for splints, padding, sheets/underpads, and stockinette.

GENERAL PROCESS

- The involved extremity should be assessed, and documentation of skin lesions, neurovascular status, soft tissue injury, and bony structures should be performed. Neurovascular status should be rechecked following immobilization by cast or splint.

- A stockinette is measured and applied to cover the area of injury and extend 10 cm beyond each end or the intended splint site. Excess is folded back to form a smooth edge once the splint or cast material has been applied. It is important to make sure the stockinette is not too tight and wrinkles are smoothed.
- Layers of padding are placed over the stockinette to prevent maceration of skin and accommodate swelling.
- Padding is wrapped circumferentially, with each new layer overlapping 50% of the previous layer. It should be two to three layers thick and extend 2–3 cm beyond the edge of the splint.
- Extra padding is placed between digits and over bony prominences. Too much padding can compromise support of the splint.
- Joints are always placed in proper position of function.
- Add 1–2 cm of splinting to each end of the splint to allow for shrinkage. Ultimately, the splint should be slightly shorter than the padding.
- The thickness or the splint depends on patient size, extremity involved, and desired strength. On average, an adult upper extremity should be splinted with 6–10 sheets; lower extremities require 12–15 sheets (4,5).
- The splinting material should be unrolled to the appropriate length; the next layer should be folded back onto itself to create subsequent layers.
- The splint material is then submerged in water until the bubbling stops. Excess water is squeezed out. The splint is then placed on a hard surface, wrinkles are smoothed out, and even wetness of all layers is ensured. The splint is placed over the padding and molded to the contours of the extremity. Stockinette and padding edges are then folded back.
- Secure the dry splint with an elastic bandage in a distal to proximal direction.
- Casting material should go over the stockinette and padding circumferentially, with each roll overlapping 50% of the previous layer. Stockinette and padding edges should be folded back before the last layer is applied.
- Avoid excess molding and indentation. If an open wound exists, a window should be cut in the cast for monitoring.

COMPLICATIONS

- Compartment syndrome is the most serious complication that involves increased pressure within a closed space that compromises blood flow, tissue perfusion, which can cause ischemia, and potential irreversible tissue damage. Symptoms may include worsening pain, tingling, numbness, and severe swelling. Immediate evaluation and prompt removal of the cast are imperative.
- Skin breakdown is the most common thermal injury that occurs during the casting or splinting process, caused by focal pressure from wrinkles or unpadded or underpadded area over bony prominences or underlying soft tissue (16).
- Bacterial and fungal infection and pruritic dermatitis can develop beneath a cast or splint and are more common with open wounds and moist and warm environments (8).
- Reflex sympathetic dystrophy (RSD), or complex regional pain syndrome, is an uncommon, late complication of a fractured extremity, resulting from vasomotor dysfunction of the sympathetic nervous system. RSD is characterized by pain, swelling, redness, and hypersensitivity often out of proportion to the initial injury. It can result in stiff joints, atrophic changes, contractures, and loss of function.
- Other complications of excessive immobilization include joint stiffness, chronic pain, and muscle atrophy.

FOLLOW-UP

- Patient education is crucial regarding cast and splinting care. Verbal and written instructions on elevation of extremity, avoiding getting splint/cast wet or pushing objects inside to scratch, precautions for compartment syndrome, pain control, and ice usage are necessary.
- Time to follow-up depends on site fracture site, type, patient age, compliance, and accessibility.
- Most require follow-up within 1–2 weeks.
- If a cast was applied to an acute fracture, a follow-up visit the next day is recommended.
- There are four broad categories of follow-up: initial cast checks, replacement of the cast, assessment for healing, and assessment of function after removal.

COMMONLY USED SPLINTS AND CASTS

- **Ulnar gutter splints** are used for nondisplaced, stable fractures of the head, neck, and shaft of the fourth and fifth metacarpal with mild angulation and no rotational deformities; nondisplaced, nonrotated shaft fractures and serious soft tissue injuries of the fourth and fifth, proximal, or middle phalanx; and boxer's fractures (distal fifth metacarpal fracture, the most common injury for which ulnar gutter splints/casts are used).
- **Ulnar gutter casts** are a definitive or alternative treatment of injuries commonly treated with an ulnar gutter splint (10).
- **Radial gutter splints** are used for nondisplaced fractures of the head, neck, and shaft of the second or third metacarpal without angulation or rotation; nondisplaced, nonrotated shaft fractures and serious injuries of the second or third proximal or middle phalanx; and initial immobilization of displaced distal radius fractures (2,7).
- **Radial gutter casts** are used as definitive or alternative treatment of fractures managed with a radial gutter splint.

- **Thumb spica splints** are used for suspected injuries to the scaphoid; stable ligamentous injuries to the thumb; initial treatment of nonangulated, nondisplaced, extraarticular fractures of the base of the first metacarpal; de Quervain tenosynovitis; and first carpometacarpal joint arthritis.

- Immobilization of the thumb with a removable splint after a ligamentous injury has equal functional results compared to those with a plaster cast (14).

- **Thumb spica casts** are used for suspected or nondisplaced, distal fractures of the scaphoid; and nonangulated, nondisplaced, extra-articular fractures of the base of the first metacarpal. These patients should also be referred for orthopedic subspecialist evaluation.

- **Buddy taping (dynamic splinting)** is used for minor finger sprains; and stable, nondisplaced, nonangulated shaft fractures of the proximal or middle phalanx (1).

- **Dorsal extension-block splints** are used for larger, middle phalangeal volar avulsions with potential for dorsal subluxation; and reduce stable proximal interphalangeal joint dorsal dislocations. Buddy taping should follow.

- **Aluminum U-shaped splints** are used for distal phalangeal fractures.

- **Mallet finger splints** are used for avulsions of the extensor tendons from the base of the distal phalanx (with or without and avulsion fracture). Continuous extension in the splint for 6–8 weeks is essential, even when changing the splint. Compliance is assessed every 2 weeks. Night splinting for an additional 2–3 weeks is recommended.

- **Volar/dorsal forearm splints** are used for soft tissue injuries of the hand and wrist and temporary immobilization of carpal bone dislocations or fractures (excluding scaphoid and trapezium). They are generally not recommended for distal radial or ulnar fractures because they do not limit forearm pronation and supination.

- Recent studies, however, have demonstrated that splinting as a definitive treatment of wrist buckle fractures in children improved physical functioning. There additionally was no difference in pain or healing rates when compared with casting (12).

- **Short arm casts** are used for nondisplaced or minimally displaced fractures of the distal wrist, such as Colles and Smith fractures or greenstick, buckle, and physeal fractures in children, and carpal bone fractures other than scaphoid or trapezium.

- **Single sugar tong splints** are used in acute management of distal radial and ulnar fractures. The sugar tong splint eliminates supination and pronation of the forearm, which is an advantage over a short arm cast for distal radial and ulna fractures.

- **Long arm posterior splints** are used in the acute and definitive management of elbow, proximal and midshaft forearm, and wrist injuries and acute management of distal radial (nonbuckle) and/or ulnar fractures in children. It is not recommended for complex or unstable distal forearm fractures (1,11).

- **Long arm casts** are used as definitive treatment of injuries initially treated with a posterior splint. They are used most often in children because of the frequency of distal radial, ulnar, and distal humeral fractures.

- **Double sugar tong splints** are used in the acute management of elbow and forearm injuries, including Colles fractures. They provide pronation and supination control and limit flexion and extension about the elbow. They are preferable with complex or unstable fractures of the distal forearm and elbow.

- **Posterior ankle splints ("post mold")** are used for acute, severe ankle sprains; nondisplaced, isolated malleolar fractures; and acute foot fractures and soft tissue injuries.

- **Stirrup splints** are used for acute ankle injuries and nondisplaced, isolated malleolar fractures.

- **Short leg casts** are used for definitive treatment of injuries to the ankle and foot. Weight-bearing recommendations are determined by the type and stability of the injury and the patient's capacity and discomfort.

- **Short leg walking casts and commercially produced high-top walking boots** are acceptable alternatives.

- Evidence favors a functional approach to inversion ankle sprain treatment with the use of a semirigid or soft lace-up brace (9).

- **Toe plate extensions** are used for toe immobilization (compared to high-top walking boot or cast shoe) and distal metatarsal and phalangeal fractures, particularly of the great toe.

- **Posterior long leg splints** are used for stabilization of acute soft tissue injuries, patellar fracture or dislocation, and other traumatic lower extremity injuries.

PROPER CODING

- Use International Classification of Diseases, Ninth Revision (ICD-9) codes for diagnosis, *e.g.*, 354.0

- Use Common Procedural Terminology (CPT) codes for procedures, *e.g.*, 29125

- Use CPT for evaluation and management service on same day as procedure, *e.g.*, 09925

- Consider using fracture care codes, *e.g.*, 26600

- Carpal tunnel syndrome ICD-9 code 354.0

- Scaphoid fracture ICD-9 code 814.01

- de Quervain tenosynovitis ICD-9 code 727.04

- Gamekeeper's thumb/skier's thumb (ulnar collateral ligament injury) ICD-9 code 842.12

- Plantar fasciitis (heel spur syndrome) ICD-9 code 728.71

- Short arm thumb spica cast CPT code 29085

- Distal fibular fracture ICD-9 code 824.8

- Avulsion fracture ICD-9 code 829.0

REFERENCES

1. Benjamin HJ, Hang BT. Common acute upper extremity injuries in sports. *Clin Pediatr Emerg Med.* 2007;8(1):15–30.

2. Boutis K, Willan A, Babyn P, Goeree R, Howard A. Cast versus splint in children with minimally angulated fractures of the distal radius: a randomized controlled trial. *CMAJ.* 2010;182(14):1507–12.

3. Bowker P, Powell ES. A clinical evaluation of plaster-of-Paris and eight synthetic fracture splinting materials. *Injury.* 1992;23(1):13–20.

4. Boyd AS, Benjamin HJ, Asplund C. Principles of casting and splinting. *Am Fam Physician.* 2009;79(1):16–22.

5. Boyd AS, Benjamin HJ, Asplund C. Splints and casts: indications and methods. *Am Fam Physician.* 2009;80(5):491–9.

6. Eiff MP, Hatch RL, Calmbach WL. *Fracture Management for Primary Care.* Philadelphia (PA): WB Saunders Company; 1998. p. 19–24.

7. Hong E. Hand injuries in sports medicine. *Prim Care.* 2005;32(1):91–103.

8. Houang ET, Buckley R, Williams RJ, O'Riordan SM. Outbreak of plaster-associated Pseudomonas infection. *Lancet.* 1981;1(8222):728–9.

9. Kerkhoffs GM, Struijs PA, Marti RK, Assendelft WJ, Blankevoort L, van Dijk CN. Different functional treatment strategies for acute lateral ankle ligament injuries in adults. *Cochrane Database Syst Rev.* 2002;3: CD002938.

10. Lee SG, Jupiter JB. Phalangeal and metacarpal fractures of the hand. *Hand Clin.* 2000;16(3):323–32, vii.

11. Overly F, Steele DW. Common pediatric fractures and dislocations. *Clin Pediatr Emerg Med.* 2002;3(2):106–17.

12. Plint AC, Perry JJ, Correll R, Gaboury I, Lawton L. A randomized, controlled trial of removable splinting versus casting for wrist buckle fractures in children. *Pediatrics.* 2006;117(3):691–7.

13. Simon RR, Koenigsknecht SJ, editors. *Emergency Orthopedics: The Extremities.* 3rd ed. Norwalk: Appleton and Lange; 1995. p. 3–20.

14. Sollerman C, Abrahamsson SO, Lundborg G, Adalbert K. Functional splinting versus plaster cast for ruptures of the ulnar collateral ligament of the thumb. A prospective randomized study of 63 cases. *Acta Orthop Scand.* 1991;62(6):524–6.

15. Wehbé MA. Plaster uses and misuses. *Clin Orthop Relat Res.* 1982; 167:242–9.

16. Yap NF, Fischer S. Burns associated with plaster of Paris. Presented at the Royal Australasian College of Surgeons Annual Scientific Congress, Perth 9–13 May 2005. Abstract no. HS101P. [cited 2010 Dec 22]. Available from: http://www.blackwellpublishing.com/RACS/abstract.asp?id=20349.

Psychological Considerations in Physical Activity, Exercise, and Sport

79

Jeffrey L. Goodie and Nicole L. Frazer

INTRODUCTION

- Physical activity, exercise, and sports influence behaviors, thoughts, and emotions. Similarly, what people do, how they think, and emotional responses influence the participation and performance of individuals in physical activity, exercise, and sports. Promoting participation in physical activity and enhancing performance in exercise and sports requires an understanding of the increasing evidence base connecting psychology with exercise and sport.

- Only 50% of U.S. adults engage in recommended physical activity levels. Healthy adults between 18 and 65 years old should engage in moderate-intensity aerobic physical activity (*e.g.*, brisk walking) for at least 30 minutes 5 days a week or vigorous-intensity aerobic physical activity (*e.g.*, jogging) for at least 20 minutes 3 days each week. Additionally, these adults should engage in physical activity that maintains or increases muscle strength and endurance at least 2 days a week (18).

- There is increasing evidence that physical activity and exercise are effective interventions for ameliorating depressive symptoms (26). For example, when those diagnosed with a major depressive disorder exercised at levels consistent with public health recommendations, their depressive symptoms decreased more than those who exercised less (11). Exercise was shown to decrease depressive symptoms as much as antidepressant medications (4). A systematic review also found at least a small positive effect for exercise-reducing depression and anxiety symptoms among children and adolescents (24).

- Exercise and physical activity may also improve behavioral and psychological concerns (*e.g.*, alcohol abuse, anxiety disorders, eating disorders) (43). Exercise can improve self-esteem in children and young adults (13) and improves cognitive functioning in older adults (2).

INITIATING AND INCREASING PHYSICAL ACTIVITY

- It is important to target physical activity early in life. Adolescents who have a more positive view of physical activity and sport engage in more physical activity 5 and 10 years later (16). Among adolescents and children, education-only interventions to increase activity are not effective (47). However, for adolescents, school-based multicomponent interventions (*i.e.*, education combined with environmental or policy changes) and interventions that include school and family or community involvement are associated with increased activity (47).

- Simple interventions can increase physical activity. For example, wearing pedometers, along with having a step goal (*e.g.*, 10,000 steps per day), is associated with significant increases in daily physical activity (6). Also, using point-of-decision prompts, such as signs placed near escalators and elevators encouraging the use of stairs, significantly increases the likelihood of stair use (42).

- In 2002, the U.S. Preventive Services Task Force concluded that there was insufficient evidence that counseling adults to increase physical activity in primary care settings results in sustained changes in physical activity (12). However, England's Public Health Interventions Advisory Committee determined in 2006 that there was sufficient evidence supporting brief counseling interventions for increasing physical activity in primary care settings (15).

  - According to the National Institute for Health and Clinical Excellence (NICE), inactive individuals should be identified in primary care settings, and the patients' specific needs, preferences, and circumstances should be considered when setting goals with them. Patients should be followed over a 3- to 6-month period to sustain physical activity increases (15).

BEHAVIORAL HEALTH CONDITIONS ASSOCIATED WITH EXERCISE

■ Although disordered eating behaviors and substance use have been studied among athletes, very little is known about other psychological concerns and disorders, including anxiety disorders, attention-deficit hyperactivity disorder (ADHD), bipolar disorder, depression, overtraining syndrome, psychosis, and suicidality (39).

Disordered Eating Behavior

■ Disordered eating behavior can range from that which meets clinical diagnostic criteria for anorexia nervosa (Table 79.1) or bulimia nervosa (Table 79.2), as established in the *Diagnostic and Statistical Manual of Mental Disorders, Fourth Edition-Text Revision* (DSM-IV-TR), to subclinical levels of disordered eating behavior, which might include occasional purging and/or laxative use or diet pill use, referred to as "eating disorder not otherwise specified" in the DSM-IV-TR.

  ■ It is important to recognize that bingeing and compensatory purging may be a feature of anorexia nervosa or bulimia nervosa.

  ■ Targeted programs may help reduce the risk of disordered eating behavior among adolescent athletes (14).

Table 79.1 | **DSM-IV-TR Criteria for Anorexia Nervosa**

A. Refusal to maintain body weight at or above a minimally normal weight for age and height (*e.g.*, weight loss leading to maintenance of body weight less than 85% of that expected; or failure to make expected weight gain during period of growth, leading to body weight less than 85% of that expected).

B. Intense fear of gaining weight or becoming fat, even though underweight.

C. Disturbance in the way in which one's body weight or shape is experienced, undue influence of body weight or shape on self-evaluation, or denial of the seriousness of the current low body weight.

D. In postmenarchal females, amenorrhea, *i.e.*, the absence of at least three consecutive menstrual cycles. (A woman is considered to have amenorrhea if her periods occur only following hormone, *e.g.*, estrogen, administration.)

Specify type:

Restricting Type: during the current episode of anorexia nervosa, the person has not regularly engaged in binge-eating or purging behavior (*i.e.*, self-induced vomiting or the misuse of laxatives, diuretics, or enemas).

Binge Eating/Purging Type: during the current episode of anorexia nervosa, the person has regularly engaged in binge eating or purging behavior (*i.e.*, self-induced vomiting or the misuse of laxatives, diuretics, or enemas).

SOURCE: American Psychiatric Association. *Diagnostic and Statistical Manual of Mental Disorders.* 4th ed., text revision. Washington (DC): American Psychiatric Association; 2000.

Table 79.2 | **DSM-IV-TR Criteria for Bulimia Nervosa**

A. Recurrent episodes of binge eating. An episode of binge eating is characterized by both of the following:

  1) Eating, in a discrete period of time (*e.g.*, within any 2-hour period), an amount of food that is definitely larger than most people would eat during a similar period of time and under similar circumstances.

  2) A sense of lack of control over eating during the episode (*e.g.*, a feeling that one cannot stop eating or control what or how much one is eating).

B. Recurrent inappropriate compensatory behavior in order to prevent weight gain, such as self-induced vomiting; misuse of laxatives, diuretics, enemas, or other medications; fasting; or excessive exercise.

C. The binge eating and inappropriate compensatory behaviors both occur, on average, at least twice a week for 3 months.

D. Self-evaluation is unduly influenced by body shape and weight.

E. The disturbance does not occur exclusively during episodes of anorexia nervosa.

Specify type:

Purging Type: during the current episode of bulimia nervosa, the person has regularly engaged in self-induced vomiting or the misuse of laxatives, diuretics, or enemas.

Nonpurging Type: during the current episode of bulimia nervosa, the person has used other inappropriate compensatory behaviors, such as fasting or excessive exercise, but has not regularly engaged in self-induced vomiting or the misuse of laxatives, diuretics, or enemas.

SOURCE: American Psychiatric Association. *Diagnostic and Statistical Manual of Mental Disorders.* 4th ed., text revision. Washington (DC): American Psychiatric Association; 2000.

■ Disordered eating behaviors may be more common among athletes than in the general population. Although there has been variability in prevalence rates of eating disorders in athletes, researchers demonstrated that in a sample of elite athletes, the overall prevalence of eating disorders was 13.5% compared to 4.6% in controls. For elite athletes meeting criteria for an eating disorder, 32.4% were men (44). Disordered eating is not confined to female athletes, and assessment of eating behavior in both females and males is important.

  ■ Anorexia nervosa signs and symptoms include increasing restrictions in food consumption, social avoidance, "excessive" physical activity, which may include maintaining a rigid posture or excessive standing, being hungry less often and being full sooner, and beliefs of being too heavy despite being thin or underweight. Emotionally, individuals may demonstrate depressive symptoms, irritability, and obsessional thoughts (23). Physically, in addition to amenorrhea in women, individuals may demonstrate constipation, headaches, fainting, dizziness, fatigue and cold intolerance, dry skin, hair loss, bradycardia, orthostatic hypotension, hypoglycemia, hypothermia, and leukopenia (38).

  ■ Signs and symptoms of bulimia nervosa include some methods of getting rid of calories and diminished perceived control over eating (23). Binge eating usually occurs very rapidly, often with self-determined "forbidden foods" and while the individual is alone. The binge may involve a total calorie count from several hundred calories to more than 10,000 calories (23). Individuals may demonstrate overly restrained eating outside of binge eating episodes (23). Physical signs and symptoms may include bloating; fullness; lethargy; gastroesophageal reflux disease; abdominal pain; knuckle calluses; dental enamel erosion; hypochloremic, hypokalemic, or metabolic alkalosis; hypokalemia; and elevated salivary amylase (38). However, none of these physical signs and symptoms may be present, and the individual may still be engaging in regular binging and compensatory behaviors.

- Risk factors for developing disordered eating include:
  - Psychological factors such as body dissatisfaction, negative affect, low self-esteem, and perfectionism; sociocultural factors promoting unrealistic thinness standards; and participation in a variety of sports, not only sports promoting lean builds (*e.g.*, gymnastics, figure skating) (21). For men, distance running, wrestling, body building, lightweight football, horseracing, rowing, and ski jumping have been associated with disordered eating.
- The National Athletic Trainers Association presented recommendations for preventing, detecting, and managing disordered eating in athletes (5). Key recommendations include the following:
  - Develop policies and plans for detecting and managing disordered eating and establish screening methods to identify disordered eating as soon as possible. It is unlikely that athletes will self-identify eating problems.
  - Screening should include measures designed specifically for athletes, interviews, observations of behavior, and monitoring of body composition. Standard eating disorder screening measures may not have been validated with athletes. The ATHLETE Questionnaire has been shown to be a valid and reliable measure of psychological predictors of disordered eating among athletes (20).
  - When disordered eating is suspected, health care providers should conduct a thorough evaluation. If treatment is indicated, medical, dietary, behavioral, and cognitive interventions are necessary for effective treatment.
- The "female athlete triad" was coined by the American College of Sports Medicine® (ACSM) in 1992 to describe three interrelated conditions of functional hypothalamic amenorrhea, premenopausal osteoporosis, and disordered eating that often occur together in female athletes (31).
  - In the most recent ACSM position stand on the female athlete triad (32), it is recommended that females are screened for symptoms at preparticipation or annual health screening exams. Athletes who demonstrate one of the triad components should be screened for the other components.
  - According to the ACSM (32), treatment for those demonstrating the female athlete triad should focus on increasing energy availability (*i.e.*, increasing energy intake and/or reducing energy expenditure) through nutritional counseling. Those who are demonstrating disordered

Table 79.3	**DSM-IV-TR Criteria for Substance Abuse**

A. A maladaptive pattern of substance use leading to clinically significant impairment or distress, as manifested by one or more of the following, occurring within a 12-month period.

  1) Recurrent substance use resulting in a failure to fulfill major role obligations at work, school, or home (*e.g.*, repeated absences or poor work performance related to substance use; substance-related absences, suspensions, or expulsions from school; neglect of children or household).

  2) Recurrent substance use in situations in which it is physically hazardous (*e.g.*, driving an automobile or operating a machine when impaired by substance use).

  3) Recurrent substance-related legal problems (*e.g.*, arrests for substance-related disorderly conduct).

  4) Continued substance use despite having persistent or recurrent social or interpersonal problems caused by or exacerbated by the effects of the substance (*e.g.*, arguments with spouse about consequences of intoxication, physical fights).

B. The symptoms have never met the criteria for substance dependence for this class of substance.

SOURCE: American Psychiatric Association. *Diagnostic and Statistical Manual of Mental Disorders.* 4th ed., text revision. Washington (DC): American Psychiatric Association; 2000.

eating and eating disorders should receive nutritional counseling and individual psychotherapy. It may be necessary to restrict athletes not adhering to treatment recommendations from training and competition.

Alcohol Use and Dependence

- In a survey of 19,676 college student athletes by the National Collegiate Athletic Association (NCAA) regarding substance use habits, 76.9% reported using alcohol in the preceding 12 months, making it the most commonly abused substance by athletes (45).
  - Alcohol use has declined since 1989; however, the number of student-athletes consuming five or more drinks in one sitting has increased (45).
  - Almost 60% of student-athletes reported that they believed that their use of alcohol had no effect on their general health or athletic performance (45).
  - According to the 2005 NCAA survey, 77.7% of college student-athletes reported they began drinking before entering college (45).
- The DSM-IV-TR delineates criteria for whether a substance abuse disorder (Table 79.3) or substance dependence disorder (Table 79.4) exists. A diagnosis of alcohol dependence requires that the criteria for alcohol withdrawal are met (Table 79.5).
- A helpful screening tool in determining whether the athlete is a problem drinker is the Alcohol Use Disorders Identification Test (AUDIT-C) (8).
  - The AUDIT-C is scored on a scale of 0–12 (scores of 0 reflect no alcohol use) by summing the circled numbers

Table 79.4 | DSM-IV-TR Criteria for Substance Dependence

A maladaptive pattern of substance use, leading to clinically significant impairment or distress, as manifested by three or more of the following, occurring within the same 12-month period.

1) Tolerance, as defined by either of the following:

   (a) Need for markedly increased amounts of the substance to achieve intoxication or desired effect.

   (b) Markedly diminished effect with continued use of the same amount of the substance.

2) Withdrawal as manifested by either of the following:

   (c) The characteristic withdrawal syndrome for the substance (refer to criteria A and B of the criteria sets for Withdrawal from the specific substances).

   (d) The same (or a closely related) substance is taken to relieve or avoid withdrawal.

3) The substance is often taken in larger amounts or over a longer period than was intended.

4) A persistent desire exists to cut down or control substance use along with many unsuccessful attempts to do so.

5) A great deal of time is spent in activities necessary to obtain the substance (*e.g.*, driving long distances), use the substance, or recover from its effects.

6) Important social, occupational, or recreational activities are given up or reduced because of substance use.

7) The substance use is continued despite knowledge of having a persistent or recurrent physical or psychological problem that is likely to have been caused or exacerbated by the substance (*e.g.*, continued drinking despite recognition that an ulcer was made worse by alcohol consumption).

SOURCE: American Psychiatric Association. *Diagnostic and Statistical Manual of Mental Disorders.* 4th ed., text revision. Washington (DC): American Psychiatric Association; 2000.

Table 79.5 | DSM-IV-TR Criteria for Alcohol Withdrawal

A. Cessation of (or reduction in) alcohol use that has been heavy and prolonged.

B. Two (or more) of the following, developing within several hours to a few days after Criterion A:

   1) Autonomic hyperactivity (*e.g.*, sweating or pulse rate greater than 100)

   2) Increased hand tremor

   3) Insomnia

   4) Nausea or vomiting

   5) Transient visual, tactile, or auditory hallucinations or illusions

   6) Psychomotor agitation

   7) Anxiety

   8) Grand mal seizures

C. The symptoms in Criterion B cause clinically significant distress or impairment in social, occupational, or other important areas of functioning.

D. The symptoms are not due to a general medical condition and are not better accounted for by another mental disorder.

SOURCE: American Psychiatric Association. *Diagnostic and Statistical Manual of Mental Disorders.* 4th ed., text revision. Washington (DC): American Psychiatric Association; 2000.

tobacco, representing a decrease in use compared to previous surveys.

- The primary reason athletes cite for using tobacco is for recreational and social purposes. The most common reason for not using tobacco or for quitting was concerns about health.

in each of the four columns and then summing the values to obtain a total severity score (see Table 79.6).

- In men, a score of 4 or more is considered positive; in women, a score of 3 or more is considered positive.

- Generally, the higher the AUDIT-C score, the more likely it is that the patient's drinking is affecting his or her health and safety.

- If the AUDIT-C score is positive, health care providers should conduct a brief intervention. This includes bringing attention to the elevated level of drinking, informing the athlete about the effects of alcohol on health, recommending limiting use or abstaining, exploring and supporting in choosing a responsible drinking goal, and follow-up and refer for specialty treatment, if indicated.

Tobacco Use and Dependence

- In 2005, the NCAA revealed that among all athletes, 14.1% had smoked cigarettes and 16.3% had used smokeless

Table 79.6 | Audit-C

1. How often do you have a drink containing alcohol?				
Never (0)	Monthly or less (1)	Two or four times a month (2)	Two to three times per week (3)	Four or more times a week (4)

2. How many drinks containing alcohol do you have on a typical day when you are drinking?				
1 or 2 (0)	3 or 4 (1)	5 or 6 (2)	7 or 9 (3)	10 or more (4)

3. How often do you have six or more drinks on one occasion?				
Never (0)	Less than monthly (1)	Monthly (2)	Weekly (3)	Daily or almost Daily (4)

SOURCE: Bush K, Kivlahan DR, McDonell MB, Fihn SD, Bradley KA. The AUDIT Alcohol Consumption Questions (AUDIT-C): an effective brief screening test for problem drinking. Ambulatory Care Quality Improvement Project (ACQUIP). Alcohol Use Disorders Identification Test. *Arch Intern Med.* 1998;158(16):1789–95.

Table 79.7	The "5 A's" Model for Treating Tobacco Use and Dependence
Ask about tobacco use	Identify and document tobacco use status for every patient at every visit.
Advise to quit	In a clear, strong, and personalized manner, urge every tobacco user to quit.
Assess willingness to make a quit attempt	Is the tobacco user willing to make a quit attempt at this time?
Assist in quit attempt	For the patient willing to make a quit attempt, offer medication and provide or refer for counseling or additional treatment to help the patient quit.
	For patients unwilling to quit, provide interventions designed to increase future quit attempts.
Arrange follow-up	For the patient willing to make a quit attempt, arrange for follow-up contacts, beginning within the first week after the quit date.
	For patients unwilling to make a quit attempt at the time, address tobacco dependence and willingness to quit at next clinic visit.

SOURCE: U.S. Department of Health and Human Services. *Treating Tobacco Use and Dependence: 2008 Update.* Rockville (MD): Public Health Service; 2008.

- Every athlete who uses tobacco products should be offered a minimal intervention. An intervention lasting less than 3 minutes can increase overall tobacco abstinence rates (46). The 5 A's model is recommended as a brief intervention (Table 79.7). Intensive tobacco cessation programs are also available to assist individuals in their quit efforts. The more effective interventions are based on a dose-response relation, with four or more sessions yielding higher abstinence rates (46).

- Other substances used by college athletes include amphetamines (4.1%), anabolic steroids (1.2%), cocaine (2.1%), ecstasy (1.1%), ephedrine (2.5%), marijuana (20.3%), and psychedelics (2.4%).
  - Overall, the use of these substances has generally decreased, except for the use of amphetamines, which has increased. The most common reason students report taking amphetamines is for the treatment of ADHD; the second most common reason is to increase energy.

Exercise Dependence and Overtraining

- Exercise dependence, sometimes described as "exercise addiction," is not a DSM-IV-TR diagnosis like alcohol and tobacco dependence. Researchers describe exercise dependence as a perceived need for physical activity associated with excessive exercise behavior with tolerance and/or withdrawal and psychological symptoms (19).
  - With tolerance, the individual must continually elevate the level of exercise in order to achieve the same state of feeling good. Withdrawal symptoms can encompass mood

symptoms, such as anxiousness, irritability, depression, and restlessness, or even physical symptoms of fatigue 24–36 hours after missing a scheduled session of exercise (27).
  - Prevalence rates have ranged from 2%–30% of the exercising population (17). Hypothesized mechanisms for exercising dependence include affect regulation (*i.e.*, exercise enhances positive affect and/or reduces negative affect), sympathetic arousal (*i.e.*, hormonal changes maintain need for repeated exercise), β-endorphins (*i.e.*, opioid peptides produce addictive behaviors), and cytokine overproduction (*i.e.*, exercise provides relief from symptoms associated with overproduction of cytokines, *e.g.*, fatigue, poor concentration, anxiety, depression) (17).
  - In a 2002 systematic review of 88 papers over 29 years, the authors concluded that the results of and conclusions associated with exercise dependence should be "interpreted cautiously" (p. 118) and "no definitive statement" can be made about exercise dependence (19).

- Overtraining involves increased training intensity and/or duration without adequate recovery (28). An example would be a runner who trains at increased distances every day without allowing a day of rest or recovery in between sessions. The ultimate result of this behavior is the opposite of what is pursued (*i.e.*, a state of staleness or a lack of performance improvement and possibly even deterioration in performance may result). There are limited data related to overtraining syndrome (39).
  - Overtraining syndrome can be characterized by fatigue, depression, restlessness, and increased resting heart rate, to name a few (28).
  - Mood disturbance is one of the key characteristics of the overtraining syndrome, and therefore, monitoring of an athlete's mood during increased stress may also be helpful (28). Additionally, athletes who participate in multiple sports and endurance athletes (*e.g.*, marathoners) should be monitored for signs of overtraining due to the nature of their sport behavior (28).
  - Having athletes maintain an exercise diary or log can assist in identifying whether their exercise behavior is excessive by examining frequency, duration, context, and type of physical activity. Additionally, consultation with the athletic coach and family members is recommended (22). Use of a pedometer is also an option if excessive exercise is suspected. Patients with excessive exercise have logged 20,000–30,000 steps/day, which is two to three times higher than needed for a healthy lifestyle (40).
  - Clinicians should also assess any functional impact from excessive exercise to include interference with important activities and whether the patient continues exercising despite a physical injury.

Performance Anxiety

- Although the exact prevalence of performance anxiety is unknown, largely due to methodologic differences across studies, performance anxiety in athletes is believed to be very common (34), and an estimated 2% of individuals experience debilitating performance anxiety (37).

■ Evidence supports the long-term effectiveness of behavioral interventions that target the thoughts and behaviors that might contribute to the maintenance of performance anxiety (34).

■ Behavioral strategies for performance enhancement include the use of visual imagery, diaphragmatic breathing, progressive muscle relaxation, biofeedback, autogenic training, yoga, meditation, and desensitization (29).

　■ Visual imagery may involve imagining a relaxing scene or mental rehearsal of one's performance and a desired course of action.

　■ Diaphragmatic breathing is a simple relaxation technique that involves taking slow, deep inhalations, concentrating on only moving the abdomen, holding each inhalation for a few seconds, and then exhaling.

　■ Desensitization is a technique in which the athlete gradually diminishes anxiety associated with certain performance aspects (*e.g.*, free-throws in basketball) or specific anxiety disorders (*e.g.*, social phobia) through gradual exposure, either imagined or in vivo, to the feared or anxiety-eliciting stimuli.

■ Cognitive strategies can also help athletes develop a greater sense of arousal control and, more importantly, improve performance. This might include encouraging the athlete to replace any sabotaging negative self-statements (*e.g.*, "I will never make this shot.") with reassuring, realistic self-statements (*e.g.*, "I have made this shot before and will try my best to make it again."). Additionally, goal setting can be an effective strategy for improving identified areas of performance weakness (20,41).

Sleep Disturbance

■ Ten to 28% of adults report moderate to severe symptoms of insomnia, and the prevalence of a primary insomnia diagnosis is 6% of the population (33). Clinical diagnostic criteria for primary insomnia as established in the DSM-IV-TR include difficulties with sleep onset, sleep maintenance, or nonrestorative sleep that last at least 1 month (1). These sleep problems must cause clinically significant impairment in functioning and must not be due to other clinical or substance use problems. In athletes, stress and jet lag can contribute to disrupted sleep; these disruptions can affect physical (*e.g.*, heart rate, $\dot{V}O_{2max}$) and cognitive (*e.g.*, attention, concentration, memory) functioning (25).

■ Management of sleep difficulties can include both nonpharmacologic and pharmacologic interventions.

　■ Cognitive-behavioral interventions, including sleep education, sleep hygiene, sleep restriction, and stimulus control strategies, have been well studied and can lead to long-term benefits (30). For athletes, use of such strategies can be helpful in both the short-term (*e.g.*, before competitions) and for long-term impacts on performance.

　　❏ Stimulus control interventions assist the patient with associating the bed with sleep. Patients are instructed

to only use the bed for sleep and sexual activity (*e.g.*, no reading or watching TV in bed), to go to bed only when sleepy, to get out of bed if not asleep within 10–15 minutes, and to stay out of bed until they are sleepy. If, when they return to bed, they still do not fall asleep within 10–15 minutes, they should again get out of bed until they are ready to fall asleep. Each morning, patients should wake at the same time and avoid naps throughout the day.

　　❏ Sleep restriction therapy requires determining the average amount of sleep an individual obtains at night, setting a consistent wake time, and then setting the time that the individual would go to sleep by working backwards based on the average sleep time and wake time. If someone typically sleeps 6 hours and wants to wake at 5:00 a.m., they would go to sleep at 11:00 p.m.

■ Pharmacologic interventions for primary insomnia are not ideal; however, they can sometimes be used as an acute intervention on a short-term basis (25).

　❏ Hypnotics, such as zolpidem and zopiclone, have been shown to improve sleep disruption, and use should generally be short term (< 4 weeks) and low dose, and the athlete should concurrently adjust sleep hygiene (25).

REHABILITATION

Injury Rehabilitation

■ Seven million U.S. children, adolescents, and adults (*i.e.*, 25.9 episodes per 1,000 persons) endure sports or recreational-related injuries each year (10). The injured athlete may not only present with a concern about the injury itself, but also with concern over the impact of the injury on present and future performance and concerns regarding the nature of the rehabilitation process (41). Injury, particularly head injury, is among the most common factors associated with suicide among athletes (3).

■ There are multiple models to guide rehabilitation, including the stages of return to sport model, the biopsychosocial model, and the self-determination theory model (36).

　■ The stages of return to sport model includes five physical and psychological stages including initial return, recovery confirmation, return of physical and technical abilities, high-intensity training, and return to competition. Movement between these stages is dependent on injury healing, physical conditioning, and psychological rehabilitation (36).

　■ The biopsychosocial model applied to injury rehabilitation among athletes requires an understanding of how the physical, behavioral, cognitive, emotional, and social factors influence each other and the recovery process. An understanding of the relations between these factors allows the health care provider to more effectively target areas for treatment (Table 79.8) (41). The provider may then choose from among several effective interventions

Table 79.8	Biopsychosocial Factors in Injury Rehabilitation
Physical factors	Where is the injury? What is the frequency, intensity, and duration of any associated pain? Are there any other current significant medical problems? What is their energy level? How is their sleep? What is their history of sports injuries?
Behavioral factors	Are they adhering to the rehabilitation program? Do they put forth their best effort at rehabilitation sessions? Are there any substance abuse issues (*e.g.*, alcohol, tobacco, excessive eating)? How have they changed their life since the injury (*e.g.*, have they skipped important responsibilities?)?
Cognitive factors	What is their attitude about the injury, the treatment they have received, and the rehabilitation process? Do they engage in predominantly positive or negative self-statements?
Emotional factors	Have they recently felt more sad, anxious, upset, and/or irritated than they would have liked? Do they have any fears about returning to their sport? Are they experiencing grief over the loss of their sport or exercise activity?
Relationship factors	Do they have an adequate social support system? Have coaches and/or teammates been constructive in the rehabilitation process? Have they changed their behavior toward family and friends (*e.g.*, more isolative)? Are they experiencing any relationship difficulties/stressors as a result of the injury?

SOURCE: Robinson CS. Psychology and the injured runner: recovery enhancing strategies. In: O'Connor FG, Wilder RP, Nirschl R, editors. *Textbook of Running Medicine.* New York: McGraw-Hill; 2001. p. 621–28.

to tailor a rehabilitation program to meet the athlete's needs. This might include the use of imagery and other mental devices, increasing social support, pain management, and/or other cognitive-behavioral techniques such as self-management training (41).

- The self-determination theory model suggests that when athletes are preparing to return to their sport, they may demonstrate competence concerns (*e.g.*, worry about reinjury and inability to perform at their preinjury level), relatedness concerns (*e.g.*, they may perceive themselves as isolated and lacking social support from their teammates and coaches), and autonomy concerns (*e.g.*, they may perceive pressure from others to return to the sport, or they may worry that others view them as unfit, unskilled, or not as good as they were prior to the injury) (21,36). Therefore, assisting athletes with anxiety management, increasing confidence, maintaining or improving social support and involvement with the sport, and fostering personal autonomy may help reduce return-to-sport concerns (35).
- Regardless of the model used for rehabilitation, goal setting and belief that the treatment will work have been shown to be important for effective rehabilitation.
  - Goal setting is particularly important in rehabilitation. Writing short- and long-term goals that are specific,

challenging, realistic, performance based, and monitored for completion can enhance injury recovery (9).

- Studies have shown that belief in the efficacy of treatment is correlated positively with adherence to the treatment plan (7).

- When determining whether an athlete is ready to return to competition, it is valuable to establish a specified process that includes discussing prospective return dates with the athlete, determining that the athlete is physically ready to return to the sport, assessing the confidence level of the athlete, and identifying who will be responsible for making the final decision about the return to the sport (36).

Referral to Specialty Behavioral Health Services

- It is important that health care providers are vigilant of symptoms that may warrant referral for more extensive behavioral health assessment and treatment and that they are aware of the appropriate professionals to consider when making referrals for athletes (41).
- The term "sport psychologist" is not well defined, and it should not be assumed that someone who describes themselves as a sport psychologist is qualified to provide clinical assessment or treatment services.
- The American Psychological Association recognizes sport psychology as a proficiency that is acquired with specialty training after doctoral training in psychology and licensure as a psychologist. Some "sport psychologists" may be primarily researchers, and other individuals may have no or limited training in psychology. When making a referral to a psychologist for clinical assessment or treatment services for behavioral health conditions in athletes, ask whether the individual is a "licensed psychologist" with specialized training in sport and performance psychology (9).

REFERENCES

1. American Psychiatric Association. *Diagnostic and Statistical Manual of Mental Disorders.* 4th ed., text revision. Washington (DC): American Psychiatric Association; 2000. 943 p.
2. Angevaren M, Aufdemkampe G, Verhaar HJ, Aleman A, Vanhees L. Physical activity and enhanced fitness to improve cognitive function in older people without known cognitive impairment. *Cochrane Database Syst Rev.* 2008;2:CD005381.
3. Baum AL. Suicide in athletes: a review and commentary. *Clin Sports Med.* 2005;24(4):853–69, ix.
4. Blumenthal JA, Babyak MA, Doraiswamy PM, et al. Exercise and pharmacotherapy in the treatment of major depressive disorder. *Psychosom Med.* 2007;69(7):587–96.
5. Bonci CM, Bonci LJ, Granger LR, et al. National athletic trainers' association position statement: preventing, detecting, and managing disordered eating in athletes. *J Athl Train.* 2008;43(1):80–108.
6. Bravata DB, Smith-Spangler C, Sundaram V, et al. Using pedometers to increase physical activity and improve health: a systematic review. *JAMA.* 2007;298(19):2296–304.

7. Brewer BW, Cornelius AE, Van Raalte JL, et al. Protection motivation theory and adherence to sport injury rehabilitation revisited. *The Sport Psychol.* 2003;17(1):95–103.

8. Bush K, Kivlahan DR, McDonell MB, Fihn SD, Bradley KA. The AUDIT alcohol consumption questions (AUDIT-C): an effective brief screening test for problem drinking. Ambulatory Care Quality Improvement Project (ACQUIP). Alcohol Use Disorders. *Arch Intern Med.* 1998; 158(16):1789–95.

9. Carr CM. Sport psychology: psychologic issues and applications. *Phys Med Rehabil Clin N Am.* 2006;17(3):519–35.

10. Conn JM, Annest JL, Gilchrist J. Sports and recreation related injury episodes in the US population, 1997–99. *Inj Prev.* 2003;9(2):117–23.

11. Dunn AL, Trivedi MH, Kampert JB, Clark CG, Chambliss HO. Exercise treatment for depression: efficacy and dose response. *Am J Prev Med.* 2005;28(1):1–8.

12. Eden KB, Orleans CT, Mulrow CD, Pender NJ, Teutsch SM. Does counseling by clinicians improve physical activity? A summary of the evidence for the U.S. Preventive Services Task Force. *Ann Intern Med.* 2002;137(3):208–15.

13. Ekeland E, Heian F, Hagen KB, Abbott J, Nordheim L. Exercise to improve self-esteem in children and young people. *Cochrane Database Syst Rev.* 2004;1:CD003683.

14. Elliot DL, Goldberg L, Moe EL, Defrancesco CA, Durham MB, Hix-Small H. Preventing substance use and disordered eating: initial outcomes of the ATHENA (Athletes Targeting Healthy Exercise and Nutrition Alternatives) program. *Arch Pediatr Adolesc Med.* 2004;158(11):1043–9.

15. Four commonly used methods to increase physical activity: brief interventions in primary care, exercise referral schemes, pedometers and community-based exercise programmes for walking and cycling (Public Health Intervention Guidance no. 2) [Internet]. National Institute for Health and Clinical Excellence; [cited 2011 Feb 12]. Available from: http://www.nice.org.uk/nicemedia/live/11373/31838/31838.pdf.

16. Graham DJ, Sirard JR, Neumark-Sztainer D. Adolescents' attitudes toward sports, exercise, and fitness predict physical activity 5 and 10 years later. *Prev Med.* 2011;52(2):130–2.

17. Hamer M, Karageorghis CI. Psychobiological mechanisms of exercise dependence. *Sports Med.* 2007;37(6):477–84.

18. Haskell WL, Lee IM, Pate RR, et al. Physical activity and public health: updated recommendation for adults from the American College of Sports Medicine and the American Heart Association. *Circulation.* 2007; 116(9):1081–93.

19. Hausenblas HA, Downs DS. Exercise dependence: a systematic review. *Psychol Sport Exerc.* 2002;3:89–123.

20. Hinton PS, Kubas KL. Psychosocial correlates of disordered eating in female collegiate athletes: validation of the ATHLETE questionnaire. *J Am Coll Health.* 2005;54(3):149–56.

21. Holm-Denoma JM, Scaringi V, Gordon KH, Van Orden KA, Joiner TE Jr. Eating disorder symptoms among undergraduate varsity athletes, club athletes, independent exercisers, and nonexercisers. *Int J Eat Disord.* 2009;42(1):47–53.

22. Kamm, RL. Interviewing principles for the psychiatrically aware sports medicine physician. *Clin Sports Med.* 2005;24(4):745–69, vii.

23. Klein DA, Walsh BT. Eating disorders: clinical features and pathophysiology. *Physiol Behav.* 2004;81(2):359–74.

24. Larun L, Nordheim LV, Ekeland E, Hagen KB, Heian F. Exercise in prevention and treatment of anxiety and depression among children and young people. *Cochrane Database Syst Rev.* 2006;3:CD004691.

25. Leger D, Biol D, Metlaine A, Choudat D. Insomnia and sleep disruption: relevance for athletic performance. *Clin Sports Med.* 2005;24(2): 269–85, viii.

26. Mead GE, Morley W, Campbell P, Greig CA, McMurdo M, Lawlor DA. Exercise for depression. *Cochrane Database Syst Rev.* 2009;3:CD004366.

27. Mellion MB, Putukian M, Madden CC. Exercise addiction. In: Mellion MB, Putukian M, Madden CC, editors. *Sports Medicine Secrets.* 3rd ed. Philadelphia: Hanley & Belfus; 2003. p. 181–3.

28. Mellion MB, Putukian M, Madden CC. Overtraining. In: Mellion MB, Putukian M, Madden CC, editors. *Sports Medicine Secrets.* 3rd ed. Philadelphia: Hanley & Belfus; 2003. p. 192–7.

29. Mellion MB, Putukian M, Madden CC. Psychological techniques to enhance performance. In: Mellion MB, Putukian M, Madden CC, editors. *Sports Medicine Secrets.* 3rd ed. Philadelphia: Hanley & Belfus; 2003. p. 188–91.

30. Morin CM, Rodrigue S, Ivers H. Role of stress, arousal, and coping skills in primary insomnia. *Psychosom Med.* 2003;65(2):259–67.

31. Nattiv A, Agostini R, Drinkwater B, Yeager KK. The female athlete triad. The inter-relatedness of disordered eating, amenorrhea, and osteoporosis. *Clin Sports Med.* 1994;13(2):405–18.

32. Nattiv A, Loucks AB, Manore MM, et al. American College of Sports Medicine position stand. The female athlete triad. *Med Sci Sports Exerc.* 2007;39(10):1867–82.

33. Ohayon MM. Epidemiology of insomnia: what we know and what we still need to learn. *Sleep Med Rev.* 2002;6(2):97–111.

34. Patel DR, Omar H, Terry M. Sport-related performance anxiety in young female athletes. *J Pediatr Adolesc Gynecol.* 2010;23(6):325–35.

35. Podlog L, Dimmock J, Miller J. A review of return to sport concerns following injury rehabilitation: practitioner strategies for enhancing recovery outcomes. *Phys Ther Sport.* 2011;12(1):36–42.

36. Podlog L, Eklund RC. The psychosocial aspects of a return to sport following serious injury: a review of the literature from a self-determination perspective. *Psychol Sport Exerc.* 2007;8(4):535–66.

37. Powell DH. Treating individuals with debilitating performance anxiety: an introduction. *J Clin Psychol.* 2004;60(8):801–8.

38. Pritts SD, Susman J. Diagnosis of eating disorders in primary care. *Am Fam Physician.* 2003;67(2):297–304.

39. Reardon CL, Factor RM. Sport psychiatry: a systematic review of diagnosis and medical treatment of mental illness in athletes. *Sports Med.* 2010;40(11):961–80.

40. Richardson CR, Newton TL, Abraham JJ, Sen A, Jimbo M, Swartz AM. A meta-analysis of pedometer-based walking interventions and weight. *Ann Fam Med.* 2008;6(1):69–77.

41. Robinson CS. Psychology and the injured runner: recovery enhancing strategies. In: O'Connor FG, Wilder RP, Nirschl R, editors. *Textbook of Running Medicine.* New York: McGraw-Hill; 1994. p. 621–8.

42. Soler RE, Leeks KD, Buchanan LR, et al. Point-of-decision prompts to increase stair use: a systematic review update. *Am J Prev Med.* 2010;38 (2 Suppl):S292–300.

43. Stathopoulou G, Powers MB, Berry AC, Smits JAJ, Otto MW. Exercise interventions for mental health: a quantitative and qualitative review. *Clin Psychol.* 2006;13(2):179–93.

44. Sundgot-Borgen J, Torstveit MK. Prevalence of eating disorders in elite athletes is higher than in the general population. *Clin J Sport Med.* 2004;14(1):25–32.

45. The National Collegiate Athletic Association. *NCAA Study of Substance Use of College Student Athletes.* Indianapolis (IN): NCAA; 2006.

46. Treating Tobacco Use and Dependence: 2008 Update. Rockville (MD): U.S. Department of Health and Human Services, Public Health Service; 2008.

47. van Sluijs EMF, McMinn AM, Griffin SJ. Effectiveness of interventions to promote physical activity in children and adolescents: systematic review of controlled trials. *Br J Sports Med.* 2008;42(8):653–7.

Complementary and Alternative Medicine

Anthony I. Beutler, David K. Gordon, and Wayne B. Jonas

80

WHAT IS COMPLEMENTARY AND ALTERNATIVE MEDICINE?

- Many different medical systems and medical practices exist in the world today including traditional Oriental medicine, Native American practices, Ayurveda, and Western biomedicine (to name only a few).

- Western biomedicine is the medicine practiced in American hospitals and taught in American medical schools. Western biomedicine is neither the oldest nor the most widely used medical system in the world today. The World Health Organization estimates that a substantial portion the world's population receives their medical care outside the Western biomedical system (43).

- The term "complementary and alternative medicine (CAM)" is Western biomedicine's term for all medical practices that lie outside its boundaries. CAM's boundaries are imprecise and constantly changing as Western scientific methods are applied to study and establish the efficacy of "outside" medical practices in the treatment of Western biomedical disease states. For instance, is massage therapy an adjunct to standard athletic care or a CAM treatment? Is glucosamine supplementation for osteoarthritis (OA) pain a Western biomedical therapy or a CAM therapy (43)? Some practices are both.

- CAM is often called "traditional" or "indigenous" medicine. Most recently, the term "integrative medicine" has been proposed for general use. Because the National Institutes of Health (NIH) still uses the CAM terminology, this chapter will refer to these diverse systems and practices as CAM.

WHO USES COMPLEMENTARY AND ALTERNATIVE MEDICINE?

- Many developing countries rely on CAM practices to provide most of the health care for their citizens.

- Americans spend more than $33 billion each year (most of it unreimbursed by insurance) on CAM practices. Visits to U.S. CAM practitioners rose from 400 million per year in 1990 to 600 million per year in 1996 and have continued to increase steadily. Approximately 40% of the U.S. population (compared with 75% of the population of France) report using a CAM practice at least once during the year (8,20).

- Among Western CAM consumers, 95% use CAM in a "complementary" fashion or in addition to Western biomedicine. Only 5% use CAM exclusively, or as an "alternative" to Western biomedicine (7).

- Studies reveal that CAM users in the United States tend to be more educated, more affluent, more holistic in their view of health care, and more likely to have chronic pain or a chronic disease than nonusers of CAM (7,12,20). Past reports indicated that some minorities, such as African Americans, were less likely to use CAM. However, a more recent study specifically designed to assess CAM use among minorities found no difference in CAM use among ethnic groups (42). Women consistently use CAM more than men, as they do all medical care.

- CAM therapies are popular for both major and minor illnesses. Roughly half of patients with human immunodeficiency virus (HIV) and half of patients diagnosed with cancer will try CAM therapies to combat their illnesses. However, CAM therapies are less commonly used to treat diseases for which Western biomedicine offers safe, effective treatments. For instance, although 57% of patients with diabetes mellitus type 2 report using CAM treatments, only 20% report trying CAM therapies to treat their diabetes (75).

DO ATHLETES USE COMPLEMENTARY AND ALTERNATIVE MEDICINE?

- No comprehensive study of CAM use among athletes is available (72). One study at a single Division I National Collegiate Athletic Association (NCAA) institution found that 56% of athletes (67% of women, 49% of men) used CAM. Eighty percent of these athletes used CAM in addition to traditional Western medicine (48). Common sense and common experience suggest that CAM use should be regarded as the rule, not the exception, in athletes.

- According to the 2002 National Health Interview Survey (NHIS), CAM use is more prevalent in adults who engage in physical activity during leisure time (8).

■ Athletes may use CAM therapies to enhance performance, decrease recovery time after workouts, or speed return to play following an injury.

■ Examples of CAM treatments commonly used by athletes to enhance performance include caffeine (guarana), creatine, ginkgo biloba, hormone supplements, and ephedra. Examples of CAM treatments typically used for pain control or accelerated return to play include iontophoresis, microcurrent, spinal manipulation, homeopathic arnica, and acupuncture.

■ The high pressure and high stakes of athletic competition, together with the exceptionally small margin that separates success from failure, demand that sports medicine physicians exercise great vigilance in protecting the athletes entrusted to their care.

WHERE CAN I FIND GOOD EVIDENCE ON COMPLEMENTARY AND ALTERNATIVE MEDICINE THERAPIES?

■ The best type of evidence to use in evaluating a CAM therapy depends on:

■ Risks posed by the therapy

■ Cost of the therapy

■ Information preference of the individual patient

■ Availability of other proven, effective, and safe therapies for the patient's condition

■ Randomized controlled trials (RCTs) are important for evaluating high-risk and/or high-cost therapies because RCTs provide essential safety and risk–benefit data. However, RCTs have some important limitations. RCTs are difficult and expensive to sustain for long periods of study. Additionally, the results of an RCT depend greatly on the careful selection of the all-important "control" group (38).

■ Clinical outcomes research is another, less recognized type of research trial that is useful in studying CAM therapies. Outcomes research is more similar to clinical practice than RCTs: It involves a wider range of patients over longer periods of time and allows for variations in care caused by interactions with multiple providers. Outcomes research examines the probability that a therapy will produce a beneficial effect and provides an estimate of how large that effect will be in everyday clinical practice. For long-term, chronic conditions and their therapies, outcomes research often provides the only relevant evidence (67).

■ Table 80.1 lists a number of sources for obtaining quality evidence on specific CAM therapies and practices.

■ The patient's individual beliefs and personality can affect the likelihood of therapeutic efficacy. If a patient believes that a specific therapy will alleviate their condition, this "prior plausibility" has its own therapeutic effect.

■ If conventional medicine offers a safe, proven therapy that is acceptable to the patient, any potential CAM therapy must pass equally stringent evidence standards for efficacy and safety before being considered as a viable treatment option.

Table 80.1	Internet Resources — Reliable Complementary and Alternative Medicine (Cam) Evidence for Physicians

The Cochrane Library
The library contains a database of systematic reviews featuring randomized controlled trials of CAM and conventional therapies, as well as a controlled trials register that provides bibliographic listings of controlled trials and conference proceedings.
Abstracts of the reviews and trials are available free of charge at http://www.cochrane.org
Full text copies of all materials are available through several subscription services including http://gateway.ovid.com

PubMed
The most comprehensive and popular medical search engine has a new "clinical queries" filter to assist in limiting your search results to CAM. The most comprehensive search is obtained by using the key words "complementary medicine."
Free access at multiple Web sites including http://www.pubmed.org

National Center for Complementary and Alternative Medicine (NCCAM)
The clinical trials section contains an index of trials by treatment or condition. The index can also be accessed via www.clinicaltrials.gov or through PubMed.
The NCCAM Web site is http://www.nccam.nih.gov

National Library of Medicine
Powerful search engine allows searches across all government guidelines, plus PubMed. "Synonym and related terms" search option is very helpful for CAM therapies with multiple common names.
The search engine may be accessed free of charge at http://hstat.nlm.nih.gov
Individual guidelines from many government agencies can be found at http://www.guideline.gov or http://www.cdc.gov/publications

Natural Medicines Comprehensive Database
The online database contains comprehensive listings and cross-listings of natural and herbal therapies, including very helpful sections on "all known uses" and "herb–drug interactions." The database also offers an extensive review of the available pharmacologic evidence.
From the publishers of *The Prescriber's Letter*, the database can be accessed via a purchased subscription at http://www.naturaldatabase.com

ePocrates Rx Pro
Listing of alternative medicines for mobile devices, but does not contain information on nonmedicinal modalities (acupuncture or manipulation). Provides names, common uses, suggested dosages, and a multicheck feature that checks the patient's medical regimen for drug–drug, herb–herb, and drug–herb interactions.
Alternative medicine content is available only with the purchase of ePocrates Rx Pro, not with the free version of ePocrates Rx. http://www.epocrates.com

HOW DO I ADVISE MY PATIENTS ABOUT COMPLEMENTARY AND ALTERNATIVE MEDICINE THERAPIES?

■ Ninety-five percent of patients who use CAM therapies also use conventional, Western biomedicine. However, over 60% of these patients do not inform their physicians of their CAM therapy use (19). This "CAM communication gap" results in a wasteful, and potentially dangerous, patient–physician environment.

■ Patients who use CAM practices possess character traits that incline them to active participation and partnering in their medical care (20). A physician who refuses to discuss and denies any knowledge of CAM treatments does not alter the patient's need for partnering, but merely forces them to seek association elsewhere — thus widening the already precipitous CAM communication gap.

■ Many effective strategies can be used to partner with patients on CAM therapies. However, we recommend the strategy proposed by Jonas (37). He suggests that depending on the specific patient and the specific treatment, physicians should **protect, permit,** or **promote** CAM therapies (37).

Protecting from Harm

■ Many CAM practices are inherently low risk when performed or prescribed by competent providers. However, herbal remedies and high-dose vitamin supplementation (both very popular CAM therapies) can cause serious or fatal consequences (17).

■ "Natural" does not equal "safe," contrary to the popular conceived connotation. Herbs and vitamins have real effects, real side effects, and real toxicities. Even without direct toxicity, herb–herb and herb–drug interactions can be severe. Other quality issues such as contamination, varying potencies, and differing absorption rates abound in the poorly regulated domain of nutritional supplements (17).

■ Biofeedback, meditation, prayer, and acupuncture pose minimal risk for direct toxicity. However, even these "safe" practices may indirectly result in harm if used in place of more effective treatments. The physician should detail the risks and benefits (both direct and indirect) of all therapeutic options.

■ Ephedra (or ma huang) especially in combination with caffeine (or guarana), chromium picolinate, and pulsed magnetic field therapy are examples of therapies from which patients should be protected. (See later section on specific CAM treatments.)

Permitting Unproven, Nontoxic Therapies

■ Physicians may experience trepidation in allowing patients to engage in unproven practices or therapies. But if the therapy has no toxicity and is not used in place of a proven effective treatment, the practice can be safely permitted and may be encouraged.

■ The physician's ultimate goal should be to relieve patient suffering. Patients welcome relief — and physicians should do likewise — even should relief come through nonquantifiable means (spiritual effect, placebo effect, belief, prior plausibility) (46).

■ Homeopathic arnica, acupuncture, spinal manipulation, ginkgo biloba supplementation, and many other CAM therapies can be safely permitted when properly administered and appropriately prescribed.

Promoting Proven Treatments

■ Physicians should promote safe, effective treatments regardless of their medical system of origin. Western biomedicine has adopted and should continue to incorporate proven techniques and therapies from other systems of medical care (37).

■ Glucosamine supplementation is a prime example of a CAM therapy that should be promoted for individuals with knee OA. Acupuncture and massage for back pain are other examples of proven CAM therapies to be promoted.

WHAT'S THE CURRENT EVIDENCE FOR OR AGAINST SOME POPULAR COMPLEMENTARY AND ALTERNATIVE MEDICINE TREATMENTS?

■ Summaries of the evidence for and against a few of the most popular CAM treatments used by athletes and the general population appear in the following sections. They are organized into the sections of **Prevent**, **Permit**, and **Promote.**

Prevent

Herbs and Supplements

■ Ephedra (ma huang, herbal ecstasy, zhong mahuang) (10,16,32,34)

■ **Primary use:** Weight loss or enhanced athletic performance, endurance. Less commonly used for respiratory conditions or asthma.

■ **Evidence:** Ephedra can potentiate a small weight loss of 2–5 kg over 6 weeks to 6 months, but only in patients with body mass index over 30. The weight loss is typically transient and often requires combination with other stimulants (*i.e.,* caffeine or guarana). Multiple studies show no performance-enhancing effect unless combined with caffeine/guarana or used in very high dosages.

■ **Toxicity:** High dosages and combination with caffeine known to increase toxicity. High dosages can cause dizziness, restlessness, anxiety, palpitations, hypertension, myocardial infarction, seizure, stroke, and psychosis, among other conditions (18,24,34,36,47,69). **Fatal events have been reported**. Newer evidence suggests that toxicity can occur with short-term use in low doses as well (24,34). Capsules have been found to contain many impurities, including banned substances.

■ **Regulated/banned:** Banned by the Food and Drug Administration (FDA) and the International Olympic Committee (IOC) (25).

■ **Conclusion:** Ephedra products, especially ephedra/guarana combinations, are banned substances, are not safe, and have been demonstrated to cause considerable harm. As negative publicity builds, "ephedra-free" versions of products appear, but there is no evidence that these will be any safer than the original formulations.

- Chromium picolinate (12,26,45,56)

  - **Primary use:** Increase lean body mass, improve glycemic control in diabetes, enhance athletic performance, and increase energy.

  - **Evidence:** While earlier, design-flawed studies suggested some beneficial effects, newer studies show no ergogenic or fat-burning effects. Some studies suggest slight, dose-dependent improvements in diabetes control and lipid profiles.

  - **Toxicity:** Tremor and cognitive, sleep, and mood changes have been reported as side effects. Concern exists for potential DNA mutations with long-term exposure to chromium supplementation.

  - **Regulated/banned:** No.

  - **Conclusion:** Although inexpensive and minimally toxic with short-term use, real concern exists for DNA mutations with long-term use or high chromium levels. Since the reported benefits are very small and the risk of long-term toxicity potentially great, patients should avoid this supplement.

Other CAM Therapies

- Pulsed electromagnetic field (PEMF) therapy (1,9,35)

  - **Primary use:** Decrease pain and stiffness in OA.

  - **Evidence:** The beneficial effect of PEMF therapy in delayed union fractures is well established. Similar magnetic fields have been found to stimulate proteoglycan production in vitro in chondrocytes. However, despite abundant anecdotal Internet reports, a recent Cochrane review found only three quality articles in the scientific literature. The review found that PEMF produced statistically significant but clinically insignificant changes in knee OA pain and disability. The optimum dosage and frequency of PEMF — as well as acceptable technical standards for the PEMF equipment — remain unknown. The cost of PEMF can exceed $200 per day.

  - **Toxicity:** Unknown. The effects of pulsed electromagnetic fields on human tissues have not been well studied.

  - **Regulated/banned:** No.

  - **Conclusion:** Patients should be advised that PEMF's small benefits in OA pain and stiffness are outweighed by uncertain side effects, incomplete technical data, and high cost. Other proven-effective, lower cost treatments for OA exist and are favored over PEMF therapy.

Permit

Herbs and Supplements

- Ginkgo leaf (49,51,62)

  - **Primary use:** Combat memory loss and slow progressive dementia. Also used to relieve vascular claudication symptoms.

- **Evidence:** Most studies suggest that ginkgo leaf can slow dementia progression and increase cognitive function in middle-aged adults without subjective memory loss. In some countries, ginkgo is the standard of care (in place of cholinesterase inhibitors) for Alzheimer dementia. However, a large NIH-funded RCT showed no benefit in slowing memory loss in early dementia whether Alzheimer or non-Alzheimer related (55). Limited evidence also suggests that ginkgo may improve walking distance in vascular claudication.

- **Toxicity:** Mild gastrointestinal (GI) upset and constipation are the most common side effects reported. However, ginkgo has anticoagulant properties and lowers the seizure threshold. Ginkgo has been linked to spontaneous bleeding. It should not be used in patients taking other anticoagulants or in those with a seizure disorder or in combination with other drugs that lower seizure threshold.

- **Regulated/banned:** No.

- **Conclusion:** In appropriately selected patients, ginkgo is a permissible complement to conventional drug treatments, especially if the patient prefers ginkgo supplementation.

- St. John's wort (SJW) (12,13,31,54,74)

  - **Primary use:** Antidepressant, anxiolytic, anti-insomnia, and adjunct to weight-loss uses are commonly described.

  - **Evidence:** Most evidence suggests SJW to be effective for mild to moderate depression. SJW may also be effective in obsessive-compulsive disorders. Severe depression is not reliably treated by SJW, and higher dosages of SJW increase the risk for severe skin reactions.

  - **Toxicity:** Insomnia, restlessness, and GI distress are common. Hypericin doses over 5 mg d^{-1} increase risk for photodermatitis. SJW has fewer side effects than tricyclic antidepressants or selective serotonin reuptake inhibitor antidepressants; however, the potential for severe herb–herb and drug–herb interactions — including serotonin syndrome — is greater with SJW. SJW can accelerate the metabolism of drugs cleared by the P450 enzyme system and should not be used by those on immunosuppressants or antiviral medications without monitoring.

  - **Regulated/banned:** Not banned by athletic regulatory agencies. However, due to the risk of serious drug interactions, the distribution of SJW was recently banned in France. The governments of Japan, the United Kingdom, and other European countries are considering similar bans.

  - **Conclusion:** In monitored patients with mild-moderate depression, SJW therapy is acceptable if the patient has a simple, compatible medical regimen and strongly prefers SJW to conventional drug treatment.

- Creatine (63,66,73)

  - **Primary use:** Decrease workout recovery time, improve muscular strength/athletic performance.

- **Evidence:** Many studies document increases in repetitive strength tasks of less than 30 seconds in duration. Certain individuals who have low baseline levels of creatine may experience a more pronounced effect.
- **Toxicity:** Common side effects include GI upset, diarrhea, and mild muscle cramping. Case reports have attempted to implicate creatine in everything from cardiomyopathy to renal failure to rhabdomyolysis, but these effects are difficult to distinguish from the effects of volume depletion and heat illness. Creatine's ergogenic effects are largely negated by caffeine consumption.
- **Regulated/banned:** Not a banned substance, but the NCAA prohibits universities from providing creatine for their athletes.
- **Conclusion:** A discussion of risks and benefits is critical to creatine. After thorough discussion with an athlete, creatine use can be permitted in otherwise healthy patients involved in strength-related events. Creatine should not be used in pediatric athletes (unclear safety), athletes with kidney disease, or athletes prone to dehydration (osmotic action of creatine predisposes to dehydration and intensifies subsequent heat illness). For most athletes, creatine has no proven benefit. In fact, the increased body mass (2–4 kg) caused by creatine supplementation may impair performance in endurance events.

- Chondroitin (40,41,58)
  - **Primary use:** Improving pain and stiffness from OA.
  - **Evidence:** Several trials suggest (size and design limiting) that chondroitin and ibuprofen are more effective than ibuprofen alone for improving OA symptoms. Additionally, the drugs have different times to onset of action. Ibuprofen reaches maximum efficacy in a matter of days; chondroitin is maximally effective over a few weeks. Chondroitin is typically sold in varying combinations with glucosamine, manganese, and magnesium. Some data suggest the combination of glucosamine and chondroitin treatment to be more effective than the single agent alone.
  - **Toxicity:** Mild GI distress is the most common side effect. Combination tablets can exceed safe daily doses of manganese and cause central nervous system irritability. Chondroitin has a heparinoid structure and may predispose to bleeding if used with other anticoagulants.
  - **Regulated/banned:** No.
  - **Conclusion:** Although less convincing than glucosamine (see later section), some evidence supports chondroitin use in OA. Several studies with 5+ years of follow-up report no adverse events related to chondroitin use. Given the moderately high cost of chondroitin tablets, a 6- to 8-week trial period is advisable. If no clinical effect is noted during this trial, chondroitin should be discontinued due to cost considerations.

- *Panax* ginseng (3,21,71,76)
  - **Primary use:** Improve cognitive function and athletic performance and increase energy.

- **Evidence:** Many studies document that ginseng supplementation has no ergogenic effects. Similarly, *Panax* ginseng has not been shown to improve memory when used alone but has been demonstrated to have efficacy when combined with ginkgo supplementation in middle-aged individuals.
- **Toxicity:** Insomnia, tachycardia, and palpitations become more common with high doses. Mastalgia, vaginal bleeding, and amenorrhea are likely related to the estrogenic effects of ginseng. Long-term use is not well studied. Ginseng will intensify the effects of other common stimulants (caffeine, guarana, and tea).
- **Regulated/banned:** No.
- **Conclusion:** Studies suggest minimal toxicity with short-term use, but long-term use is more difficult to justify since estrogenic risks may outweigh the unclear benefits. However, further studies continue to explore other possible indications for ginseng supplementation.

- Homeopathy (*Arnica*) (22,61,64,65)
  - **Primary use:** Relief of delayed-onset muscle soreness (DOMS).
  - **Evidence:** Homeopathic arnica is more properly viewed as an alternative medical system with many distinct, pharmacologic interventions. No single homeopathic treatment has been conclusively proven to be effective in reducing DOMS. Small trials of diverse remedies offer contradictory conclusions for homeopathy in DOMS. Poor design, differing methodologies, and differing definitions of DOMS predictably plague these trials.
  - **Toxicity:** No side effects above placebo levels have been reported. Reports of severe allergic reactions appear to be rare. Extreme dilution of homeopathic remedies makes direct toxicity highly unlikely.
  - **Regulated/banned:** No. A few states credential homeopathic physicians.
  - **Conclusion:** The homeopathic system of medicine is complex and has not yet been adequately evaluated. However, its costs and toxicities are low in the hands of trained professionals. Current research does not support its use for DOMS.

Other CAM Therapies

- Transcutaneous electrical nerve stimulation (TENS) (29)
  - **Primary use:** Relief of low back pain.
  - **Evidence:** While RCTs are lacking, a recent Cochrane review found that TENS is effective at providing pain relief and improving range of motion in patients suffering from chronic low back pain.
  - **Toxicity:** There is no known toxicity associated with TENS. Patients can experience mild discomfort and involuntary muscle contraction due to the electrical stimulation of the nerves.
  - **Regulated/banned:** No.
  - **Conclusion:** Early, poor-quality data indicate this treatment modality is effective with minimal side effects. The

cost of TENS devices may be prohibitive, and more studies with improved academic rigor are needed.

- Massage (27)
    - **Primary use:** Relief of low back pain and relief of DOMS.
    - **Evidence:** A recent Cochrane review found that when massage is combined with exercises and education, it might be beneficial for relief of subacute and chronic low back pain. This review found that acupuncture massage is more effective than traditional massage, but more studies are needed. A more recent study found two types of massage (deep tissue and relaxation) to be more effective than conventional therapy for low back pain (14). A review of 17 case series found no consistent evidence that massage improved exercise performance but did find a trend supporting massage as effective in relieving DOMS (11).
    - **Toxicity:** None.
    - **Regulated/banned:** No.
    - **Conclusion:** While further studies are needed, massage is a low-cost treatment modality with negligible side effects that can be used along with traditional pain relief and rehabilitation modalities for relief of subacute and chronic low back pain. Current evidence does not support massage to relieve specific sports-related injury or pain.
- The role of expectation in physical performance
    - **Primary use:** Placebo used in concert with patients' expectations on whether they expect to perform well or not.
    - **Evidence:** In a recent review, Pollo et al. (52) provide examples where physiologic or pathologic conditions are altered following the administration of an inert substance with verbal instructions that induce expectations of a change. Placebo effects can extend beyond the clinical setting, in the domain of physical performance, and have implications for sport competitions.
    - **Toxicity:** Placebo (from negative expectations) may produce adverse effects, and deception is ethically problematic.
    - **Regulated/banned:** No, but ethical issues can be associated with deception.
    - **Conclusion:** Despite very different experimental conditions and across many different outcomes measured, data strongly indicate context factors and athletes' expectations as important factors in physical performance to be taken into account in training strategies and exercises.
- Spinal manipulation (4–6,39,53,68)
    - **Primary use:** Relief of low back pain/stiffness, relief of DOMS, and speeding return to play following low back injury.
    - **Evidence:** Majority of evidence suggests spinal manipulation to be at least as effective as but not superior to conventional treatment for acute or chronic low back pain. Nine of 10 well-designed RCTs in a recent review concluded that spinal manipulation provided more pain relief than control treatments. However, differences

between manipulation techniques make conclusions difficult to generalize. Additionally, several recent Cochrane reviews have found that there is no clinically relevant difference in pain reduction between spinal manipulation and other standard therapies. Manipulation may require more physician visits than conventional care, increasing the cost of therapy. Health insurers may reimburse some of this cost.

- **Toxicity:** Rare case reports of stroke, paralysis, or spinal cord damage are mostly related to cervical spine manipulation and occur at a frequency of one per millions of manipulations. No severe complications have been reported from over 15,000 patients enrolled in monitored RCTs.
- **Regulated/banned:** No.
- **Conclusion:** Competently performed lumbar spine manipulation is safe and likely effective for low back pain, although it may be at higher cost than other therapies and may not provide any greater benefit than these lower cost therapies.

Promote

Herbs and Supplements

- Glucosamine sulfate (15,23,44,50,57,70)
    - **Primary use:** Relief of stiffness and pain in OA and temporomandibular joint dysfunction (TMJ).
    - **Evidence:** Despite a recent high-quality meta-analysis showing no benefit in glucosamine supplementation (70), multiple trials have demonstrated superior efficacy of glucosamine sulfate to placebo. So why is this issue still not settled? The issue centers around the quality of clinical trials performed to date. While the large NIH-sponsored Glucosamine/chondroitin Arthritis Intervention Trial (GAIT) trial showed no efficacy for glucosamine overall, this trial was hampered by a 60% placebo response rate, far above that seen in clinical practice. Further review of the GAIT trial shows an overenrollment of patients with very mild OA symptoms and an underenrollment of patients with more clinically relevant moderate to severe OA symptoms. The subgroup analysis of patients with moderate–severe symptoms showed glucosamine/chondroitin combination to be significantly more effective than placebo and more effective than celecoxib in relieving OA pain (15). Other studies are hampered by industry sponsorship. The results of the meta-analyses vary greatly depending on which studies they include and how heavily each study result is weighted. The upcoming results (expected mid-2012) of the Long-Term Evaluation of Glucosamine Sulphate Study (LEGS) should answer most of the lingering questions regarding glucosamine sulfate supplementation. Insufficient data exist to determine if glucosamine slows the rate of OA progression. Knee OA is the most widely studied, but efficacy data also exists for glucosamine in TMJ and OA of the hand and spine.

- **Toxicity:** Mild GI distress (comparable to placebo levels) has been reported. Concerns for exacerbations of diabetic control or reactions in patients with shellfish allergy appear to be unfounded. Despite disagreement regarding efficacy, all published data show that glucosamine sulfate supplementation is extremely safe for all adults. No data exist regarding use in pregnant women and children. Patients on renal dialysis should not use glucosamine sulfate since metabolites are cleared via the kidney.

- **Regulated/banned:** No.

- **Conclusion:** Glucosamine provides effective relief of OA symptoms for some patients with at least moderate symptoms. A 6- to 8-week trial of glucosamine supplementation should be promoted as safe and likely effective for OA pain, especially in the senior athlete population where comorbidities may limit other treatment options. Glucosamine supplementation should be discontinued if no clinical response occurs after a 6- to 8-week trial due to its moderate cost.

Other CAM Therapies

- Acupuncture (2,28,30,33,59,60)

  - **Primary use:** Relief of acute and chronic low back pain, chronic neck pain, OA, and lateral elbow pain.

  - **Evidence:** Acupuncture may be considered as a separate medical system or an adjunct to other therapies. There are conflicting data regarding the effectiveness of acupuncture for acute low back pain. However, for treatment of chronic low back pain, acupuncture has been found to be more effective than no treatment or sham treatments for short-term pain relief and functional improvement. It should be noted that acupuncture has not been found to be more effective than other complementary or alternative treatments for chronic low back pain. There is moderate evidence now showing that acupuncture is effective for immediate pain relief of chronic neck pain, and this relief persists at short-term follow-up. For lateral elbow pain, a recent Cochrane review found insufficient evidence to make any recommendations. RCTs of acupuncture for low back pain are contradictory and poorly designed. Acupuncture has been proven effective in reducing postoperative pain and relief of nausea.

  - **Toxicity:** Broken needles, pneumothorax, and infectious disease transmission are anecdotally reported, but unlikely in the hands of licensed professionals. Pain, fatigue, bleeding, and fainting are the most common side effects.

  - **Regulated/banned:** No. Over 30 states license acupuncturists. The FDA has approved acupuncture needles as experimental devices.

  - **Conclusion:** There is a growing body of clinical experience and RCT evidence indicating that acupuncture is effective for pain relief. Also, acupuncture is low cost and does not carry with it the side effects or risks of sedation, renal toxicity, GI bleeding, or addiction common to many conventional pain treatments. For these reasons,

acupuncture — under the care of a trained professional — can be recommended to patients for pain relief so long as acupuncture is not thought to be a cure for a musculoskeletal injury that needs rehabilitation or surgery. It is most advisable that patients use acupuncture as an adjunct to proven treatments for pain relief.

REFERENCES

1. Aaron RK, Ciombor DM, Jolly G. Stimulation of experimental endochondral ossification by low-energy pulsing electromagnetic fields. *J Bone Miner Res.* 1989;4(2):227–33.
2. Acupuncture. *NIH Consensus Statement Online* [Internet]. 1997 Nov 3–5 [cited 1997 Dec 30];15(5):1–34. Available from: http://consensus.nih.gov/1997/1997acupuncture107html.htm.
3. Allen JD, McLung J, Nelson AG, Welsch M. Ginseng supplementation does not enhance healthy young adult's peak aerobic exercise performance. *J Am Coll Nutr.* 1998;17(5):462–6.
4. Andersson GB, Lucente T, Davis AM, Kappler RE, Lipton JA, Leurgans S. A comparison of osteopathic spinal manipulation with standard care for patients with low back pain. *N Engl J Med.* 1999;341(19):1426–31.
5. Assendelft WJ, Koes BW, Knipschild PG, Bouter LM. The relationship between methodological quality and conclusions in reviews of spinal manipulation. *JAMA.* 1995;274(24):1942–8.
6. Assendelft WJ, Morton SC, Yu EI, Suttorp MJ, Shekelle PG. Spinal manipulative therapy for low back pain. *Cochrane Database Syst Rev.* 2009;1:CD000447.
7. Astin JA. Why patients use alternative medicine: results of a national study. *JAMA.* 1998;279(19):1548–53.
8. Barnes PM, Bloom B, Nahin RL. *Complementary and alternative medicine use among adults and children: United States, 2007. National Health Statistics Report, No. 12.* Hyattsville, MD: National Center for Health Statistics; 2008. p. 1–23.
9. Bassett CA, Pawluk RJ, Pilla AA. Augmentation of bone repair by inductively coupled electromagnetic fields. *Science.* 1974;184(4136):575–7.
10. Bell DG, Jacobs I, McLellan TM, Zamecnik J. Reducing the dose of combined caffeine and ephedrine preserves the ergogenic effect. *Aviat Space Environ Med.* 2000;71(4):415–9.
11. Best TM, Hunter R, Wilcox A, Haq F. Effectiveness of sports massage for recovery of skeletal muscle from strenuous exercise. *Clin J Sport Med.* 2008;18(5):446–60.
12. Beutler AI, Jonas WB. Complementary and alternative medicine for the sports medicine physician. In: Birrer RB, O'Connor FG, editors. *Sports Medicine for the Primary Care Physician.* 3rd ed. Boca Raton: CRC Press; in press.
13. Brenner R, Azbel V, Madhusoodanan S, Pawlowska M. Comparison of an extract of hypericum (LI 160) and sertraline in the treatment of depression: a double-blind, randomized pilot study. *Clin Ther.* 2000;22(4):411–9.
14. Cherkin DC, Sherman KJ, Kahn J, et al. Effectiveness of focused structural massage and relaxation massage for chronic low back pain: protocol for a randomized controlled trial. *Trials.* 2009;10:96.
15. Clegg DO, Reda DJ, Harris CL, et al. Glucosamine, chondroitin sulfate, and the two in combination for painful knee osteoarthritis. *N Engl J Med.* 2006;354(8):795–808.
16. Congeni J, Miller S. Supplements and drugs used to enhance athletic performance. *Pediatr Clin North Am.* 2002;49(2):435–61.
17. De Smet PA. Herbal remedies. *N Engl J Med.* 2002;347(25):2046–56.

18. Doyle H, Kargin M. Herbal stimulant containing ephedrine has also caused psychosis. *BMJ*. 1996;313(7059):756.

19. Eisenberg DM. Advising patients who seek alternative medical therapies. *Ann Intern Med*. 1997;127(1):61–9.

20. Eisenberg DM, Davis RB, Ettner SL, et al. Trends in alternative medicine use in the United States, 1990–1997: results of a follow-up national survey. *JAMA*. 1998;280(18):1569–75.

21. Ellis JM, Reddy P. Effects of Panax ginseng on quality of life. *Ann Pharmacother*. 2002;36(3):375–9.

22. Ernst E, Barnes J. Are homeopathic remedies effective for delayed-onset muscle soreness? A systematic review of placebo-controlled trials. *Perfusion*. 1998;11:4–8.

23. Foerster KK, Schmid K, Rovati LC. Efficacy of glucosamine sulfate in osteoarthritis of the lumbar spine: a placebo-controlled, randomized, double-blind study. In: *Am Coll Rheumatol. 64th Ann Scientific Mtg; 2000 Oct 29–Nov 2*: Philadelphia (PA).

24. Food and Drug Administration. Proposed rule: dietary supplements containing ephedrine alkaloids [Internet]. [cited 2000 Jan 25]. Available from: http://www.verity.fda.gov.

25. Food and Drug Administration, HHS. Final rule declaring dietary supplements containing ephedrine alkaloids adulterated because they present an unreasonable risk. Final rule. *Fed Regist*. 2004;69(28):6787–854.

26. Fox GN, Sabovic Z. Chromium picolinate supplementation for diabetes mellitus. *J Fam Pract*. 1998;46(1):83–6.

27. Furlan AD, Imamura M, Dryden T, Irvin E. Massage for low-back pain. *Cochrane Database Syst Rev*. 2010;6:CD001929.

28. Furlan AD, Van Tulder MW, Cherkin D, et al. Acupuncture and dry-needling for low back pain. *Cochrane Database Syst Rev*. 2010;6:CD001351.

29. Gadsby JG, Flowerdew M. Transcutaneous electrical nerve stimulation and acupuncture-like transcutaneous electrical nerve stimulation for chronic low back pain. *Cochrane Database Syst Rev*. 2007;1:CD000210.

30. Garvey TA, Marks MR, Wiesel SW. A prospective, randomized, double-blind evaluation of trigger-point injection therapy for low-back pain. *Spine (Phila Pa 1976)*. 1989;14(9):962–4.

31. Gaster B, Holroyd J. St John's wort for depression: a systematic review. *Arch Intern Med*. 2000;160(2):152–6.

32. Gillies H, Derman WE, Noakes TD, Smith P, Evans A, Gabriels G. Pseudoephedrine is without ergogenic effects during prolonged exercise. *J Appl Physiol*. 1996;81(6):2611–7.

33. Green S, Buchbinder R, Barnsley L, et al. Acupuncture for lateral elbow pain. *Cochrane Database Syst Rev*. 2002;1:CD003527.

34. Haller CA, Benowitz NL. Adverse cardiovascular and central nervous system events associated with dietary supplements containing ephedra alkaloids. *N Engl J Med*. 2000;343(25):1833–8.

35. Hulme J, Robinson V, DeBie R, Wells G, Judd M, Tugwell P. Electromagnetic fields for the treatment of osteoarthritis. *Cochrane Database Syst Rev*. 2002;1:CD003523.

36. Jacobs KM, Hirsch KA. Psychiatric complications of ma-huang. *Psychosomatics*. 2000;41(1):58–62.

37. Jonas WB. Alternative medicine — learning from the past, examining the present, advancing to the future. *JAMA*. 1998;280(18):1616–8.

38. Jonas WB, Levine JS. How to practice evidence-based complementary medicine. In: Jonas W, Levin J, editors. *Essentials of Complementary and Alternative Medicine*. Philadelphia: Lippincott Williams & Wilkins; 1999. p. 72–87.

39. Koes BW, Assendelft WJ, van der Heijden GJ, Bouter LM. Spinal manipulation for low back pain. An updated systematic review of randomized clinical trials. *Spine (Phila Pa 1976)*. 1996;21(24):2860–71.

40. Leeb BF, Schweitzer H, Montag K, Smolen JS. A metaanalysis of chondroitin sulfate in the treatment of osteoarthritis. *J Rheumatol*. 2000;27(1):205–11.

41. Leffler CT, Philippi AF, Leffler SG, Mosure JC, Kim PD. Glucosamine, chondroitin, and manganese ascorbate for degenerative joint disease of the knee or low back: a randomized, double-blind, placebo-controlled pilot study. *Mil Med*. 1999;164(2):85–91.

42. Mackenzie ER, Taylor L, Bloom BS, Hufford DJ, Johnson HC. Ethnic minority use of complementary and alternative medicine (CAM): a national probability survey of CAM utilizers. *Altern Ther Health Med*. 2003;9(4):50–6.

43. Marty AT. Fundamentals of complementary and alternative medicine. *Chest*. 1997;112(6):16-A.

44. McAlindon TE, LaValley MP, Gulin JP, Felson DT. Glucosamine and chondroitin for treatment of osteoarthritis: a systematic quality assessment and meta-analysis. *JAMA*. 2000;283(11):1469–75.

45. McLeod MN, Gaynes BN, Golden RN. Chromium potentiation of antidepressant pharmacotherapy for dysthymic disorder in 5 patients. *J Clin Psychiatry*. 1999;60(4):237–40.

46. Moerman DE, Jonas WB. Deconstructing the placebo effect and finding the meaning response. *Ann Intern Med*. 2002;136(6):471–6.

47. Morgenstern LB, Viscoli CM, Kernan WN, et al. Use of ephedra-containing products and risk for hemorrhagic stroke. *Neurology*. 2003;60(1):132–5.

48. Nichols AW, Harrigan R. Complementary and alternative medicine usage by intercollegiate athletes. *Clin J Sport Med*. 2006;16(3):232–7.

49. Oken BS, Storzbach DM, Kaye JA. The efficacy of ginkgo biloba on cognitive function in Alzheimer disease. *Arch Neurol*. 1998;55(11):1409–15.

50. Pavelká K, Gatterová J, Olejarová M, Machacek S, Giacovelli G, Rovati LC. Glucosamine sulfate use and delay of progression of knee osteoarthritis: a 3-year, randomized, placebo-controlled, double-blind study. *Arch Intern Med*. 2002;162(18):2113–23.

51. Pittler MH, Ernst E. Ginkgo biloba extract for the treatment of intermittent claudication: a meta-analysis of randomized trials. *Am J Med*. 2000;108(4):276–81.

52. Pollo A, Carlino E, Benedetti F. Placebo mechanisms across different conditions: from the clinical setting to physical performance. *Philos Trans R Soc Lond B Biol Sci*. 2011;366(1572):1790–8.

53. Rubinstein SM, van Middelkoop M, Assendelft WJ, de Boer MR, van Tulder MW. Spinal manipulative therapy for chronic low-back pain: an update of Cochrane review. *Spine (Phila Pa 1976)*. 2011;36(13):E825–46.

54. Schrader E. Equivalence of St. John's wort extract (Ze 117) and fluoxetine: a randomized, controlled study in mild-moderate depression. *Int Clin Psychopharmacol*. 2000;15(2):61–8.

55. Snitz BE, O'Meara ES, Carlson MC, et al. Ginkgo biloba for preventing cognitive decline in older adults: a randomized trial. *JAMA*. 2009;302(24):2663–70.

56. Speetjens JK, Collins RA, Vincent JB, Woski SA. The nutritional supplement chromium(III) tris(picolinate) cleaves DNA. *Chem Res Toxicol*. 1999;12(6):483–7.

57. Thie NM, Prasad NG, Major PW. Evaluation of glucosamine sulfate compared to ibuprofen for the treatment of temporomandibular joint osteoarthritis: a randomized double blind controlled 3 month clinical trial. *J Rheumatol*. 2001;28(6):1347–55.

58. Towheed TE, Anastassiades TP. Glucosamine and chondroitin for treating symptoms of osteoarthritis: evidence is widely touted but incomplete. *JAMA*. 2000;238(11):1483–4.

59. Trinh K, Graham N, Gross A, et al. Acupuncture for neck disorders. *Cochrane Database Syst Rev*. 2010;3:CD004870.

60. Tulder MW, van Cherkin DC, Berman B, Lao L, Koes BW. Acupuncture for low back pain. *Cochrane Database Syst Rev*. 2000;2:CD001351.

61. Tveiten D, Bruset S, Borchgrevink CF, Norseth J. Effects of the homeopathic remedy Arnica D 30 on marathon runners: a randomized, double-blind study during the 1995 Oslo Marathon. *Complement Ther Med* 1998;6:71–4.

62. van Dongen MC, van Rossum E, Kessels AG, Sielhorst HJ, Knipschild PG. The efficacy of ginkgo for elderly people with dementia and age-associated memory impairment: new results of a randomized clinical trial. *J Am Geriatr Soc.* 2000;48(10):1183–94.

63. Vandenberghe K, Goris M, Van Hecke P, Van Leemputte M, Van Gerven L, Hespel P. Long term creatine intake is beneficial to muscle performance during resistance training. *J Appl Physiol.* 1997;83:2055–63.

64. Vickers AJ, Fisher P, Smith C, Wyllie SE, Lewith GT. Homeopathy for delayed onset muscle soreness: a randomized double blind placebo controlled trial. *Br J Sports Med.* 1997;31(4):304–7.

65. Vickers AJ, Fisher P, Smith C, Wyllie SE, Rees R. Homoeopathic Arnica 30x is ineffective for muscle soreness after long-distance running: a randomised, double-blind, placebo-controlled trial. *Clin J Pain.* 1998; 14(3):227–31.

66. Volek JS, Duncan ND, Mazzetti SA, et al. Performance and muscle fiber adaptations to creatine supplementation and heavy resistance training. *Med Sci Sports Exerc.* 1999;31(8):1147–56.

67. Walach H, Jonas WB, Lewith G. The role of outcomes research in evaluating complementary and alternative medicine. In: Lewith G, Jonas W, Walach H, editors. *Clinical Research in Complementary Therapies.* London (UK): Churchill Livingston; 2002. p 29–45.

68. Walker BF, French SD, Grant W, Green S. Combined chiropractic interventions for low-back pain. *Cochrane Database Syst Rev.* 2011; 2:CD005427.

69. Walton R, Manos GH. Psychosis related to ephedra-containing herbal supplement use. *South Med J.* 2003;96(7):718–20.

70. Wandel S, Jüni P, Tendal B, et al. Effects of glucosamine, chondroitin, or placebo in patients with osteoarthritis of hip or knee: network meta-analysis. *BMJ.* 2010;341:c4675.

71. Wesnes KA, Ward T, McGinty A, Petrini O. The memory enhancing effects of a ginkgo biloba/Panax ginseng combination in healthy middle-aged volunteers. *Psychopharmacology (Berl).* 2000;152(4):353–61.

72. White J. Alternative sports medicine. *Phys Sportsmed.* 1998;26(6):92–105.

73. Williams MH, Kreider RB, Branch JD. *Creatine. The Power Supplement.* Champaign (IL): Human Kinetics; 1999.

74. Woelk H. Comparison of St. John's wort and imipramine for treating depression: randomized controlled trial. *BMJ.* 2000;321(7260):536–9.

75. Yeh GY, Eisenberg DM, Davis RB, Phillips RS. Use of complementary and alternative medicine among persons with diabetes mellitus: results of a national survey. *Am J Public Health.* 2002;92(10):1648–52.

76. Yun TK, Choi SY. Non-organ specific cancer prevention of ginseng: a prospective study in Korea. *Int J Epidemiol.* 1998;27(3):359–64.

81 Special Considerations for Postoperative Athletes

Eric W. Carson

- Prior to return to play following surgery, athletes must demonstrate resolution of pain and swelling, attainment of normal range of motion (ROM) and strength, and ability to perform sport-specific skills with normal biomechanics and be psychologically ready.
- A knowledge of postoperative rehabilitation protocols and time frames for return to training and competition will assist sports medicine physicians caring for the postoperative patient.

ANTERIOR CRUCIATE LIGAMENT RECONSTRUCTION (2,7,8)

- Preoperative restoration of ROM is important to minimize risk of arthrofibrosis postoperatively.
- Athletes generally return to running by 3 months and full sport activity by 4–6 months.

Preoperative Rehabilitation Phase

- Preoperative goals include control pain and swelling, restoration of normal ROM, and the development of muscle strength sufficient for normal gait and activities of daily living (ADLs).
- Suggested ROM exercises include the following:
  - For extension: Passive knee extension sitting in a chair with the heel on the edge of a stool or chair, heel props with a rolled towel under the heel, and the prone hang exercise.
  - For flexion: Passive knee bend while sitting on the edge of a table, wall slides, and heel slides.
- Muscle strength is developed with the stationary bicycle, elliptical cross-trainer, leg press machine, leg curl machine, and treadmill walking.

Postoperative Days 1–7

- Immediate postoperative goals include control of pain and swelling, care for the knee and dressing, early ROM exercises (with an emphasis on full passive extension), activation of the quadriceps muscles, and gait training.

- Inflammation is controlled swelling with elevation and cryotherapy. Narcotics are appropriate early postoperatively to control pain. Nonsteroidal anti-inflammatory drugs are avoided because they may decrease graft incorporation.
- Early ROM emphasizes extension. The knee immobilizer is removed every 2–3 hours while awake. The heel is positioned on a pillow or rolled blanket or towel with the knee unsupported, and the knee is allowed to sag into full extension for 10–15 minutes. Active-assisted extension is performed by using the opposite uninjured leg and contracting the quadriceps muscles to straighten the knee from the 90-degree position to 0 degrees. Passive flexion of the knee to 90 degrees is performed with the uninjured leg while sitting.
- Quadriceps exercises include isometric contractions with the knee fully extended and straight leg raises (SLRs) with the knee immobilizer on.
- Following patellar tendon graft procedures, hamstring isometric contractions are also performed.
- For patients who have had anterior cruciate ligament reconstruction using the hamstring tendons, it is important to avoid excessive stretching of the hamstring muscles during the first 6 weeks after surgery.

Postoperative Days 8–10

- Goals during postoperative days 8–10 emphasize maintenance of full extension: The athlete continues quadriceps isometrics, SLR, active flexion, and active-assisted extension exercises. It is emphasized to continue removing one's leg from the knee immobilizer four to six times a day for 10–15 minutes at a time to perform extension exercises.

Postoperative Week 3

- During postoperative week 3, goals include maintenance of full extension, achievement of 100–120 degrees of flexion, and development of enough muscular control to wean from the knee immobilizer. In addition to extension exercises and passive flexion, active flexion exercises are added.
- Additional muscular strengthening exercises include partial squats and toe raises. Stationary bike is used with no or low resistance.

■ Crutches are discontinued and the knee immobilizer is discontinued when good muscle control of quadriceps muscle is achieved.

Postoperative Weeks 3–4

■ Goals for weeks 3–4 include advancement of ROM and strengthening. Expected ROM is from full extension to 100–120 degrees of flexion. Wall slides assist with flexion. Strengthening exercises and stationary bike are continued. The elliptical machine and inclined leg presses (from 0–70 degrees) are added. For those with patellar tendon graft, seated hamstring curls are initiated (hamstring curls are avoided until week 8–10 in patients with hamstring graft). Upper body exercise machines, swimming pool walking, flutter kick, water bicycle, and water jogging promote general conditioning.

Postoperative Weeks 4–6

■ Goals for weeks 4–6 include 125 degrees of flexion pushing toward full flexion and continued strength building. The athlete continues quad sets, SLR, partial squats, toe raises, stationary bike, elliptical machine, leg presses, and leg curls. Tilt board or balance board exercises for balance and proprioception training are added.

Postoperative Weeks 6–12

■ Strengthening, general conditioning, and tilt and balance board are continued. Flexion is advanced with goal of 135 degrees of flexion. Treadmill walking without incline is commenced and road bike on flat roads permitted.

Postoperative Weeks 12–20

■ Running and agility drills are introduced. The athlete continues all of week 6–12 strengthening exercises. Straight forward and straight backward running is initiated. Athletes advance to agility drills including zig-zags and cross-over drills.

Postoperative Months 4–6

■ Athletes return to sport during this period. Criteria to return to sport include the following: resolution of swelling, stable knee examination, full ROM, quadriceps/hamstring muscle strength at least 80% of the normal leg (Cybex isokinetic dynamometer evaluation), KT 2000 arthrometric evaluation with a < 3-mm side to side difference, and the ability to complete a running program.

ARTHROSCOPIC PARTIAL MEDIAL/ LATERAL MENISCECTOMY REHABILITATION (4,15)

■ Return to run in 4 weeks. Return to sports in 4–6 weeks.
■ Preoperative rehabilitation emphasizes ROM and quadriceps strengthening.

Phase 1: Days 1–10

Postoperative Days 1–3

■ Crutches are used as needed with weight bearing as tolerated. Cryotherapy and a light compression wrap are used. Electrical stimulation is used to stimulate the quadriceps. Stretching emphasizes full extension. Flexion is permitted to tolerance. Strengthening exercises include SLR, hip adduction and abduction, and one-quarter and/or one-half squats.

Postoperative Days 4–7

■ Cryotherapy, compression wrap, and electric muscle stimulation to quadriceps are continued. Knee extension strengthening from 90–40 degrees is added. Balance and proprioceptive drills are added.

Postoperative Days 7–10

■ Leg presses with light weight, toe raises, and hamstring curls are added. Bicycling is allowed when swelling is resolved and ROM from 0 to 105 degrees is achieved.

Phase 2: Day 10 to Week 4

■ During phase 2, the athlete should achieve full nonpainful ROM, restore normal muscle strength and endurance, and return to functional activities.

Postoperative Days 10–17

■ Strengthening and coordination exercises include lateral lunges, front lunges, half squats, leg press, lateral step-ups, knee extension (90–40 degrees), hamstring curls, hip adduction and abduction, hip flexion and extension, and toe raises. Proprioceptive, balance and stretching exercises continue. Bicycle, StairMaster, and elliptical promote motion and endurance.

Postoperative Day 17 to Week 4

■ Exercises are continued. Pool program (deep water running and leg exercises) is initiated. A compression brace may be used during activities.

Phase 3: Advanced Activity Phase — Weeks 4–7

■ The athlete will return to sport during phase 3. Progression to phase 3 requires resolution of pain and effusion, full ROM, and adequate strength based on satisfactory isokinetic test. Strengthening emphasizes closed-chain exercises. Plyometrics and agility drills are added. Running commences at week 4, and the athlete progresses to sport activity.

MENISCUS REPAIR REHABILITATION PROTOCOL (12,13)

■ Return to running at 3 months; return to sports at 4 months.

Phase 1: 0–2 Weeks

■ Partial weight bearing (50%) in brace locked in extension is permitted during the first 2 weeks. While non–weight bearing, flexion to 90 degrees is permitted. Quad sets, SLRs, and hamstring isometrics are performed. Exercises are generally performed outside of the brace; however, if hamstring control is poor, exercises are performed in the brace. Patellar mobilization is performed. Special attention is given to avoiding weight bearing with flexion > 90 degrees.

Phase 2: 2–8 Weeks

■ The brace is locked to allow 90 degrees of flexion. Weight bearing as tolerated. The athlete continues phase 1 exercises.

Phase 3: 8–12 Weeks

■ Full weight bearing and full ROM. Strengthening progresses to include closed-chain activities, hamstring strength, lunges from 0 to 90 degrees, proprioception/balance program, leg press from 0 to 90 degrees of flexion only, and stationary bike.

Phase 4: 12–16 Weeks

■ Progress to single-leg hops, jogging, plyometrics, sideboard, and sports-specific drills. The athlete returns to sport during this phase.

ANKLE BROSTROM-GOULD PROCEDURE REHABILITATION (9)

■ Return to run in 4 months. Return to sports in 5–6 months.

Phase 1: 0–6 Weeks

■ During the first 6 weeks, the patient is non–weight bearing in a cast. No exercises are performed.

Phase 2: 6–12 Weeks

■ At 6 weeks, the cast is removed, and the patient is placed in a controlled ankle motion (CAM) walker. Partial weight bearing with crutches is done for 2 weeks (weeks 6–7), and then full weight bearing in the CAM walker is allowed during week 8. The CAM walker is removed at the end of week 8, and an air cast ankle splint is used for an additional 3 weeks.

■ Passive ROM is performed in dorsiflexion, plantarflexion, and eversion. Strengthening is initiated with three-way Theraband isotonics (dorsiflexion, plantarflexion, and eversion). **Inversion is avoided through 12 weeks.** Stationary bike is used for conditioning.

■ During weeks 6–8, additional exercises include seated proprioceptive drills, leg press, knee extension, and swimming.

■ During weeks 8–9, vertical squats, side and front lunges, lateral step-ups, and water walking are added.

■ During weeks 10–12, proprioceptive drills, stairclimber, and pool running are added.

Phase 3: 4–5 Months

■ Phase 2 exercises are continued. A return to running program begins. Plyometric, agility, and sport-specific training programs commence.

Phase 4: 5–6 Months

■ During this final phase, strengthening (closed chain), plyometric, running, agility, and sport-specific training continue progressing to a return to full sport activity.

HIP ARTHROSCOPY REHABILITATION: LABRAL DEBRIDEMENT/LABRAL REPAIR/ACETABULOPLASTY/ OSTEOCHONDROPLASTY (3,14)

■ Return to running in 8–9 weeks. Return to sports in 12–13 weeks.

Phase 1: 0–4 Weeks

■ Following labral debridement, patients are allowed to weight bear as tolerated. Following labral repair, osteoplasty, or capsular repair, partial weight bearing (20 lb or less) is adhered to for the first 4 weeks.

■ Following labral repair and capsular repair, flexion is limited to 90 degrees for 10 days, extension and external rotation are limited to 0 degrees for 3 weeks, and abduction is limited to 25 degrees for 3 weeks. Internal rotation is freely permitted.

■ Following osteoplasty, flexion is limited to 90 degrees for 10 days. No limits are placed on extension, abduction, internal rotation, or external rotation.

■ Exercise during week 1 includes passive ROM emphasizing internal rotation and piriformis stretch, quadriceps sets, gluteal sets, transversus abdominis isometrics, stationary bike with minimal resistance, and aquatic therapy/water walking.

■ During week 2, heel slides, quadruped rocking, hip abductor/adductor isometrics, prone internal rotation/external rotations isometrics, and uninvolved knee to chest are added.

■ During week 3, three-way leg raises (abduction, adduction, and extension), double-leg bridging (with SPRI band around knees), and water jogging are added.

■ During week 4, side-lying clams (external rotation), SLR, and leg presses (light weights) are added.

Phase 2: 4–8 Weeks

■ Criteria for progression to phase 2 include minimal pain with phase 1 exercises, ROM ≥ 75% of uninvolved side, and proper muscle firing patterns for initial exercises.

■ Crutches are weaned and weight bearing as tolerated permitted. Once patient is weight bearing without crutches, phase 2 strengthening is commenced. Full ROM is permitted.

- Precautions: No ballistic or forced stretching; no treadmill; avoid hip flexor, adductor, or piriformis inflammation.
- During week 4, the following exercises are added: one-third partial squats, side bridges, and stationary bike with resistance.
- During week 5, manual long-axis distraction and manual anterior/posterior mobilizations are performed (**delay 2 weeks with capsule repair**). Additional exercises include hip four-way/multi-hip machine, single-leg balance/stability exercises (foam/DynaDisc), and advanced bridging/lumbopelvic stabilization progression.
- During week 6, lateral shuffles (SPRI band), Euroglide skaters, lateral step downs, single-leg partial squats, and elliptical/StairMaster are added.
- During weeks 7–8, single-leg resisted rotation with cords and golf progression commence.

Phase 3: 9–13 Weeks

- Criteria for progression to phase 3 include full ROM, normal gait, hip flexion strength > 60% of the uninvolved side, and hip adduction/abduction, extension, internal rotation, and external rotation strength > 80% of the uninvolved side.
- This phase focuses on a return-to-run program, agility drills, and return to sports.

ARTHROSCOPIC ROTATOR CUFF REPAIR PROTOCOL (6)

- Philosophy: This protocol is designed to serve as a guide for the clinician to rehabilitate a patient following massive or fragile rotator cuff repair procedures. Time frames allow for optimal healing and should be used as criteria for advancement along with a patient's functional ability.
- Return to sport following rotator cuff repair generally occurs at 6 months.
- Preoperative exercises emphasize regaining as much of normal ROM and strength as possible.

Phase 1: 0–4 Weeks

- Immediately postoperatively, focus is on protection of the repair and education regarding rotator cuff repair precautions. Passive ROM is limited to forward flexion and scaption. Scapular awareness exercises are initiated.
- Precautions: The athlete must wear sling at all times except when exercising for 6 weeks. No active ROM (AROM) or active-assisted ROM (AAROM) is permitted during phase 1. No passive internal rotation stretching is allowed for 4 weeks. External rotation stretching is limited to 45 degrees only. No strengthening is performed during this phase (and is avoided for 12 weeks).
- Phase 1 exercises include PROM for flexion, scaption, and external rotation (to 45 degrees); grade II and III glenohumeral mobilizations in anterior, inferior, and posterior directions;

manual scapular resistance exercises; Codman's exercise in all directions; active elbow flexion and extension; gripping exercises for the hand; and cervical AROM in all directions.

Phase 2: 4–12 Weeks

- During phase II, passive ROM (PROM) is allowed in all directions. AAROM is initiated at weeks 4–6 and AROM at week 6.
- Precautions: No AROM is permitted until 6 weeks. Strengthening is avoided until 12 weeks. Patients must avoid abnormal scapular substitution patterns with initiation of active motion, particularly substitution pattern of the upper trapezius.
- Exercises during weeks 4–6 include PROM in all planes and AAROM for flexion, abduction, external rotation, and internal rotation (pulleys, wand, etc.), cueing for good scapular positioning/scapulohumeral rhythm. Trunk stabilization exercises are initiated. Lower extremity strengthening and cardiovascular exercises that are nonstressful to the shoulder promote general conditioning.
- During weeks 6–12, AROM commences for flexion and scaption with emphasis on scapular awareness to minimize the upper trapezius influence. Add active scapular retraction and prone Houston exercises and bicep and triceps strengthening with bands only. The extremity is used for light ADLs.

Phase 3: 12–24 Weeks

- Goals of phase 3 include achievement of full AROM in all directions with normal scapulohumeral rhythm and minimal to no shoulder pain with light to moderate ADLs.
- Shoulder strengthening is initiated.
- Precautions: All strengthening should be performed below 90 degrees until normal scapular rhythm and sufficient rotator cuff strength are achieved. Exercise bands only (no free weights) are used for first 4 weeks of strengthening.
- Exercise:
  - Continue PROM and joint mobilization as needed.
  - Initiate strengthening of rotator cuff, deltoid, and scapulothoracic musculature with exercise bands only. Can progress to free weights 4 weeks later if good control is present. General progression recommended:
    - ❏ Prone scapular program
    - ❏ Integrate functional patterns
    - ❏ Increase speed of movements
    - ❏ Integrate kinesthetic awareness drills into strengthening program
    - ❏ Progress to closed-chain dynamic stability activities
  - Initiate proprioceptive training, closed-chain exercises, proprioceptive neuromuscular facilitation patterns, and trunk stabilization/strengthening.

Phase 4: 6 Months

- At 6 months, ADLs are performed without restriction. If sufficient strength exists, the athlete may commence a return to golf and lifting program. Stretching and rotator cuff, scapulothoracic, and trunk strengthening program is continued. Plyometrics may commence.

BANKART LABRAL (ANTERIOR/POSTERIOR) REPAIR AND SUPERIOR LABRAL TEAR (SLAP LESION) REPAIR REHABILITATION PROTOCOL (1,5)

Phase 1: 0–4 Weeks

- During the first 4 weeks postoperatively, the ultra-sling/immobilizer is worn at all times except for hygiene and exercises with physical therapist.

- During this time, internal rotation is permitted as tolerated. Active and active-assisted abduction and external rotation are limited to 40 degrees. Forward flexion is limited to 140 degrees.

- Addition exercises include elbow/wrist/hand ROM, grip strengthening, and isometric abduction, external rotation, and internal rotation exercises with elbow at side.

Phase 2: 4–6 Weeks

- AROM/AAROM/PROM is increased gradually to full ROM as tolerated. Gentle joint mobilizations (grade I–II) assist with motion. Elbow and wrist exercises continue. Scapular stabilization, Theraband exercises, and prone extensions are initiated.

Phase 3: 6–12 Weeks

- During phase 3, the athlete continues scapular stabilizing exercises. Posterior capsular stretching is added. Internal/external rotation isometrics are advanced to light isotonic exercises. Theraband is advanced to lightweights.

Phase 4: 4–6 Months

- Strengthening and ROM exercises are advanced during phase 4. Sports-specific exercises prepare for a return to sports during this phase.

LATERAL EPICONDYLE DEBRIDEMENT/RELEASE REHABILITATION (10,11)

- Return to modified work activity with affected extremity after 4 weeks. Return to sports in 8–12 weeks.

Phase 1: Days 1–7

- A sling for is used for comfort. Cryotherapy three times a day controls edema. A wrist splint minimizes wrist extension. An elbow pad may be used to protect surgical site. Exercises include active shoulder ROM, periscapular exercises, and elbow/wrist/hand ROM.

Phase 2: Weeks 2–4

- The sling is discontinued. Continue cryotherapy three times a day. Tubigrip compression may be used to help control edema. PROM and AAROM are permitted to end-range of patient's tolerance. Submaximal isometrics are initiated.

Phase 3: Weeks 5–7

- Cryotherapy and ROM are continued. An elbow counterforce brace is applied. Strengthening is advanced as tolerated to include weights or Theraband with an emphasis on endurance training of wrist extensors. Gentle massage along and against fiber orientation is performed. A modified return to activity using the upper extremity is permitted.

Phase 4: Weeks 8–12

- Rehabilitative exercise is continued. A gradual return to sports and functional activities is performed.

REFERENCES

1. Blackburn TA, Guido JA. Rehabilitation after ligamentous and labral surgery of the shoulder: guiding concepts. *J Athl Train.* 2000;35(3):373–81.
2. Cascio BM, Culp L, Cosgarea AJ. Return to play after anterior cruciate ligament reconstruction. *Clin Sports Med.* 2004;23(3):395–408, ix.
3. Garrison JC, Osler MT, Singleton SB. Rehabilitation after arthroscopy of an acetabular labral tear. *N Am J Sports Phys Ther.* 2007;2(4):241–50.
4. Goodyear-Smith F, Arroll B. Rehabilitation after arthroscopic meniscectomy: a critical review of the clinical trials. *Int Orthop.* 2001;24(6):350–53.
5. Kim SH, Ha KI, Jung MW, Lim MS, Kim YM, Park JH. Accelerated rehabilitation after arthroscopic Bankart repair for selected cases: a prospective randomized clinical study. *Arthroscopy.* 2003;19(7):722–31.
6. Koo SS, Burkhart SS. Rehabilitation following arthroscopic rotator cuff repair. *Clin Sports Med.* 2010;29(2):203–211, vii.
7. Kvist J. Rehabilitation following anterior cruciate ligament injury: current recommendations for sports participation. *Sports Med.* 2004;34(4):269–80.
8. Myer GD, Paterno MV, Ford KR, Quatman CE, Hewett TE. Rehabilitation after anterior cruciate ligament reconstruction: criteria-based progression through the return-to-sport phase. *J Orthop Sports Phys Ther.* 2006;36(6):385–402.
9. Nery C, Raduan F, Del Buono A, Asaumi ID, Cohen M, Maffulli N. Arthroscopic-assisted Broström-Gould for chronic ankle instability: a long-term follow-up. *Am J Sports Med.* 2011;39(11):2381–8.
10. Nirschl RP, Ashman ES. Tennis elbow tendinosis (epicondylitis). *Instr Course Lect.* 2004;53:587–98.
11. Ollivierre CO, Nirschl RP. Tennis elbow. Current concepts of treatment and rehabilitation. *Sports Med.* 1996;22(2):133–9.
12. Pabian P, Hanney WJ. Functional rehabilitation after medial meniscus repair in a high school football quarterback: a case report. *N Am J Sports Phys Ther.* 2008;3(3):161–9.
13. Shelbourne KD, Patel DV, Adsit WS, Porter DA. Rehabilitation after meniscal repair. *Clin Sports Med.* 1996;15(3):595–612.
14. Stalzer S, Wahoff M, Scanlan M. Rehabilitation following hip arthroscopy. *Clin Sports Med.* 2006;25(2):337–57, x.
15. Vervest AM, Maurer CA, Schambergen TG, de Bie RA, Bulstra SK. Effectiveness of physiotherapy after meniscectomy. *Knee Surg Sports Traumatol Arthrosc.* 1999;7(6):360–4.

Baseball

Catherine N. Laible, Dennis A. Cardone, and Eric J. Strauss

82

OVERVIEW

- America's pastime is one of the most popular sports played today. It has been estimated that more than 8.6 million children ages 6–17 are involved in youth baseball in the United States (16).
- Although classified as a "limited contact" sport, the incidence of injury ranges between 2% and 8% of participants per year (12).
- Serious injuries are associated with blunt chest impact and head and eye trauma.
- Most injuries involve soft tissue trauma or throwing injuries.

BACKGROUND

- *Biomechanics* of overhand throwing depends on adequate transfer of momentum. This kinetic energy is produced from larger slower muscles and transferred to smaller faster body parts (9).
- *Anatomy* of the shoulder includes the sternoclavicular joint, acromioclavicular joint, glenohumeral joint, and scapulothoracic joint. The glenohumeral joint is a complex joint involving many static stabilizers including the joint capsule, glenoid labrum, glenohumeral ligaments, and dynamic stabilizers including the rotator cuff musculature.
- *Anatomy* of the elbow includes the ulnotrochlear joint, radiocapitellar joint, and proximal radioulnar joint. Further stabilizers include the medial and lateral collateral ligament complexes. Musculature of the elbow includes the biceps brachii, brachioradialis, brachialis, triceps, anconeus, supinator, and pronator teres.
- Ossification of the pediatric elbow is important to understand, because age can help determine the injury pattern. Ligaments are stronger than the physis, and therefore, the injury is more likely to involve the bone than the soft tissue. The distal humerus has four ossification centers; the radius and ulna each have one. The capitellum is the first to ossify, followed by the radius, the medial epicondyle, the trochlea, the olecranon, and finally the lateral epicondyle.
- Six phases of throwing: (1) Windup begins with initial movement of the pitcher, the deltoid abducts the arm, and ends when the hands come apart or ball leaves the nondominant hand. (2) Early cocking begins when the hands come apart, the deltoid abducts the arm, the infraspinatus and teres minor externally rotate the shoulder, and ends when the front leg is extended and strikes the ground. (3) Late cocking begins when the front foot strikes the ground, the glenohumeral joint externally rotates, and ends when the shoulder is maximally externally rotated. (4) Acceleration begins with the ball moving forward, horizontal adduction and internal rotation of shoulder, and ends when ball is released. (5) Deceleration occurs after the ball is released. (6) Follow-through ends when motion stops.
- Pitchers develop a shift in the rotational arc of motion of the shoulder, with an increase in external rotation and a compensatory decrease in internal rotation.
- *Deliveries* include overhead, three-quarters, and sidearm, each with their own specific risks of injury.

COMMON INJURIES

- *Rotator cuff injuries* vary from mild forms of tendonitis and impingement to complete tears. They are often due to overuse injuries and can be associated with joint instability. Examination findings include a positive Neer's sign, positive Hawkin's sign, and pain and weakness with resistive muscle testing. If a tear is suspected, the rotator cuff can be visualized on magnetic resonance imaging (MRI). Treatment varies from nonsteroidal anti-inflammatory drugs (NSAIDs) and physical therapy to surgery, depending on the severity of the injury.
- *Instability* can be due to labral injury, trauma, poor mechanics, overuse, or generalized joint laxity. Symptoms include pain during the acceleration phase of throwing. Physical examination findings include a positive apprehension and relocation test, a positive load-and-shift test, and possibly generalized ligamentous laxity. MRI or MRA is the diagnostic modality of choice to evaluate the status of the glenoid labrum. Treatment includes physical therapy with scapular stabilization exercises and, if severe or unresponsive to conservative treatment, may include surgical repair.
- *Superior labral injuries* may occur due to trauma, instability, poor mechanics, or changes in throwing or training. Symptoms include painful clicking, pain with overhead actions, and

pain with acceleration. *SLAP lesions* (superior labrum anterior posterior) are common in throwers. *Internal impingement* is found primarily in pitchers. It occurs during the cocking phase and is caused by repetitive contact between the undersurface of the rotator cuff insertion on the greater tuberosity and the posterosuperior glenoid with abduction and external rotation of the shoulder during the cocking phase of throwing. Examination findings include a positive clunk test, a positive grind test, and a positive O'Brien's test. MRI is the diagnostic modality of choice to evaluate the status of the superior labrum. Conservative treatment includes physical therapy, rest, and NSAIDs. For internal impingement, stretching of the posterior structures is advised. Treatment is surgery if conservative therapies fail.

- *Bennett lesion* is a region of mineralization at the posterior-inferior glenoid rim. This ossification is unique in throwing athletes and is often associated with rotator cuff injuries or instability. Symptoms are usually related to secondary shoulder pathology, and diagnosis is made with a computed tomography (CT) scan. Conservative treatment is favored over surgical intervention (3).

- *Osteochondritis dissecans* (OCD) of the humeral capitellum is often due to repetitive valgus stress across the radiocapitellar joint. Symptoms can include lateral elbow pain associated with throwing, as well as clicking and locking during elbow motion. Crepitus and limited extension may be found on examination, and loose bodies may be seen on plain films. Diagnosis can be made on x-rays or MRI; however, MRI is needed to determine whether the lesion is stable or unstable. Fractures, avascular necrosis, and accessory centers of ossification have been reported to be associated with OCD (14). Treatment depends on degree of lesion displacement and includes conservative measures such as rest, ice, and NSAIDs, as well as operative treatments including surgery.

- *Olecranon stress fracture* results from repetitive concentric firing of the triceps muscle, typically occurring during pitching. Physical examination typically shows point tenderness over the olecranon and pain during the pitching motion. Diagnosis can be made on CT or MRI and can sometimes be seen on plain x-ray. Treatment primarily consists of rest, and repeat imaging can assist with determining when the fracture is healed.

- *Ulnar collateral ligament* injury often occurs in throwing athletes from repetitive valgus stress, causing medial elbow instability and pain. Physical examination findings include decreased extension, tenderness over the course of the ulnar collateral ligament, and laxity and pain with valgus stress testing. Plain x-rays may be negative; however, ultrasound and MRI can assist with the diagnosis (13). Conservative treatment includes rest, ice, and NSAIDs. Indications for surgery include chronic instability, failed conservative treatment, or a complete third-degree tear.

- *Ulnar neuritis* can result from direct trauma to the medial elbow or repetitive overuse. Symptoms include pain at the medial elbow, as well as paresthesias in the fourth and fifth digits. Examination includes pain reproduced with cubital tunnel pressure, a positive Tinel's sign at the cubital tunnel, and distal hand weakness. Treatment includes rest, elbow range-of-motion exercises, and rarely surgery for failed conservative therapy.

- *Little leaguer's elbow* is an overuse injury found in skeletally immature pitchers, resulting from repetitive throwing. The throwing motion causes injury to the medial epicondyle apophysis. Examination is significant for medial elbow tenderness. Treatment includes rest and throwing modifications.

- *Valgus extension overload* is seen primarily in pitchers and is also known as posterior impingement of the elbow. It is caused by contact between the bone and soft tissues in the olecranon fossa during repetitive forced extension, which leads to osteophyte formation on the posteromedial olecranon. This, in turn, leads to chondromalacia of the medial aspect of the olecranon fossa, as well as injuries to the medial collateral ligament (MCL) and the radiocapitellar joint. Symptoms include pain with elbow hyperextension. Physical exam may show valgus instability if the MCL is also injured. X-rays may reveal osteophytes or loose bodies. Treatment includes rest, throwing modification, ice, and NSAIDs. Surgical treatment to resect the osteophyte may be performed arthroscopically or open.

- *Commotio cordis* is dysrhythmia or cardiac arrest occurring after a direct blow to the chest. Numerous cases of batters hit by a baseball causing sudden death have heightened awareness and controversy for safer and softer baseball use (2,6). Chest protectors may also be used for better prevention (17).

- *Head injuries* occur often in baseball due to wild pitches, swinging bats, and hit baseballs often striking fans or spectators. The most common mechanism of injury is direct ball impact to players on the field (10).

ASSOCIATED INJURIES

- *Oral cancer* is a concern in many baseball players using chewing tobacco. Education should be directed toward prevention.

- *Eye injuries* are typically the result of wild pitches and struck baseballs. Baseball is the leading cause of sports-related eye injuries in children (1). Because of this, new helmet designs feature an extended face guard, and sports goggles are recommended for runners on base.

- *Abdominal injuries* have been reported from sliding, collisions, falls, and direct impact of the baseball. Common injuries to the abdomen include muscular contusion, rectus sheath hematoma, and spleen and renal injury. Careful physical examination is important, and CT imaging is often necessary to make a final diagnosis (11).

- *Aneurysm of midaxillary artery* is rare but has been reported in baseball players and should be considered in the differential diagnosis of a throwing athlete with hand pain and paresthesias. Arterial embolization in the arm or hand may occur and is thought to be due to the forceful downward displacement of the humeral head or pectoralis minor tendon, damaging the arterial intima in throwing athletes. Treatment is often surgical revascularization (4,15).

EQUIPMENT

- Baseball equipment includes batting helmets, athletic supporters with cups, cleats, batting gloves, aluminum or wooden bats, and mouth guards.
- Position-specific equipment includes mask, chest, throat, and shin protectors for catchers; toe guards for batters and catchers; forearm batting protectors; and gloves or mitts for field players.
- Health care professionals have recently proposed the implementation of softer baseballs in Little League Baseball to reduce the risk of injury.

REHABILITATION

- Rehabilitation for a baseball player or throwing athlete is often injury specific. Physical therapy should include rehabilitation of the large lower body muscle groups and the smaller muscle groups of the upper extremity. Strengthening often needs to be directed at the rotator cuff and scapular stabilizing muscles.
- The phases of rehabilitation include the acute, recovery, and maintenance phases. The acute phase concentrates on reducing pain and swelling and improving strength. During the recovery phase, treatment is focused on pain-free range of motion, strength, and improved stability and function. The maintenance phase of rehabilitation includes increases in power, endurance, strength, and activity-specific function.
- Interval throwing programs (ITPs) are structured to increase a pitcher's strength and endurance before returning to competitive pitching. ITPs are prescribed after an injury or at the start of preseason training. Programs are designed for players to reach specific goals, often over a period of 3–4 weeks, and combine periods of exercise and rest. Throwing days start with warm-ups and stretching and are followed by throwing. Throwing distances are gradually increased throughout the program.

PREVENTION

- Prevention of injuries is directed at proper conditioning, proper mechanics, proper equipment, and avoiding overuse injuries.
- Pitchers throwing more frequent change-ups have a decreased risk of elbow pain compared to pitchers throwing more sinkers (7,8).

- Monitoring and limiting innings and pitches pitched in Little League Baseball have been implemented to decrease the incidence of overuse injuries.
- Implementing use of safer equipment including break-away bases, batting helmets with face guards, and lighter mass baseballs in youth play can also help prevent injury (5).

LITTLE LEAGUE BASEBALL

- For information on Little League Baseball, including policies, rules, and restrictions for pitchers, visit their Web site at http://www.littleleague.org.

The American Academy of Pediatrics Recommendations (18)

- Baseball and softball for children 5 through 14 years of age should be acknowledged as relatively safe sports. Catastrophic and chronically disabling injuries are rare; the frequency of injuries does not seem to have increased during the past two decades.
- Preventive measures should be used to protect young baseball pitchers from throwing injuries. These measures include a restriction on the number of pitches thrown in organized and informal settings and instruction in proper training, conditioning, and throwing mechanics. Parents, coaches, and players should be educated about the early warning signs of an overuse injury and encouraged to seek timely and appropriate treatment if evidence of an injury develops.
- Serious and potentially catastrophic baseball injuries can be minimized by the proper use of available safety equipment. This includes the use of approved batting helmets; helmets, masks, and chest and neck protectors for all catchers; and rubber spikes. Protective fencing of dugouts and benches and the use of break-away bases also are recommended, as is the elimination of the on-deck circle. Protective equipment should always be properly fitted and well maintained. These preventive measures should be used in games and practices and in organized and informal participation.
- Baseball and softball players should be encouraged to wear polycarbonate eye protectors on the batting helmets to reduce the risk of eye injury. These eye protectors should be required for functionally one-eyed athletes (best corrected vision in the worst eye of less than 20/50) and for athletes who have undergone eye surgery or experienced severe eye injuries if the ophthalmologists judge them to be at an increased risk for eye injuries. These athletes also should protect their eyes when fielding by using polycarbonate sports goggles.
- Consideration should be given to using low-impact baseballs and softballs for children 5–14 years of age. In particular, children younger than 10 years should be encouraged to use the lowest impact balls.

■ Developmentally appropriate rule modifications, such as avoidance of headfirst sliding, should be implemented for children younger than 10 years.

■ Because current data are limited, the routine use of chest protectors is not recommended for baseball players other than catchers.

■ Surveillance of baseball and softball injuries should be continued. Studies should continue to determine the effectiveness of low-impact balls for reducing serious impact injuries. Research should be continued to develop other new, improved, and efficacious safety equipment.

REFERENCES

1. Committee on Sports Medicine and Fitness. American Academy of Pediatrics: risk of injury from baseball and softball in children. *Pediatrics*. 2001;107(4):782–4.

2. Curfman GD. Fatal impact — concussion of the heart. *N Engl J Med* 1998;338(25):1841–3.

3. De Maeseneer M, Jaovisidha S, Jacobson JA, et al. The Bennett lesion of the shoulder. *J Comput Assist Tomogr*. 1998;22(1):31–4.

4. Ishitobi K, Moteki K, Nara S, Akiyama Y, Kodera K, Kaneda S. Extra-anatomic bypass graft for management of axillary artery occlusion in pitchers. *J Vasc Surg*. 2001;33(4):797–801.

5. Janda DH. The prevention of baseball and softball injuries. *Clin Orthop Relat Res*. 2003;(409):20–8.

6. Janda DH, Bir CA, Viano DC, Cassatta SJ. Blunt chest impacts: assessing the relative risk of fatal cardiac injury from various baseballs. *J Trauma*. 1998;44(2):298–303.

7. Lyman S, Fleisig GS, Waterbor JW, et al. Longitudinal study of elbow and shoulder pain in youth baseball pitchers. *Med Sci Sports Exerc*. 2001;33(11):1803–10.

8. Marshall SW, Mueller FO, Kirby DP, Yang J. Evaluation of safety and faceguards for protection of injuries in youth baseball. *JAMA*. 2003; 289(5):568–74.

9. Newsham KR, Keith CS, Saunders JE, Goffinett AS. Isokinetic profile of baseball pitchers' internal/external rotation 180, 300, 450 degrees. *Med Sci Sports Exerc*. 1998;30(10):1489–95.

10. Pasternack JS, Veenema KR, Callahan CM. Baseball injuries: a little league survey. *Pediatrics*. 1996;98(3 Pt 1):445–8.

11. Riviello RJ, Young JS. Intra-abdominal injury from softball. *Am J Emerg Med*. 2000;18(4):505–6.

12. Roberts DG. A kinder, gentler baseball. *Clin Pediatr (Phila)*. 2001; 40(4):205–6.

13. Sasaki J, Takahara M, Ogino T, Kashiwa H, Ishigaki D, Kanauchi Y. Ultrasonographic assessment of the ulnar collateral ligament and medial elbow laxity in college baseball. *J Bone Joint Surg Am*. 2002;84–A(4):525–31.

14. Takahara M, Shundo M, Kondo M, Suzuki K, Nambu T, Ogino T. Early detection of osteochondritis dissecans of the capitellum in young baseball players: report of three cases. *J Bone Joint Surg Am*. 1998;80–A(6): 892–7.

15. Todd GJ, Benvenisty AI, Hershon S, Bigliani LU. Aneurysm of the mid axillary artery in major league baseball pitchers — a report of two cases. *J Vasc Surg*. 1998;28(4):702–7.

16. USA Baseball website [Internet]. Available from: http://www.usa baseball.com

17. Viano DC, Bir CA, Cheney AK, Janda DH. Prevention of commotio cordis in baseball: an evaluation of the chest protectors. *J Trauma*. 2000;49(6):1023–8.

18. Washington RL. Risk of injury from baseball and softball in children. AAP Recommendations. *Am Acad Pediatr*. 2001;107(4):782–4.

Basketball

83

Michael Needham and Chad A. Asplund

INTRODUCTION

- Basketball has been an organized sport since the 1890s and is considered a limited contact sport. It involves a tremendous amount of running with explosive movements and rapid changes in direction and pace. Extreme stresses on the body during play result in many acute musculoskeletal injuries, whereas the ability to play year round and at most ages leads to many overuse injuries.

- With the great popularity of basketball, most teams at the high school level and beyond have associated physicians or certified athletic trainers who are responsible for injury prevention and medical care; however, care for the athlete falls to the hands of many health care providers because many injuries occur outside of organized play (21,35).

- Injury rates in basketball are increasing as popularity rises and the nature of the sport becomes more aggressive (8,35).

EPIDEMIOLOGY

- Nearly one million people are involved in basketball injuries each year in the United States. Population-based injury rates are 3.9 per 1,000, but player injury rates are seen as high as 50% in some European professional leagues (16).

- An epidemiologic study of 100 representative U.S. high schools over the 2005–2006 and 2006–2007 seasons reported an injury rate of 1.94 per 1,000 athlete exposures (AEs) (8).

- Several studies demonstrate no significant difference in the risk for injury between males and females (20,32); others have shown that females are more frequently injured than males (2.08/1,000 AEs vs. 1.83/1,000 AEs) (8).

- College injury rates are 5.7 per 1,000 athlete exposures for males and 5.6 for females (32).

- High school players are more likely to be injured during competition than college players (3.27/1,000 AEs vs. 1.4/1,000 AEs) (8). Between 62% and 64% of injuries in college basketball occur during practice (32), whereas 53%–58% of high school basketball injuries occur during practice (34). In the National Basketball Association (NBA), 49.9% of reported injuries over 17 years were sustained during games (12).

- Basketball has the highest per capita injury rate for all sports in the age group 14–25 years, ranks second in ages 5–14 years, and third in ages 25 years and up (11).

- Approximately 17.5% of sports-related emergency room visits and 13.5% of sports-related visits to primary care physicians are basketball related (11).

- Sprains are the most common type of injury in basketball. Sprains account for 32%–34% of injuries at the collegiate level (32) and 44% at the high school level (8).

- Children are more susceptible to overuse injuries due to open physes, especially at the elbow, knee, and ankle (9).

- Following European professional players over 2 years, there were 37 surgeries (8.7%) performed on a total of 423 injuries (16); 6.9%–8.1% of U.S. high school basketball injuries required surgery (8) (Table 83.1).

DERMATOLOGIC ISSUES

- Fungal infections are prevalent in athletes, and tinea pedis is the most common dermatophytosis. High-top shoes, perspiration, friction, and poor foot care contribute to recurrent problems. Drying feet, changing socks, absorbent powders (without corn starch), and over-the-counter (OTC) and prescription antifungals are effective treatment measures. Similar measures should be taken to treat tinea cruris or "jock itch," which is also common in athletes.

- Blisters are another common problem that can cause significant problems for the basketball athlete. Rigid footwear and significant movement inside of the shoe cause this to occur as the shear stresses between epidermal layers cause fluid to build up. These can be safely drained under sterile conditions if full and tense, and these areas should be protected with Vaseline, moleskin, etc., and treated with topical antibiotics if there are open lesions. Proper footwear, including cushion socks, and conditioning can prevent blisters.

CONCUSSION

- Concussion or mild traumatic brain injury (MTBI) occurs in basketball from two mechanisms — player-to-player contact or contact with the floor (8).

Table 83.1	Common Location of Basketball Injuries (8)
Location	**Frequency of Injury**
Ankle/foot	39.7%
Knee	14.7%
Head/face/neck	13.6%
Arm/hand	9.6%
Hip/thigh/upper leg	8.4%

- MTBI comprises 3.3% of injuries in male basketball players < 20 years old and 5.2% in females < 20 years old, which represents a twofold increase in males and a threefold increase in girls over a 10-year period (35) and reflects the higher incidence of MTBI in females of all age groups. Player collisions are the most likely etiology, and most of these occur in the open court, not under the basket (33).

CARDIAC

- Basketball involves significant physiologic stress as reflected in findings from professional players. Heart rates average 169 bpm and are above 85% predicted maximum for 75% of competitive playing time (26).
- Hypertension is seen in basketball, even though many players are young. Blood pressure elevation over 140 mm Hg systolic and 90 mm Hg diastolic on two separate readings should be investigated. Family history, supplement and medication use, and substance abuse should be considered while investigating other secondary causes.
- Blood pressure should be controlled before allowing exercise. In mild and moderate hypertension, exercise is often part of a treatment plan, but in severe hypertension, it is contraindicated. When choosing treatment options, medications with negative performance side effects such as diuretics and nonselective β-blockers should be a last resort (4).
- Sudden cardiac death is a rare but serious threat, with an incidence of one in 11,394 in National Collegiate Athletic Association (NCAA) basketball players. Incidence is significantly higher in males and in black athletes, with a prevalence of one in 3,000 Division I male basketball players based on a study from 2004–2008 (15). This represents a significantly higher incidence than previously estimated, and basketball players have been found to be at higher risk for sudden cardiac death than any other athletes (15,25). This could be linked to a predisposition for basketball players to be tall and thin, or Marfanoid, or to a predisposition for a higher prevalence of hypertrophic cardiomyopathy in young African American athletes (24).

- Preparticipation examination with a focus on history taking is the best method to prevent sudden death but has not been proven to improve morbidity or mortality.
- High-risk individuals with a family history of premature or sudden death, history of exercise-related syncope, or findings of Marfan syndrome should be identified for further testing.

Marfan Syndrome

- Marfan syndrome is a disorder that affects multiple organ systems, including disproportionate overgrowth of the long bones in the musculoskeletal system and valve dysfunction, dilated cardiomyopathy, and predisposition to aortic aneurysm and dissection in the cardiovascular system (18).
- Because people affected with Marfan syndrome tend to be tall with longer extremities, a higher proportion of them are found among basketball players. Family history is important because Marfan syndrome is passed on as a dominant trait, but about 25% of cases are sporadic.
- Marfan Syndrome Diagnostic Criteria is a list of features doctors use to diagnose (or decide if someone has) Marfan syndrome. The diagnostic criteria are sometimes called the "Ghent Criteria," named after the city in Belgium where doctors decided which features to include on the list (Table 83.2).
- In the 2010 revised Ghent nosology, aortic root aneurysm and ectopia lentis are now cardinal features. In absence of any family history, the presence of these two manifestations is sufficient for the unequivocal diagnosis of Marfan syndrome.
- In patients who die from Marfan syndrome, the etiology is cardiovascular (aortic dissection, congestive heart failure, or cardiac valve disease) in over 90% of cases (18).

Hypertrophic Cardiomyopathy

- Hypertrophic cardiomyopathy (HCM) accounts for 36% of sudden cardiac death in young athletes and has been noted to occur more commonly in male athletes and approximately twice as often in nonwhites, predominantly blacks (24,25).
- HCM is a relatively common disorder, with an incidence of about 1:500, and can lead to cardiac death by fatal arrhythmias, so thorough evaluation is indicated in those diagnosed with HCM to risk stratify and determine treatment (24).
- Clinical diagnosis of HCM is established most easily and reliably with two-dimensional echocardiography by imaging the hypertrophied but nondilated left ventricular (LV) chamber, in the absence of another cardiac or systemic disease (e.g., hypertension or aortic stenosis) (24).
- In clinically diagnosed patients, increased LV wall thicknesses range widely from mild (13–15 mm) to massive (≥ 30 mm) (normal LV thickness ≤ 12 mm) (24).
- However, in trained athletes, modest segmental wall thickening (i.e., 13–15 mm) raises the differential diagnosis between extreme physiologic LV hypertrophy (i.e., athlete's heart) and mild morphologic expressions of HCM; further imaging may be needed.

Table 83.2	Diagnostic Criteria for Marfan Syndrome by Body System (18)

For an *index (new) case*, diagnosis REQUIRES: Major criteria in two categories AND involvement of a third system.

For the *relative of an index case*, diagnosis REQUIRES: One major criterion in family history AND one major criterion in any organ system AND involvement in a second organ system.

Body System	Major Criteria	Minor Criteria
Skeletal	Must have 4 of the following: ■ Pectus carinatum ■ Surgical pectus excavatum ■ Arm span greater than height ■ Length of torso shorter than length of legs ■ Positive wrist sign ■ Scoliosis (> 20-degree curve) ■ Spondylolisthesis ■ Pes planus ■ Protrusion acetabulae	■ Nonsurgical pes excavatum ■ Hypermobile joints ■ High arched palate ■ Marfanoid facial appearance (long, thin face; deep set eyes)
Cardiovascular system	■ Ascending aortic dilation or aneurysm ■ Aortic dissection	■ Mitral valve prolapse ■ Enlarged pulmonary artery ■ Calcium deposits on mitral valve ■ Any aortic aneurysm ■ Any aortic dissection
Pulmonary	No major criteria	■ Spontaneous pneumothorax ■ Apical blebs
Skin	No major criteria	■ Recurrent hernia ■ Striae
Dura	■ Dural ectasia	No minor criteria

■ Magnetic resonance imaging may be of diagnostic value when echocardiographic studies are technically inadequate or in identifying segmental LV hypertrophy undetectable by echocardiography.

■ Because of this potential gray area between physiologically normal "athlete's heart" and mild HCM, clearance and return-to-play decisions should be made by a cardiologist familiar with HCM and athletes.

FACIAL AND ORAL INJURIES

■ Basketball has no accepted regulations, and few players wear face guards or mouth guards for protection against injury. There is ample contact between players, and most facial injuries result from contact with elbows or fingers from other players (5). Five to 10% of basketball injuries involve the face or scalp (33), and an estimated 7,500 eye injuries occur annually in the United States (17).

■ Most lacerations occur over bony prominences, and fractures must be suspected when significant force is applied and symptoms extend beyond local mild tenderness and ecchymosis.

■ The American Academy of Ophthalmology recommendations state that they "strongly recommend" eye protection for all athletes with risk for eye injury and that eye protection should be mandatory for functionally one-eyed athletes and for athletes after eye surgery or after eye trauma (1).

■ Of eye injuries in professional basketball players, eyelid lacerations make up 50%, periorbital contusions make up 28%, and corneal abrasions make up 12% (12,39).

■ Dental injuries are often permanent as teeth do not have much ability to heal. Mouth guards absorb force and help prevent tooth fracture, jaw injury, and even neck injury. A 10-year study of the women's basketball team showed a reduction in incidence of dental injury after instituting mandatory mouth guard use from 8.3 injuries per 100 athlete seasons to 2.8 injuries, but the reduction was not statistically significant (10). Custom-molded guards are inexpensive and preferable to off-the-shelf products.

■ Dental literature reports injury rates from 1% to 14% (22). Most dental trauma occurs to the upper anterior teeth, especially the upper lip and two central incisors.

■ In some studies, mouth guards and protective eyewear have been shown reduce rates of injury (19,39), but an estimated 1%–4% or less of players use these protections (37,39).

SPINE AND PELVIS

■ Back injuries make up more than 5.3% of all basketball injuries (27).

■ The dynamic nature of basketball, including fast changes in direction, repetitive jumping, twisting, rapid starts and stops, high velocity, and overhead arm use, produces significant strain on the spine. The vertebral column and intervertebral discs carry 70% of forces, and the posterior spine transmits 30%.

- Cervical injury from acceleration/deceleration injuries (whiplash) occurs in basketball but is less severe than in other contact sports. Pain and muscular dysfunction are common, but radicular symptoms can be a warning of more significant injury. Treatment includes relative rest, motion and strength exercises, nonsteroidal anti-inflammatory drugs, ice, heat, and modalities. If pain persists, consider facet dysfunction or intervertebral disc degeneration.

- Basketball typically involves repetitive extension and hyperextension from rebounding, guarding opponents, and shooting. This can lead to excessive forces on the lumbar spine and injury. Defects of the posterior portions of the vertebra can lead to significant low back pain exacerbated by extension and axial loading.

- Spondylolysis is the presence of a defect in the pars interarticularis from any etiology including congenital defects, chronic stress, or acute fracture. This is the most common source of back pain in people under age 26 (7). Symptoms include low back pain with radiation into buttock and hamstrings from resulting spasm. Pain is worse with standing and back extension, and there is an absence of radicular pain. Treatment involves back strengthening with a focus on flexion exercises, avoidance of back extension that produces pain, and analgesia as needed. Radiographs for suspected patients are indicated and may need to be repeated if symptoms persist to detect any instability of the spine.

- Spondylolisthesis is the resulting anterior–posterior subluxation of the one vertebra on another when bilateral defects occur. Slippage greater than 50% may need surgical attention. Otherwise, treat patients conservatively with exercise and follow them closely for development of symptoms of nerve root impingement or spinal stenosis. Many athletes can return to basketball after aggressive strengthening and rehabilitation.

- Sacroiliac (SI) dysfunction is commonly seen, misdiagnosed, and treated as muscular low back pain, and athletes fail to improve significantly. Patients usually cannot find any comfortable position for more than 10–15 minutes and have pain radiating into the posterior thigh. Pain is worse with motion that involves combined back flexion/extension and trunk rotation. Physical examination with focused attention to palpation of SI joints and functional testing (Faber's test, Gaenslen's test, Gillet's test, Trendelenburg's test) will allow identification and more appropriate treatment.

UPPER EXTREMITY

- In high school players, 10%–12% of all basketball injuries occur to the hand and wrist, and 2%–4% occur to the shoulder (8).

- The most common upper extremity injuries are sprains and dislocations of the proximal interphalangeal (PIP) joints of the finger (38,40). Radiographs should be considered when a PIP joint injury is identified, as an untreated fracture or dislocation at this location may result in significant long-term disability (29).

- Mallet finger (distal interphalangeal flexion injury) can be seen, which requires a minimum of 6 weeks of continuous splinting and can lead to swan neck deformity if untreated (29).

LOWER EXTREMITY

- Lower extremity injuries account for the majority of injuries at every level of competition. Lower extremity injuries account for 51% in recreational players (21) and between 56% and 69% in high school athletes (14,28,34).

- There is a gender difference, with 56%–64% of male injuries occurring to the lower extremity and 65%–69% of female injuries occurring to the lower extremity (8,26,32). This is thought to be due to higher female knee injury rates compared to males.

KNEE

- Twelve percent of all injuries in male collegiate athletes are knee injuries, whereas the knee accounts for 19% of injuries in women (3).

- Although knee injuries are not the most common type of lower extremity injury, they account for most of the lost playing time (12).

- Patellofemoral syndrome is a broad description that characterizes pain and dysfunction of the extensor mechanism of the knee resulting from poor biomechanics (patella tracks laterally) or inflammation that, in athletes, is usually associated with overuse of the knee. Treatment involves modification of training regimen, ice, NSAIDs, and correction of underlying muscle or bony maltracking with quadriceps strengthening and improving landing mechanics. The vastus medialis is responsible for maintaining medial patellar alignment when other forces act to move the patella laterally. If strength training does not correct the problem, taping or functional braces can be helpful.

- Two common causes of anterior shin pain in basketball players are medial tibial stress syndrome (shin splints) and tibial stress fractures. They represent two points on a continuum of muscle overuse leading to periostitis and finally bone degradation. These overuse injuries are characterized by pain on the medial border of the tibia, typically in the lower midportion. Ice, rest, NSAIDs, correcting foot and ankle biomechanics, and adjusting training regimens will usually improve shin splints.

- Stress fracture symptoms included worsening of typical pain beyond the time of activity and prolonged recovery times from episodes of intense activity or competition.

Plain films can show periostitis and stress fractures, but delayed-phase bone scans and magnetic resonance imaging (MRI) are much more sensitive. Treatment involves an initial period of rest that may include use of removable casts or crutches for pain relief. A very gradual reintroduction of activity with close symptom monitoring will allow for recovery in most cases.

- Patellar tendinitis, or jumper's knee, is common in basketball, found in 40%–50% of high-level players (20). It results from excessive forces through the extensor mechanism on the anterior knee. Symptoms include anterior knee pain just below the patella that is worse with sitting, squatting, kneeling, or climbing stairs. Point tenderness on the superior pole of the patellar tendon and pain with hyperextension of the knee are seen. An initial phase of symptom reduction with relative rest, ice, and NSAIDs can be followed by strengthening exercises with postactivity ice application. Use of infrapatellar straps or taping is common.

- Osgood-Schlatter disease is an inflammatory apophysitis resulting from excessive pull by the patellar tendon on the tibial tuberosity. It appears in young players typically age 10–15 years during a period of rapid growth combined with intense physical activity. Treatment includes relative rest and analgesia, but pain diminishes when growth ceases. Rupture is rare, so participation in sports should not be limited.

- Anterior cruciate ligament (ACL) injuries account for 10% of male basketball knee injuries and 26% of female knee injuries (35). The majority of ACL injuries are noncontact and involve the player planting and pivoting on the knee.

- ACL injury differences between males and females have been attributed to intrinsic factors such as intercondylar notch size and shape, hormone differences, ACL size, and joint laxity as well as extrinsic factors such as strength, skill, experience, shoe wear, and conditioning. The International Olympic Committee Medical Commission put together a current concepts statement identifying risk factors for female athletes suffering ACL injury that include (a) being in the preovulatory phase of menstrual cycle as opposed to the postovulatory phase, (b) having decreased intercondylar notch width, and (c) developing increased knee abduction movement during impact on landing (36).

- A prospective cohort study showed that high knee abduction movement during landing conferred increased risk of ACL injury (30). This suggests further that teaching good landing mechanics is important to reduce lower extremity injury in basketball players, particularly in females.

- Several studies, mostly relatively small, have been done assessing the efficacy of improved landing mechanics with decreased peak tibial shear force, which is a measure of axial loading. These studies have shown that modified mechanics can decrease the risk of ACL injury without compromising performance (23,31,36).

- The natural history of ACL tears is early degenerative arthritis to the affected knee. To avoid this, it is generally recommended for athletes to have ACL reconstruction using one of many accepted techniques (patellar autograft, cadaver graft, hamstring autograft, and the like). Return to play within 12 months is seen in 50%–75% of athletes status post ACL repair, although the numbers tend to be lower in women, and up to two-thirds do not return to the preinjury level of competition (2). If patients are not expecting significant continued activity on the knee, there are times when rehabilitation and bracing are appropriate.

ANKLE AND FOOT

- Ankle injuries make up 87% of lower extremity injuries and are the most common type seen in basketball (35). Inversion sprains to the anterior talofibular ligament comprise 66% of all ligamentous ankle injuries. Many injuries result from a player landing on another player's foot, putting centers and forwards at higher risk than guards.

- Ankle taping has been shown to prevent injury (13), but the concern exists that support from taping declines with time and activity.

- Lace-up and semirigid ankle braces have been shown by prospective trials to reduce incidence of ankle injury (hazard ratio, 0.32) but have not been shown to significantly reduce severity (24). Players do not like wearing ankle braces, but if given a week-long break-in period, there is no detriment to athletic performance and players feel comfortable (31).

- Ottawa ankle rules have a sensitivity of 98% for ankle fractures and should be used. Specificity of the rules varies greatly from 10%–70% (6) (Table 83.3; Fig. 83.1).

- Ankle sprains should be treated with relative rest, NSAIDs, weight bearing as tolerated, ice, bracing, and physical therapy with a focus on regaining proprioception that helps prevent repetitive injury.

- Navicular stress fractures are the most common stress fractures seen in jumping athletes and present with foot pain that is activity related and may persist to a lesser degree out of activity. Bone scan or MRI is needed for diagnosis because plain films are inadequate. Treatment involves immobilization and non–weight bearing until the navicular is nontender (19).

Table 83.3	Ottawa Foot and Ankle Rules
Ankle X-Rays Needed	**Foot X-Rays Needed**
Pain in the malleolar zone (tibia and fibula 6 cm above the articulation with the talus) AND any of the below findings: Bony tenderness at posterior tip or edge of lateral malleolus Bony tenderness at the posterior edge or tip of medial malleolus Inability to bear weight both immediately and in the emergency department	Any pain in the midfoot AND any of the below findings: Bony tenderness at the base of the fifth metatarsal Bone tenderness at the navicular Inability to bear weight both immediately and in the emergency department

Lateral View

Medial View

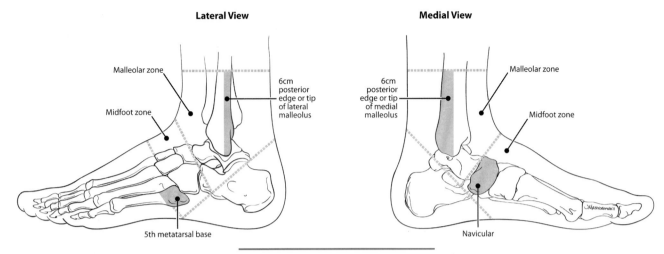

Malleolar zone

Midfoot zone

6cm posterior edge or tip of lateral malleolus

5th metatarsal base

6cm posterior edge or tip of medial malleolus

Malleolar zone

Midfoot zone

Navicular

Figure 83.1: Ottawa Foot and Ankle Rules.

REFERENCES

1. American Academy of Ophthalmology. Protective eyewear for young athletes. Joint policy statement of the American Academy of Pediatrics and American Academy of Ophthalmology [Internet]. 2003. Available from: http://one.aao.org/CE/PracticeGuidelines/ClinicalStatements_Content.aspx?cid=1fda605b-97b9-47e3-90d1-11b7a9607797.

2. Ardern CL, Webster KE, Taylor NF, Feller JA. Return to the preinjury level of competitive sport after anterior cruciate ligament reconstruction surgery: two-thirds of patients have not returned by 12 months after surgery. *Am J Sports Med.* 2011;39(3):538–43.

3. Arendt EA, Agel J, Dick R. Anterior cruciate ligament injury patterns among collegiate men and women. *J Athl Train.* 1999;34(2):86–92.

4. Asplund C. Treatment of hypertension in athletes: an evidence-based review. *Phys Sportsmed.* 2010;38(1):37–44.

5. Azodo CC, Odai CD, Osazuma-Peters N, Obuekwe ON. A survey of orofacial injuries among basketball players. *Int Dent J.* 2011;61(1):43–6.

6. Bachmann LM, Kolb E, Koller MT, Steurer J, ter Riet G. Accuracy of Ottawa ankle rules to exclude fractures of the ankle and mid-foot: systematic review. *BMJ.* 2003;326(7386):417.

7. Borenstein DG, Wiesel SW, Boden SD. *Low Back Pain: Medical Diagnosis and Comprehensive Management.* Philadelphia (PA): WB Saunders; 1995. 735 p.

8. Borowski LA, Yard EE, Fields SK, Comstock RD. The epidemiology of US high school basketball injuries, 2005–2007. *Am J Sports Med.* 2008;36(12):2328–35.

9. Caine D, DiFiori J, Maffulli N. Physeal injuries in children's and youth sports: reasons for concern? *Br J Sports Med.* 2006;40(9):749–60.

10. Cohenca N, Roges RA, Roges R. The incidence and severity of dental trauma in intercollegiate athletes. *J Am Dent Assoc.* 2007;138(8):1121–6.

11. Conn JM, Annest JL, Gilchrist J. Sports and recreation related injury episodes in the US population, 1997–99. *Inj Prev.* 2003;9(2):117–23.

12. Drakos MC, Domb B, Starkey C, Callahan L, Allen AA. Injury in the National Basketball Association: a 17-year overview. *Sports Health.* 2010;2:284–90.

13. Garrick JG, Requa RK. Role of external support in the prevention of ankle sprains. *Med Sci Sports.* 1973;5(3):200–3.

14. Gomez E, DeLee JC, Farney WC. Incidence of injury in Texas girls' high school basketball. *Am J Sports Med.* 1996;24(5):684–7.

15. Harmon KG, Asif IM, Klossner D, Drezner JA. Incidence of sudden cardiac death in national collegiate athletic association athletes. *Circulation.* 2011;123(15):1594–600.

16. Huget J. The pathology of basketball. Report by the Medical Commission of Federation of International Basketball Associations, 1999.

17. Jones NP. Eye injury in sport. *Sports Med.* 1989;7(3):163–81.

18. Judge DP, Dietz HC. Marfan's syndrome. *Lancet.* 2005;366(9501):1965–76.

19. Kerr IL. Mouth-guards for the prevention of injuries in contact sports. *Sports Med.* 1986;3(6):415–27.

20. Khan K. Lower extremity considerations. In: McKeag D, editor. *Olympic Handbook of Sports Medicine: Basketball.* Oxford (UK): Blackwell; 2003.

21. Kingma J, ten Duis HJ. Sports members' participation in assessment of incidence rate in five sports from records of hospital-based clinical treatment. *Percept Mot Skills.* 1998;86(2):675–86.

22. Kvittem B, Hardie NA, Roettger M, Conry J. Incidence of orofacial injuries in high school sports. *J Public Health Dent.* 1998;58(4):288–93.

23. Lim BO, Lee YS, Kim JG, An KO, Yoo J, Kwon YH. Effects of sports injury prevention training on the biomechanical risk factors of anterior cruciate ligament injury in high school female basketball players. *Am J Sports Med.* 2009;37(9):1728–34.

24. Maron BJ. Hypertrophic cardiomyopathy: a systematic review. *JAMA.* 2002;287(10):1308–20.

25. Maron BJ, Doerer JJ, Haas TS, Tierney DM, Mueller FO. Sudden deaths in young competitive athletes: analysis of 1866 deaths in the United States, 1980–2006. *Circulation.* 2009;119(8):1085–92.

26. McInnes SE, Carlson JS, Jones CJ, McKenna MJ. The physiological load imposed on basketball players during competition. *J Sport Sci.* 1995;13(5):387–97.

27. McKay GD, Goldie PA, Payne WR, Oakes BW, Watson LF. A prospective study of injuries in basketball: a total profile and comparison by gender and standard of competition. *J Sci Med Sport.* 2001;4(2):196–211.

28. Messina DF, Farney WC, DeLee JC. The incidence of injury in Texas high school basketball. A prospective study among male and female athletes. *Am J Sports Med.* 1999;27(3):294–9.

29. Micheo W. Head and face considerations. In: McKeag DB, editor. *Olympic Handbook of Sports Medicine: Basketball.* Oxford (UK): Blackwell; 2003.

30. Myer GD, Ford KR, Khoury J, Succop P, Hewett TE. Development and validation of a clinic-based prediction tool to identify female athletes at high risk for anterior cruciate ligament injury. *Am J Sports Med.* 2010;38(10):2025–33.

31. Myers CA, Hawkins D. Alterations to movement mechanics can greatly reduce anterior cruciate ligament loading without reducing performance. *J Biomech.* 2010;43(14):2657–64.

32. National Collegiate Athletic Association. *NCAA Injury Surveillance System for All Sports.* Overland Park (KA): National Collegiate Athletic Association; 1998.

33. Powell J. Injury toll in prep sports estimated at 1.3 million. *Athl Train.* 1989;24:360–73.

34. Powell JW, Barber-Foss KD. Sex-related injury patterns among selected high school sports. *Am J Sports Med.* 2000;28(3):385–91.

35. Randazzo C, Nelson NG, McKenzie LB. Basketball-related injuries in school-aged children and adolescents in 1997–2007. *Pediatrics.* 2010; 126(4):727–33.

36. Renstrom P, Ljungqvist A, Arendt E, et al. Non-contact ACL injuries in female athletes: an International Olympic Committee current concepts statement. *Br J Sports Med.* 2008;42(6):394–412.

37. Spinas E, Savasta A. Prevention of traumatic dental lesions: cognitive research on the role of mouthguards during sport activities in paediatric age. *Eur J Paediatr Dent.* 2007;8(4):193–8.

38. Wilson RL, McGinty LD. Common hand and wrist injuries in basketball players. *Clin Sports Med.* 1993;12(2):265–91.

39. Zagelbaum BM, Starkey C, Hersh PS, Donnenfeld ED, Perry HD, Jeffers JB. The National Basketball Association eye injury study. *Arch Ophthalmol.* 1995;113(6):749–52.

40. Zvijac J, Thompson W. Basketball. In: Caine CG, Lindner KJ, editors. *Epidemiology of Sports Injuries.* Champaign (IL): Human Kinetics; 1996. p. 86–97.

84 Boxing: Medical Considerations

Kevin deWeber

INTRODUCTION

- Acute traumatic brain injuries (TBI) and permanent and irreversible neurologic dysfunction are the primary medical concerns of boxing and the ringside physician.
- Amateur and professional boxing have unique differences in their approach to providing for the safety of the boxers.
- This chapter discusses the medical considerations required of the ringside physician.

AMATEUR VERSUS PROFESSIONAL BOXING

- Amateur and professional boxing have many similarities but also many differences (Table 84.1). An objective assessment of amateur boxing leads to the conclusion that it probably does not involve the same degree of neurologic risk as seen in the professional sport. Shorter competitions, termination of a bout for head blows, headgear, and shorter careers make this understandable.
- Rules for professional boxing vary by state; check http://www.aaprp.org for summary (American Association of Professional Ringside Physicians). Rules for amateur boxing are governed by USA Boxing; check http://www.usaboxing.org for latest Rulebook (7).

MEDICAL RESPONSIBILITIES OF THE RINGSIDE PHYSICIAN

- Prevention and treatment of acute injuries is the primary role of the physician at ringside. This is accomplished through a sound medical plan to cover all aspects of the event — the precompetition phase, the ringside observation, and the postbout examination.

PRECOMPETITION PHASE (3,5,6)

- Having two to three ringside physicians is recommended. This assures that the contest can continue on schedule when a more thorough postbout examination is necessary.

- Evaluation of the competition site by the ringside physician is mandatory. An area for prebout and postbout assessments should be secure, easily accessible, and quiet with enough room and light to perform a neurologic examination, treat an injured boxer, and place a cot or stretcher for observation or transportation.
- Identify the nearest emergency room with neurosurgical, ophthalmologic, and dental capabilities. The on-duty emergency physician and neurosurgeon (if available) should be notified of the event. Have all emergency numbers available and map out evacuation routes.
- Request and require emergency medical technician (EMT) services to be available *on site*. EMTs are a valuable asset in their support of injury care and medical assessments. They should remain on site until they are dismissed by the head physician.
- There should be a table large enough to seat the physicians at ringside. It should be situated near a neutral corner with an unobstructed view of the competition.
- A set of steps next to that corner will allow the physician quick and easy access to the ring apron (the narrow area just outside the ropes).
- Recommended items (as a minimum) for the ringside physician are the following:
  - Stretcher, cervical spine stabilization pads, and oxygen apparatus under the ring
  - A physician's emergency bag to handle cardiopulmonary resuscitation (*i.e.*, Ambu bag, oral and nasal airways) and to manage an unconscious patient
  - Sterile gauze pads for cuts and epistaxis
  - Disposable examination gloves
  - Otoscope and ophthalmoscope
  - Penlight
  - Blood pressure cuff and stethoscope
- Other supplies should be on hand, such as would be carried in a typical team physician medical bag.

Precompetition Physical Examination

- Each boxer must undergo a comprehensive history and physical examination by a licensed physician when joining a boxing club, looking for disqualifying conditions (Table 84.2) and those that need treatment prior to

| Table 84.1 | Differences in Amateur and Professional Boxing |

	Amateur	**Professional**
1. Governing body	USA Boxing; AIBA	Multiple, by state
2. Scoring	All blows equal; computerized at Nationals and above	Weighted toward knockdowns; more subjective
3. Age limit	34 years old (open division USA)	None
4. Competition	3 rounds of 1–2 minutes, based on age	4–12 rounds of 3 minutes
5. Referee	Stops contest early	Stops contest late
6. Headgear	Required	Sparring only
7. Standing 8 count	Up to 3 in 1 round, 4 in bout	Varied rules
8. Lacerations	Uncommon due to headgear; more likely to stop contest	Less likely to stop contest
9. Retinal tear	No further competition	Individual decisions
10. Medical restriction	Uniform periods	Varied rules
11. Risk of cTBI/CTE	No strong evidence of link	Low-quality evidence of link

AIBA, Association Internationale de Boxe Amateur (International Amateur Boxing Association); cTBI, chronic traumatic brain injury; CTE, chronic traumatic encephalopathy.
SOURCE: Schwartz MB. Medical safety in boxing: administrative, ethical, legislative and legal considerations. *Clin Sports Med.* 2009;28(4):505–14, v; and Zazryn TR, McCrory PR, Cameron PA. Neurologic injuries in boxing and other combat sports. *Neurol Clin.* 2008;26(1):257–70, xi.

participating in boxing. The evaluation should be updated annually. Optimally, this should be available for review by the event physician.

■ The precompetition physical examination should be conducted on the day of the scheduled bouts. It need not be comprehensive but must assure that the athlete is fully capable to box — neurologically intact, lacks febrile or contagious conditions, not under the influence of medications, and free of significant injury. The majority of amateur prebout examinations include large numbers of anxious athletes who present without a preparticipation physical

examination questionnaire. Nonetheless, the examination can be accomplished in a few minutes.

■ Important questions to be answered by the boxer that will assist the physician in evaluating for medical conditions and assessing mental status include the following:
  ■ When was your last bout?
  ■ Do you have any medical problems?
  ■ Are you using any medications, pills, or supplements, or have you had any recent injections?
  ■ Have you had any recent illness or injury?

| Table 84.2 | Amateur Boxing Disqualifying Conditions |

Lack of annual comprehensive examination

For females: pregnancy, painful pelvic disease, abnormal vaginal bleeding of unknown etiology, secondary amenorrhea of unknown etiology, recent breast bleeding/mass/dysfunction

General illnesses: acute and chronic infections; severe blood dyscrasias; sickle cell anemia; uncontrolled diabetes or thyroid disease; significant psychological disturbances or drug abuse

Eyes: uncorrected visual acuity worse than 20/400 (USA Boxing) or 20/200 (International); corrected visual acuity worse than 20/60; retinal detachment; cataract; refractive or intraocular surgery

Cardiopulmonary: significant congenital or acquired cardiovascular or pulmonary abnormalities

Musculoskeletal: significant congenital or acquired deficiencies that affect the ability to box

Neurologic: unresolved postconcussion symptoms; significant congenital or acquired intracranial mass lesions or bleeding; seizure within 3 years

Abdomen: hepatomegaly, splenomegaly, ascites

Skin: wounds of the scalp/face/nose/ears requiring external dressing (colloids okay)

Infectious: HIV infection or AIDS, hepatitis B or C; exposed open skin infections

AIDS, acquired immunodeficiency syndrome; HIV, human immunodeficiency virus.
SOURCE: References: Schwartz MB. Medical safety in boxing: administrative, ethical, legislative and legal considerations. *Clin Sports Med.* 2009;28(4):505–14, v; and USA Boxing Rulebook, 2008–2009 [Internet]. Available from: http://www.usaboxing.org/for-members/official-rulebook.

- Have you had any visual disturbances?
- Have you ever been knocked out, and if so, when?
- Do you have a headache or pain anywhere on your body?
- Have you had any recent shortness of breath, chest pain, palpitations, or light-headedness during training?
- The following examination is recommended for the prebout evaluation:
  - Vital signs.
  - Examine the eyes for corneal abrasions and hyphema. Check extraocular motion and pupil equality and reactivity. Ensure intact visual fields by confrontation to rule out possible retinal detachment. Soft contact lenses may be worn in the ring.
  - Examine the ears for cuts and drainage.
  - Examine the nose and mouth.
  - Examine the face for cuts, and palpate for facial fractures. Piercing hardware must be removed before competition.
  - Examine the skin for active infections.
  - Auscultate the heart and lungs, and compress the chest wall looking for rib fractures.
  - Palpate the abdomen for organomegaly or tenderness.
  - Examine the neurologic system to assure good balance and strength.
  - Inspect the musculoskeletal system including cervical spine and upper extremities for tenderness, range-of-motion deficit, swelling, or deformities.

RINGSIDE OBSERVATION (3,5)

- During the bout, the physician's role is to study and to observe the individual boxers and the flow of the event. One looks for signs of distress in a boxer during and between rounds. If there is concern, listen to what is being said in the corner by the coaches. The physician can go into a boxer's corner between rounds if a closer inspection is required. Generally, the following are the only things allowed in a corner: Vaseline, Adrenalin 1:1,000 topical, thrombin, water, ice, gauze pads, towels, sponges, Q-tips, chilled pressure plates for soft tissue swelling, and scissors. Artificial skin coverings, liniments, lotions, or any stimulants (such as smelling salts) are not allowed. Know these rules for the event organization.
- During the action, the boxer's stance and ring movement are key indicators of the skill level and balance. Since effective defense is necessary for safety, its absence mandates cessation of a contest. Early signs of a lapse in defense and of the onset of fatigue are lowered punch counts, lowered arms, and increasing clutches. A staggering or running boxer is a more serious sign.
- Observation of cumulative trauma is important. Facial swelling, cuts, and epistaxis can lead to impaired vision and mouth breathing, making the boxer susceptible to significant head trauma. The experienced referee will provide a level of safety by closely observing the boxers and their eyes, administering

standing 8 counts, and alerting the physicians and corner when there is a concern. If the referee is concerned, the ringside physician should be alert and ready to render care.

- The physician enters the ring on the referee's request to evaluate a boxer after a stoppage or between rounds. Even without the referee's request, if a serious injury is suspected during competition, the physician should climb the stairs onto the ring apron to suspend or terminate the bout.
- When entering the ring, the physician should do so calmly but quickly and confidently, carrying gauze pads and a penlight and wearing exam gloves. Remove the boxer's mouthpiece and assure an adequate airway. Although there may be resistance, a disabled boxer should be made to lie down (if already on the mat) or sit on a stool until fully responsive. When possible, walk the boxer to their corner. Establish a baseline neurologic evaluation. Further observation and serial examinations will be necessary by the physician to determine appropriate future care.
- If no serious conditions are present in the ring and the ringside physician feels the boxer is not at risk of serious injury, the bout can resume.

Conditions That Should Prompt Termination of the Bout

- Airway compromise by bleeding or swelling
- Significant oral bleeding or drainage of blood into posterior oropharynx from epistaxis
- Altered mental status
- Musculoskeletal injury causing significant dysfunction
- Severe facial or lip laceration, especially those overlying a nerve or involving the eyelid or vermillion border of the lip
- Impaired vision caused by swelling, bleeding, or ocular trauma
- Nasal fracture causing airway obstruction or open nasal fracture
- Obviously loose or newly missing teeth
- A boxer feeling he or she cannot continue

After medical termination of the bout and initial stabilization, escort the boxer to the medical treatment area. If recovery is not as expected, evacuate as indicated. If recovery is satisfactory, release the boxer to the supervision of the coach, family, or responsible adult and recommend appropriate follow-up care.

Management of the Unconscious ("Stricken") Boxer (3)

- The unconscious boxer presents a potential medical emergency, and the physician should enter the ring immediately and provide treatment. Obtain assistance from nearby qualified personnel as needed.
- Stabilize the cervical spine while the boxer is still unconscious to prevent spinal cord injury, and open the airway with the jaw-thrust maneuver.
- Assess the airway and breathing efforts. If not breathing, provide artificial breathing with facemask or oxygen apparatus.

If breathing spontaneously, maintain an open airway while maintaining cervical spine stabilization.

- Usually boxers regain consciousness quickly without further stimulation, but if they haven't within approximately 1 minute, stabilize on a backboard with cervical spine immobilization and transport immediately to the emergency facility.
- Once conscious, evaluate the boxer's motor function, speech, orientation, and papillary reaction. When the boxer is moving all extremities, have him or her sit upright for a few moments, and if recovery progresses well, transition to standing and move to the boxer's corner.
- A boxer who has delayed cognitive or neurologic recovery should be transported to a hospital using stretcher, supplemental oxygen, and emergency medical services.

POSTBOUT EXAMINATION (3,5,6)

- Each contestant must be examined immediately after the bout. For bouts without obvious injury, a quick evaluation can be performed as the boxer exits the ring. For a more thorough evaluation, the boxer should be taken to the predetermined medical area away from ringside or to the locker room.
- The brief examination should include observation of the boxer exiting the ring, asking questions to assess his or her orientation, noticing speech patterns and response, and performing a quick survey of the face, head, mouth, and upper extremities. If there are nonurgent but suspicious findings, have the coach bring the boxer back for a reevaluation after a determined amount of time.
- Criteria for transferring a boxer to the emergency room include airway compromise (actual or potential), worsening central nervous system symptoms (*e.g.*, worsening headache, decreasing level of consciousness, abnormal focal neurologic exam, persistent nausea/vomiting, seizures), or any injuries requiring urgent diagnostic studies or treatment care beyond your capability on site.
- The ringside physician should complete any forms required by the event governing body to document injuries sustained and any resulting mandatory bout restrictions. For instance, there are minimum restriction periods mandated by USA Boxing for any bout ending by Referee Stops Contest (Head Blows), or RSC(H). For a bout ending in RSC(H) due to three standing 8 counts in a round or four in a bout or due to stunning head blows not causing unconsciousness, 30-day restriction is mandatory. This must be documented on a Restrictions Affidavit and signed by the ringside physician and other officials (7).

EPIDEMIOLOGY OF INJURIES

- Acute TBI (of which concussion is the most common type) comprises 16%–70% of boxing injuries in professionals and 6%–52% in amateurs. Risk of concussion is 186–250 per 1,000 athletic exposures in professionals and 11–78 per 1,000 in amateurs (4,8).
- Incidence of chronic TBI or chronic traumatic encephalopathy is unknown. The risk is proven in professional boxers but not supported by good evidence in amateurs. Proven risk factors include longer career, higher age, higher number of bouts and of knockouts, and genetic factors (4,8).
- Eye trauma is common and usually minor (corneal abrasion, subconjunctival hemorrhage, lid and periocular swelling) but has the potential of causing significant injury. Pronounced and vision-threatening ocular injuries occur in 21%–58% of professional boxers over a career and include retinal tear or detachment, cataract, macular lesions, angle injuries, and globe rupture (2).
- Nasal contusion and fracture, epistaxis, facial lacerations, hand fractures, and extensor tendon dislocation at the metacarpophalangeal joint are the most common nonneurologic injuries (1).
- Renal contusion, splenic or hepatic injury, and commotio cordis are documented but rare (1).

REFERENCES

1. Coletta DF Jr. Nonneurologic emergencies in boxing. *Clin Sports Med.* 2009;28(4):579–90, vi.
2. Corrales G, Curreri A. Eye trauma in boxing. *Clin Sports Med.* 2009; 28(4):591–607, vi.
3. Goodfellow RI, editor. *Medical Handbook of Olympic Style Boxing.* 7th ed. AIBA (Association Internationale de Boxe Amateur); 2009. Available from: http://www.aiba.org/documents/site1/docs/AIBA%20Medical%20Handbook%202009%20final%20with%20foreword.pdf.
4. Jordan BD. Brain injury in boxing. *Clin Sports Med.* 2009;28(4): 561–78, vi.
5. Kelly M. Role of the ringside physician and medical preparticipation evaluation of boxers. *Clin Sports Med.* 2009;28(4):515–19, v.
6. Schwartz MB. Medical safety in boxing: administrative, ethical, legislative and legal considerations. *Clin Sports Med.* 2009;28(4):505–14, v.
7. USA Boxing Rulebook, 2008–2009 [Internet]. Available from: http://www.usaboxing.org/for-members/official-rulebook.
8. Zazryn TR, McCrory PR, Cameron PA. Neurologic injuries in boxing and other combat sports. *Neurol Clin.* 2008;26(1):257–70, xi.

85 Mixed Martial Arts: Ringside Safety

Anthony G. Alessi and Michael B. Schwartz

INTRODUCTION

- Mixed martial arts (MMA) is the fastest-growing segment of combat sports. Participants vary in age, weight, gender, and fighting styles. Combat sports are the only contests that are won solely on the basis of causing direct injury to the opponent. This diversity presents a challenge for the ringside physician.

- Common styles of MMA combat include wrestling, boxing, kickboxing, Brazilian jiu-jitsu, karate, and Muay Thai.

- There are both amateur and professional classifications but no unified governing body for the sport. Medical requirements for participation are based on individual jurisdictions without any uniformity.

- The safety of the contest is heavily dependent on the competence of the ringside physician.

RULES AND REGULATIONS (1)

- MMA contests consist of between two and five rounds, lasting 3–5 minutes.

- The contest may be held in a cage or standard boxing ring.

- A contest may end by knockout, submission (a fighter taps either his opponent or the mat three times), or technical knockout.

- It is imperative that ringside physicians have the authority to end a contest at any time if they believe a fighter is too severely injured to continue. This is not a standard rule and should be explored by the physician before agreeing to participate in an event.

RINGSIDE PHYSICIAN'S ROLE

- The responsibilities of the ringside physician are best divided into three phases: prefight, ringside, and postfight.

Prefight Responsibilities

- The preparticipation examination (PPE) is a vital aspect in determining fitness, preventing deaths, and minimizing injuries.

- The PPE consists of multiple evaluations including:
  - Review of previous fight results when available.
  - Collection and analysis of prefight medical requirements (Table 85.1). The medical requirements listed were developed by the American Association of Professional Ringside Physicians and the Association of Boxing Commissions.
  - Medical history.
  - Physical examination.

- The medical history should begin with completion of a simple but comprehensive medical history form including:
  - Family history: sudden premature death, hypertension, diabetes, lipid disorders
  - Cardiac history: chest pain, syncope, dizziness
  - Pulmonary history: wheezing, shortness of breath, coughing
  - Medications: daily medications, anti-inflammatory medications, supplements
  - Surgical history: laser-assisted in situ keratomileusis (LASIK), orthopedic, neurologic

- Physical examination: The prefight examination allows the ringside physician an opportunity to identify potential physical limitations.

- The examination must be brief and directed. Variation from these criteria may lead to disqualification. Essential elements include:
  - Vital signs: blood pressure < 140/100 mm Hg, pulse < 100, afebrile.
  - Skin: look for surgical or traumatic scars, rashes
  - Visual acuity: < 20/40 bilaterally near or < 20/100 distant
  - Eyes: signs of radial keratotomy or LASIK procedures, cataracts
  - Ears: ruptured tympanic membranes
  - Nose: rhinitis, deviation
  - Throat/glands: exudate, lymphadenopathy
  - Respiratory: prolonged expiration, wheezing
  - Cardiac: arrhythmias, murmurs
  - Abdominal: distension, tenderness
  - Genitourinary: hernias, testicular exam
  - Musculoskeletal: range of motion, joint deformities
  - Neurologic: pupils, fundi, cognitive, motor, cerebellar, sensory

Table 85.1 | Preparticipation Medical Requirements For Mixed Martial Arts

Medical Requirements	Validity
CT scan/MRI brain scan	Baseline
Dilated eye exam (ophthalmologist)	1 year
Hepatitis Bs antigen, hepatitis Ca antibody, HIV blood testing	180 days
CT, MRI, or complete neurologic exam	1 Year
Electrocardiogram (with interpretation)	Initial only (if normal)
Complete history and physical examination	1 year (commission approved form)
Final prefight mini-physical	At the venue
Serum or urine pregnancy test	14 days
Complete gynecologic examination	6 months

CT, computed tomography; HIV, human immunodeficiency virus; MRI, magnetic resonance imaging.

- Female fighters:
  - Have female present
  - Previous surgeries including breast augmentation
  - On-site urine pregnancy testing
- Special considerations include:
  - Copied medical reports: The physician must be alert to falsified documents.
  - Rapid weight loss: This is a major problem in MMA and may lead to hyperthermia, arrhythmia, seizures, or death.
  - Electrocardiogram: This is typically abnormal in many athletes with hypertrophic cardiomyopathy as a result of training. A comparative study is important along with an echocardiogram and exercise tolerance test when indicated.
  - Radial keratotomy: Can result in traumatic rupture of the cornea.
  - LASIK: May result in dislocation of the corneal flap.
  - Breast implants: May deflate or rupture with trauma.

Ringside Responsibilities

- Arrive at least 1.5–2 hours before the first bout.
- Inspect the ring/cage. Be sure the physicians working at ringside have easy access to the ring. Physicians should familiarize themselves with how the cage entry mechanisms operate. Two physicians should be present at ringside for each contest.
- Meet with the emergency medical services (EMS) personnel. No bout should be held without availability of an ambulance.

If an ambulance must leave, the fight should be delayed until it is replaced.

- Emergency equipment should be stored under the ring, thus allowing for easy access. Necessary items include:
  - Backboard.
  - Emergency kit with resuscitation equipment including Ambu bag, airways, mask, and cervical spine immobilizer. The kit should also have a blood pressure cuff, gauze, ophthalmoscope, and otoscope.
  - Oxygen tank with appropriate tubing and mask.
- Emergency egress should be planned in advance, taking into consideration the potential for confusion at ringside.
- Referees are essential to the success of the contest, and all participating referees should have their blood pressure and pulse checked before the fights begin. Upper limits of 150/100 are generally acceptable.
- The physicians should meet with the referees beforehand to discuss where each physician will be located at ringside in the event that the referee would like consultation during the fight. Communication among the physicians and referees at ringside is imperative.
- At ringside, a physician should have gloves, a flashlight, gauze, and a stethoscope on their person at all times.
- After the fight has commenced, visibility is crucial. The physician should not hesitate to move around to get a better view of the action. This is especially true in MMA where the fighters may be grappling on the mat for an extended period of time. The Jumbotron, or other projection device in the arena, can often be a useful means of observing a fighter's activity.
- "Tapping out" provides an honorable way for an MMA combatant to end a match. Experienced participants know when they are helpless and will not hesitate to tap out. Less experienced, amateur combatants require careful attention when they are subject to a chokehold. Often they will not tap out and may lose consciousness.
- The most difficult ringside decision is whether the fight should continue. This decision can be made at several points during the contest:
  - During a round:
    - A fighter's inability to adequately provide protection from an opponent's attacks, along with loss of coordinated footwork and punching, is indicative of brain injury.
    - Bleeding from a cut above the eye may obstruct vision.
  - Time out:
    - The referee may choose to call a time out and ask the physician to evaluate the fighter based on suspicion of injury.
  - Between rounds:
    - In the corner, between rounds, is a perfect time to chat with the fighter and his corner man. Asking the fighter and corner people if they wish to continue is

important. The fighter should respond to questions quickly, clearly, and accurately. Pupillary response and extraocular movements should be assessed at this time.

Postfight Evaluation

- After each bout, both fighters must be examined. The examination should take place in a private area. Having three physicians at ringside allows for one to perform a detailed examination while the next fight begins.
- The examination should include observation of the fighter's gait, ability to converse, pupillary examination, and examination of the hands and any areas suspected of injury based on the action during the bout.
- EMS personnel should accompany the physician in case transport to a facility is needed.
- Referral to a medical center is indicated for:
  - Severe lacerations
  - Musculoskeletal injuries requiring assisted ambulation or immobilization
  - Brain or spinal injury
  - Difficulty breathing
- Documentation of the postfight examination is important to determine any medical suspensions necessary. The fighter should sign off on the exam after any findings have been explained.
- Directions to a local trauma center should be provided in the event that symptoms develop later that night.

MIXED MARTIAL ARTS INJURIES

- Although MMA has been promoted as a ruthless "blood" sport, a recent study evaluated injuries over a 5-year period with 1,270 fight exposures. The study concluded that injury rates for regulated MMA competitions are similar to other combat sports. In fact, the overall risk of critical sports-related injury appears lower in MMA (2).
- The distribution of injuries is best described by a study published in 2010 reviewing MMA injuries from 1999 to 2006 in Hawaii. The study encompassed 232 exposures and 53 injuries, including 28 abrasions and lacerations, 11 concussions, five facial injuries, and 11 orthopedic injuries (3).
- Concussions are less common in MMA compared with boxing. Given the critical nature of this potentially life-threatening injury, a high level of vigilance on the part of the ringside physician is imperative.

REFERENCES

1. Mohegan Tribe Department of Athletic Regulation. *Rules and Regulations Regarding Boxing and Mixed Martial Arts.* Uncasville (CT): Mohegan Tribe Department of Athletic Regulation; 2010.
2. Ngai KM, Levy F, Hsu EB. Injury trends in sanctioned mixed martial arts competition: a 5-year review from 2002 to 2007. *Br J Sports Med.* 2008;42(8):686–9.
3. Scoggin JF 3rd, Brusovanik G, Pi M, et al. Assessment of injuries sustained in mixed martial arts competition. *Am J Orthop (Belle Mead NJ).* 2010;39(5):247–51.

Crew

Andrew D. Perron

OVERVIEW

- Whether on the water or with rowing machines (ergometers), the sport of rowing is rapidly growing at both the recreational and competitive levels. Today, competitive rowing occurs at the Olympic, elite, collegiate, club, and high school levels.

- Virtually all rowing injuries are caused by overuse, and the vast majority of these can be traced to training errors or equipment problems (4,8,10,14,15).

- The back is the most frequently injured region of the rower, thought to be due to hyperflexion coupled with excessive rotational forces (15,18). Rib stress fractures in rowers are the injury responsible for the most time lost from on-the-water training and competition (15,20).

MECHANICS AND EQUIPMENT

- Boats have one, two, four, or eight rowers, who may have either one oar (sweep rowing) or two oars (sculling). Each rower sits in a sliding seat and places his or her feet in a pair of fixed shoes. The oar is held in an outrigger that can be adjusted in multiple ways that can vary the height, position, angle, and load per stroke.

- The rowing stroke begins at the *catch,* where the back and legs are maximally flexed and the arms extended. It is at this point where the oar enters the water. During the *drive* (power) phase of the stroke, the legs are extended, the back opened, and the arms flexed to the chest. At the *finish* the oar is removed from the water and the blade feathered, or turned parallel to the water. Finally, during the *recovery* phase, the body returns to the catch position with legs and back flexed and arms extended.

- Races are usually run over 1,000- to 2,000-meter courses during the *sprint* season of spring and summer. These races are contested with boats side-by-side and are run at near maximal aerobic capacity, beginning and ending with an anaerobic sprint. A typical sprint race will last 5–8 minutes. In the fall, *head* races are normally run over a 3-mile course, where the individual boat races against the clock. These competitions are run at a lower intensity than sprint races, with the competitor staying within aerobic capacity, and generally run 15–20 minutes in duration.

TRAINING

- Rowing, acknowledged as one of the most strenuous sports (7), requires high levels of both strength and aerobic capacity. With both a sprint season and a head season, rowers train nearly year-round. A typical yearly training cycle mandates strength and distance training in the fall, weights and machine training in the winter, and anaerobic work in the spring and summer racing seasons.

- The successful rower usually has a high aerobic capacity, with elite rowers demonstrating $\dot{V}O_{2max}$ levels of 65–70 mL · kg · min^{-1} (16). The sport favors taller athletes with an extended reach, as they can cover more distance per individual stroke.

COMMON INJURIES

Low Back Pain

- The rowing stroke places a great deal of stress on the low back. It is maximally loaded at the catch, or fully flexed position, which places large forces on both the musculature of the back and the intervertebral discs (4,8,10). One review on the sport found that back and knee injuries were by far the most common injuries to collegiate rowers (1).

- With sweep (one oar) rowing, the back is not only maximally flexed at the catch, but it is also twisted prior to maximal loading in order to extend the athlete's reach. This maximal loading with the back flexed and twisted may result in even more back injury in this patient population (17), although this has been disputed (10).

- Back injury syndromes that can be seen include muscular and ligamentous strains, spondylolysis/spondylolisthesis, and lumbar disc herniation (6,10,17–19)

- Specifically for the rower, training errors of distance, technique, or intensity should be addressed. Additionally, a search for mechanical errors should occur, with modification of equipment as needed to decrease load per stroke, adjust oar/foot height, or even switch side rowed (for sweep rowers) (10,15).

Overuse Knee Injuries

- The rowing stroke maximally loads the knee when it is in the fully flexed position. As a result, patellofemoral pain is a common complaint among rowers. As with patellofemoral problems in other sports, this is more common in women and in those with anatomy that predisposes them to abnormalities in patellar tracking. Tracking problems can be further exacerbated by the position of the shoes fixed in the rowing shell. Their height, spacing, or orientation may be mechanically inappropriate for the rower's anatomy, resulting in increased symptoms (10).

■ Usual treatment of patellofemoral pain, focusing on strengthening of the vastus medialis muscle to improve patellar tracking, is recommended. Shoe position should be checked and modified if not appropriate for the athlete. Heel wedging can also be used to decrease compressive forces across the flexed knee.

Tendinopathy (Patellar, Quadriceps, and Forearm)

■ Tendinopathy can occur in the patellar or quadriceps tendon from repeated flexion/extension with the rowing stroke. Pain is noted over either tendon, worsened by use, and relieved by rest. Usual treatment modalities are employed for relief of symptoms, with a focus on modifying training and equipment errors.

■ Iliotibial band (ITB) friction syndrome can also result from repeated sliding of the ITB over the lateral condylar prominence. A varus knee alignment will exacerbate this condition. ITB friction syndrome is usually associated with a tight ITB coupled with weak hip abductors. ITB stretching and strengthening of the hip abductors are important for successful rehabilitation (10,15).

■ The rowing stroke predisposes to forearm tendinopathy in the dorsal wrist both from tightly gripping the oar during the stroke and from feathering the oar at the finish. Feathering requires rapid extension of the wrist, which further stresses an already strained forearm. Rowers will complain of pain in the dorsal wrist, specifically at the intersection of the first and third dorsal wrist compartments (4,5,10). Physical examination will reveal pain and swelling at this location, and in more severe cases, crepitance may be noted.

■ Treatment of forearm tendinopathy involves relative rest as well as technique modification. Medical modalities, such as ice, brief immobilization, nonsteroidal anti-inflammatory medications, and on occasion, local steroid injection into the affected tendon sheath, may all be employed (5). Technique modification involves stressing a looser grip on the oar, as well as a grip that places the wrist in as flat a position as possible (10).

Nerve Entrapment Syndromes

■ A number of different nerve entrapment syndromes are seen in rowers. These range from digital nerve compression in individual fingers to carpal tunnel syndrome in the upper extremity and frank sciatica in the lower extremity.

■ Digital nerve compression results from a tight grip on the oar with direct pressure on the neurovascular bundle. Equipment and grip modification can alleviate the vast majority of these cases.

■ Carpal tunnel syndrome is also frequently the result of an overly tight grip on the oar as well as repeated extension of the wrist at the finish of the stroke. In addition to standard treatment, technique modification, involving a looser grip as well as equipment modification, with shaving the oar handle to give it a smaller diameter may help with these symptoms.

■ Sciatica can result from an improperly fitted seat that places pressure on the sciatic nerve. Additionally, there are small holes in the seats of rowing shells designed to fit the ischial tuberosities as the rower moves through the rowing stroke. If the holes are improperly spaced for the individual rower, nerve compression can result with associated numbness. This is especially common if women use seats designed for men that don't accommodate their wider pelvis (10).

Rib Stress Fracture

■ Stress fractures of the ribs have been seen with increasing frequency in rowers (2,3,8,12,20). This is thought to be secondary to equipment changes that have put more loads on the oar during the stroke (9). While there is some debate as to exact etiology, it has been traditionally thought to be caused by the pull of the serratus anterior muscle on the scapula during the rowing stroke. These fractures are seen most frequently in the posterolateral region of ribs 5–9 (9,10).

■ Rib stress fracture usually presents with slow onset of chest wall pain in the posterolateral location. As with other stress fractures, pain is initially only with the inciting activity, but will progress to pain at rest if the overuse continues. Ultimately, a bony callus may be noted at the site of the stress fracture. Diagnosis may be made with a plain film demonstrating callus formation or a bone scan in questionable cases.

■ Treatment for rib stress fracture, as with most other stress fractures, involves rest, frequently for up to 6 weeks to allow complete healing (10,13). Prevention with slow progression of load and duration is ideal. Technique modification to unload the oar may also be helpful (10). Switching sides for sweep rowers is also a possibility (15).

Dermatologic Problems

■ The skin of the rower is subject to repetitive trauma in the hand, the posterior calf, and the buttock. As a consequence, the rower may have a number of dermatologic complaints referable to these locations.

■ The hands of rowers are highly susceptible to blisters, caused by friction with the oar handle. These are considered a badge of honor by experienced rowers and a rite of passage for novices. Rowers rarely wear gloves, as this is felt to interfere with the ability to feel the oar as it passes through the water.

Blisters can become secondarily infected, occasionally requiring topical or oral antibiotics in significant cases (11).

- The buttocks are susceptible to chafing, blisters, callus formation, and abrasions due to repetitive trauma from the small sliding seat. Blisters can become infected and occasionally require topical or systemic treatment. Changing the seat, use of a foam pad, and judicious use of petroleum jelly can all help to alleviate symptoms.

- *Track bite* is an injury to the skin of the posterior calves. During the rowing stroke, the legs are forcefully extended, and at the finish, the posterior lower leg contacts the metal track that the seat slides in. The repetitive trauma of the leg hitting the track can result in skin breakdown, or a track bite. Athletes who hyperextend their knees or row with shoes adjusted into a lower position are particularly at risk for these injuries. These injuries can become superinfected, requiring local or systemic antibiotics. Prevention with padding on the end of the track and/or circumferential leg taping at the point of contact can help to alleviate these injuries.

REFERENCES

1. Boland AL, Hosea TM. Rowing and sculling and the older athlete. *Clin Sports Med.* 1991;10(2):245–56.
2. Brukner P, Khan K. Stress fracture of the neck of the seventh and eighth ribs: a case report. *Clin J Sport Med.* 1996;6(3):204–6.
3. Christiansen E, Kanstrup IL. Increased risk of stress fractures of the ribs in elite rowers. *Scand J Med Sci Sports.* 1997;7(1):49–52.
4. Edgar M. Rowing injury: a physiotherapist's perspective. *Sport Care J.* 1995;2:32–5.
5. Fulcher SM, Kiefhaber TR, Stern PJ. Upper-extremity tendinitis and overuse syndromes in the athlete. *Clin Sports Med.* 1998;17(3):433–48.
6. George SZ, Delitto A. Management of the athlete with low back pain. *Clin Sports Med.* 2002;21(1):105–20.
7. Hagerman FC. Applied physiology of rowing. *Sports Med.* 1984;1(4):303–26.
8. Hickey GJ Fricker PA, McDonald WA. Injuries to elite rowers over a 10-yr period. *Med Sci Sports Exerc.* 1997;29(12):1567–72.
9. Karlson KA. Rib stress fractures in elite rowers. A case series and proposed mechanism. *Am J Sports Med.* 1998;26(4):516–9.
10. Karlson KA. Rowing injuries: identifying and treating musculoskeletal and nonmusculoskeletal conditions. *Phys Sportsmed.* 2000;28(4):40–50.
11. Knapik JJ, Reynolds KL, Duplantis KL, Jones BH. Friction blisters. Pathophysiology, prevention and treatment. *Sports Med.* 1995;20(3):136–47.
12. McKenzie DC. Stress fracture of the rib in an elite oarsman. *Int J Sports Med.* 1989;10(3):220–2.
13. Perron AD, Brady WJ, Keats TA. Principles of stress fracture management. The whys and hows of an increasingly common injury. *Postgrad Med.* 2001;110(3):115–8, 123–4.
14. Redgrave A. Rowing injuries: an overview. *Sportcare J.* 1995;2:28–31.
15. Rumball JS, Lebrun CM, Di Ciacca SR, Orlando K. Rowing injuries. *Sports Med.* 2005;35(6):537–55.
16. Secher NH. Physiological and biomechanical aspects of rowing. Implications for training. *Sports Med.* 1993;15(1):24–42.
17. Stallard MC. Backache in oarsmen. *Br J Sports Med.* 1980;14(2–3):105–8.
18. Teitz CC, O'Kane J, Lind BK, Hannafin JA. Back pain in intercollegiate rowers. *Am J Sports Med.* 2002;30(5):674–9.
19. Thomas P. Managing rowing backs. *Practitioner.* 1989;233(1465):446–7.
20. Warden SJ, Gutschlag FR, Wajswelner H, Crossley KM. Aetiology of rib stress fractures in rowers. *Sports Med.* 2002;32(13):819–36.

BACKGROUND

- Cross-country skiing is one of the three Nordic skiing disciplines along with ski jumping and Nordic combined (skiing and jumping). Most historic references to Nordic skiing discuss its military use. Indeed, the sport of biathlon (skiing and shooting) has its origin in this historic relationship.

- Cross-country skiing is generally associated with a low injury rate, and it is considered to be one of the highest aerobic demand activities. Although generally confined to the northern tier and mountain states, its popularity in the United States continues to grow.

- Cross-country skiing had remained relatively unchanged from its remote beginnings until dramatic innovations in equipment and technique were introduced over the past 30 years. Currently, two very distinct techniques are used, the diagonal stride (classic) and ski-skating (freestyle).

COMPETITION

Elite-Level Competition

- The International Ski Federation (FIS) governs international competition. The FIS establishes race rules, schedules, doping control systems, athlete injury surveillance, and most other aspects of World Cup and World Championship racing.

- The specific events held at elite competitions are varied in both distance and technique. Formats include sprint (1 km), sprint relay, middle distance (5, 10, and 15 km), team relay (4 × 5 km, 4 × 10 km), long distance (30 and 50 km), classic/skate pursuit, and others.

- One unique aspect of elite cross-country skiing is that the athletes frequently compete as both sprinters (1 km) as well as marathon skiers (30 or 50 km) within the same race schedule. Historically, most competitors trained and raced in both the classical and skating techniques. More recently, there has been some athlete specialization in terms of event distance and technique.

Nonelite Competition

- Marathon distance races are held in nearly all of the countries of Northern, Central, and Eastern Europe as well as Japan, North America, and Australia.

- In the United States, a full calendar of local, regional, and national marathon races are scheduled throughout the winter months. The largest of these, the American Birkebeiner is 52 km long with over 7,000 participants.

- High school and college cross-country ski teams are common in the Northeast, upper Midwest, and Western states. These competitions include races 5–15 km in length with both classic stride and skating formats.

BIOMECHANICS

Technique

Diagonal (Classic) Technique

- The diagonal stride technique has been used for centuries and remains a popular style for ski touring and back-country skiing.

- In the diagonal stride, forward propulsion is accomplished through alternating kick and glide actions of the skis. This requires a full stop of the kick ski to propel the skier forward. Backward slip of the planted ski is limited by the application of high-friction kick wax on the cambered portion of the ski surface. The requirement to plant the ski to generate thrust limits the maximum speeds obtainable (19).

- In the diagonal stride, the poles are used primarily for balance but can contribute up to 30% of forward thrust in higher level skiers (19). Double poling (planting both poles simultaneously) is used to maintain forward momentum as increasing tempo limits the effectiveness of the kick and glide action.

Skating Technique

- Developed in the late 1970s, this new technique has rapidly evolved and become the method of choice for most non-elite competitors. Skating is the only technique used in both biathlon and Nordic combined competitions.

- The skating technique generates forward momentum by driving the skis at an angle to the direction of travel in a motion analogous to speed skating. There is no kick phase and thus no stopping of the ski during the cycle. Several different strides (V1 skate, V2 skate, marathon skate) are used depending on terrain and skier tempo.

- Double poling is used in most skating strides to transfer upper body energy to the skiing surface and can provide up to 60% of the forward propulsive force (24).

Biomechanical Comparison of the Techniques

- Skating is much more energy efficient than the diagonal stride technique (11). In addition, with skating there is no need for a high-friction kick wax; so low-friction glide waxes can be used along the entire surface of the ski.

- These factors, combined with the use of extremely light-weight composite construction materials as well as improvements in skiing surface preparation, have resulted in a 10%–30% increase in average speed since the 1950s (11,25).

INJURY EPIDEMIOLOGY AND PATHOPHYSIOLOGY

Overall Incidence

- Historically, the injury rates in cross-country skiing are reported to be between 0.1 and 5.63 injuries per 1,000 skiers (3,23). The true incidence is difficult to determine because skiing is not generally limited to a confined venue.

- In the limited data available from more controlled circumstances, such as endurance races, the incidence was found to be substantially higher at 10–35 per 1,000 skiers (4,19). The majority of these injuries were fatigue related.

- Studies evaluating injury patterns in elite-level skiers report higher injury rates. One study reported a rate of 11% in World Cup competitors (9). In another 12-month study, the annual rate of injury in a group of elite Finnish skiers was 62%. However, the majority of the injuries occurred in non-skiing training activities (20).

Changing Injury Patterns

- As the technique and equipment have changed, several equipment–injury relationships have been suggested (2,7,13, 14,22), although data supporting these associations have been scant at best.
  - Increased pole length with the skating technique accentuates demands on the shoulder and elbow.
  - Stiffer bindings and rigid boot construction with heel-ski fixation devices in skating equipment may increase the risk of ankle and knee injuries.
- The biomechanics of the new technique are also suggested in the changing injury patterns.
  - The skating stride places significantly greater demands on the hip adductors and external rotators (19).
  - A greater emphasis on upper body strength in the double poling action has been implicated in increasing upper extremity overuse injuries (7).
  - Ski recovery at the end of the skate cycle places greater demand on the lateral and anterior compartment of the lower extremity, resulting in an exertional compartment syndrome.

Comparison of Techniques

- Initial reports suggested greater incidence of injury in the skating technique; however, this remains unsubstantiated (2,4,7).

- In one report of injuries occurring during a long-distance event where the skating technique was the dominant style used, the injury rate was found to be higher than reported for similar races in the years prior to the adaptation of the skating technique (4).

INJURY DISTRIBUTION

- Studies describing the distribution of musculoskeletal injuries in mass participation events demonstrated that lower extremity injuries are somewhat more common than upper extremity injuries (55% vs. 35%) (23).

The Types of Injuries

- Sprains/twists, 40.4%; fractures, 27.4%; contusions, 16.4%; lacerations, 9.3%; dislocations, 5.8%; and other, 0.7%

- The most frequently encountered acute orthopedic complaints include thumb ulnar collateral ligament strain, knee medial collateral ligament sprain, and plantar fascia strain.

- The most common overuse injuries include sacroiliitis, first metatarsophalangeal (MTP) degenerative joint disease/synovitis, lateral ankle pain, exertional compartment syndrome, and wrist tendinitis.

Medical Problems

- Common medical illnesses reported include exhaustion/dehydration, cold injury, gastrointestinal symptoms, photokeratitis, and bronchospasm.

COMMON MEDICAL CONDITIONS

Exercise-Induced Asthma

- **Incidence:** Exercise-induced asthma (EIA) affects up to 42% of winter sports athletes, with the highest incidence found in cross-country skiers (12,17,21,26). One study reported that 50% of elite cross-country skiers have EIA (21).

- **Pathophysiology:** EIA refers to an inflammatory-mediated bronchial response precipitated by exercise. Exercise is a common trigger of symptoms in athletes with classic asthma. There does appear to be a separate population of athletes who exhibit symptoms only with extreme exercise. Etiologic factors are low humidity and temperature of the inspired air and extremely high-minute volume.

- Typically, the athlete with true EIA will develop symptoms only in relatively extreme circumstances. The likelihood of developing symptoms increases with exercise involving a higher minute volume and cold, dry conditions.

- **History:** It is common for these athletes to exhibit symptoms intermittently. The usual symptoms include shortness of breath with exercise that is out of proportion to effort, burning chest pain, postexercise cough, and wheezing.

- Other red flags include a history of childhood asthma, frequent upper respiratory illnesses, and a chronic cough.

- **Physical examination:** When the athlete is symptomatic, he or she may demonstrate wheezing; otherwise, the examination is typically normal.

- **Diagnostic testing:** The majority of testing protocols use running as the exercise challenge with preexercise and postexercise pulmonary function test change as the measured variable, and as such, the protocols have significant limitations when evaluating the cross-country skier (see Chapter 24) (1,5,6,8,10,15,16,18,21). Ski-specific protocols have been described and are used commonly in the evaluation of elite skiers (16).

- **Treatment:** With classic asthma, the mainstay of therapy is inhaled corticosteroid with inhaled bronchodilator used for symptom management. These athletes should be identified and treated appropriately.

- With EIA, the main goal is prevention of airway irritation and bronchospasm through preexercise administration of medications. Typically a stepped approach is undertaken, beginning with a single bronchodilator prior to exercise and adding additional medications as needed.

Preventive Medications

- Short-acting β-agonists (albuterol, pirbuterol) are usually effective and have the advantage of low cost, ease of use, and high compliance.

- Long-acting β-agonists (salmeterol)

- Leukotriene inhibitors (montelukast sodium) should be reserved as a second-line treatment and should always be used with a β-agonist as a rescue medication.

- Cromolyn sodium is rarely effective when used alone.

Moderate to Severe Symptoms

- Athletes who require second-line medications should be further evaluated.

- Addition of a second medication, listed above

- Addition of inhaled corticosteroid (budesonide, fluticasone) or β-agonist/corticosteroid combinations (Advair; Glaxo Wellcome)

- Inhaled corticosteroid is effective in alleviating the postexercise cough brought on by late-phase inflammatory effects of EIA.

- **Doping control:** Care must be taken to ensure compliance with doping control measures in elite-level skiers.

- Most asthma medications are restricted, and appropriate procedures for documenting their use is required. Currently, the International Olympic Committee (IOC) and FIS require documented testing of these athletes prior to the use of asthma medications.

- The U.S. Anti-Doping Agency hotline is a useful resource for any questions regarding the use of these medications (1-800-223-0393).

COMMON MUSCULOSKELETAL PROBLEMS

Sacroiliitis

- **Pathophysiology:** The sacroiliac (SI) joint is a biconcave articulation of the hemipelvis to the sacrum. It has relatively small rotational motion but functions primarily to transmit force from the lower extremity to the spine. SI dysfunction is the most common cause of low back pain in the skier.

- Injury can result from direct trauma associated with a fall, but more commonly arises from repetitive loading. Contributing factors in this injury include SI joint hypermobility, excessive shear forces, and relative core strength deficits.

- **Clinical features:** Symptoms stem from inflammation in the SI joint and include local pain at the SI joint that is exacerbated with walking, running, or skiing.

- The athlete will often have associated lateral hip pain and pain at the gluteal prominence. Radicular symptoms are unusual and are associated with piriformis spasm, facet irritation, or concomitant disc disease.

- Examination will typically reveal the following: tenderness at the SI joint and relative hypomobility on the affected side with a standing knee-to-chest test.

- FABER test (flexion, abduction, and external rotation) will usually elicit symptoms. Neurologic examination is normal.

- **Diagnostic testing:** Radiographs may demonstrate arthrosis or degenerative disease of the lower spine.

- **Treatment:** Pain relief strategies include oral analgesics/anti-inflammatory medications, osteopathic manipulation or chiropractic treatment, ice, massage, and stretching.

- Long-term management aims at improving SI function through core stabilization and muscle balance training (Theraball program, Pilates, or similar).

- Technique and equipment issues should also be reviewed.

Greater Trochanter Bursitis

- See detailed description in Chapter 59.

Retropatellar Knee Pain (Patellofemoral Dysfunction)/Iliotibial Band Friction Syndrome

- See detailed descriptions in Chapters 62 and 63, respectively.

Exertional Anterior Compartment Syndrome

- **Pathophysiology:** In cross-country skiers, exertional compartment syndrome (ECS) typically affects the anterior or lateral compartments representing injury to the tibialis anterior or peroneus brevis muscles, respectively.

- ECS is precipitated by exercise-induced swelling of the soft tissue in the confined compartment, leading to ischemic pain in the affected muscle.

- This is most common in skating technique where the foot is dorsiflexed and everted during ski recovery.

- This injury was very prevalent when the technique was first introduced due to the excessive length of the ski and relatively soft binding used with the classic stride. As equipment has been developed specifically for the skating technique, this has become less common. It is now most commonly seen with the use of combination equipment (designed for both skating and classic technique) and with poorly fitting equipment.

- **Clinical features:** See detailed description of symptoms in Chapters 23 and 65.

- **Diagnostic testing:** Preexercise and postexercise compartment pressure testing may be helpful, although it is difficult to reproduce the specific conditions of skiing in the laboratory (see Chapter 23).

- **Treatment:** Includes decreasing compartment inflammation using anti-inflammatory medications and improving function through a balanced stretching and strengthening program.

- Equipment modifications should be made to use a skating-specific boot-binding-ski system. A stiffer binding and shorter ski may also help.

- In resistant cases, a surgical fasciotomy may be necessary (see Chapter 65).

Peroneus Tendon Injury

- **Pathophysiology:** Injury to the peroneus tendon can occur with an acute inversion dorsiflexion injury or can develop through repetitive overload that leads to tendinitis. With an acute injury, the peroneus tendon can be torn or may be subluxed from the fibular groove with disruption of the overlying retinaculum. Acute injuries occur with both classic and skating techniques, whereas chronic tendinitis is usually seen in the skating technique.

- **Clinical features:** Acute injuries will present with pain, swelling, and bruising along the posterior and inferior fibula. The athlete will often report a pop in association with an appropriate mechanism, as described earlier.

- Following the acute phase, a chronic clicking sensation may be present, representing subluxation of the peroneal tendon.

- Peroneal tendinitis will usually present with pain and swelling along the posterior and inferior fibula. Pain will be worse after skiing and will interfere with other activities, such as running and walking.

- Physical examination may demonstrate subluxation of the affected peroneus tendon when compared to the contralateral ankle. Resisted eversion of the foot will reproduce pain.

- **Diagnostic testing:** In most acute injuries, an ankle x-ray rules out associated fracture.

- In an acute peroneal tear or subluxation, magnetic resonance imaging (MRI) evaluation may be helpful to evaluate the extent of injury.

- **Treatment:** Acute strain injuries without a complete tear can be treated with immobilization (either casting or controlled ankle movement [CAM] walker boot depending on extent of injury). This is typically continued for 4–6 weeks.

- Complete tear of the tendon or avulsion of the retinaculum is best managed surgically.

- Tendinitis is managed with temporary immobilization in a CAM walker followed by active rehabilitation incorporating passive stretching and eccentric overload exercise.

- Anti-inflammatory medications may be helpful for pain management. Corticosteroid injection may also address the athlete's discomfort. This is accomplished by injecting a solution of 60 mg of triamcinolone, or equivalent injectable steroid, in 2–3 cc of 1% lidocaine into the peroneus sheath. An ankle brace or taping may allow the athlete to continue active training during the rehabilitation process.

Skier's Toe

- **Pathophysiology:** Skier's toe is a term frequently used to describe pain in the first MTP joint.

- This may represent either an acute injury (turf toe or acute sesamoid injury) or chronic problem (hallux rigidus, MTP synovitis, or sesamoiditis).

- In skiers, the chronic form stemming from degenerate joint disease and synovitis is most common and is associated almost exclusively with the classical technique. The mechanism of injury is repetitive extreme extension of the MTP joint.

- **Clinical features:** Athlete complains of pain, swelling, and limited motion at the great MTP joint.

- Symptoms are exacerbated with classical skiing, running, and other activities involving repetitive forced extension of the toe.

- Physical examination may reveal obvious degenerative changes on inspection of the joint. Tenderness and erythema are common. Pain is exacerbated with passive extension/flexion.

- **Diagnostic testing:** Radiographs typically demonstrate first MTP degenerative disease.

- If a stress fracture or sesamoiditis is suspected, a three-phase bone scan or limited MRI study may be useful.

- Analysis of joint aspirate may demonstrate uric acid crystals if degeneration is caused by gouty arthritis.

- **Treatment:** Temporary exclusion of the classic technique helps to alleviate symptoms.

- Modifying nonskiing footwear to eliminate flexion with a spring steel insert or rigid orthotic is also beneficial.

- Severe cases may require temporary use of a rocker bottom boot. Nonsteroidal anti-inflammatory drugs (NSAIDs) are often helpful.

- In cases with substantial degeneration, the athlete may benefit from surgical intervention.

UPPER EXTREMITY

de Quervain Tenosynovitis

- **Pathophysiology:** The repetitive gripping and ulnar/radial deviation motion associated with double poling can lead to tendinitis of the extensor pollicis brevis or abductor pollicis longus. Both tendons occupy the first dorsal wrist compartment and are generally both involved.

- Symptoms can be insidious in onset or may arise acutely with a traumatic event. Chronic pain is common if untreated.

- **Clinical features:** Typical symptoms include pain and swelling along the radial aspect of the wrist.

- Pain is precipitated by gripping and rotational motions (removing the lid from a jar or opening a door).

- Examination reveals tenderness along the extensor surface of the thumb, radial wrist, and forearm. Pain is precipitated with resisted thumb abduction or extension. The patient may demonstrate a positive Finkelstein's test (see Chapter 55).

- **Treatment:** Pain modification via the principles of PRICEMM (protection, rest, ice, elevation, medication, modalities).

- Corticosteroid injection may also be beneficial. Triamcinolone (60–80 mg), or equivalent injectable steroid, with 3 cc of lidocaine is injected into the tendon sheath within the first dorsal wrist compartment.

- Protective bracing with a thumb spica splint is helpful and may allow the skier to continue to ski while being treated.

- Physical or occupational therapy is often useful to address strength and flexibility issues.

- Surgical treatment (synovectomy) may be necessary in persistent cases.

- Return to skiing when symptom free or if symptom free in appropriate brace.

Skier's Thumb (Ulnar Collateral Ligament)/ Extensor Tenosynovitis/Intersection Syndrome

- See detailed descriptions in Chapter 55.

REFERENCES

1. Anderson SD, Daviskas E. The mechanism of exercise-induced asthma is. . . . *J Allergy Clin Immunol.* 2000;106(3):453–9.

2. Bovard R. The new ski-skating poles: a role in fracture risk? *Phys Sport Med.* 1994;22(1):41–7.

3. Boyle JJ, Johnson RJ, Pope MH. Cross-country ski injuries. A prospective study. *Iowa Orthop J.* 1981;1:41–8.

4. Butcher JD, Brannen SJ. Comparison of injuries in classic and skating Nordic ski techniques. *Clin J Sport Med.* 1998;8(2):88–91.

5. Carlsen KH, Engh G, Mørk M. Exercise-induced bronchoconstriction depends on exercise load. *Respir Med.* 2000;94(8):750–5.

6. de Bisschop C, Guenard H, Desnot P, Vergeret J. Reduction of exercise-induced asthma in children by short, repeated warm ups. *Br J Sports Med.* 1999;33(2):100–4.

7. Dorsen P. Overuse injuries from Nordic ski skating. *Phys Sport Med.* 1986;14:34.

8. Eggleston PA. Methods of exercise challenge. *J Allergy Clin Immunol.* 1984;73(5 Pt 2):666–9.

9. Flørenes TW, Nordsletten L, Heir S, Bahr R. Injuries among World Cup ski and snowboard athletes. *Scand J Med Sci Sports.* 2012;22(1):58–66.

10. Garcia de la Rubia S, Pajarón-Fernandez MJ, Sanchez-Solís M, Martinez-Gonzalez Moro I, Perez-Flores D, Pajarón-Ahumada M. Exercise-induced asthma in children: a comparative study of free and treadmill running. *Ann Allergy Asthma Immunol.* 1998;80(3):232–6.

11. Hoffman MD, Clifford PS. Physiological responses to different cross country skiing techniques on level terrain. *Med Sci Sports Excerc.* 1990;22(6):841–8.

12. Larsson K, Ohlsén P, Larsson L, Malmberg P, Rydström PO, Ulriksen H. High prevalence of asthma in cross country skiers. *BMJ.* 1993;307(6915):1326–9.

13. Lawson SK, Reid DC, Wiley JP. Anterior compartment pressures in cross-country skiers. A comparison of classic and skating skis. *Am J Sports Med.* 1992;20(6):750–3.

14. Lindsay DM, Meeuwisse WH, Vyse A, Mooney ME, Summersides J. Lumbosacral dysfunctions in elite cross-country skiers. *J Orthop Sports Phys Ther.* 1993;18(5):580–5.

15. Mannix ET, Manfredi F, Farber MO. A comparison of two challenge tests for identifying exercise-induced bronchospasm in figure skaters. *Chest.* 1999;115(3):649–53.

16. Ogston J, Butcher J. A sport-specific protocol for diagnosing of exercise-induced asthma in cross-country skiers. *Clin J Sport Med.* 2002;12(5):291–5.

17. Pojantähti H, Laitinen J, Parkkari J. Exercise-induced bronchospasm among healthy elite cross country skiers and non-athletic students. *Scand J Med Sci Sports.* 2005;15(5):324–8.

18. Randolph C, Fraser B, Matasavage C. The free running athletic screening test as a screening test for exercise-induced asthma in high school. *Allergy Asthma Proc.* 1997;18(2):93–8.

19. Renstrom P, Johnson RJ. Cross-country skiing injuries and biomechanics. *Sports Med.* 1989;8(6):346–70.

20. Ristolainen L, Heinonen A, Turunen H, et al. Type of sport is related to injury profile: a study on cross country skiers, swimmers, long-distance runners and soccer players. A retrospective 12-month study. *Scand J Med Sci Sports.* 2010;20(3):384–93.

21. Rundell KW, Wilber RL, Szmedra L, Jenkinson DM, Mayers LB, Im J. Exercise-induced asthma screening of elite athletes: field versus laboratory exercise challenge. *Med Sci Sports Exerc.* 2000;32(2):309–16.

22. Schelkun PH. Cross-country skiing: ski skating brings speed and new injuries. *Phys Sports Med.* 1992;20(2):168–74.

23. Sherry E, Asquith J. Nordic (cross-country) skiing injuries in Australia. *Med J Aust.* 1987;146(5):245–6.

24. Smith GA. Biomechanical analysis of cross-country skiing techniques. *Med Sci Sports Exerc.* 1992;24(9):1015–22.

25. Street GM. Technological advances in cross-country ski equipment. *Med Sci Sports Exerc.* 1992;24(9):1048–54.

26. Sue-Chu M, Larsson L, Bjermer L. Prevalence of asthma in young cross-country skiers in central Scandinavia: differences between Norway and Sweden. *Respir Med.* 1996;90(2):99–105.

Bicycling Injuries

Chad A. Asplund

88

INTRODUCTION

- Participation in bicycling is rapidly growing.
  - In 2009, 38.1 million Americans age 7 and older were estimated to have ridden a bicycle six times or more (22).
- There are many different ways to participate in bicycling: road cycling, mountain biking, touring/commuting, cyclocross, and BMX.
- With the increased participation, there has been an increase in both traumatic and overuse injuries:
  - Each year, more than 500,000 people in the United States are treated in emergency departments and more than 700 people die as a result of bicycle-related injuries (10).
- Most common areas for overuse injuries in bicycling are the knee, neck, and back (3,4).
- Many of these overuse injuries occur secondary to improper bicycle fit or to training errors.
- This chapter will outline the different ways people can participate in bicycling, the anatomy and fit of the bicycle, injury epidemiology, traumatic and overuse injuries, cycling-related equipment, and common training errors.

DIFFERENT MODES OF BICYCLING

Road Cycling

- Road racing: Open road 25–100 miles.
- Criterium: Multiple laps around a short course.
  - Very popular in America
  - High potential for crashing/injury
- Time trial: Race against the clock with wave start with 1–5 minutes between riders.

Mountain Biking

- Cross-country: Longer races over variable terrain.
- Downhill: Steep downhill race where focus is on speed; injuries occur as safety is sacrificed for speed.
- Dual slalom: Two racers compete in downhill ski-style slalom course.

Touring/Commuting

- Long-distance road riding for recreation. Rider may be carrying panniers/saddlebags.

Cyclocross

- Off-road race on road-style bike, in which riders complete multiple short (1–2 mile) loops in a set time period. Obstacles require rider to dismount, remount, and carry bicycle over the course.

BMX/Trick Cycling

- Riders compete against other riders over dirt courses of varied terrain or individually on ramps with stairs and railings, with aerial stunts. There is a high risk for injury with aerial acrobatics.
  - Fastest growing segment of U.S. cycling with 60,000 riders (14).
  - Largest portion of child and adolescent cyclists.

BICYCLE ANATOMY

- Although there are many different modes of bicycling, the general anatomy of the bicycle is similar (Fig. 88.1).

Frame Types

- Standard road: Traditional upright geometry with top tube parallel to ground.
- Compact road: Sloping top tube allows rider to fit smaller frame; this maximizes stiffness and minimizes weight.
- Mountain/hybrid: Flatter geometry, heavier bicycle, may have front and/or rear suspension to absorb shock.

Fit

- Most important attribute in the evaluation of overuse bicycling injuries.
- Bicycle fit may be done at local bike shop with bicycle purchase or available for a fee.
- Fit Kit and Serotta "Size Cycle" have been used (11).

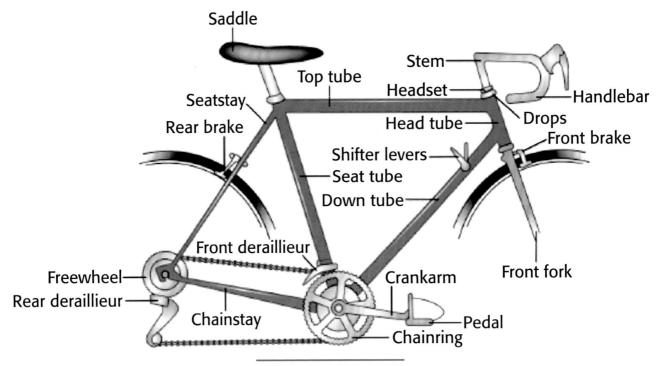

Figure 88.1: Bicycle anatomy.

- Best frame size for cyclist is as small vertically as possible with enough length horizontally to allow a stretched out relaxed upper body. This frame will be lighter and stiffer and handle better (12).

Frame Size

- Most important attribute for appropriate frame size is top tube length.

Top Tube Length

- The ideal position varies here more than anywhere else for cyclists, depending on riding style, flexibility, body proportions, and frame geometry, among others.
- Upper body position may change as riding style evolves.
- May be measured by placing the elbow at the fore end of the saddle; outstretched fingers should touch the handlebars.
- May also have rider, while in the drops, look straight down; the hub of the front wheel should be obscured by the handlebar.

Seat Height

- Optimal saddle height has been estimated based on maximal power output and caloric expenditure (9).
- Calculate height, which will be within a centimeter of 0.883 × inseam length, measured from the center of the bottom bracket to the low point of the top of the saddle. This allows full leg extension, with a slight bend in the leg at the bottom of the pedal stroke.

- When seated on the bike with the pedal at the 6 o'clock position, there should be 20–25 degrees of flexion of the knee.
- Alternatively, the seat may be raised until the hips start rocking when pedaling and then the seat is lowered until the rocking disappears.

Saddle Position

- Check the position of the forward knee relative to the pedal spindle; for a neutral knee position, you'll be able to drop a plumb line from the tibial tubercle and have it bisect the pedal spindle (knee over pedal spindle [KOPS] position) (9).

Handlebar Position

- Most cyclists select a bar that is just as wide as their shoulders.
  - A wider bar opens the chest for better breathing and more leverage but sacrifices aerodynamics.
  - A narrower bar increases aerodynamics but sacrifices stability.
- Handlebar height should be at or below the saddle height; how far below depends on the flexibility and experience of the cyclist.

Crank Arm Length

- Length is based on size and riding style. Shorter crank arm length is better for quick acceleration. Long crank arms are better for pushing larger gears at a lower cadence (12).
- To minimize oxygen consumption, crank arm length is dependent on femur length.

- 2.33 × femur length + 55.8 cm (28). This roughly translates to:
  - Frame size < 54 cm: 170-cm crank arm
  - Frame size 55–61 cm: 172.5-cm crank arm
  - Frame size > 61 cm: 175-cm crank arm

Gearing

- Chain wheels: Large chain ring (usually 53 teeth) and small chain ring (usually 39 teeth) 53/39; recently, a more compact 50/34 chain ring combination has become more popular to allow riders to climb hills and spin at higher cadence.
- Cassette: Cluster of gears (cogs) mounted to right of rear wheel.
- Gear ratio: Number of teeth on chain ring divided by number of teeth on selected cog.
- Higher ratio requires more strength, endurance, and technique.
- Lower gear ratio allows for more spinning and higher cadence; without proper technique will yield less power.

Cadence

- Optimal cadence determined by type of race (time trial, climbing, criterium), body type, muscle fiber type, and training level (8).
- Higher cadences put less strain on trained leg muscles.
- Low cadences increase intramuscular pressure, reducing blood flow to the muscles during the power phase of the pedal stroke.
- High-cadence/low-resistance training reduces the incidence of overuse injuries. Cyclists beginning a season or returning from injury should return with this type of training.
- Cadence is individual and should be determined on a rider-by-rider basis.

INJURIES

Epidemiology

- Each year, more than 500,000 bicyclists in the United States are treated in emergency departments, and more than 700 people die as a result of bicycle-related injuries (8).
- Children are at particularly high risk for bicycle-related injuries. In 2001, children 15 years and younger accounted for 59% of all bicycle-related injuries seen in U.S. emergency departments.
- Peak incidence of bicycle-related injuries is in the 9- to 15-year-old age group.
- Bicycle crashes are the second leading cause of sports-associated serious injury (riding animals is the leading cause) (26).
- Risk factors for injury include not wearing helmet, crashes involving motor vehicles, unsafe riding environment, and male sex (26).

- Conspicuous (brightly colored) clothing may reduce crash-related injury in cyclists (27).
- Mountain bikes account for 3.7% of overall injuries, but 51%–85% of mountain bikers sustain injuries each year (13,18).
- BMX bikers are frequently injured doing stunts; 6.3% of all BMX riders sustain injury in competition (26).

Traumatic Injuries

Upper Extremity
- Fall on outstretched hand:
  - Scaphoid fracture
  - Distal radius (Colles) fracture
  - Fractures of the radial head
- Acromioclavicular joint separation; usually direct trauma to shoulder:
  - First- and second-degree may resume riding as tolerated.
  - Third-degree may take 4–6 weeks to heal.
- Clavicular fracture:
  - If aligned, may resume riding in 48 hours.
  - Nonaligned may return in 4–6 weeks as bone heals or as pain dictates.
  - Fractures with > 2 cm of displacement benefit from surgical fixation (31).

Head
- Head injuries account for most bicycle-related deaths (1,000/year).
- Generally, head injuries are preventable with helmets (severity reduced 85%–90%) (25,26).
- Helmet wear reduces incidence of skull fracture and reduces severity of head injury but does not reduce the incidence of concussion.
- Mandatory legislation increases helmet use among cyclists, particularly in younger age groups (17).
- Bicycle-related mortality in children age 1–15 dropped significantly with mandatory helmet legislation (30).

Skin
- Abrasions (road rash): graded as first degree (superficial), second degree (partial thickness), or third degree (full thickness).
- Wound irrigation, debridement, protection from further trauma and bacterial contamination, creation of a moist wound environment, and judicious use of antibiotics (when indicated) will help achieve optimal outcomes.
- Treated with hydroactive dressing and silvadene or mupirocin ointment.
- Polymeric dressings may be useful for larger wounds (24).
- Large third degree: silvadene cream three times daily or wet to dry dressings.

Visceral

- Mostly caused by blunt trauma from crashes and/or impaling handlebars:
  - Abdominal wall hematomas (16)
  - Liver, spleen, pancreas hematoma
  - Bowel perforation

Overuse Injuries

- The most common site for overuse injuries in the bicyclist is the knee (3).
- Location of knee pain:
  - Anterior
    - ❑ Patellar pain syndrome, quadriceps tendinopathy, chondromalacia patella, patellar tendinopathy
      - Causes: training errors: rapid increase in mileage, high gearing, and excessive hills.
      - Bicycle fit problems: seat too low or too far forward, malpositioned cleats, crank arm too long
      - Anatomic issues: genu valgum, genu varum, hyperpronation
      - Treatment: review and adjust training program, improve bike fit, correct anatomic abnormalities as possible, quadriceps strengthening
  - Medial
    - ❑ Irritation of medial patellofemoral ligament, plica, or pes anserine bursitis
      - Causes: training errors
      - Bicycle fit problems: cleats with toes pointing out, feet too far apart
      - Treatment: review and adjust training program; adjust cleats or shorten bottom bracket axle; rehabilitation and knee strengthening
  - Lateral
    - ❑ Iliotibial band (ITB) friction syndrome/tendinopathy
      - Causes: two mechanisms have been proposed for this syndrome:
        - Excessive friction resulting as the ITB slides back and forth over the lateral femoral epicondyle.
        - Changing tension in the anterior and posterior fibers of the ITB compresses the fat between the tract and a bursa, creating inflammation and merely the illusion of movement (7).
      - Bicycle fit problems: improper cleat placement; seat too high or too posterior; anatomic—hyperpronation, genu varum, tight ITB, leg length discrepancy
      - Treatment: adjust cleats, lower seat, move saddle forward, consider cycling orthotics, ITB stretching, hip girdle strengthening

- Posterior
  - ❑ Biceps femoris tendinopathy, semimembranosus tendinopathy, posterior capsule strain
    - Causes: overly aggressive training
    - Bicycle fit problems: saddle too high or too far forward, improper cleat position
    - Treatment: review and adjust training plan, move seat up and/or back, adjust cleats; rehabilitation of hamstring, quadriceps strengthening

Neck

- Second most common location of bicycling-related overuse injuries (4).
- Common; present in among 60% of riders (20).
- Bicyclists may develop myofascial trigger points in neck (levator scapulae, splenius capitis, trapezius, sternocleidomastoid, infraspinatus, supraspinatus, and rhomboid muscles).
  - Causes: most commonly caused by increased load on the arms and shoulders necessary to support the rider and the hyperextension of the neck in the horizontal riding position (4).
  - Bicycle fit problems: saddle too far aft, effective top tube length too long, handlebars too far below saddle.
  - Treatment: may treat by raising handlebars, shortening stem to reduce hyperextension of the neck. Strength and flexibility exercises may also be used.

Back

- The low back muscles are primarily what the cyclist uses for control and generation of power.
  - Causes: chronic pain and fatigue may develop due to prolonged position on the bike. In older cyclists, may be secondary to some degree of degenerative changes.
  - Bicycle fit problems: saddle too far aft.
  - Treatment:
    - ❑ On bike: change positions frequently, push lower gears, use higher cadence, and rise from the saddle on climbs.
    - ❑ Management: strength, flexibility of lumbar musculature.
    - ❑ May need to move saddle forward (excess forward reach may exaggerate lordotic lumbar posture) (4).

Hands

- Ulnar neuropathy: ulnar nerve may be compressed in Guyon's canal; pain, numbness, tingling in lateral fourth and fifth fingers secondary to compression of the ulnar nerve
  - May be treated with padded gloves, increased handlebar padding, and frequent change of hand positions while riding
- Carpal tunnel syndrome: compression of the median nerve causing numbness and tingling in the index, middle, and ring fingers
- Tenosynovitis: tendons of the extensor pollicis brevis and abductor pollicis longus (de Quervain); caused by tight grip on handlebars (23)

Foot/Ankle

- Paresthesias: numbness/tingling in feet
  - Causes: tight shoe straps and increased pressure on pedals
  - Course: usually self-limited
  - Management: loosen straps on shoes, ride at higher cadence to reduce foot pressure
- Metatarsalgia
  - Causes: poor foot position, increased pedal pressure; may be caused by pes planus or hyperpronation
  - Management: adjust cleats or consider cycling orthotics

Hip

- Trochanteric bursitis: friction causes repetitive sliding of fascia lata over greater trochanter
- Iliopsoas tendinopathy: pain in medial proximal thigh; usually caused by saddle that is too high; may lower seat and/or evaluate frame size

Perineum

- Saddle sores: caused by friction and pressure that may then result in infection; may be prevented with chamois cream
- Crotchitis (tinea cruris): more common in women; try to minimize time off bike spent in sweat-soaked cycling shorts
- Ischial tuberosity (sit bones) tenderness: eases with continual riding; may also consider wearing padded cycling shorts or adding a padded seat cover
- Pudendal neuropathy: compression of dorsal branch of pudendal nerve between bike seat and pubic symphysis (2, 19)
  - May be prevented by adjusting seated position every 5–10 minutes, tilting saddle slightly downward, or changing saddle design

Vascular

- External iliac artery endofibrosis (1,21,29)
  - Progressive stenotic intimal thickening of the external iliac artery
  - Presents with pain/cramps in buttocks, thighs, or calves; may also present with sensation of swollen leg with maximal effort or strenuous cycling
  - Majority in men; 88% unilateral (29)
    - Diagnosis:
      - Ultrasound with continuous wave Doppler
      - Systolic humeral and posterior tibial arterial pressures with oscillometer
      - Exercise test with decrease in ankle blood pressure measurement
      - Arteriography with femoral Seldinger technique
    - Treatment: surgical endarterectomy or intravascular stent

Environmental Injuries (5,6,15)

- Cyclist may be predisposed to heat and cold injuries and altitude sickness, underscoring the importance of proper clothing, nutrition, hydration, and acclimatization.

- For more information, see Chapter 42 on environmental injuries.

Equipment and Safety

- Helmet: reduces risk of head injuries 74%–85% (25,26).
- Should be worn snugly in a horizontal position on the head with the straps forming a "V" around the ears and held in place with buckle fastened.
- Only 15%–25% of children wear helmets correctly (26).
- Helmet use increases with mandatory legislation (17).
  - Possible barriers to use of helmets: discomfort, poor fit, cost, underestimation of risk of injury, peer pressure
- Protective eyeware: protects from ultraviolet radiation, flying objects, and irritants.
- Cycling gloves: cushion hands from road shock, protect hands in falls.
- Cycling shorts: protect inner thigh, groin, and perineum from chafing and pressure trauma.

Common Training Errors Leading to Injury

- Inadequate rest: overreaching to overtraining (see Chapter 40, Overtraining Syndrome)
- Rapid increase in distance or intensity: muscle tightness or microtrauma, which may lead to tendinopathy (most commonly patellar or quadriceps tendon)
- Excessive hill work: anterior knee pain
- Pushing a high-gear ratio: anterior or medial knee pain

CONCLUSION

- Participation in bicycling is increasing.
- There are multiple different ways to enjoy bicycling.
- With this increased participation, providers will likely see more cycling-related injuries.
- With knowledge of the modes of cycling, proper bicycle fit, safety equipment, and common training errors, providers can assist cyclists to ensure safe participation.

REFERENCES

1. Abraham P, Saumet JL, Chevalier JM. External iliac artery endofibrosis in athletes. *Sports Med.* 1997;24(4):221–6.
2. Asplund C, Barkdull T, Weiss BD. Genitourinary problems in bicyclists. *Curr Sports Med Rep.* 2007;6(5):333–9.
3. Asplund C, St Pierre P. Knee pain and bicycling: fitting concepts for clinicians. *Phys Sportsmed.* 2004;32(4):23–30.
4. Asplund C, Webb C, Barkdull T. Neck and back pain in bicycling. *Curr Sports Med Rep.* 2005;4(5):271–4.
5. Bailey DM. Acute mountain sickness: the "poison of the pass." *West J Med.* 2000;172(6):399–400.

6. Baker A. *Bicycling Medicine: Cycling Nutrition, Physiology and Injury Prevention and Treatment for Riders of All Levels.* New York (NY): Simon & Schuster; 1998.

7. Barber FA, Sutker MJ. The iliotibial band syndrome: diagnosis and surgical management. *Tech Knee Surg.* 2008;7(2):102–6.

8. Burke ER. Physiology of higher pedaling cadences: is Lance on to something{qmark} *Cycle Sport Journal.* 2002;116–8.

9. Burke ER. Proper fit of the bicycle. *Clin Sports Med.* 1994;13(1):1–14.

10. Centers for Disease Control and Prevention [Internet]. [cited 2010 Aug 06]. Available from: http://www.cdc.gov/homeandrecreationalsafety/bikeinjuries.html.

11. Christiaans HH, Bremner A. Comfort on bicycles and validity of commercial bicycle fitting system. *Appl Ergon.* 1998;29(3):201–11.

12. Colorado Cyclist. Bike fit: how to fit your custom bicycle [Internet]. [cited 2004 July]. Available from: http://www.coloradocyclist.com/bikefit/.

13. Gaultrapp H, Weber A, Rosemeyer B. Injuries in mountain biking. *Knee Surg Sports Traumatol Arthrosc.* 2001;9(1):48–53.

14. Grubb C. BMX builds racers. *Velonews.* 2003;1(1):11.

15. Helzer-Julin M. Sun, heat and cold injuries in cyclists. *Clin Sports Med.* 1994;13(1):219–34.

16. Holmes JH 4th, Hall RA, Schaller RT Jr. Thoracic handlebar hernia: presentation and management. *J Trauma.* 2002;52(1):165–6.

17. Karkhaneh M, Kalenga JC, Hagel BE, Rowe BH. Effectiveness of bicycle helmet legislation to increase helmet use: a systematic review. *Inj Prev.* 2006;12(2):76–82.

18. Kronisch RL, Pfeiffer RP. Mountain biking injuries: an update. *Sports Med.* 2002;32(8):523–37.

19. Leibovitch I, Mor Y. The vicious cycling: bicycling related urogenital disorders. *Eur Urol.* 2005;47(3):277–86.

20. Mellion MB. Neck and back pain in bicycling. *Clin Sport Med.* 1994;13(1):137–64.

21. Morelli MJ, Stone DA. Bicycling. In: Fu FH, Stone DA, editors. *Sports Injuries, Mechanisms, Prevention and Treatment.* 2nd ed. Philadelphia: Lippincott Williams & Wilkins; 2001. p. 312–9.

22. National Sporting Goods Association Web site [Internet]. [cited 2010 Aug 6]. Available from: http://www.nsga.org/i4a/pages/index.cfm?pageID=3482.

23. Richmond DR. Handlebar problems in cycling. *Clin Sport Med.* 1994;13(1):165–73.

24. Seiffert JG, Ebnet T. The healing effects of polymeric dressings on road rash abrasions in a racing cyclist. *MSSE.* 2008;40(5)(Supp 1):S138–9.

25. Stephens-Stidham S, Mallonee S. The prevention of traffic deaths and injuries: the role of physicians. *J Okla State Med Assoc.* 2001;94(6):192–3.

26. Thompson MJ, Rivara FP. Bicycle-related injuries. *Am Fam Physician.* 2001;63(10):2007–14.

27. Thornley SJ, Woodward A, Langley JD, Ameratunga SN, Rodgers A. Conspicuity and bicycle crashes: preliminary findings of the Taupo Bicycle Study. *Inj Prev.* 2008;14(1):11–8.

28. Too D. Biomechanics of cycling and factors affecting performance. *Sports Med.* 1990;10(5):286–302.

29. Venstermans C, Gielen JL, Salgado R, Bouquillon P, Lauwers J. Endofibrosis of the external iliac artery. *JBR-BTR.* 2009;92(3):184–5.

30. Wesson DE, Stephens D, Lam K, Parsons D, Spence L, Parkin PC. Trends in pediatric and adult bicycling deaths before and after passage of a bicycle helmet law. *Pediatrics.* 2008;122(3):605–10.

31. Wiesel BB, Getz CL. Current concepts in clavicle fractures, malunions and non-unions. *Curr Opin Orthop.* 2006;17(4):325–30.

Dance and Performing Arts Medicine

89

Devin P. McFadden

OVERVIEW

- Performing arts medicine is a growing specialty field that focuses on the care of actors, vocalists, musicians, and dancers.
- Although millions of Americans participate in these activities at a recreational or amateur level, it is estimated that there are over 200,000 professional-level performers in the United States alone (12).
- To discover the biomechanics of injury, physicians who care for these specialized performers must commit to understanding the art form of their patients.
- Just as different sports have unique injury patterns, so to do the performing arts, with each art form, instrument, and dance step carrying with it an inherent set of risks.

EPIDEMIOLOGY

- Because there is no universally accepted governing body or centralized medical oversight in the performing arts realm, it is difficult to determine the exact incidence or prevalence of injury.
- Performing artists tend to seek medical care late in the course of an injury because many are self-employed and uninsured. Injuries are also presumably underreported due to fear of missing an audition, losing a part, or being supplanted by an understudy.
- Current medical knowledge is based primarily on smaller studies investigating a single school or dance troupe. Anecdotal reports of improved injury rates with preventative strategies have been difficult to validate due to sparsity of supporting data.
- The highest prevalence of injury, and therefore the greatest amount of injury data, is found in musicians and dancers. These populations are at increased risk for insidious, chronic, overuse injuries caused by repetitive microtrauma, rather than acute traumatic injuries with a definable onset. Diagnosis and management are more challenging in this setting, and treatment frequently requires activity modification or restriction to allow healing to occur.

MEDICAL CARE OF THE MUSICIAN

- Injury is a threat to the musician just as it is to other athletes and performers. One recent study of orchestral musicians found lifetime prevalence of music-related injuries to be 82%, with 76% experiencing a condition that negatively affected their musical performance (1).
- Historically, musicians are more prone to injury when learning a new technique, practicing a particularly challenging piece, or using a new instrument (12).
- Poor posture, excessive playing force, improperly fitting instruments, and insufficient rest between rehearsals are modifiable risk factors placing the musician at risk for injury (4).
- Environmental risk factors have also been identified, including cool temperatures decreasing circulation to the distal musculature required for fine motor control and inadequate lighting causing eyestrain and abnormal posturing in musicians struggling to read their notes (4).

Injury Specifics

- Musculoskeletal injuries and tendinopathies are common in musicians and tend to present in the same way that they would in nonmusicians. Meanwhile, neurologic injuries are vastly more prevalent than in nonmusical populations, making focal neuropathies, cervical radiculopathy, thoracic outlet syndrome, ulnar neuropathy, carpal tunnel syndrome, overuse syndrome, and focal motor dystonia important diagnoses to recognize and maintain in your differential diagnosis.
- In what has been called the "trumpet player's neuropathy," focal neuropathies of the neurovascular supply to the lip have been identified, primarily in brass and woodwind players (8). Playing woodwinds with leaky valves or pads increases the effort required to produce a note and may be a risk factor for this injury type (4).
- Due to the leftward rotation and lateral flexion of the neck required to cradle the instrument, cervical radiculopathy is common in string musicians. This posture causes loading of the facet joints and anatomic narrowing of the ipsilateral neural foramen. Upon physical examination, one should perform a Spurling test (also known as the quadrant test)

where downward pressure is placed on the top of the rotated and extended head. A positive test is defined by pain and paresthesias spreading distally in the distribution of a cervical nerve root on the side that the patient is facing. Multiple studies have shown the Spurling test to be a reliable diagnostic tool with specificities ranging from 92% to 100%. Although with sensitivities of only 28%–60%, it should not be used for screening purposes (10). Consequently, even without suggestive exam findings, a magnetic resonance imaging (MRI) or electromyography (EMG) must be pursued if clinical suspicion is high.

- Thoracic outlet syndrome results from compression of the neurovascular structures passing through the superior thoracic outlet. The brachial plexus, subclavian artery, and subclavian vein are all at risk of compression while passing between the anterior and middle scalene muscles. Compression may be functional, due to shifts of the clavicle in relation to the shoulder girdle during performance, or static, as in the case of those with a cervical rib. Symptoms typically begin as vague paresthesias and pain located in the medial forearm and hand (C7, C8, or T1 dermatomes). Multiple exam maneuvers have been developed to identify the condition, but retrospective studies have found that Adson's test, Wright's hyperabduction test, Roos test, and the costoclavicular maneuver all have high false-positive rates (10). Therefore, clinical diagnosis must be made with a thorough history guiding a focused radiographic exam. The treatments of choice are postural training and physical therapy. However, when conservative methods fail, surgical decompression is sometimes required.

- With the elbow maintained in a constant state of flexion during prolonged periods of play, ulnar neuropathy at the elbow is a common injury resulting from the strain of supporting a string instrument. Diagnosis is suspected based on history and can be confirmed if a Tinel sign is present at the cubital tunnel. Conservative management with nonsteroidal anti-inflammatory drugs (NSAIDs), avoidance of aggravating activities, and splinting typically leads to resolution of symptoms within weeks.

- Often seen in pianists, carpal tunnel syndrome can result from repetitive flexion and extension of the wrist. The condition can also develop in the bow or pick hand of string instrumentalists and is common in keyboardists as well. Typical symptoms include numbness, tingling, pain, and, in severe cases, weakness of the lateral three and a half fingers, which are supplied by the median nerve. The Phalen test is a good screening exam with poor specificity reported but a sensitivity of about 80%. Meanwhile, a positive Tinel sign at or just distal to the carpal tunnel is virtually diagnostic with specificities approaching 100%, but it should not be used for screening due to poor sensitivity (11). Treatment options include avoiding provocative activities, night splinting, NSAIDs, steroid injections, and surgical release if conservative management fails.

- Overuse syndrome is a controversial and poorly understood condition that spares sensory function but causes pain, weakness, and loss of fine motor coordination in the affected extremity. It is believed to be the most common medical problem in musicians, with prevalence approaching 50% (2). The pathophysiology of the syndrome is not understood, but theories have suggested that pain may develop as a protective mechanism when tissues are stressed beyond their physiologic limits (9). Histologic data have not demonstrated an inflammatory component to this syndrome. Interestingly, an association with complex regional pain syndrome (formerly reflex sympathetic dystrophy) and focal motor dystonia has been proposed (9). Treatment of overuse syndrome focuses on relative rest with a graduated return to performance. As rehearsal times are extended and muscular fatigue develops, the musician, teachers, and musical colleagues must all help ensure maintenance of the necessary postural and ergonomic adjustments that have been adopted, lest symptoms recur (10).

- Focal motor dystonia commonly affects instrumentalists requiring rapid, coordinated fine motor movement. The condition is characterized by painless movement and involuntary spasm of the affected extremity. As with overuse syndrome, the pathogenesis of this disorder is also unknown. The fourth and fifth digits are the most commonly affected joints, with keyboard players, string musicians, and woodwind players being at the highest risk in one study (11).

- In contrast to overuse syndrome, where rest and conservative treatment result in complete resolution of symptoms in over 80% of patients (7), focal dystonia has a very poor prognosis regardless of the therapeutic approach to treatment. A multitude of treatments have been studied in an investigational setting with universally poor outcomes, meaning that a diagnosis of focal dystonia frequently represents the end of the patient's musical career.

MEDICAL CARE OF THE DANCER

- Dance is a sport that is growing in popularity and recognition across the nation, with participation in ballet alone now surpassing that of Little League Baseball and Pop Warner Football (16).

- Currently, there are an estimated 11,000 dance schools, 2,500 professional dance companies, and 38,000 professional dancers and choreographers in the United States (13).

- Elite dancers typically begin training as young as 3 or 4 years old and retire from performance by their mid-30s.

- Dance techniques and styles are limitless and include acro, ballet, ballroom, ceremonial, Highland, hip-hop, Irish, jazz, Latin, lyrical, modern, sequence, and tap, to name a few.

- Because it is one of the most popular and most demanding forms of dance, most injury data involve studies of ballet dancers.

- The majority of dance injuries are found in the lower extremity. Foot and ankle injuries represent approximately 40%

of dance injuries, while knee and back injuries each represent approximately 20% (13).

Dance Terminology

- In order to communicate with ballet dancers, it is necessary to understand the terminology they use. A few high-yield terms are listed below.
- Plié: A slow, fluid movement involving bending of the knees while the hips are maintained in maximal external rotation (turnout). Depth of the dip is determined by the prefix, with *demi* indicating half and *grand* indicating full.
- Pirouette: A whirling turn on a single leg.
- Pointe: A term indicating performance of the dance on the tip of the toes. Dancing en pointe requires special blocked-toe ballet shoes.
- Turnout: A rotation of the legs from the hips in which the knee should remain in line with the hips and ankles. In proper turnout, the feet point in exactly opposite directions.

Dance Injuries

- A dancer's fracture is a spiral fracture of the shaft of the fifth metatarsal. It is the most common acute, traumatic fracture encountered in dancers and frequently results from an inversion injury while dancing en pointe.
- Lisfranc joint injuries typically occur when a downward force is applied simultaneously to a twisting motion of the foot, resulting in a sprain injury with or without an associated fracture/dislocation to the ligaments between the first and second metatarsals and the medial and middle cuneiforms. Diagnosis requires bilateral weight-bearing films so that the injured joint space can be compared to the contralateral side. Sprains can usually be managed conservatively with 6 weeks of immobilization in a controlled ankle movement (CAM) walker boot, whereas fractures/dislocations require open reduction and internal fixation.
- Anterior impingement syndrome affects the anterior ankle during dorsiflexion or plié in ballet. Impingement occurs between the anterior tibia and the dorsum of the talus and is sometimes associated with radiographically visible spurring of the tibial ridge and talar neck. Conservative treatment, which is usually effective, involves activity modification and graduated return to dance. Surgical intervention can be pursued to remove spurs if conventional therapy fails.
- Posterior impingement syndrome, conversely, is characterized by posterolateral ankle pain during plantarflexion as during pointe work in ballet. Symptoms occur when full plantarflexion is not achieved because of a fixed obstruction such as an os trigonum, which causes increased stress on the tendinous structures and bony impingement. An os trigonum occurs when the posterolateral process of the talus does not fuse during puberty. It is a congenital variant that is found in 7%–11% of the population. Presence of an os trigonum, however, does not inevitably lead to impingement,

as many dancers with this variant are asymptomatic (3). In this setting, an ankle sprain and the resulting shift in ankle mechanics can unmask a previously asymptomatic anomaly. Conservative treatment with activity modification, NSAIDs, and therapeutic injections is nearly always successful, and surgical intervention is rarely warranted.

- Flexor hallucis longus (FHL) tendonitis, or dancer's tendonitis, occurs from overuse and microtrauma resulting from repetitive dorsiflexion and plantarflexion. The FHL travels through the fibro-osseous tunnel above the posterior talar tubercle and can be injured by compressive forces during full plantarflexion and stretching between the talar tubercle and sustentaculum tali during dorsiflexion. Over time, cumulative stress leads to posteromedial ankle pain, inflammatory changes, nodular tendinopathy, and potentially tissue degeneration.
- Achilles tendinopathy is another commonly encountered diagnosis in dancers and is considered a chronic inflammatory process rather than an acute inflammatory injury. The Achilles tendon arises from the gastrocnemius-soleus complex and is subject to excessive forces during activities such as dance (6). Previous studies have demonstrated forces of up to six times the body weight transmitted through the Achilles during running and dance, while a study in 2010 showed ankle contact forces of 14 times body weight during the "rock step" in Irish dancers (2,14). Another study of Irish dancers demonstrated that 75% had evidence of pathologic changes to the Achilles on MRI, with only half of those demonstrating radiologic changes actually manifesting symptoms (17). This suggests that the impact of dancing causes subclinical injury in the majority of participants even when not perceived by the dancer. As in other overuse injuries, the onset of Achilles tendinopathy is insidious, with pain most commonly experienced at the insertion of the Achilles tendon onto the calcaneus. Treatment can be difficult but should focus on progressive eccentric loading exercises to improve tendon vascularity and collagen synthesis thereby promoting healing (17).
- Snapping hip syndrome, or dancer's hip, is characterized by a snapping sensation and frequently an audible pop as the hip is flexed and extended. The cause in dancers is usually friction of the iliopsoas tendon as it passes over the anterior inferior iliac spine, lesser trochanter of the femur, or iliopectineal ridge. This should be differentiated from the more common form of snapping hip syndrome, most frequently encountered by runners, which results from the iliotibial band or tensor fascia lata snapping over the greater trochanter of the femur. Rest, stretching of the hip flexors and rotators, and strengthening exercises are the mainstays of conservative treatment. Corticosteroid injections can also be employed if there is an associated bursitis.
- Spondylolysis is a common and potentially disabling injury in dancers, causing low back pain with strenuous exercise, rotation, and hyperextension. It is thought to be caused by the cumulative stress of repetitive hyperextension, which results in a stress fracture of the pars interarticularis.

Spondylolysis can occur bilaterally, compromising anterior-posterior stability of the spine. If bilateral pars defects are found, spondylolisthesis or anterior slippage of the superior vertebrae can occur. Nearly 90% of spondylolistheses occur at the L5–S1 level, whereas the next most common site of injury is the L4–L5 level (4). Injury is graded according to the degree of slippage. Grade 1 and 2 injuries are typically managed conservatively with rest, spine-strengthening exercises, and occasionally bracing. Meanwhile, grade 3 and 4 injuries, which represent a minimum of a 50% slippage, are usually managed surgically.

PSYCHOLOGICAL DISORDERS

- Female athletes are under extreme pressure to perform athletically while also maintaining an aesthetically pleasing appearance. Women falling prey to these societal pressures frequently maintain a distorted body image and can suffer long-term consequences to health. The prevalence of the female athlete triad in competitive athletes is difficult to determine due to the fact that underreporting is common. Estimates of prevalence have reached 65% in some studies, and rates in dancers are among the highest of any athletes (15). The triad is a spectrum of disorders that affect a woman's physical and psychological well-being. The underlying cause is thought to be an energy imbalance resulting from disordered eating and resulting in menstrual dysfunction and potentially osteopenia or osteoporosis. Disordered eating can manifest in the forms of anorexia or bulimia; however, less severe forms of caloric restriction and excessive exercise can be equally detrimental. Similarly, menstrual dysfunction can manifest as amenorrhea, delayed menarche, oligomenorrhea, anovulation, or luteal phase deficiency. Treatment optimally involves a multidisciplinary team to focus on the medical, nutritional, and psychological aspects of the disease (5).

- The lifestyle of a performing artist can lend itself to other psychological disorders as well. High-level performing artists are typically identified for training very early in life and grow up in a world with a narrow focus and constant pressure to perform. Although the prevalence of these disorders has yet to be determined, performance anxiety, depression, panic disorder, and personality disorders have all been reported in performing artists. Identifying these issues early and addressing them proactively with the help of a sports psychologist, if available, can lead to improved performance and quality of life.

SUMMARY

- Performing artists are complex and often difficult to treat.
- They tend to present for care late in the course of disease and are frequently mistrusting of medical professionals (13).

Injuries are usually overuse rather than traumatic in nature and tend to have a good prognosis if managed conservatively with alterations in workload and a graduated return to activity.

- Working to understand the vocabulary and art form of each individual artist and coordinating with a multidisciplinary team including the patient's teachers, coaches, therapists, dieticians, and agents is often the best way to achieve success in caring for these unique and talented individuals.

REFERENCES

1. Fishbein M, Middlestadt SE, Ottati V, Ellis A. Medical problems among ICSOM musicians: overview of a national survey. *Med Probl Performing Art.* 1988;3(1):1–8.
2. Fry HJH. Incidence of overuse syndrome in the symphony orchestra. *Med Probl Perform Art.* 1986;1(2):51–5.
3. Hamilton WG. Posterior ankle pain in dancers. *Clin Sports Med.* 2008; 27(2):263–77.
4. Hansen PA, Reed K. Common musculoskeletal problems in the performing artist. *Phys Med Rehabil Clin N Am.* 2006;17(4): 789–801.
5. Herring SA, Bergfeld JA, Boyajian-O'Neill LA, et al. Female athlete issues for the team physician: a consensus statement. *Med Sci Sport Exerc.* 2003;35(10):1785–93.
6. Hodgkins CW, Kennedy JG, O'Loughlin PF. Tendon injuries in dance. *Clin Sports Med.* 2008;27(2):279–88.
7. Knishkowy B, Lederman RJ. Instrumental musicians with upper extremity disorders: a follow up study. *Med Probl Perform Art.* 1986;1:85–99.
8. Lederman RJ. Peripheral nerve disorders in instrumentalists. *Ann Neurol.* 1989;26(5):640–6.
9. Lockwood AH, Lindsay ML. Reflex sympathetic dystrophy after overuse: the possible relationship to focal dystonia. *Med Probl Perf Art.* 1989;4(3):114–7.
10. Malanga GA, Nadler SF. Physical examination of the hip. In: *Musculoskeletal Physical Examination — An Evidence-Based Approach.* Philadelphia: Elsevier Mosby; 2006.
11. Newmark J, Hochberg FH. Isolated painless manual incoordination in 57 musicians. *J Neurol Neurosurg Psychiatry.* 1987;50(3):291–5.
12. Ostwald PF, Baron BC, Byl NM, Wilson FR. Performing arts medicine. *West J Med.* 1994;160(1):48–52.
13. Shah S. Determining a young dancer's readiness for dancing on pointe. *Curr Sports Med Rep.* 2009;8(6):295–9.
14. Shippen JM, May B. Calculation of muscle loading and joint contact forces during the rock step of Irish dance. *J Dance Med Sci.* 2010;14(1):11–8.
15. Smolak L, Murnen SK, Ruble AE. Female athletes and eating problems: a meta-analysis. *Int J Eat Disord.* 2000;27(4):371–80.
16. Solomon R, Micheli LJ, Ireland ML. Physiologic assessment to determine readiness for pointe work in ballet students. *Impulse.* 1993;1(1):21–38.
17. Walls RJ, Brennan SA, Hodnett P, O'Byrne JM, Eustace SJ, Stephens MM. Overuse ankle injuries in professional Irish dancers. *Foot Ankle Surg.* 2010;16(1):45–9.

Dive Medicine

James H. Lynch

90

BACKGROUND

- Recreational scuba diving is a growing sport with some unique considerations for the sports medicine team.
  - The number of annual diving certifications has tripled in the past 20 years worldwide (38).
  - There are roughly 3 million sport divers in the United States alone (38).
  - Divers may seek medical care for a disorder acquired in a remote location with injuries or illnesses unique to diving and the underwater environment.
- Improper diagnosis and treatment of some diving injuries can result in catastrophic outcomes, particularly involving the brain and spinal cord.
- The sports medicine physician must be aware of "fitness to dive" recommendations for patients of all ages who are seeking medical clearance to dive.
- In contrast to most other sports, recreational diving places athletes at increased risk of injury or illness primarily due to environmental extremes and hazards in the underwater setting.
- The most significant environmental exposure in diving is the increased ambient pressure.
  - Pressure increases in a linear fashion with depth underwater (Table 90.1) (28).
  - Exposure to increased pressure can result in several pathophysiologic changes as described by the common gas laws outlined later (47).

DIVE PROFILE TERMINOLOGY (34)

- Descent: Diving deeper involves increases in pressure of 1 atmosphere per 33 feet of sea water. Equilibration of pressure in gas-filled spaces is critical during this phase.
- Bottom time: The amount of time spent underwater (traditionally referred to time spent at lowest depth). Bottom time influences amount of gas absorption in tissues.
- Ascent: Moving up toward the surface involves decreases in pressure and the release of absorbed gas back into local tissues and the bloodstream.

- Surface interval: Time between dives. This time allows the body to reacquire homeostasis, especially with respect to tissue gas concentration. Dive injuries may not present until the diver surfaces.
- Decompression stop: A pause in ascent following a deep dive that allows for absorbed inert gas bubbles to be safely eliminated from tissues.
- No-decompression dive: A dive profile that does not require decompression based on limited depth and bottom time. Most sport divers perform no-decompression dives to mitigate risk of decompression sickness.

EAR AND SINUS BAROTRAUMA

- Barotrauma is defined as the tissue damage that results from an inability to equalize pressure in a gas-filled space (e.g., middle ear).
- During ascent and descent, the body is exposed to changes in ambient pressure.
  - According to Boyle's law, as ambient pressure increases during descent, the volume of gas-filled spaces decreases.
  - In the ear, the tympanic membrane is deflected inward to the point of rupture unless air is allowed to enter the middle ear via the eustachian tube (24).
- Middle ear barotrauma ("middle ear squeeze") is the most common diving injury, occurring in 30% of first-time divers and 10% of experienced divers.
  - Manifests as acute onset of ear pain.
  - Is sometimes associated with vertigo and conductive hearing loss.
  - Clinical findings range from injection of the tympanic membrane to hemotympanum, with or without ruptured tympanic membrane (15).
- Sinus barotrauma ("sinus squeeze") is another common diving injury usually resulting from transient nasal pathology or chronic sinusitis.
  - A relative negative pressure in a sinus cavity is caused by blockage of the sinus ostium during descent.
  - Negative pressure is followed by engorgement and mucosal edema, which may cause bleeding into the sinuses.
  - Manifests as acute onset of facial pain with epistaxis (39).

Table 90.1	Effects of Depth on Ambient Pressure		
fsw	**ata**	**mm Hg**	**psi**
0 (sea level)	1	760	14.7
33	2	1,520	29.4
66	3	2,280	44.1
99	4	3,040	58.8
132	5	3,800	73.5

ata, absolute pressure in atmospheres; fsw, feet of sea water; mm Hg, millimeters of mercury; psi, pounds per square inch.
SOURCE: Reproduced, with permission, from Lynch JH, Bove AA. Diving medicine: a review of current evidence. *J Am Board Fam Med.* 2009;22:399–407. Available from: doi:10.3122/jabfm.2009.04.080099. Copyright © 2012 American Board of Family Medicine. All Rights Reserved.

- Treatment for middle ear and sinus barotrauma includes:
  - Decongestants and analgesics.
  - Systemic antibiotics for prophylactic treatment of otitis media may be considered in middle ear barotrauma with tympanic membrane perforation.
  - Tympanic membrane rupture must be allowed to heal completely prior to diving again.
- Prevention of middle ear and sinus barotrauma consists of:
  - Careful attention to pressure equilibration using the Valsalva maneuver during descent.
  - Slow, feet-first descent.
  - Nasal and/or systemic decongestants such as oxymetazoline and pseudoephedrine prior to diving may be helpful. They must be used with caution to avoid the rebound effect sometimes associated with a reverse block during ascent at the end of the dive. As the medication effect diminishes, nasal passages may become congested and allow for sinus ostial blockage and pain with ascent (25).
  - Avoid diving with an upper respiratory infection or rhinosinusitis, which contribute to ostial insufficiency and may increase risk for barotraumas (14).
- Inner ear barotrauma is a condition related to middle ear barotrauma.
  - Forceful attempts to equalize the middle ear with the Valsalva maneuver may rupture the round or oval window causing perilymph leakage.
  - Manifests as acute sensorineural hearing loss, tinnitus, and vertigo.
  - Treatment is not recompression therapy, but rather bed rest, head elevation, avoidance of straining, and referral to an otolaryngologist.
  - A detailed dive history is helpful in distinguishing inner ear barotrauma from inner ear decompression sickness (24).

PULMONARY BAROTRAUMA

- According to Boyle's law, during ascent, as ambient pressure is reduced, gas inside the lungs will expand.
- If a diver breathing compressed air at depth does not allow the compressed air in the lungs to escape by exhaling, or if air empties slowly from a lung segment due to obstructive pulmonary conditions, then the gas will expand on ascent (as ambient pressure falls). This causes alveoli to rupture.
- After alveolar rupture, the air under pressure will then escape the alveoli and rush into surrounding tissues resulting in mediastinal or subcutaneous emphysema or pneumothorax.
- In the most severe cases, air will enter the bloodstream via pulmonary veins, traveling through the left heart as an arterial gas embolism (AGE).
  - Air bubbles distribute throughout the arterial circulation and reach the brain where they occlude blood flow, compromise the blood–brain barrier, and result in stroke-like events (36).
  - Almost all cases of AGE present within 5 minutes of ascent.
  - AGE manifests as gross neurologic deficits including stupor, bilateral or unilateral motor and sensory changes, unconsciousness, visual disturbances, vertigo, convulsions, and (in about 5%) complete cardiovascular collapse (Table 90.2) (37).
  - Treatment of AGE consists of advanced cardiac life support, 100% oxygen, hydration, and immediate recompression using the U.S. Navy Diving Manual Table 6 algorithm — a standard protocol that involves recompression to 60 feet in a hyperbaric chamber while breathing oxygen (Fig. 90.1) (16,37).
- The greatest change in lung volume per change in depth occurs nearest the surface.
- It is possible for divers breathing compressed air in a pool as shallow as 4 feet to develop pulmonary barotrauma if they ascend to the surface while breath-holding at maximum lung volume (7).
- The majority of individuals with AGE fully recover with prompt recompression therapy (36).

DECOMPRESSION SICKNESS

- Decompression sickness (DCS) is caused by bubble formation in blood and tissues.
- As ambient pressure increases at depth, the partial pressures of inspired gases increase proportionately.
- Inert gas, primarily nitrogen, is dissolved in tissues, creating a supersaturated state in the body.
- If ascent is too rapid, the dissolved nitrogen in blood and tissues will become supersaturated and form bubbles.

Table 90.2 | Summary of Diving-Related Conditions

Condition	Presentation	Dive History	Prevention/Treatment
Barotrauma			
Middle ear	Acute ear pain, vertigo, tympanic membrane rupture	Usually during descent	Slow equalization on descent; decongestants, consider antibiotics for tympanic membrane perforation
Inner ear	Acute vertigo, nausea, vomiting, hearing loss	Usually during descent	Bed rest, elevated head, avoidance of Valsalva, otolaryngology consult
Sinus	Acute facial pain, epistaxis	Usually during descent	Slow equalization on descent; decongestants
Arterial gas embolism	Stupor, coma, focal weakness, visual disturbances	Immediately upon surfacing or during ascent	100% oxygen, supportive care, U.S. Navy Table 6 Algorithm
Decompression sickness			
Type I	Poorly localized joint pain, rash, itching	Significant time at depth; 50% develop symptoms within 1 h of surfacing, 90% within 6 h	100% oxygen, supportive care, U.S. Navy Table 6 Algorithm
Type II	Numbness, dizziness, weakness, gait abnormality, hypoesthesia	Significant time at depth; 50% develop symptoms within 1 h of surfacing, 90% within 6 h	100% oxygen, supportive care, U.S. Navy Table 6 Algorithm

SOURCE: Reproduced, with permission, from Lynch JH, Bove AA. Diving medicine: a review of current evidence. *J Am Board Fam Med.* 2009;22(4):399–407. Copyright © 2012 American Board of Family Medicine. All Rights Reserved.

Treament Table 6

1. Descent rate - 20 ft./min.

2. Ascent rate - Not to exceed 1 ft/min. Do not compensate for slower ascent rates. Compensate for faster rates by halting the ascent.

3. Time on oxygen begins on arrival at 60 feet.

4. If oxygen breathing must be interrupted because of CNS Oxygen Toxicity, allow 15 minutes after the reaction has entirely subsided and resume schedule at point of interruption (see paragraph 20-7.11.1.1).

5. Table 6 can be lengthened up to 2 additional 25-minute periods at 60 feet (20 minutes on oxygen and 5 minutes on air), or up to 2 additional 75-minute periods at 30 feet (15 minutes on air and 60 minutes on oxygen), or both.

6. Tender breathes 100 percent O_2 during last 30 min. at 30 fsw and during ascent to the surface for an unmodified table or where there has been only a single extension at 30 or 60 feet. If there has been more than one extension, the O_2 breathing at 30 feet is increased to 60 minutes. If the tender had a hyperbaric exposure within the past 18 hours an additional 60-minute O_2 period is taken at 30 feet.

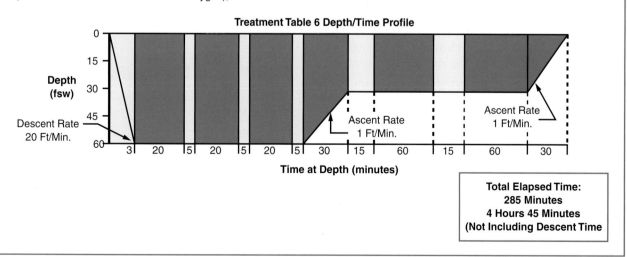

Figure 90.1: U.S. Navy diving manual.

- Bubbles cause tissue injury through mechanical effects, vascular occlusion, and activating the clotting cascade and inflammatory mediators.
- Bubbles are often detected initially in the venous system and may pose a further risk for systemic injury by entering the arterial circulation through a patent foramen ovale (PFO), which produces a right-to-left cardiac shunt.
- Bubbles entering the arterial circulation via a shunt will produce symptoms similar to AGE (48).
- The incidence of DCS among recreational scuba divers is approximately 2–3 cases per 10,000 dives (41).
- DCS manifests with a wide array of signs and symptoms and is typically classified into type I and type II DCS (see Table 90.2).
  - Type I (nonsystemic or musculoskeletal DCS) is characterized by the absence of neurologic and other systemic symptoms and usually manifests as:
    - ❏ Musculoskeletal symptoms, such as pain that is often dull or throbbing and poorly localized around a joint; the shoulder and elbow are the most common sites.
    - ❏ Cutaneous manifestations such as skin rash and pruritus. Less common is cutis marmorata or skin marbling, which may be a harbinger of more serious symptoms requiring recompression therapy.
    - ❏ In 95% of those affected, type I DCS presents within 6 hours of surfacing.
    - ❏ Treatment for type I or musculoskeletal DCS is recompression (see Fig. 90.1).
    - ❏ Joint pain is rapidly relieved with recompression therapy.
    - ❏ Cutaneous manifestations usually resolve spontaneously in 12–24 hours (31).
  - Type II (neurologic or systemic DCS) describes DCS, which affects the neurologic, vestibular, or pulmonary systems.
    - ❏ Neurologic involvement is most common among sport divers and can be due to either spinal cord or cerebral involvement.
      - Half of patients develop symptoms within 1 hour of surfacing, and 90% report symptoms within 6 hours.
      - The most common presenting neurologic symptoms include numbness, dizziness, weakness, gait abnormality, and hypoesthesia (37).
    - ❏ Inner ear DCS (the "staggers") may be due to bubble formation in the semicircular canals and presents as acute vertigo, nystagmus, tinnitus, and nausea with vomiting.
    - ❏ Pulmonary DCS (the "chokes") is a rare condition likely caused by a massive pulmonary gas embolism.
      - This usually follows a rapid or uncontrolled ascent.
      - Manifests as immediate substernal pain, cough, and cardiovascular shock resembling adult respiratory distress syndrome (ARDS) (20).

- ❏ Treatment for type II DCS is hydration, 100% oxygen, and immediate transport to a recompression facility for treatment (see Fig. 90.1). If the patient must be flown to a chamber, altitude must be limited to less than 1,000 feet, or employ an aircraft that can be pressurized to sea level to prevent exacerbation of symptoms.

DECOMPRESSION ILLNESS

- "Decompression illness" (DCI) is a term that encompasses DCS and AGE.
- This term was introduced because treatment of either DCS or AGE is recompression.
- Distinction between the two is important for prognosis in future diving exposures.
- For clinical management, the greatest challenge may be to distinguish between DCI and nondiving conditions due to the vague nature of symptoms.
  - There are no specific diagnostic tests for DCI.
  - Diagnostic certainty is not required.
  - Divers with suspected DCI should be recompressed if there are no medical contraindications (such as untreated pneumothorax or seizures) and a chamber is available (49).

FLYING AFTER DIVING

- The Divers Alert Network (DAN) 2002 Consensus Guidelines for Flying After Recreational Diving are summarized below. They apply to air dives followed by flights at cabin altitudes of 2,000–8,000 ft for divers without DCS symptoms.
  - For a single no-decompression dive, one should wait at least 12 hours prior to flying.
  - For multiple dives per day or multiple days of diving, 18 hours are suggested.
  - For any decompression dives, "substantially longer than 18 hours appears prudent" (46).

MARINE LIFE EXPOSURES (4)

- Coral abrasions:
  - Coral scrapes and lacerations are the most common diving injuries from marine life.
  - The sharp surface of coral is covered by soft living material that is deposited into scrapes causing inflammation, infection, and delayed wound healing.
  - Treatment:
    - ❏ Vigorous scrubbing and irrigation with soap and water.
    - ❏ Topical antibiotics and wet-to-dry dressings.
    - ❏ For any signs of infection, systemic antibiotics including coverage for *Vibrio* species should be used.

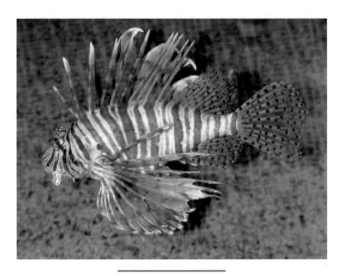

Figure 90.2: Lionfish.

- Sea urchins:
  - Sea urchin spines are venom-filled and cause painful punctures primarily on the hands and feet.
  - Spines are brittle and can break off in the skin.
  - Treatment:
    - Immerse the wound in nonscalding hot water (110–113°F).
    - Remove any visible spines without digging around in the skin. Retained spines near joints may require surgical removal.
    - For any signs of infection, systemic antibiotics including coverage for *Vibrio* species should be used.
    - One- to 2-week course of nonsteroidal anti-inflammatory drug (NSAID) for pain and inflammation.
- Poisonous fish envenomation:
  - Lionfish (Fig. 90.2), scorpion fish, and stonefish have venomous spines that cause painful puncture wounds, some of which are blistering.
  - These fish are found in coastal waters of the tropics primarily in the Indo-Pacific region but recently extending to the Bahamas and Southeastern United States.
  - Some toxins are heat labile.
  - Stonefish stings can be life-threatening.
  - Treatment:
    - If the injured diver appears intoxicated, weak, vomiting, or short of breath, provide advanced emergent care as indicated, which may include treating for DCS if definitive diagnosis is uncertain.
    - An antivenin is available for stonefish stings, which may also be helpful for scorpion fish stings, but unlikely to help with lionfish stings. Emergency departments in endemic areas should have access to these medications and are trained in their use.
    - Immerse the wound in nonscalding hot water (110–113°F).

- Standard wound care including topical antibiotics may be required for weeks to months for some of these wounds.
- Sea bather's eruption:
  - Caused by stings from nematocysts from certain anemones and thimble jellyfish.
  - Confluent, erythematous papular rash involving the bathing suit–covered areas of the skin (Fig. 90.3).
  - Tingling may be noticed under the suit, which is exacerbated by freshwater shower.
  - This may progress to severe and painful itching, usually lasting 3–5 days.
  - Treatment:
    - Immediate application of vinegar or rubbing alcohol for decontamination.
    - Topical low-potency steroids twice a day.
    - Systemic corticosteroids may be required for severe reactions.
    - Thorough cleaning of swimwear with alcohol or vinegar and soap and water.
- Seaweed dermatitis:
  - Caused by the blue-green algae *Microcoleus lyngbyaceus* — a hairlike plant that gets inside the bathing suit — commonly found in Hawaii and Florida waters during the summer months.
  - Widespread erythematous, pruritic (sometimes vesicular) rash involving the bathing suit–covered areas of the skin.
  - Treatment:
    - Vigorous soap and water scrub followed by rinse with rubbing alcohol.
    - Topical low-potency steroids twice a day.
    - Systemic corticosteroids may be required for severe reactions.

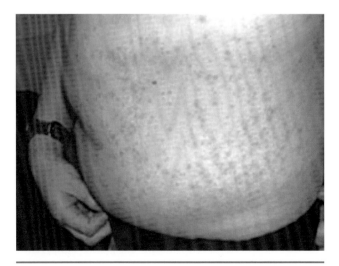

Figure 90.3: Seabather's eruption. From Studdiford JS, Bonat J. Pruritic rash after an ocean swim. *Am Fam Physician*. 2007;76(3):425–6, with permission.

- Jellyfish stings:
  - Depending on the species, jellyfish stings can range in severity from mild burning and skin redness to excruciating pain and severe blistering with generalized illness.
  - A sting from the tiny box jellyfish (*Chironex fleckeri*) of Australia, which contains one of the most potent animal venoms known to man, can induce death in minutes.
  - Most jellyfish are not fatal but can inflict a painful sting when a diver comes in contact with their tentacles.
  - Treatment:
    - If the sting is from a box jellyfish, immediately flood the wound with vinegar and soak it at least 10 minutes. Seek advanced supportive care as soon as possible. Antivenin is available as an intramuscular injection.
    - For all other stings, briskly rinse the skin with sea water.
    - Liberally apply to the skin any of the following decontaminants: vinegar, rubbing alcohol, one-quarter–strength household ammonia, or baking soda.
    - Scrape or shave the skin carefully to remove the nematocysts (stinging cells), and then reapply the decontaminant for 15 minutes.
    - Be prepared to treat an allergic reaction following any jellyfish sting. Immediately administer injectable epinephrine and an oral antihistamine for any signs of anaphylaxis.
- Ciguatera poisoning (3,4):
  - Caused by ingesting warm-water reef fish that have accumulated toxins from microscopic dinoflagellates that produce ciguatoxin.
  - Ciguatoxin-carrying fish most commonly ingested include the jack, barracuda, grouper, and snapper. In the United States, these are found in Hawaii and Florida.
  - Ciguatoxin is heat stable and unaffected by cooking method.
  - Symptoms, which begin roughly 6–12 hours after eating the contaminated fish, include:
    - Abdominal pain, nausea, vomiting, diarrhea
    - Tongue and throat numbness, tooth pain
    - Ataxia, weakness, fasciculation, incoordination
    - Blurred vision, rash, pruritus, lacrimation
    - Reversal of hot and cold sensation (hot liquids seem cold, and vice versa)
  - Signs include hypotension, bradycardia, neurologic deficits, and altered mental status.
  - Ciguatera poisoning is seldom lethal; mortality rate is 0.1%.
  - Treatment is mostly symptom-driven supportive care.
    - Gastrointestinal decontamination with activated charcoal if performed within 4 hours of ingestion.
    - Medications used to treat ciguatera poisoning include osmotic diuretics, serotonin-norepinephrine reuptake inhibitors, antihistamines, analgesics, antipyretics, and anti-inflammatories.
  - Recovery may be protracted, but prognosis is excellent for full recovery.

COMMON MEDICAL DISORDERS AND DIVING

- Some of the more controversial topics in diving medicine are covered below, including coronary artery disease, PFO, asthma, diabetes, spontaneous pneumothorax, and the elderly.
- Detailed fitness to dive considerations for a more comprehensive list of conditions can be found in:
  - Guidelines for Recreational Scuba Diver's Physical Examination (45)
  - DAN Web site at https://www.diversalertnetwork.org/default.aspx (17)
  - Standard texts such as *Diving Medicine* or *Bennett and Elliott's Physiology and Medicine of Diving* (8,11)
- DAN is available for phone consultation during business hours at (800) 446-2671 or for emergency calls 24 hours a day, 7 days a week at (919) 684-9111 (17).

CORONARY DISEASE

- According to 2006 American Heart Association statistics (2):
  - Seventeen million Americans have coronary heart disease — the single leading cause of death in the United States.
  - An estimated 1.3 million Americans will suffer an acute coronary syndrome this year.
  - Over 150,000 Americans killed by cardiovascular disease in 2006 were under age 65.
- DAN fatality surveillance data reveal cardiac conditions as the number 2 cause of death (second only to drowning) for the 75 U.S. and Canadian recreational diving-related deaths in 2006 (41).
  - Approximately 80% of fatalities were 40 years or older.
  - Hypertension and heart disease were the most common conditions reported.
- Diving places the following unique stresses on the heart:
  - Increased myocardial oxygen demands from swimming.
  - Preload is increased due to immersion-induced increased central venous return.
  - Afterload is increased from cold-induced peripheral vasoconstriction.
- The Recreational Scuba Training Council (RSTC), Undersea and Hyperbaric Medical Society (UHMS), and DAN recommend that divers over 40 undergo risk assessment for coronary artery disease.
  - Exercise stress testing may be recommended for asymptomatic divers with multiple cardiac risk factors (23).
  - Routine screening would not be advised for young, low-risk divers due to the low positive predictive value of exercise stress testing in these individuals (27).

- Fitness to dive is optimal when a diver can reach a maximum capacity of 13 METS (metabolic equivalents) or stage 4 of the Bruce protocol. This peak capacity allows a diver to exercise comfortably at 8–9 METS (40).
- Individuals with known coronary artery disease (including those with previous heart attacks and those with revascularization procedures) may dive with proper evaluation. After 6–12 months of healing and stabilization, if a thorough cardiovascular evaluation, including stress testing, determines that age-adjusted cardiopulmonary fitness is not impaired, then clearance for low-stress sport diving may be granted (13).

PATENT FORAMEN OVALE

- The foramen ovale is open during fetal life to allow for right to left shunting. For most people, this opening is closed at birth by a flap that seals against the atrial septum.
    - The flap is not sealed in about one-third of the population and can open with changes in intrathoracic pressure (29).
    - Ultrasound examination of divers has demonstrated that venous gas bubbles, which are common after diving and usually filtered by the pulmonary vasculature, can pass through a PFO and embolize the arterial circulation (33).
    - Shunting through a PFO may occur during times of certain respiratory movements, such as the period following a Valsalva maneuver, which may take place with straining to lift heavy objects (*i.e.*, scuba tanks after a dive).
- The relationship between PFO and DCS is controversial.
    - Although causality is still unproven, there appears to be an increased relative risk of developing DCS with a PFO versus without.
    - The most widely quoted odds radio for serious DCS with PFO versus without PFO is 2.52 (95% confidence interval, 1.5–4.25) as determined by a meta-analysis published in 1998 (9).
        - In 2003, a review of 145 peer-reviewed journal articles related to PFO found no clear agreement regarding the role of PFO in DCS (19).
        - Other authors have concluded that PFO increases the risk for DCS between 2.6 and 5.5 times (12,21,43).
    - In terms of the absolute increased risk, DCS in recreational divers is extremely rare, occurring after only 0.005%–0.08% of dives.
    - DAN Project Dive Exploration recorded three cases of DCS in approximately 15,000 dives (41).
- Evidence supports that the average recreational sport diver need not be screened for PFO.
    - For those already diagnosed as having a PFO, this is not an absolute contraindication for diving.
    - A safe strategy would be to reduce the venous bubble load when diving by avoiding dives that require

decompression stops, by limiting bottom time, or by the appropriate use of oxygen-enriched breathing mixes (32).

ASTHMA

- More than 22 million Americans have asthma, which is roughly 7% of the total population (35).
    - Several surveys have revealed the prevalence of active asthmatic disease among divers from 4% to 7% (26).
- Historically, asthma was considered an absolute contraindication to diving.
    - Pulmonary obstruction, air trapping, and hyperinflation that accompany an acute asthma attack would seemingly place the asthmatic diver at increased risk for pulmonary barotrauma.
    - Conditions such as cold and exercise serve as triggers for many asthmatics (36).
- Despite the theoretical risk, the evidence for actual risk of pulmonary barotrauma or DCS among divers with asthma is equivocal.
    - A comprehensive review of the literature in 2003 found no epidemiologic evidence for an increased relative risk of pulmonary barotrauma, DCS, or death among divers with asthma (26).
- When considering fitness to dive, asthma should not be viewed as a single disease.
    - With such variation among patients of precipitating factors, pulmonary function, degree of airway obstruction, and reversibility, this condition demands individualized consideration based on each specific diver's history and disease syndrome (36).
    - Several published guidelines for diving with asthma are summarized below:
        - In Australia, all divers with asthma should be considered for provocative lung function testing prior to certification (22).
        - In the United Kingdom, well-controlled asthmatics (excluding cold-, exercise-, or emotion-induced asthmatics) may dive as long as they do not require a bronchodilator within 48 hours (10).
        - Among experts and other major diving organizations, the consensus is that lung function must be normal before an asthmatic can dive.
        - The RSTC and UHMS recommend that carefully selected mild to moderate well-controlled asthmatics with normal screening spirometry (preexercise and postexercise) may be considered candidates for diving (18).
            - Medication used to maintain normal spirometry is not a contraindication to diving.
            - Inhalation challenge tests using methacholine are not recommended.

- Provocation testing with exercise or hypertonic saline inhalation may be more specific for evaluating the effects of asthma on diving (45).
  - Management is the same for chronic obstructive pulmonary disease (COPD). Because most COPD patients will have persistent abnormal laboratory studies, they should be advised not to dive.

DIABETES MELLITUS

- Diabetics have historically been prohibited from diving because of the potential for underwater hypoglycemic events (44).
- The RSTC, UHMS, and DAN consider diabetes a severe risk condition in accordance with the Scuba Schools International guidelines (45).
  - This guideline warns that a rapidly changing level of consciousness associated with hypoglycemia can contribute to drowning and specifies that "diving is therefore generally contraindicated, unless associated with a specialized program that addresses these issues" (45).
- Multiple studies have demonstrated that select diabetics can safely participate in recreational diving and that evidence is lacking for a widespread ban on diving for all diabetics (44).
- Diabetic divers must be held to a very high standard of physical fitness and experience in diabetes management, to include monitoring daily glucose patterns and the effects of strenuous exercise and exclude divers with any significant systemic diabetic sequelae, recent history of hypoglycemia, or poorly controlled blood glucose (23,44).
- A workshop jointly sponsored by the UHMS and DAN in 2005 published guidelines for diabetes and recreational diving.
  - These guidelines stipulate that adults with diabetes may qualify as fit to dive during their annual physician's review if they have:
    - Been on a stable dose of insulin for 1 year or oral hypoglycemic agents for 3 months
    - Hemoglobin A1c ≤ 9%
    - No significant episodes of hypoglycemia or hyperglycemia for 1 year
    - No secondary complications of diabetes
    - No hypoglycemia unawareness
  - Additionally, these guidelines provide scope of diving limitations and recommendations for glucose management on the day of diving (42).

SPONTANEOUS PNEUMOTHORAX

- Some individuals have weak areas (blebs) in the pleural lining of the lung that can rupture without provocation, resulting in pneumothorax.

- In diving, these blebs predispose a diver to pulmonary barotrauma because they are weaker than normal lung tissue, empty their air slowly during exhalation, and can build up pressure during ascent causing rupture.
- About half of those who suffer a spontaneous pneumothorax are likely to have another (5).
- Individuals who have experienced spontaneous pneumothorax should not dive under any circumstances (37).
  - Even if computed tomography (CT) scanning shows no evidence of underlying lung disease, patients with a history of spontaneous pneumothorax are recommended not to dive (30).
  - Even after pleurodesis, designed to prevent recurrent spontaneous pneumothorax, recommendations remain to avoid diving (45).

ELDERLY AND DIVING

- The diving population is aging, along with the U.S. population at large.
- There is no upper age limit for recreational scuba diving.
- Recommendations for diving in the elderly are based on the presence of acute or chronic illness and especially on the physical conditioning of the individual.
- Physical capacity is known to decline with age, yet there are many older athletes who have attained a higher level of fitness than many of their younger counterparts.
- Some physiologic responses to aging should be considered when reviewing fitness to dive for older individuals (6).
  - Known cardiovascular changes with age include:
    - Increases in blood pressure and peripheral vascular resistance
    - Decreases in oxygen uptake, work capacity, and maximal heart rate
  - Coronary artery disease, frequently found in the elderly, is a major contributor to diving-related deaths in North America.
  - Emphasis is placed on assessing physical capacity and screening for coronary disease during evaluation for fitness to dive.
    - Individuals 40 years of age or older should undergo risk assessment for coronary artery disease, which may require formal exercise testing.
    - A maximum capacity of 13 METS is the suggested criteria for stress testing to allow a diver to swim comfortably with diving gear in a 1-knot current expending 8–9 METS (45).
  - Other physiologic changes with age include breathing difficulties from increased dead space, glucose intolerance, heat and cold intolerance, decreased range of motion from changes in collagen structure, and alterations of neurologic function.

■ With careful evaluation, some elderly athletes in good health can undertake a safe recreational diving program that should not be as rigorous as programs recommended for their younger counterparts (1,6).

REFERENCES

1. American College of Sports Medicine Position Stand. Exercise and physical activity for older adults. *Med Sci Sports Exerc*. 1998;30(6): 992–1008.

2. American Heart Association Web site [Internet]. Cardiovascular disease statistics. Dallas: American Heart Association; [cited 2011 Jan 9]. Available from: http://www.americanheart.org/presenter.jhtml? identifier=4478.

3. Arnold T. Ciguatera toxicity. *eMedicine* [Internet]. 2010 [cited 2011 Jan 9]. Available from: http://emedicine.medscape.com/article/813869-overview.

4. Auerbach PS. Marine life trauma. *Alert Diver* [Internet]. 1998 [cited 2011 Jan 9]. Available from: https://www.diversalertnetwork.org/medical/articles/article.asp?articleid=10.

5. Bove AA. Asthma and diving. *Scubamed* [Internet]. 2007 [cited 2011 Jan 9]. Available from: http://www.scubamed.com/divmed.htm.

6. Bove AA. Diving in the elderly and the young. In: Bove AA, Davis JC, editors. *Diving Medicine*. 4th ed. Philadelphia: Saunders; 2004. p. 411–20.

7. Bove AA. Medical aspects of sport diving. *Med Sci Sports Exerc*. 1996;28(5):591–5.

8. Bove AA. Medical evaluation for sport diving. In: Bove AA, Davis JC, editors. *Diving Medicine*. 4th ed. Philadelphia: Saunders; 2004. p. 519–32.

9. Bove AA. Risk of decompression sickness with patent foramen ovale. *Undersea Hyperb Med*. 1998;25(3):175–8.

10. British Sub-Aqua Club Web site [Internet]. Asthma. Ellesmere Port (UK): British Sub-Aqua Club; [cited 2011 Jan 9]. Available from: http://www.bsac.com/core/core_picker/download.asp?id=10093&filetitle=Asthma.

11. Brubakk AO, Neuman TS, Bennett PB, Elliot DH. *Bennett and Elliott's Physiology and Medicine of Diving*. 5th ed. London (UK): Saunders; 2003. 800 p.

12. Cartoni D, De Castro S, Valente G, et al. Identification of professional scuba divers with patent foramen ovale at risk for decompression illness. *Am J Cardiol*. 2004;94(2):270–3.

13. Caruso J. Cardiovascular fitness and diving. *Alert Diver* [Internet]. 1999 [cited 2010 Dec 27]. Available from: https://www.diversalertnetwork.org/medical/articles/article.asp?articleid=11.

14. Cheshire WP. Headache and facial pain in scuba divers. *Curr Pain Headache Rep*. 2004;8(4):315–20.

15. Clenney TL, Lassen LF. Recreational scuba diving injuries. *Am Fam Physician*. 1996;53(5):1761–74.

16. Diagnosis and treatment of decompression sickness and arterial gas embolism. U.S. Navy Diving Manual, Rev 6 [Internet]. 2008;5:20–41 [cited 2008 Apr 15]. Available from: http://www.supsalv.org/00c3_publications.asp.

17. Divers Alert Network Web site [Internet]. Durham (NC): Divers Alert Network; [cited 2011 Jan 9]. Available from: https://www.diversalertnetwork.org/default.aspx.

18. Elliott DH. *Are Asthmatics Fit to Dive?* Kensington (MD): Undersea and Hyperbaric Medical Society; 1996. 81 p.

19. Foster PP, Boriek AM, Butler BD, Gernhardt ML, Bové AA. Patent foramen ovale and paradoxical systemic embolism: a bibliographic review. *Aviat Space Environ Med*. 2003;74(6 Pt 2):B1–64.

20. Francis TJ, Mitchell SJ. Pathophysiology of decompression sickness. In: Bove AA, Davis JC, editors. *Diving Medicine*. 4th ed. Philadelphia: Saunders; 2004, p. 165–83.

21. Germonpré P. Patent foramen ovale and diving. *Cardiol Clin*. 2005; 23(1):97–104.

22. Gorman D, Veale A. SPUMS policy on asthma and fitness for diving. South Pacific Underwater Medicine Society [Internet]. 1995 [cited 2010 Dec 27]. Available from: http://www.spums.org.au/page/spums-policy-asthma-and-fitness-diving.

23. Harrison D, Lloyd-Smith R, Khazei A, Hunte G, Lepawsky M. Controversies in the medical clearance of recreational scuba divers: updates on asthma, diabetes mellitus, coronary artery disease, and patent foramen ovale. *Curr Sports Med Rep*. 2005;4(5):275–81.

24. Hunter SE, Farmer JC. Ear and sinus problems in diving. In: Bove AA, Davis JC, editors. *Diving Medicine*. 4th ed. Philadelphia: Saunders; 2004. p. 431–59.

25. Kay E. Prevention of middle ear barotrauma. *Doc's Diving Medicine* [Internet]. 2000 [cited 2010 Dec 23]. Available from: http://faculty.washington.edu/ekay/MEbaro.html.

26. Koehle M, Lloyd-Smith R, McKenzie D, Taunton J. Asthma and recreational SCUBA diving: a systematic review. *Sports Med*. 2003;33(2):109–16.

27. Lauer M, Froelicher ES, Williams M, Kligfield P; American Heart Association Council on Clinical Cardiology, Subcommittee on Exercise, Cardiac Rehabilitation, and Prevention. Exercise testing in asymptomatic adults: a statement for professionals from the American Heart Association Council on Clinical Cardiology, Subcommittee on Exercise, Cardiac Rehabilitation, and Prevention. *Circulation*. 2005;112(5):771–6.

28. Lynch JH, Bove AA. Diving medicine: a review of current evidence. *J Am Board Fam Med*. 2009;22(4):399–407.

29. Lynch JJ, Schuchard GH, Gross CM, Wann LS. Prevalence of right-to-left atrial shunting in a healthy population: detection by Valsalva maneuver contrast echocardiography. *Am J Cardiol*. 1984;53(10): 1478–80.

30. Moon RE. Scanning for blebs. *Divers Alert Network* [Internet]. 2000 [cited 2011 Jan 9]. Available from: https://www.diversalertnetwork.org/medical/articles/article.asp?articleid=40.

31. Moon RE. Treatment of decompression illness. In: Bove AA, Davis JC, editors. *Diving Medicine*. Philadelphia: Saunders; 2004. p. 195–217.

32. Moon RE, Bove AA. Transcatheter occlusion of patent foramen ovale: a prevention for decompression illness? *Undersea Hyperb Med*. 2004;31(3):271–4.

33. Moon RE, Camporesi EM, Kisslo JA. Patent foramen ovale and decompression sickness in divers. *Lancet*. 1989;1(8637):513–4.

34. Morris G. Scuba diving. In: Madden C, Putukian M, Young C, McCarty E, editors. *Netter's Sports Medicine*. Philadelphia: Saunders; 2010. p. 538–45.

35. National Asthma Education and Prevention Program (National Heart Lung and Blood Institute). Third Expert Panel on the Management of Asthma, and National Center for Biotechnology Information (U.S.). *Expert Panel Report 3 Guidelines for the Diagnosis and Management of Asthma. NIH Publication No. 07-4051*. Bethesda (MD): U.S. Department of Health and Human Services, National Institutes of Health, National Heart, Lung, and Blood Institute; 2007.

36. Neuman TS. Pulmonary barotrauma. In: Bove AA, Davis JC, editors. *Diving Medicine*. Philadelphia: Saunders; 2004. p. 185–94.

37. Newton HB. Neurologic complications of scuba diving. *Am Fam Physician*. 2001;63(11):2211–8.

38. PADI Worldwide Certification History [Internet]. Rancho Santa Margarita (CA): Professional Association of Diving Instructors;

[cited 2010 Dec 23]. Available from: http://www.padi.com/padi/en/footerlinks/certhistorynum.aspx.

39. Parell GJ, Becker GD. Neurological consequences of scuba diving with chronic sinusitis. *Laryngoscope.* 2000;110(8):1358–60.

40. Pendergast DR, Tedesco M, Nawrocki DM, Fisher NM. Energetics of underwater swimming with SCUBA. *Med Sci Sports Exerc.* 1996;28(5):573–80.

41. Pollock N. *DAN Annual Diving Report: 2008 Edition.* Durham (NC): Divers Alert Network; 2008. 139 p.

42. Pollock NW, Uguccioni DM, Dear G. Diabetes and recreational diving: guidelines for the future. In: *Proceedings of the Undersea Hyperbaric Medical Society/Divers Alert Network Workshop: June 19, 2005.* Durham (NC); 2005.

43. Schwerzmann M, Seiler C, Lipp E, et al. Relation between directly detected patent foramen ovale and ischemic brain lesions in sport divers. *Ann Intern Med.* 2001;134(1):21–4.

44. Scott DH, Marks AD. Diabetes and diving. In: Bove AA, Davis JC, editors. *Diving Medicine.* 4th ed. Philadelphia: Saunders; 2004. p. 507–18.

45. Scuba Schools International. *Guidelines for Recreational Scuba Diver's Physical Examination.* Jacksonville (FL): Recreational Scuba Training Council; 2002. 4 p.

46. Sheffield P, Vann R. Flying after diving. In: *Proceedings of the DAN Flying after Diving Workshop.* Durham (NC); 2004.

47. Taylor L. Diving physics. In: Bove AA, Davis JC, editors. *Diving Medicine.* 4th ed. Philadelphia: Saunders; 2004. p. 11–35.

48. Vann RD. Mechanisms and risks of decompression. In: Bove AA, Davis JC, editors. *Diving Medicine.* 4th ed. Philadelphia: Saunders; 2004. p. 127–64.

49. Vann RD, Moon RE, Freiberger JJ, et al. Decompression illness diagnosis and decompression study design. *Aviat Space Environ Med.* 2008;79(8):797–8.

Figure Skating

Roger J. Kruse and Jennifer Burke

91

SCOPE OF PARTICIPATION

- The U.S. Figure Skating Association (USFSA), a member of the International Skating Union (ISU) and U.S. Olympic Committee (USOC), is the national governing body for figure skating and includes more than 740 member clubs and over 176,000 members (21).

DISCIPLINES

- *Singles skaters* combine the highest level of athleticism and artistry. These skaters complete multirevolution jumps and spins with rapid footwork sequences, spiral sequences, and connecting moves.
- *Pairs skaters* skate as a traditional couple, performing not only multirevolution jumps and spins, but also numerous high-risk maneuvers such as throw jumps and overhead lifts.
- *Ice dancers* skate as a traditional couple, concentrating on speed, body lean, edges, and precise technique. The rules of the sport limit jumps, spins, and lifts, and partner separations.
- *Synchronized skating* is a technical form of team skating characterized by speed, intricate formations, and transitions. It is currently the fastest-growing discipline in figure skating with approximately 570 registered teams nationally. Teams are typically composed of 16 skaters, most often female skaters.

COMPETITION

- In the United States, the competition levels for men and women are preliminary, prejuvenile, juvenile, intermediate, novice, junior, senior, and adult. Participation in each level is generally determined not by age, but by accomplishment of the specific skill tests.
- In competition, singles, pairs, dance, and synchronized skaters perform two programs, the components of which are dictated by level.
- The *short program* varies in length with competition level, but not as a function of gender. Senior competitors perform required elements to music that cannot exceed 2 minutes and 40 seconds in length.
- The *long program* is performed to music that for senior skaters cannot exceed 4 minutes and 30 seconds and is more difficult.

SPORT SCIENCE

Athlete Attributes

Physical

- Figure skaters are generally shorter, lighter, and leaner than average (11,12). At the most elite levels, shortness, leanness, and linearity of physique are particularly noted in the female ice dancers and pair skaters. Most figure skaters are right-leg dominant, rotate counter-clockwise, and land on their right leg.

Physiology

- Physiologic testing, including $\dot{V}O_{2max}$, flexibility, vertical jump, body composition, strength, and power evaluations, are useful in planning and monitoring training programs. Off-ice training and periodization of training are necessary in order to optimize these elements. While performing a program, a figure skater will reach 90%–100% of their maximal heart rate within 30–60 seconds and then sustain that level of intensity for the duration of the program. Figure skating can be compared to tennis with regard to the necessity of a well-developed anaerobic and aerobic energy system. The effort required for a long program in figure skating can be compared to running a 4-minute mile. The increasing complexity of the technical elements being performed in all disciplines of skating is approaching the acrobatics of gymnastics.

Nutrition

- Skaters, particularly female figure skaters, eat with the goal of achieving or maintaining the lean athletic body type demanded by the sport. Female pair skaters must be lightweight for successful completion of increasingly complex lifts and throw jumps. Female ice dancers are judged on an aesthetically pleasing body line, particularly at higher levels of competition.
- The most common dietary issues encountered are inadequate caloric intake and hydration, as well as suboptimal food choices and poor timing of nutrition (25,26).

- Total energy intake and intake of dietary fiber and fat (females) are often below dietary recommendations.

- Intake of some micronutrients, including vitamin D, vitamin E, magnesium, potassium, folate, pantothenic acid, phosphorous, and calcium, in females was shown to be less than two-thirds of the recommended daily allowance (6).

- Approximately 50% of elite figure skaters use dietary supplements, with multivitamins being the most commonly consumed supplement (27).

Bone Mass

- Prepubertal figure skaters' bone mineral density of the spine and lower extremities has been shown to be significantly higher than in nonskaters, suggesting that intense weight-bearing exercise may protect bone mass in younger athletes, despite inadequate nutritional intake (19).

- Postmenarchal skaters with a history of stress fracture do not typically have lower bone mineral density as compared to nonathletic controls but do have significantly lower bone mineral density compared to skaters without fractures (14).

Psychology

- More than 85% of the most successful elite skaters are using sports psychology techniques year-round; almost every elite athlete in the United States uses visualization and imagery.

- The abilities to concentrate and refocus are positive predictors of how well athletes will perform. Negative thinking and lack of emotional control are significant issues.

- The relationship of the skater, parent, and coach is a very close one, and the treating physician must communicate with each to optimize treatment compliance and outcome. Addressing the psychological impact of an injury is very important to the recovery process.

- As a team sport, team dynamics and team building in synchronized skating are integral to success and must be included in training programs.

Equipment

Boots and Blades

- The skating boot is made primarily from leather. A skater's ankles are plantarflexed in the skate due to the height of the boot heel. Some manufacturers make a boot with heat-molded parts in order to customize the fit.

- The design of the skating boot has changed over the past 25 years. The boots have become increasingly stiff in response to requests from skaters and coaches to enhance support, slow break down, and accommodate skaters with suboptimal ankle strength and proprioception to improve jump landing success rates.

- Over-the-counter or stock boots and blades are less expensive and less rigid and can be variable in construction. They are sold as a single unit, with the blade screwed or riveted to the boot. Most elite athletes wear stiff custom-made boots bought separately from the blades.

- New skates and blades can cost well over $1,000 and are usually replaced every year. Skaters typically replace boots when the ankle support breaks down. Stock boots are available for half the price of custom-made boots but must be replaced more often.

- More recently, to improve the biomechanical advantage of plantarflexion in performing jumps, to facilitate increasingly complex and technical elements, and to perhaps decrease injury rates, boot designs such as the "hinged boot" or articulated band lighter-weight synthetic boots have been introduced with mixed success. Off-ice analysis of skaters jumping using the articulated boots showed evidence of decreases in peak heel forces and loading rate. Analysis of on-ice jumps did not demonstrate the same decrease in landing forces (3). Most recently, inserts and blade mounting techniques are being introduced to help decrease/improve impact forces.

- Optimal boot fit is necessary to prevent boot-related injuries. The boot should be lightweight ($< 5\%$ of skater's body weight). It should have a broad forefoot, a well-fitted heel, and a well-padded tongue. New boots should be introduced at the end of the competitive season and never be worn alternately with old boots. There is little room in boots to accommodate orthoses, although increasingly, stock and custom options are commercially available. The plantarflexed position in which the boot holds the foot must be accounted for in orthotic construction.

Biomechanics

Jumps

- Shoulder abductor strength and knee extensor strength are two main predictors of jump height (16). An athlete's upper body strength and consequent ability to pull arms against centrifugal forces, attaining a tight air position, when initiating jump rotation are correlated positively with the athlete's ability to perform the more difficult jumps.

- To perform the increasingly difficult triple and quadruple jumps, the athletes are rotating faster, not necessarily jumping higher (7). Flight times for single, double, and triple jumps are very similar due to nearly identical vertical velocity at takeoffs (7). However, athletes who have mastered higher revolution jumps, such as triple and quadruple jumps, generate greater vertical velocity at takeoff of lower revolution jumps (9).

- Impact forces are greater on landing higher revolution jumps as a result of delayed landing and the need for the athlete to forcefully extend his or her landing leg toward the ice from a shorter distance (9).

Spins

- It is important to be aware that spinning typically requires a greater energy expenditure than jumping. The athlete rotates three to six revolutions per second, creating 200–300 pounds of centrifugal force (13), and when the athlete changes position during the spin, these forces can go up. Upper body, lower body, and core strength are all required to keep the arms and legs close to the axis of rotation to counteract the centrifugal force.

Throws and Lifts

- Pair skaters and ice dancers and, to a lesser degree, synchronized skaters are continuing to push technical boundaries and are increasingly performing more complex, creative, and acrobatic elements.
- To perform the increasingly difficult throw double and triple twists, similar to triple and quadruple jumps, the pair teams use primarily increased rotational rates and, to a lesser degree, increased flight time due to delayed or lower catches (8).

Training

General

- Figure skaters often begin rigorous training as early as 5 years of age, and some are performing jumps requiring two or three revolutions by the age of 8. The more elite athletes can spend up to 45 hours a week dedicated to their sport: roughly 15–30 hours per week on the ice and 5–15 hours performing off-ice conditioning. Additional time is spent on choreography, attention to nutritional plan, sport psychology, music selection, and costume design and fitting.
- Periodized training schedules run virtually year-round with only a small break during the early spring, significantly increasing the risk of overuse injury, particularly during times of rapid growth.
- The level of training required of a developing and certainly an elite figure skater requires singular focus and high demands, so many of these athletes pursue concurrent home schooling.

On-Ice

- A typical on-ice training regimen includes two to three 45-minute on-ice sessions throughout the day. Training programs are usually most intense from late spring through summer. During the competitive seasons, less time is spent conditioning, and more time is spent perfecting choreography.

Off-Ice

- Athletes who participate in off-ice programs are stronger, have better developed aerobic and anaerobic energy systems, jump higher, have more consistent jump landings, have tighter and faster spins, and feel more confident on the ice. Additionally, these athletes may have decreased injury rates for level of participation.
- Off-ice conditioning is mandatory for success at the preelite and elite levels.
- Off-ice programs should include core strengthening, plyometrics, and attention to symmetry of limb flexibility and strength, especially hip, ankle, and foot, as well as cardiovascular fitness, including both aerobic and anaerobic fitness. As the athlete spends more time taking part in off-ice conditioning programs, it is important to adjust the time spent on the ice. It is also important to consider and account for both off-ice and on-ice training when determining injury mechanisms and returning the athlete to sport.

MEDICAL ISSUES

Musculoskeletal Issues

General

- The musculoskeletal problems of skaters primarily affect the lower extremity: the knee, foot, and ankles. However, the rates of lower extremity stress injuries, particularly in female athletes (5), as well as back injuries and perhaps, most notably, pelvic injuries have progressively increased over the past 15–20 years. Since the elimination of figures in 1990 and the introduction of a new scoring system in 2004, the focus of the sport has shifted to achieving points based on technical feats. A large majority of the athlete's training is spent practicing jumps, throws, lifts, complex spins, and footwork sequences.
- The incidence of injury in figure skating has been calculated to range from 1.37 to 3 per 1,000 hours of training (2,10). The nature of injuries often varies with the skater's discipline (20). At least half of all injuries in singles skaters are attributed to overuse mechanisms (2,5,10) and may be preventable with attention to optimizing flexibility, symmetry of strength and power, attentiveness to periodization of training, and being mindful of the number of times an athlete is landing a jump or a throw, particularly during times of rapid growth and new skill development. These data, however, precede the change in the scoring system and do not reflect the increasing rate of injuries observed.
- Pairs skaters and ice dancers have a higher risk of acute injuries than singles skaters due to falls from lifts and throw jumps (5).
- Synchronized skaters have an increasing number of acute injuries affecting: lower extremities > upper extremities > head injuries (4).

Boot- and Blade-Related Issues

- The boot and blade are the most important pieces of equipment of the figure skater and are likely contributors to most injuries.
- Boot stiffness, fit, alignment, weight, and blade mount and alignment are issues that can contribute to injury.

Lower Extremity

Foot

- *Bursitis* is the most common skating problem related to the foot and is caused by boot pressure points causing excessive compression and shear forces. Both malleoli can be affected, although medial malleolar bursitis is more common.

The fibula at the boot top and the area over the anterior tibialis tendon are also commonly affected. Bursitis is generally well tolerated but can easily become inflamed with minor irritation or boot changes. These types of injuries are treated by operating on the boot, not the skater. Focal stretching/punching out of boot in rub areas and/or padding placed to distribute compressive forces around the malleoli will typically alleviate the problem. Aspiration and subsequent injection with cortisone and a compressive wrap are tempting, although *infrequently* indicated or beneficial. *Rarely* is surgery required (1).

- A *pump bump or Haglund deformity of the calcaneal tuberosity* is caused by a boot heel that is too wide for the skater's heel. This allows the skater's heel to slide up and down within the boot, resulting in callus and bursa inflammation. For nearly all cases, the skate fit should be addressed. It is important that the heel of the boot be sufficiently narrow to prevent up and down motion of the heel. This can be done with padding medial and lateral to the Achilles tendon region, paying special attention not to compress that structure. Small heel lifts may also be helpful to hold the calcaneal tuberosity firmly against the upper part of the skate heel as it curves forward.

- *Tibialis anterior and extensor hallux tendinosis or tenosynovitis* are caused by repetitive dorsiflexion and plantarflexion of the ankle, excessive compression of crossing laces, and abnormal creasing of the boot tongue across the anterior foot. Crepitus over the tendon structure and nodules are not uncommon clinical findings. To prevent anterior compression injuries, the boot tongue should be in a neutral position or slightly medial, especially when the boots are being broken in. If the tongue is properly centralized, tibialis anterior tendinosis can still occur, but it can be prevented by padding the boot tongue with closed cell foam or thermoplastic material. A more flexible boot may be preventative.

- *Sinus tarsi pain* is less common and is typically caused by the break-in crease.

- *Achilles tendinosis, partial tears and nodules of the Achilles tendon,* can occur from compression of the tendon with plantarflexion of the foot against the boot and can also occur during off-ice training with running and jumping. The Achilles tendon is generally protected by the height of the boot heel, although in some cases, the posterior portion of the boot can be inappropriately angled forward. Boot modifications may be helpful. Ice dancers often have boots with low cutout areas for the Achilles tendon to improve their line and ability to bend their knees. This modification may be helpful for any skater.

- *Plantar fasciitis* is very common in figure skaters because of the repetitive pounding. It is treated in the usual manner with ice, relative rest, stretching, night splinting, and physical therapy.

- *Stress fractures* commonly occur in the tarsal navicular and the metatarsals and are caused primarily by the cumulative effect of jumping, repetitively training a new element, and the position of the foot in the boot.

- Other areas that can be irritated include the base of the fifth metatarsal and the tarsal navicular. Corns and calluses on the toes are seen frequently. Typically, these are all issues that occur as a result of improper boot fit and can be treated with donut pads, punching out the boot, and other modifications to the boot.

Ankle

- Poor ankle proprioception, inversion, and eversion strengths are significant issues among skaters due to the stiffness of the boot and the many hours skaters spend on the ice. Over the past 10–15 years, however, attention has been placed on optimizing foot and ankle strength in off-ice programs.

Lower Leg

- Posterior medial tibial syndrome, peroneal tendinitis, and/or fibular stress syndrome may develop at the level of the top of the boot, extending above and below the level of the boot. These syndromes are typically attributed to weakness of the tibialis posterior and peroneal muscles. They can also be due to relative inflexibility of the gastrocnemius–soleus complex. Continued training with such symptoms can culminate in tibial and/or fibular stress fractures. Treatment and prevention include optimizing flexibility in the gastrocnemius–soleus complex, strengthening of the ankle inverters and everters, evaluation of the boot and the skater's position within the boot, and attention to repetitions of jump and throw landings, particularly suboptimal landings. Orthoses, blade mounting, and padding of the top of the boot may be beneficial.

Knee

- Anterior knee pain is one of the most frequent problems and typically occurs in the "landing leg." The etiologies are multiple and include relative hip weakness, quadriceps weakness, inadequate flexibility of the hip and thigh musculature, patella shape, and tracking issues. Skaters may also experience patellar compression injuries from falling but rarely experience patellar fracture.

- Infrapatellar tendinosis and patellar tendinosis are seen in elite skaters and are often very difficult to treat because of the lengthy competitive season. In addition to activity modification, strapping, and physical therapy, platelet-enriched plasma injections with ultrasound guidance have been used with encouraging results.

- Meniscus and ligament injuries are relatively rare in figure skaters, likely due to the lack of fixation of the blade in the ice. Jumps are typically landed as the athlete is skating backward, and co-contraction of the quadriceps and hamstring muscles is necessary for control of the landing. However, with increasing technical demands and complexity of pair and ice dance elements, in particular, the rate of these injuries is increasing.

Core, Hip, and Pelvis

- Athletes continue to present with an increasing rate of groin, hip flexor, adductor complex, and external and internal oblique injuries. These types of injuries are some of the most common and debilitating injuries sustained by the most elite athletes. More than 25% of the elite athletes from the United States and Canada have been affected by these injuries during their careers. These injuries occur more often during times of rapid growth as a result of fatigue or suboptimal conditioning as new technical elements are introduced and due to the lack of attention to complexities of periodized training.

- The increase in these types of injuries is attributed to the focus on triple and quadruple revolution jumps, the increasingly complex choreography, and the dynamic foot work sequences. The mechanisms are multifaceted. Skaters perform upwards of 45–60 practice jumps daily. They often have tight hip flexors and asymmetrically strong hip flexors. Additionally, skaters can have relatively weak or asymmetrically strong core musculature and hip stabilizers. Combined, these issues increase the potential for overuse injury.

- Avulsion fractures of the ischium, lesser tuberosity, and crest of the ilium have increasingly been reported in singles and pair skaters, as well as synchronized skaters. These occur during early phases of growth spurts and have markedly increased in athletes who perform the more difficult double, triple, and quadruple axel jumps. These injuries are slow to heal and often recur. Proactive evaluation of the athlete for hip strength asymmetry, flexibility, and endurance can be preventive. Additionally, it is important to ensure that an athlete has adequate strength to initiating training for such jumps.

Spine

- Many skating elements and jump landings require an arched or hyperextended back, placing the posterior elements of the lumbar spine at increased stress and causing potential for lumbar strain, facet pain, posterior iliac crest injury, spondylolysis, and spondylolisthesis. This is compounded by the increasing technical complexities rewarded by the point-based scoring system requiring the athlete to jump more, land more throws, spin in compromised positions, and perform more dynamic footwork sequences that place a cumulative load on the posterior elements of the spine. The rigidity of the boot and restricted plantarflexion of the ankle limit adequate knee flexion; therefore, the athlete is unable to maintain normal alignment of the spine with jump and throw landings, during some spin positions, and during some complex choreography.

- Spondylolysis is often missed by clinicians, and a high level of suspicion is important to diagnose this injury in skaters. A young skater with persistent back pain should be evaluated with x-rays, followed by a single photon emission computed tomography bone scan or magnetic resonance imaging with attention to the pars articularis.

- Appropriate therapy includes strengthening of the core musculature to provide control of the trunk and pelvis and to assist in maintaining the alignment of the body during jumps, spins, and lifts, as well as strengthening of the ankle-supporting musculature, which may give the skater an option to consider the use of a more flexible boot that accommodates greater dorsiflexion during landing.

Upper Extremities

- Upper body strength is essential to both jumping and spinning and pair elements. Many elite skaters have inadequate shoulder stabilizers.

- Male pair skaters are at the highest risk of chronic rotator cuff dysfunction and scapular stabilizer insufficiency.

- Synchronized skaters are at increased risk of shoulder and wrist injuries because they often hold onto each other throughout their programs.

MEDICAL CONCERNS

Exercise-Induced Bronchospasm

- The incidence of exercise-induced bronchospasm (EIB) ranges from 33% to 50% in elite skaters in the United States, with greater prevalence among females and younger skaters (17,23).

- Relatively cold air temperatures in combination with exposure to carbon monoxide and nitrogen dioxide in enclosed ice rinks (15), questionable air quality from ice resurfacer exhaust fumes, inadequate ventilation systems, and mold in many rinks contribute to ambient pollution that produces a significant environmental trigger for EIB (13,23). Repetitive bouts of extremely vigorous exercise, where heart rate often reaches 90%–100% of predicted maximums during the first minute of a 4- to 5-minute program, also put athletes at increased risk for symptoms of EIB.

- Ideally, screening for EIB in elite athletes should be carried out using spirometry in a sport-specific environmental setting and under competition level of exertion (18).

- Because spirometry is not easily available at most ice rinks, an athlete can be educated to check their peak flows while at the rink. Peak flows should be obtained before a performance of a long program and at 1 and 5 minutes after the program is completed. A 10%–15% decrease in peak flow can be suggestive of EIB.

- Most skaters respond well to preexercise treatment with an inhaled quick-acting β-agonist. Some skaters need to use inhaled steroids prophylactically to moderate their EIB symptoms.

- Vocal cord dysfunction is an important alternative consideration in the differential diagnosis of EIB in figure skaters.

Disordered Eating

- Disordered eating patterns and eating disorders, as in any sport that emphasizes a leaner body with linearity of physique, are of a significant risk among figure skaters. It is unclear what the prevalence is and whether the risk of eating disorders increases as the skaters climb through the ranks of national and international levels.

Menstrual Dysfunction

■ Later age of menarche is not uncommon among female figure skaters, particularly in elite pair skaters (22). Later onset of menarche and irregularities of menstrual cycle can be attributed to familial resemblance (22), as well as to a high level of training, which is associated with inadequate caloric intake with relation to activity level (24).

THE FEMALE ATHLETE TRIAD

■ As in any sport in which appearance is judged, clinicians must maintain a high level of suspicion for the potential of the continuum of the female athlete triad.

CONCUSSIONS, LACERATIONS, AND CONTUSIONS

■ Skaters involved in pairs skating, ice dancing, and synchronized skating suffer a higher rate of concussions, contusions, and lacerations as compared with single skaters. Frequently, multiple skaters are injured at the same time in synchronized skating.

THE FUTURE

■ In summary, at least half of all figure skating injuries appear to be preventable and are due to overuse mechanisms and/or boot and blade issues. New boot designs have been introduced with mixed success, and future considerations in boot and blade development continue to include flexibility, comfort, support, durability, cushioning of landing impact, lighter weight, ability to plantarflex and dorsiflex foot to assist with shock absorption from jumping and to assist in power for jump takeoffs, affordability, blade alignment and mounting, weight of boot and blades, and adaptability to orthoses.

■ Figure skating is a demanding sport that requires athletes to begin training at a young age and be able to successfully perform jumps of increasing difficulty. The new scoring system, introduced in 2004, rewards increasingly difficult and complex jumps, spins, footwork sequences, and transitions. The athletes are performing more elements and more technically demanding elements in each of their programs. Unfortunately, many prepubescent athletes train using a large number of jumps daily, and these athletes, particularly while going through puberty, are at a high risk of being injured. It is likely that reported injury rates underestimate the rate of injury observed subsequent to the introduction of the new scoring system. Like gymnastics, the longevity of the most elite athletes is increasingly fleeting. It is unlikely that we will see another athlete like Michelle Kwan, who has nine national titles.

■ In order to prevent injuries, studies need to be done incorporating the age and the development of the athletes, to determine optimal training programs that can address relative jump counts (similar to Little League pitch counts) and frequency of training new and more complex choreography that places the young athlete's body in functionally comprised positions. Factors that should be considered include type of jump, level of mastery, physical issues such as strength and symmetry, hours of on-ice and off-ice training, recovery time between sessions, and time in training cycle.

■ The level of performance required of the successful elite athlete is escalating. In order to decrease the risk of injury and optimize the health and performance of the athlete, planning and continued careful attention to complexities of a detailed, periodized training plan are necessary. Communication between the skater, the skater's parents and coaches, the off-ice support group, and the medical support staff is imperative.

REFERENCES

1. Bradley MA. Prevention and treatment of foot and ankle injuries in figure skaters. *Curr Sports Med Rep.* 2006;5(5):258–61.
2. Brock RM, Striowski CC. Injuries in elite figure skaters. *Phys Sports Med.* 1986;14:111–5.
3. Bruening DA, Richards JG. The effects of articulated figure skates on jump landing forces. *J Appl Biomech.* 2006;22(4):285–95.
4. Dubravcic-Simunjak S, Kuipers H, Moran J, Simunjak B, Pecina M. Injuries in synchronized skating. *Int J Sports Med.* 2006;27(6):493–9.
5. Dubravcic-Simunjak S, Pecina M, Kuipers H, Moran J, Haspl M. The incidence of injuries in elite junior figure skaters. *Am J Sports Med.* 2003;31(4):511–7.
6. Jonnalagadda SS, Ziegler PJ, Nelson JA. Food preferences, dieting behaviors, and body image perceptions of elite figure skaters. *Int J Sport Nutr Exerc Metab.* 2004;14(5):594–606.
7. King DL, Arnold AS, Smith SL. A kinematic comparison of single, double and triple axels. *J Appl Biomech.* 1994;10:51–60.
8. King DL, Smith SL, Brown MR, McCrory JL, Munkasy BA, Scheirman GI. Comparison of split double and triple twists in pair figure skating. *Sport Biomech.* 2008;7(2):222–37.
9. King DL, Smith SL, Higginson BK, Muncasy B, Scheirman GL. Characteristics of triple and quadruple toe-loops performed during the Salt Lake City 2002 Winter Olympics. *Sports Biomech.* 2004;3(1):109–23.
10. Kjaer M, Larsson B. Physiological profile and incidence of injuries among elite figure skaters. *J Sports Sci.* 1992;10(1):29–36.
11. Leone M, Lariviere G, Comtois AS. Discriminant analysis of anthropometric and biomotor variables among elite adolescent female athletes in four sports. *J Sports Sci.* 2002;20(6):443–9.
12. Monsma DV, Malina RM. Anthropometry and somatotype of competitive female figure skaters 11–22 years. Variation by competitive level and discipline. *J Sports Med Phys Fitness.* 2005;45(4):491–500.
13. Nash HL. U.S. Olympic figure skaters: honing their performances. *Phys Sports Med.* 1988;6:181–5.
14. Oleson CV, Busconi BD, Baran DT. Bone density in competitive figure skaters. *Arch Phys Med Rehabil.* 2002;83(1):122–8.
15. Pelham TW, Holt LE, Moss MA. Exposure to carbon monoxide and nitrogen dioxide in enclosed ice arenas. *Occup Environ Med.* 2002;59(4):224–33.

16. Podolsky A, Kaufman KR, Cahalan TD, Aleshinsky SY, Chao EY. The relationship of strength and jump height in figure skaters. *Am J Sports Med.* 1990;18(4):400–5.

17. Provost-Craig MA, Arbour KS, Sestili DC, Chabalko JJ, Ekinci E. The incidence of exercise-induced bronchospasm in competitive figure skaters. *J Asthma.* 1996;33(1):67–71.

18. Rundell KW, Wilber RL, Szmedra L, Jenkinson DM, Mayers LB, Im J. Exercise-induced asthma screening of elite athletes: field versus laboratory exercise challenge. *Med Sci Sports Exerc.* 2000;32(2):309–16.

19. Slemenda CW, Johnston CC. High intensity activities in young women: site specific bone mass effects among female figure skaters. *Bone Miner.* 1993;20(2):125–32.

20. Smith AD. Skating injuries: a guide to prevention and management. *J Musculoskel Med.* 1997;14:10–29.

21. US Figure Skating Web site [Internet]. Colorado Springs (CO): US Figure Skating. Available from: http://www.usfsa.org.

22. Vadocz EA, Siegel SR, Malina RM. Age at menarche of competitive figure skaters: variations by competency and discipline. *J Sports Sci.* 2002;20(2):93–100.

23. Wilber RL, Rundell KW, Szmedra L, Jenkinson DM, Im J, Drake SD. Incidence of exercise-induced bronchospasm in Olympic winter sport athletes. *Med Sci Sports Exerc.* 2000;32(4):732–7.

24. Williams NI, Young JC, McArthur JW, Bullen B, Skrinar GS, Turnbull B. Strenuous exercise with caloric restriction: effect on luteinizing hormone secretion. *Med Sci Sports Exerc.* 1995;27(10):1390–8.

25. Ziegler PJ, Jonnalagadda SS, Lawrence C. Dietary intake of elite figure skating dancers. *Nutr Res.* 2001;21(7):983–92.

26. Ziegler PJ, Jonnalagadda SS, Nelson JA, Lawrence C, Baciak B. Contribution of meals and snacks to nutrient intake of male and female elite figure skaters during peak competitive season. *J Am Coll Nutr.* 2002;21(2):114–9.

27. Ziegler PJ, Nelson JA, Jonnalagadda SS. Use of dietary supplements by elite figure skaters. *Int J Sport Nutr Exerc Metab.* 2003;13(3):266–76.

92 Football

John M. MacKnight

INTRODUCTION

- Sports medicine coverage of American football places unique demands on the sports medicine practitioner. A wide variety of football-specific conditions demand that those responsible for the care of football teams be well versed in an array of both medical and orthopedic issues.
- Appropriate planning can minimize the likelihood of athlete injury and help to ensure that athletes are protected and returned to play safely and in a timely manner.

MUSCULOSKELETAL INJURIES

- Fifty percent of football players at all levels will be injured to some degree in any given season. The majority of these injuries involve the lower extremity, with sprains, contusions, and strains being most common. Fractures account for approximately 10% of injuries.

Lower Extremity Injuries

Medial Collateral Ligament Sprain, Knee

- The most common knee injury seen in football, resulting from a valgus load to the knee by another player during blocking or tackling.
- Grading of medial collateral ligament (MCL) sprains:
  - Grade I injuries have stretched but not disrupted the ligament, and the knee examination (valgus loading of the knee at 0 and 30 degrees of flexion) reveals no laxity compared to the uninjured side.
  - Grade II injuries have partial ligament disruption with discernible laxity and increased excursion on valgus testing but preservation of an endpoint.
  - Grade III injuries represent full ligament tears with gross laxity and no discernible endpoint.
- All three grades are generally managed conservatively with icing, nonsteroidal anti-inflammatory drugs (NSAIDs), and protective bracing. Even athletes with grade III injuries may resume sport in protective braces if symptoms allow.
- Many football programs now use protective medial stabilizing braces to decrease the incidence of MCL injury,

particularly in interior linemen. Although data have not clearly proven their efficacy, braces may enhance proprioceptive function (and thus allow the player to avoid high-risk knee positions) and are a reasonable preventative measure for at-risk players.

Meniscal Tears

- An injury to the medial or lateral meniscal cartilage typically resulting from a rotational injury applied to the flexed knee.
- Pain may be acute or chronic, and the athlete commonly complains of mechanical symptoms including a sense of locking or giving way of the knee.
- Meniscal tears are classically characterized by small effusions, focal joint line tenderness to palpation, normal ligament testing, and positive McMurray and Apley grind tests. Pain and dysfunction may also be elicited by squatting.
- Definitive diagnosis is usually via magnetic resonance imaging (MRI), which demonstrates characteristic signal changes in the affected meniscus.
- Most meniscal tears are amenable to arthroscopic debridement with resumption of football activities in as few as 2 weeks.

Anterior Cruciate Ligament Tear

- The most devastating knee injury commonly seen in football, anterior cruciate ligament (ACL) tears, generally result from valgus loading of the slightly flexed knee, creating significant shear forces on the ACL with resultant tearing. The majority are noncontact injuries, but the ACL may be torn in a similar contact mechanism to that of the MCL noted earlier. As such, simultaneous injury of both ligaments is not uncommon.
- The injury is accompanied by significant pain, often an audible "pop" or a sense of tearing inside the knee, immediate swelling, subjective instability of the knee, and laxity on the Lachman or anterior drawer test.
- For competitive athletes, ACL tears generally require surgical reconstruction. Graft options include patellar tendon, hamstring tendon, or cadaveric grafts. Patellar tendon grafts are generally preferred in athletes but may lead to earlier patellofemoral arthritis than the alternatives. Caution must also be used with patellar grafting in athletes with prior patellar tendon dysfunction. After 6–9 months of aggressive rehabilitation, functional bracing to protect the reconstructed ACL is generally desirable to aid safe return to full football activities.

Hamstring Strain

- A common injury typically of the midsubstance of the hamstring musculature characterized by partial tearing, edema, and ecchymosis.

- Clinically presents with acute onset of posterior thigh pain in association with sprinting, explosive acceleration or deceleration, or change in direction.

- Physical exam reveals focal tenderness over the injured muscle belly. There may be a discernible muscular defect present. Mild warmth and edema may be present. Ecchymosis is common and can be impressive.

- The athlete typically limps, holds the knee in mild flexion, and has obvious loss of knee extension range of motion.

- Management focuses on acute injury modalities followed by general restoration of range of motion and full strength before resuming running or football activities.

- Significant hamstring strains may take up to 6 weeks to heal.

Thigh/Quadriceps Contusion

- The most common soft tissue injury in football, resulting from blunt trauma.

- Treatment focuses on limitation of hemorrhage and inflammation while maintaining range of motion and strength. Ice and NSAIDs are appropriate initial interventions. Some practitioners advocate immobilizing the knee in 120 degrees of flexion to limit hemorrhage and hematoma formation.

- Massage and ultrasound should be avoided early in the treatment course to allow for early stabilization of the damaged muscle and to minimize the risk of developing myositis ossificans. This complication is characterized by calcific changes in areas of damaged muscle and occurs in up to 20% of cases if treated inadequately.

- Athletes may return to play when they have full range of motion and strength equivalent to that of the uninjured leg.

Turf Toe

- A sprain of the plantar–capsular ligament complex with associated articular cartilage damage to the metatarsal heads or base of the proximal phalanx.

- The first metatarsophalangeal (MTP) joint is the primary area of injury, typically resulting from forced dorsiflexion of the planted toe on the turf. Athletes experience significant pain, have local swelling, and often limp.

- Artificial turf surfaces and lighter, more flexible shoes have been implicated in a rising incidence of turf toe injuries.

- Management centers on protection of the area with a rigid insert in the shoe to protect against dorsiflexion, donut padding, taping, ice, and NSAIDs. Activity status is as dictated by pain.

Hip Pointer

- Contusion or separation of attached muscle fibers at the superior aspect of the iliac crest as a result of blunt trauma, generally resulting in a significant degree of pain and dysfunction.

- X-rays are generally unnecessary at the time of diagnosis but should be strongly considered for symptoms that are prolonged or increasing.

- Management includes aggressive icing, stretching of the low back and flank muscles, and additional protective padding at the time of return to play.

- Local modalities such as ultrasound, corticosteroid injections, or platelet-rich plasma injections may speed the healing response as well.

Upper Extremity Injuries

Glenohumeral Instability

- Glenohumeral instability is a common shoulder malady in football athletes occurring when the glenohumeral joint is partially or completely destabilized as a result of repetitive blows to the shoulder or the unique acute loading that may arise with blocking and tackling.

- Frank dislocations occur anteriorly in 95% of cases and result from excessive abduction, extension, and external rotational forces.

- Physical examination classically reveals apprehension when the humeral head is moved anteriorly or posteriorly in the glenoid.

- Instability events should prompt an early x-ray evaluation to assess for bony injury to the glenoid labrum (Bankart lesion) or impaction injury to the humeral head from sliding across the glenoid (Hills-Sachs lesion).

- Single or recurrent instability episodes may predispose to labral cartilage tears. These typically arise in the **Superior** portion of the **Labrum** and extend **Anterior** to **Posterior**. This common pattern gives rise to the term "SLAP" tear.

- Although surgery to correct shoulder instability is a frequent consideration because the recurrence rate for subluxations or dislocations is 50%, aggressive rotator cuff strengthening coupled with functional bracing may provide excellent results.

- Open stabilization surgery, rather than arthroscopy, is a more predictable means of restoring shoulder stability with excellent maintenance of range of motion and postoperative stability (14).

- SLAP tears in association with mild instability may be addressed arthroscopically without performing a stabilization procedure.

- Offensive linemen may also develop posterior instability from blocking with outstretched arms and repetitively loading the posterior capsule of the glenohumeral joint. Except in extreme cases, aggressive rehabilitation and modification of weightlifting techniques are generally adequate for management.

Acromioclavicular Sprain

- This common shoulder injury, also referred to as a "separated shoulder," is a sprain of the supporting ligaments of the acromioclavicular (AC) joint.

- The typical mechanism of injury is either striking another player with the point of the shoulder or landing directly on the point of the shoulder, often when being tackled.

- Initial presentation reveals exquisite point tenderness over the AC joint. A bony "step-off" with inferior displacement of the acromion relative to the clavicle may be appreciated.

- X-rays are indicated to evaluate for concomitant clavicle fracture and to assess the degree of AC separation. Weighting of the injured arm may help to determine if there is widening of the AC joint with downward distraction.

- Management focuses on control of inflammation and pain, protection of the AC joint via padding, early restoration of active shoulder range of motion, and preservation of shoulder strength.

- Even high-grade AC sprains generally do not require surgery, and most heal completely in 6 weeks. Elite athletes may opt for surgical stabilization to speed their return to play.

Mallet Finger

- Force applied to the distal interphalangeal (DIP) joint of the finger may result in a flexion injury, which either results in injury to the extensor tendon or in a fracture at its attachment point on the dorsal aspect of the distal phalanx.

- Mallet finger classically presents as an "extension lag" of the DIP with drooping and an inability to fully actively extend the DIP joint.

- X-rays may reveal a fracture of the dorsal base of the distal phalanx on lateral view or may be normal with a pure tendon injury.

- Standard management is to splint the DIP joint in mild hyperextension **continuously** for 6 weeks using a Stax splint or equivalent.

- If recognized and managed early, surgery is often unnecessary.

Jersey Finger

- Forced extension of the actively flexed finger, as in attempting to grasp an opponent for a tackle, may result in avulsion of the flexor digitorum profundus from its insertion on the volar side of the distal phalanx.

- The ring finger is most commonly involved, followed by the middle finger.

- The athlete will feel a pop, and the retracted tendon may be palpable proximally in the finger. Examination will demonstrate loss of independent flexion of the DIP joint.

- Early surgical repair is the treatment of choice.

SPINAL AND NEUROLOGIC INJURIES

Cervical Spine Injury

Mechanism

- Historically, head trauma had been the most common source of morbidity and mortality in football, most commonly from subdural hematomas. Better helmet construction decreased

such head injuries but fostered technique changes in play that favored leading with the head and neck for tackling and blocking, so-called "spearing." This dangerous technique led to a marked increase in cervical spine injuries until rule changes were instituted to outlaw spearing in football.

- A review of 1,300 cervical spine injuries from the National Football Head and Neck Injury Registry has documented *axial loading of the cervical spine* as the major mechanism of catastrophic cervical spine injuries (22).

- The normal cervical spine is comprised of an arc of vertebral bodies that is able to withstand substantial loading by dissipating forces evenly across each vertebral level. However, when the neck is flexed forward 30 degrees, it becomes a straight segmented column of bones that cannot dissipate force evenly. Axial loading of the neck in this flexed position may then result in excessive forces on the vertebral bodies, leading to bony failure, fracture, and cervical spinal cord injury.

Cervical Cord Neurapraxia

- Transient, reversible deformation of the spinal cord resulting from significant trauma to the neck.

- The etiology of transient quadriplegia.

- Athletes may experience transient *bilateral* (differentiating this entity from a brachial plexus neurapraxia—see next section) sensory changes, frank sensation loss, and variable motor changes including complete paralysis.

- Episodes typically last less than 15 minutes but may persist up to 2 days.

- A ratio of spinal canal to vertebral body widths (as determined by lateral radiographs of the cervical spine) of < 0.8 has been found reliably in athletes suffering cervical cord neurapraxia (15). Although this measure has a high sensitivity for cervical cord neurapraxia, it has a low specificity and low positive predictive value and should not be used as a screening tool. In addition, caution must also be used in the interpretation of this ratio in football players because their large vertebral bodies may falsely decrease the ratio in the absence of true cervical spinal stenosis.

- The average rate of recurrence for players who returned to football was 56% (19).

- Management of the football player with known cervical spinal stenosis remains controversial because leading authorities in this area have expressed differing opinions with respect to return-to-play criteria. Some authorities have suggested that cervical spinal stenosis is an absolute contraindication to return to contact sport. This belief is based on a known predisposition to spinal cord injury in these patients and a higher incidence of permanent neurologic sequelae in this group as compared to those with normal spinal canal volumes (2,3).

- Others contend that, despite its association with transient quadriplegia, cervical spinal stenosis is not reliably associated with catastrophic spinal cord injury and does not mandate exclusion from participation in all cases (20). The following guidelines have been proposed for participation in this group of athletes:

- Canal to vertebral body ratio of 0.8 or less in asymptomatic individuals—*no contraindication*
- Ratio of 0.8 or less with one episode of cervical cord neurapraxia—*relative contraindication*
- Documented episodes of cervical cord neurapraxia associated with intervertebral disc disease and/or degenerative changes—*relative contraindication*
- Documented episode of cervical cord neurapraxia associated with MRI evidence of cord defect or cord edema—*relative/absolute contraindication*
- Documented episode of cervical cord neurapraxia associated with ligamentous instability, symptoms of neurologic findings lasting more than 36 hours, and/or multiple episodes—*absolute contraindication*

Brachial Plexus Neurapraxia

- Commonly referred to as a "stinger" or "burner," brachial plexus neurapraxia results from traction or compression of the brachial plexus with violent lateral flexion of the neck.
- The most common nerve injury in football, with defensive players most commonly affected.
- Athletes note *unilateral* burning or stinging pain, numbness, or tingling radiating from the supraclavicular area down to the fingers, most commonly in a C5 or C6 distribution. There may be weakness, most commonly of the deltoid, but *no neck pain*. Symptoms typically resolve in minutes. Symptoms that persist suggest more substantial injury to the brachial plexus, including cervical root avulsion, and mandate imaging and appropriate neurologic consultation.
- Athletes may resume competition when they demonstrate full range of motion, full strength, and a normal neurologic examination of the upper extremity.
- Prospective analysis of college football players revealed that a favorable overall spinal canal to vertebral body ratio (> 0.9) is associated with a low initial incidence of brachial plexus injury (4). Players with multiple such injuries had significantly smaller ratios than those suffering only one event (0.75 vs. 0.87, respectively).

Spear Tackler's Spine

- Characterized by developmental narrowing of the cervical canal (a canal to vertebral body ratio of < 0.8), straightening or reversal of the normal cervical lordosis, and posttraumatic radiographic abnormalities.
- These individuals are at such great risk for permanent spinal cord injury that they should be precluded from participation in tackle football (21).

Management of the Potential Cervical Spine Injury

- All unconscious athletes and any conscious athlete complaining of neck pain must have the cervical spine immobilized prior to removal from the playing field. This is accomplished by coordinated sports medicine care with a lead care provider at the head and neck to provide traction and stability, particularly if the athlete must be rolled onto their back prior to receiving additional care.
- The helmet should never be removed on the field because the presence of shoulder pads will favor passive hyperextension of the cervical spine and may contribute to further cervical spine or spinal cord injury. The face mask should be removed to allow control of the athlete's airway. *Only in an appropriate acute care setting should the helmet and shoulder pads be removed.*
- Evaluation includes cervical spine x-rays in several planes and may require computed tomography (CT) scanning to rule out fracture in equivocal cases. Football padding has been shown to compromise proper cervical imaging in the hospital setting (6). Consequently, efforts may be undertaken, once in a controlled setting, to remove the helmet and shoulder pads so as not to compromise the quality of cross-table lateral and odontoid view cervical spine x-rays.
- Every potential cervical spine injury must be treated with the same conservative approach and proper technique to prevent unnecessary neurologic compromise.

Lumbar Spine Injury

Spondylolysis

- Stress injury to the pars interarticularis in the posterior aspect of the spine as a result of repetitive extension loading. Offensive and defensive linemen are most commonly affected.
- Athletes complain of deep pain in the low back, which is exacerbated by active or passive extension, particularly when standing on one leg. X-rays may reveal a fracture in the pars interarticularis on oblique views, although bone scan or MRI is often required to make the diagnosis definitively.
- Most athletes respond well to conservative management including rest and rehabilitative activities. Thoracolumbar bracing may be used for additional spinal stability but is often unnecessary.
- Most athletes may return in 6–8 weeks if asymptomatic.

Spondylolisthesis

- Displacement ("slippage") of one vertebral body over another as a result of a stress injury to the pars interarticularis (spondylolysis).
- Approximately 1% of both professional and collegiate football players have a spondylolisthesis (17).
- The presence of a spondylolisthesis is not a contraindication to playing football but may predispose to pain and associated dysfunction and may also lead to further worsening of the anatomic changes in the spine over time.
- Pathologic forces on both lumbar discs and pars interarticularis have been demonstrated in blocking linemen (8). The mechanics of repetitive blocking, most notably loaded extension of the lumbar spine, may be responsible for the increased incidence of such injuries in football linemen.

Concussion

General

- Concussion is defined as a complex pathophysiological process affecting the brain, induced by traumatic biomechanical forces.

- Concussion is estimated to occur at a rate of at least 250,000 events per year in football players. Concussion incidence has been found to be highest at the high school (5.6%) and Division III collegiate levels (5.5%) (10), suggesting an association between level of play and risk of injury.

  - Mechanisms of injury include a direct blow to the head by an opposing player, whip-like motion of the head and neck in response to a blow delivered to another part of the body, or a blow to the head from hitting the ground. Brain shearing and acceleration/deceleration forces result in a cascade of neurochemical changes including local glucose depletion, edema, and local vascular effects.

    - Many athletes either do not realize they have suffered a concussion or fail to report it to their sports medicine staff.

- Tight ends and defensive linemen are most commonly affected (7).

- The majority of concussed football players suffer recurrent concussive injuries, which may place them at risk for long-term neurologic complications.

Evaluation

- Concussed athletes are dazed and disoriented and may have loss or alteration in consciousness. These manifestations may be mild and transient or prolonged and profound. They may complain of dizziness, headache, vision disturbance, and nausea, and they often display changes in personality and behavioral patterns.

- Physical examination is generally within normal limits. In addition to an abbreviated neurologic examination to rule out gross neurologic dysfunction (cranial nerve assessment and gross motor, sensory, and cerebellar testing), sideline neuropsychological tests should be performed to screen for impairment in general orientation (person, place, time of day, and situation — game, game location, quarter, score, and opponent), short- and long-term memory/recall, and complex processing tasks such as reciting the months of the year in reverse order. Athletes should always be assessed for the presence of antegrade (since the time of injury) or retrograde (prior to the injury) amnesia. Antegrade amnesia is generally considered to be a more worrisome finding.

- Commonly applied sideline tools to assess these parameters include the Standardized Assessment of Concussion (SAC) and the Sport Concussion Assessment Tool 2 (SCAT-2).

- There is no consistent correlation between the degree of impairment in neuropsychological testing and the anticipated time to return to play from a concussive injury. For example, loss of consciousness had previously dictated a lengthy period of disqualification. It is now generally accepted that *brief* loss of consciousness (< 15 seconds) does not necessarily indicate a concussion of greater severity. Previously published concussion guidelines and grading systems (*e.g.*, Cantu, Colorado Medical Society, American Academy of Neurology) are no longer used.

- Emphasis should be placed on the description of the concussion's characteristics (presence and duration of antegrade or retrograde amnesia, headache, vomiting, vision change, persisting confusion or disorientation, sleep disturbance) as opposed to a specific grade, which had previously dictated a rigid course of management. Concussions are sufficiently heterogeneous that they require flexibility in their diagnosis and management, particularly with respect to contact sports such as football.

- Brain imaging via CT scan or MRI is generally unnecessary in the evaluation of an uncomplicated concussion. Clinical factors that warrant urgent imaging, typically via CT scanning, include initial prolonged (> 15 seconds) loss of consciousness, progressive decline in level of consciousness, worsening headache, development of a frank neurologic deficit, or refractory nausea and vomiting. In these circumstances, imaging should be used to assess for epidural or subdural hematomas and skull fractures.

Management

- As outlined in recently updated consensus statements (13), return to play from concussion should follow a consistent algorithm.

- It is now standard of care to remove any football player with a concussion from participation for the remainder of the game or practice. *No concussed player should return to play on the day of injury regardless of circumstances.*

- Complete absence of symptoms both at rest and with exertion, normal neurologic examination, and return to baseline neurocognitive and emotional states are the key features to the determination of suitability to return to play.

- Using these guidelines in a stepwise fashion ensures that the concussed football player has adequate time to heal from the event prior to resuming contact activities.

- Once asymptomatic at rest, the athlete must then demonstrate a return to normal baseline of their neurocognitive status. This is ideally shown by comparative testing with baseline data obtained prior to the concussion, generally before preseason workouts begin.

- Balance testing has also been shown to aid in the evaluation and management of concussion (9). This testing modality is again most powerful when compared to a preinjury baseline.

- Once symptom and neurocognitive criteria are satisfied, the athlete is allowed to advance noncontact activity in a stepwise fashion over several days. If the athlete remains asymptomatic with increasing activity, the athlete is then released to resume full football activities.

Complications

- The most feared complication of concussion is the "second-impact syndrome," a generally fatal cascade of cerebral hemorrhage and edema resulting from a second concussive blow following incomplete resolution of a first concussive event. Although exceedingly rare, the potential for second-impact syndrome absolutely dictates disqualification from football until the concussed athlete has completely recovered from their initial injury.

- Neuropsychological testing has demonstrated the presence of lower cognitive function in collegiate football players with a history of multiple concussions (5), and it has been shown that prior National Football League (NFL) players have a higher rate of cognitive dysfunction than the general population.

- Repeated head trauma from sport has increasingly been associated with chronic traumatic encephalopathy (CTE), which is manifest by progressive pathologic changes including deposition of tau protein within the brain and a clinical presentation consistent with dementia.

- Studies have linked the presence of apolipoprotein E (apoE4) genotype and risk for cognitive impairment with head injury (12). The resultant cognitive status of such athletes with repeated head trauma appears to be influenced by this genetic predisposition as well as age and cumulative exposure to contact.

- Although its utilization as a screening tool is still under study, apoE4 and similar genetic markers may become a practical means of determining an athlete's relative risk for permanent neurocognitive loss in association with head injury in sport.

Headache

- Football-related headache is common, with 85% of sampled high school and college football players reporting a history of headache as a result of hitting (16).

- Defensive backs (25%), defensive linemen (19%), and offensive linemen (18%) were most likely to have headache related to hitting. Given the high rate of headache and the low rate of serious complications (cerebral hemorrhage, second-impact syndrome), the presence of headache, unless persistent or accompanied by other symptoms, does not mandate disqualification from competition.

Heat Illness

- Heat-related illness in football is common as a result of practice and play in warm weather months coupled with impaired heat dissipation from extensive body coverage with heavy padding and helmets.

- Heat illness may manifest as a broad spectrum of conditions including heat cramps, heat syncope, heat exhaustion, and potentially lethal heat stroke.

- Heat cramps, syncope, and exhaustion are characterized by heat-associated physiologic changes that do not result in significant elevations in core body temperature or in central nervous system dysfunction. Heat cramps and syncope may be treated safely with aggressive oral hydration, external cooling measures, electrolyte supplementation, and rest.

- Heat exhaustion is heralded by complaints of dizziness, headache, nausea and vomiting, and generalized weakness and malaise. Core body temperature (measured rectally) is below 104°F, and athletes generally continue to sweat to dissipate heat. Management includes removal from participation, removal of helmet and padding, external cooling measures (cool water immersion, fanning), and intravenous fluids. Resolution of associated symptoms, normal hydration status, and restoration of baseline body weight are necessary prior to resumption of physical activity.

- Heat stroke is defined as core body temperature in excess of 104°F coupled with central nervous system dysfunction characterized by disorientation, confusion, personality change, and even coma. Although the pathophysiology of classic heat stroke includes absence of sweating, athletes with exertional heat stroke may sweat profusely, an important fact to be remembered by care providers.

- Heat stroke is a medical emergency requiring immediate cooling measures such as ice bath immersion and immediate activation of the emergency medical system for rapid transport to a hospital setting where additional aggressive cooling measures may be employed. Consequences of heat stroke may include irreversible brain damage, renal failure, rhabdomyolysis, and death.

- Stimulant supplements and "energy drinks" containing stimulants have been implicated in precipitating heat stroke and death in highly competitive athletes. Their detrimental effects are the result of sympathomimetic activity and resultant vasoconstriction during activities that require vasodilation for appropriate heat dissipation.

- *Football players must have free access to water.* Thirst is a poor measure of hydration status, so athletes must consume fluids regularly during activity regardless of their sense of need to drink.

- The general hydration goal is for fluid consumption sufficient to prevent decreases in total body weight (BW) of 2% or more (1).

- Before exercise, players should consume 5–7 mL/kg BW at least 4 hours prior to exercise. Consumption of beverages with sodium (20–50 mEq/L) and/or small amounts of salted snacks or sodium-containing foods at meals will help to stimulate thirst and retain the consumed fluids (18).

- During exercise, the goal is to prevent excessive dehydration (> 2% BW loss from water deficit) and excessive changes in electrolyte balance that may compromise exercise performance. It is recommended that individuals monitor their body weight changes during training/competition to estimate their sweat losses during particular exercise tasks and weather conditions. Use of preexercise and postexercise body weights is useful for determining sweat rates and customized fluid replacement programs. Differences in metabolic requirements, exercise duration, clothing, equipment, and weather all influence sweat rate and fluid loss.

- American football players wearing full equipment in hot weather may have sweat losses > 8 L/day.

- After exercise, the consumption of normal meals and snacks with sufficient volume of plain water will restore euhydration, provided the food contains sufficient sodium to replace sweat losses (11). More rapid restoration may be accomplished with consumption of 1.5 L of fluid per kilogram of BW lost (18).

- Diet can be used to ensure adequate salt and electrolyte replacement, which will aid in overall water balance.

- Weights should be monitored to screen for subclinical dehydration, and participation should be precluded for athletes who are greater than 1%–2% below their preexercise baseline weight.

- Appropriate guidelines for practice duration and attire should be based on wet bulb globe temperature (WBGT), which accounts for the heating effects of temperature, humidity, and intensity of sunlight exposure.

SUDDEN DEATH

- Sudden death in football players is a rare but devastating occurrence.

- The primary causes of nontraumatic death in athletes include hypertrophic cardiomyopathy, malignant cardiac arrhythmias, heat stroke, asthma, and complications of sickle cell disease.

- Screening measures should focus on the identification of such potential conditions or a familial predisposition to them, accepting that such screening methods at present are limited in their yield.

- The presence of an automated external defibrillator (AED) and appropriate training for its use by the sports medicine staff may be crucial in enhancing survival for athletes with cardiac etiologies of sudden death.

- AEDs and trained staff to use them should be present at all football practices and games whenever logistically feasible.

REFERENCES

1. American College of Sports Medicine, Sawka MN, Burke LM, et al. American College of Sports Medicine position stand: exercise and fluid replacement. *Med Sci Sports Exerc.* 2007;39(2):377–90.
2. Cantu RC. Cervical spinal injuries in the athlete. *Semin Neurol.* 2000; 20(2):173–8.
3. Cantu RC. Stingers, transient quadriplegia, and cervical spinal stenosis: return to play criteria. *Med Sci Sports Exerc.* 1997;29(7 Suppl):S233–5.
4. Castro FP Jr, Ricciardi J, Brunet ME, Busch MT, Whitecloud TS 3rd. Stingers, the Torg ratio, and the cervical spine. *Am J Sports Med.* 1997;25(5):603–8.
5. Collins MW, Grindel SH, Lovell MR, et al. Relationship between concussion and neuropsychological performance in college football players. *JAMA.* 1999;282(10):964–70.
6. Davidson RM, Burton JH, Snowise M, Owens WB. Football protective gear and cervical spine imaging. *Ann Emerg Med.* 2001;38(1): 26–30.
7. Delaney JS, Lacroix VJ, Leclerc S, Johnston KM. Concussions among university football and soccer players. *Clin J Sport Med.* 2002;12(6): 331–8.
8. Gatt CJ Jr, Hosea TM, Palumbo RC, Zawadsky JP. Impact loading of the lumbar spine during football blocking. *Am J Sports Med.* 1997;25(3):317–21.
9. Guskiewicz KM. Balance assessment in the management of sport-related concussion. *Clin Sports Med.* 2011;30(1):89–102, ix.
10. Guskiewicz KM, Weaver NL, Padua DA, Garrett WE Jr. Epidemiology of concussion in collegiate and high school football players. *Am J Sports Med.* 2000;28(5):643–50.
11. Institute of Medicine. Water. In: *Dietary Reference Intakes for Water, Potassium, Sodium, Chloride, and Sulfate.* Washington (DC): National Academies Press; 2005. p. 73–185.
12. Kutner KC, Erlanger DM, Tsai J, Jordan B, Relkin NR. Lower cognitive performance of older football players possessing apolipoprotein E epsilon4. *Neurosurgery.* 2000;47(3):651–7, discussion 657–8.
13. McCrory P, Meeuwisse W, Johnston K, et al. Consensus statement on concussion in sport: 3rd International Conference on Concussion in Sport held in Zurich, November 2008. *Clin J Sport Med.* 2009;19(3): 185–200.
14. Pagnani MJ, Dome DC. Surgical treatment of traumatic anterior shoulder instability in american football players. *J Bone Joint Surg Am.* 2002;84-A(5):711–5.
15. Pavlov H, Torg JS, Robie B, Jahre C. Cervical spinal stenosis: determination with vertebral body ratio method. *Radiology.* 1987;164(3):771–5.
16. Sallis RE, Jones K. Prevalence of headaches in football players. *Med Sci Sports Exerc.* 2000;32(11):1820–4.
17. Shaffer B, Wiesel S, Lauerman W. Spondylolisthesis in the elite football player: an epidemiologic study in the NCAA and NFL. *J Spinal Disord.* 1997;10(5):365–70.
18. Shirreffs SM, Maughan RJ. Volume repletion after exercise-induced volume depletion in humans: replacement of water and sodium losses. *Am J Physiol.* 1998;274(5 Pt 2):F868–75.
19. Torg JS, Corcoran TA, Thibault LE, et al. Cervical cord neurapraxia: classification, pathomechanics, morbidity, and management guidelines. *J Neurosurg.* 1997;87(6):843–50.
20. Torg JS, Ramsey-Emrhein JA. Suggested management guidelines for participation in collision activities with congenital, developmental, or postinjury lesions involving the cervical spine. *Med Sci Sports Exerc.* 1997;29(7 Suppl):S256–72.
21. Torg JS, Sennett B, Pavlov H, Leventhal MR, Glasgow SG. Spear tackler's spine. An entity precluding participation in tackle football and collision activities that expose the cervical spine to axial energy inputs. *Am J Sports Med.* 1993;21(5):640–9.
22. Torg JS, Vegso JJ, O'Neill MJ, Sennett B. The epidemiologic, pathologic, biomechanical, and cinematographic analysis of football-induced cervical spine trauma. *Am J Sports Med.* 1990;18(1):50–7.

Golfing Injuries

Benjamin J. Ingram and Gregory G. Dammann

93

BACKGROUND

- Golf was invented in the 12th century in Northern Europe (16).
- The first golf course was built in the United States in 1888 (4). At the beginning of the 21st century, 29.5 million golfers played on 15,000 golf courses in the United States. In total, 55 million golfers play on 30,000 golf courses worldwide (1,3).
- The National Sporting Goods Association estimates that 18–20 million Americans play golf at least two times per year.
- As a sport, golf is classified as a noncontact, low-intensity sport; therefore, only moderate cardiovascular fitness is required.
- Most injuries result from the golf swing, the equipment, or objects, including the ball, on the course.

THE GOLF SWING

- For definition in this chapter, for the right-handed golfer, the dominant side is the right or trailing side and the nondominant side is the left or leading side. The left-handed golfer would reverse left and right in regard to dominance.
- There are two types of swings in golf: "modern" (in common use since the 1960s) and "classic" (5).
- The modern swing is comprised of multiple coordinated movements of different parts of the body: the hands, wrists, arms, trunk, and legs.
- There are four phases:
  - Backswing or take away: Rotation of the trunk, raising the arms, and cocking the wrists while drawing the club head away from the ball. This is often called *coiling*.
  - Downswing or forward swing: Movement of the club head toward the ball using the shoulders and uncocking of the wrists. Often called *uncoiling*.
  - Acceleration and ball strike: The arms and trunk continue to rotate back toward the ball and the wrists are uncocked. The leading wrist also supinates while the trailing wrist pronates. This is the fastest portion of the swing.
  - Follow through: Momentum of the swing continues with rotation of the shoulders and trunk while raising the arms (5).

EPIDEMIOLOGY

- Annual injury rate is around 40% (2).
- Injuries are different for professional and amateur golfers.
- Amateur golfers most often injure the lower back and elbow with conflicting evidence on the most common site (15,21,23).
- In amateurs, 25% of injuries are from overuse, 21% are from hitting the ground with the club during the swing, and 19% are from poor swing mechanics (13).
- Professional golfers most frequently injure the lower back, followed by nondominant wrist and shoulder injuries. Professional golfers report fewer elbow injuries than their amateur counterparts (15,21).
- Eighty percent of professional injuries occurred secondary to overuse, 12% occurred from hitting the ground during the swing, and 5% occurred from twisting the trunk (excessive torque) during the swing (12).
- It is unclear whether stretching for increased flexibility prevents golf injury (2).
- Golfers walk approximately 3 miles during 18 holes of golf (2).

LOWER BACK INJURIES

- The lower back is the most common injury in professional and amateur golfers (23.7%–34.5% of all injuries) (15).
- The professional golfer has a more efficient and smoother swing than amateur counterparts, but professional golfers still have the highest incidence of low back pain of all professional sports (21).
- The lumbar spine rotates, side bends, compresses, flexes, and hyperextends during the golf swings. These movements result in lateral bending, shear, compression, and torque forces. The shear and torque forces are 80% significantly higher in the amateur compared to the professional golfer (4,21).
- The modern swing ends the follow-through phase in the "reverse C" (lumbar hyperextension) (18). "Crunch factor" describes the lumbar lateral bending that takes place during the swing (5). Reverse C and crunch factor can be more pronounced in amateur golfers. Explanations for this difference

include inadequate weight transfer during the swing, a more varied stance, leaning away from the ball at impact and follow-through, and less hip turn than allowed in the classic swing (4,5,15,21). The professional's swing is more smooth and refined from repetition, which results in coordinated muscle firing throughout the swing and a more upright stance at the end of follow-through (5,17).

- These forces put golfers at risk for muscle strains, herniated nucleus pulposus (HNP), facet arthropathies, and spondylosis/spondylolisthesis.
  - Lumbosacral strains typically occur during activity and are relieved with rest. There is tenderness over the affected soft tissue area and no radiologic abnormalities.
  - HNP and sciatica are almost always associated together. Ninety-five percent of all HNPs occur at L4–L5 or L5–S1, and these nerve roots provide sensory and motor functions to the lower extremity (4).
  - Facet arthropathies and spinal stenosis are related as a dysfunction that develops at the posterior facet joints producing a narrowing of the spinal foramen. The pain is often increased with extension and side bending to the affected side.
  - Spondylolysis (defect in pars interarticularis) can occur from the significant torque produced during the coiling and uncoiling of the lumbar spine. This torque causes fractures at the pars interarticularis. With a pars defect, especially bilateral, there is the potential for spondylolisthesis (anterior displacement or sliding of the affected vertebrae) (18). This displacement can cause impingement of the spinal nerve roots or cord.
- Additionally, golf bags are traditionally carried on one shoulder, leading to asymmetric loading (2). Newer bags have the ability for two-shoulder carry or use of a rolling pull cart. Additionally, most golf carts have an area for carry of golf bags.
- Most injuries can be managed conservatively because greater than 90% of patients recover in 4 weeks after injury (4); however, some "red flags" should alert the clinician of underlying pathology: back pain in a patient over 50 or less than 20 years old; a history of cancer; constitutional symptoms of fever, night sweats, weight loss, and the like; bowel and/or bladder dysfunction; and saddle anesthesia. If any of these are positive, a more complete workup with imaging studies would be indicated. If no red flags are present, the patient should be encouraged to perform activities that their pain tolerance allows (active rest) and to use ice and acetaminophen and/or nonsteroidal anti-inflammatory drugs (NSAIDs) as required (5,18). Additionally, consider core-strengthening exercises (18) with or without formal physical therapy and have golf swing mechanics reviewed on return to play. Care by a physician, therapist, and professional golf instructor at return to play has been shown to produce a 98% rate of no new golf injuries at 1 year upon return (18). Consideration of changing to a more classic swing may also remove some of the problematic forces that result from the modern swing (5).

- Stress fractures of the ribs, attributed in literature to weakness of the serratus anterior, have been reported in golfers (18,21).

SHOULDER INJURIES

- Shoulder injuries account for 8%–12% of golf injuries, with overuse injuries predominating (8,15). The nondominant shoulder is typically affected due to its range of motion during the swing. The nondominant shoulder goes through internal rotation, adduction, abduction, and external rotation.
- The acromioclavicular (AC) joint is the most often injured area followed by impingement and rotator cuff tendinopathy, posterior glenohumeral subluxation, rotator cuff tears, and glenohumeral arthritis (10,15).
- The AC joint is compressed during the backswing on the nondominant side and may cause shoulder pain. This is especially true in older golfers (21).
- Treatment of the degenerative AC joint includes shortening the backswing and weight training with a focus on the rotator cuff muscles. Reviewing swing mechanics may also be beneficial (21).
- The nondominant shoulder is more sensitive than the dominant shoulder to impingement and rotator cuff damage that will negatively affect the golf swing. The supraspinatus of the nondominant shoulder is more active than the dominant side during all phases of the swing except take away, where the dominant supraspinatus shows more activity. The nondominant subscapularis is active during all phases of the swing (21).
- There is evidence that golfers with arthroplasty to either the dominant or nondominant shoulder or both shoulders can resume playing golf safely and with decreased pain (15).
- Shoulder instability is a rare problem in golfers and is usually found in the younger golfer with generalized joint laxity (1).

ELBOW INJURIES

- Amateur golfers are more likely to have elbow injuries compared to professionals.
- The term "golfer's elbow" refers to medial epicondylitis, usually in the dominant hand, despite the fact that most amateur golfing elbow injuries occur in the lateral nondominant elbow ("tennis elbow") (21). Eighty-five percent of all golf elbow injuries occur in the lateral aspect (15).
- Medial epicondylitis, involving the epicondyle of the humerus at the origin of the wrist and finger flexor muscles and pronator muscles, can occur for a variety of reasons, including striking the ground before the ball and hitting off of hard surfaces and practice mats (21).
- Tennis elbow, involving the lateral epicondyle of humerus, wrist and finger extensor muscles, and supinator muscles,

is associated with gripping the club too tightly (21) and forceful contraction of left elbow extensors during impact phase of swing (17).

- Reasons for injury include overuse, poor swing mechanics, and contact with objects other than the ball such as the ground and rocks (15).

- Radiographs are often not needed, and diagnosis is made with history and examination (1).

- Three common therapies for these elbow injuries are counterforce bracing, equipment modification, and physical therapy.

  - Counterforce bracing can help provide a reactive force against the contractile muscle and either spread the force over a wider area or decrease the contractile pull on the epicondyle (11,21).

  - Equipment changes such as graphite shafts can help to decrease the force applied to the forearm by decreasing the amount of vibration at impact.

  - Physical therapy can focus on forearm muscle strength, flexibility, and endurance (11).

- Additional treatments include use of injected steroids, sclerosing agents, or platelet-rich plasma, although the latter two are new treatments and not well studied. Surgery is generally reserved for symptoms lasting over 6 months and nonresponsive to other therapies (1).

HAND AND WRIST INJURIES

- Tendinopathies are the most common problems seen in the golfer's wrist and are typically secondary to the repetitive movements generated during the golf swing and stress at impact.

- Professional golfers tend to have more wrist injuries compared to their amateur counterparts.

- The nondominant wrist is injured more frequently than the dominant wrist because of increased stress with more forceful contact with the ground at impact (1,13).

- de Quervain tenosynovitis involving the first dorsal compartment is a common condition affecting golfers. Ulnar deviation of the leading wrist at ball impact and repeated impact between the club and the ground may trap the nondominant thumb between the trailing hand and shaft thus stressing the tendons in the first dorsal compartment. Poor swing mechanics in a golfer may also lead to premature uncocking of the wrist at the beginning of the downswing rather than during acceleration and ball striking, resulting in ulnar deviation of the nondominant wrist too early in the swing (11). However, the nature of the swing places those even with good swing mechanics at risk for de Quervain tenosynovitis (1).

- Treatment of de Quervain tenosynovitis usually involves conservative therapy including rest, analgesia, therapy, and consideration of immobilization. Injected corticosteroids and surgery are also options if conservative measures have failed (1).

- Other tendon groups that may be injured by improper swing mechanics are the extensor carpi ulnaris of the nondominant arm and flexor carpi radialis and ulnaris of the dominant arm (1,15). Amateurs are more likely to hit a "fat" shot, defined as the club head striking the ground too far behind the ball, specifically impacting these tendon groups (15).

- Hook of the hamate fractures, the most common fracture in golf, occur with impingement between the hand and the club handle (butt of the club), more common in the nondominant hand (15).

- Accounting for only 2% of all wrist fractures, 33% of hamate fractures are found in golfers (1,11).

- The "carpal tunnel view" is the best x-ray view to visualize this fracture. If it is not visible on plain film, then computed tomography (CT) scan is the image of choice (1,15,17). Preventive measures include proper club length with the butt of the club extending slightly beyond the palm of the leading hand rather than digging into the hypothenar eminence.

HIP INJURIES

- There is minimal literature on hip injuries in golf.

- In one study of a survey design involving 703 professional and amateur golfers, hip injuries accounted for only 2.8% of all injuries reported. The study did not comment further on the nature of those injuries (6).

- Golf can be safely played following total hip arthroplasty (20).

KNEE INJURIES

- Knee injuries make up only 6% of golf injuries. The dominant knee receives peak force during the back swing followed by transfer of force to the nondominant knee during the impact and follow-through (15).

- Given that many golfers are older, osteoarthritis of the knees needs to be taken into consideration with evaluation of knee pain (15).

- There is evidence that golf can safely be played with decreased pain following knee arthroplasty (15).

- Other knee injuries, such as strains, can be caused by a combination of environmental factors, such as hilly terrain and wet grass causing a player to slip while walking.

EYE AND HEAD INJURIES

- Golf accounts for only 1.5%–6% of sports-related eye injuries (7), making them relatively uncommon but potentially devastating when they do occur.

- The usual mechanism of injury to the eye is a stray ball or the head of a club of another golfer during their swing (15).

- The word "fore" is typically yelled by golfers to alert to the potential that a ball is heading the way of another golfer. The typical response, which is to turn toward the person yelling "fore," is not recommended. Turning away and crouching down with the hands covering the face is recommended (15).
- Pediatric eye and head golf-related injuries are typically club related, mostly secondary to unsupervised play (7,9).

SKIN DISORDERS

- Golf is a sport played in the outdoor setting with minimal sun protection available on the course. Golfers spend the majority of their time in sunny locations and often play in the middle of the day when the ultraviolet (UV) light is most damaging to the skin. Skin cancer is more likely to occur in individuals with fair skin, who sunburn easily, and who have increased exposure to UV light. Prevention recommendations are that golfers protect their exposed skin with sunscreens and clothing that block these harmful rays.

PSYCHOLOGICAL DISORDERS

- The *yips* or "golfer's cramps" are an involuntary motor disturbance that affects some golfers, especially during putting. This disorder is described as jerking, tremors, freezing of the hands, or spasm of the arms. It is believed that performance anxiety contributes to the cause of this disorder. No medications have been proven to be of benefit. One case report from 2010 of a golfer given a series of acupuncture treatments showed continued symptom relief from yips at 24 months (19).

GOLF CART INJURIES

- Golf carts for use in sport are unique to golf, although use of golf carts for nongolf purposes is increasing. In 2007 alone, golf cart trauma led to 17,107 injuries (2). The most common location (45%) for golf cart–related injury to occur is the golf course (14). The lack of safety equipment on golf carts, such as seat belts and front brakes, along with newer models achieving greater speeds contribute to their potential for danger (22).
- A study by Watson et al. (22) analyzing data from the National Electronic Injury Surveillance System revealed that in golf cart injuries the mean and median ages for injury were 33.6 and 28 years, respectively, although injuries to children < 16 years old involved 31.3% of cases. Falls from the carts were the most common mechanism of injury (38.3%), with soft tissue injury being the most common diagnosis (47.7%). Head injuries involving golf carts have also been reported (14,22).

OTHER

- Golf is an outdoor sport; therefore, heat and cold injuries can and do occur on the course.
- Lightening results in an average of 30–500 deaths per year with more than 1,000 nonlethal injuries (2).

REFERENCES

1. Bayes MC, Wadsworth LT. Upper extremity injuries in golf. *Phys Sportsmed*. 2009;37(1):92–6.
2. Brandon B, Pearce PZ. Training to prevent golf injury. *Curr Sports Med Rep*. 2009;8(3):142–6.
3. Farrally MR, Cochran AJ, Crews DJ, et al. Golf science research at the beginning of the twenty-first century. *J Sports Sci*. 2003;21(9):753–65.
4. Fu FH, Stone DA. *Sports Injuries*. 2nd ed. Philadelphia (PA): Lippincott Williams & Wilkins; 2001. 1264 p.
5. Gluck GS, Bendo JA, Spivak JM. The lumbar spine and low back pain in golf: a literature review of swing biomechanics and injury prevention. *Spine J*. 2008;8(5):778–88.
6. Gosheger G, Liem D, Ludwig K, Greshake O, Winkelmann W. Injuries and overuse syndromes in golf. *Am J Sports Med*. 2003;31(3):438–43.
7. Hink EM, Oliver SC, Drack AV, et al. Pediatric golf-related ophthalmic injuries. *Arch Ophthalmol*. 2008;126(9):1252–6.
8. Jobe FW, Pink MM. Shoulder pain in golf. *Clin Sports Med*. 1996;15(1):55–63.
9. Macgregor DM. Golf related head injuries in children. *Emerg Med J*. 2002;19(6):576–7.
10. Mallon WJ, Colosimo AJ. Acromioclavicular joint injury in competitive golfers. *J South Orthop Assoc*. 1995;4(4):277–82.
11. McCarroll JR. Overuse injuries of the upper extremity in golf. *Clin Sports Med*. 2001;20(3):469–79.
12. McCarroll JR, Gioe TJ. Professional golfers and the price they pay. *Phys Sportsmed*. 1982;10(7):64–70.
13. McCarroll JR, Rettig AC, Shelbourne KD. Injuries in the amateur golfer. *Phys Sportsmed*. 1990;18(3):122–6.
14. McGwin G Jr, Zoghby JT, Griffin R, Rue LW 3rd. Incidence of golf cart-related injury in the United States. *J Trauma*. 2008;64(6):1562–6.
15. McHardy A, Pollard H, Luo K. Golf injuries: a review of the literature. *Sports Med*. 2006;36(2):171–87.
16. Mellion MB, Walsh WM, Shelton GL. *The Team Physician's Handbook*. 2nd ed. Philadelphia (PA): Mosby; 1996. 910 p.
17. Metz JP. Managing golf injuries: technique and equipment changes that aid treatment. *Phys Sportsmed*. 1999;27(7):41–56.
18. Reed JJ, Wadsworth LT. Lower back pain in golf: a review. *Curr Sports Med Rep*. 2010;9(1):57–9.
19. Rosted P. Acupuncture for treatment of the yips? A case report. *Acupunct Med*. 2005;23(4):188–9.
20. Swanson EA, Schmalzried TP, Dorey FJ. Activity recommendations after total hip and knee arthroplasty: a survey of the American Association for Hip and Knee Surgeons. *J Arthroplasty*. 2009;24(6 Suppl):120–6.
21. Wadsworth LT. When golf hurts: musculoskeletal problems common to golfers. *Curr Sports Med Rep*. 2007;6(6):362–5.
22. Watson DS, Mehan TJ, Smith GA, McKenzie LB. Golf cart-related injuries in the U.S. *Am J Prev Med*. 2008;35(1):55–9.
23. Wiesler ER, Lumsden B. Golf injuries of the upper extremity. *J Surg Orthop Adv*. 2005;14(1):1–7.

Gymnastics

John P. DiFiori and Dennis J. Caine

94

INTRODUCTION

- Gymnastics is an extremely popular sport in the United States and worldwide. There are an estimated 90,000 competitive gymnasts and an additional three million recreational gymnasts in the United States (78). Almost 1,500 athletes participate in National Collegiate Athletic Association (NCAA) gymnastics each year (60).

- Gymnastics training begins at very young ages. The average age at onset is 5–6 years for girls and 6–7 years for boys (52). Most girls reach their highest competitive level by age 16 due to the biomechanical demands for a small, lean, prepubertal physique (3). Peak performance for males is often at a later age because of the requirements for greater levels of strength that occur after puberty.

- Physicians caring for gymnasts must be familiar with the requirements of the sport, common and unique injuries, and potential methods to prevent such injuries.

GYMNASTICS FACTS

- Current-day gymnastics at the Olympic level includes men's artistic gymnastics, women's artistic gymnastics, rhythmic gymnastics, and trampoline gymnastics. The focus of this chapter will be artistic gymnastics.

- Male and female gymnasts compete in different individual events. Male gymnasts compete in floor exercise, still rings, horizontal bar, parallel bars, pommel horse, and vault. Female gymnasts compete in floor exercise, uneven parallel bars, beam, and vault. Most gymnasts train for all of the events. Gymnasts acquire new skills for each event via repetition of individual elements and series (groups of elements).

- The competitive levels in women's gymnastics are levels 1–10 and elite, with level 10 and elite being the most advanced. Collegiate gymnasts are typically the equivalent of level 9 or higher. Male gymnasts currently compete in classes 1–7; class 1 is the most advanced. There are also over 150 elite male gymnasts in the United States (78).

- The *code of points* dictates the degree of difficulty for each skill. There is a specific list of requirements for each level of competition. The *code of points* evolves with the sport and is revised every 4 years, essentially increasing the required levels of difficulty with each revision.

- The training regimen for gymnastics is rigorous. An advanced or elite level gymnast practices an average of 25–35 hours per week throughout the year. Even young, beginning level gymnasts may train 10 hours per week or more.

- Special equipment used by gymnasts includes grips with or without wooden dowels for the bars, beam shoes, and wrist supports. Gymnasts may also train using crash mats, foam pits, beam and bar pads, low balance beams, and twisting or spotting belts.

INCIDENCE OF INJURY

- During 1988–2004, gymnastics had the highest incidence rate of practice-related injury among all women's intercollegiate sports, followed by soccer. Women's gymnastics had the second highest injury rate during competition, preceded by women's soccer (31).

- The incidence of injury in women's club gymnastics ranges from 0.5 to 5.4 injuries per 1,000 hours of participation, with practice and competition exposures combined (39,43). During 1988–2004, practice and competition injury rates for NCAA women gymnasts were 15.84 and 7.96 injuries per 1,000 athletic exposures, respectively (48). A more than twofold increased risk of injury in competition versus practice has also been reported in girls' club-level gymnastics (2). This finding may be explained by the fact that gymnasts are better protected in training because of landing in foam pits, spotting, and softer mats (71).

- There is a paucity of epidemiologic research on injuries affecting male gymnasts. Most of the club-level studies were carried out in the 1980s and 1990s and were reported with reference to participant seasons, which do not account for differences in exposure to injury risk (26). Available injury surveillance data for male collegiate gymnasts are also dated. During 1985–1994, NCAA male gymnasts incurred an overall injury rate of 5.33 injuries per 1,000 athletic exposures (57).

INJURY CHARACTERISTICS

Injury Onset

■ High-level performance in artistic gymnastics requires long hours of training and the practice and performance of high-risk skills. As a result, it is not unexpected that both acute and overuse injuries will occur. Generally, studies involving male and/or female gymnasts and reporting on injury onset report a slightly greater proportion of acute versus overuse injuries (15). This likely reflects the different types of apparatus used in men's gymnastics that place greater demands on the upper body (14).

Anatomic Location

■ The lower extremity is the most frequently injured body region among female and male gymnasts, followed by the upper extremity and spine/trunk (15). However, Dixon and Fricker (22) examined injuries among top-level gymnasts over a 10-year period and found that the upper extremity was the site of a greater proportion of injuries for males (53.4% of injuries) than females (32.7% of injuries).

■ A more specific look at body regions reveals that injuries to the knee are most common among female gymnasts, followed by those to the ankle and lower back. Among male gymnasts, the shoulder and wrist are more commonly injured, likely reflecting the different kinds of apparatus and related training in men's gymnastics. However, male gymnasts also experience a high rate of ankle and knee injuries (15).

Injury Severity

■ **Pain:** Many gymnasts continue training with pain. Studies have found that as many as 71% of female gymnasts train with an injury (71). Wrist pain, for example, is a common complaint among gymnasts, with prevalence estimates ranging from 46% to 87.5% (11,19–21). Gymnastics may be unique in that the injured gymnast can alter his or her workout depending on the injury; for example, a gymnast with an ankle injury can continue full training on the uneven bars, provided he or she avoids the dismount.

■ **Time loss:** Severity of injury has been assessed by calculating the duration of restricted training. While most injuries are minor, resulting in less than a week away from training, 12.5% (2) to 25.9% (5) result in a time loss of greater than 3 weeks. One study found that the average time until full participation resumed was almost 4.5 weeks per injury (43). Several studies involving female gymnasts have reported that mean time loss per injury was greater for advanced than for lower level gymnasts (2,38,40). Similarly, Caine (8) found that advanced level participants experience a greater proportion of severe injury ($\geq$ 21 days of time lost) than beginning level gymnasts (37.5% vs. 10.2%). Among NCAA female gymnasts followed for 16 years, 39% of competition

injuries and 32% of training injuries resulted in a time loss of 10 days (48).

■ **Catastrophic injury:** Although direct catastrophic injuries are relatively rare in most sports, including gymnastics, the risk of these injuries appears to be greater in gymnastics than in other sports. Rates for nonfatal catastrophic injuries (*i.e.*, permanent severe functional disability such as quadriplegia) were highest for male and female gymnasts at both the high school and college levels during 1982–2007 (56). Data on catastrophic injuries are unfortunately lacking for club-level gymnasts, where most competitive gymnasts participate.

■ **Nonparticipation:** An important reason for participation in sports is of course the health benefits that can be accrued from physical activity. An important question and concern that arises, therefore, is how many athletes drop out of their sport due to injury. In their study of Australian elite gymnasts over 10 years, Dixon and Fricker (22) reported that 9.5% of gymnasts retired as a result of injury. Three studies reported that between 16.3% and 52.4% of club-level gymnasts were injured at the time they withdrew (2,42).

■ **Residual effects:** Despite the high incidence and severity of injury among gymnasts, very little research has examined the long-term effects of these injuries. One survey of former collegiate gymnasts found that 45% of previous injuries were still symptomatic (79). Despite the large number of young gymnasts with back pain, a study comparing former elite gymnasts with age-matched controls concluded that fewer former gymnasts (27%) had subjective back problems than did the controls (38%) (77). The lack of follow-up research on the residual effects of gymnastics injuries is a concern given evidence of a link between youth sports injuries, particularly of the knee or ankle, and early-onset osteoarthritis (13).

COMMON INJURIES IN GYMNASTICS

■ Sprains are the most common types of injury in women's gymnastics, followed by strains. Other types of injuries that are common include contusions, fractures, and inflammatory conditions (15). Common injuries are discussed in more detail below.

■ **Ankle ligament sprains:** Typically caused by inversion injuries, ankle ligament sprains are the most common acute injuries in gymnastics (5,22,43). They are usually the result of an incorrect landing or fall. One study found an alarming number of ankle injuries from gymnasts landing with their foot inside a crack in the floor or between mats (45). Evaluation and treatment of gymnasts' ankle injuries are similar to those in other athletes (see Chapter 65).

1. Once the gymnast has completed a functional rehabilitation program, he or she should initially attempt to return to sport with the use of an ankle brace or tape for support. However, many gymnasts do not tolerate long-term use of

ankle braces since the brace may cause slipping from the apparatus, and it alters their form and appearance. Flesh-colored tape is typically the best-tolerated intervention.

2. There is little information on the use of prophylactic bracing and taping in gymnasts.

■ **Low back pain:** Back pain caused by lumbar strain and sprain injuries is common in gymnasts. Gymnasts place demands on the lower back that are unparalleled in most other sports. Demands on the gymnast's back include flexion and hyperextension postures during vaulting, dismounts, and somersaults. In addition to the hyperlordotic postures, vertical impact loading occurs as the gymnast lands on both feet during dismount activities. Low back pain should be managed as with other athletes (see Chapter 45). However, care should be taken to exclude spondylolysis as a cause of the symptoms (see below). Strengthening and core stability are especially important in gymnasts.

■ **Spondylolysis:** Spondylolysis (or stress fracture of the pars interarticularis) is a common cause of lower back pain in young gymnasts, especially those between the ages of 9 and 13. It occurs in gymnasts secondary to repetitive flexion and hyperextension of the spine: backbends, walkovers, tumbling, and high-impact landings (28). The prevalence of spondylolysis is higher in gymnasts (range, 5.9%–33.8%) than in the general population (5%–6%) (15,25,33).

1. Gymnasts with spondylolysis typically have unilateral back pain that localizes to the lumbar area. The pain increases with activity (especially hyperextension) and decreases with rest. Physical examination may find tenderness to palpation at the lower lumbar spine. A single-leg standing hyperextension test (stork test) is sensitive and specific for spondylolysis (34).

2. Diagnostic testing begins with plain radiographs, which may show the classic pars interarticularis fracture on the oblique view: the "collared Scottie dog." Single photon emission computed tomography (SPECT) bone scans are highly sensitive for diagnosing active spondylolysis. The study should be performed to confirm the diagnosis of an active lesion because spondylolysis seen radiographically may be asymptomatic (51). Thin-sliced computed tomography (CT) is more specific than bone scan and can also be used to confirm the diagnosis. CT is especially helpful in determining the healing potential of an active spondylolysis and is typically used in conjunction with SPECT once an active lesion has been identified. Magnetic resonance imaging (MRI) with thin slices has been reported to be effective in visualizing the pars interarticularis (16). MRI is perhaps most helpful in identifying other causes of lower back pain when a SPECT scan is negative for active spondylolysis (51).

3. Treatment initially involves modification of activity (no running, jumping, or gymnastics activities that cause pain) for at least 4–6 weeks (51,54). Physical therapy should target spine stabilization, abdominal muscle strengthening, and hamstring flexibility. The use of bracing is controversial. Some recommend the use of bracing if a SPECT scan demonstrates an active lesion (51). A CT scan can also be used to help guide the decision regarding bracing. If the CT demonstrates that an active lesion has healing potential, bracing may be the preferred initial intervention. Decisions regarding bracing should be made on an individual basis (54). The role of bone stimulators to potentially aid in healing of active lesions is not well defined (51).

4. Return to sport depends on progress with activity modification and physical therapy. Many gymnasts can return to an initially low level of participation after 4–6 weeks (51). Activity is then advanced as tolerated. Maintenance exercises should be continued for the remainder of the gymnast's career.

■ **Traumatic knee injuries:** Knee injuries can be severe and disabling (50). The typical mechanism is a landing or fall while the gymnast is still completing a twisting rotation. Anterior cruciate ligament (ACL), medial collateral ligament (MCL), and meniscal injuries are the most common and may predispose the gymnast to early-onset osteoarthritis (13). Most gymnasts require surgical reconstruction of an ACL tear in order to continue gymnastics. In young athletes, this procedure may be delayed until after physeal closure. Whether early or delayed ACL reconstruction results in the best outcome in skeletally immature patients is not yet clear (55). Gymnasts do not tolerate large knee braces because bulky braces impair the gymnasts' form and appearance. See Chapters 60 and 61 for further description of the evaluation and treatment of acute knee injuries.

■ **Overuse injuries of the knee:** These injuries result from the repetitive running, jumping, and landing required in gymnastics. Common diagnoses include Osgood-Schlatter disease, patellofemoral pain syndrome, and patellar tendinopathy. The differential diagnosis for knee pain may also include stress-related injury to the distal femoral and/or proximal tibial epiphyseal plate (12). Treatment involves relative rest and physical therapy, including strengthening exercises (see Chapters 62 and 63).

■ **Sever's injury:** This was the most common overuse injury in one survey (45). It typically occurs between ages 7 and 14. The main finding on examination is tenderness at the insertion of the Achilles tendon onto the calcaneus. However, many patients have tenderness of the medial or lateral aspect of the calcaneal body. Traditionally considered a traction apophysitis, newer evidence has indicated that Sever's injury may actually result from repetitive compression to the actively remodeling metaphysis (61). Sever's injury is a self-limited condition. Treatment includes relative rest, ice, heel lifts used on a short-term basis, stretching, and strengthening exercises (27).

■ **Dorsal wrist pain:** Chronic wrist pain affects 46%–87% of young gymnasts (11,21). Cross-sectional surveys indicate that approximately 45% of gymnasts report pain of at least 6 months in duration (19,21). Painful dorsiflexion while supporting body weight and dorsal wrist pain, without acute trauma or swelling, characterize gymnast's wrist (50). Factors associated with wrist pain include training hours, skill level, and age at initiation of training (21). It appears to be more common during the adolescent growth spurt. Dorsal wrist pain can be associated with radiographic findings of distal radial physeal injury (19). Cases of stress-related premature closure of the distal radial physis have been reported (1,6,7,12).

1. The mainstay of treatment is reduction of loading to the wrist. Strengthening of the wrist and upper extremity may be helpful. Use of a brace with a hyperextension block may decrease symptoms (62). Premature closure of the distal radial growth plate may result in symptomatic positive ulnar variance (2,20,21).

2. In skeletally mature gymnasts, if ulnar-sided wrist pain develops as a result of positive ulnar variance, an ulnar shortening procedure may be required to treat this condition.

- **Elbow dislocations:** Elbow dislocations in gymnasts are typically the result of a fall on outstretched hand (FOOSH) injury (62). As a result, gymnasts are taught not to reach down with their hands when they fall. Elbow joint dislocations require a thorough neurovascular examination, x-rays, and, in most cases, closed reduction (see Chapter 52).

INJURIES UNIQUE TO GYMNASTICS

- **Clavicular stress fractures:** Clavicular stress fractures are rare but have been described in gymnasts, presumably because of the repetitive forces to which the upper extremity is exposed in activities such as tumbling and vaulting. The injury can be diagnosed with plain radiographs, CT, or MRI. An MRI is also useful to rule out pathologic causes, such as a tumor. Treatment is conservative. In one report, full training was resumed after 8 weeks of upper extremity rest (24).

- **Osteochondritis dissecans of the capitellum:** This is believed to be underrecognized in gymnasts (62). Although there were several case series of this condition affecting female and male gymnasts reported in the 1980s and 1990s (32,46,73), there has been no follow-up to determine the prevalence or incidence of osteochondritis dissecans of the capitellum in this population. It occurs in young gymnasts with open growth plates, typically aged 10–15, from repeated valgus stress to the elbow. Symptoms include the gradual onset of lateral elbow pain that worsens with activity, inability to fully extend the elbow, and possibly locking or clicking. Management depends on the severity of symptoms and imaging results (see Chapter 53).

- **Forearm fracture:** *Griplock* is an entity unique to gymnastics. Gymnasts wear leather handgrips for bar and ring work. With griplock, the grip accidentally catches on the bar, and while the athlete's momentum carries him or her around the bar, the hand and forearm are kept in a locked position. The result is a serious forearm fracture that may require surgery (69). Griplock is more common in male gymnasts, who use a bar with a smaller circumference, and in gymnasts whose grips are overused and stretched out.

- **Hand blisters/rips:** Gymnasts frequently train with blisters or *rips* on their hands caused by the friction created between skin and bars. These are difficult to treat and prevent, because usual treatments such as tape or moleskin will not adhere to the hands while practicing. The friction of the bars will usually cause the blister to pop as soon as it arises. These areas should be kept clean to avoid infection. Once an open lesion has dried, the application of a topical antibiotic ointment can be used at night in order to prevent both infection and painful cracking of the lesion.

- **Abdominal wall contusion:** Female gymnasts may develop severe bruising around the lower abdomen and anterior superior iliac spine by doing a beat maneuver on the uneven bars. Gymnasts at the lower competitive levels typically perform this skill, which involves hanging from the high bar and dropping the anterior pelvis and hips onto the low bar. Use of padding may prevent repetitive injury (53). Although painful, the prognosis of this injury is good. Ice and avoidance are generally required for treatment.

- **Vulvar hematomas:** Vulvar hematomas result from a straddle injury on the balance beam. On most occasions, these falls do not result in significant injury. When a vulvar hematoma develops, incision and drainage can be performed if the hematoma is very large or is expanding (66). In minor cases, ice and relative rest are recommended.

- **Heel pad contusions:** Heel pad contusions develop after trauma to the fat pad, usually from a hard landing onto the beam or unpadded floor. If symptoms continue to worsen, radiographs and/or MRI should be performed to rule out an occult fracture or a calcaneal stress fracture. Management of heel pad contusions is conservative: ice, rest, anti-inflammatory medications, and a heel cushion.

RISK FACTORS FOR INJURY

- Factors that may contribute to the occurrence of gymnastics injury may be classified as either intrinsic or extrinsic. Intrinsic risk factors are individual anatomic and psychosocial characteristics predisposing a gymnast to the outcome of injury. Extrinsic risk factors are factors that have an impact on the gymnast while he or she is participating, for example training methods or equipment.

Intrinsic Risk Factors

- **Adolescent growth spurt:** Two studies indicate an increased risk of gymnastics injury during age or maturity periods associated with rapid growth (5,19). However, the findings of these studies await confirmation from a comparison of growth velocity with individual injury rates. The rapid change in height alters the moment of inertia for certain skills, requiring gymnasts to make gradual changes in technique. Growth-related changes affecting the articular cartilage and physes may also contribute.

- **Age:** Singh et al. (74) reported that upper extremity injuries were more common in the 6- to 11-year age group (relative risk [RR], 1.46; 95% confidence interval [CI], 1.37–1.56) than in the 12- to 17-year age group and that lower extremity injuries were more common in the 12- to 17-year age group (RR, 1.69; 95% CI, 1.56–1.83).

- **Gender:** As discussed earlier, the distribution of injuries varies by gender, with male gymnasts having a higher percentage of upper extremity injuries and female gymnasts having a greater proportion of lower extremity injuries (22). This variation is likely the result of differences in the events: Most men's events, such as the parallel bars, high bar, rings, and pommel horse, primarily require use of the upper extremities. In other sports, adolescent female athletes are at increased risk of sustaining a knee injury, and the injury is more likely to require surgery or to involve the ACL compared to males (10). However, this relationship has not been fully evaluated in young gymnasts.

- **Motor characteristics:** Lindner and Caine (43) reported less speed, poorer balance, and higher endurance and flexibility as predicting injury among club-level gymnasts. However, these predictors were not significant at all age and competitive levels studied, and the sample size in the subgroups was small.

- **Physical characteristics:** Greater body size and body fat percentage have been correlated with higher risk of injury (3,75); however, these studies did not control for such variables as training hours and age (3). It is also possible that factors such as greater height and weight characterize older gymnasts who are competing at higher levels of competition (4). Older gymnasts may be more likely to sustain injury because of more complex and difficult skills and greater accumulated participation exposure.

- **Previous injury:** The reinjury rate in gymnastics is high: 32.7% in 1 year (5). As many as one in four injuries is a reinjury (3). Previous injury was reported as a significant predictor of overuse injury among young female gymnasts (Injury Rate Ratio [IRR], 2.12; 95% CI, 1.61–2.78) (12). The lower back was the most common site of recurrent injury in one study of female gymnasts (5). The high rates of reinjury in gymnasts are felt to be due to premature return to training and inadequate rehabilitation (5).

- **Psychosocial factors:** Two studies reported that increased levels of life stress were associated with the number and severity of injuries (35,37). In both studies, however, the psychosocial measures were taken after the injury occurred. It is possible, therefore, that the stress profiles of the gymnasts were different at the time of injury (15). In a prospective study, female gymnasts who were injured reported a higher negative life stress than their noninjured counterparts (63). Advanced gymnastics training involves many hours and years of commitment. A gymnast who has created a sense of self-worth primarily on the basis of successes in gymnastics may continue to train long after losing interest in the sport (76). In such cases, gymnasts may create an injury (either imaginary or self-inflicted) in order to discontinue the sport without disappointing family, coaches, or themselves (76).

Extrinsic Risk Factors

- **Level of competition:** Although two reports indicate lower injury rates for elite than subelite gymnasts (38,40), several other studies have found that gymnasts at advanced or elite levels suffer more injuries (2,5,8,43,48). This is felt to be due to an increased number of training hours, increased skill difficulty, and perhaps less supervision (5,2). The high prevalence of chronic injuries in this group has been associated with more time spent in the gym (65).

- **Competition:** Although most injuries occur while training, the incidence when calculated per exposure is two to three times higher for competition (2,8,48). This is especially true among advanced level gymnasts (2). The timed warm-up period before a competition may be an especially high-risk time for injuries (2), perhaps because the gymnasts are in a stressful and hurried situation.

INCITING EVENTS FOR INJURY

- Very few studies provide incidence rates related to the action or activity leading to injury in gymnastics. Additionally, most available data do not distinguish between overuse and acute injuries. As a result, it is difficult to determine risk related to specific events or inciting events and whether gradual-onset injuries are specifically related to maneuvers in a given event.

- **Event:** Caine (2) found that floor exercise was the event most likely to lead to acute injury in women's club-level gymnastics. Floor exercise was also associated with the highest frequency of injury during international competitions (41). In men's gymnastics, one study reported that 52.9% of all knee injuries and 43.8% of all ankle injuries occurred during floor exercise (36).

- **Action:** In a 16-year study of women's collegiate gymnastics injuries, 70.7% of competition injuries resulted either from landings in floor exercise or when dismounting from other apparatus (48). The majority of both practice and competition injuries in this study involved contact with the floor, the mat, or equipment.

- **Gymnast behavior:** One study reported that the most common gymnast behavior related to acute injury was a missed move, followed by falls from an apparatus and dismounts (43).

OTHER GYMNASTICS-RELATED CONCERNS

Female Athlete Triad

- The female athlete triad refers to the relationships between adequate nutrition in the form of energy availability, menstrual function, and bone mineral density (BMD), which can manifest in the clinical conditions of eating disorders, amenorrhea, and osteoporosis (58). This important issue is discussed in detail in Chapter 115.

- Although the exact prevalence is unknown, female gymnasts, like other female athletes in sports where aesthetics and leanness are emphasized, are at risk for developing the female athlete triad or related conditions within the spectrum of the triad (58,59,62).

- Losing weight to enhance performance is an important reason for dieting among adolescent elite athletes (49). The prevalence of disordered eating among gymnasts is not well established. Some studies of gymnasts have found a high prevalence of disordered eating behaviors and weight control behaviors (64,68). Recent studies, however, found that self-reported disordered eating prevalence may be no greater among adolescent young athletes than controls (30,49).

- The focus on body image may begin at an early age: Girls involved in aesthetic sports such as gymnastics reported higher weight concerns at ages 5–7 than control groups (17).

  - Nutrition studies on female gymnasts consistently report mean energy intakes that are 275–1,200 kilocalories lower than national recommendations (4,9). Female gymnasts also have correspondingly inadequate intakes of essential micronutrients such as zinc, iron, and calcium that may impact upon growth and skeletal development (4,9).

  - When compared with age-matched controls, gymnasts have a later onset of menarche (42). Menstrual dysfunction occurs more commonly in athletes (range, approximately 3%–70%) than in the general population (range, 2%–5%) (58). The specific prevalence in gymnasts is unknown. The etiology of menstrual dysfunction in athletes is felt to be related to inadequate caloric intake relative to energy expenditure, termed "negative energy balance" (44,58).

- The repetitive impact-loading characteristic of gymnastics training appears to have a salutary effect on BMD (67). Studies of prepubertal and peripubertal and college-aged and retired gymnasts show greater total-body and regional BMD and bone mineral content when compared to other athletic and nonathletic controls (23). However, athletes in weight-bearing sports are known to have a higher BMD than nonathletes, and this must be considered when evaluating athletes for the triad (58). In general, a BMD Z-score of < -1.0 may warrant further investigation in gymnasts (58).

- Coaches, parents, and athletes, as well as medical support staff, should be educated regarding the symptoms, signs, and potentially serious health consequences of the triad.

PREVENTION OF INJURY

Prevention Research

- Although there is evidence that the rate and severity of gymnastics injuries are high compared to other sports, there is surprisingly little research in gymnastics that has tested preventive measures (29,47). In contrast, there has been promising research in other sports (*e.g.,* team handball, soccer, basketball) supporting the use of injury prevention strategies that include preseason conditioning, functional training, education, and strength and balance programs that are continued throughout the playing season (72).

Suggestions for Prevention

- Preparticipation screening and periodic rescreening should be performed to include an assessment of injury history, ensure adequate recovery from prior injury, assess general health, and screen for disordered eating and menstrual dysfunction.

- Protective equipment may decrease the incidence of injury and should be used when possible. This includes crash mats, pits, low beams, and foam beam and bar covers. Floor mats and pads should be checked often to ensure that there are no cracks that could lead to an ankle injury.

- Some changes aimed at injury prevention in gymnastics have already been made. A safer vault horse was instated at the senior levels in 2001 in order to decrease injuries. Padded mats are now allowed on the floor exercise at college competitions. Certain high-risk skills, such as the Yurchenko (round-off entry) vault, are restricted to only the most advanced levels.

- Coaches should receive ongoing education in the technical aspects of the sport, as well as those pertaining to conditioning and injury prevention and recognition.

- Training should be in a cyclically progressive manner to allow for accommodation to overall increases in repetitive loading. Quality of training rather than volume should be emphasized, especially when a given skill has been mastered (70).

- Consideration should be given to alternating loading types during workouts. For example, alternating swinging and support-type movements may reduce loading of the wrist (70).

- Larger gymnastics programs should consider adding sports medicine support staff such as a certified athletic trainer, even on a part-time basis, to assist in monitoring for injuries, early intervention, and guidance of rehabilitation and return to competition.

- Increases in training loads should be very gradual and perhaps reduced during periods of rapid growth (18).

- As a result of the high rate of recurrent injury, gymnasts should not return to full training until rehabilitation is completed (5).
- Primary rehabilitation, or prehab, may help to avoid common overuse injuries, such as those to the Achilles tendon or knee (45).

REFERENCES

1. Albanese SA, Palmer AK, Kerr DR, Carpenter CW, Lisi D, Levinsohn EM. Wrist pain and distal growth plate closure of the radius in gymnasts. *J Pediatr Orthop.* 1989;9(1):23–8.
2. Caine D. Injury and growth. In: Sands WA, Caine DJ, Borms J, editors. *Scientific Aspects of Women's Gymnastics. Vol. 45.* Basel (Switzerland): Karger; 2003. p. 46–71.
3. Caine D. Injury epidemiology. In: Sands WA, Caine DJ, Borms J, editors. *Scientific Aspects of Women's Gymnastics. Vol. 45.* Basel (Switzerland): Karger; 2003. p. 72–104.
4. Caine D, Bass S, Daly R. Does preparation of children and adolescents for elite gymnastics place them at risk of reduced growth and delayed maturation? Quit possibly. *Pediatr Exerc Sci.* 2003;15:360–72.
5. Caine D, Cochrane B, Caine C, Zemper E. An epidemiologic investigation of injuries affecting young competitive female gymnasts. *Am J Sports Med.* 1989;17(6):811–20.
6. Caine D, DiFiori J, Maffulli N. Physeal injuries in children's and youth sports: reasons for concern? *Br J Sports Med.* 2006;40(9):749–60.
7. Caine D, Howe W, Ross W, Bergman G. Does repetitive physical loading inhibit radial growth in female gymnasts? *Clin J Sport Med.* 1997;7(4):302–8.
8. Caine D, Knutzen K, Howe W, et al. A three-year epidemiological study of injuries affecting young female gymnasts. *Phys Ther Sport.* 2003;4:10–23.
9. Caine D, Lewis R, O'Connor P, Howe W, Bass S. Does gymnastics training inhibit growth of females? *Clin J Sport Med.* 2001;11(4):260–70.
10. Caine D, Maffulli N, Caine C. Epidemiology of injury in child and adolescent sports: injury rates, risk factors, and prevention. *Clin Sports Med.* 2008;27(1):19–50, vii.
11. Caine D, Roy S, Singer KM, Broekhoff J. Stress changes of the distal radial growth plate. A radiographic survey and review of the related literature. *Am J Sports Med.* 1992;20(3):290–8.
12. Caine DJ, Daly RM, Jolly D, Hagel BE, Cochrane B. Risk factors in young competitive female gymnasts. *Br J Sports Med.* 2006;40:90–1.
13. Caine DJ, Golightly YM. Osteoarthritis as an outcome of paediatric sport: an epidemiological perspective. *Br J Sports Med.* 2011;45(4):298–303.
14. Caine DJ, Lindner KJ, Mandelbaum BR, et al. Gymnastics. In: Caine DJ, Caine CG, Lindner KJ, editors. *Epidemiology of Sports Injuries.* Champaign (IL): Human Kinetics; 1996. p. 213–46.
15. Caine DJ, Nassar L. Gymnastics injuries. *Med Sport Sci.* 2005;48:18–58.
16. Campbell RS, Grainger AJ. Routine thin slice MRI effectively demonstrates the lumbar pars interarticularis. *Clin Radiol.* 2000;55(12):984.
17. Davison KK, Earnest MB, Birch LL. Participation in aesthetic sports and girls' weight concerns at ages 5 and 7 years. *Int J Eat Disord.* 2002; 31(3):312–7.
18. DiFiori JP, Caine DJ, Malina RM. Wrist pain, distal radial physeal injury, and ulnar variance in the young gymnast. *Am J Sports Med.* 2006;34(5):840–9.
19. DiFiori JP, Puffer JC, Aish B, Dorey F. Wrist pain, distal radial physeal injury, and ulnar variance in young gymnasts: does a relationship exist? *Am J Sports Med.* 2002;30(6):879–85.

20. DiFiori JP, Puffer JC, Mandelbaum BR, Dorey F. Distal radial growth plate injury and positive ulnar variance in nonelite gymnasts. *Am J Sports Med.* 1997;25(6):763–8.
21. DiFiori JP, Puffer JC, Mandelbaum BR, Mar S. Factors associated with wrist pain in the young gymnast. *Am J Sports Med.* 1996;24(1):9–14.
22. Dixon M, Fricker P. Injuries to elite gymnasts over 10 yr. *Med Sci Sports Exerc.* 1993;25(12):1322–9.
23. Erlandson MC, Kontulainen SA, Baxter-Jones AD. Precompetitive and recreational gymnasts have greater bone density, mass, and estimated strength at the distal radius in young childhood. *Osteoporos Int.* 2011;22(1):75–84.
24. Fallon KE, Fricker PA. Stress fracture of the clavicle in a young female gymnast. *Br J Sports Med.* 2001;35(6):448–9.
25. Fredrickson BE, Baker D, McHolick WJ, Yuan HA, Lubicky JP. The natural history of spondylolysis and spondylolisthesis. *J Bone Joint Surg Am.* 1984;66(5):699–707.
26. Garrick JG, Requa RK. Girls' sports injuries in high school athletics. *JAMA.* 1978;239(21):2245–8.
27. Gillespie H. Osteochondroses and apophyseal injuries of the foot in the young athlete. *Curr Sports Med Rep.* 2010;9(5):265–8.
28. Goldberg MJ. Gymnastic injuries. *Orthop Clin North Am.* 1980;11(4): 717–26.
29. Harringe ML, Renström P, Werner S. Injury incidence, mechanism and diagnosis in top-level teamgym: a prospective study conducted over one season. *Scand J Med Sci Sports.* 2007;17(2):115–9.
30. Hoch AZ, Pajewski NM, Moraski L, et al. Prevalence of the female athlete triad in high school athletes and sedentary students. *Clin J Sport Med.* 2009;19(5):421–8.
31. Hootman JM, Dick R, Agel J. Epidemiology of collegiate injuries for 15 sports: summary and recommendations for injury prevention initiatives. *J Athl Train.* 2007;42(2):311–9.
32. Jackson DW, Silvino N, Reiman P. Osteochondritis in the female gymnast's elbow. *Arthroscopy.* 1989;5(2):129–36.
33. Jackson DW, Wiltse LL, Cirincoine RJ. Spondylolysis in the female gymnast. *Clin Orthop Relat Res.* 1976;117:68–73.
34. Keene JS. Low back pain in the athlete. From spondylogenic injury during recreation or competition. *Postgrad Med.* 1983;74(6):209–12, 13, 17.
35. Kerr GA, Minden H. Psychological factors related to the occurrence of athletic injuries. *J Sport Exerc Psychol.* 1988;10:167–73.
36. Kirialanis P, Malliou P, Beneka A, Giannakopoulos K. Occurrence of acute lower limb injuries in artistic gymnasts in relation to event and exercise phase. *Br J Sports Med.* 2003;37(2):137–9.
37. Kolt G, Kirkby R. Injury in Australian female competitive gymnasts: a psychological perspective. *Aust J Physiother.* 1996;42(2):121–6.
38. Kolt G, Kirkby RJ, Lindner H. Coping processes in competitive gymnasts: gender differences. *Percept Mot Skills.* 1995;81(3 Pt 2):1139–45.
39. Kolt GS, Hume PA, Smith P, Williams MM. Effects of a stress-management program on injury and stress of competitive gymnasts. *Percept Mot Skills.* 2004;99(1):195–207.
40. Kolt GS, Kirkby RJ. Epidemiology of injury in elite and subelite female gymnasts: a comparison of retrospective and prospective findings. *Br J Sports Med.* 1999;33(5):312–8.
41. Leglise M. Limits on young gymnast's involvement in high-level sport. *Technique.* 1998;18:8–14.
42. Lindholm C, Hagenfeldt K, Ringertz BM. Pubertal development in elite juvenile gymnasts. Effects of physical training. *Acta Obstet Gynecol Scand.* 1994;73(3):269–73.
43. Lindner KJ, Caine DJ. Injury patterns of female competitive club gymnasts. *Can J Sport Sci.* 1990;15(4):254–61.
44. Loucks AB, Verdun M, Heath EM. Low energy availability, not stress of exercise, alters LH pulsatility in exercising women. *J Appl Physiol.* 1998; 84(1):37–46.

45. Mackie SJ, Taunton JE. Injuries in female gymnasts. Trends suggest prevention tactics. *Phys Sportsmed*. 1994;22:40–5.

46. Maffulli N, Chan D, Aldridge MJ. Derangement of the articular surfaces of the elbow in young gymnasts. *J Pediatr Orthop*. 1992;12(3):344–50.

47. Marini M, Sgambati E, Barni E, Piazza M, Monaci M. Pain syndromes in competitive elite level female artistic gymnasts. Role of specific preventive-compensatory activity. *Ital J Anat Embryol*. 2008;113(1):47–54.

48. Marshall SW, Covassin T, Dick R, Nassar LG, Agel J. Descriptive epidemiology of collegiate women's gymnastics injuries: National Collegiate Athletic Association Injury Surveillance System, 1988–1989 through 2003–2004. *J Athl Train*. 2007;42(2):234–40.

49. Martinsen M, Bratland-Sanda S, Eriksson AK, Sundgot-Borgen J. Dieting to win or to be thin? A study of dieting and disordered eating among adolescent elite athletes and non-athlete controls. *Br J Sports Med*. 2010;44(1):70–6.

50. McAuley E, Hudash G, Shields K, et al. Injuries in women's gymnastics. The state of the art. *Am J Sports Med*. 1987;15(6):558–65.

51. McCleary MD, Congeni JA. Current concepts in the diagnosis and treatment of spondylolysis in young athletes. *Curr Sports Med Rep*. 2007;6(1):62–6.

52. McNitt-Gray JL. Gymnastics. In: Garrett WE, Lester GE, McGowan J, et al., editors. *Women's Health in Sports and Exercise*. Rosemont (IL): AAOS; 2001. p. 209–28.

53. Mellion MB, Walsh WM, Shelton GL. Gymnastics. In: Mellion MB, Walsh WM, Shelton GL, editors. *The Team Physician's Handbook*. 2nd ed. Philadelphia: Hanley & Belfus; 1997. p. 770.

54. Moeller JL, Rifat SF. Spondylolysis in active adolescents: expediting return to play. *Phys Sportmed*. 2001;29(12):27–32.

55. Mohtadi N, Grant J. Managing anterior cruciate ligament deficiency in the skeletally immature individual: a systematic review of the literature. *Clin J Sport Med*. 2006;16(6):457–64.

56. National Center for Catastrophic Sports Injury Research. *National Center for Catastrophic Sports Injury Research – Twenty-Fifth Annual Report: Fall of 1982 – Spring of 2007* [Internet]. [cited 2008 August 14]. Available from: http://www.unc.edu/depts/nccsi/AllSports.htm

57. National Collegiate Athletic Association 1993–94 men's and women's gymnastics injury surveillance system. *NCAA Report*. Kansas City (KS): National Collegiate Athletic Association; 1994.

58. Nattiv A, Loucks AB, Manore MM, et al. American College of Sports Medicine position stand. The female athlete triad. *Med Sci Sports Exerc*. 2007;39(10):1867–82.

59. Nattiv A, Mandelbaum BR. Injuries and special concerns in female gymnasts. *Phys Sport Med* [Internet]. 1993 [cited 2003 May 14];21:66–82. NCAA Online: Available from: http://www.ncaa.org!sports3cience.

60. NCAA Sports Sponsorship and Participation Rates Report: 1981–2007 [Internet]. [cited 2010 December 20]. Available from: http://www.ncaapublications.com/productdownloads/PR2008.pdf

61. Ogden JA, Ganey TM, Hill JD, Jaakkola JI. Sever's injury: a stress fracture of the immature calcaneal metaphysis. *J Pediatr Orthop*. 2004;24(5):488–92.

62. Ott SM. Gymnastics. In: Ireland ML, Nattiv A, editors. *The Female Athlete*. Philadelphia (PA): Saunders; 2002. p. 669.

63. Petrie TA. Psychosocial antecedents of athletic injury: the effects of life stress and social support on female collegiate gymnasts. *Behav Med*. 1992;18(3):127–38.

64. Petrie TA, Stoever S. The incidence of bulimia nervosa and pathogenic weight control behaviors in female collegiate gymnasts. *Res Q Exerc Sport*. 1993;64(2):238–41.

65. Pettrone FA, Ricciardelli E. Gymnastics injuries: the Virginia experience 1982–1983. *Am J Sports Med*. 1987;15(1):59–62.

66. Propst AM, Thorp JM Jr. Traumatic vulvar hematomas: conservative versus surgical management. *South Med J*. 1998;91(2):144–6.

67. Robinson TL, Snow-Harter C, Taaffe DR, Gillis D, Shaw J, Marcus R. Gymnasts exhibit higher bone mass than runners despite similar prevalence of amenorrhea and oligomenorrhea. *J Bone Miner Res*. 1995;10(1):26–35.

68. Rosen DS, Hough DO. Pathogenic weight-control behavior of female college gymnasts. *Phys Sportsmed*. 1988;16:141–4.

69. Samuelson M, Reider B, Weiss D. Griplock injuries to the forearm in male gymnasts. *Am J Sports Med*. 1996;24(1):15–8.

70. Sands WA. Injury prevention in women's gymnastics. *Sports Med*. 2000;30(5):359–73.

71. Sands WA, Shultz BB, Newman AP. Women's gymnastics injuries. A 5-year study. *Am J Sports Med*. 1993;21(2):271–6.

72. Schiff M, Caine D, O'Halleron R. Injury prevention in sports. *Am J Lifestyle Med*. 2010;4:42–64.

73. Singer KM, Roy SP. Osteochondrosis of the humeral capitellum. *Am J Sports Med*. 1984;12(5):351–60.

74. Singh S, Smith GA, Fields SK, McKenzie LB. Gymnastics-related injuries to children treated in emergency departments in the United States, 1990–2005. *Pediatrics*. 2008;121(4):e954–60.

75. Steele VA, White JA. Injury prediction in female gymnasts. *Br J Sports Med*. 1986;20(1):31–3.

76. Tofler IR, Stryer BK, Micheli LJ, Herman LR. Physical and emotional problems of elite female gymnasts. *N Engl J Med*. 1996;335(4):281–3.

77. Tsai L, Wredmark T. Spinal posture, sagittal mobility, and subjective rating of back problems in former elite gymnasts. *Spine (Phila Pa 1976)*. 1993;18(7):872–5.

78. USA Gymnastics Online [Internet]. [cited 2010 December 20]. Available from: http://www.usa-gymnastics.org/pages/aboutus/pages/about_usag.html

79. Wadley GH, Albright JP. Women's intercollegiate gymnastics. Injury patterns and "permanent" medical disability. *Am J Sports Med*. 1993; 21(2):314–20.

Ice Hockey Injuries

Peter H. Seidenberg

95

INTRODUCTION

- Ice hockey is an extremely fast-paced, high-contact game that requires the mastery of many skills (22,49). Many of these skills (skating, stick handling, body checking, shooting, and goal tending) are unique to the sport (41).
- The sport dates back to the 1850s, with formal rules first established in Canada in 1881 (48).
- It is a National Collegiate Athletic Association (NCAA), international, and Olympic sport that made its debut in the Antwerp Olympic Games in 1920 (48).
- It is increasing in popularity yearly in the United States. During the 2009–2010 season, there were 580,714 registered players, coaches, and officials in USA Hockey. This includes 61,612 girls' and women's players (48).
  - USA Hockey is the governing body for amateur hockey in the United States.
- Women are active participants in all roles in ice hockey (22,48).
  - Females were involved in Canada as early as 1892.
  - The International Ice Hockey Federation coordinated women's world ice hockey tournaments in 1992, 1994, and 1997, and it first appeared as a medal sport in the 1998 Olympic Games.
  - Today, the NCAA considers female ice hockey an emerging sport, and USA Hockey registrants include 42,292 female players and 1,684 exclusive women's teams.
  - Many women are playing on men's teams, even up to the minor league level.
- The physician providing medical care for ice hockey athletes needs to be proficient in treating a wide variety of traumatic and atraumatic problems that range in severity from mild to life threatening.

EQUIPMENT

- All leagues now require helmets, which should fit snugly and use a four-point fit (like football helmets) (22,49).
  - The hockey helmet must be able to withstand low-mass, high-velocity impacts from the puck and high-mass, low-velocity forces from running into the boards (6).
- USA Hockey recommends the use of Hockey Equipment Certification Council (HECC)–approved helmets, full face masks, and full mouthpieces for all players during both practices and games (14,49).
- The mouthpiece should be internal and should cover all the remaining teeth of one jaw. It is required to be colored (not clear) in age 19 and under leagues. A form-fitting mouthpiece is recommended (49).
  - International play does not require mouthpieces; however, they are still highly encouraged (22).
  - The purpose of mouthguards is to protect dentition (23).
  - They may also prevent or decrease the severity of concussion (6,20,23), although this is controversial.
- Full face masks are mandatory for all youth and college leagues (49) and are slowly gaining popularity on the professional level.
- Kevlar throat protectors are required in many leagues and countries (22).
- Gloves, elbow pads, shin pads, shoulder pads, hip pads or padded hockey pants, and protective cup are recommended (49).
  - There has been a recent trend of wearing hockey gloves with shorter cuffs for the purpose of allowing increased wrist motion (22).
    - This may be at the cost of increased risk of wrist and forearm injury.
  - Hockey pants have padding to protect from the hips to the top of the knees (22,49).
  - Shin pads should cover from the top of the knees to the ankles (22).
- All protective equipment except helmets, face masks, padded hockey gloves, padded hockey pants, and goalie leg pads are worn under the uniform (49).
- Goalkeeper protective equipment (49)
  - Blocker worn on stick hand.
  - Trapper glove worn on the nonstick hand. Looks similar to a baseball mitt with protective padding extending up the forearm.
  - Leg guards up to 12 inches in width on each leg.
  - Full masks are required. Form-fitting masks are not recommended and are illegal except in adult leagues. Use in adults requires signing a waiver.

- Approved HECC helmets are required unless the above form-fitting mask includes a back skull plate.
  - Throat protector
  - Chest protector
  - Cup
  - Goalie skates
- Skates have a protective heel tip (not required for the goalie)(49).
  - Probably the most important piece of equipment used by the hockey player (13).
  - Speed skates are prohibited (49).
  - Many players prefer leather skates that have external plastic shields for ankle support and protection (18).
  - Athletes usually prefer ice skates to be snugly fit and may not wear socks so as to improve the feel of the ice (22).
- The puck is made of vulcanized rubber and weighs between 5.5 and 6.0 ounces. It is 1 inch thick and 3 inches in diameter (49).
  - For midget league play, a 4.0- to 4.5-ounce puck is recommended.
- Equipment that is in poor repair or that has been altered for the purpose of causing harm to other players is prohibited. Use of such equipment results in penalization of the offending player (49).

PHYSIOLOGY OF ICE HOCKEY

- Skating during a game involves repeated accelerations, decelerations, turning, and stopping (18,41).
- The players skate forward, backward, and side to side, often with sudden changes in direction (18,41).
- During competition, players will typically work at $> 70\%$ of their $\dot{V}O_{2max}$ with a substantial amount of play at $> 90\%$ $\dot{V}O_{2max}$ (16,18).
  - However, with the frequent stoppage of play per shift (on average 2–3) and with 3–4 minutes of rest between shifts, the resulting mean $\dot{V}O_2$ consumed per game is 55%–66% of maximum.
- Players can lose 4.5–6.5 pounds via sweat per game (41).
- If games are played in consecutive days, glycogen stores are often not replenished (41).
- Elite ice hockey players average 10% body fat (41).
- Physiologic differences by position (41)
  - Energy expenditure
    - Playing time
    - Goalies have the least number of substitutions and may play an entire game.
    - Defensemen have more playing time than forwards and typically have less rest time between shifts.
    - Goal tending requires quick, short explosive movements interspersed with periods of relative rest.

- High reliance on adenosine triphosphate (ATP)–phosphocreatine system.
- Forwards and defensemen have a high reliance on both glycolytic and aerobic metabolism.
- During games, adult forwards and defensemen skate greater than 4 miles.
- Energy expenditure is one-third aerobic and two-thirds anaerobic; postgame lactate increases over eight times the pregame level.
- Forwards have greater anaerobic activity and typically skate faster than defensemen or goalies.
- Despite the above differences by position, muscle fiber composition remains equivalent between positions.
- Flexibility (41)
  - Goalkeepers are significantly more flexible than forwards or defensemen.
  - Forwards and defensemen have been found to have equal flexibility.
- Shooting (4,5,41)
  - Properly coordinated acceleration and deceleration of motion of body segments produces maximal velocity.
  - Motion is concentrated in the lower arm.
  - However, maximal velocity is produced through maximal use and full rotation of the trunk.
  - Accuracy of the shot is enhanced via trunk stabilization and restricted use of body segments.

EPIDEMIOLOGY OF INJURIES

- Ice hockey is classified as a collision sport by the American Academy of Pediatrics (39).
- There are many opportunities for injury in this aggressive, fast-paced sport.
  - Contact/collision occurs with the hard ice surface, unpadded boards, goal posts, equipment from other players (skate blades, sticks), the puck, and the bodies and, at times, fists of opponents (41).
    - In elite hockey, the puck can travel at speeds up to 120 miles per hour, producing impact forces $> 1,250$ pounds.
    - Professional players can skate at speeds up to 30 miles per hour.
    - Sliding on the ice after a fall can occur at speeds up to 15 miles per hour.
- Fatigue appears to be a risk factor for injury (28,31,42,43).
- Equipment that is in poor repair also places the athlete at increased risk for injury; however, even when adequate protection is worn, injury is still possible. Studies have found that 58% of injuries occur on body parts that were covered with protective equipment (31).

- Overall injury rates
  - Aggregation of injury data is limited by varying definitions and methods for reporting in the literature.
  - Data from injuries presenting to U.S. emergency departments demonstrate the following distribution of injury location (15,21):
    - Upper extremity: 36.0%–43.8%
    - Head: 12.3%–16.3%
    - Lower extremity: 16.1%–19.1%
    - Trunk: 9.3%–13.8%
    - Face: 10.0%–23.0%
    - The above data are limited by the fact that not all ice hockey injuries result in a visit to the local emergency department.
  - Overall injury rate is 5.6 injuries per 1,000 player-hours (1.5 per 1,000 hours in practice, 54 per 1,000 hours in games) (31). Due to difficulty quantifying player-hours, many studies will instead describe injury rates per athletic exposure.
  - Injury is more common in the game setting (76%) than in practice (23%), even though practice represents significantly more time. Injuries are thus 5–25 times more common in game settings (1–3,31,43).
  - Acute and traumatic injures account for 85% of injuries, whereas overuse injuries represent 15% of all injuries (47).
  - Approximately 16% of injures are related to rule infractions (31).
  - During games, Pelletier et al. (36) found that 27.1% of injuries occurred during the first period, 35.6% occurred during the second period, and 26.6% occurred during the third period. In contrast, other investigators suggest that third-period injuries are roughly equal to first- and second-period injuries combined (31) or that injures are twice as common in the third period (43).
- Age-specific injury rates: Injuries appear to increase with increasing age, with a peak in early adulthood (Table 95.1).
- Studies suggest that injury rates in youth hockey show a dramatic increase during the first year that body checking is permitted, regardless of the age that checking is instituted (27,51).

Table 95.1	Injury Rates by Age of Athlete (43)	
	Rate of Injury per 1,000 Player-Hours	
Age of Athlete	**Practice Time**	**Game Time**
Youth		
Squirt (age 9–10)	1.2	0
Pee Wee (age 11–12)	2.2	0
Bantam (age 13–14)	2.5	10.9
Junior A (age 17–19)	3.9	96.1
Intercollegiate (age 18–21)	2.3	84.3
Swedish Elite (age 19–33)	1.4	78.4

- Mechanisms of injuries
  - Collisions — 14%–65% of all injuries, with one study showing that 29% are caused by unintentional or accidental collisions. The majority of collisions that resulted in injury involved player-to-player contact, whereas collisions with the boards only account for roughly 10% of all injuries (1,2,25,26,28,31,40–43,47).
  - Puck — 3%–20% of injuries (25,26,28,31,36,40–43,47). Puck velocity may reach 120 miles per hour at professional levels.
  - Stick — 8%–29% of injuries (31,36,43). It should be noted that many of the injuries caused by the stick are to the face, the majority of which may be prevented with proper protective gear.
  - Skate — 5%–11% of injuries, often related to lacerations from sharp steel blades (25,26,43)
  - Fighting — 3%–6.5% of injuries (37,43)
  - Overuse — 14.6% (47)
  - Falls — 4%–7% (31,43)
  - Foul play or illegal play — 9%–16% (31)
  - Noncontact injuries — 2.2% (36)
- Type of injury (15,36)
  - Sprain/strain — 16.9%–42.3%
    - Average number of days lost from play due to sprains = 13.61
  - Contusion — 21.0%–23.6%
  - Laceration —13.0%–27%
  - Fracture — 10.2%–17.3%
    - Average number of days lost from play due to fractures = 22.22
  - Concussion — 7%–7.5%
  - General trauma — 5.9%
- Rates of injury per anatomic site are listed in Table 95.2.

Table 95.2	Anatomic Location of Hockey Injuries (36)
Anatomic Site of Injury	**Percentage of Total Injuries Reported**
Head and neck	10.6%
Face, eye, ear, jaw, teeth	17.6%
Shoulder and clavicle	14.9%
Chest and back	4.8%
Arm, elbow	3.7%
Forearm, wrist, hand	6.9%
Hip, groin, abdomen	6.4%
Hamstring, thigh	9.0%
Knee	18.6%
Ankle	3.2%
Foot	1.6%

- Injuries related to position on ice (31)
  - Goalkeeper — 5.8%
  - Defensemen — 31.2%
  - Center — 18.5%
  - Wing — 36.0%
  - Missing position data — 8.5%
  - However, position played has no statistical relationship to days lost from an injury.
- Injuries by sex: NCAA injury data analysis shows the following differences between injury rates in male versus female ice hockey athletes (1–3):
  - Rate of injury in games was eight (males) and five (females) times higher than in practice.
  - Preseason practice injury rates were approximately twice those of in-season practice injury rates (males and females).
  - Most common injuries in games:
    - Male = knee internal derangement (13.5%), concussion (9.0%), acromioclavicular joint injury (8.9%)
    - Female = concussion (21.6%), knee internal derangement (12.9%), acromioclavicular joint injury (6.8%)
  - Most common injuries in practice:
    - Male = pelvis and hip strain (13.1%), knee internal derangement (10.1%), ankle ligament sprains (5.5%)
    - Female = concussion (13.2%), pelvis and hip strains (12.0%), foot contusion (7.2%)
  - More research is needed to determine why women hockey players have a higher rate of concussion than men.

INJURIES BY LOCATION

- **Ocular:** Thirty-eight to 47% of sports-related eye injuries occur in hockey (35).
  - Most common injuries are soft tissue (34%), hyphema (27%), other intraocular injuries (23%), corneal damage (9%), orbital fracture (4%), and ruptured globes (3%).
  - Pashby (35) found that approximately 15% of all eye-injured hockey athletes were left with an injury resulting in a legally blind eye.
  - However, 58% of these injuries would have been preventable with face shields.
- **Concussions:** Management should be as in any other sport. No concussed athlete should be allowed to return to competition.
  - Hockey players sustain head trauma and impact forces from axial loading in a similar mechanism as football players (14).
  - Unlike football, the hockey athlete is also at risk for traumatic brain injury through contact with the hockey puck, which as previously mentioned can reach speeds up to 120 miles per hour (41).

- Concussions account for 7.5% of all hockey injuries (36).
  - This percentage is likely underestimated, because many injury-reporting studies have only looked at injuries that have resulted in time lost from play (25,26,47). Additionally, it is suggested that, especially in youth hockey organizations, there is a trend of underreporting concussion (52). As such, many concussions may not have been identified.
- Benson et al. (10) included mild concussions in their head and neck injury study and found a concussion incidence of 1.53–1.57 per 1,000 athlete exposures.
- National Hockey League (NHL) studies have found the concussion rate to be 1.04–1.81 per 1,000 athlete exposures (50).
- NCAA data show a concussion rate of 0.72 per 1,000 athlete exposures for men and 0.82 per 1,000 athlete exposures for women (3).
- Emergency department data suggest that the percentage of traumatic brain injuries increases as age decreases (15,21).
- **Maxillofacial:** When abrasions and lacerations are excluded, maxillofacial trauma represents 11.5% of hockey injuries (40).
  - Blows from the stick represent 54.1% of maxillofacial and dental injuries, whereas contact with the puck only represents 14.2% of injuries to this same area (40).
  - Of these injuries, 69.9% occur during games with the remainder occurring during practice sessions (40).
  - Injury to teeth and alveolar processes represents 84.5% of injuries (40).
  - Ice hockey accounts for roughly 40% of all sports-related dental injuries (19).
  - Maxillofacial injuries have been drastically reduced since the introduction of mandatory face masks in many levels of the sport (40).
  - Of the previously reported facial injuries, 47% may have been preventable through the use of protective visors (25,26).
  - Studies have shown that the use of helmets with face masks significantly reduces (but does not completely eliminate) the incidence of facial lacerations (Table 95.3) (10,24,33).

Table 95.3	Rate of Hockey-Induced Facial Lacerations (10,24–26,33)	
Situation	**Number of Facial Lacerations per 1,000 Player-Hours**
Game play, no face mask	70.0
Game play, with face mask	14.7–15.1
Practice, no face mask	21.8
Practice, with face mask	0.0–0.2

- Despite face masks, facial lacerations still occur, and the team physician should be prepared to evaluate and repair these injuries appropriately.
- **Cervical spine**
  - The number of catastrophic cervical spine injuries in ice hockey is low compared to other sports; however, the incidence per 1,000 participants is relatively high (32).
  - The effect of helmet and face mask use on cervical spine injury is controversial.
    - ❑ After the increased use of helmets with face masks in ice hockey, there retrospectively appeared to be an increasing incidence of cervical spine injury. Several investigators hypothesize that this is caused as a result of the player wearing a helmet adopting a more aggressive style of play, resulting in more cervical injury. It has been proposed that the protective devices have also altered how officials perceive game situations, leading them to be more lenient in penalization. The net result has been an increase in illegal and injurious behaviors, such as checking from behind (an activity associated with catastrophic cervical spine injury) (33,37).
    - ❑ However, the prospective study by LaPrade et al. (24) of intercollegiate athletes and face mask use showed no increase in head and neck injuries (24).
  - Mechanism of injury is axial loading caused by a blow to the head from collision with the boards, other players, the ice, or the goal post (44).
  - The majority of these injuries occurred when the injured player was checked from behind, throwing the athlete horizontally into the boards (45).
  - Many of the reported cervical spine injuries were a result of either illegal play or high-risk aggressive behavior. New rules have been instituted by both the Canadian Amateur Hockey Association and USA Hockey in an attempt to reduce the number of spinal cord injuries. These new rules have moved the action away from the boards and restricted checking; preliminary results appear successful in limiting the incidence of complete spinal cord injuries (45,46).
  - During the management of a cervical spine–injured athlete, the physician may carefully remove the helmet if necessary. As opposed to football, the shoulder pads of hockey are much less bulky, and the unhelmeted hockey player's cervical spine can still be easily stabilized with shoulder pads in place.
- **Shoulder:** Clavicle fractures, acromioclavicular joint separations, and glenohumeral subluxation/dislocation are relatively common in ice hockey (8,9,30). They usually are high-velocity injuries that result from the shoulder being driven into the boards following aggressive body checks.
- **Elbow:** A player who does not wear elbow pads may receive a traumatic olecranon bursitis and/or elbow fracture during collision with the ice or the boards.

- **Wrist, hand:**
  - When hockey players fight (which occurs frequently at higher levels of play), the gloves are typically thrown down, and blows are exchanged using bare hands. The typical street fighter hand injuries can then occur.
  - Gamekeeper's thumb (ulnar collateral ligament injury) has been reported (41) and is typically due to the player's thumb being hyperabducted when the stick handle is suddenly forced toward the body during a collision with the boards.
  - Wartenberg syndrome (34): In hockey, direct trauma to the superficial radial nerve at the wrist can occur when an opponent strikes the distal forearm with the stick. The athlete will complain of pain and/or paresthesias shooting up the thumb and dorsal wrist in a radial distribution. Players who use gloves with shorter cuffs (so as to increase wrist mobility) are at increased risk for this injury.
  - Scaphoid fracture: Mechanism of injury usually is fall on outstretched hand or a dorsiflexed wrist colliding with the boards. The gloves provide some protection against this injury.
- **Chest:** Commotio cordis has been reported in youth ice hockey. League organizers and physicians should consider having an automated external defibrillator (AED) available at the rink because there is a 16% survival with rapid defibrillation (29).
- **Back:**
  - Back strain and sprain — Players skate in a forward flexed position. This position, combined with the frequent trunk rotation that accompanies shooting and passing, can place the player at risk for these injuries.
  - Spondylolysis has been reported in ice hockey athletes.
- **Abdomen:**
  - Because of the abrupt and sudden changes in movement, hockey players are at risk for abdominal muscle strain (22,41).
  - Athletes can sustain traumatic abdominal injury, especially when the handle of the stick is forced into the abdomen during a collision into the boards (which is typically the result of illegal checking).
- **Thigh, groin:**
  - Anterior thigh hematomas may occur as a result of collision with the boards or of blocking a shot puck. These hematomas are at risk for myositis ossificans (41), and treatment should be directed at preventing this complication.
    - ❑ If the hematoma is identified immediately after the game, the athlete can be placed in fixed knee flexion for 24 hours in an attempt to tamponade the bleeding, thereby decreasing the size of the hematoma.
    - ❑ Old hematomas should not be passively stretched, as this may increase the risk of myositis ossificans.

- Adductor strains are common enough that studies have been performed in an attempt to determine if certain players are at increased risk for this injury and to ascertain what prevention measures can be implemented in an attempt to decrease lost playing time. Hockey players are at risk for this injury as a result of the explosive starts and changes in direction (22).

- Osteitis pubis has also been reported in hockey players. There is thought to be an increased risk for this disorder due to abrupt and sudden changes in movement.

- **Knee:** Most common significant lower extremity injury.
  - Although anterior cruciate ligament (ACL) and meniscal injury has been reported, medial collateral ligament (MCL) injury is 14 times more common (31).
  - The ACL appears to be spared because the foot does not lock in position on the ice.
  - The mechanisms for MCL injury are both contact and noncontact valgus stress to the knee.

- **Ankle:** Ankle sprain — Mechanism of injury is dorsiflexion, eversion, and external rotation (43), producing deltoid ligament sprain.
  - This is in contrast to most other sports where the typical mechanism is plantarflexion, inversion, and internal rotation, producing lateral ligament (especially anterior talofibular ligament) injury.
  - The mechanism of injury also places the hockey athlete at risk for syndesmotic injury and Maisonneuve fracture (due to transmittal of the force out through the fibula).
  - Ankle sprains result in 10% of major injuries in ice hockey (defined as absence from sport > 28 days) (31).
  - In an attempt to prevent these debilitating injuries, many hockey players prefer skates that have added external ankle support (18).
  - Boot lace lacerations — The ice skate blade is essentially a 10- to 12-inch scalpel. The anterior ankle is at risk for laceration of tendons and neurovascular structures because of its proximity to the skates of others. A relatively small laceration can cause damage to these underlying superficial structures (44).
    - However, most athletes are relatively protected from this injury because of the thickly padded skate tongue over the anterior ankle. Athletes who turn their skate tongue downward (out of personal preference) place themselves at increased risk.

- **Foot:** Lace bite (18,22) is nagging dorsal foot pain and/or paresthesias.
  - Players often do not wear socks and prefer tight-fitting skates because this is thought by athletes to improve performance and speed on the ice. The compression of the laces in such situations can cause extensor tendon and nerve injuries of the dorsum of the foot.
  - To prevent this injury, the tongue of the boot should remain in a neutral position.

MEDICAL ILLNESSES

- Indoor ice rinks have ice-resurfacing machines, commonly referred to as Zambonis, that are gas or propane powered. The emissions from the machine coupled with poor ventilation can create increased carbon monoxide levels on the ice.

- Nitrogen dioxide–induced lung injury and other indoor air quality syndromes

- Cold-induced vasomotor rhinitis (7,11)
  - Profuse watery rhinorrhea that typically begins within minutes of skating on the ice. It is thought to be the result of an overly sensitive cholinergic reflex in response to exposure to cold air and changes in humidity.
  - The athlete has little nasal itching, ocular pruritus, or sneezing, but increased nasal secretions, postnasal drip, sinus headaches, anosmia, and sinusitis are common.
  - It is a diagnosis of exclusion. Rhinitis caused by infection, allergy, anatomic abnormalities, and eosinophilia should first be ruled out.
  - Many athletes self-medicate with decongestants for this disorder; however, this category of medicines is on the banned substances list for the International Olympic Committee (IOC). There has been some promise in treating this disorder with ipratropium bromide nasal spray, a medication that is not on the prohibited list.

PREVENTION

- Youth hockey programs need to educate players, coaches, and parents of the importance of knowing and following the rules (39).

- Body checking should not be allowed in youth hockey for children ages 15 and under (12,39).

- Fair-play rules should be used to decrease the incidence of injury in youth hockey. This system gives teams credit for sportsmanship in the final standings of league and tournament play. Teams have points added to their totals for staying under a preestablished limit of penalties per game, whereas teams that rely on intimidation and foul play have points subtracted. Implementation of this style of play was shown to reduce the number of high school hockey injuries (38).

- Players, coaches, parents, and officials should be educated on the dangers of checking another player from behind (39).

- The officials and coaches should be encouraged to strictly enforce the rules against illegal body checking.
  - These forms of checking include boarding, charging, checking from behind, cross-checking, elbowing, and roughing.

- Contact with an opposing player made above the shoulder using the fist, forearm, elbow, shoulder, knee, or stick must be penalized. If such an act was deliberate, the stiffest sanctions should be used.

- Deliberate attempts to injure other players are illegal and should be heavily penalized.
- Rules against high sticking should be strictly enforced.
  - Frequently occurs during a slap shot or when attempting to bat down airborne puck
    - During a slap shot, it is considered high sticking if the stick comes above the level of the waist on the back swing; slap shots are illegal in midget play.
    - Batting a puck down with the stick above the shoulders is also considered high sticking.
- Fighting needs to be discouraged by officials, coaches, players, and players' parents.
- Players should be encouraged or mandated to wear helmets with full-coverage face masks at any level of play for both game and practice situations.
- Ensure adequate ventilation and monitoring of air quality in indoor ice rinks.
- The medical team providing coverage for ice hockey should have the availability of medical equipment for the stabilization of potentially devastating injury at the ice rink. This should include a spine board, cervical collar, and cardiopulmonary resuscitation equipment (17). The logistics of how to get this equipment to the injured athlete on the ice should be preestablished. The emergency plan should be in place and practiced prior to the beginning of the season so that in the event of a devastating injury, morbidity due to delay in stabilization can be reduced.

REFERENCES

1. Agel J, Dick R, Nelson B, Marshall SW, Dompier TP. Descriptive epidemiology of collegiate women's ice hockey injuries: National Collegiate Athletic Association Injury Surveillance System, 2000–2001 through 2003–2004. *J Athl Train.* 2007;42(2):249–54.

2. Agel J, Dompier TP, Dick R, Marshall SW. Descriptive epidemiology of collegiate men's ice hockey injuries: National Collegiate Athletic Association Injury Surveillance System, 1988–1989 through 2003–2004. *J Athl Train.* 2007;42(2):241–8.

3. Agel J, Harvey EJ. A 7-year review of men's and women's ice hockey injuries in the NCAA. *Can J Surg.* 2010;53(5):319–23.

4. Alexander JF, Drake CJ, Reichenback PJ Haddow JB. Effect of strength development on speed of shooting in varsity ice hockey players. *Res Q.* 1964;35:101–6.

5. Alexander JF, Haddow JB, Schultz GA. Comparison of the ice hockey wrist and slap shots for speed and accuracy. *Res Q.* 1963;34:259–66.

6. Arheim DD, Prentice WE. Protective sports equipment. In: *Principles of Athletic Training.* Chicago (IL): Mosby Yearbook; 1996. p. 116.

7. Ayars G. Nonallergic rhinitis. *Immun and Allergy Clin.* 2000;20(2):179–92.

8. Bahr R, Bendiksen F, Engerbretsen L. Tis the season: diagnosing and managing ice hockey injuries. *J Musculoskel Med.* 1995;12(2):48–56.

9. Behrman RE, Kliegman R, Jenson HB. Bone and joint disorders: sports medicine. In: Behrman RE, Kliegman R, Jenson HB, editors. *Nelson Textbook of Pediatrics.* Philadelphia: WB Saunders; 2000. p. 2111.

10. Benson BW, Mohtadi NG, Rose MS, Meeuwisse WH. Head and neck injuries among ice hockey players wearing full face shields vs half face shields. *JAMA.* 1999;282(24):2328–32.

11. Bousquet J, Van Cauwenberge P, Bachert C, et al. Requirements for medications commonly used in the treatment of allergic rhinitis. European Academy of Allergy and Clinical Immunology (EAACI), Allergic Rhinitis and Its Impact on Asthma (ARIA). *Allergy.* 2003;58(3):192–7.

12. Brust JD. Children's ice hockey injuries. *Am J Dis Child.* 1992;146(6):741–7.

13. Clanton T, Wood R. Etiology of injury to the foot and ankle. In: DeLee JC, Drez D, Miller M, editors. *DeLee and Drez's Orthopaedic Sports Medicine.* Philadelphia (PA): Saunders; 2003. p. 2265–7.

14. Cross KM, Serenelli C. Training and equipment to prevent athletic head and neck injuries. *Clin Sports Med.* 2003;22(3):639–67.

15. Deits J, Yard EE, Collins CL, Fields SK, Comstock RD. Patients with ice hockey injuries presenting to US emergency departments, 1990–2006. *J Athl Train.* 2010;45(5):467–74.

16. Ferguson RJ, Marcotte GG, Montpetit RR. Maximal oxygen uptake test during ice skating. *Med Sci Sports Exerc.* 1969;1:207–11.

17. Ghiselli G, Schaadt G, McAllister DR. On-the-field evaluation of an athlete with a head or neck injury. *Clin Sports Med.* 2003;22(3):445–65.

18. Green H, Bishop P, Houston M, McKillop R, Norman R, Stothart P. Time-motion and physiological assessments of ice hockey performance. *J Appl Physiol.* 1976;40(2):159–63.

19. Häyrinen-Immonen R, Sane J, Perkki K, Malmström M. A six-year follow-up study of sports-related dental injuries in children and adolescents. *Endod Dent Traumatol.* 1990;6(5):208–12.

20. Hickey JC, Hickey JC, Morris AL, Carlson LD, Seward TE. The relation of mouth protectors to cranial pressure and deformation. *J Am Dent Assoc.* 1967;74(4):735–40.

21. Hostetler SG, Xiang H, Smith GA. Characteristics of ice hockey-related injuries treated in US emergency departments, 2001–2002. *Pediatrics.* 2004;114(6):e661–6.

22. Joyner D, Snouse S. Skiing, speed skating, ice hockey. In: Ireland M, Nattiv A, editors. *The Female Athlete.* Philadelphia: Saunders; 2002. p. 769–75.

23. Labella CR, Smith BW, Sigurdsson A. Effect of mouthguards on dental injuries and concussions in college basketball. *Med Sci Sports Exerc.* 2002;34(1):41–4.

24. LaPrade RF, Burnett QM, Zarzour R, Moss R. The effect of the mandatory use of face masks on facial lacerations and head and neck injuries in ice hockey. A prospective study. *Am J Sports Med.* 1995;23(6):773–5.

25. Lorentzon R, Wedrèn H, Pietilä T. Incidence, nature, and causes of ice hockey injuries. A three-year prospective study of a Swedish elite ice hockey team. *Am J Sports Med.* 1988;16(4):392–6.

26. Lorentzon R, Wedrèn H, Pietilä T, Gustavsson B. Injuries in international ice hockey. A prospective, comparative study of injury incidence and injury types in international and Swedish elite ice hockey. *Am J Sports Med.* 1988;16(4):389–91.

27. Macpherson A, Rothman L, Howard A. Body-checking rules and childhood injuries in ice hockey. *Pediatrics.* 2006;117(2):e143–7.

28. Mair SD, Seaber AV, Glisson RR, Garrett WE Jr. The role of fatigue in susceptibility to acute muscle strain injury. *Am J Sports Med.* 1996;24(2):137–43.

29. Maron BJ, Gohman TE, Kyle SB, Estes NA 3rd, Link MS. Clinical profile and spectrum of commotio cordis. *JAMA.* 2002;287(9):1142–6.

30. Minkoff J, Varoltta G, Simonson B. Ice hockey. In: Fu F, Stone D, editors. *Sports Injuries: Mechanisms-Prevention-Treatment.* Baltimore (MD): Williams & Wilkins; 1994. p. 397–444.

31. Mölsä J, Airaksinen O, Näsman O, Torstila I. Ice hockey injuries in Finland. A prospective epidemiologic study. *Am J Sports Med.* 1997;25(4):495–9.

32. Mueller FO, Cantu RC. *National Center for Catastrophic Sports Injury Research: Twentieth Annual Report, Fall 1982-Spring 2002.* Chapel Hill (NC): National Center for Catastrophic Sports Injury Research; 2002. p. 1–25.

33. Murray TM, Livingston LA. Hockey helmets, face masks, and injurious behavior. *Pediatrics.* 1995;95(3):419–21.

34. Nuber GW, Assenmacher J, Bowen MK. Neurovascular problems in the forearm, wrist, and hand. *Clin Sports Med.* 1998;17(3):585–610.

35. Pashby TJ. Ocular injuries in hockey. *Int Ophthalmol Clin.* 1988;28(3):228–31.

36. Pelletier RL, Montelpare WJ, Stark RM. Intercollegiate ice hockey injuries. A case for uniform definitions and reports. *Am J Sports Med.* 1993;21(1):78–81.

37. Reynen PD, Clancy WG Jr. Cervical spine injury, hockey helmets, and face masks. *Am J Sports Med.* 1994;22(2):167–70.

38. Roberts WO, Brust JD, Leonard B, Hebert BJ. Fair-play rules and injury reduction in ice hockey. *Arch Pediatr Adolesc Med.* 1996;150(2):140–5.

39. Safety in youth hockey: the effects of body checking. American Academy of Pediatrics. Committee on Sports Medicine and Fitness. *Pediatrics.* 2000;105(3 Pt 1):657–8.

40. Sane J, Ylipaavalniemi P, Leppänen H. Maxillofacial and dental ice hockey injuries. *Med Sci Sports Exerc.* 1988;20(2):202–7.

41. Sim FH, Simonet WT, Melton LJ 3rd, Lehn TA. Ice hockey injuries. *Am J Sports Med.* 1988;16(Suppl 1):S86–96.

42. Smith RW, Reischl SF. Metatarsophalangeal joint synovitis in athletes. *Clin Sports Med.* 1988;7(1):75–88.

43. Stuart MJ, Smith A. Injuries in Junior A ice hockey. A three-year prospective study. *Am J Sports Med.* 1995;23(4):458–61.

44. Tator CH. Neck injuries in ice hockey: a recent, unsolved problem with many contributing factors. *Clin Sports Med.* 1987;6(1):101–14.

45. Tator CH, Carson JD, Edmonds VE. Spinal injuries in ice hockey. *Clin Sports Med.* 1998;17(1):183–94.

46. Tator CH, Prowidenza C, Cassidy JD. Spinal injuries in Canadian ice hockey: an update to 2005. *Clin J Sports Med.* 2009;19(6):451–6.

47. Tegner Y, Lorentzon R. Ice hockey injuries: incidence, nature and causes. *Br J Sports Med.* 1991;25(2):87–9.

48. USA Hockey Web site [Internet]. 2011 [cited 2011 Sept 1]. Available from: http://www.usahockey.com.

49. USA Hockey: 2011–2013 Official Rules of Ice Hockey, from the USA Hockey Web site [Internet]. 2011 [cited 2011 Sept 1]. Available from: http://www.usahockey.com.

50. Wennberg RA, Tator CH. Concussion incidence and time lost from play in the NHL during the past ten years. *Can J Neurol Sci.* 2008;35(5):647–51.

51. Willer B, Kroetsch B, Darling S, Hutson A, Leddy J. Injury rates in house league, select, and representative youth hockey league. *Med Sci Sports Exerc.* 2005;37(10):1658–63.

52. Williamson IJ, Goodman D. Converging evidence for the under-reporting of concussions in youth ice hockey. *Br J Sports Med.* 2006;40(2):128–32.

Climbing Injuries, Treatment, and Injury Prevention

96

Katrina D. Warme and Winston J. Warme

BRIEF HISTORY OF CLIMBING

- Initially, climbing was about ascending the available summits. Mt. Everest, the tallest peak on the planet at 29,035 feet, finally succumbed to Sir Edmund Hillary and Tenzing Norgay in 1953. Subsequently, climbers turned their attention to the most difficult lines on mountains and often the most direct line (directissima) or the steepest, most sustained face. This desire to achieve increasingly technically difficult climbs led to focused and sport-specific training in preparation for climbing, rather than just maintaining good aerobic conditioning and overall fitness. Climbers took to the gyms and developed novel indoor training techniques. As time has progressed, these exercises and protocols have become more and more sophisticated. With the genesis of professional climbers (alpine guides, World Cup competitors, and sponsored climbers), athletes are able to climb and train for climbing full time. This has allowed for subspecialization in climbing, with subspecialists pushing the limits in each discipline.

EVOLUTION OF CLIMBING

- In the past 25 years, the sport of climbing has increased in its popularity, and the numbers of participants has greatly expanded. The stigma of climbers being a reckless fringe element of extreme risk takers has changed, and climbing has become more acceptable as its participants include a broad spectrum of the population from kids to executives. Females can often climb as well as men and make up about a quarter of the participants.
- With the advent of climbing gyms in populous cities, more people are introduced to climbing in a safe and supervised setting. The first climbing gym in the United States was established in Seattle in 1987. At the time of this writing, there are over 233 climbing gyms in the United States, not including those on college campuses, in camps, or in fitness clubs.

Many recreational (casual) climbers have joined the sport, and serious climbers are spending more time training.

- In 1989, the estimated number of active climbers in the United States was 100,000 (1). As of 2008, it estimated to be approaching 2 million.
- The sport of climbing is categorized into different subspecialties or disciplines:
  - **Bouldering:** Shorter routes, usually 15–20 feet in height, are undertaken without any ropes, usually to train more difficult moves. Thick foam pads are commonly placed below the route to cushion falls, and participants will often spot the climber.
  - **Traditional climbing:** Longer routes, 50 to several hundred feet in length, where the climber must use the features of the rock itself, such as a crack, to place protection. Initially, these were metal pitons that were hammered into cracks, which have largely been replaced with removable stoppers and camming devices. These are designed to resist pull out and shorten the climber's fall by catching the rope, which is secured by the belayer.
  - **Sport climbing:** Routes where protection such as bolts and anchors are already present in the rock face; makes protecting the climb easier. This approach allows the climber to push his physical limits more with more robust fixation available should a fall occur. Additionally, climbers can protect sheer walls without options for natural protection, opening up new and often challenging terrain to other climbers.
  - **Alpine climbing:** Climbing style where only the bare essentials are taken; usually describes longer endeavors (days to weeks) to reach the summits of mountains, and includes all the disciplines of climbing; rock climbing, ice climbing, and glacier travel are often carried out at high elevations and in severe weather conditions.
  - **Ice climbing:** A style of climbing that involves ascending ice formations, such as frozen waterfalls, icefalls, and rock faces that are covered in ice, using ice axes and crampons (spikes that are fastened to mountaineering boots). Ice screws (hollow metal tubes with threads) are placed into

the ice as the climber ascends. These are used to protect the climber as the rope can be clipped in, such that the belayer can catch a fall. This form of protection can be weak or strong depending on the quality of the ice.

- **Speed climbing:** A style of climbing where the ultimate goal is speed; often aspiring to break exisiting records. This is done to some degree in subspecialties, by a small elite percentage of climbers. Extra risks are taken to save time, such that this can be a very dangerous practice.

- **Solo climbing:** Also known as "soloing." A style of climbing without someone else belaying. There are four subcategories, listed in ascending level of risk:
  - ❏ Top-roping: climbing the rock with a fixed rope and with a self-locking device as back up should a fall occur.
  - ❏ Lead climbing alone with a rope and a self-locking device to stop a fall.
  - ❏ Deep-water soloing/psicobloc: climbing over water without a rope, using the water as a landing substrate to cushion falls.
  - ❏ Free solo climbing: climbing without a rope or other forms of protection.

- **Aid climbing:** A form of climbing where one inserts devices in the cracks in the rock to pull up on or to step up on rather that just using the rock itself to hold on to. Sometime aiders, or étriers (short stepladders made of webbing), are used to clip into the protection and then the climber can stand in them. This is a slow form of climbing that is very gear intensive. Often climbers will take haul bags full of gear and folding cot-like "portaledges" to sleep on during multiday ascents.

- Focused training: As climbers have become more subspecialized, they have developed different training techniques that allow for plyometric and dynamic movements, which can yield impressive strength gains but can also generate high loads and place climbers at greater risk of injury.
  - Bouldering:
    - ❏ John Gill: The father of modern bouldering, circa 1950s. He was a gymnast who eschewed concentrated gymnastic-type effort to overcome short climbs on boulders. He used gymnastic training techniques to increase strength, especially hand and core strength, for climbing (*e.g.,* one-finger one-arm pull-ups and front levers) and introduced the use of chalk (to improve the climbers grip) and dynamic movements to climbing.
  - Rock climbing:
    - ❏ Wolfgang Gullich: A German climber circa 1980s who pushed the limits and trained specifically in the off-season to be able to do certain climbs; invented the "campus board." This device is a series of holds placed horizontally a fixed distance one above the other on an overhanging piece of plywood. These rungs were of various widths, and this device was used to develop finger strength and the ability to develop "lock off," or

hold one's body at the top of a pull up with one hand. This built both strength and endurance for physically taxing climbs.
  - ❏ John Bachar: Very instrumental in the 1980s when he was pushing the limits of roped climbing in Yosemite and also began pushing the limits of soloing. As part of his training, he developed an upside-down rope ladder that he often climbed with weights to develop upper body strength and endurance, known as the "Bachar ladder."
  - ❏ Chris Sharma: Probably still the top rock climber today, amazingly staying at the forefront of rock climbing for over 10 years, and has pushed technical difficulties into the 5.15a/b range, along with other climbers. (See rating scale below.)
  - ❏ Climbing difficulty has a variety of rating schemes; the Yosemite Decimal System most commonly used in this country rates a climb as 5.0 where a rope should be used or a serious fall could occur. A 5.4 or 5.5 climb could be done by most athletes, but after that, practice, composure and sports-specific strength are needed. Serious experienced climbers climb in the 5.10–5.12 range with subdivisions of a, b, c, and d separating climbing difficulty above 5.10. A very select few climbers ever manage to climb above 5.13.
- Mountaineering:
  - ❏ Reinhold Messner: A German visionary for traveling fast and light in the mountains; he renounced the conventional siege approach to the biggest mountain and made his mark in the 1970s and 1980s as the first to summit all of the 8,000-meter peaks. He was not afraid to climb these peaks solo and without supplemental oxygen and was renowned for his hardcore "deprivation training" to prepare him physically and psychologically for the rigors of climbing in the "death zone." This term is used to describe the region above an altitude of 26,000 feet or 8,000 meters where the human body cannot adapt or acclimatize, such that the human body cannot survive here for more than a few days (10).
  - ❏ Ueli Steck: Took a scientific approach to training at a new level in the 21st century and brought speed climbing to the high mountains. Known for speed ascents of the Trilogy of North Faces of the Alps (Eiger, Grand Jorasses, and Matterhorn), each in under 3 hours, as well as similar exploits in the Himalayas.

INJURIES

- Because of the extreme nature of the sport, injuries in climbing are common, and around half of all climbers surveyed in one study had sustained an injury within the last year (11). Throughout several studies conducted, overuse injuries were found to be the most prevalent of all climbing injuries.

Overuse injuries accounted for 93% of injuries reported, and 28% of climbers reported at least one such injury (2). Dedicated and experienced climbers are more susceptible to overuse injuries, whereas casual and new climbers more often experience fall-related injuries (11,15). Contributing risk factors associated with increase in injuries include climbing frequency and technical difficulty (2,11).

- Rock climbing has a spectrum of sport-specific injuries, almost half involving the wrist and hand (12). Understanding these injuries, the types of training techniques, and the obsession of many climbers to train can help physicians deliver optimal care and advice in an appropriate way such that their patients will have the best chance of healing and preventing further injury.

- "A series of repetitive high torque movements of the upper limbs are needed to ascend a wall or rock face. These movements subject the hand and wrist to large forces, potentially resulting in ligament and tendon sprains or rupture" (12). Contrary to popular belief, descending is not more risky than ascending; 69% of injuries occur during ascending (1).

- Injuries in rock climbers are common. During their climbing career, 83%–89% of climbers reported a history of least one acute injury symptomatic for 10 days or more (7). "These acute injuries are mainly the result of a sudden tendon/ligament strain or a fall, with almost half occurring while training and two-thirds during the ascent. Overuse injuries are also common and occur in more than 40% of indoor rock climbers. Hand and wrist injuries account for almost half of all acute climbing injuries" (12).

- **Accident/fall-related injuries**

  - Many of these injuries are covered in different chapters because falls are not unique to climbing, but can be sustained in a variety of sports. The injuries from falls are not necessarily readily classified as climbing related because they are similar to those experienced by skiers, parachutists, or hikers.

  - However, due to the advent of climbing gyms, international speed climbing competitions, World Cup climbing events, and other competitions with monetary rewards, as well as the individual climber's drive to climb at the highest level physiologically possible, overtraining injuries have far surpassed fall-related injuries in terms of incidence (23). These competitions have accelerated participants' interest in training, subsequently resulted in overtraining, and have increased the public's awareness of and interest in climbing.

  - Contrary to conventional wisdom, some types of climbing are relatively safe. "Overall, climbing sports had a lower injury incidence and severity score than many popular sports, including basketball, sailing or soccer; indoor climbing ranked the lowest in terms of injuries of all sports assessed" (16).

  - Compared to overuse injuries, fall-related injuries are relatively infrequent, although do still occur (11).

  - However, with regard to cases seen in emergency rooms between 1990 and 2007, three-quarters of rock climbing–related injuries were a result of falls. These falls were twice as likely to involve injury to the torso (15). Severity of injury is found to be directly related to the length of the fall (24).

  - "It is not found that the riskier forms of climbing (traditional leading and soloing) predicted fall-related injuries. This may reflect the comparatively infrequent nature of fall-related injuries, for example only four [in a small series] climbers reported sustaining a fracture (2%)" (11).

  - "Falls while climbing represent one of the more common causes of serious injury, although acute and chronic musculoskeletal injuries of the hands and extremities are also frequent afflictions" (19).

  - In a survey of the British Climber's Club in 2003, one-fifth of hand injuries were fractures. These included wrist (12%) and phalangeal/metacarpal bone fractures (7%), which are usually a result of falls or rock falls. "Phalangeal and thumb dislocations were common, accounting for 13% of the total number of hand injuries" (12).

  - "In the United States, head injuries are the leading cause of death in both mountaineering and rock climbing. Most of the rock climbers sustained their injuries as a result of falls while leading, with lower extremity injuries predominating" (24). Helmet use in climbers is increasing, but is far from standard such as seen in cyclists. Physicians can certainly help encourage the use of helmets in their patients who climb.

- **Overuse injuries**

  - Overuse injuries account for 75%–90% of indoor climbing injuries. Although supervision, crash mats, and proper equipment help reduce rates of traumatic injuries in indoor climbing, these precautions also allow climbers to climb beyond their ability. Moreover, the easy access, controlled climate, and social nature of these clubs provide climbers with unlimited opportunities to overtrain. Thus, the same factors that reduce traumatic injuries are also contributors to the prevalence of overuse injuries, especially in indoor climbers. A2 pulley rupture, also known as "climber's finger," is particularly prevalent in the elite competition climbers (2,23).

  - Similar to other athletes, climbers are increasingly affected by overuse injuries (22). In fact, 44% of climbers report having an overuse injury at some time, most commonly in the fingers (32%) (11).

  - Overexertion injuries (compared to other mechanisms) are more than five times as likely to occur to the upper extremities as to other parts of the body. Injuries especially to the hand and wrist predominate (15,11,22). In climbers who participate in sport climbing or bouldering, these injuries are seen even more often, especially in dedicated climbers (2,11).

  - More experienced climbers tend to have a lower reinjury risk, whereas climbers with a higher body mass index (BMI) tend to have a higher reinjury risk (2).

- **A2 pulley injury**
  - ❏ Grips
    - ▪ Two primary grips used by climbers are the open and crimp grips; the latter is very prone to causing injury.
    - ▪ In the open grip, the distal interphalangeal (DIP) joint is flexed to about 30 degrees, and the proximal interphalangeal and metacarpophalangeal joints are slightly flexed or straight. No force vectors are pointed at the pulleys, which are well protected with this hold.
    - ▪ The crimp grip is particularly problematic because it biomechanically applies the highest loads to the A2–A4 pulleys. In this grip, the DIP is extended while the PIP is flexed often to more than 90 degrees. Climbers preferentially use this grip because it is the most secure way to hold onto small edges. This security can come at a cost.
  - ❏ "The A2 pulley injury was only first described in 1990 and appears to be unique to rock climbers", with only a few cases reported from windsurfing and industrial accidents (3,13). "It is easy to understand how the injury may occur, considering the huge forces involved as a climber pulls up on a finger flexed at the proximal interphalangeal joint" (24). These grip-specific loads on the pulley system can reach as high as 700 N (6).
  - ❏ "In a situation where the weight of the body is suddenly placed on one finger, as in a one finger pull-up, the force almost at right angles to the A2 pulley has been calculated to be in the region of 450 Newton. This is greater than that required to tear the A2 pulley under experimental conditions" (9).
    - ▪ When the A2 pulley is ruptured, "the tendon is bowstrung and active flexion of the distal phalanx is limited" (20).
  - ❏ Approximately 69% of hand injuries occur to the A2 pulley of the ring finger or middle finger (23). Surprisingly, few cases of pulley injuries are reported for the index and the little fingers (21).
  - ❏ A2 pulley injuries occur most often when the crimp/cling grip is used, especially if associated with a foothold slip suddenly increasing the force on the pulley and causing a rupture. The middle and ring fingers are most often involved," because they are the strongest fingers for climbers (12).
  - ❏ The greater the climbing intensity calculated over a climber's career, the greater is the likelihood of sustaining injuries to the finger tendons or pulleys (12).
- Too small or unnaturally shaped climbing shoes cause the majority of climbing foot injuries, even greater than the number of injuries from falls (14). Climbers at a higher level of ability show more deformities and injuries than casual climbers as a result of wearing shoes that are significantly smaller sizes than normal street wear. Smaller shoes are worn by experienced climbers to eliminate foot slippage in the shoe, maximize the feel of the rock, and improve performance.
  - ❏ Young climbers are especially at risk with too small shoes, particularly while their feet are still growing. Difficulties reaching full growth potential and onset of localized chronic pain, injury, or deformity have been noted (14).
- Climber's back is a postural adaptation characterized by an increased kyphosis of the thoracic spine along with a compensatory increase in lumbar lordosis. This deformity was closely correlated with increased climbing ability level especially seen in elite male climbers. As such, it is probably a biomechanical adaptation to intensive climbing that may actually facilitate elite climbing kinetics. It has no known downside, but may with greater follow-up. It emphasizes the need for regular flexibility and cross-training to prevent this deformity and balance the biomechanical stresses that can lead to the development of "climber's back" (5).
- **Training**
  - ❏ "The risks involved with climbing increase in proportion to the skill-level of the climber: the higher the skill-level, the more hours are required for training and on more difficult routes" (8). Furthermore, "the longer and harder a climber has climbed, the greater the likelihood of exposure to a situation that may result in injury" (12).
  - ❏ The level of training of a climber often dictates the types of injuries seen. Elite climbers are most at risk for overuse injuries of their fingers, whereas recreational climbers typically have a wider variety of injuries (15).
  - ❏ "Climbing frequency and technical difficulty are associated with climbing injuries occurring at both indoor and outdoor venues, particularly cumulative trauma to the upper extremities" (11).
- **Types of climbing**
  - ❏ "The types of injuries sustained from rock climbing differ between elite and recreational climbers and by types of climbing (indoor vs. outdoor; bouldering vs. lead or top-roping; traditional vs. sport)" (15).
  - ❏ Because of the increasing popularity and availability of climbing walls, "it is likely that sprains, tendon, and pulley injuries are more common in the modern climber. . .both in and out of season" (12).
  - ❏ "Handholds in rock climbing generate large forces in the flexor digitorum profundus and superficialis tendons and the associated interphalangeal joints. The distribution of forces often depends on the type of hold adopted. This can result in acute rupture or acute episodes of tendonitis. Soft tissue sprains of the wrist are likely to have occurred following repetitive undercling hand holds" (12).
  - ❏ Elite climbers who engage in difficult training for indoor speed climbing are at greater risk for strain injuries than casual climbers. (12).

- Climbers who boulder or lead more than they top-rope have a higher probability of sustaining an injury. There is a direct and linear relationship between lead grade and climbing injury (23). Additionally, climbers who participate in traditional or solo climbing typically report more injuries than casual or sport climbers (7).
- **Health and drug influences**
  - "A higher BMI was related to an increased injury risk for climbers who participated in bouldering. This can be explained by the nature of competitive disciplines, as they are designed to challenge the climbers' ability to ascend particularly difficult routes that often have small footholds and handholds" (2)
  - Climbers who reported climbing under the influence of drugs or alcohol also documented more injuries than climbers without these substances (7).
- **Gender and age**
  - Gender
    - "Men accounted for 71.8% of all rock climbing-related injuries and are more likely to sustain lacerations and fractures. Men are also more than twice as likely as women to fall more than 20 feet." Consequently, men are twice as likely as women to be hospitalized for climbing-related injuries. Men were also noted to sustain more lacerations and fractures, whereas women sustained more sprains or strains (15). In Europe, the third most common complaint from male climbers and the most common from female climbers is elbow pain (9).
    - "The majority of rock climbing–related injuries occurred among those aged 20–39 years. Research indicates that those aged 16–24 years make up the majority of climbing participants (56%), with 20% aged >35 years" (15).
    - "The probability of sustaining an overuse injury was higher in men, those who had climbed for more than 10 years, those climbing harder routes, and those who boulder or lead more than they top rope" (11).
    - However, gender as an independent predictor of injury disappears, likely because of its relation to lead grade. There are relatively few women climbing at the highest difficulty, and they are thus not as susceptible to the same risks as the men who lead at those high difficulty levels (23).
  - Age
    - Young climbers (up to the age of 17) have more varied risks than older climbers. "The critical age is between 14 and 15 years old, when skeletal mass increases approximately twofold and is at greater risk of injury" (14).
    - However, observed injuries in young climbers still represent the range of expected injury in rock and competition climbing. Rates of injury were not higher than among junior athletes of other sports (18).

TREATMENT

- A2 pulley injury
  - If an isolate pulley rupture is diagnosed, closed treatment with a supportive brace and rest from climbing for 6–8 weeks will usually be sufficient. Severe pulley injuries should be referred to a hand surgeon with experience treating climbers. The patients who are treated nonoperatively often report mild pain while climbing, whereas those who had surgery were free of pain. Additionally, bowstringing was completely reduced in four of five patients who underwent pulley reconstruction in one small series (4).
  - "Full-sport activities can be performed after 3 months but taping should be continued for at least 6 months" (17).
  - "The injuries are graded according to a system to define therapeutic standards. Grade I to III injuries (strains, partial ruptures, single ruptures) are treated conservatively with initial immobilization and early functional therapy under pulley protection. Grade IV injuries (multiple ruptures) require a surgical repair" (17).
- Elbow pain in climbers
  - This is typically lateral epicondylitis, although medial epicondylitis is also seen. Standard treatments includes stretching the common extensor and flexor tendons, ice, relative rest, nonsteroidal anti-inflammatory drugs, and counterforce braces."
  - Early recognition and intervention with a specific amount of rest from climbing, such as 4 weeks, with refocus on core and aerobic training will usually allow climbers to return to climbing, as long as they do so gradually.

PREVENTION

- Physicians
  - Practitioners dealing with climbers who sustain injuries should familiarize themselves with the range of climbing-specific injuries that can occur, as well as the management of these injuries. Educating climbers about the nature of climbing injuries and proper strategies for prevention is likely the most realistic opportunity to intervene effectively (11,24).
  - "The stoical nature of climbers, sportsmen [and women] accustomed to minor injuries, results in underestimation of their injuries, accounting for the high rate of missed fractures. The late or missed diagnosis of fractures may have unfortunate consequences. Doctors should be aware of the large forces involved in any rock climbing fall and be suspicious of significant injury" (24).
  - Suggesting that climbers choose a less strenuous activity, climb only easier routes, or retire after 10 years is an ineffective strategy because of their high commitment level

to the sport. Perhaps the best impact that practitioners can have is to make the results of studies widely available. In doing so, inform climbers about their risks for sport-specific injuries, heightened risk factors, and the signs and symptoms of overuse (8,23).

- Climbers
  - Climbers younger than age 16 should limit the intensity of training (14,18). They should not train excessively for nor should they participate in international bouldering competitions and should also avoid intensive finger strength training because they are at risk for physeal injuries.
  - In an effort to avoid overuse injuries, climbers should gradually and systematically increase climbing loads and hours, after appropriate training (2). Reports of swelling of joints, aching, or finger tenderness that does not completely resolve before the next workout should be interpreted as an impending injury, and rest/cross-training should be instituted until that signal resolves.
  - Taping is widely used by climbers. Typically, athletic tape is applied to the back of hands to protect them when extended amounts of crack climbing are done. Additionally, climbers will often tape the fingers to "reinforce" the pulleys, wishfully protecting them against injury, despite the experimental literature that has not been able to demonstrate a significant protective effect (22).
  - Risks of rock climbing would be reduced if lead climbers would consistently arrange protection at earlier stages of climbs. Adequately protecting lower heights can help prevent and reduce the trauma of lengthy falls, as are more common in lead climbing (24). This is the ideal solution, but often climbs do not present opportunities to place protection ad libitum, thus increasing the odds of longer and potentially more injurious falls.
  - "Ensure adequate strength of the brachialis muscle by using pull-ups in a forearm-pronated rather than forearm-supinated position when training" (9). Clearly, a balanced approach to training flexor and extensor groups makes sense to climbers and physicians alike.
  - Levels of climbing that require either single- or double-finger pull-ups should be avoided until after regularly training in climbing for 6–8 years (9).
  - The use of campus boards and Bachar ladders should be undertaken with great discipline and limited to once or twice a week at the most.
  - As in other sports, periodicity of training and block training focusing on building blocks of endurance, power, and aerobic capacity are helpful to make gains in these areas as well as to give body parts much needed rest.
  - Furthermore, to help limit damage to the climber's feet, climbing shoes should be removed between climbs, especially by elite and experienced climbers who wear excessively restrictive shoes (14).

- Equipment
  - Advances in both climbing equipment and technique have greatly reduced the potential risks to both climber and belayer; however, the risks are still present (24). Participants should regularly inspect and repair safety equipment, replace equipment as necessary, and wear helmets.
- Age-appropriate training
  - "Practice schedules designed for experienced competitive athletes in a variety of upper extremity weight-bearing sports are inappropriate for novices, and in particular adolescents whose bones and ligaments are not fully developed" (2).
- Injury-specific training
  - "Since pulley injuries are largely acquired as a function of the finger position, the most significant prophylactic intervention that can be made is to avoid using the crimp grip in repetitive training exercises and when an open grip will suffice" (22).

REFERENCES

1. Addiss DG, Baker SP. Mountaineering and rock-climbing injuries in US National Parks. *Ann Emerg Med.* 1989;18(9):975–9.
2. Backe S, Ericson L, Janson S, Timpka T. Rock climbing injury rates and associated risk factors in a general climbing population. *Scand J Med Sci Sports.* 2009;19(6):850–6.
3. Bollen SR. Injury to the A2 pulley in rock climbers. *J Hand Surg Br.* 1990;15(2):268–70.
4. Bowie WS, Hunt TK, Allen HA Jr. Rock-climbing injuries in Yosemite National Park. *West J Med.* 1988;149(2):172–7.
5. Förster R, Penka G, Bösl T, Schöffl VR. Climber's back — form and mobility of the thoracolumbar spine leading to postural adaptations in male high ability rock climbers. *Int J Sports Med.* 2009;30(1):53–9.
6. Gabl M, Rangger C, Lutz M, Fink C, Rudisch A, Pechlaner S. Disruption of the finger flexor pulley system in elite rock climbers. *Am J Sports Med.* 1998;26(5):651–5.
7. Gerdes EM, Hafner JW, Aldag JC. Injury patterns and safety practices of rock climbers. *J Trauma.* 2006;61(6):1517–25.
8. Haas JC, Meyers MC. Rock climbing injuries. *Sports Med.* 1995;20(3):199–205.
9. Holtzhausen LM, Noakes TD. Elbow, forearm, wrist, and hand injuries among sport rock climbers. *Clin J Sport Med.* 1996;6(3):196–203.
10. Huey RB, Eguskitza X. Limits to human performance: elevated risks on high mountains. *J Exp Biol.* 2001;204(Pt 8):3115–9.
11. Jones G, Asghar A, Llewellyn DJ. The epidemiology of rock-climbing injuries. *Br J Sports Med.* 2007;42(9):773–8.
12. Logan AJ, Makwana N, Mason G, Dias J. Acute hand and wrist injuries in experienced rock climbers. *Br J Sports Med.* 2004;38(5):545–8.
13. Mallo GC, Sless Y, Hurst LC, Wilson K. A2 and A4 flexor pulley biomechanical analysis: comparison among gender and digit. *Hand.* 2008;3(1):13–6.
14. Morrison AB, Schöffl VR. Physiological responses to rock climbing in young climbers. *Br J Sports Med.* 2007;41(12):852–61.

15. Nelson NG, McKenzie LB. Rock climbing injuries treated in emergency departments in the U.S., 1990–2007. *Am J Prev Med.* 2009;37(3):195–200.

16. Schöffl V, Morrison A, Schwarz U, Schöffl I, Küpper T. Evaluation of injury and fatality risk in rock and ice climbing. *Sports Med.* 2010;40(8):657–79.

17. Schöffl V, Schöffl I. Injuries to the finger flexor pulley system in rock climbers: current concepts. *J Hand Surg Am.* 2006;31(4):647–54.

18. Schöffl VR, Hochholzer T, Imhoff AB, Schöffl I. Radiographic adaptations to the stress of high-level rock climbing in junior athletes: a 5-year longitudinal study of the German Junior National Team and a group of recreational climbers. *Am J Sports Med.* 2007;35(1):86–92.

19. Smith LO. Alpine climbing: injuries and illness. *Phys Med Rehabil Clin N Am.* 2006;17(3):633–44.

20. Tropet Y, Menez D, Balmat P, Pem R, Vichard P. Closed traumatic rupture of the ring finger flexor tendon pulley. *J Hand Surg Am.* 1990;15(5):745–7.

21. Vigouroux L, Quaine F, Paclet F, Colloud F, Moutet F. Middle and ring fingers are more exposed to pulley rupture than index and little during sport-climbing: a biomechanical explanation. *Clin Biomech.* 2008;23(5):562–70.

22. Warme WJ, Brooks D. The effect of circumferential taping on flexor tendon pulley failure in rock climbers. *Am J Sports Med.* 2000;28(5):674–8.

23. Wright DM, Royle TJ, Marshall T. Indoor rock climbing: who gets injured? *Br J Sports Med.* 2001;35:181–5.

24. Wyatt JP, McNaughton GW, Grant PT. A prospective study of rock climbing injuries. *Br J Sports Med.* 1996;30(2):148–50.

97 Lacrosse

Thad J. Barkdull

INTRODUCTION

- History (17)
  - Considered to be the oldest sport in North America.
  - Derived from *baggataway*, a game French observed Native Americans playing in 17th century Canada.
  - Stick, or *lacrosse*, used in game comes from appearance similar to bishop's crosier or crosse.
  - In 1879, Canada formed the National Lacrosse Association (now the Canadian Lacrosse Association).
  - Eleven U.S. men's college and club teams formed the National Lacrosse Association in 1879.
  - By 1950, over 200 teams existed in the United States.
  - Lacrosse is still the National Summer Sport of Canada.
- Demographics (U.S. Lacrosse)
  - Estimated that 568,021 people played organized lacrosse in 2009.
    - Over 340,000 men
    - Over 220,000 women
  - Nearly 19,000 men participated in over 250 universities with sanctioned programs.
  - Over 136,000 men at 1,600 high schools now have varsity programs.
  - Over 250 universities have sanctioned women's programs for 12,868 women athletes.
  - As of 2010, lacrosse was a sanctioned sport in 19 state high school athletic associations.
  - There are currently two professional leagues: Major League Lacrosse (indoor or box) and the National Lacrosse League (outdoor or field).
- The game
  - Men's field lacrosse (16)
    - Ten players per side:
      - Three attackmen (offense), three defensemen (defense), three midfielders (both), and one goalie (defense)
      - Teams may allow a maximum of six players on the offensive half and seven on the defensive half.
    - The field is 110 × 60 yards.
    - Goals are 6-feet square with a 9-feet diameter circular *crease* around them.
    - Substitutions may occur during play stoppage or during play (similar to hockey).
    - Players may pass the ball or run while cradling the ball in their stick, or *crosse*.
    - The object is to score more points than the opponent by putting the ball into the opposition's goal.
    - Players may hit an opposing player who controls the ball or is within 5 yards of ball.
    - Players may hit an opponent's stick or gloved hand with their own stick.
  - Women's field lacrosse (14)
    - Twelve players: One goalie, four attackers, four defenders, and three midfielders
    - The field is 120 × 70 yards.
    - No contact between players
    - Restraining Line Rule — only seven offensive and eight defensive players in 30-yard area around goal
  - Box lacrosse
    - Six players per side
    - Played in enclosed area
    - More contact allowed than field lacrosse
- Equipment (13)
  - *Crosse* or stick
    - Length varies by position.
    - Made of wood, laminated wood, or synthetic material.
    - Attackmen's and midfielders' sticks must be 40–42 inches long.
    - Defensemen's sticks must be 52–72 inches long.
    - The head must be 6.5–10 inches wide, or 10–12 inches for the goalie.
  - Ball
    - Made of solid rubber
    - 7.75–8 inches in circumference
    - 5–5.25 ounces
  - Personal equipment
    - Varies by different game and position played
    - Required equipment

- All players are required to wear mouthguards.
- In men's game, helmet with full face mask and padded gloves.
- Women are currently only required to wear mouthguards and eye protection, although some wear soft helmets (goalies are a notable exception, see below).
  - Goalies
    - Both men's and women's games require head, chest, and throat protection.
    - The stick has a significantly larger net than sticks of other players.
    - Athletic cup is optional but highly recommended.
  - Attackmen
    - Frequently wear elbow pads, shoulder pads, and rib protectors.
    - Sticks tend to be shorter.
  - Defensemen
    - Frequently wear less protective gear in the men's game, often only the required helmet, mouthguard, and gloves.
    - Have a much longer stick than other players.
  - Midfielders
    - Often wear less protection than attackmen.
    - May have longer or shorter stick depending on specialty (defensive midfielders have longer sticks).

INJURY EPIDEMIOLOGY (NCAA INJURY SURVEILLANCE SYSTEM)

- The Injury Surveillance System (ISS) was developed by the National Collegiate Athletic Association (NCAA) in 1982 to monitor collegiate athlete injury patterns (3).

- The latest data were presented in 2007 as a summary of injury patterns from the 1988–1989 season through the 2003–2004 season in all three NCAA divisions, focusing on 15 different sports (4).
- Monitors type of injury, body part injured, severity of injury, field type, field condition, and special equipment worn.
- Data are collected by certified athletic trainers at NCAA-sanctioned schools.
- Reportable injuries must meet specific criteria (5).
  - Occurs during practice or contest.
  - Requires medical attention by athletic trainer or physician.
  - Causes the student-athlete to miss one or more days of participation beyond the day of injury.
  - In 1994, ISS expanded to include data regarding any dental injury, regardless of time lost.
- Injury rate
  - Men's overall (7)
    - Game — 12.6 per 1,000 athlete exposures (A-E); eighth
    - Practice — 3.2; twelfth
  - Women's overall (7)
    - Game — 7.2; twelfth
    - Practice — 3.3; eleventh
- Frequency by body part
  - Men's (5) (Figs. 97.1 and 97.2)
    - Game
      - Head/neck: 11.7%
      - Upper extremity: 26.2%
      - Trunk/back: 11.9%
      - Lower extremity: 48.1%
      - Other: 2.2%
    - Practice
      - Head/neck: 6.2%
      - Upper extremity: 16.9%

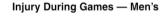

Injury During Games — Men's

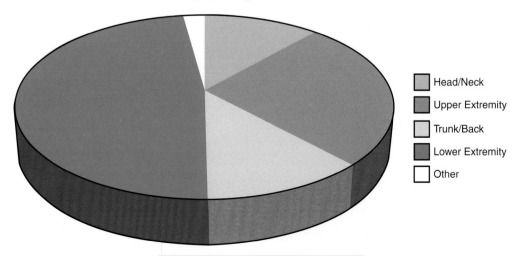

Head/Neck

Upper Extremity

Trunk/Back

Lower Extremity

Other

FIGURE 97.1: Injury during games — men.

Injury in Practice — Men's

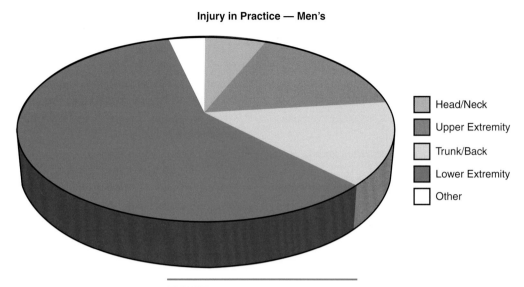

Legend:
- Head/Neck
- Upper Extremity
- Trunk/Back
- Lower Extremity
- Other

FIGURE 97.2: Injury in practice — men.

- Trunk/back: 14.4%
- Lower extremity: 58.7%
- Other: 3.8%
- Women's (14) (Figs. 97.3 and 97.4)
  - Game
    - Head/neck: 21.9%
    - Upper extremity: 8.9%
    - Trunk/back: 6.1%
    - Lower extremity: 61.0%
    - Other: 2.2%
  - Practice
    - Head/neck: 12.2%
    - Upper extremity: 5.9%
    - Trunk/back: 12.0%

- Lower extremity: 64.3%
- Other: 5.9%
- Men experienced injury rates almost four times as frequently in game situations than practice.
- Injury during practice occurred twice as often during the pre-season compared with in-season practice for men and women.
- Women had more than twice as many injuries in games than practice.
- Specific injury patterns
  - Men's (5)
    - Ankle ligament sprain (0.53 A-E), upper leg muscle tendon strain (0.37), knee internal derangement (0.23), pelvis/hip muscle tendon strain (0.18), and concussion (0.12) were the most common injuries during practices.

Injury During Games — Women's

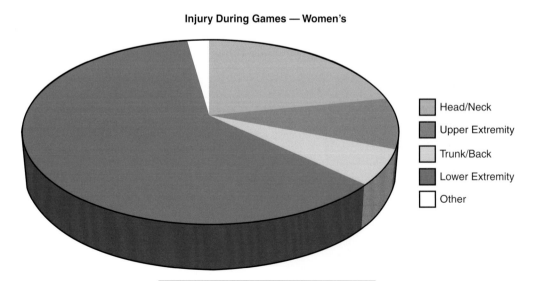

Legend:
- Head/Neck
- Upper Extremity
- Trunk/Back
- Lower Extremity
- Other

FIGURE 97.3: Injury during games — women.

Injury During Practice — Women's

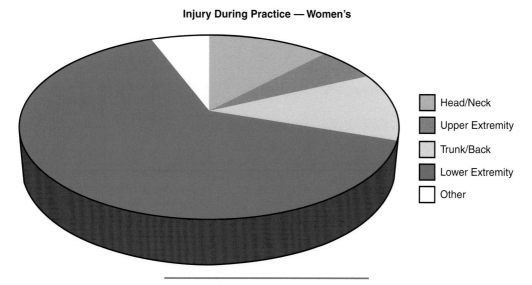

FIGURE 97.4: Injury in practice — women.

❏ Ankle ligament sprain (1.43 A-E), knee internal derangement (1.14), concussion (1.08), upper leg contusion (1.00), and upper leg muscle tendon strain (0.94) were the most common injuries in game situations.

❏ Players were most likely to be injured while engaging in noncontact activity during practice (50%), whereas player contact (45.9%) accounted for the most common time period to be injured during competition.

■ Women's (14)

❏ Ankle ligament sprain (0.51 A-E), upper leg muscle tendon strain (0.39), knee internal derangement (0.20), pelvis/hip muscle tendon strain (0.16), and concussion (0.15) were the most common injuries during practices.

❏ Ankle ligament sprain (1.62 A-E), knee internal derangement (1.00), concussion (0.70), upper leg muscle tendon strain (0.52), and nasal fracture (0.18) were the most common injuries in game situations.

❏ Players were most likely to be injured while engaging in noncontact activity during practice (62%), as well as during competition (44.3%).

■ Injuries resulting in 10+ days of activity time loss (Fig. 97.5)

❏ Men's

■ Game (21.0% of all injuries)

– Internal derangement of knee (27.3%)

– Acromioclavicular (AC) joint injury (7.3%)

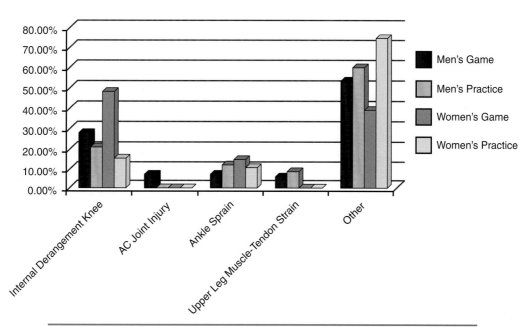

FIGURE 97.5: Injuries resulting in 10 days or greater loss of participation. AC, acromioclavicular.

- – Ankle sprain (7.1%)
- – Upper leg muscle tendon strain (5.6%)
- – Other (52.8%)
  - Practice (21% of all injuries)
    - – Internal derangement of knee (20.5%)
    - – Ankle sprain (11.9%)
    - – Upper leg muscle tendon strain (8.3%)
    - – Other (59.2%)
- ❏ Women's
  - Game (21.9% of all injuries)
    - – Internal derangement of knee (47.6%)
    - – Ankle sprain (14.2%)
    - – Other (38.2%)
  - Practice (23.9% of all injuries)
    - – Lower leg stress fracture (15.8%)
    - – Internal derangement of knee (15.1%)
    - – Ankle sprain (10.6%)
    - – Other (58.5%)
- Catastrophic injuries (12)
  - ❏ Data collected from 1982 to 2009.
  - ❏ In men's high school lacrosse, there have been only two fatalities (0.21 fatalities per 100,000 participants), four nonfatal (permanent severe functional disability) injuries (0.42), and seven serious injuries (0.63) (significant injury without permanent disability) reported as a result of direct competition or practice.
  - ❏ Seven fatalities (0.73) have occurred as a result of indirect contact while playing lacrosse (exertional injury or complication of a nonfatal injury).
  - ❏ In men's collegiate lacrosse, there have been only four fatalities (2.49 fatalities per 100,000 participants), five nonfatal (permanent severe functional disability) injuries (1.86), and two serious injuries (1.24) (significant injury without permanent disability) reported as a result of direct competition or practice.
  - ❏ Two fatalities (1.24) have occurred as a result of indirect contact while playing lacrosse (exertional injury or complication of a nonfatal injury).

INJURIES IN LACROSSE

Noncontact (1,2,9,16)

- Lower extremity
  - Groin, hamstring, and low back strains
    - ❏ Associated with twisting motion of the torso
    - ❏ Common motion during passing, shooting, checking, and scooping ground balls
    - ❏ Performed at high speeds and with rapid changes in direction

- ❏ Cryotherapy and strengthening of affected regional musculature key in return to play and reducing repeat injuries
- Knee
  - ❏ Similar to other field sports, anterior cruciate ligament (ACL) and medial collateral ligament (MCL) injuries are not uncommon.
    - Account for fewer than 20% of injuries.
    - MCL more commonly affected than lateral collateral ligament.
    - Because of the MCL's deep attachment to the medial meniscal periphery, meniscal tears should be suspected with higher grade MCL injuries.
    - Typically the result of force on the lateral aspect of knee at full extension, with foot planted.
    - May be the result of a lateral blow, but more often the result of planting and directional change, resulting in intolerable stresses on ligaments.
    - Grades I and II may be treated nonsurgically.
    - Cryotherapy, hinged braces, and hamstring and quad strengthening are mainstays of rehabilitation.
    - Recovery may take up to 6 weeks, with hinged brace used in competition for 1–2 months for protection.
  - ❏ Patellofemoral syndrome
    - Often seen in female players age 12–15, due to anatomic stresses.
    - Typically presents as anterior knee pain without any physical findings (*i.e.*, instability or effusion).
    - Theoretic risk factors include foot pronation, genu valgus, rotated or tilted patellae, or an increased dynamic Q-angle.
    - In the past, focus has been on strengthening of medial quadriceps (vastus medialis oblique) and hamstrings for prevention and treatment, but now it is recognized that excessive femoral anteversion as the result of relatively weak hip external rotators and adductors may also contribute to maltracking of the patella, particularly in women.
    - Some significant anatomic abnormalities may require surgical intervention to alleviate symptoms.
- Ankle
  - ❏ Accounts for 16.2% of total injuries in NCAA lacrosse (1994–1996 ISS).
  - ❏ Majority are inversion injuries.
  - ❏ Slight inversion and plantarflexion is the state of least stability and the point when injury most often occurs.
  - ❏ Ligamentous injuries are most common.
    - Anterior talofibular ligament, followed by calcaneofibular ligament, and then posterior talofibular ligament.
    - Deltoid ligament injuries are associated with eversion mechanism.

- Avulsion fractures should be suspected with higher grade ligamentous injuries (grade II or higher).
  - ❏ Early mobilization for nonfractures is the key to rapid return to healthy play.
    - Consider non–weight-bearing exercises (*i.e.*, aqua jogging).
    - Strengthening of evertors, invertors, plantarflexors, and dorsiflexors, as well as hip abductors and adductors and extensors.
    - Final rehabilitation should include dynamic strengthening focusing on proprioception (*i.e.*, slide board, figure-eight running drills).
    - Most sprains will recover in 1–3 weeks.
- Upper extremity
  - Much less common
  - Blocker's exostosis
    - ❏ Most often occurs with repetitive stick-to-body contact at deltoid insertion.
    - ❏ Use of appropriate shoulder protection (deltoid cup) is important in prevention.
    - ❏ Monitoring for myositis ossificans is important (see later Contact section).
  - Medial and lateral epicondylitis
    - ❏ Usually result of cradling motion in the throwing arm.
    - ❏ Cradling of the ball requires rapid pronation/supination and flexion/extension of the arm.
    - ❏ Stretching of affected muscle groups along with braces to reduce strain at tendinous insertions have proven effective in treating this injury.
- Others
  - Exertional heat illness (EHI)
    - ❏ May occur in both field, usually a spring sport, and box lacrosse.
    - ❏ Players with more protective equipment (*i.e.*, goalies) are at higher risk.
    - ❏ Hydration is essential.
    - ❏ Monitor players for signs/symptoms of EHI.
    - ❏ Provide appropriate water and electrolytes to players during games.
    - ❏ Avoid conditions where EHI is more likely.
      - Anticipate problems with acclimation in different climates/altitudes.
      - Identify players at greater risk (higher body mass index, slower long-distance run times).
      - Consider screening for sickle cell trait in higher risk ethnicities, because mortality is higher in EHI with those carrying the trait.
      - Players showing signs of EHI should be immediately removed from play, equipment should be removed, and measures should be taken to decrease body temperature.

- Abrasions/turf burns
  - ❏ More common in box lacrosse or competition on artificial surfaces.
  - ❏ Padding and lubrication with petroleum jelly on at-risk areas may reduce incidence.
  - ❏ Ensure antiseptic cleansing of wound and clean dressings to reduce infection risk.
  - ❏ Prepatellar bursitis is a common complication, especially in adolescent athletes.
- Blisters
  - ❏ Occur in areas of increased friction.
  - ❏ Petroleum jelly, powders, moleskin, and nylon socks under thick socks may all help to reduce friction.
  - ❏ Treatment with donut pads to distribute forces away from blister; appropriate cleansing of blister (especially if it has opened).
- Anterior tibial shin splints
  - ❏ Overuse injury.
  - ❏ Associated with fatiguing tibialis anterior that spasms with eccentrically decelerating forefoot.
  - ❏ Irritation of fascia or anterior border of tibia results.
  - ❏ Prevention revolves around proper stretching.
- Turf toe
  - ❏ Hyperextension of first metatarsal.
  - ❏ Associated with rapid deceleration, commonly on artificial turf.
  - ❏ Results in a sprain of the plantar capsuloligamentous complex of the hallux metatarsophalangeal joint.
  - ❏ Prevention with proper shoe fit allowing some toe and forefoot movement.
  - ❏ Limiting hyperextension by taping is appropriate treatment to allow for return to play.

Contact

- Lower extremity
  - Much less common
  - Most often associated with stick-to-body or ball-to-body contact
  - Contusions are common
    - ❏ May result from contact with hard rubber ball, which may be propelled at up to 100 miles per hour.
    - ❏ Player controlling the ball is often repeatedly hit in the upper torso and extremities by the defender's stick.
    - ❏ Treated by standard PRICEMM (protection, rest, ice, compression, elevation, modalities, medication); may cover area with donut protection to distribute future forces to area around injury.
    - ❏ May be complicated by *myositis ossificans*.
      - Inflammatory bony deposition in muscle from repetitive trauma.

- Often occurs in vastus lateralis and deltoid insertion of humerus.
- Areas receiving repeated trauma should be protected with donut and hard plate over area.

■ Upper extremity

▨ Olecranon bursitis
  ❑ Often stick-to-body or body-to-ground contact
  ❑ Many players do not wear elbow pads and are thus more susceptible to this injury.
  ❑ Drainage of bursal fluid allows for improvement of symptoms and may respond to steroid injection into bursal sac; protective gear (*i.e.*, elbow pads) reduces risk of further complications.

▨ AC separation
  ❑ Associated with checks into the boards (box lacrosse), stick-to-body contact with a downward blow to the outer aspect of the shoulder, and fall on the outstretched hand (FOOSH) mechanisms.
  ❑ Specific taping systems have been used to allow for reduction in pain with movement to encourage earlier mobilization.
  ❑ AC immobilizers can be helpful in limiting movement of the joint to reduce pain.
  ❑ Activity without pain is key factor in determining return to play.

▨ Clavicular fracture
  ❑ Frequently the result of a direct blow from an opponent's *crosse*.
  ❑ Usually can be treated with a sling for comfort, although some experts encourage fixation, especially when significant shortening (> 1.5 cm) has occurred. External fixation is rarely successful and discouraged (15).

▨ Scaphoid fracture
  ❑ Most often from FOOSH injury.
  ❑ Immobilization is appropriate treatment.

▨ Hamate fracture (8)
  ❑ Typically the "hook" of the hamate.
  ❑ Results from sudden deceleration of the *crosse* stick within the grip of the hand, such as when a player's stick is stopped by another's while shooting or passing.
  ❑ Best identified with a "carpal tunnel view" on plain film or computed tomography.
  ❑ Often heals with time and symptomatic treatment, but cases with chronic pain may improve with surgical excision of the avulsed tip.

▨ Metacarpal, phalangeal, and interphalangeal joint dislocations
  ❑ Immediate traction and reduction are ideal.
  ❑ Often associated with stick checking or falls where the stick traps the hand/fingers in pathologic manner.

▨ Gamekeeper's or skier's thumb
  ❑ Associated typically with falls in which the thumb is trapped by the stick.
  ❑ Hyperextension results in a tear of the ulnar collateral ligament.
  ❑ May be complicated by retraction of the ulnar collateral ligament under the adductor aponeurosis, thus impairing reattachment to the proximal phalanx (Stener lesion).

▨ Forearm fractures
  ❑ Either from stick-to-body contact during checking or from FOOSH injuries.
  ❑ Immobilization is mainstay of treatment.
  ❑ Surgical reduction and fixation may be required depending on severity of injury.

▨ Shoulder subluxation/dislocation
  ❑ Anterior instability is the most common and most often occurs when a significant force is applied to an abducted and externally rotated shoulder (as when a player is passing or shooting).
  ❑ Although rare (2%–4% of dislocations), posterior instability can also occur, especially when a force is applied as the shoulder is flexed, adducted, and internally rotated, which occurs especially with defensive players as they push an attacker out of position (11).
  ❑ An experienced practitioner may attempt a manual relocation on the sideline, as this may be easier prior to the posttraumatic spasming of the musculature. It is essential to assess for neurovascular integrity after relocating the joint, and it is highly advisable to get plain films to assess for any bony fracture (*i.e.*, Hill-Sachs deformity or bony Bankart lesion).
  ❑ Treatment should start with aggressive physical therapy to strengthen the stabilizing muscles around the joint, although some surgeons have recommended surgical stabilization even for first-time dislocators, because the rate of redislocation is high. Risks and benefits should be discussed with the patient.

▨ Shoulder burners (stingers)
  ❑ Commonly result from stick-to-body contact with a check to the shoulder or a fall onto head or shoulder.
  ❑ Downward, forward depression of the shoulder.
  ❑ Often present with acute, shooting, shock-like pain in extremity.
  ❑ May have some transient motor deficits.
  ❑ Typically resolve without complication.
  ❑ Bilateral burners are almost exclusively the result of a more central spinal cord injury and should be evaluated as such.

■ Others

▨ Lacerations
  ❑ Pressure, hemostasis, and suturing if needed

▨ Nose bleeds
  ❑ Hold head forward (player may choke on own blood).
  ❑ Put pressure on lower two-thirds of nostrils.

- Packing may aid in tamponading bleed.
  - Packing may be soaked with a vasoconstrictor (*i.e.*, oxymetazoline) to aid in hemostasis.
- Concussions (10)
  - Head injuries account for 8.6% of game-time men's lacrosse injuries (5).
  - Lacrosse helmets are designed to deflect blows from a stick or ball but are not meant to protect against high-velocity impacts, like being thrust into the boards (box lacrosse) or impact into the ground.
  - Also common when players are crouched down for scooping ground balls and are struck by another player.
  - Most recent recommendations for concussion management encourage abandoning prior grading of concussions.
  - When in doubt, withhold player from play until symptom-free and a graded exercise progression is completed without resumption of symptoms.
- Eye injuries (18,19)
  - Much more common in women's lacrosse due to minimal protective gear.
    - It is felt that appropriate enforcement of the rules for contact will minimize eye and facial injuries.
    - Eye protection recently has been mandated by the NCAA, significantly reducing the number of injuries (14).
  - May be the result of contact with ball or inadvertent stick contact.
  - Traumatic eye injuries should be referred for immediate ophthalmologic examination.
    - Sunken eyes or extraocular muscle deficiencies may represent periorbital skull fractures.
    - Assessment for associated closed head injury may be warranted.
- Rib fractures and abdominal trauma
  - Most commonly from stick checking.
  - Injuries to abdominal organs are uncommon but should be entertained in cases of significant abdominal pain.
  - Rib padding may offer some protection.
- Throat trauma
  - Usually the result of the ball striking the throat.
  - Goalies are most at risk.
  - Throat deflectors significantly reduce the incidence of injury.
- Goalkeeper's thumb (6)
  - Fracture of distal or proximal phalanx of thumb.
  - Typically results from impact of ball directly on extending thumb as goalie is attempting to save shot on goal.
  - May require surgical fixation or immobilization.
  - May be prevented with rigid covering over distal end of thumb.

REFERENCES

1. Bartlett B, Cress D, Bull RC. Lacrosse. In: Bull RC, editor. *Handbook of Sports Injuries.* New York: McGraw-Hill, Health Professions Division; 1991. p. 423–51.
2. Casazza BA, Rossner K. Baseball/lacrosse injuries. *Phys Med Rehabil Clin N Am.* 1999;10(1):141–57, vii.
3. Dick R, Agel J, Marshall SW. National Collegiate Athletic Association Injury Surveillance System commentaries: introduction and methods. *J Athl Train.* 2009;44(2):173–82.
4. Dick R, Lincoln AE, Agel J, Carter EA, Marshall SW, Hinton RY. Descriptive epidemiology of collegiate women's lacrosse injuries: National Collegiate Athletic Association Injury Surveillance System, 1988–1989 through 2003–2004. *J Athl Train.* 2007;42(2):262–9.
5. Dick R, Romani WA, Agel J, Case JG, Marshall SW. Descriptive epidemiology of collegiate men's lacrosse injuries: National Collegiate Athletic Association Injury Surveillance System, 1988–1989 through 2003–2004. *J Athl Train.* 2007;42(2):255–61.
6. Elkousy HA, Janssen H, Ferraro J, Levin LS, Speer K. Lacrosse goalkeeper's thumb. A preventable injury. *Am J Sports Med.* 2000;28(3):317–21.
7. Hootman JM, Dick R, Agel J. Epidemiology of collegiate injuries for 15 sports: summary and recommendations for injury prevention initiatives. *J Athl Train.* 2007;42(2):311–9.
8. Ingari JV. Wrist and hand. In: DeLee JC, Drez D, Miller MD, editors. *DeLee & Drez's Orthopaedic Sports Medicine: Principles and Practice.* New York: Saunders; 2009. p. 1340–7.
9. Matthews LS, Hinton RY, Burke N. Lacrosse. In: Fu FH, Stone DA, editors. *Sports Injuries: Mechanisms, Prevention and Treatment.* Philadelphia: Lippincott Williams & Wilkins; 2001. p. 568–82.
10. McCrory P, Meeuwisse W, Johnston K, et al. Consensus statement on Concussion in Sport 3rd International Conference on Concussion in Sport held in Zurich, November 2008. *Clin J Sport Med.* 2009;19(3):185–200.
11. McMahon PJ, Debski RE. Shoulder. In: DeLee JC, Drez D, Miller MD, editors. *DeLee & Drez's Orthopedic Sports Medicine: Principles and Practice.* New York: Saunders; 2009. p. 924–6.
12. National Center for Catastrophic Sport Injury [Internet]. Chapel Hill (NC): NCCSIR Data Tables; [cited 16 May 2011]. Available from: http://www.unc.edu/depts/nccsi/index.htm.
13. NCAA Web site [Internet]. Indianapolis (IN): NCAA Publications; [cited 14 May 2011]. Available from: http://www.ncaapublications.com/productdownloads/LC12.pdf.
14. NCAA Web site [Internet]. Indianapolis (IN): NCAA Publications; [cited 16 May 2011]. Available from: http://www.ncaapublications.com/productdownloads/WLC09.pdf.
15. Ring D, Jupiter JB. Injuries to the shoulder girdle. In: Browner BD, Jupiter JB, Levine AM, Trafton PG, Krettek C, editors. *Skeletal Trauma: Basic Science, Management and Reconstruction.* New York: Saunders; 2008. p. 1767–9.
16. Sherbondy PS. Lacrosse. In: Mellion MB, Walsh WM, Madden C, Putukian M, Shelton GL, editors. *Team Physician's Handbook.* 3rd ed. Philadelphia: Hanley & Belfus; 2002. p. 759–65.
17. US Lacrosse Web site [Internet]. Baltimore (MD): US Lacrosse; [cited 14 May 2011]. Available from: http://www.lacrosse.org.
18. Waicus KM, Smith BW. Eye injuries in women's lacrosse players. *Clin J Sport Med.* 2002;12(1):24–9.
19. Webster DA, Bayliss GV, Spadaro JA. Head and face injuries in scholastic women's lacrosse with and without eyewear. *Med Sci Sports Exerc.* 1999;31(7):938–41.

98 Rugby Injuries

Peter H. Seidenberg and Rochelle M. Nolte

INTRODUCTION

- Rugby union is a fast-paced contact-collision game with the continuous pace of soccer combined with contact situations similar to those seen in American football.
- It is the fastest growing amateur sport in the United States.
  - There are greater than 90,000 members in USA Rugby (the governing body for Rugby Union in the United States) (30).
  - There are 7 territorial unions and 34 local area unions.
  - The USA national men's team (the Eagles) was established in 1976, and the women's team was established in 1987.
- Rugby is played in over 150 countries worldwide and has a strong tradition in Great Britain, New Zealand, Australia, and South Africa.
  - Its popularity is second only to soccer in the world (14).
- World Cup competition occurs every 4 years.
- There are similar sports that are sometimes confused with rugby union such as rugby league and Australian Rules football, which will not be discussed in this chapter.

HISTORY

- Invented in 1832 when William Webb Ellis picked up the ball and advanced it in a soccer match at Rugby College in England. The only way to stop the runner was to tackle him or her (6).
- American football is thought to have been birthed from rugby in the late 19th century.
- It was an Olympic sport from 1900 to 1924 (27).
  - The United States won the gold medal in 1920 and 1924.
- After 1924, it was no longer an Olympic sport, and this was followed by decreased popularity in the United States (27).
- In October 2009, the International Olympic Committee announced that rugby sevens (the seven-a-side version of the game) will appear in the 2016 Olympic Games (27).

MATCH

- **Goals (12)**
  - Whereas American football is a game of yardage, rugby union is a game of possession.
  - The player with possession of the ball is the front-most player on the attacking team. He or she may advance the ball by running with the ball, kicking it forward, or passing it backward or laterally to another player on his or her team.
    - ❏ All teammates are behind the ball carrier in support.
    - ❏ Unlike American football, blocking for the ball carrier is not permitted and is penalized as obstruction.
  - The objective is to maintain control of the ball and touch it down in the try zone (the rugby equivalent of the American football end zone).
    - ❏ Once crossing the try line, the player must touch the ball down on the ground in order to register a try, which is worth 5 points.
    - ❏ The try entitles the scoring team to attempt to kick the ball through the goal posts directly back from the point the ball was touched down in the try zone, which is worth another 2 points.
  - An offensive player may also attempt to drop-kick the ball through the goal posts during open play, which is worth 3 points.
  - If a penalty occurs, an attempt to kick to the ball through the goal posts is allowed from a ball placed at the point of the foul.
  - The team with the maximum points at the end of the match is the victor.
  - A typical game requires the athlete to cover a distance of 5–8 km, running at speeds up to 5–8 m · s^{-1} (comparable to soccer) (5).
  - In addition, the rugby player is involved in more than one to two episodes of collision contact per minute (5).
    - ❏ These equate to approximately 40 tackles and up to 70 rucks and mauls per game.
    - ❏ The forwards sustain an additional 30 scrums and 40 line outs per game.

- There are few substitutions allowed. The mean duration of high-intensity work (sprinting or contact) is 38 seconds per minute, with an average workload of 51 minutes per 80-minute match. In comparison, the average American football game has only 10 minutes of contact or significant exertion per game (5).
- **Pitch:** The rugby field is called the pitch (12).
  - The rectangular field of play (which excludes the goal zones) does not exceed 70 meters in width and 100 meters in length.
  - Each try zone is the same width as the remainder of the pitch and is between 10 and 22 meters in depth.
  - The pitch has the following solid lines:
    - ❏ Halfway line or midfield line (half the distance between the try lines)
    - ❏ Ten-meter lines on each side of the halfway line
    - ❏ Twenty-meter lines (22 meters from the try lines)
    - ❏ Try lines
    - ❏ Dead ball lines (at the deepest portion of the try zone)
    - ❏ Touch lines (side lines)
  - Dashed lines
    - ❏ Positioned 5 and 15 meters parallel to the touch lines
  - The goal posts are on the goal line and are in the field of play.
    - ❏ The distance between the posts is 5.6 meters in width with a minimum height of 3.4 meters.
    - ❏ The crossbar is 3.0 meters from the ground.
    - ❏ The posts should be padded (because players can collide with them as they are in the field of play).
- **Rules (12)**
  - The match is divided into two 40-minute halves with a 5- to 10-minute half time.
  - A player who leaves the match and is substituted may not return to the match.
    - ❏ Exception: A player may be substituted for a maximum of 15 minutes for control of bleeding from an injury. After bleeding is controlled, he or she may then return to play. This is commonly referred to as a blood sub.
    - ❏ Exception: A referee may permit a substituted tight five player to return to the match to replace an injured player if no eligible player on the team is experienced in these skilled positions.
  - The play clock runs continuously.
  - There is one referee to monitor play.
    - ❏ Play is stopped only for a penalty, the ball leaving field of play, a score, or a serious injury (in the referee's judgment).
    - ❏ The referee may summon a medical attendant onto the pitch or may allow the player to temporarily leave the pitch for medical evaluation.

- ❏ Even though a medical attendant may be on the pitch evaluating an injured player, the referee may allow play to continue around the injured player.
- ❏ The medical attendant does not have the power to stop play but does have the ability to determine whether an injured player is allowed to continue to play.
- Rules have been instituted to decrease the incidence of neck injury in rugby union. The following actions are illegal:
  - ❏ High tackles above the level of the shoulders.
  - ❏ Spearing.
  - ❏ Leaving your feet to make a tackle.
  - ❏ Tackling a player who is in the follow-through phase of kicking a ball.
  - ❏ Tackling a player who has jumped in the air to catch a ball.
  - ❏ The tackler must wrap the opposing ball carrier with arms or grasp the player with hands. Tacklers cannot merely hit the opponent with a shoulder or shove him or her.
  - ❏ This rule separates rugby union from other contact-collision sports.
  - ❏ Laws are periodically reviewed and revised by the international rugby board to enhance safety and improve the flow of the game.
- **Positions (12)**
  - There are 15 players on each team with specific positions and responsibilities (12).
  - Each team ideally has at least five to seven substitutes available.
  - The players numbered 1 through 8 are the forwards.
    - ❏ They are generally responsible for gaining and maintaining possession of the ball.
  - Players numbered 9 through 15 are the backs.
    - ❏ They are generally responsible for advancing the ball down the field and defending the open field.
  - Props
    - ❏ Position no. 1 — Loose head prop
    - ❏ Position no. 3 — Tight head prop
    - ❏ One of three people of the front row, which includes two props on either side of a hooker
    - ❏ They are responsible for the stability and strength of the front row.
    - ❏ They are generally the stoutest and least aerobically fit players on the pitch (25).
  - Hooker
    - ❏ Position no. 2
    - ❏ Responsible for hooking (securing the ball with feet) during the scrum
    - ❏ Hooker is in the middle position of the front row of the scrum and is tightly supported by the props on

either side, who support the hooker so his or her feet are off the ground. This enables the hooker to hook the ball backward during the scrum.

- ❏ Hooker is usually slightly shorter and lighter than the props to provide a stable front row platform; however, at elite levels, this stereotype is not necessarily true.

- ■ Second row/locks
  - ❏ Positions no. 4 and 5
  - ❏ They are responsible for providing the driving force to the front row of the scrum.
  - ❏ Typically, they are the jumpers for the line out.
  - ❏ Generally, they are the tallest players on the pitch.
  - ❏ The second and first rows make up the tight five.

- ■ Flanker/wing forward
  - ❏ Positions no. 6 and 7
  - ❏ Together with the eightman, they make up the loose forwards.
  - ❏ Typically, they are the first players to leave a scrum.
  - ❏ Generally, they are the best tacklers and all-around athletes on the team.
  - ❏ Ideal flanker has both size and speed.

- ■ Eightman
  - ❏ Position no. 8
  - ❏ Eightman is at the rear end of the scrum and has his or her head between the second row players.
  - ❏ He or she is responsible for providing stability and drive to the scrum.
  - ❏ Generally, the eightman is the tallest loose forward.
  - ❏ He or she needs to be able to reach around the locks to hold them securely together.
  - ❏ The eightman is responsible for controlling the ball at the rear of the scrum until the scrumhalf retrieves the ball.

- ■ Scrumhalf
  - ❏ Position no. 9
  - ❏ Acts as the quarterback of the forwards.
  - ❏ Responsible for offensive and defensive strategy of the forwards during loose play.
  - ❏ Secures the ball from the scrum, rucks, mauls, and tackles.
  - ❏ Responsible for delivering the ball to the backs for open-field play.
  - ❏ Responsible for placing the ball in the tunnel (see scrum below).
  - ❏ The scrumhalf is usually smaller and quicker than the other forwards and has a fast and accurate pass.

- ■ Flyhalf
  - ❏ Position no. 10
  - ❏ Acts as the quarterback of the backs and is the first player in the back line.

- ❏ Is responsible for calling back plays.
- ❏ Generally, the flyhalf is smaller and lighter than other backs with good passing and kicking ability.

- ■ Centers
  - ❏ Position no. 12 — inside center
  - ❏ Position no. 13 — outside center
  - ❏ Generally the larger and more physical backs.
  - ❏ They are often called upon to crash into the competition by intentionally running into defenders to establish a ruck or maul.

- ■ Wings
  - ❏ Positions no. 11 and 14
  - ❏ Generally the players who are the quickest and most elusive on the team. They are required to outrun the opposition in open-field play.

- ■ Fullback
  - ❏ Position no. 15
  - ❏ The last line of defense in rugby.
  - ❏ Has responsibilities similar to the safety, punter, and punt returner of American football.
  - ❏ Essential skills include being able to field a kicked ball, kick for distance and accuracy, and consistently tackle in the open field.

- ■ **Formations**
  - ■ Scrum
    - ❏ This aspect of the game is tightly controlled by the referee to prevent injury.
    - ❏ In preparation for the scrum, each pack assembles under the directions of their individual hooker.
    - ❏ After both teams are assembled and stable in the crouched position, the referee will call "Engage!"
      - ▪ Engagement is when the two scrums come together forming a tunnel between the front row players.
      - ▪ The referee calling "engage" is a recent change to enhance safety in the scrum. Previously, the scrums would come together at the end of a cadence called by the hooker of the attacking team. This change was in response to cervical spine injuries that were being reported as result of a powered engagement.
    - ❏ The scrumhalf introduces the ball into the tunnel.
    - ❏ The hookers attempt to hook (kick) the ball backward to their own team.
    - ❏ After the ball has traveled to the rear of the scrum, the ball can be picked up for advancement.
    - ❏ The scrum is used to restart play after the referee has stopped play for minor infringements and at other points in the match.
    - ❏ Strategically, it is used both offensively and defensively (21).
      - ▪ Offense → base for attacking play
      - ▪ Defense → denying the opponents clean possession

- The stability of the scrum is determined by the front row's ability to use their strength to transmit the force to their opponents (21).
- Line out
  - Used to restart play after the ball has gone into touch (out of bounds).
  - There are two to seven forwards from each team arranged in parallel lines that are perpendicular to the touch line.
  - The hooker throws the ball into the tunnel formed by the standing forwards of both teams.
  - Each team has jumpers who will fight for possession of the thrown ball.
  - The jumper is assisted by lifters — two players who grab the jumper above the knees (usually by the shorts) and lift him or her into the air. The lifters also ensure a controlled return to the ground after the jumper has caught the ball. Afterward, a maul (see below) is usually formed.
- Maul
  - Is formed when the ball carried is stopped by a defender but not taken to the ground.
  - Players from both teams attempt to drive the maul down the field by binding to each other and giving a unified push.
  - Both sides attempt to grab the ball out of the maul to restart open-field play.
- Ruck
  - Is formed when a player is tackled and brought to the ground.
  - The tackled player releases the ball on the ground.
  - The opposing teams come together over the top of the ball in an attempt to drive the other team backward away from the ball.
  - One team must drive the other team completely off the ball before the ball can be picked up.
- **Equipment**
  - Ball: ovoid ball that is somewhat larger and rounder than a football
  - Boots: the rugby cleats
    - Typically have removable studs or molded multistudded rubber soles and have cleats similar to soccer. Single-toe cleats (as in baseball) are not permitted.
  - No braces containing metal or hard plastic of any kind (including knee braces) are permitted.
  - Unlike American football, casts or splints are not permitted to be worn during play.
  - No jewelry, earrings, hair devices (other than elastic bands), or eye wear (other than contact lenses) are permitted.
  - Optional equipment:
    - Shoulder pads: Generally a padded pull over top with a maximum thickness of 1/2 inch of foam padding.
    - Mitts: Fingerless gloves
    - Soft headgear: Scrumcap for ear protection to prevent ear trauma
    - Mouthguard
      - Highly suggested
      - Mandatory for high school and below
    - Shin guards: Thin, 0.5-cm soft padding only (no hard plastic) may be worn under the rugby socks.
    - Women may wear chest pads; generally similar to shoulder pads, except padding extends down the front of the chest.
    - Some authors suggest that a lack of regulation mandating protective equipment has resulted in an injury rate three times that of American football (17). This statement, however, does not take into account the vastly differing styles of play between the two sports. Other studies have found a lesser injury rate than American football (10).

EPIDEMIOLOGY

- In rugby union, estimated injury incidence has doubled in the last 40 years (7).
- However, current studies on rugby injury incidence demonstrate a lack of a standardized definition for injury, resulting in the discrepancies seen in the literature with reports ranging from 32 to 218 injuries per 1,000 player-hours of exposure (1–3,9,11,20,29) or an incidence of injury of 1.45 per 100 player appearances (6).
- Injury rates in collegiate and men's club teams range from 13 to 30 per 1,000 game hours.
- Injury rate for youth rugby (< 18 years old) is generally 8–10 per 1,000 game hours (5,16).
  - Concussion is the most common head or neck injury, with an incidence of 4 per 1,000 game hours, and is responsible for approximately 25% of all injuries in this age group. There is a mandatory 21-day recovery period for concussion unless the athlete is asymptomatic and cleared prior to that time period by a physician.
- Injuries in women occur with less frequency. The ratio of injures in men to women is 4:3.
  - The exception may be anterior cruciate ligament (ACL) injury (13).
- Game play produces a greater number and severity of injuries compared to practice (1,3,29).
- Higher body mass index has been associated with a higher injury rate (22).
- Tackling has been cited as the major cause of injury (1,3,6,8,28,29).
  - The player being tackled has twice the injury incidence of the tackler (3).

- The player with the lower momentum is four times more likely to be injured than the player with the higher momentum (3).
- There is a higher rate of tackling injury when two or more tacklers simultaneously make contact with the ball carrier (19).

■ Sprains, strains, contusions, abrasions, and lacerations are to be expected in rugby (1,3,6,9,29).

■ The New Zealand Injury and Performance Project found that the location of injuries in this sport is widespread throughout the entire body (8). The following are the percentages of players who reported an injury at each of the following sites in the previous 12 months.

  - Head/skull/inner ear: 10%
  - Face/outer ear/eye: 19%
  - Neck: 11%
  - Shoulder/clavicle: 21%
  - Back: 17%
  - Chest and abdomen: 4%
  - Arm/elbow: 1%
  - Wrist/hand/finger: 4%
  - Pelvis/hip/groin: 2%
  - Thumb: 18%
  - Upper leg: 19%
  - Knee: 17%
  - Lower leg: 17%
  - Ankle: 24%
  - Heel/foot/toe: 1%

■ The same study examined the total number of rugby injuries in a year and found the following total distribution of injuries (8):

  - Sprains, strains, and other soft tissue injury: 74%
  - Laceration or abrasion: 10%
  - Fracture: 7%
  - Closed head injury: 5%
  - Other: 4%

■ Australia, New Zealand, South Africa, and the United Kingdom have published papers on the incidence of injuries in rugby for varying age and skill levels (1,3,6–9,22, 23,25,26,29,31). The following is an attempted aggregate of the data compiled by Brooks and Kemp (4). The reader should note that this is limited by lack of standardized methods for defining injury.

  - Lower limb injuries: 41%–55%
    - ❏ The lower limb accounts not only for the highest number of injuries, but also the most severe injuries (measured by time lost from participation).
    - ❏ The knee seemed to have the most injuries of the lower limb, with medial collateral ligament (MCL), meniscus, and extensor mechanism injuries being the most common. However, ACL and MCL injuries resulted in the longest periods of absence from sport.
    - ❏ The thigh injuries were predominantly hematomas and hamstring strains.
    - ❏ Ankle injuries were mostly lateral ligament sprains and Achilles tendon injuries.

  - Head and noncatastrophic neck injuries: 12%–33%
    - ❏ Lacerations and concussions were the most common, followed by facial fractures.
    - ❏ However, it should be noted that concussion is often underreported due to a lack of knowledge of the symptoms of concussion and/or due to a delay in diagnosis (14).

  - Upper limb injuries: 15%–24% (4)
    - ❏ The shoulder experienced the greatest number of upper limb injuries, and the damage was disproportionately severe. Acromioclavicular (AC) joint sprain and rotator cuff strain were the most common, but shoulder instability and dislocation caused the longest absences from participation.

■ In the United States, Wetzler et al. (32) published a retrospective study of cervical spine injuries that occurred during the rugby scrum from 1970 to 1996.

  - Fifty-eight percent of rugby cervical spine injuries occurred during the scrum.
  - Sixty-four percent of the above injuries occurred during engagement.
  - Only 36% of the above injuries occurred when the scrum collapsed.
  - Hookers accounted for 78% of injured players, and props accounted for 19% of injured players. Second row players accounted for the remaining 3%.

■ In the United States, 47.5% of all rugby cervical spine injuries occurred in hookers versus 18.6% outside of the United States.

■ There were 57.6% of U.S. catastrophic rugby injuries that occur in the scrum, in contrast to 41.5% outside of the United States (6,32).

■ It is theorized that the discrepancy may be due to the fact that most rugby players in the United States learn to play the sport at college age or older. This is in contrast to other countries where rugby skills and techniques are learned at a much younger age (32).

■ Swain et al. (28) prospectively evaluated neck injury in Australian amateur rugby. Their data show that the majority of neck injuries (42.5%) occur in the tackling phase of play.

  - This was true of all positions, with the exception of the front row (especially hooker), which had the majority of neck injuries during the scrum.
  - There was no statistical difference between the phase of play and the severity of neck injury.
  - The greatest number of neck injuries occurred during game play (85.6%).

- In the United States, there is not a good database for rugby injuries other than catastrophic injuries. USA Rugby is attempting to compile injury data through a standardized reporting system (30).

INJURIES BY POSITION

- The front row is most susceptible to injury during a scrum.
  - When the ball is put into play during a scrum, the necks of the front row are already in a position of slight flexion.
  - The two opposing scrums are applying an axial force on the cervical spines that is equivalent to 0.5–1.5 tons (6,21).
  - Collapse is often related to the following (21):
    - ❏ Inappropriately vertical force vectors during engagement
    - ❏ Poor field conditions with poor traction
    - ❏ Inexperience
    - ❏ Fatigue
    - ❏ Playing with injury
    - ❏ Opposing scrum mismatch in terms of size, ability, strength, and experience
- The second row is susceptible to the following injuries:
  - Neck injury — for the same reasons as the front row but to a lesser extent
  - Auricular hematomas, ear avulsions, and head lacerations, because their heads are positioned between the thighs of the front row players
  - Often wear scrumcaps or an electrical tape headband to secure their ears to the side of their head
  - Susceptible to injuries when they are being lifted during line outs
- Flanker/wing forward
  - Susceptible to injuries in the tackling situation
  - High incidence of AC joint injuries
- Eightman: susceptible to similar head and facial injuries as the locks because of his or her head position between the locks.
- Scrumhalf: susceptible to contact injuries while attempting to secure the ball.
- Pack (positions 1–9): at risk for contact knee injuries (6).
- Backs (positions 10–15) (6)
  - At risk for contact and noncontact knee injuries
  - Susceptible to injury of the head, neck, and shoulders during tackling
- In rucks, the players on the ground are at risk for abrasions, lacerations, contusions, and orofacial trauma from the cleats of other players.
- In mauls and rucks, all players are susceptible to hand and finger injuries from binding to each other's jerseys.

- During tackling, players are at risk for the same injuries as other collision sports.

PREVENTION

- Locks often wear scrumcaps or electrical tape headbands to secure their ears to the side of their head to prevent ear injuries.
- Some players wear shoulder pads to attempt to prevent AC joint injuries.
- There are currently limited studies to date that show the above measures have prevented injury. Marshall et al. (15) found that mouthguards and padded headgear prevented orofacial and scalp injuries.
- Unfortunately, the use of padded headgear has no effect on concussion incidence (15,18).
- Marshall et al. (15) also found that support sleeves may decrease sprains and strains.
- It is apparent that more prospective research is needed on injury prevention.
- On the rugby boots, no toe cleats (like baseball cleats) are allowed.
  - Tackled players are frequently on the ground underneath players from both teams who are attempting to secure the ball with their feet. As such, toe cleats would increase the risk of lacerations to players on the ground.
- The referee conducts a safety inspection of the pitch and all players prior to the match.
  - The referee may prohibit a player from participating if unsafe footwear, uniform, illegal equipment, or long fingernails are found.
  - Medical personnel are encouraged to join the referee for the inspection.
- Because *tight five* players have the highest incidence of cervical spine injury in the United States, they should have extensive practice and instruction prior to competition.
- Depowering the scrum or having uncontested scrums in less experienced play may decrease the risk of cervical spine injury.
- Because fatigue is thought to be a risk factor for injury, all players should maintain a high level of fitness (21).
- USA Rugby encourages all coaches to complete a series of coaching clinics. These clinics will arm coaches with techniques to provide proper instruction on some of the more complex skills and techniques of the game.
- A standardized coach and referee educational program has been shown in New Zealand to decrease catastrophic neck injuries (24). Similar initiatives should be instituted internationally to prevent neck injury in rugby union.
- More evidence-based research is needed on injury epidemiology and injury prevention.

SIDELINE PREPAREDNESS

- Because the spectrum of injury in rugby union is wide, the physician covering this sport must be well rounded and prepared to handle the variety of acute injuries.

- The nature of the substitution rules of rugby places more pressure on a sideline physician to make a timely decision on fitness to play. Prompt and accurate evaluation is therefore critical. The game continues without a substitution while the physician is evaluating the injured athlete. If another player replaces the injured rugger, he or she cannot return to the match, even if physically capable. Therefore, the coach relies on the physician to tell him or her whether to play one man down until the injured person returns or whether a permanent substitution needs to be made.

- There is a delicate balance between not prematurely removing an athlete from play versus minimizing the time the team competes one man short while the physician is performing the evaluation.

- Lacerations deserve special mention because the team physician's proficiency in attending to a bleeding wound within the allotted "blood sub" time of 15 minutes will determine whether an athlete is able to return to play.

- Although rare, catastrophic injury has been reported in rugby union play. An emergency response plan should be preestablished in case of such a situation.

- The USA Rugby and the International Rugby Board Web sites have sections for medical providers that provide good information for those interested in providing sideline coverage for rugby union (http://www.usarugby.org and http://www. irbplayerwelfare.com).

REFERENCES

1. Bathgate A, Best JP, Craig G, Jamieson M. A prospective study of injuries to elite Australian rugby union players. *Br J Sports Med.* 2002;36(4):265–9.
2. Best JP, McIntosh AS, Savage TN. Rugby World Cup 2003 injury surveillance project. *Br J Sports Med.* 2005;39(11):812–7.
3. Brooks JH, Fuller CW, Kemp SP, Reddin DB. A prospective study of injuries and training amongst the England 2003 Rugby World Cup squad. *Br J Sports Med.* 2005;39(5):288–93.
4. Brooks JH, Kemp SP. Recent trends in rugby union injuries. *Clin Sports Med.* 2008;27(1):51–73, vii–viii.
5. Dexter WD. Rugby. In: Mellion MB, Putukian M, Madden C, editors. *Sports Medicine Secrets.* Philadelphia: Hanley and Belfus; 2003.
6. Dietzen CJ, Topping BR. Rugby football. *Phys Med Rehabil Clin N Am.* 1999;10(1):159–75.
7. Garraway WM, Lee AJ, Hutton SJ, Russell EB, Macleod DA. Impact of professionalism on injuries in rugby union. *Br J Sports Med.* 2000;34(5):348–51.
8. Gerrard DF, Waller AE, Bird YN. The New Zealand rugby injury and performance project: II. Previous injury experience of a rugby-playing cohort. *Br J Sports Med.* 1994;28(4):229–33.
9. Jakoet I, Noakes TD. A high rate of injury during the 1995 Rugby World Cup. *S Afr Med J.* 1998;88(1):45–7.
10. Kaplan KM, Goodwillie A, Strauss EJ, Rosen JE. Rugby injuries: a review of concepts and current literature. *Bull NYU Hosp Jt D.* 2008;66(2):86–93.
11. Kemp SP, Hudson Z, Brooks JH, Fuller CW. The epidemiology of head injuries in English professional rugby union. *Clin J Sport Med.* 2008;18(3):227–34.
12. Laws of the Game Rugby Union. International Rugby Board Web site [Internet]. [cited 2011 Sept 1]. Available from: http://www.irblaws.com/EN/.
13. Levy AS, Wetzler MJ, Lewars M, Laughlin W. Knee injuries in women collegiate rugby players. *Am J Sport Med.* 1997;25(3):360–2.
14. MacQueen AE, Dexter WW. Injury trends and prevention in rugby union football. *Curr Sports Med Rep.* 2010;9(3):139–43.
15. Marshall SW, Loomis DP, Waller AE, et al. Evaluation of protective equipment for prevention of injuries in rugby union. *Int J Epidemiol.* 2005;34(1):113–8.
16. Marshall SW, Spencer RJ. Concussion and rugby: the hidden epidemic. *J Athl Train.* 2001;36(3):334–8.
17. Marshall SW, Waller AE, Dick RW, Pugh CB, Loomis DP, Chalmers DJ. An ecologic study of protective equipment and injury in two contact sports. *Int J Epidemiol.* 2002;31(3):587–92.
18. McIntosh AS, McCrory P, Finch CF, Best JP, Chalmers DJ, Wolfe R. Does padded headgear prevent head injury in rugby union football? *Med Sci Sports Exerc.* 2009;41(2):306–13.
19. McIntosh AS, Savage TN, McCrory P, Fréchède BO, Wolfe R. Tackle characteristics and injury in a cross section of rugby union football. *Med Sci Sports Exerc.* 2010;42(5):977–84.
20. McManus A. Validation of an instrument for injury data collection in rugby union. *Br J Sports Med.* 2000;34(5):342–7.
21. Milburn PD. Biomechanics of rugby union scrummaging. Technical and safety issues. *Sports Med.* 1993;16(3):168–79.
22. Quarrie KL, Alsop JC, Waller AE, Bird YN, Marshall SW, Chalmers DJ. The New Zealand rugby injury and performance project. VI. A prospective cohort study of risk factors for injury in rugby union football. *Br J Sports Med.* 2001;35(3):157–66.
23. Quarrie KL, Cantu RC, Chalmers DJ. Rugby union injuries to the cervical spine and spinal cord. *Sports Med.* 2002;32(10):633–53.
24. Quarrie KL, Gianotti SM, Hopkins WG, Hume PA. Effect of nationwide injury prevention programme on serious spinal injuries in New Zealand rugby union: ecological study. *BMJ.* 2007;334(7604):1150.
25. Quarrie KL, Handcock P, Toomey MJ, Waller AE. The New Zealand rugby injury and performance project. IV. Anthopometric and physical performance comparisons between positional categories of senior A rugby players. *Br J Sports Med.* 1996;30(1):53–6.
26. Quarrie KL, Handcock P, Waller AE, Chalmers DJ, Toomey MJ, Wilson BD. The New Zealand rugby injury and performance project: III. Anthropometric and physical performance characteristics of players. *Br J Sports Med.* 1995;29(4):263–70.
27. Scher AT. Rugby injuries to the cervical spine and spinal cord: a 10-year review. Clin Sports Med. 1998;17(1):195–206.
28. Swain MS, Pollard HP, Bonello R. Incidence, severity, aetiology and type of neck injury in men's amateur rugby union: a prospective cohort study. *Chiropr Osteopat.* 2010;18:18.
29. Targett SG. Injuries in professional Rugby Union. *Clin J Sport Med.* 1998;8(4):280–5.
30. USA Rugby Web site [Internet]. Colorado Springs (CO): USA Rugby; [cited 1 Sept 2011]. Available from: http://www.usarugby.org.
31. Waller AE, Feehan M, Marshall SW, Chalmers DJ. The New Zealand rugby injury and performance project: I. Design and methodology of a prospective follow-up study. *Br J Sports Med.* 1994;28(4):223–8.
32. Wetzler MJ, Akpata T, Laughlin W, Levy AS. Occurrence of cervical spine injuries during the rugby scrum. *Am J Sports Med.* 1998;26:(2):177–80.

Running

Robert Wilder and Francis G. O'Connor

EPIDEMIOLOGY OF RUNNING INJURIES (160)

- There are over 30 million runners, of whom more than 10 million run on more than 100 days per year.
- One million enter competitive races per year (39,68,155).
- Yearly injury incidence rate ranges from 29.5% to 56% (39,68, 87,145,155,157).
- Injury rate ranges from 2.5 to 5.8 injuries per 1,000 hours of running (39,87,155). The lower rate of 2.5 per 1,000 hours is seen in long-distance and marathon runners. Sprinters have the highest rate of 5.8 injuries per 1,000 hours, and middle-distance runners are between the two at 5.6 injuries per 1,000 hours (87).
- Despite the relatively high incidence rate of running injuries per runner per year, this incidence rate is still two to six times lower than in other sports (39,155).

Common Injury Sites

- Most running injuries are musculoskeletal overuse syndromes (Table 99.1); 70%–80% occur from the knee down.
- Back: 5%
  - Hip and groin: 15%
  - Knee: 40%
  - Lower leg: 20%
  - Foot and ankle: 20%
- Although there are no age- or gender-related differences, there are differences in injury pattern between sprinters, middle-distance runners, and long-distance runners. Hamstring strains and tendinitis are more commonly seen in sprinters; backache and hip problems are more commonly seen in middle-distance runners; and foot problems are more common among long-distance and marathon runners (87,121).

Risk Factors for Running Injuries (26,27,44, 72,88,146,154,159,160,165)

- Important risk factors (for which a clear association with injury has been identified)
  - Training miles per week (risk increases at 19 miles per week and increases more sharply at 40 miles per week) (44,88)
  - Previous running injury (within past 12 months) (88)

- Inexperienced runner (running < 3 years)
  - Recent transition in training
  - Training intensity
  - Cavus feet
- Equivocal risk factors (for which evidence demonstrating a clear link with injury is unclear)
  - Hyperflexibility or hypoflexibility
  - Stretching exercises (3,148)
  - Running shoes
  - Shoe orthotics
  - Roadside running
  - Malalignment problems (genu varum and valgus, high Q-angle, femoral neck anteversion, pelvic obliquity, knee and patella alignment, rearfoot valgus, leg length discrepancy)
  - Body morphology (slight protective effect in men with body mass index > 26 kg · m²)
  - Age
- Unrelated risk factors (have not been associated with increase in running injuries)
  - Gender
  - Running surface
  - Cross-training
  - Time of day
  - Warm-up or cool-down periods

BIOMECHANICS OF RUNNING

The Running Gait Cycle

- During walking, the stance phase occupies 40% of the gait cycle. The stance phase is decreased to approximately 30% while running and 20% while sprinting (18).
- Walking differs from running in that walking has two double support periods in stance, whereas running has two periods of double float in swing. Running does not have a period of double support (18).

Kinematics

- Generally, there is an increase in joint range of motion (ROM) as velocity increases. However, there are no major differences

Table 99.1 | **Top Running Injuries (42,124,156)**

Diagnosis	Percentage
Patellofemoral pain syndrome	32.2
Tibial stress syndrome, "shin splints"	17.3
Achilles tendinitis	7.2
Stress fractures	7.2
Patellar tendinitis	5.7
Iliotibial band syndrome	6.3
Metatarsal stress syndrome	3.3
Adductor strain	3
Hamstring strain	2.6
Posterior tibial tendinitis	2.6
Ankle sprain	2.4
Peroneus tendinitis	1.9
Iliac apophysitis	1.6

between walking and running kinematics in the coronal and transverse planes. Most kinematic differences occur in the sagittal plane (18,112). The body lowers its center of gravity with increased speed by increasing flexion at the hips and knees and by increased dorsiflexion at the ankle (18,92).

- The hip
  - The hip demonstrates an overall increase in ROM as velocity increases. The most significant motion occurs in the sagittal plane. Most of this increase occurs in flexion, and the amount of extension actually decreases slightly. Overall ROM was determined to be 43 degrees with maximum flexion and extension, measuring 37 and 6 degrees, respectively, for normal walking. In running, however, overall ROM was increased to 46 degrees, with the hip flexing and never quite returning past neutral into extension (18,113).

- The knee
  - As in the hip, the most significant motion occurs in the sagittal plane. The knee joint demonstrates increased flexion as velocity increases, but extension is, as in the hip, decreased. Maximum flexion in walking reaches 64 degrees, and extension is −8 degrees (8 degrees of flexion). In running, maximum flexion reaches 79 degrees, and extension is −16 degrees (16 degrees of flexion) (18,92).

- The ankle and foot
  - Overall ROM at the ankle during walking is estimated to be 30 degrees, with maximum plantarflexion of 18 degrees and maximum dorsiflexion of 12 degrees. Running produces a greater overall ankle ROM of 50 degrees due to increased hip and knee flexion during running (18).
  - At initial contact, due to the increased hip and knee flexion, the ankle undergoes rapid dorsiflexion during the absorption phase. In running, because the ankle

never quite reaches the amount of plantarflexion that it undergoes while walking, the amount of supination in the subtalar joint is limited, but the degree of pronation is increased (18).

- Subtalar motion is determined by muscular activity as well as response to ground reactive forces. Midtarsal joint motion, however, is determined by subtalar position (18).

- When the calcaneus and the talus are supinated, the axis is such that an increased obliquity is produced across the oblique and longitudinal midtarsal joints. This serves to lock the midtarsal joint functionally, thereby resulting in a decrease in available motion and allowing the foot to become a "rigid lever." This occurs during late terminal stance and preswing. When the calcaneus and talus are pronated, the axis is such that an increased parallelism exists between the oblique and longitudinal midtarsal joints. This results in an increased available motion in these joints, serving to unlock the midtarsal joint and allowing an increased ROM for adaptation to the ground surface as well as absorbing the ground reactive forces, which lets the foot become a "mobile adapter." This occurs during the midstance (18).

- As the foot makes contact with the floor, the pelvis, femur, and tibia begin the process of internal rotation. This internal rotation lasts through loading response and into midstance, resulting in eversion and unlocking of the subtalar joint. This results in subtalar pronation, which allows unlocking of the oblique and longitudinal midtarsal joints, resulting in further pronation. The pelvis, femur, and tibia then begin to rotate externally, which causes inversion and locking of the subtalar joint (18).

Kinetics

- Walking produces vertical ground reactive forces equal to 1.3–1.5 times body weight. During running, vertical ground reactive forces spike sharply at contact to produce an impact peak, may slightly decrease, and then continue to an active peak measuring 2.2–2.6 times body weight. It is thus during midstance when ground reactive forces are greatest, with peak internal joint moments generating peak mechanical stress on tissues (35,132).

- It is unclear whether increased impact forces lead to injury or impact peak performance (35,62,63,105,108).

- The percentage of muscle activity increases throughout stance phase during running. It is rare to see a muscle group active for more than 50% of the stance phase during walking, but in running, activity is noted for 70%–80% of the stance phase (91).

- During walking, the **gluteus maximus** is active from the end of the swing phase until the foot is flat on the floor. This serves to decelerate the limb and stabilize the hip joint for initial contact. During running, however, it is active from terminal swing through 40% the stance phase. This helps to produce hip extension (18).

- The **hip abductors** function during the terminal swing and throughout 50% of the stance phase during walking and running. This serves to stabilize the stance leg pelvis at initial contact, which prevents excessive sagging of the swing leg (18,67).

- The **hip adductors** are active during the last one-third of the stance phase during walking. During running, they are active during the entire stance and swing phases (18,91).

- The **quadriceps** are active at the end of the swing phase to bring about terminal knee extension and to aid in hip flexion, through a concentric contraction. They also help stabilize the knee joint at initial contact, through an eccentric contraction. In running, they are highly active during the absorption phase of stance to deal with the greater requirements of weight acceptance. They are continually active throughout knee flexion eccentrically to limit the rate at which knee flexion occurs. They are active for 50%–60% of the running stance phase and for only 25% of the walking stance phase (18).

- During walking, the **hamstrings** are active at the end of swing phase and into stance phase until the foot is in full contact with the ground. This occurs in about 10% of the walking gait cycle. During running, they are active during the last third of the swing phase during hip and knee extension. Here they are acting concentrically across the hip joint but eccentrically across the knee joint. This action initiates hip extension and resists knee extension simultaneously (18).

- During walking, the **anterior tibial muscle** group is active from late stance phase through the swing phase and then for the first 10%–15% of the next stance phase. This produces dorsiflexion of the ankle during the swing phase through concentric contraction. It also helps to control plantarflexion by initial contact through eccentric contraction, thereby preventing foot slap. During running, these muscles are active from late stance phase through the swing phase and for the first 50%–60% of the next stance phase. For their duration of activity, they are undergoing concentric contraction. During walking, they decelerate foot plantarflexion at initial contact; however, during running they appear to accelerate movement of the leg over the fixed foot. In heel strikers, a greater degree of activity is found in the anterior tibial muscle group than in midfoot strikers (18).

- Activity of the **posterior leg musculature** begins during terminal swing of gait. During walking, these muscles act to resist forward movement of the tibia over the fixed foot during the stance phase. They are active from 25% to 50% of the stance phase through mostly eccentric contraction. During their last 25% of activity, they undergo concentric contraction to initiate active plantarflexion. During running gait, initial contact is a period of rapid dorsiflexion. Here the triceps undergo eccentric contraction, again to resist this motion. They are active for approximately 60% of the stance phase. Initially they serve to stabilize the ankle joint at initial contact, and then to provide for propulsion (18).

COMMON RUNNING INJURIES

Patellofemoral Syndrome (6,32,36,49,50)

- Definition
  - Pain associated with the articular surface of the patella and femoral condyles
  - "Runner's knee"; number 1 presenting complaint to runners' clinics
  - Number 1 cause of lost time in basic training in military recruits
- Diagnosis (25,49)
  - Anterior, peripatellar, subpatellar pain
  - Increased pain following prolonged sitting (theatre sign) as well as running downhill and walking downstairs
  - Apprehension (shrug) sign
  - Abnormal patella tilt (tilt < 5 degrees in males and < 10 degrees in females)
  - Abnormal patella glide (medial glide < two quadrants, lateral glide > three quadrants)
- Contributing factors (6,25,49,97,150)
  - Femoral dysplasia
  - Patellar facet asymmetry
  - Malalignments contributing to excessive pronation
    - ❏ Femoral anteversion
    - ❏ External tibial torsion
    - ❏ Varus ankle, foot
  - Patella alta, baja
  - Increased Q-angle
  - Muscle and soft tissue imbalances
    - ❏ Weak vastus medialis oblique (VMO)
    - ❏ Tight lateral structures (iliotibial band [ITB], lateral retinaculum)
    - ❏ Weakness of hip abductors, extensors, external rotators
- Treatment (25,107)
  - Correct biomechanical factors that lead to compensatory subtalar pronation and obligatory internal tibial rotation: genu valgum, tibia vara, hindfoot varus, forefoot pronation
  - Flexibility: ITB, hamstrings, quadriceps, gastrocnemius
  - Manual therapy to stretch tight retinaculum: medial glide and tilt
  - Strengthening: quadriceps with emphasis on VMO, hip abductors, extensors, external rotators
  - McConnell taping
  - Bracing (patellar straps and braces) (126)
  - With persistent symptoms, consider:
    - ❏ Magnetic resonance imaging (MRI) (osteochondritis, cartilage injury)

❏ Injections (steroid, viscosupplementation)

❏ Surgery: lateral release if tight retinaculum; realignment

Iliotibial Band Syndrome (6,46,47,48,51,57)

■ Definition

- An overuse tendinopathy of the ITB most commonly as it passes over the lateral femoral condyle.

- ITB syndrome is the most common cause of lateral knee pain in runners, accounting for up to 12% of all running-related overuse injuries (10,23,85,106).

- ITB syndrome results from repetitive friction of the ITB at the lateral femoral epicondyle. The ITB moves anterior to the epicondyle as the knee extends and posterior as the knee flexes, remaining tense in both positions (41,48,111). Specifically, the posterior edge of the ITB impinges against the lateral femoral epicondyle of the femur just after foot strike. This "impingement zone" occurs at or at slightly less than 30 degrees of knee flexion (111). Fairclough et al. (42) have alternatively proposed that ITB syndrome results from compression of the ITB against the lateral femoral epicondyle as a consequence of internal tibial rotation after foot strike as opposed to friction. Repetitive irritation can lead to chronic inflammation, especially beneath the posterior fibers of the ITB, which are thought to be tighter against the lateral femoral condyle than the anterior fibers (48,111).

- The ITB is a continuation of the tendinous portion of the tensor fascia lata (TFL) muscle, with some contribution from the gluteal muscles. It is connected to the linea aspera via the intermuscular septum. Distally, the ITB spans out and inserts on the lateral border of the patella, the lateral retinaculum, and Gerdy's tubercle of the tibia. The ITB is free from bony attachment between the superior aspect of the lateral femoral epicondyle and Gerdy's tubercle (48,93,147).

- Functioning as abductors during open-chain activity, the TFL, gluteus medius, and gluteus minimus provide important function through the support phase of the gait cycle, eccentrically lengthening while stabilizing the pelvis and controlling femoral adduction (48,56).

■ Diagnosis

- Lateral pain and crepitus at lateral femoral condyle (or insertion at Gerdy's tubercle)

- Tight ITB on Ober's test

- Abductor weakness

■ Contributing factors (10,46,48,85,89,98,99)

- Varus positioning of knee, tibia, and foot

- Increased hip adduction and internal rotation

- Internal tibial torsion

- Excessive supination or pronation

- Abductor tightness and weakness

- Higher knee flexion at heel strike

- Downhill running

- Running on crowned roads

- Excessive running in same direction on track

■ Treatment

- PRICEMM (protection, rest, ice, compression, elevation, modalities, medication); iontophoresis

- ITB strap or dual-action strap

- Foam roller exercise for soft tissue work

- Myofascial release

- Flexibility and strength (hip abductors, adductors, rotators, flexors, extensors)

■ With persistent symptoms, consider:

- Injection (steroid)

- MRI to rule out lateral meniscus, other

Shin Splints

■ Definition

- Shin splints, or medial tibial stress syndrome, is a clinical entity characterized by diffuse tenderness over the posteromedial aspect of the distal third of the tibia. Shin splints have been reported to account for 12%–18% of running injuries (21,58,69) and to occur in 4% of all military recruits in basic training (5). Women appear more frequently affected than men.

- Medial tibial stress syndrome should be differentiated from stress fractures and exertional compartment syndrome. Although different entities, they may coexist. Plain films are negative (except in cases of previous or coexistent stress fracture). Bone scans will demonstrate characteristic vertical linear increased activity along the tibial periosteum, which differs from the more focal fusiform increased radiotracer uptake exhibited by stress fractures.

- Medial tibial stress syndrome is felt by most to represent a periostalgia or tendinopathy along the tibial attachment of the tibialis posterior or soleus muscles. Other proposed etiologies have included posterior compartment syndrome and fascial inflammation. Detmer (33) proposed a classification scheme for medial tibial stress syndrome based on etiology. Type 1 includes local stress fractures, type 2 includes periostitis/periostalgia, and type 3 includes deep posterior compartment syndrome.

■ Diagnosis

- Dull ache in medial shaft with activity

- Tenderness to palpation along shaft

- Normal neurovascular exam and x-ray

■ Contributing factors

- Factors that increase valgus forces and pronation, which then increase eccentric contraction of the soleus and tibialis posterior: femoral anteversion, genu varum, tibia and forefoot varus, excessive Q-angle.

- Excessive pes planus or cavus
- Tarsal coalition
- Leg length inequality
- Muscle imbalances: inflexibility of plantarflexors; weakness of dorsiflexors, plantarflexors, invertors
- Extrinsic risk factors include improper shoe wear, a rapid transition in training, inadequate warm-up, running on uneven or hard surfaces, running in cold weather, and low calcium intake.
- Treatment (5)
  - Flexibility: gastrocnemius-soleus, tibialis posterior
  - Strength: concentric and eccentric, including tibialis posterior soleus, tibialis anterior, flexor hallucis, flexor digitorum longus
  - Orthotic to control compensatory pronation
  - Shin sleeve
- With persistent symptoms, consider:
  - Bone scan/MRI to rule out stress fracture
  - Compartment testing to rule out compartment syndrome
  - Consider lumbar radiculopathy

Exertional Compartment Syndrome

- Definition
  - Chronic exertional compartment syndrome is defined as reversible ischemia secondary to a noncompliant osseofascial compartment that is unresponsive to the expansion of muscle volume that occurs with exercise. Most commonly seen in the lower leg, exertional compartment syndrome in athletes has also been described in the thigh and medial compartment of the foot (17,100,128).
  - There are four major compartments in the leg. Each is bound by bone and fascia, and each contains a major nerve.
    - The anterior compartment contains the extensor hallucis longus, extensor digitorum longus, peroneus tertius, and anterior tibialis muscles, as well as the deep peroneal nerve.
    - The lateral compartment contains the peroneus longus and brevis as well as the superficial peroneal nerve.
    - The superficial posterior compartment contains the gastrocnemius and soleus muscles and the sural nerve.
    - The deep posterior compartment contains the flexor hallucis longus, flexor digitorum longus, and posterior tibialis muscles, as well as the posterior tibial nerve. Some authors believe that the posterior tibialis should be considered a separate compartment because it is surrounded by its own fascia (2).
  - Anterior compartment syndrome is most common (45%), followed by the deep posterior compartment (40%), lateral compartment (10%), and superficial posterior compartment (5%) (38).

- Diagnosis
  - Recurrent exercise-induced leg discomfort that occurs at a well-defined and reproducible point and increases if the training persists. Pain is usually described as a tight, cramp-like, or squeezing ache over a specific compartment of the leg. Relief of symptoms only occurs with discontinuation of activity. Examination may or may not demonstrate fascial hernias. In some cases, the classic exertional component is not as evident, and patients complain of pain at rest or with daily activities as well.
  - A neurologic and vascular examination should also be performed with reproduction of the symptoms. Understanding the distribution of nerves and functions of muscles in relation to symptoms can help identify the affected compartment in cases where the pain is not well localized to one specific compartment, or it may help determine which compartments are more severely affected in cases where more than one compartment is involved.
    - Anterior compartment: weakness of dorsiflexion or toe extension; paresthesias over the dorsum of the foot; numbness in the first web space; or even transient or persistent foot drop.
    - Lateral compartment: sensory changes over the anterolateral aspect of the leg and weakness of ankle eversion. An inversion and equinus deformity may also be present.
    - Superficial posterior compartment: dorsolateral foot hypoesthesia and plantarflexion weakness.
    - Deep posterior compartment: paresthesias in the plantar aspect of the foot and weakness of toe flexion and foot inversion.
  - The gold standard diagnostic tool is intracompartment pressure monitoring (66).
  - One or more of the following pressure criteria must be met in addition to a history and physical examination that is consistent with the diagnosis of chronic exertional compartment syndrome: preexercise pressure ≥ 15 mm Hg; 1-minute postexercise pressure ≥ 30 mm Hg; or 5-minute postexercise pressure ≥ 20 mm Hg. Diagnosis may require the **sport-specific activity** to induce symptoms and raise intracompartment pressure (116).
  - Other tools that have been used in the diagnosis of compartment syndrome include the triple-phase bone scan, MRI, near-infrared spectroscopy, methoxyisobutylisonitrile (MIBI) perfusion imaging, and thallous chloride scintigraphy (4,8,20,40,61,71,75,95,96,114,136,137,161,162).
- Contributing factors
  - Enclosure of compartmental contents in an inelastic fascial sheath, increased volume of the skeletal muscle with exertion due to blood flow and edema, muscle hypertrophy as a response to exercise, and dynamic contraction factors due to the gait cycle.
  - It has also been proposed that myofiber damage as a result of eccentric exercise causes a release of protein-bound

ions and a subsequent increase in osmotic pressure within the compartment. The increase in osmotic pressure increases capillary relaxation pressure, thus decreasing the blood flow.

- Rapid increases in muscle size due to fluid retention are also believed to play a role in the development of chronic exertional compartment syndrome in athletes taking the popular supplement creatine (55).

- Treatment (162)

  - Conservative measures include relative rest (limiting activity to that level that avoids any more than minimal symptoms), anti-inflammatories, stretching and strengthening of the involved muscles, and orthotics (particularly in cases of excessive pronation).

  - Should symptoms persist despite 6–12 weeks of conservative care, in cases of extreme pressure elevation or progressive neurologic deficit, surgical remediation (fasciotomy of the involved compartments with or without fasciectomy) should be undertaken (84,103,129,142,152,164).

  - Single and double incision as well as endoscopic techniques have been described. Regardless of the technique, any fascial hernias must be included in the fascial incision. Surgical treatment generally has good success with return to running without significant symptoms. Anterior compartment fasciotomy success rates usually exceed 85%. Deep posterior success rates are lower, approximately 70%. Due to a high rate of coexistence, some authors advocate release of the lateral compartment whenever a procedure for anterior compartment syndrome is performed. Others have stated that this dual release may not be necessary if clinical evaluation and compartment pressure testing fail to demonstrate lateral compartment involvement. When performing a deep posterior compartment release, attention must be given to adequate decompression of the tibialis posterior (30,138,161).

Achilles Tendinopathy

- Definition (7,70,73,79,115,127,141,162)
  - A spectrum of tissue disorders involving the Achilles tendon and sheath: tendinitis, tendinosis, peritendinitis, tear
- Diagnosis
  - Tenderness at myotendinous junction or insertion
- Contributing factors
  - Pronation
  - Lower extremity varus
  - Tight heel cord
  - Weak dorsiflexors/plantarflexors
  - Ankle instability
- Treatment (79)
  - Heel lifts
  - Control pronation
  - Flexibility (include gastrocnemius and soleus)

- Strength (particularly eccentric strength) (90,141)
- Modalities (iontophoresis, cross-friction massage)
- If persistent, consider:
  - Retrocalcaneal bursitis
  - MRI (evaluate tears)
  - Immobilization
  - Lidocaine injections for peritendinitis
  - Nitro-Dur patches (65,117)
  - Platelet-rich plasma (controversial) (34,101)

Plantar Fasciitis

- Definition
  - An overload injury including inflammation, degeneration, and tearing of the plantar fascia, most commonly at its calcaneal insertion
- Contributing factors (24,45,80,120,131)
  - Tight gastrocnemius-soleus, plantar fascia
  - Rigid rear foot
  - Overpronation or oversupination
  - Decreased ankle strength
  - Obesity
  - Excessive time on one's feet
- Diagnosis (24,37,54,149)
  - Pain in plantar heel worse in morning and with activity
  - Tenderness in plantar medial heel
  - Normal neurologic exam
  - No bony (calcaneal) tenderness
- Treatment
  - Phase 1: nonsteroidal anti-inflammatory drugs, Medrol (if severe)
    - ❏ Device (*i.e.*, Counterforce (CTF) arch brace) or low dye taping
    - ❏ Stretch (gastrocnemius-soleus, plantar fascia, hamstrings, ITB)
    - ❏ Strength (foot intrinsic, ankle, lower quarter stability)
  - Phase 2: Physical therapy (phonophoresis/iontophoresis, massage, manual therapy to improve ankle and subtalar mobility)
    - ❏ Continue exercise
    - ❏ Different device (*i.e.*, heel cushion)
    - ❏ Night splint or sock (11,13,28,118,125)
  - Phases 3 and 4: Injections (three maximum) (1,22,28, 74,82), orthotics (76,119,135,163)
- If persistent, consider:
  - MRI to rule out calcaneal stress injury
  - Electromyography/nerve conduction studies to rule out medial calcaneal, plantar neuropathy (first branch of lateral plantar nerve), radiculopathy
  - Immobilization (151)

- Emerging therapies: shockwave therapy (symptoms > 12 months) (19,59,102,109,110,133,134,143,158), platelet-rich plasma/autologous blood (89), Botox injection (9,86,122)
- Surgery if conservative care fails (6–12 months)

Stress Fractures

- Definition
  - Failure of bone to adapt adequately to mechanical loads (ground reaction forces and muscle contraction) experienced during physical activity
  - Tibial stress fractures predominate in distance runners. Navicular stress fractures predominate in track athletes.
- Diagnosis (60)
  - Focal tenderness
  - Recent transition in training
  - X-ray (often negative, especially early)
  - Bone scan (all three phases with increased uptake)
  - MRI (periosteal and marrow edema T2 > T1)
- Contributing factors
  - Rapid transition in training (144)
  - Low bone mineral density (in women) (14,15,77)
  - Menstrual irregularities; in particular, amenorrhea > 6 months
  - Smaller cross-sectional bone geometry (29,43,123)
  - Low calcium and vitamin D intake (83,104,153)
  - Lesser thigh and calf muscle size (14,16)
  - Leg length difference > 0.5 cm (16)
  - Excessive pes cavus (femoral, tibial) or pes planus (metatarsals)
  - Varus forefoot (64,81,94)
  - Higher loading rate, but not peak force magnitude of ground reaction force (31)
  - Femoral anteversion
  - Hip adduction, rearfoot eversion (tibial)
  - Poor shoe wear (shoes > 5 months old) (53)
- Treatment
  - Noncritical: Noncritical stress fractures can be treated with 6–8 weeks of relative rest and include the following: medial tibia, metatarsals 2, 3, and 4; fifth metatarsal avulsion. Athletes may benefit from a short period (*i.e.*, 3 weeks) in a walking boot.
  - Critical stress fractures require more specific attention due to slower healing and higher rates of nonunion and include the following: femoral neck, anterior tibia, medial malleolus, navicular, base of fifth metatarsal.
    - Femoral neck (52)
      - Normal x-ray, no cortical break: conservative treatment, partial weight bearing to weight bearing as tolerated. Follow clinically and serial MRI 8–12 weeks. Cortical break: orthopedic referral.
      - Superior (distraction) fractures have a higher incidence of worsening and nonunion than inferior (compression) fractures.
    - Anterior tibia (12,130)
      - Conservative care can take up to 6–8 months. Options include pneumatic leg brace +/− bone stimulator, casting, and relative rest.
      - If no healing: orthopedic referral (transverse drilling, grafting, medullary fixation)
    - Medial malleolus (139,140)
      - Nondisplaced: boot or air cast for 6 weeks
      - Displaced or nonunion: orthopedic referral
    - Navicular (78)
      - Non–weight bearing for 6–8 weeks
      - Progressive activity over 6 more weeks
    - Proximal fifth metatarsal (124,156,166)
      - Jones fracture of proximal diaphysis: cast, non–weight bearing for 6–10 weeks
      - Nonunion: orthopedic referral consider orthopedic early in competitive athletes.

SOME PRACTICAL GUIDELINES FOR CLINICIANS

- Certain injuries require the runner to refrain from running (stress fractures, radiculopathy). With most overuse injuries, however, some level of training may be permitted following the "Relative Activity Modification Guidelines" (Wilder RP; The Runner's Clinic at University of Virginia).
  - Pain/discomfort should not exceed the mild level (< 3/10 on the 10-point pain scale).
  - Pain that eases after a warm-up is generally benign. Do not run if pain progressively worsens.
  - Do not run if you are limping or changing your gait mechanics.
- Supplement lost run training with cross-training (aqua running, bike, elliptical).
- Do not increase mileage more rapidly than 10% per week.
- Long run of the week increases no more than 2 miles per week and should not exceed 30% of one's weekly mileage.
- Change shoes every 350–400 miles.

REFERENCES

1. Acevedo JI, Beskin JL. Complications of plantar fascia rupture associated with corticosteroid injection. *Foot Ankle Int.* 1998;19(2):91–7.
2. Albertson KS, Dammann GG. The leg. In: O'Connor FG, Wilder RP, editors. *The Textbook of Running Medicine.* New York: McGraw-Hill; 2001. p. 647–54.

3. Amako M, Oda T, Masuoka K, Yokoi H, Campisi P. Effect of static stretching on prevention of injuries for military recruits. *Mil Med*. 2003;168(6):442–6.

4. Amendola A, Rorabeck CH, Vellett D, Vezina W, Rutt B, Nott L. The use of magnetic resonance imaging in exertional compartment syndromes. *Am J Sports Med*. 1990;18(1):29–34.

5. Andrish JT, Bergfeld JA, Walheim J. A prospective study on the management of shin splints. *J Bone Joint Surg Am*. 1974;56(8):1697–700.

6. Arroyo J, McConnell J, Fredericson M. The knee. In Wilder RP, O'Connor FG, Magrum E, editors. *The Textbook of Running Medicine*. Philadelphia: Human Kinetics; in press.

7. Aström M, Rausing A. Chronic Achilles tendinopathy. A survey of surgical and histopathologic findings. *Clin Orthop Relat Res*. 1995;316: 151–64.

8. Awbrey BJ, Sienkiewicz PS, Mankin HJ. Chronic exercise-induced compartment pressure elevation measured with a miniaturized fluid pressure monitor. A laboratory and clinical study. *Am J Sports Med*. 1988;16(6):610–5.

9. Babcock MS, Foster L, Pasquina P, Jabbari B. Treatment of pain attributed to plantar fasciitis with botulinum toxin A: a short-term, randomized, placebo-controlled, double-blind study. *Am J Phys Med Rehabil*. 2005;84(9):649–54.

10. Barber FA, Sutker AN. Iliotibial band syndrome. *Sports Med*. 1992;14(2):144–8.

11. Barry LD, Barry AN, Cher Y. A retrospective study of standing gastrocnemius-soleus stretching versus night splinting in the treatment of plantar fasciitis. *J Foot Ankle Surg*. 2002;41(4):221–7.

12. Batt ME, Kemp S, Kerslake R. Delayed union stress fractures of the anterior tibia: conservative management. *Br J Sports Med*. 2001;35(1):74–7.

13. Batt ME, Tanji JL, Skattum N. Plantar fasciitis: a prospective randomized clinical trial of the tension night splint. *Clin J Sports Med*. 1996;6(3):158–62.

14. Beck TJ, Ruff CB, Shaffer RA, Betsinger K, Trone DW, Brodine SK. Stress fracture in military recruits: gender differences in muscle and bone susceptibility factors. *Bone*. 2000;27(3):437–44.

15. Bennell KL, Malcolm SA, Thomas SA, et al. Risk factors for stress fractures in track and field athletes. A twelve-month prospective study. *Am J Sports Med*. 1996;24(6):810–8.

16. Bennell KL, Malcolm SA, Thomas SA, Wark JD, Brukner PD. The incidence and distribution of stress fractures in competitive track and field athletes. A twelve-month prospective study. *Am J Sports Med*. 1996;24(2):211–7.

17. Birnbaum J. Recurrent compartment syndrome in the posterior thigh. *Am J Sports Med*. 1983;11(1):48–9.

18. Birrer RB, Buzermanis S, DellaCorte MP, Grisalfi PJ. Biomechanics of running. In: O'Connor F, Wilder R, editors. *The Textbook of Running Medicine*. New York: McGraw-Hill; 2001.

19. Böddeker R, Schäfer H, Haake M. Extracorporeal shockwave therapy (ESWT) in the treatment of plantar fasciitis — a biometrical review. *Clin Rheumatol*. 2001;20(5):324–30.

20. Breit GA, Gross JH, Watenpaugh DE, Chance B, Hargens AR. Near-infrared spectroscopy for monitoring of tissue oxygenation of exercising skeletal muscle in a chronic compartment syndrome model. *J Bone Joint Surg Am*. 1997;79(6):838–43.

21. Briner WW Jr. Shin splints. *Am Fam Physician*. 1988;37(2):155–60.

22. Chandler TJ. Iontophoresis of 0.4% dexamethasone for plantar fasciitis. *Clin J Sport Med*. 1998;8(1):68.

23. Clement DB, Taunton JE, Smart GW, McNicol KL. A survey of overuse running injuries. *Phys Sportsmed*. 1981;9(5):47–58.

24. Cole C, Seto C, Gazewood J. Plantar fasciitis: evidence-based review of diagnosis and therapy. *Am Fam Physician*. 2005;72(11):2237–42.

25. Collado H, Fredericson M. Patellofemoral pain syndrome. *Clin Sports Med*. 2010;29:379–98.

26. Cowan DN, Jones BH, Frykman PN, et al. Lower limb morphology and risk of overuse injury among male infantry trainees. *Med Sci Sports Exerc*. 1996;28(8):945–52.

27. Cowan DN, Jones BH, Robinson JR. Foot morphologic characteristics and risk of exercise-related injury. *Arch Fam Med*. 1993;2(7):773–7.

28. Crawford F, Thomson C. Interventions for treating plantar heel pain. *Cochrane Database Syst Rev*. 2003;3:CD000416.

29. Crossley K, Bennell KL, Wrigley T, Oakes BW. Ground reaction forces, bone characteristics, and tibial stress fracture in male runners. *Med Sci Sports Exerc*. 1999;31(8):1088–93.

30. Davey JR, Rorabeck CH, Fowler PJ. The tibialis posterior muscle compartment. An unrecognized cause of exertional compartment syndrome. *Am J Sports Med*. 1984;12(5):391–7.

31. Davis IF, Milner CE, Hamill JF. Does increased loading during running lead to tibial stress fractures? A prospective study. *Med Sci Sports Exerc*. 2004;36:S58.

32. Davis IS, Powers CM. Patellofemoral pain syndrome: proximal, distal, and local factors, an international retreat, April 30-May 2, 2009, Fells Point, Baltimore, MD. *J Orthop Sports Phys Ther*. 2010;40(3):A1–A16.

33. Detmer DE. Chronic shin splints. Classification and management of medial tibial stress syndrome. *Sports Med*. 1986;3(6):436–46.

34. deVos RJ, Weir A, ven Schie HT, et al. Platelet-rich plasma injection for chronic Achilles tendinopathy: a randomized controlled trial. *JAMA*. 2010;303(2):144–9.

35. Dicharry J. Kinematics and kinetics of gait: from lab to clinic. *Clin Sports Med*. 2010;29(3):347–64.

36. Dierks TA, Manal KT, Hamill J, Davis IS. Proximal and distal influences on hip and knee kinematics in runners with patellofemoral pain during a prolonged run. *J Orthop Sports Phys Ther*. 2008;38(8):448–56.

37. DiMarcangelo MT, Yu TC. Diagnostic imaging of heel pain and plantar fasciitis. *Clin Podiatr Med Surg*. 1997;14(2):281–301.

38. Edwards P, Myerson MS. Exertional compartment syndrome of the leg: steps for expedient return to activity. *Phys Sportsmed*. 1996;24(4):31–46.

39. Epperly T, Fields KB. Epidemiology of running injuries. In: O'Connor FG, Wilder RP, editors. *Textbook of Running Medicine*. New York: McGraw-Hill; 2001.

40. Eskelin MK, Lötjönen JM, Mäntysaari MJ. Chronic exertional compartment syndrome: MR imaging at 0.1 T compared with tissue pressure measurement. *Radiology*. 1998;206(2):333–7.

41. Evans P. The postural function of the iliotibial tract. *Ann R Coll Surg Engl*. 1979;61(4):271–80.

42. Fairclough J, Hayashi K, Toumi H, et al. Is iliotibial band syndrome really a friction syndrome? *J Sci Med Sport*. 2007;10(2):74–6.

43. Franklyn M, Oakes B, Field B, Wells P, Morgan D. Section modulus is the optimum geometric predictor for stress fractures and medial tibial stress syndrome in both male and female athletes. *Am J Sports Med*. 2008;36(6):1179–89.

44. Fredericson M. Common injuries in runners. Diagnosis, rehabilitation, and prevention. *Sports Med*. 1996;21(1):49–72.

45. Fredericson M, Bergman AG. A comprehensive review of running injuries. *Crit Rev Phys Med Rehab*. 1999;11:1–34.

46. Fredericson M, Cookingham CL, Chaudhari AM, Dowdell BC, Oestreicher N, Sahrmann SA. Hip abduction weakness in distance runners with iliotibial band syndrome. *Clin J Sport Med*. 2000;10(3): 169–75.

47. Fredericson M, Weir A. Practical management of iliotibial band friction syndrome in runners. *Clin J Sport Med*. 2006;16(3):261–8.

48. Fredericson M, Wolf C. Iliotibial band syndrome in runners: innovations in treatment. *Sports Med*. 2005;35(5):451–9.

49. Fredericson M, Yoon K. Physical examination and patellofemoral pain syndrome. *Am J Phys Med Rehabil.* 2006;85(3):234–43.

50. Fulkerson JP. Diagnosis and treatment of patients with patellafemoral pain. *Am J Sports Med.* 2002;30(3):447–56.

51. Fulkerson JP, Kalenak A, Rosenberg TD, Cox JS. Patellofemoral Pain. *Instr Course Lect.* 1992;6:57–71.

52. Fullerton LR Jr. Femoral neck stress fractures. *Sports Med.* 1990;9(3):192–7.

53. Gardner LI Jr, Dziados JE, Jones BH, et al. Prevention of lower extremity stress fractures: a controlled trial of shock absorbent insole. *Am J Public Health.* 1988;78(12):1563–7.

54. Gill LH. Plantar fasciitis: diagnosis and conservative management. *J Am Acad Orthop Surg.* 2004;350:2159–66.

55. Glorioso J, Wilckens J. Exertional leg pain. In: O'Connor F, Wilder R, editors. *The Textbook of Running Medicine.* New York: McGraw Hill; 2001. p. 181–98.

56. Gottschalk F, Kourosh S, Leveau B. The functional anatomy of tensor fasciae latae and gluteus medium and minimus. *J Anat.* 1989;166:179–89.

57. Grau S, Krauss I, Maiwald C, Axmann D, Horstmann T, Best R. Kinematic classification of iliotibial band syndrome in runners. *Scand J Med Sci Sports.* 2011;21(2):184–9.

58. Gudas CJ. Patterns of lower-extremity injury in 224 runners. *Compr Ther.* 1980;6(9):50–9.

59. Haake M, Buch M, Schnoellner C, et al. Extracorporeal shock wave therapy for plantar fasciitis: randomised controlled multicentre trial. *BMJ.* 2003;327(7406):75.

60. Harrast MA, Colonno D. Stress fractures in runners. *Clin Sports Med.* 2010;29(3):399–416.

61. Hayes AA, Bower GK, Pitstock KL. Chronic (exertional) compartment syndrome of the legs diagnosed with thallous chloride scintigraphy. *J Nucl Med.* 1995;36(9):1618–24.

62. Hreljac A. Impact and overuse injuries in runners. *Med Sci Sports Exerc.* 2004;36(5):845–9.

63. Hreljac A, Marshall RN, Hume PA. Evaluation of lower extremity overuse injury potential in runners. *Med Sci Sports Exerc.* 2000;32(9):1635–41.

64. Hughes LY. Biomechanical analysis of the foot and ankle for predisposition to developing stress fractures. *J Orthop Sports Phys Ther.* 1985;7(3):96–101.

65. Hunte G, Lloyd-Smith R. Topical glyceryl trinitrate for chronic Achilles tendinopathy. *Clin J Sport Med.* 2005;15(2):116–7.

66. Hutchinson MR, Ireland ML. Chronic exertional compartment syndrome: gauging pressure. *Phys Sportsmed.* 1999;27(5):101–2.

67. Inman VT. Functional aspects of the abductor muscles of the hip. *J Bone Joint Surg Am.* 1947;29(3):607–19.

68. Jacobs SJ, Berson BL. Injuries to runners: a study of entrants to a 10,000 meter race. *Am J Sports Med.* 1986;14(2):151–5.

69. James SL, Bates BT, Osternig LR. Injuries to runners. *Am J Sports Med.* 1978;6(2):40–50.

70. Järvinen M, Józsa L, Kannus P, Järvinen TL, Kvist M, Leadbetter W. Histopathological findings in chronic tendon disorders. *Scand J Med Sci Sports.* 1997;7(2):86–95.

71. Jimenez C, Allen T, Hwang I. Diagnostic imaging of running injuries. In: O'Connor F, Wilder R, editors. *The Textbook of Running Medicine.* New York: McGraw-Hill; 2001. p. 67–84.

72. Jones BH, Cowan DN, Tomlinson JP, Robinson JR, Polly DW, Frykman PN. Epidemiology of injuries associated with physical training among young men in the army. *Med Sci Sports Exerc.* 1993;25(2):197–203.

73. Kader D, Saxena A, Movin T, Maffulli N. Achilles tendinopathy: some aspects of basic science and clinical management. *Br J Sports Med.* 2002;36(4):239–49.

74. Kane D, Greaney T, Bresnihan B, Gibney R, FitzGerald O. Ultrasound guided injection of recalcitrant plantar fasciitis. *Ann Rheum Dis.* 1998;57(6):383–4.

75. Kaplan PA, Helms CA, Dussault R. *Musculoskeletal MRI.* 1st ed. Philadelphia (PA): WB Saunders; 2001.

76. Karageanes SJ. What type of orthosis is most effective in treating chronic plantar fasciitis? *Clin J Sports Med.* 2007;17(3):227–8.

77. Kelsey JL, Bachrach LK, Procter-Gray E, et al. Risk factors for stress fracture among young female cross-country runners. *Med Sci Sports Exerc.* 2007;39(9):1457–63.

78. Khan KM, Brukner PD, Kearney C, Fuller PJ, Bradshaw CJ, Kiss ZS. Tarsal navicular stress fracture in athletes. *Sports Med.* 1994;17(1):65–76.

79. Khan KM, Cook JL, Bonar F, Harcourt P, Astrom M. Histopathology of common tendinopathies. Update and implications for clinical management. *Sports Med.* 1999;27(6):393–408.

80. Kibler WB, Goldberg C, Chandler TJ. Functional biomechanical deficits in running athletes with plantar fasciitis. *Am J Sports Med.* 1991;19(1):66–71.

81. Korpelainen R, Orava S, Karpakka J, Siira P, Hulkko A. Risk factors for recurrent stress fractures in athletes. *Am J Sports Med.* 2001;29(3):304–10.

82. Kruse RJ, McCoy RL, Erickson T. Diagnosing plantar fascia rupture. *Phys Sports Med.* 1995;23:65–9.

83. Lappe J, Cullen D, Haynatzki G, Recker R, Ahlf R, Thompson K. Calcium and vitamin D supplementation decreases incidence of stress fractures in female navy recruits. *J Bone Miner Res.* 2008;23(5):741–9.

84. Leversedge FJ, Casey PJ, Seiler JG 3rd, Xerogeanes JW. Endoscopically assisted fasciotomy: description of technique and in vitro assessment of lower-leg compartment decompression. *Am J Sports Med.* 2002;30(2):272–8.

85. Lidenburg G, Pinshaw R, Noakes TD. Iliotibial band friction syndrome in runners. *Phys Sports Med.* 1984;12(5):118–30.

86. Logan LR, Klamar K, Leon J, Fedoriw W. Autologous blood injection and botulinum toxin for resistant plantar fasciitis accompanied by spasticity. *Am J Phys Med Rehabil.* 2006;85(8):699–703.

87. Lysholm J, Wiklander J. Injuries in runners. *Am J Sports Med.* 1987;15(2):168–71.

88. Macera CA, Pate RR, Powell KE, Jackson KL, Kendrick JS, Craven TE. Predicting lower-extremity injuries among habitual runners. *Arch Intern Med.* 1989;149(11):2565–8.

89. MacMahon JM, Chaudhari AM, Adriacchi TP. Biomechanical injury predictors for marathon runners: striding towards iliotibial band syndrome injury prevention [abstract]. Hong Kong (HK): International Society of Biomechanics; 2000.

90. Mafi N, Lorentzon R, Alfredson H. Superior short-term results with eccentric calf muscle training compared to concentric training in a randomized prospective multicenter study on patients with chronic Achilles tendinosis. *Knee Surg Sports Traumatol Arthrosc.* 2001;9(1):42–7.

91. Mann RA. Biomechanics of running. In: Nicholas JA, Hershman EB, editors. *The Lower Extremity and Spine in Sports Medicine*, vol. 1. St. Louis: The C.V. Mosby Company; 1986. p. 395–411.

92. Mann RA, Hagy J. Biomechanics of walking, running, and sprinting. *Am J Sports Med.* 1980;8(5):345–50.

93. Martens M, Libbrecht P, Burssens A. Surgical treatment of iliotibial band friction syndrome. *Am J Sports Med.* 1989;17(5):651–4.

94. Matheson GO, Clement DB, McKenzie DC, Taunton JE, Lloyd-Smith DR, Macintyre JG. Scintigraphic uptake of 99mTc at non-painful sites in athletes with stress fractures. The concept of bone strain. *Sports Med.* 1987;4(1):65–75.

95. Matin P. Basic principles of nuclear medicine techniques for detection and evaluation of trauma and sports medicine injuries. *Semin Nucl Med.* 1988;18(2):90–112.

96. Mattila KT, Komu ME, Dahlström S, Koskinen SK, Heikkilä J. Medial tibial pain: a dynamic contrast-enhanced MRI study. *Magn Reson Imaging*. 1999;17(7):947–54.

97. Messier SP, Davis SE, Curl WW, Lowery RB, Pack RJ. Etiologic factors associated with patellofemoral pain in runners. *Med Sci Sports Exerc*. 1991;23(9):1008–15.

98. Messier SP, Edwards DG, Martin DF, et al. Etiology of iliotibial band friction syndrome in distance runners. *Med Sci Sports Exerc*. 1995;27(7):951–60.

99. Messier SP, Pittala KA. Etiologic factors associated with selected running injuries. *Med Sci Sports Exerc*. 1988;20(5):501–5.

100. Mollica MB, Duyshart SC. Analysis of pre- and post-exercise compartment pressures in the medial compartment of the foot. *Am J Sports Med*. 2002;30(2):268–71.

101. Monto R. Platelet-rich plasma effectively treats chronic Achilles tendinosis. *AAOS Annual Meeting*. 2010.

102. Moretti B, Garofalo R, Patella V, Sisti GL, Corrado M, Mouhsine E. Extracorporeal shock wave therapy in runners with a symptomatic heel spur. *Knee Surg Sports Traumatol Arthosc*. 2006;14(10):1029–32.

103. Mouhsine E, Gorofalo R, Moretti B, Gremion G, Akiki A. Two minimal incision fasciotomy for chronic exertional compartment syndrome of the lower leg. *Knee Surg Sports Traumatol Arthrosc*. 2006;14(2):193–7.

104. Nieves JW, Melsop K, Curtis M, et al. Nutritional factors that influence change in bone density and stress fracture risk among young female cross-country runners. *PMR*. 2010;2(8):740–50.

105. Nigg BM. The role of impact forces and foot pronation: a new paradigm. *Clin J Sport Med*. 2001;11(1):2–9.

106. Noble CA. Iliotibial band friction syndrome in runners. *Am J Sports Med*. 1980;8(4):232–4.

107. Noehren B, Davis I. The effect of gait retraining on hip mechanics, pain and function in runners with patello-femoral pain syndrome. *PFPS Retreat*. Baltimore (MD): University of Delaware; 2009 May.

108. O'Connor JA, Lanyon LE, MacFie H. The influence of strain rate on adaptive bone remodeling. *J Biomech*. 1982;15(10):767–81.

109. Ogden JA, Alvarez R, Levitt R, Cross GL, Marlow M. Shock wave therapy for chronic proximal plantar fasciitis. *Clin Orthop Relat Res*. 2001;387:47–59.

110. Ogden JA, Alvarez RG, Marlow M. Shockwave therapy for chronic proximal plantar fasciitis: a meta-analysis. *Foot Ankle Int*. 2002;23(4):301–8.

111. Orchard JW, Fricker PA, Abud AT, Mason BR. Biomechanics of iliotibial band friction syndrome in runners. *Am J Sports Med*. 1996;24(3):375–9.

112. Ounpuu S. The biomechanics of running: a kinematic and kinetic analysis. *Instr Course Lect*. 1990;39:305–18.

113. Ounpuu S. The biomechanics of walking and running. *Clin Sports Med*. 1994;13(4):843–63.

114. Owens S, Edwards P, Miles K, Jenner J, Allen M. Chronic compartment syndrome affecting the lower limb: MIBI perfusion imaging as an alternative to pressure monitoring: two case reports. *Br J Sports Med*. 1999;33(1):49–51.

115. Paavola M, Kannus P, Järvinen TA, Khan K, Józsa L, Järvinen M. Achilles tendinopathy. *J Bone Joint Surg Am*. 2002;84-A(11):2062–76.

116. Padhiar N, King JB. Exercise induced leg pain-chronic compartment syndrome. Is the increase in intra-compartment pressure exercise specific? *Br J Sports Med*. 1996;30(4):360–2.

117. Paoloni JA, Appleyard RC, Nelson J, Murrell GA. Topical glyceryl trinitrate treatment of chronic noninsertional Achilles tendinopathy. A randomized, double-blind, placebo-controlled trial. *J Bone Joint Surg Am*. 2004;86-A(5):916–22.

118. Petrizzi MJ, Petrizzi MG, Roos RJ. Making a tension night splint for plantar fasciitis. *Phys Sportsmed*. 1998;26(6):113–4.

119. Pfeffer G, Bacchetti P, Deland J, et al. Comparison of custom and prefabricated orthoses in the initial treatment of proximal plantar fasciitis. *Foot Ankle Int*. 1999;20(4):214–21.

120. Pfeffer GB. Plantar heel pain. In Baxter DE, editor. *The Foot and Ankle in Sport*. St. Louis: Mosby-Year Book; 1995. p. 195–206.

121. Pinshaw R, Atlas V, Noakes TD. The nature and response to therapy of 196 consecutive injuries seen at a runners' clinic. *S Afr Med J*. 1984;65(8):291–8.

122. Placzek R, Deuretzbacher G, Meiss AL. Treatment of chronic plantar fasciitis with botulinum toxin A: preliminary clinical results. *Clin J Pain*. 2006;22(2):190–2.

123. Popp KL, Hughes JM, Smock AJ, et al. Bone geometry, strength, and muscle size in runners with a history of stress fracture. *Med Sci Sports Exerc*. 2009;41(12):2145–50.

124. Portland G, Kelikian A, Kodros S. Acute surgical management of Jones' fractures. *Foot Ankle Int*. 2003;24(11):829–33.

125. Powell M, Post WR, Keener J, Wearden S. Effective treatment of chronic plantar fasciitis with dorsiflexion night splints: a crossover prospective randomized outcome study. *Foot Ankle Int*. 1998;19(1):10–8.

126. Powers CM, Shellock FG, Beering TV, Garrido DE, Goldbach RM, Molnar T. Effect of bracing on patellar kinematics in patients with patellofemoral joint pain. *Med Sci Sports Exerc*. 1999;31(12):1714–20.

127. Puddu G, Ippolito E, Postacchini F. A classification of Achilles tendon disease. *Am J Sports Med*. 1976;4(4):145–50.

128. Raether PM, Lutter LD. Recurrent compartment syndrome in the posterior thigh. Report of a case. *Am J Sports Med*. 1982;10(1):40–3.

129. Raikin SM, Rapuri VR, Vitanzo P. Bilateral simultaneous fasciotomy for chronic exertional compartment syndrome. *Foot Ankle Int*. 2005;26(12):1007–11.

130. Rettig AC, Shelbourne KD, McCarroll JR, Bisesi M, Watts J. The natural history and treatment of delayed union stress fractures of the anterior cortex of the tibia. *Am J Sports Med*. 1988;16(3):250–5.

131. Riddle DL, Pulisic M, Pidcoe P, Johnson RE. Risk factors for plantar fasciitis: a matched case-control study. *J Bone Joint Surg Am*. 2003;85-A(5):872–7.

132. Rodgers MM. Dynamic biomechanics of the normal foot and ankle during walking and running. *Phys Ther*. 1988;68(12):1822–30.

133. Rompe JD, Decking J, Schoellner C, Nafe B. Shock wave application for chronic plantar fasciitis in running athletes. A prospective, randomized placebo-controlled trial. *Am J Sports Med*. 2003;31(2):268–75.

134. Rompe JD, Schoellner C, Nafe B. Evaluation of low-energy extracorporeal shock-wave application for treatment of chronic plantar fasciitis. *J Bone Joint Surg Am*. 2002;84-A(3):335–41.

135. Roos E, Engström M, Söderberg B. Foot orthoses for the treatment of plantar fasciitis. *Foot Ankle Int*. 2006;27(8):606–11.

136. Rowden GA, Abdelkarim B, Vaca F. Compartment syndromes. *eMedicine from WebMD, Medscape* [Internet]. 2008 [cited 2008 Oct 29]. Available from: http://emedicine.medscape.com.

137. Samuelson DR, Cram RL. The three-phase bone scan and exercise induced lower-leg pain. The tibial stress test. *Clin Nucl Med*. 1996;21(2):89–93.

138. Schepsis AA, Gill SS, Foster TA. Fasciotomy for exertional anterior compartment syndrome: is lateral compartment release necessary? *Am J Sports Med*. 1999;27(4):430–5.

139. Schils JP, Andrish JT, Piraino DW, Belhobek GH, Richmond BJ, Bergfeld JA. Medial malleolar stress fractures in seven patients: review of the clinical and imaging features. *Radiology*. 1992;185(1):219–21.

140. Shelbourne KD, Fisher DA, Rettig AC, McCarroll JR. Stress fractures of the medial malleolus. *Am J Sports Med*. 1988;16(1):60–3.

141. Silbernagel KG, Thomeé R, Thomeé P, Karlsson J. Eccentric overload training for patients with chronic Achilles tendon pain — a randomised controlled study with reliability testing of the evaluation methods. *Scand J Med Sci Sports.* 2001;11(4):197–206.

142. Slimmon D, Bennell K. Burkner P, Crossley K, Bell SN. Long-term outcome of fasciotomy with partial fasciectomy for chronic exertional compartment syndrome of the lower leg. *Am J Sports Med.* 2002; 30(4):581–8.

143. Speed CA, Nichols D, Wies J, et al. Extracorporeal shock wave therapy for plantar fasciitis. A double blind randomised controlled trial. *J Orthop Res.* 2003;21(5):937–40.

144. Sullivan D, Warren RF, Pavlov H, Kelman G. Stress fractures in 51 runners. *Clin Orthop Relat Res.* 1984;187:188–92.

145. Taunton JE, Ryan MB, Clement DB, McKenzie DC, Lloyd-Smith DR, Zumbo BD. A prospective study of running injuries: the Vancouver Sun Run "In Training" clinics. *Br J Sports Med.* 2003;37(3):239–44.

146. Taunton JE, Ryan MB, Clement DB, McKenzie DC, Lloyd-Smith DR, Zumbo BD. A retrospective case-control analysis of 2002 running injuries. *Br J Sports Med.* 2002;36(2):95–101.

147. Terry GC, Hughston JC, Norwood LA. The anatomy of the iliopatellar band and iliotibial tract. *Am J Sports Med.* 1986;14(1):39–45.

148. Thacker SB, Gilchrist J, Stroup DF, Kimsey CD Jr. The impact of stretching on sports injury risk: a systematic review of the literature. *Med Sci Sports Exerc.* 2004;36(3):371–8.

149. The diagnosis and treatment of heel pain. *J Foot Ankle Surg.* 2001;40(5):329–40.

150. Thomeé R, Renström P, Karlsson J, Grimby G. Patellofemoral pain syndrome in young women. I. A clinical analysis of alignment, pain parameters, common symptoms and functional activity level. *Scand J Med Sci Sports.* 1995;5(4):237–44.

151. Tisdel CL, Harper MC. Chronic plantar heel pain: treatment with a short leg walking cast. *Foot Ankle Int.* 1996;17(1):41–2.

152. Tzortziou V, Maffuli N, Padhiar N. Diagnosis and management of chronic exertional compartment syndrome (CECS) in the United Kingdom. *Clin J Sport Med.* 2006;16(3):209–13.

153. Välimäki VV, Alfthan H, Lehmuskallio E, et al. Risk factors for clinical stress fractures in male military recruits: a prospective cohort study. *Bone.* 2005;37(2):267–73.

154. van Gent R, Siem D, van Middelkoop M, van Os AG, Bierma-Zeinstra SM, Koes BW. Incidence and determinants of lower extremity running injuries in long distance runners: a systematic review. *Br J Sports Med.* 2007;41(8):469–80.

155. van Mechelen W. Running injuries. A review of the epidemiological literature. *Sports Med.* 1992;14(5):320–35.

156. Vu D, McDiarmid T, Brown M, Aukerman DF. Clinical inquiries. What is the most effective management of acute fractures of the base of the fifth metatarsal? *J Fam Pract.* 2006;55(8):713–7.

157. Walter SD, Hart LE, McIntosh JM, Sutton JR. The Ontario cohort study of running-related injuries. *Arch Intern Med.* 1989;149(11): 2561–4.

158. Weil LS Jr, Roukis TS, Weil LS, Borrelli AH. Extracorporeal shock wave therapy for the treatment of chronic plantar fasciitis: indications, protocol, intermediate results, and a comparison of results to fasciotomy. *J Foot Ankle Surg.* 2002;41(3):166–72.

159. Wen DY, Puffer JC, Schmalzried TP. Lower extremity alignment and risk of overuse injuries in runners. *Med Sci Sports Exerc.* 1997;29(10): 1291–8.

160. Wilder R, O'Connor F. Epidemiology of running injuries. In: Wilder R, O'Connor F, Magrum E, editors. *Textbook of Running Medicine.* Philadelphia: Human Kinetics; in press.

161. Wilder RP, Magrum E. Exertional compartment syndrome. *Clin Sports Med.* 2010;29(3):429–35.

162. Wilder RP, Sethi S. Overuse injuries: tendinopathies, stress fractures, compartment syndrome and shin splints. *Clin Sports Med.* 2004;23(1): 55–81, vi.

163. Winemiller MH, Billow RG, Laskowski ER, Harmsen WS. Effect of magnetic vs sham-magnetic insoles on plantar heel pain: a randomized controlled trial. *JAMA.* 2003;290(11):1474–8.

164. Wittstein J, Moorman CT 3rd, Levin LS. Endoscopic compartment release for chronic exertional compartment syndrome. *J Surg Orthop Adv.* 2008;17(2):119–21.z

165. Yeung EW, Yeung SS. Interventions for preventing lower limb soft-tissue injuries in runners. *Cochrane Database Syst Rev.* 2001;3: CD001256.

166. Zwitser EW, Breederveld RS. Fractures of the fifth metatarsal; diagnosis and treatment. *Injury.* 2010;41(6):555–62.

100 Alpine Skiing and Snowboarding

Devin P. McFadden

OVERVIEW

- Alpine skiing and snowboarding are two of the most popular winter sports throughout the world.
- Injury patterns are distinct to each specific sport, with predominantly lower extremity injuries in skiing and predominantly upper extremity injuries in snowboarding.
- A recent focus on injury prevention has led to the development of helmets and wrist guards that have been proven to be effective in preventing injury. However, these technologic advancements have not yet been universally adopted by mainstream athletes.

EPIDEMIOLOGY

- The popularity of skiing and snowboarding continues to grow throughout the world, with 200 million participants worldwide and 12 million in the United States alone (11,13).
- Snowboarders tend to be younger and have a reputation for greater risk taking.
- Historical injury rates of 7.6 per 1,000 skier days were quoted as early as the 1950s (7,13).
- Although modern equipment has led to a reduction in injury volume, the severity of injuries has increased because new equipment allows for greater speeds and sharper turns.
- Current data suggest injury rates of about 1–6 per 1,000 skier days, with improved injury rates attributed to hard-shelled ski boots, release bindings, and better grooming of slopes (4).
- Catastrophic injuries still occur, however, with an average of 20–30 deaths yearly in the United States alone, or 0.5 deaths per 1 million skier days (9).

BIOMECHANICS

- The different biomechanics and equipment of skiing and snowboarding result in their vastly different injury patterns.

- Snowboarders have both feet strapped to the board, resulting in less torsion injury to the knees. Also, the large surface area of the board and comparative difficulty making sharp turns result in lower velocity falls that allow the athlete to extend his arms and brace for impact. Subsequently, snowboarders have a significantly increased risk of injury to the hand, wrist, and arm.
- Skiers, on the other hand, are capable of sharp, quick turns and high-velocity collisions. Fall on outstretched hand (FOOSH) injury is relatively uncommon, leading to a greater percentage of lower extremity injuries. In addition, a skier who has lost control can find his skis advancing in diverging directions, which causes a rotational torque and leads to a high incidence of knee injuries.
- Snowboarders most often injure their backs while falling backward after a missed jump, causing axial loading and an increased incidence of compression fractures in the thoracolumbar spine. Conversely, skiers tend to fall forward after losing control or colliding with something and have a greater incidence of burst fractures (13).
- Finally, lacerations, which are rarely found in snowboarders, have been noted to account for 8% of all injuries in skiers, where release bindings expose athletes to the sharpened ski edge (1).

SKI INJURIES

- As discussed, upper extremity injuries are uncommon in skiing, representing only an estimated 20%–35% of alpine ski injuries (14).
- Shoulder injuries occur at a rate of 0.2–0.5 per 1,000 skier days and represent 4%–11% of alpine ski injuries, with the most common injury types being glenohumeral joint subluxations, rotator cuff strains, acromioclavicular joint separations, and clavicle fractures (16).
- Although less common than in snowboarders, wrist and hand injuries do occur in skiing, typically as a consequence of a FOOSH injury. The most common fracture in the forearm is the distal radius or Colles fracture, named after the Irish surgeon who first described it in 1814. The diagnosis

is usually made based on plain radiographs, and immobilization is all that is needed if the fracture is not displaced. However, if the joint space is compromised, the neurovascular supply is injured, or the fracture is displaced, surgical intervention is often required.

- The thumb is the most frequently injured digit of the hand in skiing, and the injury almost universally results from the traction caused when an isolated thumb is pulled away from the rest of the hand in a skier using poles, resulting in extension and forced abduction at the metacarpophalangeal (MCP) joint. The aptly named skier's thumb is a sprain injury to the ulnar collateral ligament (UCL) of the first MCP joint. It is characterized by pain and tenderness to palpation over the ulnar aspect of the thumb and is diagnosed when laxity is noted on clinical exam. Conservative management with thumb spica casting followed by splinting is recommended when less than 30 degrees of valgus laxity are noted. A complete disruption of the UCL with retraction of the ligament to the adductor aponeurosis is known as a Stener lesion and is characterized by a palpable mass. In this case, or if a bony avulsion is present, surgical management is preferred. The UCL can also be injured through chronic stress rather than an acute, violent force and, in this case, is commonly referred to as "gamekeeper's thumb." Although UCL injury is undoubtedly the most common and most recognized injury pattern, dislocations, subluxations, and Bennett fractures of the base of the first metacarpal are also quite common in skiers (16).

- Representing 35% of all injuries and injured at a rate of 1.14 per 1,000 skier days, the traumatic knee injury is the most frequently reported ski injury (4,6). The classic explanation for these injuries focuses on the torque generated by the diverging skis of a skier who has lost control and the resultant external rotation and valgus stress placed on the knee as the primary causes of medial collateral ligament and anterior cruciate ligament (ACL) injury. Other injury patterns have also been noted, however, such as an airborne skier landing with his center of gravity too far back, resulting in the anterior displacement of the tibia when levered against the static ski boot in what has been referred to as an "anterior drawer effect." Finally, a skier whose weight is too far back on his skis will experience simultaneous flexion and internal rotation at the knee joint if he catches his inside edge on the snow, yielding perhaps the most common cause of ACL disruption (5).

- Tibia and fibula fractures, as well as boot-top hematomas, can occur due to the continued momentum of the lower legs if the skis are rapidly slowed or stopped. Achilles tendon ruptures can also result from a similar mechanism, as the force is translated through the stronger proximal tibia distally to the ankle (16).

- Ankle and foot injuries remain possible but are now relatively rare since the advent of hard-shelled boots.

SNOWBOARDING INJURIES

- Snowboarders are 13 times more likely than skiers to sustain a wrist injury (19), and wrist injuries represent 40% of all snowboarding injuries (17).

- Ankle injuries are also much more common in snowboarders, with a more than twofold increase in risk compared to skiers (11).

- Snowboarder's ankle is a rare but potentially disabling fracture of the lateral process of the talus and can lead to vascular necrosis and chronic nonunion if mistaken for a routine ankle sprain. While the exact mechanism of injury is not clearly understood, a high-energy axial load of the lateral ankle is required and results in pain of the anterolateral ankle that can mimic a severe ankle sprain (5). Up to 50% of these lesions are missed by standard radiography; thus, diagnosis requires a high index of suspicion and can often only be made by computed tomography scan (15,19). Treatment for fractures with displacement of less than 2 mm is casting, whereas comminuted fractures or those with a greater degree of displacement should be referred for possible surgical management.

HEAD AND SPINAL CORD INJURY

- The leading cause of death in both skiing and snowboarding is traumatic brain injury, usually following a collision with a tree, chairlift pole, or another person (2).

- Studies indicate that head injuries make up 9%–19% of all snowsport injuries reported by ski patrols and emergency departments, with neck and spinal cord injuries representing 1%–4% (18).

ENVIRONMENTAL AND ALTITUDE INJURY

- Exercise-induced bronchospasm (EIB), acute mountain sickness (AMS), and hypothermia can all be encountered when skiing or snowboarding.

- EIB is a transient, reversible narrowing of the distal airways caused by strenuous activity. EIB is more common in cool conditions, as cold air itself can trigger airway hyperresponsiveness. Rapid respiratory rates, cool air temperatures, and low-humidity environments contribute to airway drying and bronchial spasm. Some estimate that EIB affects up to 50% of winter athletes (3). Common symptoms include postexercise dyspnea, cough, burning chest pain, and rarely wheezing. Symptoms peak 10–20 minutes after exercise, with a late phase occurring at 2–12 hours and lasting up to 2 days in some athletes. The eucapnic voluntary hyperventilation challenge (EVHC) seems to be the most accurate method of making a diagnosis, although a laboratory-based or sport-specific competition-based exercise challenge is also a viable alternative. Treatment is similar to that of mild asthma, with albuterol used as a rescue medication at onset of symptoms or 20–40 minutes prior to activity as a prophylactic measure. Physicians of competitive athletes must be aware of the World Anti-Doping Agency (WADA) regulations, which require validated testing to confirm the diagnosis if albuterol or other asthma medications are used during competition or training (3).

- AMS, or altitude sickness, is the pathologic response of the human body to acute increases in elevation to levels greater than 2,500 meters. Oxygen levels decrease as altitude increases, leading to elevated respiratory rates, heart rates, and stroke volumes. Common symptoms include throbbing headaches, anorexia, nausea, fatigue, dizziness, and insomnia and can easily be mistaken for a viral illness, hangover, or allergic response. Potentially fatal if not recognized and treated, AMS can progress to high-altitude pulmonary edema (HAPE) and high-altitude cerebral edema (HACE). Improper hydration, fitness, and rate of ascent are risk factors for developing symptoms, and proper acclimatization can take up to a week (8).

- Hypothermia, defined as a core body temperature less than 35°C, is a rare cause of injury in recreational skiers, but due to its potential morbidity, it deserves mention here. With every 1,000 meters of altitude ascended, the temperature drops by 5.5°C. Death by hypothermia is usually a secondary sequela of an injury, avalanche, or altitude sickness that prevents the athlete from escaping from the elements (22). When hypothermic patients are evacuated, they should immediately be dressed in warm, dry clothing. A Bair Hugger is one way to provide external rewarming, whereas heated intravenous fluids and exposure to heated, humidified air have been show to be effective in rewarming even severely obtunded patients. Mortality rate from hypothermia is estimated to be 0.18 deaths per 1 million skier days (20).

INJURY PREVENTION

- Many studies have investigated the effect of helmet use on head injuries in skiing and snowboarding, with mixed results reported. However, a well-designed meta-analysis of 12 previous studies suggested that helmet use could potentially prevent 35% of all head injuries without increasing the risk of neck injury (18).

- The effectiveness of wrist guards in preventing snowboarding injuries has also been evaluated and has demonstrated a promising 85% reduction in hand, wrist, and forearm injuries in those who wore protection. The benefit may be partially offset, however, because a twofold increase in elbow, upper arm, and shoulder injuries was also found in one case-control study (10).

- Educational campaigns focusing on alpine sport safety and sun protection use have been met with moderate success but are resource intensive and thus unlikely to find widespread acceptance (12,21).

SUMMARY

- Skiing and snowboarding are fun yet potentially dangerous snowsports.

- Injuries usually involve the upper extremity in snowboarders and the lower extremity in skiers.

- Environmental injuries are frequently overlooked due to the prevalence of orthopedic trauma; nonetheless, their importance within the sport cannot be underestimated by the treating physician.

- Preventative measures and improvements in equipment have come a long way in helping to reduce injury rates; however, helmets and wrist guards can only be effective to the extent that they are used.

REFERENCES

1. Abu-Laban RB. Snowboarding injuries: an analysis and comparison with alpine skiing injuries. *CMAJ.* 1991;145(9):1097–103.

2. Ackery A, Hagel BE, Provvidenza C, Tator CH. An international review of head and spinal cord injuries in alpine skiing and snowboarding. *Inj Prev.* 2007;13(6):368–75.

3. Butcher JD. Exercise-induced asthma in the competitive cold weather athlete. *Curr Sports Med Rep.* 2006;5(6):284–8.

4. Davidson TM, Laliotis AT. Alpine skiing injuries. A nine-year study. *West J Med.* 1996;164(4):310–4.

5. Deady LH, Salonen D. Skiing and snowboarding injuries: a review with a focus on mechanism of injury. *Radiol Clin North Am.* 2010;48(6): 1113–24.

6. Demirag B, Oncan T, Durak K. [An evaluation of knee ligament injuries encountered in skiers at the Uludag Ski Center]. *Acta Orthop Traumatol Turc.* 2004;38(5):313–6.

7. Earle AS, Moritz JR, Saviers GB, Ball JD. Ski injuries. *JAMA.* 1962; 180:285–8.

8. Eichner ER. Sports medicine pearls and pitfalls: going higher. *Curr Sports Med Rep.* 2008;7(6):310–1.

9. Fu HF, Stone DA. *Sports Injuries: Mechanisms — Prevention — Treatment.* Baltimore (MD): Williams & Wilkins; 1994.

10. Hagel B, Pless IB, Goulet C. The effect of wrist guard use on upper-extremity injuries in snowboarders. *Am J Epidemiol.* 2005;162(2): 149–56.

11. Hunter RE. Skiing injuries. *Am J Sports Med.* 1999;27(3):381–9.

12. Josse MJ, Cusimano M. The effect of a skiing/snowboarding safety video on the increase of safety knowledge in Canadian youths — a pilot study. *Int J Circumpolar Health.* 2006;65(5):385–8.

13. Kary JM. Acute spine injury in skiers and snowboarders. *Curr Sports Med Rep.* 2008;7(1):35–8.

14. Kocher MS, Dupré MM, Feagin JA Jr. Shoulder injuries from alpine skiing and snowboarding: aetiology, treatment and prevention. *Sports Med.* 1998;25(3):201–11.

15. McCrory P, Bladin C. Fractures of the lateral process of the talus: a clinical review. "Snowboarder's ankle." *Clin J Sport Med.* 1996;6(2):124–8.

16. Pecina M. Injuries in downhill (alpine) skiing. *Croat Med J.* 2002; 43(3):257–60.

17. Roberts WO. *Bull's Handbook of Sports Injuries.* 2nd ed. New York (NY): McGraw-Hill; 2004.

18. Russell K, Christie J, Hagel BE. The effect of helmets on the risk of head and neck injuries among skiers and snowboarders: a meta-analysis. *CMAJ*. 2010;182(4):333–40.

19. Sacco DE, Sartorelli DH, Vane DW. Evaluation of alpine skiing and snowboarding injury in a northeastern state. *J Trauma*. 1998;44(4):654–9.

20. Sherry E, Richards D. Hypothermia among resort skiers: 19 cases from the Snowy Mountains. *Med J Aust*. 1986;144(9):457–61.

21. Walkosz BJ, Buller DB, Anderson PA, et al. Increasing sun protection in winter outdoor recreation a theory-based health communication program. *Am J Prev Med*. 2008;34(6):502–9.

22. Windsor JS, Firth PG, Grocott MP, Rodway GW, Montgomery HE. Mountain mortality: a review of deaths that occur during recreational activities in the mountains. *Postgrad Med J*. 2009;85(1004):316–21.

101 Rodeo Injuries

Craig R. Denegar and Richard M. Blyn

INTRODUCTION

- Rodeo, unlike most of the sports addressed in this section, is not a single sport or event. In rodeo, cowboys and cowgirls compete in one or more individual competitions that constitute a performance.

- A rodeo is often made up of several performances over several days. Rodeo is not solely a professional sport.

- Youth, high school, college, and professional rodeo organizations sponsor competitions. Although rodeo is associated with the American West, there are rodeos across the United States and Canada as well as South America, Central America, and Australia.

- The events in *professional* rodeo include the rough stock competitions and timed events. Rough stock competitions consist of bareback riding, saddle bronc riding, and bull riding. The timed events include tie-down calf roping, steer wrestling, team roping, and barrel racing.

- In *youth, high school, and college rodeo*, additional timed events may be on a schedule, but our focus will be on the primary events listed in Table 101.1. For the most part, the rough stock events, tie-down roping, steer wrestling, and team roping are cowboy events, whereas women compete in barrel racing. However, these gender roles are not absolute across all levels of rodeo.

- Serious injuries, including fractures, concussions, and sprains are common, with more injuries occurring in rough stock competitions (2,3,5,7).

- In the only report of its kind, the incidence of catastrophic and fatal injuries has been reported to be 9.45 and 40.5 per 100,000 exposures, respectively, with the greatest risk occurring in bull riding (3).

HISTORY

- Rodeo did not begin as an athletic competition but grew from the work of cowboys and cowgirls working with livestock on ranches. The events of bareback and saddle bronc riding are the extension of work done to break horses at a time when the horse was the fastest means of transportation. The care of cattle required the roping and tying of the animal to administer medical care. Tie-down calf roping and steer wrestling are offshoots of this work.

- Bull riding, however, emerged from the cowboy spirit rather than the work of the cowboy. At the end of the trail or a long day of work, cowboys began to develop competitions among themselves or cowboys from other outfits to see who the best rider, best roper, and all-around best ranch hands were. From these informal competitions and our fascination with the life of the cowboy, Wild West shows and true rodeo competitions evolved.

- Although the Wild West shows have vanished, rodeo has grown into a business, drawing large crowds to events and allowing the professional to earn a living through rodeo competition.

COWBOYS, COWGIRLS, RODEOS, AND ORGANIZATIONS

- As noted, there are rodeos for young cowboys and cowgirls, high school and college athletes, and professionals. Below is a partial list of the organizations that sponsor or sanction rodeos. There are a number of youth and state high school, college, and professional associations, including those listed below. The Web sites are provided to assist in locating information on age groups, rules, and events.
  - Youth Rodeo Association. (http://www.yratx.com/)
  - National High School Rodeo Association (http://www.nhsra.com/)
  - National Intercollegiate Rodeo Association (http://www.collegerodeo.com/)
  - Professional Rodeo Cowboys Association (http://www.prorodeo.com/)
  - Women's Professional Rodeo Association (http://www.wpra.com/)
  - Professional Bull Riders (http://www.pbrnow.com/)

- Unlike many sports where athletes are a part of a team or identified athletic organization, the rodeo athlete stands alone. The rodeo athlete usually must pay an entry fee to compete and earns only what they win in competition or through sponsorship. In reality, the opportunity to earn money requires that the rodeo athlete compete. These athletes travel extensively, and the sports medicine provider often has little knowledge of medical history and little opportunity for follow-up care.

Table 101.1	Events of Professional Rodeo and Associated Injuries	
Event	**Description**	**Injuries and Risk**
Rough stock	Must ride 8 seconds, scored 0–100, 50 points for animal performance, 50 points for cowboy. Protective vests common or required in bull riding and bareback riding.	Accounts for approximately 85% of injuries. Concussion and fractures account for large portion of serious injuries.
Bull riding	Cowboy maintains position on animal using a bull rope. Helmets worn by some contestants.	Accounts for nearly half of injuries and large portion of fatalities. High incidence of concussion and fractures.
Bareback	Cowboy maintains position on animal with a handle-shaped rigging. Cowboys wear protective vests but not helmets.	Second highest risk of serious injury. Injuries to the elbow caused by hyperextension are common.
Saddle bronc	Cowboy sits in a saddle and maintains control holding a bronc rein (rope). Considered most technically demanding rough stock event. Cowboys wear protective vests but not helmets.	Lower risk of serious injury of rough stock events. Knee injuries (posterior cruciate ligament) occur with landing on fully flexed knee following dismount.
Timed events	Performance is judged on time to complete event.	Lower risk of injury, especially concussion and crush/impact mechanism injury, compared to rough stock events.
Tie-down roping	Cowboy must rope calf, dismount, flank (lay on side) calf, and tie 3 legs.	Thumb, shoulder, and lower extremity injuries during dismount most common.
Steer wrestling	Cowboy dismounts grabbing the horns of a running steer and then throws the steer with all four legs pointed in same direction.	Shoulder and lower extremity sprains most common injuries.
Team roping	Two cowboys attempt to rope the head and hind legs of steer.	Shoulder and hand injuries most common.
Women's barrel racing	Horses run cloverleaf pattern around 3 barrels.	Primary risk or serious injury is from crush mechanism when horse falls on rider.

RODEO SPORTS MEDICINE

- The history of rodeo sports medicine is as unique as the sport itself. Although local practitioners may have provided care to cowboys who came to town to compete, a formal program to provide and coordinate care only appeared in the United States through a program developed in 1980 with the support of the Justin Boot Company.

- Mobile Sports Medicine Systems, Inc. grew from the support of Justin Boots, Co. and now coordinates care at major rodeos across the United States. In Canada, the Canadian Pro Rodeo Sport Medicine Team (CPRSMT) has grown over the past 25 years to coordinate volunteer coverage of Canadian Professional Rodeo Association events.

- Of the more than 800 Professional Rodeo Cowboys Association–sanctioned rodeos annually, the Mobile Sports Medicine Systems Inc. is present at fewer than 200. Similarly, CPRSMT is not present at all professional rodeo events in Canada.

- At many professional and other rodeo competitions at all levels, care for the rodeo athlete is dependent on local providers.

- Bull riding is the event in rodeo that draws the most attention. In 1994, a group of rodeo cowboys formed Professional Bull Riders (PBR). The associated risks of this single event led to efforts to provide well-coordinated care to bull riders at the top level in their sport.

- Through the Justin Sports Medicine program and more recently Extreme Sports Medicine Inc., the PBR has brought increased attention to medical care. There has also been an increased focus on injury prevention through improved safety equipment and conditioning. Today, the growing network of providers has greatly improved sports medicine care for the rodeo athlete.

EVENTS AND RULES

- The rules and equipment differ between the seven events in professional rodeo, although there are some commonalities.

- In the rough stock events, cowboys must stay on the animal for 8 seconds without touching the animal with their free arm. Cowboys are awarded a score from 0 to 100 by a team of judges if they are successful in staying on for the 8 seconds. One-half of the score is based on the performance of the animal and one-half on the ability of the rider.

  - In bareback and saddle bronc events, the cowboy must mark out the animal, meaning that the cowboy's spurs must be in contact with the point of the horse's shoulder until the horse's front feet hit the ground once the chute gate is opened.

  - In bareback riding, the cowboy's hand is inserted into a rigging that resembles the handle of a suitcase, whereas in saddle bronc, the cowboy holds onto a rein attached to a halter.

- In bull riding, there is no requirement for a mark out. The bull rider wraps one hand in a bull rope wrapped around the chest of the bull. In bull riding, the cowboy wears a protective vest, and the use of helmets has become widespread in the past decade.

- The first National Operating Committee on Standards for Athletic Equipment–rated helmet for bull riders (Phoenix Performance Products Inc., Vaughan, Ontario, Canada) recently became available. Many bareback and saddle bronc riders wear protective vests, but beyond the vests, helmets, and a mouthpiece, the cowboys have little to protect them from injury.

- In the timed events, the goal is to complete the required task in the shortest amount of time. In the roping events and steer wrestling, the animal is given a head start into the arena.

  - In tie-down calf roping, the cowboy must rope the calf from the back of his horse, dismount and reach the calf, flank or throw the calf to the ground, and tie any three legs.

  - The steer wrestler must chase and ride alongside the steer. The hazer, a cowboy riding on the opposite side of the steer, guides the animal into position. The cowboy dismounts onto the head of the steer, grasping around the horns. The cowboy must stop the steer and throw it to the ground with all four feet pointing in the same direction.

  - In team roping, two cowboys, a header and heeler, chase the steer. The header's job is to rope the steer around the head and turn the steer so that the heeler can throw his rope around the two back feet. The clock is stopped when the slack is removed from the rope of the header and heeler.

  - In barrel racing, the cowgirl rides her horse in a cloverleaf pattern around three barrels. Penalties are assessed if a barrel is knocked over, with the fastest total time winning.

INJURIES AND EPIDEMIOLOGY

- Working around livestock carries inherent risks, and the medical team providing care at a rodeo must anticipate the possibility of injury to rodeo athletes, bull fighters, and those who handle and manage the horses, bulls, calves, and steers.

- Of the rodeo events, the rough stock events pose the greatest risk and also are associated with the greatest variety of injuries (2,5–7). Rough stock events accounted for 76.6% of all injuries at the national high school rodeo finals between 1996 and 2005 and 88.2% of injuries in professional rodeo between 1981 and 2005 (5).

- Of the rough stock events, bull riding is by far the most dangerous, and many injuries are severe (2). In fact, bull riding accounted for nearly 50% of rough stock event injuries based on data collected from 1981 to 2005 (5). The incidence rate

of injury in professional and high school rodeo has been estimated to be 32.2 (2) and 28.5 (7) per 1,000 exposures, respectively, in bull riding. The incidence rate in bareback and saddle bronc riding is between 17.5 and 31.9 per 1,000 exposures, with higher rates in high school athletes (2,7).

- Concussions (6) were the most common major injuries reported in the 1981–2005 summary of professional rodeo injuries. Fractures involving the extremities and trunk as well as glenohumeral dislocations make up a large portion of nonconcussion major injuries. These injuries are often caused by being stepped on by the animal or being thrown to the ground or against the bucking chute (1,4).

- Although the vest worn by bull riders offers protection, internal injuries and fractures can result from being stepped on.

- Injuries to the hand, wrist, elbow, and shoulder may result from a cowboy being "hung-up" where their hand does not release from the bull rope or bareback rigging.

- In rough stock events, injury to the cervical spine can occur when the cowboy is thrown from the animal. More than one-third of the injuries in rodeo occur in bareback and saddle bronc events (5). Like bull riding, the mechanisms of injury in these events involve being thrown from or stepped on by the animal.

- Elbow injuries are very common in bareback riders because of the stresses to the joint during the ride.

- In saddle bronc riding, there is a greater risk of injuries to the knee, particularly the cruciate ligaments during the dismount.

- Injuries in tie-down calf roping and steer wrestling often involve the lower extremity, with the knee being most susceptible.

- Team roping and barrel racing carry the lowest risk of injury.

- Rodeo athletes are also susceptible to muscle strains, particularly involving the groin.

- Roping cowboys can suffer from nontraumatic or repetitive use injuries to the shoulder and arm.

- A significant concern in rodeo is the care of open wounds. These can occur at any point before, during, and after a rodeo. The sports medicine team must recognize that the rodeo arena and livestock holding areas are inherently dirty. All wounds must be thoroughly cleansed and closely monitored for infection.

EVENT PREPARATION

- Providing sports medicine care to rodeo athletes is a unique experience. The first reaction when one witnesses an injury to an athlete is to wait until play stops and run to the assistance of the athlete. Bulls and horses do not stop play when an injury occurs. The livestock in and around the arena pose a risk of injury to sports medicine personnel, and the provider must be certain that the arena is safe to enter before attending to an injury. DO NOT BECOME THE SECOND VICTIM!!

- Rodeo athletes are a unique breed. The cowboy culture is one of toughness bread from the demands of the working ranch where medical assistance was often far off and care for the livestock paramount.
- Rodeo athletes are not likely to complain and may not seek attention for an injury. Moreover, the rodeo athlete is often stubborn and may choose not to follow the advice of the sports medicine professional. The expansion of rodeo sports medicine has increased the bond of trust between athlete and provider, but developing a professional relationship can take time.
- Once one is aware of the environment and culture of rodeo, planning for sports medicine coverage is similar to other sports that pose a high risk of traumatic injury. The provider must be prepared to assess injuries that are orthopedic and nonorthopedic in nature.
- The data collected on major injuries in rodeo from 1981 to 2005 (6) provide an overview of what one can anticipate. Concussion and fractures are common, but injuries to the viscera, teeth, and eyes also occur.
- Some of these injuries can be life threatening, so a well-planned and practiced emergency response must be in place.
- The sports medicine team should practice caring for a rodeo athlete wearing a protective vest and helmet.
- The rodeo ground is often rough, and access by emergency medical assistance can be limited by fencing and seating. A plan for the equipment to be brought to the injured athlete should also be developed. It is usually not possible to roll a stretcher over the soft ground found in a well-prepared arena.
- A plan to transport an injured athlete from the arena must be developed at each venue.
- Emergency medical personnel should be reminded of the danger posed by livestock. These professionals should only enter the arena when directed by the medical staff in charge.

INJURY PREVENTION

- Unlike team sports and individual sports where coaches and strength and conditioning specialists are available to athletes, rodeo athletes rely on themselves and fellow athletes for management of their conditioning and rehabilitation from minor injuries.
- These athletes often ask event medical staff for advice and recommendations. In general, the sports medicine team should promote the use of safety equipment and be prepared

to provide recommendations regarding strength and flexibility training. The safety equipment requirements differ between rodeo organizations, and helmets are not required for bull riders at the professional level. Of note, none of the athletes who died of head injuries (3) were reported to have been wearing a helmet.

- Rodeo athletes earn their living on the road and may not have access to strength training and other exercise equipment. The sports medicine provider may need to adapt recommended exercises to the athlete's schedule and environment. Moreover, the sport-specific demands of the athlete's event must be considered.

CONCLUSION

- Rodeo is an exciting sport, and the rodeo athlete is genuinely appreciative of sports medicine professionals willing to learn about the sport and provide care. There is certainly a need to continue to expand and coordinate care of the rodeo athlete.
- Although the rodeo arena is a unique setting, these athletes and the officials for the rodeo are very willing to share their knowledge and help the sports medicine professional understand rodeo and feel welcome in what is often a new world of athletic health care.

REFERENCES

1. Butterwick DJ, Brandenburg MA, Andrews DM, et al. Agreement statement from the 1st international rodeo research and clinical care conference: Calgary, Alberta, Canada (July 7–9, 2004). *Clin J Sport Med.* 2005;15(3):192–5.
2. Butterwick DJ, Hagel B, Nelson DS, LeFave MR, Meeuwisse WH. Epidemiologic analysis of injury in five years of Canadian professional rodeo. *Am J Sports Med.* 2002;30(2):193–8.
3. Butterwick DJ, Lafave MR, Lau BH, Freeman T. Rodeo catastrophic injuries and registry: initial retrospective and prospective report. *Clin J Sport Med.* 2011;21(3):243–8.
4. Butterwick DJ, Meeuwisse WH. Bull riding injuries in professional rodeo: data for prevention and care. *Phys Sportsmed.* 2003;31(6):37–41.
5. Justin Sportsmedicine Team Web site [Internet]. Fort Worth (TX): Justin Sportsmedicine Team; [cited 2010 Aug 16]. Available from: http://www.justinboots.com/News/InjuriesperEvent_25yr_1195854968_7097.pdf.
6. Justin Sportsmedicine Team Web site [Internet]. Fort Worth (TX): Justin Sportsmedicine Team; [cited 2010 Aug 16]. Available from: http://www.justinboots.com/News/MajorInjuries_25yr_1195854968_1324.pdf.
7. Sinclair AJ, Smidt C. Analysis of 10 years of injury in high school rodeo. *Clin J Sport Med.* 2009;19(5):383–7.

102 Soccer

Nicholas A. Piantanida

INTRODUCTION

- The global success of soccer as a worldwide attraction actively involves an estimated 270 million people or 4% of the world's population (4).
- The increases in participation, with some countries such as Canada reporting a mean rate of increase in excess of 27% from 1998 to 2008 (7), draws attention to the importance of this sport's specific injury pattern and the effective methods of injury prevention.

HISTORICAL PROSPECTIVE

- The rules of soccer (football) were officially codified by Great Britain in 1863. In 1869, Princeton and Rutgers played the first American intercollegiate football game played by "soccer" rules.
- The enactment of Title IX in 1972 within the National Collegiate Athletic Association (NCAA) formed the initial American catalyst of soccer growth with the direct effect on the creation of female soccer programs. More recently, the 1991 U.S. women's soccer team World Cup victory in China was a second stimulus for growth.
- The World Cup of Soccer was held in the United States for men and women in 1994 and 1999, respectively. This local spectacle of sport propelled and elevated the caliber of play of soccer in the United States, which culminated in strong World Cup men's performances in 2002 and Olympic Gold Medal performances for women's soccer in 1996, 2004, and 2008.
- The U.S. Soccer Federation is the governing body of soccer in the United States. The professional first divisions for men's and women's soccer in the United States are Major Soccer League (MSL) and Women's Professional Soccer (WPS), respectively. Currently, the MSL is composed of 16 teams, and the WPS is composed of 7 teams.

PHYSICAL DEMANDS OF SOCCER

- Soccer is classified as a high- to moderate-intensity contact/collision sport by the American Academy of Pediatrics.

- The 26th Bethesda Conference classifies soccer as a low-static, high-dynamic sport.
- Soccer demands change of direction or cutting maneuvers followed by deceleration and jumping with major muscle movement and proprioception through the trunk and lower extremity.
- The aerobic challenges of soccer infuse the endurance requirements of a distance runner with the abrupt acceleration demands of a sprinter. The average distance covered by an elite midfield male player is in the 10-km range, with the strikers, fullbacks, and center backs covering less distance. Sprinting makes up significantly 10% of the total distance (31).
- The physiologic demands of soccer present unique challenges to hydration. In 2006, the U.S. Soccer Federation published its "Youth Soccer Heat Stress Guidelines" based on research conducted at the University of Connecticut (34). Several sport-specific factors expose soccer players to heat injury, including limited stoppage times with periods of intense aerobic activity, large fields with limited to no shade, and numerous games or practice sessions occurring in a day with limited attention to environmental stressors of heat and/or humidity.
- As little as 2% body weight drop in young competitors in hot conditions not only generates impairments in performance but also causes a compounded reduction in the ability to dissipate heat, resulting in accelerated heat-related injury. In temperate to cool environments, research shows greater tolerance for body weight drops in these same ranges. Most experts agree that a 5% drop in body weight during or following a soccer match or practice should sideline that athlete for 24 hours to recuperate fluid losses and to identify an intrinsic etiology such as poor acclimatization, supplement usage, or illness (8,27).
- It has been demonstrated that 30–60 mg of carbohydrate ingestion in the fluids before and during soccer activity can delay muscle glycogen depletion. In one study, Foster et al. (18) demonstrated that indoor soccer athletes who drank a glucose polymer enhanced work output and increased time to exhaustion when compared to controls.

SOCCER INJURY RATES

- The overall injury incidence in soccer varies across studies because of differences in study designs, populations, and injury definitions.

- Soccer has a higher injury rate than many contact sports, including field hockey, rugby, basketball, and football (26).

- Injury rates within the sport of soccer increase with participant age and correlate with the increased intensity of the match. More injuries occur during competitive games than during practice. Over a complete season, girls and boys may expect 4.0 and 3.5 injuries per season, respectively. When a correction is incorporated for exposure rates, senior athletes (age > 18) sustain 15–30 times as many injuries as youths, but when analyzing the National Electronic Injury Surveillance System, approximately 80% of these injuries affected participants younger than 24 years old (24,26,33).

- Female youths can have soccer injury rates more than twice as high as male youths. Engström et al. (16) published an incidence per 1,000 player-hours of 12 for girls versus 5 for boys. Schmidt-Olson et al. (32) documented an incidence per 1,000 player-hours of 17.6 for girls versus 7.4 for boys.

- Lower extremity injuries are the most common, with nonbody contact composing the majority of the injuries (16,24,26,29,32). Ankle injuries represent 16%–29% of these injuries and predominate among male players. Knee injuries occur in 16%–29% of players and occur more frequently in females (24,26,29,32).

- Ankle sprain is the single leading injury in soccer and is implicated as a reinjury 56% of the time (15).

- Soccer injury rates reported by the NCAA use an established Injury Surveillance System to follow male and female collegiate injuries (29).

- Head injuries represent 1.2%–8% of all injuries, depending on the study. The higher head injury rates in youth soccer are thought to be attributed to underdeveloped neck muscles to absorb the impact shock, increased ball weight to head weight ratio, and, more importantly, improper head ball technique (33).

- Serious anterior cruciate ligament (ACL) tear injury and concussion-type injuries follow gender differences. Women soccer players sustain more concussions than men, at a ratio of 4.3:1, and more ACL injuries, at ratios of 1.8:1 (practice) and 5.78:1 (games) (2,15,22,25).

- Indoor versus outdoor soccer injury rates are similar in severity and type (14).

- Soccer in the competitive ranks has migrated to artificial turf. In 2005, Fédération Internationale de Football Association (FIFA) accepted the use of third-generation artificial turf for official tournaments. Research on injury risk on third-generation artificial turf is limited but indicates small differences in injury pattern between artificial turf and natural grass (19).

SOCCER INJURY CHARACTERISTICS

Ankle Injury

- The mechanism of a lateral ankle sprain is often an inversion stress as the subtalar joint tilts in plantarflexion to manage tasks such as pivoting, jumping, and hard turns with the ball. In this position, the anterior talofibular ligament (ATFL) is at maximal tension and most vulnerable to injury because the stability of the subtalar joint is deviated from the neutral mortise position. The calcaneal fibular ligament (CFL) and posterior talofibular ligament follow in order of injury as the magnitude of stress is increased to the ATFL. The spectrum of severity spans from a lateral ankle ligament stretch (grade 1) to partial tear (grade 2) to complete tear (grade 3).

- Medial ankle ligament injuries are uncommon due to the dominant strength of the deltoid ligament. Therefore, a medial ankle disruption denotes a high-energy impact injury mechanism and will possibly demonstrate ankle mortise alteration requiring surgical repair and extensive rehabilitation.

- The mechanism of injury for high ankle injuries in soccer players occurs during collisions or player-to-player impact for contested balls. The ankle position during impact can be in the talar neutral position, with or without a slight lateral talar tilt. This predisposes the athlete to greater stresses across the CFL and the inferior anterior tibiofibular ligament. On clinical exam, performing a proximal tibial-fibular "squeeze test" with distal referred pain at the ankle or instability with external foot rotation is sensitive for a high ankle sprain.

- Talar dome lesions such as osteochondral fractures or a fracture to the lateral process of the talus must be considered in the ankle with persistent pain and swelling beyond 2 weeks. If clinical suspicion is high, magnetic resonance imaging (MRI) can assist in assessing this injury.

- Chronic anterior ankle pain extending on to the midfoot in an injured soccer player who had an acute axial loading of the forefoot and midfoot (kick into the turf) should be evaluated for a bifurcate ligament injury, impingement syndrome (especially for repeat ankle injuries), or Lisfranc fracture. If weight-bearing x-rays of the ankle/foot are normal, then an MRI of the ankle/foot should be done.

- Sever disease and, more commonly, retrocalcaneal bursitis are seen in young indoor soccer players with ankle pain or hindfoot pain (15,26,32,33) secondary to a pattern of repetitive heel trauma against the sideboards. Achilles tendinopathy and medial calf strain are typically seen in soccer players older than 18. Achilles tendinopathy differs from the above two conditions by presenting several centimeters proximally to the tendon insertion into the calcaneus.

- Chronic posterior ankle pain should raise concern for a calcaneal stress fracture as evident by calcaneal squeeze test or an os trigonum fracture. Both are verified by triple-phase nuclear bone scan.

Knee Injury

- Soccer players can experience the spectrum of overuse and acute knee problems. Youth players are susceptible to Osgood-Schlatter disease or any other patellofemoral anterior knee tracking maladies seen in all running sports. Senior soccer players will incur collateral ligament and meniscal injuries, along with the pain of degenerative osteoarthritis or patellar chondromalacia.

■ Meniscal and/or knee ligament injuries are vulnerable during dynamic passing sequences as the grounded cleats of the soccer shoe fixate the leg and support both rapid rotational and flexion changes of the trunk or lower leg. This sports-specific motion produces a sudden rotation of the femur relative to the fixed leg. As mentioned earlier, tackling is a high-risk maneuver where knee ligament strain often occurs when a player is tackled with the loaded leg secured to the ground.

■ Soccer athletes tear their ACL through direct contact or noncontact. Noncontact/noncollision ACL tears are the predominant means for ACL injury in most sports other than skiing. However, Arendt and Dick (2) reported that male collegiate soccer players have an equal rate of contact versus noncontact ACL injuries. As previously mentioned, the female collegiate soccer ACL injury rate dominates the male ACL injury rate, but follows the usual trend for noncontact ACL injury.

■ Understanding the injury mechanism is critical to preventing noncontact ACL injuries. The literature is rich with well-designed and well-executed studies analyzing ACL loading stresses. Most conclusions characterize the mechanism for noncontact ACL injury as following the common pattern of advancing anterior shear force at the proximal tibia produced as the knee is loaded through deceleration and accentuated by knee pivoting with internal or external rotation or the awkward landing of a varus or valgus collapsed knee. Researchers have found that ACL loading mechanisms are further elevated by a small knee flexion angle (15–30 degrees) and/or a strong quadriceps muscle contraction or a great posterior ground reaction force (6,12,35).

■ Contact ACL injuries in male soccer players follow a pattern of collision with a valgus stress to the knee. These injuries are often complicated by associated injuries to the menisci, the collateral ligaments, and the articular cartilage.

■ In chondral injuries, soccer maneuvers that require repetitive pivoting and deceleration produce extreme stress on the articular cartilage, generating abrasive wear or the acute disruption of the deep cartilage ultrastructure by large shear forces. Chondral lesions are more often found on the femoral condyle. Acute x-ray imaging for a swollen knee should include tunnel views to investigate an osteochondral fracture, and if present, the fracture should be staged by knee MRI and co-managed with an orthopedic surgeon.

Lower Leg Injury

■ A soccer player's lower leg is vulnerable to abrasions, contusions, and fractures. Shin guards have become the only mandatory protective devices in soccer, but serve primarily to protect the leg from minor soft tissue injuries. Soccer tibial and fibular fractures occur at high rates despite athletes wearing shin guards (5).

■ The soccer player with both a tibia and fibula fracture is sidelined, on average, for 40 weeks. Players with individual fibula and tibia fractures return to competitive play on average in 18 and 35 weeks, respectively (5).

■ The broad differential for exertional lower leg pain incorporates many overuse injuries to the lower extremity. The more common exertional lower leg ailments include compartment syndrome, medial tibial stress syndrome (MTSS), and stress fractures.

■ Anterior tibial compartment syndrome is insidious and effort dependent, with running pain that reduces performance over several months to years. Conversely, acute compartment syndrome may occur when a player sustains a high-velocity kick to the protected or unprotected anterior or lateral lower leg. In both cases, the player typically describes lower leg pain with tingling and/or weakness extending to the dorsum of the foot. Diagnostic compartment testing with a handheld device and co-management with an orthopedic surgeon should follow.

■ Connective tissue recovery and bone adaptation occur in a normal pattern of cyclic recovery provided rest, time, and nutrition are balanced. Injury patterns for MTSS and stress fractures are multifactorial (intrinsic or extrinsic sources of overuse) and represent maladaptive versions of cyclic tissue and bone recovery.

■ Stress fractures and MTSS are best differentiated by triple-phase bone scan or MRI and treated with phased degrees of activity modification. MRI results depicting a stress fracture have both diagnostic and prognostic recovery parameters.

Groin Injury

■ Soccer groin and torso injuries are less commonly seen but may serve to be the most challenging to treat.

■ The mechanism of groin injury in the soccer athlete is associated with a strain at the groin while the hip is abducted and externally rotated, sometimes against an opposing force such as the ground or the opponent. This process of strain or overstretching compromises the adolescent's apophyseal pelvic ring or pubic attachments or, in the case of the senior player, the muscular–tendinous attachments.

■ Adductor muscle tendinopathy is a form of overuse strain where groin pain gradually develops after advancing play intensity or frequency of workouts. These cases should be differentiated from osteitis pubis and "sports hernias," which can present with a similar pain pattern.

■ Hip flexor strain to the iliopsoas/bursitis is seen in soccer and is clinically defined by deep groin pain with an occasional slapping hip sensation or pain extension onto the anterior thigh. Treatment consists of relative rest with a prescribed stretching program for hip flexors and rotators. Additionally, an iliopsoas strengthening program should precede the return to competitive play (28).

■ Gilmore groin, or groin disruption, was clinically defined in 1980 following the successful treatment of three professional soccer players who had been sidelined with pain for

3 months. Clinical symptoms of groin disruption include insidious unilateral pain in the adductor region that progresses with activity and follows a course of postactivity aggravation getting out of bed or the car. Exam findings are evasive and variable but may include tenderness and dilation of the internal inguinal ring on scrotal hernia palpation. The anatomic features of this condition include torn external oblique aponeurosis, torn conjoined tendon, conjoined tendon tear from the pubic tubercle, dehiscence between conjoined tendon and inguinal ligament, and no hernia. Diagnosis should include Stork radiographs to evaluate pelvic stability, and treatment failures after a 2- to 4-week rehabilitative process should proceed to surgery for repair (20).

Head Injury

- The head functions as a significant physical contributor in the play of soccer. The heading technique is a learned skill when executed properly. The complex synchronized motion whereby the head strikes forcefully through the ball as the trunk goes into flexion requires coaching and practice. Maintaining a rigid neck during impact diminishes potential injury from angular head and neck acceleration.

- The challenge with mild traumatic brain injury or concussion is that 70% of collegiate football and soccer players experienced concussion symptoms during a defined season, but only 20% were aware that they sustained an injury (11). Furthermore, researchers are intrigued as to the risk of successive head balls over an extended career of playing soccer. Such subclinical concussions may predispose soccer athletes to advancing brain injury analogous to the "punch drunk" syndrome of chronic progressive traumatic encephalopathy seen in career boxers.

- In a study by Haglund and Eriksson (21) (level of evidence A, controlled clinical trial), "typical header" soccer players and a control group were studied using neuropsychiatric, radiologic, and electroencephalogram (EEG) data, and no differences between the groups were found.

- Jordan et al. (23) (level of evidence A, controlled clinical trial) analyzed U.S. National Soccer Team players with brain MRI and a head injury questionnaire. This study found no differences in brain anatomy when comparing soccer player MRIs with age-matched controlled track athletes, but remarkably, the questionnaire further reinforced the concern for the higher incidence of unrecognized concussions in soccer athletes.

- Therefore, currently with limited research, the data suggest that heading the ball is safe; however, many studies are under way, and the American Youth Soccer Organization recommends that children under the age of 10 should not head the soccer ball.

- Regarding concussions in soccer, they occur many times without acknowledgement from the player. Concussions in soccer are a result of impact with another player, the ground, or the goal posts. Soccer players require coach- or team physician–directed instruction on the symptoms of a concussion.

- Any soccer athlete with a history of concussion will objectively perform worse on neurocognitive testing, such as ImPact. Baseline preseason neurocognitive testing is encouraged for position players on the offensive line, the goalie, and any player with a prior concussion history. Female soccer players with concussion perform more poorly than males in neurocognitive testing and have more symptoms (9).

- Assessment and management of a head-injured soccer athlete should be no different from any other athlete. Diagnostic studies and return-to-play criteria are discussed in another section.

Facial and Oral Injuries

- The mechanism for eye injuries is usually blunt trauma caused by a kicked ball or the kicking foot. A hyphema is the most common injury type and can occur in up to 50% of all blunt eye traumas in soccer (24). A hyphema should be co-managed with an ophthalmologist.

- The frequency of eye injuries in soccer has prompted the recommendation by the American Academy of Pediatrics Committee on Sports Medicine and Fitness and the American Academy of Ophthalmology Committee on Eye Safety and Sports Ophthalmology that protective sports eye equipment using polycarbonate lenses be worn during both soccer practice and competition (1).

- Orofacial and dental injuries in soccer rank second behind basketball (17) but are exceedingly rare events. Widespread use of protective mouthguards has been advocated in the dental literature to reduce the number of such injuries (30), but this practice is not supported in the sports medicine literature.

PREVENTION

- Ekstrand and Gillquist (13) (level of evidence A, prospective controlled study) found that soccer injuries can be reduced by 75% by the implementation of a multilevel preventative approach.

- A skilled coaching staff must marginalize training errors and recognize that quality is more important than quantity.

- Attention to equipment utilization, including shin guards and mouthguards, and optimal field conditions pays dividends on injury prevention. Wet bulb globe temperature (WBGT) guidelines in accordance with American College of Sports Medicine guidelines should direct periods of play or practice and hydration standards.

- Prophylactic ankle taping or bracing benefits players with clinical instability or history of previous ankle strain (13).

- Arnason et al. (3) (level of evidence A, prospective controlled study) have demonstrated a significant reduction in hamstring strains in elite soccer players through eccentric hamstring strengthening.

- Players with serious knee instability will not benefit from bracing, and to avoid the risk of ACL injury, exclusion from soccer participation is worthy of discussion.

- Educate soccer players on the importance of disciplined play and proper technique, especially with head balls.

- No head balls should be performed by children under age 10. Meticulous attention to technique must be the focus of training.

- Soccer headgear is under development to reduce the risk that an athlete will sustain head injury by reducing impact acceleration. Researchers are still defining parameters for evidenced applications of headgear, but women stand to benefit more than males (10).

- Educate players and staff on the early identification and management of concussions. Preseason standardized neuropsychological testing should be done in patients at risk by history or by position (goalie or forward). Pad goal posts.

- Team physicians must prescribe a supervised and progressive rehabilitative process. Return-to-play decisions after injury should come directly from the team physician and physical therapist. End-state rehabilitation and functional goals include full range of motion, 90% strength, and dynamic agility testing.

CONCLUSION

- Soccer is one of the most popular sports played in the world today.

- The present injury profile for soccer is considered safe. Clinicians should be well versed in the many unique injury challenges that span the spectrum of age and gender to draw attention to soccer's sport-specific injury presentations and management goals.

- To make soccer safer, research should address advancing needs to prevent ankle and noncontact ACL injuries and answer the question regarding the long-term cognitive effects of the sport in relation to head injuries.

REFERENCES

1. American Academy of Pediatrics, Committee on Sports Medicine and Fitness. Protective eyewear for young athletes. *Pediatrics.* 2004;113 (3 pt 1):619–22.

2. Arendt E, Dick R. Knee injury patterns among men and women in collegiate basketball and soccer. NCAA data and review of literature. *Am J Sports Med.* 1995;23(6):694–701.

3. Arnason A, Andersen TE, Holme I, Engebretsen L, Bahr R. Prevention of hamstring strains in elite soccer: an intervention study. *Scand J Med Sci Sports.* 2008;18(1):40–8.

4. Big Count 2006: statistical summary report by gender/category/region, FIFA Communications Division, Information Services [Internet]. 2007 [cited 2010 Oct 18]. Available from: http://www.fifa.com/aboutfifa/media/newsid=529882.html.

5. Boden BP. Leg injuries and shin guards. *Clin Sports Med.* 1998;17(4): 769–77, vii.

6. Boden BP, Dean GS, Feagin JA Jr, Garrett WE Jr. Mechanisms of anterior cruciate ligament injury. *Orthopedics.* 2000;23(6):573–8.

7. Canadian Soccer Association. 2008 demographics report: player registrations [Internet]. 2008 [cited 2010 Oct 12]. Available from: http://www.canadasoccer.com/documents/demographics/2008_demographics_report.pdf.

8. Casa DJ, Armstrong LE, Hillman SK, et al. National athletic trainers' association position statement: fluid replacement for athletes. *J Athl Train.* 2000;35(2):212–24.

9. Colvin AC, Mullen J, Lovell MR, West RV, Collins MW, Groh M. The role of concussion history and gender in recovery from soccer-related concussion. *Am J Sports Med.* 2009;37(9):1699–704.

10. Delaney JS, Al-Kashmiri A, Drummond R, Correa JA. The effect of protective headgear on head injuries and concussions in adolescent football (soccer) players. *Br J Sport Med.* 2008;42(2):110–5.

11. Delaney JS, Lacroix VJ, Leclerc S, Johnston KM. Concussion among university football and soccer players. *Clin J Sport Med.* 2002;12(6):331–8.

12. Delfico AJ, Garrett WE Jr. Mechanisms of injury of the anterior cruciate ligament in soccer players. *Clin Sports Med.* 1998;17(4):779–85, vii.

13. Ekstrand J, Gillquist J. Soccer injuries and their mechanisms: a prospective study. *Med Sci Sports Exerc.* 1983;15(3):267–70.

14. Emery CA, Meeuwisse WH. Risk factors for injury in indoor compared with outdoor adolescent soccer. *Am J Sports Med.* 2006;34(10):1636–42.

15. Emery CA, Meeuwisse WH, Hartmann SE. Evaluation of risk factors for injury in youth soccer. *Am J Sports Med.* 2005;33(12):1882–91.

16. Engström B, Johansson C, Törnkvist H. Soccer injuries among elite female players. *Am J Sports Med.* 1991;19(4):372–5.

17. Flanders RA, Bhat M. The incidence of orofacial injuries in sports: a pilot study in Illinois. *J Am Dent Assoc.* 1995;126(4):491–6.

18. Foster C, Thompson NN, Dean J, Kirkendall DT. Carbohydrate supplementation and performance in soccer players. *Med Sci Sport Exerc.* 1986;18(Suppl 8):12.

19. Fuller CW, Dick RW, Corlette J, Schmalz R. Comparison of the incidence, nature and cause of injuries sustained on grass and new generation artificial turf by male and female football players. Part 2: training injuries. *Br J Sports Med.* 2007;41(Suppl l):i27–32.

20. Gilmore J. Groin pain in the soccer athlete: fact, fiction and treatment. *Clin Sport Med.* 1998;17(4):787–93, vii.

21. Haglund Y, Eriksson E. Does amateur boxing lead to chronic brain damage? *Am J Sports Med.* 1993;21(1):97–109.

22. Hewett TE, Myer GD, Ford KR. Anterior cruciate ligament injuries in female athletes: part 1, mechanisms and risk factors. *Am J Sports Med.* 2006;34(2):299–311.

23. Jordan SE, Green GA, Galanty HL, Mandelbaum BR, Jabour BA. Acute and chronic brain injury in United States National Team soccer players. *Am J Sports Med.* 1996;24(2):205–10.

24. Junge A, Rösch D, Peterson L, Graf-Baumann T, Dvorak J. Prevention of soccer injuries: a prospective intervention study in youth amateur players. *Am J Sports Med.* 2002;30(5):652–9.

25. Kiani A, Hellquist E, Ahlqvist K, Gedeborg R, Michaëlsson K, Byberg L. Prevention of soccer-related knee injuries in teenaged girls. *Arch Intern Med.* 2010;170(1):43–9.

26. Koutures CG, Gregory AJ; American Academy of Pediatrics. Council on Sports Medicine and Fitness. Injuries in youth soccer. *Pediatrics.* 2010;125(2):410–4.

27. Maughan RJ, Shirreffs SM, Merson SJ, Horswill SA. Fluid and electrolyte balance in elite male football (soccer) players training in a cool environment. *J Sports Sci.* 2005;23(1):73–9.

28. Morelli V, Smith V. Groin injuries in athletes. *Am Fam Physician.* 2001;64(8):1405–14.

29. National Collegiate Athletic Association. *NCAA Injury Surveillance System*. Indianapolis (IN): NCAA; 2000.

30. Powers JM, Godwin WC, Heintz WD. Mouth protectors and sports team dentists. Bureau of Health Education and Audiovisual Services, Council on Dental Materials, Instruments, and Equipment. *J Am Dent Assoc*. 1984;109(1):84–7.

31. Reilly T, Thomas V. An analysis of work-rate in different positional roles in professional football match-play. *J Hum Movement Sci*. 1976; 2:87–97.

32. Schmidt-Olsen S, Jørgensen U, Kaalund S, Sørensen J. Injuries among young soccer players. *Am J Sports Med*. 1991;19:273–5.

33. Sullivan JA, Gross RH, Grana WA, Garcia-Moral CA. Evaluation of injuries in youth soccer. *Am J Sports Med*. 1980;8(5):325–7.

34. U.S. Soccer's Youth Soccer Heat Stress Guidelines [Internet]. 2007 [cited 2010 Oct 12]. Available from: http://onthepitch.org/wp-content/uploads/2007/08/ussf_hydration_guide.pdf.

35. Yu B, Garrett W. Mechanisms of non-contact ACL injuries. *Br J Sports Med*. 2007;41(Suppl 1):i47–51.105

103

Softball Injuries

Lindsay J. DiStefano and Jeffrey M. Anderson

INTRODUCTION

- This chapter is focused on competitive fast-pitch softball injuries in women. Fast-pitch softball is a sport played predominantly by women, but there are many men's or coed leagues as well. Slow-pitch softball is also frequently played across the world. However, the majority of the literature surrounding softball-related injuries is in regard to competitive women's fast-pitch softball, which provides the rationale for this chapter's focus.

- Fast-pitch softball has grown tremendously in popularity over the past several decades. During a 15-year period between the 1988–1989 and 2003–2004 seasons, National Collegiate Athletic Association (NCAA) softball added 362 schools, causing participation to increase by over 70% (9,389 participants in 1988–1989 to 16,079 participants in 2003–2004) (15).

- Softball has been an NCAA sport since 1982 and was an Olympic sport from 1996 to 2012.

- During the 2009–2010 academic year, high school fast-pitch softball was the fourth most popular sport, with 378,211 participants (17).

RULES AND REGULATIONS

- Comparisons between softball and baseball are constantly made due to the similar general nature of the games. Where appropriate, references to the rules and regulations of baseball are provided.

- Similar to baseball, softball plays with nine field positions: pitcher, catcher, first base, second base, shortstop, third base, right field, center field, and left field.

- Regulation games consist of seven innings. *(Baseball: nine innings)*

- Distance between bases: 18.29 meters (60 ft). *(Baseball: 60 ft [Little League] to 90 ft)*

- Distance between the pitcher's mound and home plate: 13.11 meters (43 ft) (14 and under: 12.19 m [40 ft]; 12 and under: 10.66 m [35 ft]). *(Baseball: 46 ft [Little League] to 60.5 ft)*

- In contrast to baseball, the pitching mound in softball is not elevated.

- The ball size is 30.5 cm (12 in). *(Baseball: 23 cm [9 in])*

INJURY EPIDEMIOLOGY

- Softball has a relatively low rate of injuries compared to other sports. However, costs for medical care of baseball and softball injuries still exceeded $1 billion in 2009 (1).

- Table 103.1 shows game and practice injury rates per 1,000 athlete exposures (AE) for both intercollegiate and high school softball with comparisons to baseball and women's soccer, which usually has the highest injury rate for a female sport.

  - The intercollegiate injury data come from studies using the NCAA Injury Surveillance System (ISS) over a 16-year period (1988–1989 to 2003–2004) (5,12).

  - The high school injury data come from studies using High School RIO (Reporting Information Online; The Research Institute at Nationwide Children's Hospital, Columbus, OH) during the 2005–2006 academic year (21).

NCAA Softball Epidemiology

- Softball has the lowest game injury rate of NCAA female sports (8,15) and the fourth lowest practice injury rate (8).

- A softball athlete is 1.6 times more likely to sustain an injury during a game than during a practice. This is a relatively low difference between game and practice injury rates compared to sports like women's ice hockey, where athletes are 5 times more likely to sustain an injury during a game than practice (8). This small difference is probably due to a low amount of player contact in softball games (15).

- Only 22% of softball game and practice injuries result in more than 10 days lost from activity (15).

High School Softball Epidemiology

- Softball has one of the lowest injury rates among high school sports, second to volleyball (12,18,21).

- Softball injuries do not tend to be severe. In a study using injury data from North Carolina high schools, 77% of injuries resulted in less than 8 days lost from activity, whereas

Table 103.1	Practice/Game Injury Rate Comparisons	
Sport	**Game Injury Rate (per 1,000 AE)**	**Practice Injury Rate (per 1,000 AE)**
NCAA		
Softball	4.3	2.7
Baseball	5.8	1.9
Women's soccer	16.4	5.2
High school		
Softball	1.78	0.79
Baseball	1.77	0.87
Women's soccer	5.21	1.1

AE, athlete exposures.

only 7% resulted in more than 21 days lost [12]. The High School RIO data revealed a similar trend, with almost 60% of all softball injuries resulting in less than 1 week lost from activity [21].

- High school softball injuries have one of the lowest rates of injuries that require surgery (0.57/10,000 AE) [20].

TYPES OF INJURIES

- Table 103.2 illustrates the injury percentages by body part in high school and collegiate softball [15,21].
- Rechel et al. [21] reported similar injury percentages by body part between high school softball and baseball.
- The most common injuries in collegiate softball are:
  - Ankle sprains (games: 0.44 injuries/1,000 AE; practices: 0.25 injuries/1,000 AE) [15]

Table 103.2	Injury Percentages by Body Part	
Body Part Injured	**High School (%)**	**NCAA (%)**
Lower extremity		
Practice	35.0	40.8
Game	49.1	43.3
Upper extremity		
Practice	40.7	33.0
Game	32.3	33.1
Head/face/neck		
Practice	22.4	9.6
Game	17.1	13.4
Trunk		
Practice	1.9	1.9
Game	1.5	1.1

NCAA, NAtional Collegiate Athletic Association.

- Knee internal derangement (games: 0.37 injuries/1,000 AE; practices: 0.14 injuries/1,000 AE) [15]
- The NCAA ISS data revealed that head or neck injuries are more likely to occur during a game, but trunk or back injuries are more common during practice [15].
- In contrast to the NCAA ISS data, the High School RIO data show that concussions are more common in high school softball practice (8.9%) than games (0.4%) [21].

MECHANISM OF INJURIES

- Marshall et al. [15] reported game injuries by position from the NCAA ISS data:
  - Base runner: 28%
  - Batter: 13%
  - Pitcher: 11%
  - Catcher: 9%
  - Outfielders: 4% average
  - Infielders: 5% average
- The most common mechanism of injury during games is contact with something (*i.e.*, ground, base, ball, wall) other than a person [15,19] and usually is due to base running in high school softball [19].
- The majority of practice injuries are due to noncontact mechanisms (no contact with anything external to the body) (*i.e.*, throwing, running) [15,19].
- Sliding accounts for 23% of game injuries in collegiate softball. The injury rate in softball due to sliding is 12.76 injuries/1,000 AE [9]. *(Baseball: 6.2 injuries/1,000 AE)*
- Base running is responsible for 10% of all collegiate game injuries and 32.7% of all high school game injuries [19].
- Being hit by a ball during a collegiate game leads to 11% of game injuries [15].

SPECIFIC INJURIES

Shoulder

- Softball is responsible for one of the highest shoulder injury rates (1.10/10,000 AE) in high school girls' sports. *(Baseball: 1.90/10,000 AE)* [13]
- High school softball athletes are more likely to sustain a shoulder injury due to chronic/overuse mechanisms and contact with another player compared with baseball athletes [13].
- In high school softball, 51% of shoulder injuries result in less than 1 week lost from participation [4].
- Throwing accounts for a higher incidence of shoulder injuries during high school softball practices compared with pitching [13].
- The most common shoulder injuries in high school softball are muscle strains/incomplete tears [13].

Pitching

- Pitching is the most common mechanism of a shoulder injury that lasts more than 9 days (13).
- Softball is unique because it involves the windmill pitch, which requires the pitcher to circumduct his or her extended arm around the body and release the ball below the hip with an underarm motion.
- The windmill pitching motion results in higher biceps muscle activity compared to overhead throwing, especially during the deceleration phase (22).
- Despite longer pitching distances in baseball, distraction forces are similar between baseball and softball pitchers (25).
- Bogenschutz et al. (2) studied young adult softball athletes for bone mass, bone size, and bone strength adaptations in the humerus. The authors concluded that overhead throwing causes greater skeletal adaptations in the humerus than windmill throwing, which may be a result of less torsional forces during the windmill technique.
- Softball pitchers may pitch 1,200–2,000 times over 3 days compared to pitchers in baseball, who pitch approximately 100–150 times, but baseball has higher rates of injury in pitchers than softball (8,19,26).
- Shanley et al. (23) conducted a prospective study with high school baseball and softball pitchers for upper extremity injury risk factors. The authors reported that passive glenohumeral range-of-motion restrictions predicted injury in baseball pitchers, but not softball pitchers.

Concussions

- Although concussions are not extremely common in softball, softball demonstrated an injury rate twice as high as baseball in the NCAA (8) and nearly twice as high as baseball in high school sports practice (5,14,18).
- The reason for this higher incidence of injury may be due to possible sex differences in concussion pathology or the closer distances between bases and the pitcher's position relative to home plate.
- Concussions in softball typically occur due to catching, fielding, or pitching. A much lower proportion of concussions occurs during batting compared to baseball (5).

Anterior Cruciate Ligament and Ankle Sprain Injuries

- Similar to concussions, the incidence rates of anterior cruciate ligament (ACL) injuries (0.08/1,000 AE) and ankle sprain injuries (0.32/1,000 AE) in softball are relatively low compared to other intercollegiate sports (8).
- However, both injuries are more frequent in softball compared to baseball (ACL injuries: 0.02/1,000 AE; ankle sprains: 0.23/1,000 AE).
- These data suggest that a sex discrepancy in ACL injuries between softball and baseball does exist, which agrees with other sports such as basketball and soccer (7).

- Despite the overall relatively low injury rate for ACL injuries in softball, knee internal derangement injuries still account for nearly 10% of overall injuries in the sport (ACL injuries account for 33% of these injuries) (15).

SPECIFIC INJURIES IN SOFTBALL

- Although no injuries are specifically unique to the sport of softball, the unique motion of the softball windmill pitch can predispose an individual to specific forearm, hand, and upper extremity neurologic injuries.
  - Ulnar diaphyseal stress fractures
    - ❏ Several case studies of these injuries have been published (6,16,24).
    - ❏ The postulated mechanism of development of the stress injury includes repetitive flexion of the wrist (16) or recurrent pronation of the wrist (24).
    - ❏ The recurrent pronation mechanism is consistent with the proposed mechanism of the development of similar injuries in tennis (3).
    - ❏ Athletes with ulnar diaphyseal stress fractures present with pain in the region of the ulnar shaft associated with their specific activity. On examination, they are tender in the area of the stress injury, and pain is reproduced with resisted motion, including pronation, wrist flexion, and flexion of the ulnar-sided digits of the hand (6).
    - ❏ Diagnostic modalities include plain radiographs, which may be normal or show evidence of new periosteal bone formation at the site of the injury. Radionuclide bone scans and magnetic resonance imaging have been used to make the definitive diagnoses in the cases reported earlier.
    - ❏ Management of the injury has included cessation of pitching along with protective bracing.
  - A fifth metacarpal stress fracture case study involving a softball pitcher has been reported in the literature (11).

WAYS TO REDUCE INJURIES IN SOFTBALL

Training

- Proper conditioning must be emphasized in all levels of softball due to the high prevalence of overuse injuries and preseason injuries.
- Neuromuscular training programs, such as ACL injury prevention programs, have demonstrated success with other sports but have yet to be studied in softball. These programs may be beneficial for reducing muscle strains, ankle sprains, and knee pathologies.
- The windmill method of pitching does not reduce the stress on pitchers' shoulders, so pitch counts and interval-throwing programs should be used to help reduce shoulder injuries.

■ Core strengthening should be encouraged to reduce low back strains, which are common injuries in softball. This type of strengthening may help avoid other common upper and lower extremity injuries and may be beneficial for performance.

■ The American Academy of Orthopaedic Surgeons has recommended the following regarding sliding (1), which is the cause of almost a quarter of all game-related injuries:

  ■ Sliding is prohibited with players under 10 years old.

  ■ Proper instruction in sliding technique should be provided, and players should practice their technique using a sliding bag.

  ■ The runner should slide to avoid a collision at home plate.

Field Equipment

■ Breakaway bases should be encouraged in all levels of softball.

  ■ Traditional stationary bases are bolted to a metal post and sunk into the ground. In contrast, breakaway bases are snapped onto grommets attached to anchored rubber mats, which hold it in place. Sliding will dislodge this attachment but normal running will not disrupt the attachment.

  ■ Janda et al. (10) demonstrated that breakaway bases in recreational softball games reduced sliding injuries by 98% and associated medical costs by 99%.

  ■ These bases are currently allowed by most softball governing bodies (NCAA, National Federation of State High School Associations[NFHS], Amateur Softball Association of America [ASA]) but are not mandatory.

  ■ The American Academy of Orthopaedic Surgeons has supported the use of breakaway bases to prevent injuries and reduce health care costs (1).

■ A double-base for first base (runner's base) should be considered for all levels of softball.

  ■ Currently required in International Softball Federation championships and the ASA, allowed by the NFHS, but not allowed by the NCAA.

  ■ The American Academy of Orthopaedic Surgeons recommends the double-base to prevent ankle and foot injuries (1).

■ Pitch distance was recently increased from 40 to 43 feet by NFHS and ASA for high school softball to reduce pitching injuries.

Player Equipment

■ Head and face injuries account for just over 7% of collegiate injuries, and contact with a pitched or batted ball is the common mechanism of injury (15).

■ Batting helmet face masks should be encouraged, if not mandated, by all levels of softball to protect the batter and base runner.

  ■ These face masks are currently required by the NFHS, but not by the NCAA.

■ Face masks for fielders should also be considered to help prevent facial injuries in the field.

  ❏ May be most beneficial for pitchers

  ❏ Currently allowed but not required by the NFHS, NCAA, and ASA

REFERENCES

1. American Academy of Orthopaedic Surgeons. *Position Statement: Use of Breakaway Bases in Preventing Recreational Baseball and Softball Injuries.* Rosemont (IL): American Academy of Orthopaedic Surgeons; 2010.

2. Bogenschutz ED, Smith HD, Warden SJ. Midhumerus adaptation in fast pitch softballers and the effect of throwing mechanics. *Med Sci Sports Exerc.* 2011;43(9):1698–706.

3. Bollen SR, Robinson DG, Crichton KJ, Cross MJ. Stress fractures of the ulna in tennis players using a double-handed backhand stroke. *Am J Sports Med.* 1993;21(5):751–2.

4. Bonza JE, Fields SK, Yard EE, Dawn Comstock R. Shoulder injuries among United States high school athletes during the 2005–2006 and 2006–2007 school years. *J Athl Train.* 2009;44(1):76–83.

5. Gessel LM, Fields SK, Collins CL, Dick RW, Comstock RD. Concussions among United States high school and collegiate athletes. *J Athl Train.* 2007;42(4):495–503.

6. Grossfeld SL, Van Heest A, Arendt E, House J. Pitcher's periostitis. A case report. *Am J Sports Med.* 1998;26(2):303–7.

7. Hewett TE, Shultz SJ, Griffin LY. Incidence of ACL injury. In: Hewett TE, Shultz SJ, Griffin LY, editors. *Understanding and Preventing Non-contact ACL Injuries/American Orthopaedic Society for Sports Medicine.* Champaign (IL): Human Kinetics; 2007. 344 p.

8. Hootman JM, Dick R, Agel J. Epidemiology of collegiate injuries for 15 sports: summary and recommendations for injury prevention initiatives. *J Athl Train.* 2007;42(2):311–9.

9. Hosey RG, Puffer JC. Baseball and softball sliding injuries. Incidence, and the effect of technique in collegiate baseball and softball players. *Am J Sports Med.* 2000;28(3):360–3.

10. Janda DH, Wojtys EM, Hankin FM, Benedict ME, Hensinger RN. A three-phase analysis of the prevention of recreational softball injuries. *Am J Sports Med.* 1990;18(6):632–5.

11. Jowett AD, Brukner PD. Fifth metacarpal stress fracture in a female softball pitcher. *Clin J Sport Med.* 1997;7(3):220–1.

12. Knowles SB, Marshall SW, Bowling JM, et al. A prospective study of injury incidence among North Carolina high school athletes. *Am J Epidemiol.* 2006;164(12):1209–21.

13. Krajnik S, Fogarty KJ, Yard EE, Comstock RD. Shoulder injuries in US high school baseball and softball athletes, 2005–2008. *Pediatrics.* 2010;125(3):497–501.

14. Lincoln AE, Caswell SV, Almquist JL, Dunn RE, Norris JB, Hinton RY. Trends in concussion incidence in high school sports: a prospective 11-year study. *Am J Sports Med.* 2011;39(5):958–63.

15. Marshall SW, Hamstra-Wright KL, Dick R, Grove KA, Agel J. Descriptive epidemiology of collegiate women's softball injuries: National Collegiate Athletic Association Injury Surveillance System, 1988–1989 through 2003–2004. *J Athl Train.* 2007;42(2):286–94.

16. Mutoh Y, Mori T, Suzuki Y, Sugiura Y. Stress fractures of the ulna in athletes. *Am J Sports Med.* 1982;10(6):365–7.

17. National Federation of State High School Associations. High school sports participation tops 7.6 million, sets record [Internet]. 2011. Available at: http://www.aledotimesrecord.com/newsnow/x2125230601/High-school-sports-participation-tops-7-6-million-sets-record.

18. Powell JW, Barber-Foss KD. Injury patterns in selected high school sports: a review of the 1995–1997 seasons. *J Athl Train.* 1999;34(3):277–84.

19. Powell JW, Barber-Foss KD. Sex-related injury patterns among selected high school sports. *Am J Sports Med.* 2000;28(3):385–91.

20. Rechel JA, Collins CL, Comstock RD. Epidemiology of injuries requiring surgery among high school athletes in the United States, 2005 to 2010. *J Trauma.* 2011;71(4):982–9.

21. Rechel JA, Yard EE, Comstock RD. An epidemiologic comparison of high school sports injuries sustained in practice and competition. *J Athl Train.* 2008;43(2):197–204.

22. Rojas IL, Provencher MT, Bhatia S, et al. Biceps activity during windmill softball pitching: injury implications and comparison with overhand throwing. *Am J Sports Med.* 2009;37(3):558–65.

23. Shanley E, Rauh MJ, Michener LA, Ellenbecker TS, Garrison JC, Thigpen CA. Shoulder range of motion measures as risk factors for shoulder and elbow injuries in high school softball and baseball players. *Am J Sports Med.* 2011;39(9):1997–2006.

24. Tanabe S, Nakahira J, Bando E, Yamaguchi H, Miyamoto H, Yamamoto A. Fatigue fracture of the ulna occurring in pitchers of fast-pitch softball. *Am J Sports Med.* 1991;19(3):317–21.

25. Werner SL, Guido JA, McNeice RP, Richardson JL, Delude NA, Stewart GW. Biomechanics of youth windmill softball pitching. *Am J Sports Med.* 2005;33(4):552–60.

26. Werner SL, Jones DG, Guido JA Jr, Brunet ME. Kinematics and kinetics of elite windmill softball pitching. *Am J Sports Med.* 2006;34(4):597–603.

Surfing

104

C. Joel Hess and Paul T. Diamond

INTRODUCTION

- Surfing is an ancient sport originating in the South Pacific that eventually became an integral part of Hawaiian culture. The practice of surfing in Hawaii was discouraged by missionaries in the 1800s but was subsequently revived as a sport by Hawaiian Olympic swimmer Duke Kahanamoku who introduced the sport to California and Australia in the 1920s (13).

- There are 1.7 million surfers in the United States and 18 million worldwide (13).

- The Association for Surfing Professionals (ASP) is the leading governing body for professional surfing and is responsible for sanctioning surfing contests and tours throughout the world.

- Surfing competitions involve 20- to 40-minute elimination heats in which surfers are scored by a group of judges with high scorers advancing on to further rounds. Athletes are judged on degree of difficulty, control, power, speed, style, and originality. Points for individual surfing contests are accumulated throughout the year to determine the overall tour rankings.

ACTIVITY PROFILE

- Surfing is an intermittent sport that is characterized by periods of high-intensity exercise interspersed with low-intensity activity and rest periods (5).

- Surfing first involves paddling away from shore. While paddling out, a maneuver called "duck diving" is used to dive nose first under oncoming waves in order to continue away from shore. When a suitable wave is identified, surfers attempt to match the speed of the oncoming wave in order to ride along the wave front. Once the surfer is pulled toward shore by the wave, they explosively transition from a prone to a standing position and ride down the face of the wave. In big-wave surfing, surfers may be towed to the wave front by a motorized watercraft in order to match a larger wave's higher velocity.

- Paddling is performed with the surfer lying in the prone position with the back and neck in hyperextension and with the arms alternating, pulling through the water alongside the board. Paddling biomechanics differ from freestyle swimming because long axis rotation is diminished while lying prone on the board and kicking is eliminated as a means of forward propulsion.

- During competition, surfers spend 51% and 42% of the time paddling and resting, respectively. Wave riding only accounts for 4% of the total time (11).

ATHLETE ATTRIBUTES

- Females account for only 5%–22% of surfers in the United States (21).

- The mean age of professional surfers is 27.5 and 26.7 years old for men and women, respectively (10).

- Elite male and female surfers tend to be shorter and lighter when compared to age-matched swimmers and water polo players. Shorter stature may be an advantage because a lower center of gravity allows for greater dynamic balance (10).

- Elite surfers have aerobic fitness, as measured by maximal oxygen consumption during arm exercise, that is significantly greater than untrained subjects and comparable to athletes in other aquatic endurance sports (6,9,11).

- Lactate threshold during arm exercise is significantly greater in elite versus nonelite surfers. Higher lactate threshold has a positive correlation with surfing performance (11).

EQUIPMENT

- Surfboards are categorized as shortboards or longboards based on length. Some overlap exists, but in general, shortboards are 6–7 feet long, and longboards are 9–10 feet long. Shortboards have a pointed nose, whereas longboards have a rounded nose. Longboards are more buoyant but less maneuverable. Most surfboards are affixed with fins on their underside that act as stabilizing struts.

- Modern surfboards are constructed with an inner core of polyurethane or polystyrene foam with a fiberglass shell. The naturally slippery surface is treated with surfwax for traction.

- Soft rubber tips that can be attached to the tip or tail and flexible fins made of urethane rubber can all help reduce the chance of board-induced injury (24).

707

- Ankle leashes are elastic ropes that tether the surfboard to the surfer via ankle strap. Shorter leashes increase the risk of board-induced self-injury via a recoil mechanism, whereas longer leashes increase the risk of the board injuring other surfers.

- Helmets consist of shatterproof plastic shells with a molded foam lining that is secured with a chin strap. Other protective amenities include shatterproof, ultraviolet protectant visors and ear cups to protect against tympanic membrane rupture.

- Surfers recognize the risk of head injury as high to moderate, but only 2% of surfers wear protective headgear. The most commonly cited reason for not wearing a helmet is "no need." Other reasons include discomfort, claustrophobia, and effects on balance (17).

INJURY EPIDEMIOLOGY

- Surfboard-related injuries are the most common cause of injury in recreational surfers, accounting for 67% of acute surfing injuries with 82% of these injuries occurring when the rider is struck by their own board (13).

- Acute injuries occur at a rate of 2.2–3.5 injuries per 1,000 surfing days (7,18).

- For recreational surfers, lacerations are the most common form of acute injury, accounting for 41%–46% of injuries (7,13,18). The most common locations are the face and lower extremity.

- In contrast, among competitive surfers, sprains and strains are the most common form of acute injury during competition, accounting for 39% of injuries, with the most commonly injured body part being the lower extremity (12). Knee strains account for a majority of these injuries and occur during aggressive turning and aerial maneuvering.

- Chronic musculoskeletal injuries account for 39% of all chronic surfing-related health problems. Neck and back injuries are the most common locations, followed by shoulder, knee, and elbow (18).

SPECIFIC INJURIES

Lacerations

- Common pathogens involved in marine soft tissue injuries include *Streptococcus* species, *Escherichia coli*, *Pseudomonas aeruginosa*, *Mycobacterium marinum*, *Staphylococcus aureus*, and *Vibrio* species (1).

- Wounds should be cultured for aerobic, anaerobic, and marine organisms.

- Outpatient oral antibiotic therapy directed at *Vibrio* species includes ciprofloxacin or trimethoprim–sulfamethoxazole. Parenteral choices include cefotaxime, ceftazidime, and tobramycin (1).

- When lacerations are secondary to envenomation, they should be allowed to heal by secondary intention or delayed primary closure (8).

Tympanic Membrane Rupture

- Tympanic membrane rupture occurs with head trauma from a strong wave or when the head contacts the water during a fall.

- Symptoms and signs include ear pain, conductive hearing loss, tinnitus, vertigo, and bloody otorrhea (15).

- Antibiotic therapy is only indicated with concomitant infection (3).

- Athletes should be advised not to return to play until the perforation is healed. If necessary, ear plugs can be placed to keep out water while the healing process continues (19).

Surfer's Myelopathy

- Surfer's myelopathy refers to spinal cord infarction that occurs exclusively in novice surfers. Overall prevalence is unknown, but 10 case reports exist in the literature.

- The mechanism of infarction is thought to be related to prolonged hyperextension during paddling in novice, unconditioned athletes that leads to either avulsion of the artery of Adamkiewicz, inferior vena cava obstruction, or fibrocartilaginous embolism (20).

- Surfers most commonly complain of low back pain, paresthesias, and urinary retention that progresses rapidly over several hours. Prior to discharge, 4 of 10 reported patients had completely recovered and 2 remained paraplegic (2,20).

- Magnetic resonance imaging (MRI), including T2 and diffusion-weighted imaging, is the most sensitive study for finding areas of spinal cord infarction. In published cases, ischemic MRI changes were localized to the distal thoracic watershed zone (20).

- Initial management entails rapid evaluation with MRI, empiric intravenous steroid administration, aggressive hydration, and allowable hypertension.

- Patients with incomplete resolution of symptoms will likely benefit from acute inpatient rehabilitation after medical stabilization. Long-term care may include intermittent catheterization and urodynamic studies, scheduled bowel regimens, pressure relief, deep vein thrombosis prophylaxis, and physical and occupational therapy.

MEDICAL ISSUES

Surfer's Ear (External Auditory Exostoses)

- External auditory exostoses (EAEs) typically present as multiple, bilateral broad-based growths of lamellar bone obstructing the external auditory canal leading to complications such as cerumen impaction, conductive hearing loss, and otitis externa.

- Overall, the prevalence of EAE among surfers is 38%–73% (4,22).
- A dose-dependent relationship between exposure to cold water and the prevalence of EAE has been identified. Cold water surfers are 2.6 times more likely to have EAE than warm water surfers (4).
- If medical management of EAE complications fails, surgical excision can be performed.
- Prevention of EAE entails decreasing exposure to cold water by means of ear plugs, ear molds, or hoods.

Otitis Externa

- EAE, trauma, and chronic moisture make surfers susceptible to recurrent otitis externa.
- Common organisms include *P. aeruginosa* and *S. aureus*, whereas fungal species such as *Candida* and *Aspergillus* may be found in diabetics (23).
- Treatment includes a 1-week course of topical antibacterial drops with systemic antibiotics indicated if a persistent case develops or if otitis media is suspected (16).
- Prevention includes application of acetic acid into the external canal after surfing and use of ear plugs (23).

Gastroesophageal Reflux Disease

- Gastroesophageal reflux disease (GERD) is significantly more prevalent in surfers (21%) than in nonsurfing athletes (7%). Higher surfing frequency is correlated with higher prevalence of GERD symptoms (14).
- Mechanisms that lead to a higher risk of GERD in the surfing population include increased intra-abdominal pressure secondary to lying prone on a hard surface during heavy exertion (14).
- Shortboard surfing has a higher prevalence of GERD than longboard surfing. Longboards have a greater surface area, allowing surfers to distribute their body mass over a greater area and thus allowing less pressure to be focused along the abdomen (14).
- A small meal of 400–500 kcal 2–4 hours prior to surfing that is free of fatty foods, peppermint, chocolate, alcohol, and acidic beverages will help maintain glycogen stores while decreasing the risk of GERD.
- If refractory to lifestyle modifications, a trial of a proton pump inhibitor or H_2 blocker should be initiated for acid suppression.

Envenomation

- Seabather's eruption
  - Seabather's eruption is a hypersensitivity reaction to larval toxins of certain coelenterates in Bermuda, the Caribbean region, and the East Coast of the United States.
  - Symptoms include a urticarial maculopapular rash in the area covered by a swimsuit that appears immediately or may be delayed by 1.5 days (23).
  - Treatment includes topical corticosteroids, oral antihistamines, and if necessary, oral steroids. Bathing suits should be thoroughly washed to avoid reenvenomation (23).
- Coelenterates
  - Coelenterates are marine invertebrates including jellyfish, Portuguese man-of-war, and box jellyfish that have tentacles filled with venomous cells called nematocysts that typically cause a local response but can rarely cause multiorgan damage (23).
  - Jellyfish stings present with burning pain, erythema, edema, urticaria, and bullae formation, which may progress to skin necrosis (23).
  - Tentacles and other retained animal parts should be removed. No consensus exists for appropriate jellyfish toxin treatment, but anecdotal evidence exists for application of hot or cold packs and irrigation with ethanol, vinegar, urine, baking soda, or methylated spirits (23).
  - An antivenom exists for the box jellyfish toxin.
- Stingrays
  - Stingrays are commonly encountered when entering or exiting the water. Their sting is caused by a sharp spine located on their tail that can penetrate wet suits and booties (19).
  - Patients present with pain out of proportion to wound appearance (19).
  - Treatment includes removing retained animal parts and hot water immersion to inactivate the heat-labile toxin (19).
  - Prevention involves shuffling through the sand to scare away stingrays and avoiding areas and times of day known to have high concentrations of stingray (19).
- Corals
  - Coral envenomation usually consists of toxins from multiple sources such as urchins and sea cucumbers (19).
  - Acetic acid can alleviate the pain associated with coral envenomation (1).

REFERENCES

1. Auerbach PS. Marine envenomations. *N Engl J Med.* 1991;325(7): 486–93.
2. Avilés-Hernández I, García-Zozaya I, DeVillasante JM. Nontraumatic myelopathy associated with surfing. *J Spinal Cord Med.* 2007;30(3): 288–93.
3. Kerr AG. Trauma and the temporal bone. The effects of blast on the ear. *J Laryngol Otol.* 1980;94(1):107–10.
4. Kroon DF, Lawson ML, Derkay CS, Hoffmann K, McCook J. Surfer's ear: external auditory exostoses are more prevalent in cold water surfers. *Otolaryngol Head Neck Surg.* 2002;126(5):499–504.
5. Lowden BJ. Fitness requirements for surfing. *Sports Coach.* 1983;6:35–8.

6. Lowdon BJ, Bedi JF, Horvath SM. Specificity of aerobic fitness testing of surfers. *Aust J Sci Med Sport.* 1989;21:7–10.

7. Lowdon BJ, Pateman NA, Pittman AJ. Surfboard-riding injuries. *Med J Aust.* 1983;2(12):613–6.

8. McGoldrick J, Marx JA. Marine envenomations; part 1: vertebrates. *J Emerg Med.* 1991;9(6):497–502.

9. Meir RA, Lowdon BJ, Davie AJ. Heart rates and estimated energy expenditure during recreational surfing. *Aust J Sci Med Sport.* 1991;23:70–4.

10. Mendez-Villanueva A, Bishop D. Physiological aspects of surfboard riding performance. *Sports Med.* 2005;35(1):55–70.

11. Mendez-Villanueva A, Bishop D, Hamer P. Activity profile of world-class professional surfers during competition: a case study. *J Strength Cond Res.* 2006;20(3):477–82.

12. Nathanson A, Bird S, Dao L, Tam-Sing K. Competitive surfing injuries: a prospective study of surfing-related injuries among contest surfers. *Am J Sports Med.* 2007;35(1):113–7.

13. Nathanson A, Haynes P, Galanis D. Surfing injuries. *Am J Emerg Med.* 2002;20(3):155–60.

14. Norisue Y, Onopa J, Kaneshiro M, Tokuda Y. Surfing as a risk factor gastroesophageal reflux disease. *Clin J Sport Med.* 2009;19(5):388–93.

15. Richmond DR, Yelverton JT, Fletcher ER, Phillips YY. Physical correlates of eardrum rupture. *Ann Otol Rhinol Laryngol Suppl.* 1989;(140):35–41.

16. Sander R. Otitis externa: a practical guide to treatment and prevention. *Am Fam Physician.* 2001;63(5):927–36, 941–2.

17. Taylor DM, Bennett D, Carter M, Garewal D, Finch C. Perceptions of surfboard riders regarding the need for protective headgear. *Wilderness Environ Med.* 2005;16(2):75–80.

18. Taylor DM, Bennett D, Carter M, Garewal D, Finch CF. Acute injury and chronic disability resulting from surfboard riding. *J Sci Med Sport.* 2004;7(4):429–37.

19. Taylor KS, Zoltan TB, Achar SA. Medical illnesses and injuries encountered during surfing. *Curr Sports Med Rep.* 2006;5(5):262–7.

20. Thompson TP, Pearce J, Chang G, Madamba J. Surfer's myelopathy. *Spine (Phila Pa 1976).* 2004;29(16):E353–6.

21. Warshaw M. *The Encyclopedia of Surfing.* Orlando (FL): Harcourt; 2005. 605 p.

22. Wong BJ, Cervantes W, Doyle KJ, et al. Prevalence of external auditory canal exostoses in surfers. *Arch Otolaryngol Head Neck Surg.* 1999;125(9):969–72.

23. Zoltan TB, Taylor KS, Achar SA. Health issues for surfers. *Am Fam Physician.* 2005;71(12):2313–7.

24. Zoumalan CI, Blumenkranz MS, McCulley TJ, Moshfeghi DM. Severe surfing-related ocular injuries: the Stanford Northern California experience. *Br J Sports Med.* 2008;42(10):855–7.

Swimming

Nancy E. Rolnik

105

EPIDEMIOLOGY/GENERAL

- Swimming is a popular activity, with participation from all ages. Young children start competitively swimming around 6 years of age.

- Competitive swimming includes four strokes: freestyle, backstroke, breaststroke, and butterfly.

- For competitive athletes, swimming is an all-year sport with little rest time. Many swimmers engage in two workouts a day, averaging between 8,000 and 20,000 yards per day. In addition, collegiate and elite training programs include cross-training and strength-training programs that can affect injury patterns.

- Swimming provides many health benefits without age limitations such as in other competitive sports. It is a great option for cardiovascular exercise for our aging population. There is evidence in masters swimmers showing that both men and women have a modest rate of performance decline until they reach the age of 70 (2,3). This indicates that physiologic changes attributed to aging alone may be more due to disuse than age.

- Masters swimmers age rules include athletes 25 years old and older (4). Individual events include athletes in 5–year age intervals (*e.g.*, 25–29, 30–34). Relay events are based on total age of team members in whole years (*e.g.*, 100–119, 120–159, 160–199) continued in 40-year increments as high as is necessary.

- The majority of injuries in swimming are due to overuse, with the most frequently injured body part being the shoulder. A study of competitive U.S. swimmers demonstrated that 47% of 13- and 14-year-old swimmers, 66% of 15- and 16-year-old swimmers, and 73% of elite swimmers had a history of interfering shoulder pain (8). A recent study of National Collegiate Athletic Association (NCAA) I-A swimmers showed that shoulder and upper arm injuries accounted for 31% of injuries in males and 36% in females. Back and neck injuries were the second most frequent areas injured (17).

STROKE MECHANICS

- Breakdown in stroke mechanics can predispose swimmers to injury, so it is important for the clinician and coach to focus attention on fundamental stoke mechanics. Some older masters swimmers were taught to swim "flat" and with one-sided breathing. By clarifying old-style stroke mechanics and adjusting mechanical stressors, athletes can limit repetitive injury.

- Regardless of the swimmer's chosen stroke event, most training is done in freestyle or drills alternating with freestyle such as freestyle/backstroke combos.

- Freestyle stroke phases include a catch, pull-through, and recovery period. During the out-of-water phase, the torso rotates on the body's longitudinal axis as the shoulder exits the water in an abducted and externally rotated position. The elbow should remain high above the hand until the hand enters the water fingers first in front and just outside the line of the shoulder. At the water entry point, the swimmer extends his or her arm to its maximum length. To keep the elbow high, the swimmer must roll the body approximately 45 degrees on the swimmer's long axis. In mechanical studies, the body roll angle can vary due to the athlete's fatigue or breathing side (11). It is not clear whether altering this angle could enhance performance or reduce injury. During the underwater phase, the shoulder internally rotates and adducts as the arm follows an S-shaped path to propel the body forward (9). The elbow should point toward the sidewall during this phase. The upper trapezius, rhomboids, supraspinatus, and deltoid all function in combination to position the scapula and humerus for hand entry and exit. It is important that the neck be extended around 30–45 degrees to decrease drag and reduce cervical strain. The athlete looks forward with the hairline just cresting the water surface. Some have advocated that the athlete look straight down without much cervical extension at all.

- The flutter kick helps stabilize the swimmer's trunk. This kick starts at the hip and simulates a motion similar to kicking off a loose shoe. The knees should flex only 30–40 degrees. Flexion at the hip is minimal.

- The swimmer must focus on the coordinated motion of both the upper and lower extremity. If the swimmer fails to kick throughout the stroke, the body will lose some of its buoyancy, and more drag is created. The upper extremity will then compensate, placing more stress at the shoulders.

- Bilateral breathing helps the swimmer develop equal pulling strength in both arms and helps ensure equal body roll on each side (6).

- When stroke mechanics need correction, the use of an underwater video can help clarify the errors. Working with a qualified coach is important.

UPPER EXTREMITY INJURIES

Swimmer's Shoulder

- Shoulder pain is the most common complaint in competitive swimmers. Nearly 50% of collegiate and masters swimmers report shoulder pain lasting at least 3 weeks (13).

- Swimmer's shoulder refers to shoulder tendinopathy or impingement. Typically, the swimmer feels maximum pain at the beginning of the pull-through phase. Often, the swimmer will swim through this pain for weeks until the pain is present throughout the entire freestyle stroke.

- Fatigue, muscle imbalance, and shoulder laxity contribute to the development of swimmer's shoulder. Land and in-water training can each play a factor in injury development.

- Typical treatment includes ice, training regimen modification, anti-inflammatory medication, and occasionally subacromial corticosteroid injection. Rarely is surgery necessary.

- The swimmer should limit the total weekly mileage and swim with various strokes.

- Kickboard workouts can allow the swimmer to maintain their fitness level while resting the shoulders. The elbow should be flexed to minimize irritation at the shoulder.

- The serratus anterior, a scapular stabilizer, is one of the most important muscles involved in the freestyle stroke, and therapy should be aimed to increase its strength (10).

- Swimmers have been shown to have greater shoulder adduction and internal rotation strength, which can lead to an imbalance in the shoulder. The swimmer should focus on creating a balance by strengthening the external rotators (16).

- Aggressive injury management and quick determination of early overuse injury decrease the swimmer's time out of the water. Coaches, parents, and trainers should encourage the athlete to notice the difference between pain and soreness and seek medical evaluation earlier to help make a more narrowed diagnosis and limit time out of the water.

- Freshman NCAA I-A swimmers have a higher rate of injury, so coaches and team physicians should observe these entering athletes for signs of overuse and fatigue. The level of training in duration and intensity is typically much greater than most of these athletes are used to at a club or high school level.

- Prevention of future injury includes correcting stroke mechanic problems by working with a swimming coach while strengthening the rotator cuff and scapular stabilizing muscles. The article "Shoulder Injury Prevention" reviews exercises for the uninjured athlete (14).

SHOULDER INSTABILITY

- In the swimmer, excessive shoulder mobility can functionally allow the athlete to have a more powerful stroke, but it is just this excessive motion that could also lead to overstretch of the supporting shoulder structures, ultimately resulting in pain and decreased performance. It is a fine balance. A stretched shoulder capsule can lead to subluxation and repeat injury, keeping the athlete poolside.

- Instability can be anterior, posterior, inferior, or a combination. The more unstable the glenohumeral joint, the greater is the risk of developing a labral tear, a Hill-Sachs lesion, or a Bankart lesion. Radiographs, including an axillary view, should be obtained. If a labral tear is suspected, a magnetic resonance imaging (MRI) arthrogram can be ordered, but some of the newer MRI machines can identify labral injury without an injection.

- The mainstay of treatment is rotator cuff muscle strengthening and scapular stabilization.

- If instability is persistent despite rehabilitation, surgery to tighten the capsule may be warranted. Warn the swimmer that a more stable shoulder may limit his or her performance, as the arm reach likely will be reduced.

- Indication for stretching is limited. If the shoulder capsule is overstretched, the risk for instability and injury is increased (10).

Elbow

- Triceps tendinitis can develop as a result of the full extension necessary in the backstroke.

- The ulnar collateral ligament may be stressed in the recovery phase of the freestyle leading to sprain.

- Treatment is with rest, nonsteroidal anti-inflammatory drugs (NSAIDs), and ice as appropriate.

LOWER EXTREMITY INJURIES

Breaststroker's Knee

- The unique whip kick done in the breaststroke places a valgus stress at the knee. Due to these mechanics, breaststrokers have more knee complaints than swimmers competing in the other strokes.

- The valgus force created at the knee may contribute to medial collateral ligament sprain (12). The swimmer needs instruction on proper technique for prevention.

- The mainstays of treatment include rest, ice, and anti-inflammatory medications.

Patellofemoral Pain

- The symptoms typical of patellofemoral syndrome also occur in swimmers usually due to the flutter kick, dolphin kick used in the butterfly stroke, and wall push off after flip turns.

- Treatment includes rest, ice, NSAIDs, and quadriceps strengthening. Swimmers should be encouraged to train using a foam buoy between the thighs in order to rest the knees.

- Some swimmers may benefit from a neoprene patella stabilizing brace, which would substitute for McConnell taping.

Foot/Ankle Problems

- Extensor tendinitis may occur from the flutter kick or dolphin kick. Treatment includes rest, ice, and NSAIDs. Rest from the flutter kick is best achieved using a foam buoy. A lower extremity stretching program focusing on improved range of motion at the ankle will help in the recovery and also in prevention.

- Local foot injury can occur if the swimmer kicks the side of the pool or gutter. This usually results in abrasions or contusions but occasionally may cause a fracture. Proper flip-turn technique will prevent foot injuries.

BACK INJURIES

Low Back Strain

- The butterfly and breaststroke require hyperextension of the lower back to maintain body position and complete the stroke. The body roll done by freestyle and backstroke swimmers can also cause strain, especially when the swimmer fatigues. The athlete will tend to roll less at the hip and more at the shoulder, increasing the strain at the lumbar spine. High-level swimmers or masters swimmers have shown to have an increased risk of developing degenerative disc disease (7). Treatment includes core strengthening and return to fundamental stroke techniques.

Cervical Strain

- Swimmers can develop strain at the neck if head rotation is exaggerated during the breathing cycle. Proper body roll reduces excess rotation at the neck during breathing cycles.

- The head rotation during the breathing cycle should only be enough to allow a breath, not bringing the face fully out of the water as some athletes do. As the swimmer moves forward, the water edge next to the mouth is cupped, allowing minimal rotation to achieve a sufficient breath.

- The athlete should maintain head position along the long axis without lifting the head or tucking the chin down when taking a breath.

- During the breaststroke, the head and neck should remain in the same position throughout the stroke. The cervical spine should be aligned with the back.

Spondylolysis/Spondylolisthesis

- The hyperextension of the back required specifically in the butterfly and breaststroke can predispose a swimmer to the development of a spondylolysis. The swimmer will often complain of pain during flip turns and starts. Spondylolysis rarely progresses to spondylolisthesis.

- Rest is the mainstay of treatment. Rarely will the athlete require bracing or surgery.

MEDICAL PROBLEMS COMMON IN SWIMMERS

Asthma

- In most of the world, swimmers train in enclosed pools that are both warm and humid.

- Asthma diagnosis is more likely to be found in elite swimmers than other competitive sports athletes. It appears that athletes with asthma may gravitate to this environment because it is less asthmagenic (5). However, there is some evidence that inhaling chlorine by-particles causes bronchospasm.

- A study involving the 1998 Winter Olympic Games swimmers revealed that 22.4% of swimmers reported either use of asthma medications or diagnosis of asthma or both (15).

- Coaches and trainers need to be aware of the asthmatic swimmer and have appropriate emergency treatment at the pool.

Otitis Externa

- Otitis externa, or "swimmer's ear," is one of the most common medical problems encountered by daily swimmers. The many hours swimmers spend submerging their ears in pool or open water may lead to ear canal maceration and infection.

- Topical treatment is effective. The swimmer should remain out of the pool for 2–3 days.

- Preventive measures include drying the ear with a drying agent such as Vosol otic drops or a homemade mixture of 50% vinegar and 50% alcohol. Using a hair dryer on cool setting is another option. Advise the swimmer to avoid traumatizing the ear canal with Q-tips.

Conjunctivitis

- Bacterial conjunctivitis and chemical conjunctivitis present similarly as a red eye. The pool chlorine kills most bacteria, so transmission via pool is rare. Goggle wear will help prevent chemical conjunctivitis, which is a self-limiting problem.

Sun Damage

- For swimmers training in open water, close attention to the skin is important to prevent sunburn.

- Twenty to 30 minutes prior to swimming, waterproof sunscreen should be liberally applied. There is no consensus on timing of reapplication of sunscreen.

Swimmer's Xerosis

- After hours submersed in the water, the skin becomes dehydrated and pruritic. Prevention is the key. Swimmers should apply lotion or body oil to their lightly patted skin after showering. The postswim shower should be short and with warm instead of hot water (1).

Green Hair

- Although not harmful, green hair can cause the swimmer undue anxiety. Application of 2% hydrogen peroxide to the hair and rinsing this out in 30 minutes will help remove the discoloration.

LIFE-THREATENING ISSUES

Drowning

- Drowning is a global problem, with more than 388,000 global drowning fatalities in the year 2004 as estimated by the World Health Organization (18).
- Prevention includes teaching people how to swim, encouraging swimming in lifeguarded areas, avoiding swimming in dangerous conditions such as where rip tides or a strong undertow are present, and limiting exposure to very cold water.
- Most resuscitations occur at the water side, so it is important that lifeguards are taught field resuscitative techniques. Ideally, skills such as the use of the bag-valve mask, oral and nasopharyngeal airways, and the laryngeal airway could be taught to further reduce deaths. Anesthesiologists have been involved in teaching advanced training to first responders with the results ultimately leading to saved lives.

REFERENCES

1. Basler RS, Basler GC, Palmer AH, Garcia MA. Special skin symptoms seen in swimmers. *J Am Acad Dermatol.* 2000;43(2 Pt 1):299–305.
2. Cooper LW, Powell AP, Rasch J. Master's swimming: an example of successful aging in competitive sport. *Curr Sports Med Rep.* 2007; 6(6):392–6.
3. Donato AJ, Tench K, Glueck DH, Seals DR, Eskurza I, Tanaka H. Declines in physiological functional capacity with age: a longitudinal study in peak swimming performance. *J Appl Physiol.* 2003;94(2): 764–9.
4. Federation Internationale de Natation Web site [Internet]. Available from: http://www.fina.org.
5. Goodman M, Hays S. Asthma and swimming: a meta-analysis. *J Asthma.* 2008;45(8):639–47.
6. Johnson JN, Gauvin J, Fredericson M. Swimming biomechanics and injury prevention: new stroke techniques and medical considerations. *Phys Sportsmed.* 2003;31(1):41–6.
7. Kaneoka K, Shimizu K, Hangai M, et al. Lumber intervertebral disk degeneration in elite competitive swimmers: a case control study. *Am J Sports Med.* 2007;35(8):1341–5.
8. McMaster WC, Troup J. A survey of interfering shoulder pain in United States competitive swimmers. *Am J Sports Med.* 1993;21(1):67–70.
9. Pink M, Perry J, Browne A, Scovazzo ML, Kerrigan J. The normal shoulder during freestyle swimming. An electromyographic and cinematographic analysis of twelve muscles. *Am J Sports Med.* 1991;19(6): 569–76.
10. Pink MM, Tibone JE. The painful shoulder in the swimming athlete. *Orthop Clin North Am.* 2000;31(2):247–61.
11. Psycharakis SG, Sanders RH. Body roll in swimming: a review. *J Sports Sci.* 2010;28(3):229–36.
12. Rodeo S. Knee pain in competitive swimming. *Clin Sports Med.* 1999;18(2):379–87, viii.
13. Stocker D, Pink M, Jobe FW. Comparison of shoulder injury in collegiate- and master's- level swimmers. *Clin J Sport Med.* 1995;5(1):4–8.
14. USA Swimming Web site [Internet]. Shoulder injury prevention. [cited 2002 Apr]. Available from: http://usaswimming.com.
15. Weiler JM, Ryan EJ 3rd. Asthma in United States Olympic athletes who participated in the 1998 Olympic Winter Games. *J Allergy Clin Immunol.* 2000;106(2):267–71.
16. Weldon EJ 3rd, Richardson AB. Upper extremity overuse injuries in swimming. A discussion of swimmer's shoulder. *Clin Sports Med.* 2001;20(3):423–38.
17. Wolf BR, Ebinger AE, Lawler MP, Britton CL. Injury patterns in Division I collegiate swimming. *Am J Sports Med.* 2009;37(10):2037–42.
18. World Health Organization Web site [Internet]. Drowning fact sheet. [cited 2010 Nov]. Available from: http://www.who.int.

Musculoskeletal Injuries in the Tennis Player

106

Marc R. Safran and Geoff Abrams

INTRODUCTION

- Tennis is a sport that is enjoyed by tens of millions of people worldwide, with total participation continuing to increase over the past 30 years. It is estimated that in the United States, total tennis participation exceeds 30 million people annually (51). Tennis is a sport for a lifetime, with competitive tournaments available for those as young as 8 years old and those older than 90 years old.

- The mechanics of tennis, a predominantly unilateral arm-dominant sport with repetitive motions, place the body at unique risk for injury.

INJURY INCIDENCE

- The exact incidence of injury in tennis has been elusive, because definitions, methodologies, and populations vary widely between individual studies. A number of investigations have reported tennis injury incidence to be anywhere from 2 to 20 injuries per 1,000 hours of tennis played (4,19,48).

- In a comprehensive review of 28 epidemiologic studies on tennis injury that have been published since 1966, Pluim et al. (42) reported the incidence as ranging from 0.04 to 21.5 injuries per 1,000 hours played (42).

- This same investigation found that most injuries occurred in the lower extremity (31%–67%), followed by the upper extremity (20%–49%), and lastly the trunk (3%–21%). The anatomic location of injuries was supported by a recent investigation of the injury profile of Swedish tennis players over a 2-year period (20). Other studies have confirmed that lower extremities predominate for the acute injuries, whereas chronic complaints are more common in the upper extremity.

- The senior author investigated elite junior tennis players (15–18 years of age) at the United States Tennis Association (USTA) National Junior Championships (23). Based on a questionnaire, only 23% of girls and 45% of boys reported no injury that kept them from playing for 1 week or more, whereas 53% of girls and 29% of boys noted more than one injury in the past.

- Low back pain was the most common ailment for both genders (47% of girls, 31% of boys) followed by shoulder pain. Thirty-five percent of junior tennis players complained of shoulder pain at some point in time, whereas more than 50% of older players and elite athletes note shoulder pain at some point in their career (23,24).

- Although there was no significant difference in the overall injury rate between boys and girls, there was a difference in the distribution of injuries. Girls sustained more injuries to the feet, leg, and wrist, whereas boys more commonly injured the ankle, groin, and hand (23).

BACK INJURIES

- Back pain is very common in tennis players and was identified as the most common injury in junior tennis players (20). Forty-seven percent of female and 31% of male tennis players reported low back pain (currently or in the past), and low back pain has been reported in up to half of all professional players (24).

- Many cases of low back pain in players are muscular in nature. These players often complain of a shorter duration of pain, with discomfort usually being located in the paraspinal musculature away from the midline.

- Rest, physical therapy, and anti-inflammatory medications are appropriate treatment options for muscular discomfort in the back.

- Neurologic complaints, such as numbness, tingling, or weakness of the legs, are not seen with muscular-type discomfort and should warrant further investigation if noted. Persistent back pain or back pain that is not responsive to conservative measures should also be investigated.

- In the younger player, spondylolysis or spondylolisthesis is more common, whereas in the older player, intervertebral disc degeneration, disc herniation, and facet arthrosis may occur.

- Overuse is the major contributor to back injury in tennis players. In particular, back extension, such as seen during the service motion, is thought to be a main contributor to the development of pars lesions. The reported incidence of symptomatic defects of the pars ranges from 15% to 47% in the younger athletic population (13).

Spondylolysis

- Players with spondylolysis will often complain of axial/midline low back pain, and some will report radiation to the gluteal area or proximal lower extremity. The onset of pain may begin after an acute injury; however, it is more often gradual, with mild symptoms being present for some time. Pain is often exacerbated by back extension during the service motion.

- Treatment of spondylolysis and low-grade spondylolisthesis in the tennis player is typically nonoperative and includes prolonged periods of rest in addition to physical therapy. Some clinicians prefer to place athletes with spondylolysis in a thoracolumbosacral orthosis or Boston brace to immobilize the low back to theoretically improve healing rates. This is controversial, however, because some evidence does support improved healing rates, whereas other studies do not, and compliance can be challenging in this group (see Chapter 45, Thoracic and Lumbar Spine). Players who do not respond to nonoperative treatment, as well as those with high-grade spondylolisthesis, may be surgical candidates.

ABDOMINAL MUSCLE STRAINS

- Abdominal muscle strains are one of the most tennis-specific injuries and occur at all levels of competition.

- Most injuries in tennis involve the rectus abdominis contralateral to the dominant arm (30), usually occurring during the tennis serve.

- With the open stance strokes now prevalent in tennis, there is an increased incidence of oblique muscle injuries reported as well (29).

- Trunk rotation and flexion and lumbar extension are critical components of the serve, placing large forces on the abdominal wall musculature. Consequently, the most common injury mechanism of the abdominal muscles in tennis players involves a forced concentric contraction of the abdominal musculature when the spine is completely hyperextended, as seen during the tennis serve (29).

- With current open stance mechanics, more abdominal muscle activity is used for racquet speed generation and force to hit the ball harder, placing great strain on the abdominal muscles, putting these muscles at risk of strain injury.

- The typical presentation for an abdominal wall muscle injury is a competitive player complaining of acute nondominant abdominal wall pain worsened by the service motion.

- Treatment of abdominal muscle injury in the tennis player includes rest with or without cryotherapy followed by rehabilitation exercises (30).

SHOULDER

- Of upper extremity injuries, the shoulder is the most commonly injured in tennis (10).

- The shoulder has the most motion of any major joint in the body, and this motion comes at the expense of stability. A careful balance between mobility and stability is necessary to maximize performance. Increased range of motion, particularly shoulder external rotation for serving, is beneficial for the tennis player who is trying to generate maximal velocity and spin with their strokes. Too much motion may result in increased reliance on soft tissues for stability, which may break down and result in shoulder instability. Many structures about the shoulder may be injured in tennis.

- Rotator cuff inflammation is common in tennis players of all levels (10). It usually occurs as a result of repetitive overhead serving motions.

- Symptoms include lateral shoulder pain with activity or at rest, pain with active arm abduction, or pain with internal/external rotation of the shoulder. Tennis players particularly complain of pain while serving and hitting overheads or high volleys.

- Although rotator cuff inflammation may be the result of overuse, or outlet impingement, it may also be seen in other situations, such as rotator cuff tears, instability or microinstability, superior labral anterior to posterior (SLAP) injuries, internal impingement, glenohumeral internal rotation deficit (GIRD), SICK scapula (see later section, "The Tennis Player's Shoulder"), shoulder stiffness, os acromiale, or scapular dyskinesis.

- It is incumbent upon the tennis physician to determine the cause of rotator cuff inflammation and correct the cause. As such, if the cause is treated, the symptoms of rotator cuff inflammation will go away.

- Initial treatment includes rest and rehabilitation, with specific emphasis not only shoulder motion (usually posterior capsular tightness), but also on rotator cuff strengthening and scapular stabilization muscle exercises (discussed later). Nonsteroidal anti-inflammatory medications may help with the pain to assist in rehabilitation, as can injectable corticosteroids.

- Aggressive treatment of rotator cuff tears is important in tennis players; Sonnery-Cottet et al. (49) have shown that repair of smaller rotator cuff tears results in a higher rate of return to tennis play as compared with players who have undergone repair of larger rotator cuff tears.

- Biceps tendonitis is another common complaint in tennis players and may be due not only to the overhead service motion but also the pronation/supination motions of the forearm required for forehands and backhands. The biceps may also become inflamed when the rotator cuff is inflamed and/or there is rotator cuff dysfunction as a result of strain, tendinopathy, or tearing. The biceps may become impinged by the humeral head and acromion or due to its proximity to the inflamed rotator cuff. The biceps may also become inflamed when there is a concomitant SLAP lesion and/or coracoid impingement.

- Players may complain of pain in the anterior aspect of the shoulder and be point tender in this area.

- Treatment again consists of rest and shoulder rehabilitation. Oral anti-inflammatory medications have a role in the treatment of biceps tendonitis, whereas the use of injectable corticosteroids remains controversial.

The Tennis Player's Shoulder

- Although scapular dyskinesis and capsulolabral changes within the overhead athlete's shoulder usually do not directly cause symptoms, they can combine in various ways to cause dysfunction and pathology in the shoulder.

- These changes take time to develop and are therefore usually seen in players who participate in tennis on a frequent basis and over a long period of time.

- Alterations in scapular motion or position can significantly affect overall glenohumeral biomechanics, as the scapula is critical in shoulder function.

- The term "SICK scapula" was introduced to describe a pathologic state of the scapula seen in overhead athletes that is characterized by (a) **s**capular malposition, (b) **i**nferior medial border prominence, (c) **c**oracoid pain and malposition, and (d) **k**inesis abnormalities of the scapula (9,22).

- Clinically, this syndrome can be recognized by a drooping shoulder on the player's dominant side, along with scapular asymmetry on inspection. The scapular asymmetry can be further elucidated by slowly adducting the abducted shoulder or with repeated slow forward elevation as the hands are brought from the side to eye level and back down again.

- Players may complain of anterior, posterior, or superolateral shoulder pain.

- A careful history and physical exam should be undertaken to recognize these constellation of findings instead of attributing the player's pain to other isolated lesions.

- It has been recognized that tennis players develop an increase in external rotation of the dominant shoulder at the expense of internal rotation, leaving the total arc of shoulder rotation unchanged (5).

- When there is a greater loss of internal rotation than gain in external rotation *and* the difference between the dominant and nondominant arm in internal rotation is greater than 25 degrees, then the potential for injury is considered greater and falls under the umbrella of GIRD (8,9).

- Kvitne and Jobe (25) initially proposed that repetitive loading in the 90/90 position (late cocking phase of the tennis serve) caused microtrauma to the anterior shoulder capsular structures and the anterior labrum, causing subtle anterior instability. This instability allows the humeral head to translate anteriorly, bringing the greater tuberosity of

the humerus and the rotator cuff in close proximity to the posterior glenoid.

- This was one theoretical etiology of internal impingement (56), where the undersurface of the posterosuperior rotator cuff (supraspinatus and infraspinatus) may impinge between the humeral head and the posterosuperior rim of the glenoid. This damages the rotator cuff tendons and may also lead to posterior superior labral pathology.

- Players usually complain of pain in the posterior shoulder with overhead activity.

- Alternatively, this anterior instability could also cause overuse of the rotator cuff by trying to maintain shoulder stability.

- More recently, basic science research has shown that posterior capsular contracture results in posterior shoulder tightness and internal rotation contracture and this contracture results in altered humeral head motion, resulting in internal impingement (7).

- Posterior capsular contracture as a result of posterior rotator cuff inflammation or hypertrophy of the posterior inferior glenohumeral ligament (IGHL) results in altered humeral head motion in the 90/90 position.

- The humeral head moves in a posterior and superior direction in the 90/90 position with posterior IGHL contracture, leading to increased posterior superior labral wear (including SLAP tears), internal impingement, and possibly SLAP tears through the "peel back" mechanism (7,8).

- The time of greatest risk for progression of pathology is when the player's GIRD exceeds the external rotation gain (8).

- Treatment of these shoulder pathologies is usually nonoperative initially.

- Rehabilitation exercises should focus on the inciting factors, such as the posterior capsular tightness and any scapular dyskinesis that may be present. Posterior capsular stretching exercises include the "sleeper stretch" and "cross-body stretch" (12), whereas scapular dyskinesis can be addressed by a number of exercises that specifically target the scapular stabilizers (9).

- Restoration of rotator cuff muscle balance and proprioceptive exercises are also important parts of the rehabilitation protocol (12).

- Should nonoperative management fail to improve symptoms, surgical management includes repairing the SLAP lesions, if present (8), and possibly cutting the posterior IGHL to gain internal rotation.

- One investigation reported good outcomes in patients undergoing combined SLAP and rotator cuff repair (55).

ELBOW

Lateral Epicondylitis

- The common term for lateral epicondylitis is "tennis elbow," although tennis is only involved in approximately 5%–10% of cases (17).

- The pathology is caused by degeneration of the deeper fibers of the extensor carpi radialis brevis (ECRB) and is attributable to overuse of wrist extension and excessive pronation/supination.

- There is no inflammation, and thus "epicondylitis" is a misnomer (57).

- Causes of lateral epicondylitis in tennis include overuse of wrist extensors, weak forearm and shoulder muscles, vibration resulting from string tension and racquet stiffness effects, undersized or oversized grips, and use of a one-handed backhand with poor form.

- Treatment of lateral epicondylitis is primarily nonoperative, with 90% of patients responding to conservative measures (34). These measures include rest, anti-inflammatory medications, cock-up wrist splints, physical therapy focusing on stretching and eccentric strengthening of the wrist extensor, and use of counterforce bracing when returning to activity.

- Injection of corticosteroids has been a mainstay of treatment for some time (26), but the senior author uses them as an adjunct to physical therapy — reducing the pain so the player can perform the rehabilitation exercises.

- Corticosteroid injections alone have not been shown to be efficacious in prospective randomized trials.

- Iontophoresis has been shown to have benefit in the management of the player with tennis elbow (36), and there has been some interest in topical nitric oxide as preliminary prospective randomized control trials have supported both these therapies (37).

- There is also some recent interest in platelet-rich plasma (PRP), although the evidence to support PRP use in lateral epicondylitis is lacking.

- Recalcitrant cases may be treated with debridement of the disease tissue either through an open technique (35) or arthroscopically (3,27).

Medial Epicondylitis

- Although tennis elbow is common in the recreational tennis player, medial epicondylitis is seen more often in the high-level player. This is likely the result of overuse of the wrist flexor/pronator muscles from hitting top spin and snapping the wrist into flexion during the service motion. Also, repeatedly hitting the ball late can result in increased stresses to the medial elbow.

- The flexor carpi radialis and pronator teres are most frequently affected, and the pathology looks the same as lateral epicondylitis.

- Treatment is similar to lateral epicondylitis, although caution should be taken with a counterforce brace, because that may compress the ulnar nerve.

Ulnar Collateral Ligament Injury

- Tennis players place tremendous tensile strain on the medial elbow, particularly the ulnar collateral ligament (UCL),

although injuries in these areas are uncommon in tennis. These forces are highest during the late cocking and early acceleration phases of the service motion and may also be notable during the forehand groundstroke, especially when hitting the ball late (15).

- The most common causes of UCL injury in the tennis player is chronic attenuation due to repetitive performance of the service motion.

- However, UCL injuries may occur as a result of altering kinematics due to pain or injury proximally in the kinetic chain, such as the shoulder, back, or hip.

- A detailed history and examination of the player with medial elbow pain is important because pain in this location may be due to a number of pathologies.

- Players with UCL injuries will typically complain of a loss of "pop" or "zip" on the serve (loss of power/velocity) and have pain during the late cocking or early acceleration phases.

- Most tears in adults are within the midsubstance of the ligament, whereas in adolescents, they often are avulsions from the humerus.

- Treatment of UCL injury may include both operative and nonoperative measures.

- Nonoperative measures include rest/cessation of overhead sport activities, anti-inflammatory medications, and physical therapy. Physical therapy includes an intensive elbow program that excludes exercises that place valgus stress on the elbow.

- Average rates of return to sport with nonoperative treatment range from 42% to 50% (44).

- Operative treatment consists of reconstruction of the torn ligament, usually using a free graft. There have been many modifications since the original technique described by Jobe et al. (21).

- Return to sport (including tennis) following operative intervention has been reported to be 80%–90% (14).

Valgus Extension Overload

- Valgus extension overload (VEO), an elbow condition that is almost exclusively seen in overhead athletes, involves the formation of posteromedial osteophytes, posteromedial chondromalacia, and risk of olecranon stress fractures.

- During the serving or overhead throwing motion, the medial aspect of the elbow (UCL) experiences tensile forces while compressive forces are seen in the lateral portion of the elbow (radiocapitellar joint), and posteriorly, the olecranon is compressed within the tight-fitting olecranon fossa.

- Repetitive and forceful shearing and abutting of the olecranon within its fossa leads to VEO and can be exacerbated by forceful elbow extension in follow-through and/or UCL insufficiency (2).

- Athletes commonly complain of posteromedial elbow pain during both the acceleration and follow-through phases of the overhead motion. Complaints of locking or catching and an inability to straighten the elbow fully may also be encountered due to loose bodies.

- Although VEO may occur as an isolated phenomenon, it more often occurs in the presence of laxity due to UCL attenuation; thus, the clinician should have a high index of suspicion for UCL injury.

- Initial treatment begins with rest and anti-inflammatory medications, followed by an evaluation of serving or throwing mechanics to identify areas for technique improvement (1).

- Failure of nonoperative management is an indication for surgery in those with VEO. Classically, an open procedure to remove olecranon osteophytes and loose bodies was performed; however, an increasing proportion of VEO is now being treated arthroscopically because this is less invasive and allows assessment of the anterior elbow as well (2).

- Assessment of the UCL is mandatory, and reconstruction (if needed) should be considered in the setting of a torn or severely attenuated ligament.

WRIST

Tendonitis

- Wrist complaints are common in tennis players (23). Nondominant wrist pain is particularly common in players using a two-handed backhand.

- One investigation of female junior tennis players found 29% and 25% prevalence rates of dominant and nondominant wrist pain, respectively (24).

- Tendonitis of the wrist may develop in tennis players who place large amounts of spin and/or velocity on the ball because this places extra demand on the muscles and tendons of the upper extremity.

- Improper technique in novice players may also be a contributing factor to the development of tendonitis.

- Wrist extensors are more commonly involved, but wrist flexor tendonitis may also be present.

- Of the wrist extensors, the extensor carpi ulnaris (ECU) is often involved. This presents as ulnar-sided wrist pain, and as with other forms of wrist tendonitis, overuse and/or improper technique is usually the cause.

- Subluxation or complete rupture of the ECU tendon can also be seen in the tennis player (32). As such, one should elicit a history of snapping about the wrist.

- ECU subluxation and/or ECU rupture usually requires surgical correction for return to play.

- ECU tendonitis is frequently associated with triangular fibrocartilage complex (TFCC) tears (the ECU subsheath is a part of the TFCC) or ulnocarpal abutment (24).

- Other tendons involved in the development of wrist tendonitis in the tennis player include extensor pollicis brevis (EPB)/ abductor pollicis longus (APL) (de Quervain tenosynovitis), extensor digitorum communis (EDC), and wrist flexors.

- de Quervain tenosynovitis likely develops from mechanical irritation of the EPB and APL tendon sheaths near the radial styloid of the radius.

- Treatment involves cessation of activity, anti-inflammatory medication, thumb spica immobilization, corticosteroid injection, and, in recalcitrant cases, surgical debridement with release of the sheath.

- Rest, anti-inflammatory medications, and immobilization are typically also successful in the treatment of EDC and wrist flexor tendonitis.

Triangular Fibrocartilage Complex Injury

- Triangular fibrocartilage complex injuries in tennis players remains a well-recognized cause of ulnar-sided wrist pain in racquet sport athletes (33).

- Players may report ulnar-sided wrist pain of a mechanical nature, swelling, weakness, or a sense of instability that is increased with the performance of forehands or backhands. The nondominant wrist may also be involved in players with two-handed backhands.

- Although somewhat controversial, most clinicians recommend a magnetic resonance imaging (MRI) arthrogram to confirm the diagnosis of a TFCC tear.

- Occasionally, TFCC tears are accompanied by instability of the distal radioulnar joint (DRUJ). Piano key assessment of the DRUJ for side-to-side instability can help confirm this diagnosis.

- When a TFCC tear is seen with a DRUJ instability, acute surgical treatment is needed.

- Without DRUJ instability, initial management of TFCC injury is nonsurgical, although high-level athletes may opt for initial surgical management in order to return to play more quickly.

- Standard nonsurgical treatments include temporary splint immobilization of the wrist and forearm, oral nonsteroidal anti-inflammatory medication, corticosteroid joint injection, and physical therapy (18).

- Surgical management includes arthroscopic techniques of repair or debridement, depending on the pathology present. Open techniques may be needed when ligament reconstruction is indicated in the setting of DRUJ instability.

- Prognosis for return to play is excellent following treatment of TFCC injuries (31).

Miscellaneous Causes of Wrist Pain

- Other causes of wrist pain may include fracture of the hook of the hamate (from impaction of the wrist against the bottom of the racquet handle), chondromalacia of the pisiform, radiocarpal arthritis, triquetrolunate ligament injury, ulnar nerve compression in Guyon canal, medial nerve entrapment at the wrist (carpal tunnel syndrome), and ulnar artery thrombosis.

- A recent report has also documented a group of tennis players with stress injury to the lunate (28).

- Lastly, stress fractures of the nondominant ulna (two-handed backhand players) and stress fractures of the distal radius and ulna of the dominant wrist may also present as wrist pain.

- Falling on an outstretched hand in tennis may result in any number of acute injuries to the hand and wrist.

HIP/THIGH

Muscle Strain

- Hip and thigh injuries account for anywhere between 6%–14% and 11%–29% of all tennis injures, respectively (24). Most of these injuries are muscle strains, with hip adductor muscles and hamstrings being the most commonly involved.

- Adductor muscle strains are usually caused by sudden lateral changes in direction or sliding on clay courts when players' legs may be at maximum abduction ("doing the splits"). These movements place the adductors on maximum stretch and thus predispose them to strains or tears.

- Those with decreased hip range of motion have been shown to be at increased risk for groin injury (53,54).

- Among the adductor group, the adductor longus is most commonly injured (52).

- Hamstring injuries may occur at either the proximal or distal end of the muscle and are usually associated with explosive accelerations.

- Although less common, hip flexor and quadriceps strains/tears may also occur. As with quadriceps, Achilles, and rotator cuff tears in the general population, older players are more susceptible to these tendon ruptures.

- Players may present with medial thigh or groin pain and may or may not recall a specific inciting event.

- In cases where the history and physical examination are equivocal, MRI may be helpful to confirm the diagnosis and differentiate between other causes of groin pain such as osteitis pubis and sports hernia (47).

- Management of adductor strains is almost always nonoperative, with rest, ice, and physical therapy when tolerated.

- There is controversy about the treatment of the acute rupture/avulsion, although currently, the pendulum favors nonoperative management.

Femoroacetabular Impingement

- Since the initial description in 1994, femoroacetabular impingement (FAI) has become an increasingly recognized cause of hip pain in athletes and tennis players in particular (39).

- The typical presentation is that of a tennis player reporting groin pain or anterolateral hip pain that is worsened during activity. Onset is usually insidious without a specific precipitating event.

- Players may complain of pain when putting on their socks/shoes, as well as lunging for a low ball. Eventually, the pain may affect the power of their serve, putting other structures in the kinetic chain at risk.

- Examination for FAI includes limited hip internal rotation (as measured in 90 degrees of flexion), as well as pain in flexion (to 90 degrees), adduction, and internal rotation. Labral stress or scour tests also may result in pain and/or clicking.

- Initial imaging should include plain radiographs, which may show the presence of the cam or pincer lesion. Further imaging should include a magnetic resonance arthrogram (MRA) of the involved hip to delineate intra-articular pathology, such as labral tears, that may be present. Many clinicians also inject anesthetic into the hip at the time of MRA.

- If patients have pain relief following injection, then intra-articular hip pathology can be confirmed as the source of pain. Intra-articular sources of pain in tennis players include labral tears, chondral injury, synovitis, and ligamentum teres tears, which may be the result of FAI, hip instability, or trauma. Rarely, do atraumatic labral tears occur without bony dysmorphology or instability.

- Treatment of confirmed FAI with intra-articular pathology is usually surgical. The key to surgical treatment is to address the cause of the pathology (either the cam and/or pincer lesions), as well as any damage to the cartilage or labrum that has resulted, which may be done through open surgical dislocation or arthroscopically (11,16).

- Return to sport for professional athletes, including tennis players, after FAI treatment has been documented (39).

KNEE

Knee Pain

- Knee pain in the tennis player is common. This stems from the fact that there is a lot of stopping and starting in tennis, with sudden changes in direction, lunging, straightening the bent knee when serving, and the ready position with the knee bent.

- Statistics from the USTA national teams show that 19% of all injuries are knee injuries, with 70% of the injuries being traumatic and 30% being overuse (24).

- In middle-aged and elderly players, the most common injuries are meniscus injuries and degenerative cartilage problems.

- In younger individuals, patellofemoral pain syndromes are the most frequent problems (43).

- Acute knee injuries, such as meniscus tears and ligament sprains, are less common in the tennis player but do occur due to the twisting demands of the knee during play (41).

- The patellofemoral joint in particular is susceptible to overuse injuries. These injuries include patellar tendonitis (jumper's knee), patellar instability, and patellofemoral syndrome or chondromalacia patellae.

- Players with patellar tendonitis typically relate a history of a recent period of increased playing time or intensity. Discomfort is usually during sports participation but may occur with activities of daily living as the disease progresses.

- Treatment for patellar tendonitis incorporates cessation or limitation of play, anti-inflammatory medication, and physical therapy for strengthening of the muscles about the knee (38).

- Although an acute patellar dislocation is typically dramatic, patellar instability is another subtle cause of anterior knee pain in the tennis player.

- Athletes may not be able to recall a discrete dislocation event but rather multiple individual episodes of anterior knee pain. Players may complain of pain near the medial facet of the patella or on the lateral aspect of the medial femoral condyle if the medial patellofemoral ligament (MPFL) has been compromised (50).

- Initial treatment of patellar instability and nonspecific patellofemoral pain in the tennis player is nonoperative and should focus on quadriceps (especially vastus medialis oblique) and hip external rotator strengthening.

- Patellar stabilization braces, particularly those with an active system to prevent lateral subluxation, and/or McConnell taping may be beneficial. For those with pes planus, orthotics (usually off-the-shelf) should also be considered to help dynamic, weight-bearing alignment.

- If physical therapy is not successful and chronic instability or dislocation occurs, a number of surgical options exist, including lateral release, MPFL repair/reconstruction, tibial tubercle osteotomy, and/or trochleoplasty, although these latter bony procedures may affect the ability to return to high-level play.

LEG/ANKLE/FOOT

Tennis Leg

- Tennis leg is described as a strain or partial tear of the medial head of the gastrocnemius muscle (6). The condition typically occurs when a player forcefully pushes off to begin a sprint to the ball.

- Players will report an acute episode of pain in the back of the lower leg at the calf muscle, and some have described it as though they were hit with a tennis ball on the back of the calf.

- Treatment involves rest, ice, elevation, and physical therapy. Specifically, stretching of the injured muscle is initiated, and as pain allows, strengthening of the gastrocnemius muscle is begun. Walking with a heel lift is used initially, and then the lift is worn when first returning to play. Return to play is guided by resolution of symptoms.

Ankle Sprains

- Ankle sprains are the most common macrotrauma injury occurring in tennis due to the frequent starting, stopping, and pivoting motions required (24).

- The term "ankle sprain" is a general term and may refer to injury to the lateral, medial, or syndesmotic ankle ligaments. Injuries to the syndesmotic ligaments are termed "high ankle sprains."

- Of these types, injuries to the lateral ankle ligaments are most common (45). The lateral ankle ligaments include the anterior talofibular ligament (ATFL), calcaneofibular ligament (CFL), and the posterior talofibular ligament (PTFL).

- Those with previous ankle sprains are at highest risk of sustaining another. In addition, those with incompletely rehabilitated ankle sprains are at higher risk of recurrent sprain than those who have undergone a complete rehabilitation program that includes strengthening and proprioception exercises.

- Players will note an acute event where the foot usually becomes plantarflexed and experiences a supination moment, therefore placing stretch on the lateral ankle ligaments and the ATFL in particular. They will often report immediate swelling and pain in the area depending on the severity of the injury.

- Initial treatment of ankle sprains includes a combination of rest, ice, elevation, compression, immobilization, and initiation of physical therapy to restore ankle strength, flexibility, and proprioception (46).

- Although this is the general treatment for all grades of ankle sprains in the United States, there is a trend in some European countries to treat acute grade III sprains operatively with ligament repair (40).

- Taping or bracing of players who sustained a previous ankle sprain may help reduce a recurrence of ankle sprain.

- High ankle sprains take longer to heal, and those with instability of the distal tibiofibular joint may require surgery to stabilize this joint.

Tennis Toe

- The feet are subject to many maladies in tennis, including plantar fasciitis, metatarsalgia, metatarsal stress fractures, blisters, and corns. Another foot injury in tennis is the tennis toe. Although it is not seen only in tennis, we will discuss it here, especially because it is named after the sport.

- Tennis toe is an injury to the great toe or second toe from forceful and repetitive abutment of these toes against the toe box of the shoe.

- This can lead to subungual hematomas, nail bed injuries, or injury to the interphalangeal or metatarsophalangeal (MTP) joints.

- This injury is more common when the shoe is too big or too small for the player's foot. Severe hematoma may result in the nail falling off the toe.

- In some cases, decompression of the hematoma, usually by drilling (or burning) a hole in the toenail, is beneficial when there is significant pain.

- Adequate padding of the toe box and well-fitting shoes are important in prevention of this problem.

ADOLESCENT TENNIS INJURIES

- Muscle and ligament strains and sprains from overuse are the predominate injuries in the young player.
- Injuries to the lower extremity are twice as common as injuries to the spine and upper extremity.
- Injuries to the foot, leg, and wrist prevail in the female adolescent player, whereas injuries to the ankle, groin, hand, abdomen, and back prevail in the male adolescent player.
- Overall predominance of injury pattern: strains > inflammation > sprain.

Physeal Injuries

- Wrist epiphysitis:
  - Repeated hyperextension and rotation of the wrist causing inflammation of the distal radius epiphysis.
  - This is commonly seen in adolescent players who attempt to put top spin on the ball.
  - Premature closure of the growth plate is a potential complication of this process.
  - Players note a warm, swollen bump on distal radius that is tender to palpation.
  - Radiographs of the distal radius may assist in making the diagnosis.
  - Treatment strategies range from activity modification and wrist immobilization to surgery for treatment of an associated fracture or for premature physeal closure.
  - Players with wrist epiphysitis should avoid push-ups and flatten strokes, avoiding top spin.
- Traction to the apophysis at the greater/lesser tuberosity of the humerus:
  - Rest and activity modification are the mainstays of treatment.
  - Upon return to play, the player should start with ground strokes only. High volleys and serves should be gradually incorporated.
- Humeral medial epicondyle apophysitis (adolescent medial tennis elbow):
  - Overuse injury resulting from the repetitive muscular contractions of the forearm and wrist flexors during forehands and serves.
  - Players note a mildly swollen, tender prominence of the medial elbow.
  - Players may sense a decrease in their ability to serve at full speed and to fully straighten the elbow.
  - Use of a racquet with vibratory dampening characteristics, an oversized/light/stiff head, flexible shaft, a large cushioned grip (that is comfortable to the player), and low-tensioned strings of gut or high-quality synthetic strings is recommended.
  - Activity modification with limitations on the intensity of conditioning/play and amount of serving, overhead play, throwing, and heavy lifting is encouraged.
- Osgood-Schlatter disease:
  - Shoe wear modification for increased shock absorption and stability, stretching of the quadriceps and hamstring musculature to decrease the tension of the muscles pulling on the patellar tendon, training on soft surfaces (clay or sandy surfaces), and use of a patellar tendon strap are recommended.
- Sever disease:
  - Most common cause of heel pain in the adolescent player.
  - Prevention and treatment entail proper stretching and use of a heel support that provides cushioning, shock absorption, and decreased tension on the Achilles tendon.

CONCLUSION

- Tennis is a sport enjoyed by millions of people around the world. There are a multitude of injuries that are particular to tennis and overhead sports athletes. Back injuries are quite prevalent in tennis players.
- Although lower extremity injuries, such as ankle sprains, are the most common acute injuries, upper extremity injuries are the more frequent chronic injuries, with GIRD being a major cause of shoulder problems.
- Tennis elbow is more common in recreational players, whereas medial epicondylitis is more common in high-level tennis players.

REFERENCES

1. Aguinaldo AL, Chambers H. Correlation of throwing mechanics with elbow valgus load in adult baseball pitchers. *Am J Sports Med.* 2009;37(10):2043–8.
2. Ahmad CS, Park MC, Elattrache NS. Elbow medial ulnar collateral ligament insufficiency alters posteromedial olecranon contact. *Am J Sports Med.* 2004;32(7):1607–12.
3. Baker CL Jr, Murphy KP, Gottlob CA, Curd DT. Arthroscopic classification and treatment of lateral epicondylitis: two-year clinical results. *J Shoulder Elbow Surg.* 2000;9(6):475–82.
4. Beachy G, Akau CK, Martinson M, Olderr TF. High school sports injuries. A longitudinal study at Punahou School: 1988 to 1996. *Am J Sports Med.* 1997;25(5):675–81.
5. Bigliani LU, Codd TP, Connor PM, Levine WN, Littlefield MA, Hershon SJ. Shoulder motion and laxity in the professional baseball player. *Am J Sports Med.* 1997;25(5):609–13.
6. Blue JM, Matthews LS. Leg injuries. *Clin Sports Med.* 1997;16(3):467–78.
7. Burkhart SS, Morgan CD, Kibler WB. The disabled throwing shoulder: spectrum of pathology. Part I: pathoanatomy and biomechanics. *Arthroscopy.* 2003;19(4):404–20.

8. Burkhart SS, Morgan CD, Kibler WB. The disabled throwing shoulder: spectrum of pathology. Part II: evaluation and treatment of SLAP lesions in throwers. *Arthroscopy.* 2003;19(5):531–9.

9. Burkhart SS, Morgan CD, Kibler WB. The disabled throwing shoulder: spectrum of pathology. Part III: the SICK scapula, scapular dyskinesis, the kinetic chain, and rehabilitation. *Arthroscopy.* 2003;19(6):641–61.

10. Bylak J, Hutchinson MR. Common sports injuries in young tennis players. *Sports Med.* 1998;26(2):119–32.

11. Byrd TW, Jones KS. Prospective analysis of hip arthroscopy with 10-year followup. *Clin Orthop Relat Res.* 2010;468(3):741–6.

12. Cools AM, Declercq G, Cagnie B, Cambier D, Witvrouw E. Internal impingement in the tennis player: rehabilitation guidelines. *Br J Sports Med.* 2008;42(3):165–71.

13. Debnath UK, Freeman BJ, Gregory P, de la Harpe D, Kerslake RW, Webb JK. Clinical outcome and return to sport after the surgical treatment of spondylolysis in the young athletes. *J Bone Joint Surg Br.* 2003;85(2):244–9.

14. Dines JS, ElAttrache NS, Conway JE, Smith W, Ahmad CS. Clinical outcomes of the DANE TJ technique to treat ulnar collateral ligament insufficiency of the elbow. *Am J Sports Med.* 2007;35(12):2039–44.

15. Elliott B, Fleisig G, Nicholls R, Escamilia R. Technique effects on upper limb loading in the tennis serve. *J Sci Med Sport.* 2003;6(1):76–87.

16. Ganz R, Parvizi J, Beck M, Leunig M, Nötzli H, Siebenrock KA. Femoroacetabular impingement: a cause for osteoarthritis of the hip. *Clin Orthop Relat Res.* 2003;417:112–20.

17. Gruchow HW, Pelletier D. An epidemiologic study of tennis elbow. Incidence, recurrence, and effectiveness of prevention strategies. *Am J Sports Med.* 1979;7(4):234–8.

18. Henry MH. Management of acute triangular fibrocartilage complex injury of the wrist. *J Am Acad Orthop Surg.* 2008;16(6):320–9.

19. Hjelm N, Werner S, Renstrom P. Injury profile in junior tennis players: a prospective two year study. *Knee Surg Sports Traumatol Arthrosc.* 2010;18(6):845–50.

20. Hutchinson MR, Laprade RF, Burnett QM 2nd, Moss R, Terpstra J. Injury surveillance at the USTA Boys' Tennis Championship: a 6-yr study. *Med Sci Sports Exerc.* 1995;27(6):826–30.

21. Jobe FW, Stark H, Lombardo SJ. Reconstruction of the ulnar collateral ligament in athletes. *J Bone Joint Surg Am.* 1986;68(8):1158–63.

22. Kibler WB. The role of the scapula in athletic shoulder function. *Am J Sports Med.* 1998;26(2):325–37.

23. Kibler WB, Safran MR. Musculoskeletal injuries in the young tennis player. *Clin Sports Med.* 2000;19(4):781–92.

24. Kibler WB, Safran MR. Tennis injuries. *Med Sport Sci.* 2005;48:120–37.

25. Kvitne RS, Jobe FW. The diagnosis and treatment of anterior instability in the throwing athlete. *Clin Orthop Relat Res.* 1993;291:107–23.

26. Lewis M, Hay EM, Paterson SM, Croft P. Local steroid injections for tennis elbow: does the pain get worse before it gets better? Results from a randomized controlled trial. *Clin J Pain.* 2005;21(4):330–4.

27. Lo MY, Safran MR. Surgical treatment lateral epicondylitis: a systematic review. *Clin Orthop Relat Res.* 2007;463:98–106.

28. Maquirriain J, Ghisi JP. Stress injury of the lunate in tennis players: a case series and related biomechanical considerations. *Br J Sports Med.* 2007;41(11):812–5.

29. Maquirriain J, Ghisi JP. Uncommon abdominal muscle injury in a tennis player: internal oblique strain. *Br J Sports Med.* 2006;40(6):462–3.

30. Maquirriain J, Ghisi JP, Kokalj AM. Rectus abdominus muscle strains in tennis players. *Br J Sports Med.* 2007;41(11):842–8.

31. McAdams TR, Swan J, Yao J. Arthroscopic treatment of triangular fibrocartilage wrist injuries in the athlete. *Am J Sports Med.* 2009;37(2):291–7.

32. Montalvan B, Parier J, Brasseur JL, Le Viet D, Drape JL. Extensor carpi ulnaris injuries in tennis players: a study of 28 cases. *Br J Sports Med.* 2006;40(5):424–9.

33. Nagle DJ. Triangular fibrocartilage complex tears in the athlete. *Clin Sports Med.* 2001;20(1):155–66.

34. Nirschl RP, Ashman ES. Elbow tendinopathy: tennis elbow. *Clin Sports Med.* 2003;22(4):813–36.

35. Nirschl RP, Pettrone FA. Tennis elbow. The surgical treatment of lateral epicondylitis. *J Bone Joint Surg Am.* 1979;61(6A):832–9.

36. Nirschl RP, Rodin DM, Ochiai DH, Maartmann-Moe C; DEX-AHE-01-99 Study Group. Iontophoretic administration of dexamethasone sodium phosphate for acute epicondylitis. A randomized, double-blinded, placebo-controlled study. *Am J Sports Med.* 2003;31(2):189–95.

37. Paoloni JA, Appleyard RC, Nelson J, Murrell GA. Topical nitric oxide application in the treatment of chronic extensor tendinosis at the elbow: a randomized, double-blinded, placebo-controlled clinical trial. *Am J Sports Med.* 2003;31(6):915–20.

38. Peers KH, Lysens RJ. Patellar tendinopathy in athletes: current diagnostic and therapeutic recommendations. *Sports Med.* 2005;35(1):71–87.

39. Philippon M, Schenker M, Briggs K, Kuppersmith D. Femoroacetabular impingement in 45 professional athletes: associated pathologies and return to sport following arthroscopic decompression. *Knee Surg Sports Traumatol Arthrosc.* 2007;15(7):908–14.

40. Pijnenburg AC, Bogaard K, Krips R, Marti RK, Bossuyt PM, van Dijk CN. Operative and functional treatment of rupture of the lateral ligament of the ankle. A randomised, prospective trial. *J Bone Joint Surg Br.* 2003;85(4):525–30.

41. Plancher KD, Steadman JR, Briggs KK, Hutton KS. Reconstruction of the anterior cruciate ligament in patients who are at least forty years old. A long-term follow-up and outcome study. *J Bone Joint Surg Am.* 1998;80(2):184–97.

42. Pluim BM, Staal JB, Windler GE, Jayanthi N. Tennis injuries: occurrence, aetiology, and prevention. *Br J Sports Med.* 2006;40(5):415–23.

43. Renström AF. Knee pain in tennis players. *Clin Sports Med.* 1995;14(1):163–75.

44. Rettig AC, Sherrill C, Snead DS, Mendler JC, Mieling P. Nonoperative treatment of ulnar collateral ligament injuries in throwing athletes. *Am J Sports Med.* 2001;29(1):15–7.

45. Safran MR, Benedetti RS, Bartolozzi AR 3rd, Mandelbaum BR. Lateral ankle sprains: a comprehensive review: part 1: etiology, pathoanatomy, histopathogenesis, and diagnosis. *Med Sci Sports Exerc.* 1999;31(7 Suppl):S429–37.

46. Safran MR, Zachazewski JE, Benedetti RS, Bartolozzi AR 3rd, Mandelbaum BR. Lateral ankle sprains: a comprehensive review: part 2: treatment and rehabilitation with an emphasis on the athlete. *Med Sci Sports Exerc.* 1999;31(7 Suppl):S438–47.

47. Schilders E, Bismil Q, Robinson P, O'Connor PJ, Gibbon WW, Talbot JC. Adductor-related groin pain in competitive athletes. Role of adductor enthesis, magnetic resonance imaging, and etheseal pubic cleft injections. *J Bone Joint Surg Am.* 2007;89(10):2173–8.

48. Silva RT, Takahashi R, Berry B, Cohen M, Matsumoto MH. Medical assistance at the Brazilian juniors tennis circuit — a one-year prospective study. *J Sci Med Sport.* 2003;6(1):14–8.

49. Sonnery-Cottet B, Edwards TB, Noel E, Walch G. Rotator cuff tears in middle-aged tennis players: results of surgical treatment. *Am J Sports Med.* 2002;30(4):558–64.

50. Steensen RN, Dopirak RM, McDonald WG 3rd. The anatomy and isometry of the medial patellofemoral ligament: implications for reconstruction. *Am J Sports Med.* 2004;32(6):1509–13.

51. Tennis Industry Association. Executive summary 2008. *The Tennis Marketplace.* 2008;9:1–16.

52. Tibor LM, Sekiya JK. Differential diagnosis of pain around the hip joint. *Arthroscopy.* 2008;24(12):1407–21.

53. Vad VB, Gebeh A, Dines D, Altchek D, Norris B. Hip and shoulder internal rotation range of motion deficits in professional tennis players. *J Sci Med Sport.* 2003;6(1):71–5.

54. Verrall GM, Slavotinek JP, Barnes PG, Esterman A, Oakeshott RD, Spriggins AJ. Hip joint range of motion restriction precedes athletic chronic groin injury. *J Sci Med Sport.* 2007;10(6):463–6.

55. Voos JE, Pearle AD, Mattern CJ, Cordasco FA, Allen AA, Warren RF. Outcomes of combined arthroscopic rotator cuff and labral repair. *Am J Sports Med.* 2007;35(7):1174–9.

56. Walch G, Boileau P, Noel E, Donnel ST. Impingement of the deep surface of the supraspinatus tendon on the posterosuperior glenoid rim: an arthroscopic study. *J Shoulder Elbow Surg.* 1992;1:238–45.

57. Wittenberg RH, Schaal S, Muhr G. Surgical treatment of persistent elbow epicondylitis. *Clin Orthop Relat Res.* 1992;278:73–80.

Triathlon

Shawn F. Kane and Fred H. Brennan, Jr

107

TRIATHLONS

- A triathlon is a unique multidisciplinary event, consisting of sequential swim, bike, and run legs. The concept was initially developed as an alternative to standard marathon or 10-km training programs. In 1974, members of the San Diego Track Club hosted a first of its kind swim-bike-run event in and around the waters of California's Mission Bay. That three-event race was called a triathlon, and to this day, the triathlon remains one of the most popular participation and spectator endurance events worldwide.

  - John Collins, a veteran of the first Mission Bay Triathlon, was influential in the further development of the sport. He is responsible for combining three endurance events — the Waikiki Rough Water Swim, the Around-Oahu Bike Ride, and the Honolulu Marathon — into one of the world's most recognized and demanding competitions, The Ironman.

  - Popularity and growth led to the establishment of the International Triathlon Union and the inaugural World Triathlon Championship competition in 1980. International recognition resulted in the continued growth of the sport through the 1990s into the new century, with inaugural triathlon competitions in the 1994 Goodwill Games in Leningrad, 1995 Pan Am Games in Argentina, and the 2000 summer Olympic Games in Sydney.

    - ❏ The popularity and growth of triathlons continue. USA Triathlon (USAT) recorded a sixfold rise in membership from 1999 to 2009 and now reports 115,000 members. The International Triathlon Union has 122 member nations, and Australia alone has over 160,000 Australians participating annually in the sport (12).

- Triathlons are a unique sport that encompass all fitness-related variables: cardiorespiratory endurance, body composition, muscular strength, endurance, and flexibility.

- Triathlon governing bodies recognize four standard race types based on distance (17). The races are sometimes listed by the total number of kilometers (*e.g.*, Ironman is a 225.8).

  - Sprint (0.75-km swim, 22-km bike, 5-km run)
  - Olympic (1.5-km swim, 40-km bike, 10-km run)
  - Half-Ironman (1.9-km swim, 90-km bike, 21-km run)
  - Ironman (3.8-km swim, 180-km bike, 42-km run)

- The popularity of the sport has led to the introduction of short- or fun-distance triathlons, usually about half the distance of a sprint triathlon (12).

VOCABULARY

- Like all sports, triathlons and triathletes have a unique vocabulary. A few of the more common terms are included here to aid in the understanding of these athletes.

  - Bonking — a reference to when a competitor begins to lose the ability to concentrate, feels disoriented and overly fatigued, and at times, is unable to continue on in a race. Bonking occurs when energy intake does not meet energy expenditure and glycogen stores are depleted. The regular intake of carbohydrates during prolonged competitions can prevent this condition from occurring.

  - Transition zone — an area of controlled chaos where athletes change from swimmer to cyclist and from cyclist to runner (T1 and T2, respectively).

  - Traumatic tattooing — skin discoloration resulting from debris that was deeply embedded in the skin following an abrasion from skidding on pavement.

  - Brick (Bike-Run-Ick) — a training method or workout used to simulate race conditions. It involves training on the bike and running in the same day and is used to simulate the bike–run transition, which many feel is the toughest part of the race.

INJURY EPIDEMIOLOGY

- Triathletes compete and train in three distinct events, each of which predisposes the athlete to its own set of injuries. Injuries specific to an individual component event of the triathlon will be covered in that specific chapter.

- Theoretically, it is possible that triathletes would have fewer overuse injuries compared to other one-sport endurance athletes because triathletes spend much of their time cross-training. The contrary may also be true; triathletes suffer from the cumulative effect of three distinct injury-producing events and are susceptible to more injuries (7).

- Injuries are defined as any musculoskeletal problem that causes a cessation of training for at least 1 day, a reduction in training mileage, the taking of pain medication, or the seeking of medical aid.
- Cycle and run training may have a cumulative stress influence on injury risk. The tendency of triathletes to modify the training regimen by increasing the load in another discipline from that which the injury occurred rather than stop training when injured increases the risk of injury recurrence and the time until full rehabilitation (27).

- Research has demonstrated injury rates among triathletes to be anywhere from 37% to 90% annually, with roughly 50% of injuries occurring solely during the preseason, 37% occurring in-season, and the remainder overlapped between seasons.

  - Overuse injuries are the primary reason for triathlete injury and comprise 68% and 78% of the injuries sustained during preseason and in-season, respectively. Acute injuries due to trauma make up the difference.

- Injury incidence: 2.5–5.4 injuries per 1,000 hours of triathlon training and 4.6–20.1 injuries per 1,000 hours of triathlon competition have been reported. These rates are higher than the reported incidences of 3.9 and 2.5 injuries per 1,000 hours of training for track and field and marathon running, respectively (5,6,7,12).

  - Running injuries account for 65%–78% of the total injuries, cycling injuries account for 16%–37% of the total injuries, and swimming accounts for 11%–21% of the injuries experienced by triathletes (17).

    - Iliotibial band syndrome, patellofemoral pain syndrome, and patellar and Achilles tendinosis are common injuries from running.

    - Aeroneck — neck pain and stiffness caused by prolonged sitting with the shoulders hunched, the neck hyperextended, and the arms tucked tightly in underneath the chest. This is a complaint that many triathletes have after or during the cycling portion of the race.

    - Patellofemoral pain, quadricep strains, and calf strains are common cycling injuries (2).

    - Corneal abrasions frequently result from having the goggles kicked off the face at the congested start of the swim phase (15).

  - Despite differences in the number of training sessions, weekly total mileage, and workout duration, there has been no reported difference in the injury prevalence, distribution, or severity among triathletes who vary in skill from elite to recreational (27).

  - Predictors of injury:

    - Total weekly training distance, weekly cycling distance, swimming distance, and total number of workouts (swimming, cycling, and running) per week, but surprisingly not running distance per week, are all associated with an increased incidence of running injuries (15,28).

    - The total amount of time spent running and cycling, but not total distance, negatively influences the incidence of cycling injuries (29).

    - The most significant predictor of injury in the preseason is number of years of experience in triathlons. More experienced triathletes have a higher injury rate (17).

    - The most significant predictor of injury during the season was a history of previous injury and high preseason running mileage (> 20 miles per week) (9,30).

    - Training errors, most specifically improper technique, have been frequently associated with injuries related to cycling and swimming.

  - Running-related injuries are the most prevalent injuries seen in triathletes. Athletes who spend greater amounts of time training in cycling and swimming are at higher risk for running-related injuries. This may be because there is less time for overall muscle recovery (30).

- Specific injury rates

  - Cardiovascular — Cardiac muscle fatigues and is stressed while performing endurance events, similarly to skeletal muscle. Troponin T levels are elevated in 27% of Ironman Triathlon finishers, and echocardiograms have demonstrated a 24% reduction in postrace ejection fractions compared to prerace values. There are no published data concerning the rate of fatal cardiac complications in triathletes. We do know from the marathon literature that fatal cardiac complications are uncommon (1 in 50,000 competitors) (14,19). The published fatality rate in triathlons is 1.5 in 100,000, with 13 of 14 deaths occurring during the swim. Drowning was the declared cause of death in all swimming deaths, but autopsies revealed a high prevalence of cardiovascular abnormalities (15).

  - Gastrointestinal bleeding — 8%–30% of marathoners have evidence of intrarace or postrace gastrointestinal bleeding. Blood shunting to exercising muscles causes relative intestinal ischemia and, combined with elevated core body temperatures, leads to cellular death and gastrointestinal bleeding.

  - Abdominal cramping — May be associated with competitors who consume a diet high in fiber before the race. Also seen with the excess consumption of carbohydrates before or during the race.

  - Diarrhea (runner's trots) — Abdominal pain and diarrhea associated with prolonged running or biking. This condition is caused by ischemic changes in the bowel due to the shunting of blood to exercising muscles. This may occur during or shortly after the completion of the race.

- Nausea and vomiting — Eating 30 minutes before a triathlon is highly associated with vomiting during the swim. A diet high in fat or protein and the consumption of hypertonic beverages result in a higher rate of nausea and vomiting among competitors.

- Hematology — 30% of triathletes demonstrate microscopic hematuria and 95% have a decrease in haptoglobin after an event. These numbers demonstrate that foot-strike hemolysis, renal ischemia, and bladder contusions are frequent occurrences.

- Infectious diseases — Fresh water swimming in high-risk areas has resulted in triathletes developing leptospirosis. Lyme disease in endemic areas may also raise the potential risk to triathletes competing in extreme-course triathlons.

- Sunburn — Sun protection factor (SPF) sunscreen of at least 15, a hat or visor, SPF-rated clothing, and ultraviolet protective sunglasses are recommended to prevent the burning effects of the sun during training and competition.

TRAINING CONSIDERATIONS

- Triathlons are unique and demanding events that require a dedicated, well-organized training program. Proper training will prepare a competitor for successful completion of the race and minimize the risk of injury while training and competing.

  - Training programs need to be customized to meet the competitors' needs; what works for one athlete may not work for another. We recommend that novice competitors consider hiring a USAT-certified coach to learn the sport and maximize available training time. There are also training-related resources on the Web and in triathlon magazines to help develop a suitable and safe program. Advice from more experienced athletes can be helpful.

  - Manipulation of the swim discipline (specifically the swimming velocity) provides a metabolic reserve and has been shown to significantly impact performance in the subsequent disciplines. The overall triathlon time is statistically significantly faster when the swim is completed at 80%–90% of maximum velocity (25).

- General triathlon training recommendations

  - Increase training distance and time by no more than 10% per week.

  - Although there is no evidence to demonstrate improved performance or decreased injury rates, consider incorporating a regular stretching program as part of training.

  - Ensure proper amounts of sleep and appropriate nutrition.

  - Listen to your body; if you start a workout and feel tired or run down, change it to a shorter distance. Pushing yourself through fatigue (a sign of overtraining) and completing the longer workout may do you more harm in the long run.

  - Swim, bike, and run distances a little further than the race distance; this builds confidence that you will be able to complete the race.

  - Open-water swimming is much different than lap swimming in a pool, and race day is not the best time to try it for the first time. Training will require some extra personnel because solo open-water swimming is not recommended.

  - Train on the actual race course if possible.

  - Do not train hard the 2 weeks prior to the triathlon; you will not make enough of an improvement to notice, but you may hamper your performance.

  - Get plenty of sleep two nights before the race and the night before the race. Prerace sleep may be of a lesser quality due to anticipation of the race.

- Brick training

  - A combination bike–run workout that is used to help train for the toughest part of the race — getting off the bike and running.

  - Bricks are demanding workouts that push the triathlete and are thought to have a positive training effect.

  - Brick workouts are very demanding and should not be a routine parts of a triathlete's workout.

- Overtraining

  - A state of persistent mental and/or physical fatigue and a feeling of "staleness" that leads to a decline in training and race performance.

  - Symptoms include loss of interest, insomnia, fatigue, irritability, depression, loss of appetite and weight fluctuations, increased muscle soreness, illness, and a persistent increase in resting pulse rate.

  - Multiple theories exist, including glycogen depletion theory (due to a negative energy balance from inadequate nutrition), autonomic imbalance theory, neuroendocrine dysfunction, and many more.

  - Prevention is the best treatment. Structured training programs with built-in relative rest cycles every 4 weeks of training help minimize the risk of overtraining.

  - A short decrease in training intensity or up to a 2-week cessation of all training may be the best treatment depending on the severity of symptoms. If this fails to improve the situation, a referral to a sports psychologist may be warranted.

- Transition zone training

  - "One sport, three disciplines, and two transitions" has been used to define triathlons. This is meant to imply that the two transitions — T1 (transition from swim to bike) and T2 (transition from bike to run) — are just as much part of the competition as the swim, bike, and run.

- The T1 transition has been shown to have negligible impact on race outcome. The T2 transition has been shown to impact the final race outcome, especially in the longer races. Biomechanics and breathing are the two areas that impact the triathletes' performance in the transition zones. It is recommended that triathletes incorporate transition zone training into their program (20).

NUTRITIONAL CONSIDERATIONS

- The gut plays an important role in training, competition, and recovery that few athletes take into consideration. Proper training and nutrition can help minimize the negative impact of gastrointestinal issues while participating in endurance events.
  - Gastric emptying is impeded by high-intensity exercise (70% of $\dot{V}O_{2max}$) and further impeded by dehydration and hyperthermia. Gastric emptying is believed to be responsible for most exercise-related gastrointestinal complaints. The gut can be trained to maximize fuel and fluid absorption (21).
- Energy expenditure depends on the duration, frequency, and intensity of the exercise. Energy expenditure and energy intake need to be balanced and appropriate for the specific activity and level of training or competition.
  - Triathlons require tremendous energy expenditure, with the average male Ironman competitor using 9,000 kcal during a race and 3,000–6,000 kcal during each training session (10).
- Of a triathlete's energy expenditure, 99% is from the body's endurance or aerobic system. After approximately 2 minutes of exercise, the body switches from anaerobic systems to aerobic systems for energy. Adenosine triphosphate (ATP)–creatine phosphate, glucose, and muscle glycogen provide rapid energy to exercising muscle but are unsustainable over prolonged periods. If carbohydrates are not continued during endurance activities, glycogen stores are depleted in approximately 60–90 minutes. The aerobic or endurance system through the utilization of fats via the Krebs cycle and the electron transport chain can produce the large amounts of ATP required for prolonged activity. More than one energy system may be used concurrently and the process is dynamic.
  - The conversion of energy systems from anaerobic to aerobic is not abrupt, and the intensity, duration, frequency, type of activity, and fitness level of the individual all play a role in determining the conversion point.
  - Training does not impact the total amount of energy expended during practice or competition. However, it can affect the fuel source used for energy. A well-trained athlete uses a higher percentage of fat, with long-chain fatty acids being the preferred fuel source. Overall carbohydrates in the stored form of glycogen are used as the major fuel source for exercising muscles.

- The diet of the triathlete should be the same generally well-rounded, balanced diet that is recommended for all adults with some specific changes based on the energy demands of the sport.
  - The average endurance athlete requires approximately 55 kcal · kg^{-1} body weight while training. The daily requirements are as follows:
    - 55%–70% (6–10 g · kg^{-1} body weight or 8–10 kcal · kg^{-1} body weight) of the diet should be in the form of carbohydrates.
    - 25%–30% of the diet should be from fats.
    - 12%–15% (1.0–1.5 g · kg^{-1} body weight) of the diet should be high-quality protein (3).
- Athletes are always looking for something that will give them an advantage over their competitors. There are many ergogenic aids that are available, both legal and illegal, to athletes in an attempt to improve their performance. Carbohydrate loading has been shown to improve performance for endurance events. Caffeine ingestion of 3–5 g · kg^{-1} also improves endurance performance for many athletes. This dose typically has an ergogenic effect without exceeding serum levels banned in competition by the International Olympic Committee (24).
  - Carbohydrate loading has been shown to increase the glycogen stores in the muscles being exercised and improve performance in events that last longer than 90 minutes.
  - The older method of depleting glycogen stores, which involved 1 week of exhaustive exercise in conjunction with 3 days of a low-carbohydrate (< 100 g · d^{-1}) diet prior to 3 days of carbohydrate loading with minimal exercise, is no longer recommended due to significant undesired side effects (irritability, hypoglycemia, stiffness and heaviness of muscles, diarrhea, dehydration, and chest pain in older athletes) (10).
  - The current recommendations for muscle loading simply include ingesting a 60%–70% carbohydrate diet, combined with a decrease in training volume and intensity for 3 days prior to competition.
- Athletes need to experiment with an individualized preevent and intraevent "performance fuel source" that will minimize glycogen depletion and dehydration. Triathletes should never initiate a new hydration/nutrition regimen on race day.
  - 200–300 g of carbohydrate ingested in any form are recommended 3–4 hours prior to the race, and high-fat and high-protein foods should be avoided in this time frame. Some competitors recommend, based on anecdote, up to 1 g · kg^{-1} of body weight of carbohydrate 1 hour before competition, but there is no evidence that this will improve performance, and individual competitors may experience the possible detrimental effects of rebound hypoglycemia and hyperinsulinemia (26).
    - The consumption of foods and/or fluids with low glycemic indices may provide more sustained blood glucose and insulin responses, reducing the potential

metabolic disturbances associated with a rapidly absorbed carbohydrate load.

- During events that last longer than 1 hour, ingestion of $30–60 \text{ g} \cdot \text{h}^{-1}$ of carbohydrate has a proven beneficial effect on performance. Glucose and sucrose should be the primary carbohydrates ingested because they provide more energy with fewer side effects than fructose. Newer studies suggest that ingesting a small amount of protein along with the carbohydrates may have a synergistic effect on endurance performance (8).

- After postevent rehydration, ingestion of foods high in carbohydrates, along with a moderate amount of protein, will help with the repair of muscle and other tissue damaged by exercise.

- Hydration

  - Hydration is the most important factor affecting performance. As little as 2%–4% dehydration has been shown to negatively affect performance.

  - Water loss occurs primarily through sweat. Ambient temperature, relative humidity, exercise intensity, acclimatization, and rate of fluid intake all play a role in the overall hydration status of a competitor. Competitors can lose 2%–6% of their body weight during a race as a result of sweating. Athletes, both trained and untrained, can lose 0.5–2.0 L of sweat per hour (2).

    - Typical, nonelite competitors do not consume enough fluid to negate the fluid lost. Consuming beverages while biking is a little easier and more productive than drinking while running. Elite runners may consume as little as 200 mL of fluid during distance events that last over 2 hours.

    - Minimal dehydration (> 2% body weight) increases core temperature, heart rate, and perceived exertion and decreases aerobic capacity and cognitive and mental performance. Worsening dehydration, especially in a hot environment, predisposes an athlete to more serious and possibly life-threatening conditions such as exertional heat stroke (2).

  - Starting an event hydrated or slightly overhydrated will be beneficial to the competitor, because we know that by the end they will be dehydrated. Competitors need to hydrate themselves the day prior to the competition and consume 400–600 mL up to 2 hours prior to the event (8).

  - Ideally, athletes will replace fluids at a rate that nearly approximates their loss. A loss of 500 mL of fluid equates to about a 1-lb decrease in body weight. This can be an excellent guide to postcompetition fluid replacement needs (11).

  - The frequency and amount of fluid consumed by an endurance athlete is a topic of great interest, with recommendations changing as more research on the topic is published. Underhydration or overhydration may result in symptomatic hypovolemia or hyponatremia, respectively.

Consuming the proper amount of fluids at the right time is paramount to maximizing performance.

- American College of Sports Medicine® guidelines recommend that competitors replace adequate fluids to nearly match sweat losses. An athlete sweating $400–1,000 \text{ mL} \cdot \text{h}^{-1}$ would consume 150–300 mL every 20 minutes of exercise (1). Slower competitors with lower sweat rates may overhydrate, and conversely, athletes with a high sweat rate or who consume less than 200 mL of fluid an hour during a standard endurance event may develop severe and symptomatic hypovolemia (8).

- Noakes (22) proposes that all competitors drink *ad libitum* (no more than $400–800 \text{ mL} \cdot \text{h}^{-1}$) instead of the traditional "drink as much as possible/ forced hydration" model. In his opinion, this method will maintain competitors' vascular status and minimize their risk for dilutional hyponatremia. The International Marathon Medical Directors Association guidelines, authored by Noakes (23), recommend limiting fluid intake to $400–800 \text{ mL} \cdot \text{h}^{-1}$ when thirst is not an adequate guide.

- Which fluids should be consumed by athletes while training or competing?

  - Competitions lasting less than 1 hour: Water is the best replacement fluid.

  - Competitions lasting greater than 1 hour: A carbohydrate/electrolyte replacement beverage will improve performance.

    - A 4%–8% carbohydrate solution is optimal to maximize the quick absorption of carbohydrates and minimize potential side effects, with 10% carbohydrates being the maximum, but often intolerable, concentration.

COMPETITION COVERAGE CONCERNS

- A well-organized medical team should have the ability to handle any emergencies that arise during the competition, as well as the generally expected injuries associated with the event. Adequate staffing and coordination, cooperation, flexibility, and communication are the keys to a successfully executed medical plan.

  - Most race-day injuries will be minor and self-limited, but it is important to quickly diagnose and treat the more serious problems, such as heat stroke, hyponatremia, rhabdomyolysis, dehydration, and cardiac disorders.

- There needs to be a clear delineation of the roles and responsibilities among the race and medical staff (13,18).

  - Race director — Overall responsible for all aspects of the race from the initial planning meetings to the postrace review.

  - Medical director — A physician who is responsible for organizing and coordinating the medical support for the event, from any prerace planning to the close of the medical facility (13).

❑ Ensure that local emergency medical services and local emergency rooms are notified and aware of the race date and time.

❑ Develop and review a prerace medical questionnaire that must be completed by all athletes. This will provide the medical team with insight into any competitors who have serious underlying medical problems.

❑ In conjunction with the race director, develop patient transportation guidelines and criteria for transport.

❑ In conjunction with the race director, develop a race crisis plan with cancellation parameters.

❑ Monitor environmental issues (ambient temperature, humidity level, wet bulb globe temperature [WBGT], lightening, etc.) that may impact the health and safety of the competitors, and make recommendations to the race committee.

❑ If the WBGT index is above 28°C (82°F) or if the ambient dry bulb temperature is below −20°C (−4°F), then it is recommended that consideration be given to rescheduling the event (3).

❑ Develop treatment algorithms for anticipated conditions that will allow for the same standard of care for each patient and allow for nurses and paraprofessionals to begin caring for patients when a physician is not readily available (16).

■ Medical tent director — Physician who is responsible for the organization and control of the medical tent. This physician should not have any direct patient care responsibilities, as he or she needs to be able to move through the entire tent to continuously assess medical issues.

■ Volunteer medical staff — Primary care and emergency medical providers are critical components of the medical team. Other critical care specialties (cardiology, anesthesia, pulmonary) can also augment the medical team. Skilled nurses are also critical to the success of the medical team.

■ Volunteer paramedical staff — Emergency medical technicians, medics, respiratory therapists, pharmacy technicians, physical therapists, athletic trainers, and clerks are essential for a successful medical support operation.

■ The size of the medical staff depends on the number of competitors, type of events, distances covered, and length of time competitors are on the course.

■ Two to three physicians and seven to eight nurses/other paramedical volunteers per every 100 athletes is a reasonable planning guide to support a triathlon.

■ One ambulance per 1,000 competitors is a reasonable guide when estimating support for an endurance event (6).

■ Location of medical services — After the proper resources have been secured, they need to be placed in a location where they are most accessible and effective.

■ Main medical tent — Located near the finish line. Most medical incidents occur shortly after the finish line.

■ Transition area medical tent — A small, modestly equipped team, able to handle routine injuries as well as stabilize and transport severe injuries, located where the competitors change disciplines, is recommended.

■ Mobile medical teams — Depending on the course length and layout, it may be advisable to have teams out on the course that can handle situations that arise a prolonged distance away from medical care.

■ Recommended supplies: An all-inclusive list of the required supplies is beyond the scope of this chapter and needs to be customized based on race conditions. The following items are some basic recommendations.

■ Monitors — Automated external defibrillator/Lifepak, portable (battery operated) electrocardiogram, blood pressure cuffs, pulse oximeters, thermometers (rectal), glucometer, point-of-care chemistry analyzer, and urinalysis strips.

■ Equipment — Cots, stretchers, intravenous poles, two-way radios, oxygen regulators, airway management items, nebulizers, blankets, ace wraps, ice packs, fluid warmers, heaters, trashcans, regulated medical waste containers, sharp containers, tapes, bandages, splinting materials, blister care, and trauma care (cervical collars, backboards, etc.).

■ Medications — Advanced cardiac life support (ACLS) drugs, intravenous fluids (normal saline), epinephrine, β-agonists, diazepam, naloxone, rapid sequence intubation drugs, acetaminophen, and other drugs based on provider preference.

■ Medical considerations

■ Review historical casualty data/numbers from previous events.

❑ Historically, during Ironman-distance triathlons, 25%–30% of starters receive medical attention; one in four competitors require transport to a higher level of care (17).

■ Hypothermia and water temperature — Colder water and longer swim distances increase the risk of developing hypothermia during the swimming phase. Age-group triathletes are allowed to wear a wetsuit without penalty in water temperatures up to 78°F; between 78 and 84°F, they can wear a wetsuit but are not eligible for an award; and at temperatures greater than 84°F, wetsuits are not permitted. Professional triathletes are allowed to wear wetsuits when the water temperature is less than 61.0°F and 71.6°F in races less than and greater than 3,000 m, respectively. All wetsuits must be less than 5 mm thick (28).

■ Exercise-associated collapse (EAC) — EAC is the most common medical problem experienced at the finish line and is believed to be the result of significant postural hypotension and secondary tachycardia, not hyperthermia or dehydration. Treatment consists of elevating the legs and encouraging competitors to keep moving after finishing.

■ Hyponatremia — Hyponatremia with serum sodium less than 135 mg · dL^{-1} is believed to occur in 10%–40% of endurance athletes. Serum sodium above 130 mg · dL^{-1} is usually asymptomatic. Serum sodium levels measuring less than 125 mg · dL^{-1} are more concerning and may manifest with altered mental status, lethargy, cramps, or seizures. Excessive water intake before or during competition may lead to symptomatic hyponatremia, which is a medical emergency. A rapid intravenous infusion of 100 mL of 3% hypertonic saline will begin to correct the symptomatic hyponatremia, although more than one bolus may be required. Seizures are treated with 3% NaCl and sometimes benzodiazepines. Patients with persistent hyponatremia or severe hyponatremia will require transfer to a higher level medical treatment facility (17,23).

■ Heat illness — Heat stroke, a potentially fatal condition characterized by a rectal temperature of greater than 40°C and mental status changes, is a medical emergency. Athletes tend to develop heat stroke toward the middle to end of the run portion of the triathlon. Cooling should be initiated immediately with whatever means is available. Cold water immersion is the most effective form of treatment for exertional heat stroke. An ice slurry bath from the nipple level on down to the abdomen and the legs is the most effective method of cooling. Cold water dousing with concomitant massage of large ice bags over major muscle groups also provides effective cooling. Additionally, placing six to eight ice water towels over the entire body can be a highly transportable (just need cooler, ice, and water) cooling method (need to rotate towels back to cooler every few minutes). Sprinkled or aerosolized water with fanning is also effective if the water content of the air is very low, as in an air-conditioned facility. Ice packs applied to the groins and armpits may also augment evaporative cooling methods. Patients demonstrating signs of severe heat exhaustion or heat stroke will require transfer to a higher level of care after immediate on-site cooling (4).

■ Rhabdomyolysis — Extreme muscle breakdown due to intense, prolonged exercise. It is often exacerbated by dehydration and hyperthermia. Elevated serum creatine kinase with brown or reddish (cola colored) urine and a urine dipstick positive for blood without red blood cells on microscopy makes the diagnosis likely. Elevated serum or urine myoglobin levels help confirm the diagnosis. Intravenous fluids administered to maintain a urine output of $200–300 \text{ mL} \cdot \text{h}^{-1}$ are recommended to help prevent acute tubular necrosis and subsequent renal failure. Patients with rhabdomyolysis or patients who you are concerned may have or may develop rhabdomyolysis will require transfer.

REFERENCES

1. American College of Sports Medicine, American Dietetic Association, Dietitians of Canada. Joint position statement: nutrition and athletic performance. *Med Sci Sports Exerc.* 2000;32(12):2130–45.

2. American College of Sports Medicine; Sawka MN, Burke LM, et al. American College of Sports Medicine position stand. Exercise and fluid replacement. *Med Sci Sports Exerc.* 2007;39(2):377–90.

3. Armstrong LE, Epstein Y, Greenleaf, et al. American College of Sports Medicine position stand. The female athlete triad: heat and cold illnesses during distance running. *Med Sci Sports Exerc.* 1996;28(10):139–48.

4. Bouchama A, Knochel JP. Medical progress: heat stroke. *N Engl J Med.* 2002;346(25):1978–88.

5. Burns J, Keenan AM, Redmond AC. Factors associated with triathlon-related overuse injuries. *J Orthop Sports Phys Ther.* 2003;33(4):177–84.

6. Cianca JC, Roberts WO, Horn D. Distance running: organization of the medical team. In: O'Connor FG, Wilder RP, editors. *Textbook of Running Medicine.* New York (NY): McGraw-Hill; 2001. p. 489–504.

7. Collins K, Wagner M, Peterson K, Storey M. Overuse injuries in triathletes. A study of the 1986 Seafair Triathlon. *Am J Sports Med.* 1989;17(5):675–80.

8. Convertino VA, Armstrong LE, Coyle EF, et al. American College of Sports Medicine position stand. Exercise and fluid replacement. *Med Sci Sports Exerc.* 1996;28(10):i–ix.

9. Cosca DD, Navazio F. Common problems in endurance athletes. *Am Fam Physician.* 2007;76(2):237–44.

10. DiMarco NM, Samuels M. Nutritional considerations. In: O'Connor FG, Wilder RP, editors. *Textbook of Running Medicine.* New York (NY): McGraw-Hill; 2001. p. 477–89.

11. Fieseler CM. The ultramarathoner. In: O'Connor FG, Wilder RP, editors. *Textbook of Running Medicine.* New York (NY): McGraw-Hill; 2001. p. 469–77.

12. Gosling CM, Forbes AB, McGivern J, Gabbe BJ. A profile of injuries in athletes seeking treatment during a triathlon race series. *Am J Sports Med.* 2010;38(5):1007–14.

13. Grange JT. Planning for large events. *Curr Sports Med Rep.* 2002;1(3):156–61.

14. Harris KM, Henry JT, Rohman E, Haas TS, Maron BJ. Sudden death during the triathlon. *JAMA.* 2010;303(13):1255–7.

15. Hellemans J. Maximizing Olympic distance triathlon performance — a sports medicine perspective [Internet]. [cited 2010 Sep 23]. Available from: http://fulltext.ausport.gov.au/fulltext/1999/triathlon/john.hellemans.pdf.

16. Hew-Butler T, Ayus JC, Kipps C, Maughan RJ, et al. Statement of the Second International Exercise-Associated Hyponatremia Consensus Development Conference, New Zealand, 2007. *Clin J Sport Med.* 2008;18(2):111–21.

17. Korkia PK, Tunstall-Pedoe DS, Maffulli N. An epidemiological investigation of training and injury patterns in British triathletes. *Br J Sports Med.* 1994;28(3):191–6.

18. Martinez JM, Laird R. Managing triathlon competition. *Curr Sports Med Rep.* 2003;2(3):142–6.

19. Mayers LB, Noakes TD. A guide to treating ironman triathletes at the finish line. *Phys Sportsmed.* 2000;28(8):35–50.

20. Millet GP, Vleck VE. Physiological and biomechanical adaptations to the cycle to run transition in Olympic triathlon: review and practical recommendations for training. *Br J Sports Med.* 2000;34(5):384–90.

21. Murray R. Training the gut for competition. *Curr Sports Med Rep.* 2006;5(3):161–4.

22. Noakes T. Hyponatremia in distance runners: fluid and sodium balance during exercise. *Curr Sports Med Rep.* 2002;1(4):197–207.

23. Noakes T; International Marathon Medical Directors Association. Fluid replacement during marathon running. *Clin J Sports Med.* 2003;13(5):309–18.

24. Paluska SA. Caffeine and exercise. *Curr Sports Med Rep.* 2002;2(4):213–9.

25. Peeling PD, Bishop DJ, Landers GJ. Effect of swimming intensity on subsequent cycling and overall triathlon performance. *Br J Sports Med.* 2005;39(12):960–4.

26. Robins A. Nutritional recommendations for competing in the ironman triathlon. *Curr Sports Med Rep.* 2007;6(4):241–8.

27. Thompson MJ, Rivara FP. Bicycle-related injuries. *Am Fam Physician.* 2001;63(10):2007–14.

28. USA Triathlon Competitive Rules (n.d.) [Internet]. Available from: http://www.usatriathlon.org/about-multisport/rulebook.

29. Vleck VE, Bentley DJ, Millet GP, Cochrane T. Triathlon event distance specialization: training and injury effects. *J Strength Cond Res.* 2010;24(1):30–6.

30. Williams MM, Hawley JA, Black R, Freke M, Simms K. Injuries amongst competitive triathletes. *N Z J Sports Med.* 1988:2–6.

108 Volleyball

Emily A. Darr

OVERVIEW

- Volleyball has become an incredibly popular sport, both recreationally and competitively. It is now one of the big five international sports (soccer, cricket, field hockey, tennis, and volleyball), and the Fédération Internationale de Volleyball (FIVB) claims it is the largest international sporting federation in the world with 220 affiliated national federations. Volleyball became an Olympic sport in 1964, and beach volleyball was added in 1996 (14).

- Volleyball skills require quick, forceful movements of the entire body all at once in multiple planes, making injuries inevitable. Although considered a noncontact sport, the rate of injury had been found to be 2.6 in 1,000 hours of play. Fortunately, the incidence of serious injury is relatively low (15).

- Players on the volleyball court engage in many different sport-specific skills, each with its own typical activity-related injuries. Serving, passing, and setting have not been associated with high numbers of injuries. Spiking, or attacking, has been associated with a fairly high incidence of injury, and blocking has been implicated in causing the highest rate of injury. The hand, shoulder, knee, and ankle are among the most commonly injured areas (4).

- Consideration must also be given to certain injuries common to specific surfaces because volleyball is played on a variety of surfaces, such as wood, grass, concrete, and the increasingly popular sand.

LOWER EXTREMITY

- Many lower extremity injuries in volleyball are due to repetitive motions, such as jumping, landing, and twisting during play. These repetitive stresses seem to be often implicated because a player may jump 150 times in the course of a match (13).

- The majority of lower extremity injuries occur when the athletes are playing in the front three positions. Studies suggest that 63% of the musculoskeletal injuries result from jumping and landing, which most often occur in these positions (15). Lower extremity injuries account for the majority of volleyball injuries. In a recent review of collegiate women's

volleyball players, the lower extremity accounted for more than 55% of all game and practice injuries, with ankle ligament sprains representing 44.1% of game injuries and 29.4% of practice injuries (1).

Knee

- The most commonly seen overuse injury in volleyball is patellar tendonitis or jumper's knee. Players tend to have pain at the lower pole of the patella and, less frequently, at the upper pole and tibial tuberosity. It often has an insidious onset with pain seen with hyperextension of the knee. Initial treatment should include rest, ice, compression with a neoprene sleeve, and nonsteroidal anti-inflammatory drugs (NSAIDs). Long-term management should include vastus medialis strengthening (10).

- Acute knee injuries ranging from mild sprains of the collateral ligaments to more serious anterior cruciate ligament and meniscal tears tend to be caused by quick changes in direction with landing, cutting, and pivoting on the court. This most frequently occurs while landing near the net after an attack.

- For unclear reasons, these acute ligamentous injuries occur more often in females than in males. Immediate treatment includes ice and removal from play (6).

Leg

- "Shin splints" or tibial periostitis can be seen in players early in the season when a sudden increase in training can cause an inflammation of the anterior and posterior tibialis muscles. Ice, rest, NSAIDs, and adjusting training regimens will typically improve the symptoms.

- Prolonged or worsening typical anterior shin pain beyond the time of intense activity is concerning for stress fracture. Delayed-phase bone scans and magnetic resonance imaging (MRI) are the most sensitive tests for diagnosing this.

Foot and Ankle

- Ankle injuries are the most common acute volleyball injury and account for 44% of all volleyball-related injuries according to a recent study (15). They are typically inversion sprains involving the lateral ligaments and are often a result of a blocker landing on the foot of an attacker from the opposing team under the net (12).

- Treatment of an acutely injured ankle will vary based on the severity. Ottawa ankle rules should be used to determine if an x-ray is warranted. The player should be removed from play if there is a suspected fracture or excessive swelling or the athlete is unable to bear weight.

- Ankle injury rehabilitation should include physical therapy, with a focus on regaining joint proprioception to prevent re-injury, in addition to relative rest, NSAIDs, ice, and bracing.

- Some volleyball teams use ankle braces prophylactically to prevent inversion-type ankle sprains at all levels of competition. However, studies show that ankle injuries still occur in athletes wearing braces (2).

- Identifying attackers who tend to land close to the centerline and coaching them to focus on more vertical travel can help to decrease the incidence of ankle sprains occurring under the net (4).

- Metatarsal, navicular, and sesamoid stress fractures can occur and require removal from participation until they are healed.

- "Sand toe" is an injury unique to beach volleyball, which is played barefoot. It involves a hyperplantarflexion injury to the metatarsophalangeal joint. Pain typically occurs with motions involving running, jumping, and pushing off. Treatment should include relative rest, ice, NSAIDs, and toe strengthening (7).

UPPER EXTREMITY

Shoulder

- The shoulder accounts for 8%–20% of volleyball injuries. The majority of shoulder injuries are related to chronic overuse, especially of the rotator cuff and long head biceps tendons. Frequent motions involving abduction and external rotation followed by forceful extension and internal rotation during the spiking motion are often the cause of these chronic injuries. An imbalance between the muscles of internal rotation and the muscles of external rotation appears to be strongly associated with shoulder injury in volleyball players and should be addressed in rehabilitation with a stretching program for internal rotators (4).

- Rotator cuff injuries are caused by repetitive overhead hitting of the ball and/or joint instability. They can vary from mild forms of tendinitis and impingement to complete tears. Treatment can vary from NSAIDs and physical therapy focusing on scapular stabilization to surgery, depending on the severity.

- Impingement syndrome occurs when the supraspinatus tendon becomes irritated and painful as it passes through the subacromial space. Players with anatomic variances, such as a "hooked acromion," may be more prone to problems. In addition, further narrowing of the space may be secondary to depression of the dominant shoulder caused by capsular instability and muscular imbalance in volleyball attackers.

Painful shoulder motion, in addition to night pain, is a result of these muscular imbalances, overuse, and variances. Surgical decompression may be necessary if conservative therapy fails to allow return to play. In some instances, a subacromial corticosteroid injection is beneficial (9).

- Suprascapular neuropathy is encountered on a surprisingly frequent basis in elite volleyball players. The nerve is typically compressed at the spinoglenoid notch where the terminal branch comes off, resulting in isolated atrophy and weakness of the infraspinatus muscle. Up to 25% loss of external rotation strength may be seen in the affected shoulder. The mechanism of injury for this neuropathy may be the "floater" serve, which is achieved by stopping follow-through immediately after contact with the ball to prevent the ball from spinning in its course to the other side of the court. Electromyography is useful in diagnosis, and conservative treatment is generally effective. Rehabilitative exercises should be aimed at strengthening external rotation. Surgery may be considered in cases of persistent pain, because ganglion cysts may also cause a similar presentation (5).

Finger, Hand, and Wrist

- Wrist injuries are commonly related to passing and digging the ball and to contacting the floor after diving. Fractures of the pisiform can be diagnosed on axial or "carpal tunnel" views on radiograph and would require casting.

- Kienböck disease, or aseptic necrosis of the lunate, can be seen with repetitive wrist trauma in volleyball players. MRI will provide the best information as to whether conservative or surgical treatment is necessary (8).

- Most injuries to the fingers and hands occur as a result of contact with the ball during play at the net, especially during blocking. Sprains and strains are most frequently seen, followed by fractures and contusions. The thumb metacarpophalangeal (MCP) joint is a frequently injured joint, and more specifically, the radial collateral ligament is often injured during the hyperextension stresses from ball impact during blocking (4).

- Most finger sprains are minor and can be managed conservatively with taping and splinting. Collateral ligament injuries to the interphalangeal joints should be "buddy taped" to an adjacent finger for adequate support.

Low Back

- Lumbar spine strains and sprains can happen in volleyball players due to the extension followed by forced flexion and rotation, and then landing, when a player attacks a ball.

- Suspicion should be high for stress fracture in cases of prolonged pain despite conservative treatment.

- Athletes with radiating leg symptoms in the setting of low back pain should be held from play until further evaluation is completed.

OTHER INJURIES

- Contusions over the anterior superior iliac spines or "hip pointers," in addition to contusions over the medial and anterior aspect of the knee, are frequently noted after defensive diving onto a hard court. Kneepads, more often than hip pads, are typically worn for protection. Icing and anti-inflammatory medications can be used in reducing pain and swelling.
- Traumatic brain injury is reported as being infrequent in volleyball players, with a rate of 0.14 per 100 injuries (11).

BEACH VOLLEYBALL

- Recognized as an Olympic sport in 1996, beach volleyball has grown immensely over the past decade. Because of its new popularity, very little is known about injuries specific to beach volleyball.
- Beach volleyball differs from indoor volleyball in many ways, including the surface played on, the number of athletes on the court, and the size of the court. Beach volleyball is played barefoot on sand, with two players on each team with no substitutions allowed. The court is smaller for beach volleyball (16 m × 8 m) compared with indoor volleyball (18 m × 9 m).
- The injuries sustained during beach and indoor volleyball are overall similar; however, there appear to be fewer time-loss injuries in beach volleyball. The three most common overuse injuries in beach volleyball are low back pain, knee pain, and shoulder problems (3).
- Similar to indoor volleyball, the ankle, knee, fingers, and low back have the highest rate of acute injury in beach volleyball. However, the rate of ankle sprains in beach volleyball is almost half that of indoor volleyball. This most likely is related to less players blocking and to a softer court surface (3).
- Acute finger injuries are as common in beach volleyball as they are in indoor volleyball; however, more finger injuries are a result of overhand digging in sand volleyball, which is a common defensive tactic against hard driven attacks (3).

- Consideration should also be given to weather conditions, which play a factor in beach volleyball.

REFERENCES

1. Agel J, Palmieri-Smith RM, Dick R, Wojtys EM, Marshall SW. Descriptive epidemiology of college women's volleyball injuries: National Collegiate Athletic Association Injury Surveillance System, 1988–1989 through 2003–2004. *J Athl Train*. 2007;42(2):295–302.
2. Bahr R, Karlsen R, Lian O, Ovrebø RV. Incidence and mechanisms of acute ankle inversion injuries in volleyball. A retrospective cohort study. *Am J Sports Med*. 1994;22(5):595–600.
3. Bahr R, Resser JC; Fédération Internationale de Volleyball. Injuries among world-class professional beach volleyball players. The Fédération Internationale de Volleyball beach volleyball injury study. *Am J Sports Med*. 2003;31(1):119–25.
4. Briner WW Jr, Kacmar L. Common injuries in volleyball. Mechanisms of injury, prevention and rehabilitation. *Sports Med*. 1997;24(1):65–71.
5. Ferretti A, De Carli A, Fontana M. Injury of the suprascapular nerve at the spinoglenoid notch. The natural history of infraspinatus atrophy in volleyball players. *Am J Sports Med*. 1998;26(6):759–63.
6. Ferretti A, Papandrea P, Conteduca F, Mariani PP. Knee ligament injuries in volleyball players. *Am J Sports Med*. 1992;20(2):203–7.
7. Frey C, Andersen GD, Feder KS. Plantarflexion injury to the metatarsophalangeal joint ("sand toe"). *Foot Ankle Int*. 1996;17(9):576–81.
8. Howse C. Wrist injuries in sport. *Sports Med*. 1994;17(3):163–75.
9. Kugler A, Krüger-Franke M, Rininger S, Trouillier HH, Rosemeyer B. Muscular imbalance and shoulder pain in volleyball attackers. *Br J Sports Med*. 1996;30(3):256–9.
10. Lian OB, Engebretsen L, Bahr R. Prevalence of jumper's knee among elite athletes from different sports: a cross-sectional study. *Am J Sports Med*. 2005;33(4):561–7.
11. Powell JW, Barber-Foss KD. Traumatic brain injury in high school athletes. JAMA. 1999;282(10):958–63.
12. Reeser JC, Verhagen E, Briner WW, Askeland TI, Bahr R. Strategies for the prevention of volleyball related injuries. *Br J Sports Med*. 2006;40(7):594–600.
13. Schafle MD, Requa RK, Patton WL, Garrick JG. Injuries in the 1987 national amateur volleyball tournament. *Am J Sports Med*. 1990;18(6):624–31.
14. The Game [Internet]. [cited 2011 Jan 15]. Available from: http://www.fivb.org/TheGame/index.htm.
15. Verhagen EA, Van Der Beek AJ, Bouter LM, Bahr RM, Van Mechelen W. A one season prospective cohort study of volleyball injuries. *Br J Sports Med*. 2004;38(4):477–81.

Water Polo Injuries

109

Dean M. Brewer, Richard P. Eide, III, and Michelle E. Szczepanik

INTRODUCTION (3,4,8,10,12)

- Water polo is a team aquatic sport played throughout the United States and in many countries around the world, particularly in Europe.
- It is a fast-paced, physically demanding game requiring both strength and skill as a swimmer combined with excellent hand–eye coordination to facilitate ball handling, passing, and scoring.
- During a typical match, a player will swim short distances with high-energy bursts lasting 10–18 seconds. For some players, these short distances can add up to 1,000 m. These sprints are separated by 30- to 40-second intervals of "eggbeater" leg work.
- Statistics from the 2004 Olympic Games demonstrated that an injury occurred once in every two to three matches, with the total incidence being 21 injuries per every 1,000 player matches. All injuries were caused by contact with another player, with the head and upper extremities being the most affected.
- Water polo had the highest incidence of injury in the 2009 Fédération Internationale de Natation Amateur (FINA) World Aquatic Championships.

HISTORY

- Although the exact origins are unclear, the first documented rules were codified in 1877 by William Wilson, a Scottish aquatics enthusiast. Initially, the game more closely resembled an aquatic form of rugby football.
- The game was altered into its modern-day form by the turn of the 20th century, when it was incorporated into the modern Olympic Games in Paris, France in 1900.
- Water polo is governed internationally by FINA and within the United States by USA Water Polo, a not-for-profit organization under the aegis of the U.S. Olympic Committee.

REQUIRED EQUIPMENT (8)

- Although it could be played in any suitably sized body of water, water polo is most often played in swimming pools. Known as "the field," the dimensions of the pool will vary depending on the age and gender of the players, ranging from 20–30 m long by 10–20 m wide by 2–4 m deep.
- The goals are rectangular, centered at both ends of the field, and 3 m wide by 0.9 m high.
- The ball is spherical, weighing approximately 1 lb, roughly equivalent in size to a volleyball, and coated with a high-friction rubber to facilitate grip.
- Individual equipment includes a swimsuit and a swim cap with cupped ear protectors.

GAME PLAY (8)

- The object is to throw the ball into the opposing team's goal, thereby scoring 1 point. The ball may be passed around the field in any direction, but a team may not possess the ball for more than 30 seconds without attempting a shot on goal, or else they forfeit the ball. The team that scores the most number of points before regulation time has expired is the winner.
- Teams are composed of seven players, six in the field of play and one goalkeeper; teams are designated by the required uniform swim caps, which also serve to protect players' ears.
- All players, with notable exception of the goaltender, may use either hand but must use only one hand at a time to handle, pass, and shoot the ball. Players will use the "eggbeater" kick, which combines the clockwise motion by one leg and a counterclockwise motion of the other leg in order to stay afloat.
- The game is divided into four quarters, which are 8 minutes in length for collegiate and professional play; youth leagues through high school have shorter periods, which range from 5–7 minutes.

FOULS (8)

- There are three types of fouls: ordinary, penalty, and exclusion.
  - Ordinary fouls are minor infractions of game play. They include holding the ball underwater or tucking inside one's swimsuit, using two hands, pushing off of the pool floor (except shallow-end goalkeeper), striking the ball with a closed fist, swimming within 2 m of the opposing

goal ahead of the ball, and impeding the free movement of an opposing player who is not holding the ball, including pushing or pushing off. Ordinary fouls result in a change of possession by means of a free throw.

■ Penalty fouls are ordinary fouls committed within the 5-m goal area and result in a penalty throw (exclusion fouls in this area also result in a penalty throw).

■ Exclusion fouls are more grievous violations and include using two hands to block a pass or shot, exiting the pool without permission, intentionally splashing water in an opponent's face, or intentionally striking an opponent (elbow, punch, kick). The penalty for exclusion fouls is removal from play for 20 seconds. The official may determine if there was malicious intent to harm another player, in which case the player is removed from the game and the team must play one man down for 4 minutes.

■ In general, water polo is an intensely physical game, with players swimming at a sprint pace in immediate proximity to one another for control of the ball and for defensive maneuvers. The result of such activity and a limited amount of protective equipment is a propensity for many different types of injuries.

■ Injuries to the head and face are among the most common (15.5%–53.0%) acute injuries in water polo due to the relative exposure above water.

EYE INJURIES (1,2,4,7,12,13)

■ Annett et al. found that eye injuries accounted for 6.1% of acute injuries in water polo.

■ The most common eye complaints in water polo are eye irritation or lacerations from direct trauma. Due to the severity of some uncommon injuries, they are also included in this section.

■ Corneal abrasion
  ❑ Signs/symptoms: Severe eye pain and photophobia
  ❑ Common mechanism: Excoriation from fingernail, toenail, or trapping of debris under contact lens
  ❑ Treatment: If you suspect corneal abrasion, you should transfer the patient to a higher center of care to confirm diagnosis with fluorescein dye and slit lamp examination, especially looking for any foreign body remnants. The athlete should be advised to keep eye closed and to avoid rubbing/touching. Topical anesthetic drops may be used initially to relieve pain and facilitate exam; however, long-term use is discouraged because these drops will delay healing of the corneal epithelium and can lead to a pseudo-addiction state by the patient, resulting in corneal ulceration, scarring, and blindness. Treatment ultimately consists of topical antibiotic ointment (*e.g.*, erythromycin) or drops (*e.g.*, Polytrim, ciprofloxacin, ofloxacin) four times a day for 3–5 days. Athlete should not be allowed to return to play until the abrasion has healed.

■ Laceration of eyelid, eyebrow, lip, cheek (*most common acute injury*)
  ❑ Signs/symptoms: Bleeding from laceration, pain
  ❑ Common mechanism: Direct trauma to skin overlying bone
  ❑ Treatment: Cleanse/irrigate wound, assess depth/severity of laceration, and repair via approximation of skin edges. The primary care provider should be skilled in simple laceration repair, although if there is concern about cosmetic result or involvement of eyelid, consultation with plastic surgeon and/or ophthalmologist is warranted. Sterile adhesive bandages (*e.g.*, Steri-strips) and adhesive glue (*e.g.*, Dermabond) may be used for small, superficial repairs with minimal active bleeding.

■ Chemical irritation
  ❑ Signs/symptoms: Discomfort/burning of eyes, scleral injection
  ❑ Common mechanism: Excessive exposure to chlorine or other disinfectant
  ❑ Treatment: Saline eye drops, limit exposure to chlorinated water

■ Hyphema (hemorrhage into anterior chamber from ruptured trabecular blood vessels)
  ❑ Signs/symptoms: Blood pooling in inferior portion of iris
  ❑ Common mechanism: Direct trauma to globe from fist, elbow, ball, etc.
  ❑ Treatment: EMERGENCY. Protect eye with loose, occlusive dressing (*e.g.*, Fox shield) and seek immediate evaluation by ophthalmology; if untreated, it could result in glaucoma or permanent corneal staining.

■ Blowout fracture of orbital floor (orbital floor is weaker relative to surrounding bones)
  ❑ Signs/symptoms: Periorbital hematoma, protruding or sunken globe; herniation of inferior contents can cause entrapment, which will manifest as an inability to gaze upward in affected eye, producing diplopia and/or maxillary numbness
  ❑ Common mechanism: Direct trauma to globe resulting in fracture of orbital floor
  ❑ Treatment: EMERGENCY. Protect eye with loose, occlusive dressing (*e.g.*, Fox shield) and seek immediate evaluation by ophthalmology to rule out intraocular trauma. It is essential to perform a thorough neurologic exam to rule out entrapment of inferior orbital contents.

EAR INJURIES (4,7,9,12,14–16)

■ Many ear injuries, especially traumatic auricular hematoma ("cauliflower ear"), can be avoided through the proper wear of special cupped ear protector swim caps, which are a required part of personal equipment.

- Commonly reported ear injuries include the following:
  - Otitis externa (swimmer's ear)
    - Signs/symptoms: Inflamed, erythematous, tender external auditory canal; exudates may be present
    - Common mechanism: Bacterial infection (often *Pseudomonas* species) from excessive moisture in external auditory canal, which removes cerumen and creates optimal pH for bacterial growth.
    - Treatment: *Best treatment is prevention* with alcohol-based drops, which provide antiseptic treatment via desiccation. If infection is present, use antibiotic ear drops with or without steroids for severe inflammation. There are a number of available preparations, but fluoroquinolones such as ofloxacin and ciprofloxacin have the broadest coverage and are typically only dosed twice daily as opposed to three or four times daily for other otic antibiotic preparations. Proper technique is important to increase effectiveness. The athlete should tilt his or her head to the shoulder opposite the affected ear, and the auricle is then grasped and pulled superiorly and posteriorly. Instill drops until the external auditory canal is filled, and then have the athlete lay on his or her side for 15–20 minutes with the affected ear still facing upward to allow for maximal time and surface area exposure.
  - Traumatic perforation of tympanic membrane (TM)
    - Signs/symptoms: Immediate pain and loss of hearing in affected ear; bleeding from ear may be present; ruptured TM will be evident on otoscopic exam.
    - Common mechanism: Compression of external ear via slap on the side of the head with a cupped hand producing a transient high pressure within the canal.
    - Treatment: The athlete should be reassured that the TM will heal spontaneously and without hearing loss; however, the athlete *should not* be allowed to swim/submerge head in water until healed. Individually tailored wax earplugs can be manufactured and used to completely occlude the external auditory canal from water entry in cases where clinical judgment would deem it reasonable for the athlete to return to play before the injury has completely healed.

UPPER EXTREMITY INJURIES

Shoulder (4,5,7,9,11,17)

- Shoulder pain is the most common musculoskeletal complaint in water polo. Studies have reported a shoulder injury rate of 11.5 per 100 injuries per year, with female players reporting more injuries than males.
- A systemic review of the literature showed that the incidence of shoulder injuries can range anywhere from 24%–80%. The majority of shoulder injuries that occur are from overuse or are minor injuries such as impingement or bursitis, compared to major injuries involving tears or requiring surgery.
- No other throwing athlete deals with water as their sole base of support for throwing. Unlike other throwing athletes, the water polo player has no fixed point from which to throw. The forceful abduction and external rotation of glenohumeral joint to achieve the "cocked" throwing position followed by the throw itself places a great strain on the anterior shoulder stabilizing muscles.
- McMaster et al. (11) demonstrated isokinetic torque imbalances in the rotator cuff of water polo players. The study showed that elite water polo players have significant adductor and internal rotator muscle strength when compared to muscles for abduction and external rotation. This imbalance within the rotator cuff likely increases the propensity for shoulder injuries.
- Webster et al. (17) performed a systemic review of the literature showing that shoulder injuries in water polo players resulted from a variety of factors, including increased mobility, muscle strength imbalance, and altered throwing techniques.
- Subacromial/coracoacromial impingement and bursitis, biceps tendinitis, acromioclavicular joint sprains or arthritis, dislocations, rotator cuff injuries, and tears are common shoulder injuries among water polo players.
- The majority of shoulder injuries can be rehabilitated or fixed through physical therapy, rest, and anti-inflammatory medications; however, full-thickness tear or failure of rehabilitation usually requires surgery to repair.
- Traumatic dislocations and subluxations are not common injuries in water polo. When they do occur, these injuries will result during the act of shooting or passing the ball.

Elbow (5,6,9)

- The majority of elbow pain in water polo players occurs along the medial aspect of the elbow.
- The overhead throwing motion of a water polo player places great stress on the ulnar collateral ligament complex. The ligament can fail at an average load of 260 N or 58 lb. This tension load can be exceeded in elite water polo competition.
- Most common injuries include ulnar collateral ligament (UCL) injuries, valgus extension overload syndrome with olecranon osteophytes and posteromedial impingement, and osteochondritis dissecans of the capitellum.
- Mild pain after throwing or a change in activity level is most often associated with overuse injuries. If a "pop" sensation is felt, a UCL injury should be suspected. Mechanical symptoms of catching, locking, or giving way are often caused by osteophytes and loose bodies.
- Part of the workup for elbow pain should include anteroposterior, lateral, and axial olecranon x-ray views. Magnetic resonance imaging is the study of choice for evaluating potential damage to the UCL complex.

- The majority of elbow injuries can be treated through nonoperative measures, including rest, ice, immobilization with a splint, and physical therapy. Any physical therapy should include core body strengthening exercises, with arm flexibility and secondary dynamic stabilizer strengthening.

- Upon completion of physical therapy, athletes should be enrolled in a throwing program to effectively rehab the elbow. Overuse injuries can take anywhere from 3–6 months before an athlete is ready for full competition, whereas an injury that involves UCL instability or reconstructive surgery can result in 9–18 months of rehabilitation before an athlete is able to return.

Hand and Fingers (5,7,9)

- A player's hand and arm are considered part of the ball during active play and are often hit by opposing players in an attempt to gain possession of the ball. The hand and fingers are also used for shot blocking and grabbing onto other players to maintain position. With the ball being thrown, grabbed for, and caught at high speeds, hand and finger injuries are common.

- The most common injuries include lacerations, dislocations, fractures, and overuse injuries.

- Commonly reported hand and finger injuries include the following:
  - Web space tear (the most common laceration in water polo)
    - Signs/symptoms: Notable tear and pain between two fingers
    - Common mechanism: Occurs when two fingers are forcibly abducted apart. This can occur when players attempt to block or catch balls thrown at high speeds.
    - Treatment: Small tears will heal with time and conservative treatment. The lacerations involving ligaments of the fingers may require reconstructive surgery.
  - Dislocations of the fingers and hand
    - Signs/symptoms: A dislocated finger is usually obvious. The finger appears crooked and swollen and is very painful. It may be bent upward or at strange angles. Bending or attempted straightening of the finger may be difficult.
    - Common mechanism: Due to a hyperextension of the joint.
    - Treatment: Athletes and trainers are usually successful with reducing these dislocations poolside. X-rays after a dislocation are recommended to rule out fractures. A protective splint may be placed on the finger, or the finger may be "buddy taped" to the healthy finger next to it.
  - "Gamekeeper's thumb"
    - Signs/symptoms: Pain at the base of the thumb in the web space between thumb and index finger; noted swelling or ecchymosis of the thumb or inability to grasp using the thumb and index finger; often tenderness to touch along the index finger side of the thumb.
    - Common mechanism: Involves injury to the UCL. This can occur when the ball strikes the thumb, causing a hyperabduction of the joint and injuring or tearing the UCL.
    - Treatment: May include a thumb spica brace or cast, with some injuries requiring surgery.

- As in other sports, water polo players are susceptible to mallet fingers and de Quervain tenosynovitis.

LOWER EXTREMITY INJURIES

Thigh and Hips (7)

- Injuries to the thigh and hips are not as common as upper extremity injuries but can still occur in water polo players. The majority of injuries stem from the "eggbeater" kick that is unique to the game of water polo and can cause overuse adductor tendinopathies and muscle strains.

- Injury to the thigh muscles can occur during the act of throwing when a player is trying to propel out of the water to gain a height advantage over the opposing player. Most often, this involves the adductors, given the mechanism of propelling out of the water.

- Physical play among players can often result in bruised quadriceps and hamstring muscles.

- Almost all thigh and hip injuries can be managed with conservative treatment, including RICE (rest, ice, compression, elevation) treatment, physical therapy, and massage.

Knee (5,7,9)

- Medial knee pain in water polo players has been reported by Kenal to be as high as 73%. These injuries may include patellofemoral pain syndrome, medial collateral ligament sprains, ligament tears, and meniscus tears.

- As previously stated, water polo players will often use the "eggbeater" kick, which combines the clockwise motion of one leg and the counterclockwise motion of the other leg in order to stay afloat.

- This eggbeater movement causes a significant valgus force along the medial aspect of the knee joint, especially to the medial collateral ligament and medial patellar retinaculum.

- The force from the eggbeater kick with compression on the medial aspect of the joint can cause degenerative changes that can be visible on radiographs.

- The majority of knee injuries can be rehabilitated using RICE treatment and physical therapy focusing on strengthening the core muscles of the quadriceps, hamstrings, and pelvis.

SPINAL INJURIES (4)

- Although not common, spinal cord injuries can occur. All pools should have spine boards and neck collars available, along with qualified personnel to remove players suspected of such injuries from the water.
- Medical personnel should recognize key red flags, including profound muscle weakness and/or reflex loss, bowel and/or bladder incontinence or retention, and saddle numbness and/or sensory changes when dealing with patients complaining of back pain.

Cervical (4,9)

- Given that players constantly rotate their cervical spine when either breathing in freestyle swimming or for rotation to follow the game, degenerative cervical spine changes or complaints can occur.
- Water polo players will often have to keep their heads afloat with periods of sustained extension and protraction, causing common muscle aches, cervicalgias, and radiculopathies.
- Players are trained to alternate the rotation of their head when swimming, so symptoms are often bilateral.
- Acceleration and deceleration injuries and whiplash can also be common cervical injuries with physical play.
- Conservative treatment and physical therapy are often successful in rehabilitation of cervical injuries.

Lumbar (4)

- The lumbar spine can see significant force during throwing and passing of the ball. This can cause many athletes to have hypertrophied latissimus muscles along the dominant arm side.
- Lower back pain can include many different types of injuries, with examples being facet joint syndromes, lumbar disc slips, muscle strains, and overuse injuries.
- Physicians must first rule out red flag symptoms before prescribing treatment. Plain film x-rays are usually not required with acute injuries. The majority of low back pain can be rehabilitated with physical therapy and analgesics. Pain that worsens or is not improved with physical therapy may warrant further imaging and testing.

ENVIRONMENTAL AND MISCELLANEOUS INJURIES

Environmental Injuries (4)

- These injuries can include sunburns, hypothermia, warts, and swimmer's exanthema.
- Sunburns, which are a risk for skin cancer, can occur with outside water polo matches. International water polo rules forbid players from wearing sunblock or sunscreen during play due to causing the ball to be greasy and slippery. Players should make all attempts to wear protective agents during practice.
- Hypothermia is defined as having a core body temperature less than 95°F or 35°C. Exhaustion, wind, and wetness are all risk factors for hypothermia. Depending on the competition environment, hypothermia can occur in all water sports, including water polo.
- A wart is a small painless skin growth caused by a viral infection. Swimming is a known risk factor for warts. There are numerous treatments for warts, including medications, ointments, cryotherapy, burning (electrocautery), surgical removal, and laser treatment.
- Swimmer's xerosis can be caused by hours of submersion in the water, causing the skin to become dehydrated and pruritic. Treatment includes using mild soaps when bathing, avoiding rubbing the skin dry after a shower or bath, and applying an oil-based protective emollient shortly after a shower or bath.

Lacerations (4,7,9)

- Lacerations to face, forehead, and hands are very common in water polo.
- As previously mentioned, the web space tear (when two fingers are forcibly abducted apart) is the most common laceration in water polo.
- Most lacerations can be repaired with Steri-strips or plastic-based waterproof spray. Some lacerations may require stitches.
- Players' fingernails and toenails are usually inspected by the referee before the start of the game in hopes of decreasing the amount of lacerations.

REFERENCES

1. Annett P, Fricker P, McDonald W. Injuries to elite male waterpolo players over a 13 year period. *New Zeal J Sports Med*. 2000;28(4):78–83.
2. Barr A, Baines PS, Desai P, MacEwen CJ. Ocular sports injuries: the current picture. *Br J Sports Med*. 2000;34(6):456–8.
3. Barr D. *A Guide to Water Polo*. London (UK): Sterling Publishing; 1981.
4. Brooks JM. Injuries in water polo. *Clin Sports Med*. 1999;18(2):313–9, vi.
5. Colville JM, Markman BS. Competitive water polo. Upper extremity injuries. *Clin Sports Med*. 1999;18:305–12, vi.
6. Creighton RA, Bach BR, Bush-Joseph CA. Evaluation of the medial elbow in the throwing athlete. *Am J Orthop (Belle Mead NJ)*. 2006;35(6): 266–9.
7. Dominguez RH. Water polo injuries. *Clin Sports Med*. 1986;5:169–83.
8. FINA/USA Water Polo Rules, 2009–2013 [Internet]. [cited 2009 Sep 16]. Available from: http://www.usawaterpolo.org.
9. Franić M, Ivković A, Rudić R. Injuries in water polo. *Croat Med J*. 2007;48(3):281–8.
10. Junge A, Langevoort G, Pipe A, et al. Injuries in team sport tournaments during the 2004 Olympic Games. *Am J Sports Med*. 2006;34(4):565–76.

11. McMaster WC, Long SC, Ciaozzo VJ. Isokinetic torque imbalances in the rotator cuff of the elite water polo player. *Am J Sports Med.* 1991;19(1):72–5.

12. Mountjoy M, Junge A, Alonso JM, et al. Sports injuries and illnesses in the 2009 FINA World Championships (Aquatics). *Br J Sports Med.* 2010;44(7):522–7.

13. Rodriguez JO, Lavina AM, Agarwal A. Prevention and treatment of common eye injuries in sports. *Am Fam Physician.* 2003;67(7): 1481–8.

14. Rybak LP, Johnson DW. Tympanic membrane perforations from water sports: treatment and outcome. *Otolaryngol Head Neck Surg.* 1983;91(6):659–62.

15. Schelkun PH. Swimmer's ear: getting patients back in the water. *Phys Sportsmed.* 1991;19:85–8.

16. Wang MC, Liu CY, Shiao AS, Wang T. Ear problems in swimmers. *J Chin Med Assoc.* 2005;68(8):347–52.

17. Webster MJ, Morris ME, Galna B. Shoulder pain in water polo: a systematic review of the literature. *J Sci Med Sport.* 2009;12(1):3–11.

Weightlifting

110

Joseph M. Hart, Christopher D. Ingersoll, and Christopher M. Kuenze

BASIC MUSCLE PHYSIOLOGY

Skeletal Muscle Contraction

- Several bundles of muscle fibers, called fascicles, comprise a skeletal muscle. A muscle fiber is composed of several myofibrils bundled together. Myofibrils contain a series of sarcomeres arranged end-to-end (20).

- Sarcomeres are the functional and contractile component of skeletal muscle through a dynamic interaction between the proteins actin and myosin.

- According to the sliding filament theory, actin and myosin slide past each other to produce sarcomere shortening. Ca^{++} is released in the sarcomere in response to an action potential that exposes myosin crossbridge binding sites on actin. Myosin crossbridges bind to actin and pull actin filaments closer to the center of each sarcomere, producing force and stiffness within the skeletal muscle (20).

- Force production by a skeletal muscle can be voluntarily graded. However, the muscle fibers innervated by one motor neuron (*i.e.*, a motor unit) act in an all-or-none fashion. As more motor units are recruited in a particular skeletal muscle, the muscle produces more force (20).

Skeletal Muscle Fiber Types

- There are several different muscle fiber types based on structure and function. These include Type I, Type IIA, and Type IIB.

- Type I muscle fibers (slow-twitch, oxidative fibers) have high mitochondria content and a rich blood supply. These fibers are generally smaller in size (diameter) and innervated by smaller diameter axons. Type I fibers contract slowly and are resistant to fatigue because their method of energy metabolism is aerobic. However, Type I fibers produce less tension, resulting in less force production.

- Type IIA muscle fibers (fast-twitch, oxidative-glycolytic fibers) also have high mitochondria content and are moderately capable of performing aerobic and anaerobic metabolism. This fiber type exhibits performance and metabolic characteristics of both Type I and IIB fibers.

- Type IIB muscle fibers (fast-twitch, glycolytic fibers) have sparse mitochondria content and blood supply. They fatigue easily but are capable of producing higher force and tension. Type IIB fibers act in an anaerobic capacity during activity.

- All muscle fibers within a motor unit have the same metabolic characteristics (fiber type). Therefore, motor units can be classified as slow contracting/fatigue resistant (Type I), fast contracting/fatigue resistant (Type IIA), and fast contracting/fatigable (Type IIB). In general, fast-twitch/fatigable motor units are largest (contain the greatest number of innervated fibers) and are highest threshold, whereas slow-twitch/fatigue-resistant motor units are smallest (contain the fewest number of innervated fibers) and are lowest threshold.

- Muscle fiber type composition in a particular human skeletal muscle is genetically determined (20). There is little information regarding muscle fiber type transformations in response to training or exercise.

- Specific training programs have been shown to be effective in targeting improvements in performance of specific fiber types. Heavy resistance training has been shown to cause increased Type IIA fibers and decreased Type IIB fibers, whereas Type I fiber composition in human skeletal muscle was unchanged (1). Low-resistance, high-volume training caused improved muscular endurance, which is thought to indicate an improvement in Type I fiber performance (2,8).

- Structural and genetic characteristics of muscle fiber types have been modulated with fiber-specific stimulation in vitro (19). However, it is unknown whether such changes occur in all muscle fiber types or if the transformation will be sustained over time in vivo.

- Because muscle fiber composition is genetically determined, athletes may participate in sports or activities that involve muscle contractions that are more "natural." Whether a distance runner can train to be a successful power lifter or vice versa is an issue that has not yet been clearly elucidated.

Types of Skeletal Muscle Contraction

- Skeletal muscle can produce joint movements through concentric and eccentric contractions. Skeletal muscle contractions produce muscle tension and control body and joint movement.

- Concentric contractions describe a movement that involves shortening of a muscle against a load, whereas eccentric contractions involve controlled lengthening of a muscle against a load.

741

■ Eccentric muscle contractions produce greater muscle force and more myofibrillar disruption than concentric exercise (9,10).

■ Eccentric muscle contractions (often referred to as "negatives" in weightlifting) are more effective in producing strength gains and hypertrophy than concentric contractions, but they are more likely to cause delayed-onset muscle soreness (7,10,11). However, both eccentric (negative) and concentric (positive) contractions elicit gains in skeletal muscle strength and size (11).

■ Isometric muscle contractions produce muscle tension without joint movement — for example, pushing against a wall or contracting the quadriceps muscle while holding the knee motionless at a particular point in the knee range of motion.

■ Isotonic muscle contractions produce muscle tension and joint movement against a constant load where rate of movement is variable. For example, a dumbbell curl is a contraction against a constant load that can be voluntarily moved at a self-selected rate. This is the most typical contraction in weightlifting.

■ Isokinetic muscle contractions involve a constant rate of joint displacement that is maintained by varying amounts of resistance based on muscle effort. This is uncommon in weightlifting or athletic settings. Isokinetic exercise requires expensive machinery and is usually most applicable in the rehabilitation setting.

■ Isotonic and isokinetic muscle movements can be performed through concentric or eccentric muscle contractions.

Muscle Response to Resistance Training

■ Improvements in muscle strength, power, or endurance are best achieved by overloading the muscle(s) being trained.

■ The *overload* principle states that when a muscle is exposed to a stress or load that is greater than what it usually experiences, it will adapt so that it is able to handle the greater load (17,20,29).

■ Similarly, the *SAID* principle (specific adaptations to imposed demands) states that a muscle or body tissue will adapt to the specific demands imposed on it. For example, if a muscle is overloaded, its fibers will grow in size so it is able to produce enough force to overcome the imposed load (20,29).

■ Observed strength gains within the first few weeks of a weightlifting program are mostly due to neuromuscular adaptations (6). As exercise intensity increases and muscles begin to fatigue, the nervous system recruits larger motor units with faster contraction rates and higher tension-production capabilities to provide the force necessary to overcome the imposed resistance (20).

■ Muscular strength has been defined as the maximum force or tension output generated by a muscle or muscles during a specific task. Related to muscle strength, muscular power refers to not only the ability of a muscle or muscles to generate force, but also the rate at which force can be developed.

■ Early strength gains and increased muscle tension production from training result from a more efficient neural recruitment process, as well as more densely packed protein filaments within the skeletal muscle (24).

Muscle Hypertrophy

■ Human skeletal muscle hypertrophy occurs when the cross-sectional area of a muscle fiber increases (5,24). As a skeletal muscle hypertrophies, contractile proteins are synthesized (6), and the muscle is therefore capable of producing more tension.

■ Type IIA fibers exhibit the greatest growth, whereas Type IIB and Type I fibers exhibit the least amount of growth in response to heavy resistance training (6). Muscle hypertrophy is more common in fast-twitch than slow-twitch muscles.

■ Strength training leads to muscle hypertrophy, which increases muscle mass (24).

■ Muscle hypertrophy is typically observed with resistance training after 6–7 weeks of strength training (6,17).

■ There appears to be a gender difference in the rate at which muscles hypertrophy favoring males (12). Additionally, females lose muscle mass quicker than males when detrained (12).

■ Resistance-trained muscles hypertrophy in order to adapt to greater imposed loads (15). Hypertrophy of individual muscle fibers contributes to changes in muscle cross-sectional area (22). Muscle fiber hyperplasia does not appear to play a role in increased muscle cross-sectional area or strength gains in resistance-trained men (22).

■ In general, it is thought that strengthening exercises using a resistance that is greater than the 6-repetition maximum (RM) are best for muscle hypertrophy, whereas those at a resistance of less than the 20-RM are best for endurance training (16). Simply stated, fewer repetitions using higher weights are best for strength gains, whereas more repetitions using lower weights are best for endurance gains.

BASIC WEIGHTLIFTING PROGRAMS

■ There are several different weightlifting programs that can be customized to an individual or their strength training and athletic goals. An effective program balances muscle overloading with recovery time to facilitate strength gains. Sample weightlifting sets based on the DeLorme and daily adjusted progressive resistance exercise (DAPRE) methods are presented in Table 110.1.

The DeLorme Method

■ The DeLorme method is a progressive resistance exercise program based on the overload principle (6,26). This method is based on the 10-RM. First, a weight that the athlete is able to lift 10 times (with the desired muscle group[s]) is determined. A total of three sets of 10 repetitions are performed per session for each muscle at 50%, 75%, and

	DeLorme (26)	DAPRE (13,14)
Table 110.1	**Weightlifting Programs**	
Set 1	50% 10-RM* × 10 reps	50% 6-RM† × 10 reps
Set 2	75% 10-RM × 10 reps	75% 6-RM × 6 reps
Set 3	100% 10-RM × 10 reps	100% 6-RM to failure
Set 4	—	Adjusted‡ weight to failure

*10-RM = maximum amount of weight with which one can perform 10 consecutive repetitions.

†6-RM = maximum amount of weight with which one can perform 6 consecutive repetitions.

‡Adjusted weight: Add 5 lb if > 7 repetitions in third set; subtract 5 lb if < 4 repetitions in third set; no change if 4–7 repetitions performed in third set.

100% of the 10-RM. The athlete is encouraged to perform more than 10 repetitions during the third set to serve as an overload to the muscle group being trained. As the athlete's 10-RM increases, so does the resistance in each set (see Table 110.1).

Daily Adjusted Progressive Resistance Exercise (DAPRE)

- The DAPRE method of strength training guides the athlete through four sets of exercise per muscle group or other desired task. DAPRE guidelines provide recommendations for when to increase resistance and how much added resistance is appropriate based on individual performance (see Table 110.1) (13,14).

- A total of four sets of repetitions are performed per muscle group.

  - First and second sets: Perform 10 repetitions at 50% and 6 repetitions at 75% of the predetermined 6-RM (the maximum weight that can be successfully "lifted" for 6 repetitions). The 6-RM is termed the "working weight."

  - Third set: 100% of the working weight is used, and repetitions are performed until failure is reached (as many repetitions as safely possible).

  - Fourth set: An "adjusted weight" is used, and repetitions are performed until failure is reached. To calculate the "adjusted weight" for the fourth set in this program, the number of repetitions performed in the third set is considered. If five to seven repetitions were performed in the third set, "adjusted" resistance for the fourth set remains the same. If less than five repetitions were performed, the adjusted weight is reduced for the fourth set; if more than seven repetitions were performed, the adjusted weight in the fourth set is increased. For example, if the athlete performs 12 repetitions of 100 lb in the third set, the weight for the fourth set can be increased to 105 lb. If only three repetitions are performed in the third set using 100 lb, the fourth set adjusted weight should be reduced to 90 or 95 lb.

- Next session guidelines: The "working weight" for the next day of resistance training is adjusted based on the number of repetitions achieved in the fourth set similar to the method used to adjust the weight for the fourth set. Using the example above, if the athlete can perform 10 repetitions during the fourth exercise set using 105 lb, he or she can adjust the working weight for the next day to 105 or 110 lb.

- The DAPRE method can be adjusted for each individual based on his or her training goals. Manipulating the amount of weight added to the adjusted weight for the fourth set or the modified working weight for the next day's lift can change the pace of individual programs.

Periodization

- Periodization (6,17,29) is a specific approach to strength training and conditioning that is intended to bring about peak performance at a desired time, typically at the time of competition.

- A macrocycle is a long-term plan of exercise progression with the goal of achieving peak performance at the time of competition. Commonly, macrocycles are composed of preparation, competitive, and transition phases. For seasonal sports participants, a macrocycle will include a calendar year that is divided into the following mesocycles: preseason, in-season, and off-season.

- A mesocycle is a shorter phase of training that makes up a portion of a macrocycle with variable length depending on the training goals and length of the macrocycle. The volume and intensity of an activity during these cycles should be determined by the goals of the macrocycle and response of the individual.

- Over the course of an athlete's macrocycle of periodization, training intensity, volume, and mode will change to allow for maximum performance and minimum risk for injury and overuse. For an Olympic athlete, a macrocycle may be 4 years, where periodized training regimens are tailored to maximize performance at the desired time(s).

- In preparation for athletic competition, linear periodization begins in the athletic off-season, where training volume is high but intensity is low. Initially, strength gains and muscle hypertrophy are the goals of this phase. As training intensity gradually increases through the postseason and into the preseason, training volume decreases. This progression continues through the preseason where sport-specific skill training is maximized to facilitate the transition to competition.

- Undulating periodization has been shown to be more effective in producing strength gains and muscle hypertrophy when compare with traditional linear paradigms. This method includes the use of varied resistance (*e.g.*, 3- to 5-RM, 8- to 10-RM, and 12- to 15-RM) while completing multiple sets of the same exercise within a single training session (3). It remains unclear how implementation of this paradigm may affect functional performance goals or the transition from preseason training to in-season performance (3).

SAMPLE EXERCISES FOR MAJOR MUSCLE GROUPS

■ There are several exercises that can be used for each muscle group. The appropriate exercise depends on equipment availability, experience or preference of the weightlifter, and training goals. Isolated muscle exercises are appropriate for toning and strengthening muscles. Whole-body strength exercises that require coordinated, multiple body segment movements are appropriate to develop power and athletic skill.

Upper Body/Trunk

■ Seated military press (deltoid): In the seated position, weighted dumbbells or a bar is lifted above the head and then returned to the anterior shoulders/upper chest.

■ Bench press (pectoralis major): While supine on a bench, weighted dumbbells or a bar is lifted off the chest until the arms are fully extended and then lowered slowly back to the chest.

■ Bicep curls (biceps brachii): In the seated or standing position, weighted dumbbells or a bar is lifted through the full elbow range of motion from the extended to flexed position and then returned slowly back to the extended position

■ Triceps extension (triceps brachii): While in the supine position, with shoulders flexed to 90 degrees and elbows extended, resistance is lowered by flexing the elbow, followed by concentric elbow extension.

■ Rows (trapezius/rhomboids): In the seated or standing position and with shoulders flexed to 90 degrees, arms are drawn back by extending the shoulders and flexing the elbows. Visualize "squeezing" the back blades (scapula) together. This exercise can be done with free-weights, resistive bands, or a machine.

Lower Body

■ Squats (quadriceps): In the standing position with resistance fixed at the shoulders, the body is lowered by flexing the hips and knees while maintaining upright upper body posture.

■ Hamstring curls (hamstrings): In the prone position, resistance fixed at the distal lower leg is curled toward the hips by flexing the knee. This is usually done with the assistance of a pulley-style machine, or it can be done in standing with ankle weights.

■ Calf raises (triceps surae): In the standing or seated position, the body, with added resistance (if desired), is elevated by plantarflexing the ankle joint.

GUIDELINES FOR EXERCISE PRESCRIPTION (TABLE 110.2)

Training Volume and Intensity

■ It is important to consider training volume and intensity of training when designing an effective weightlifting program. The goal of a weightlifting program is to achieve maximal or desired gains while allowing for an appropriate amount of time between sets and between sessions for muscle and body recovery.

■ Training volume is determined by multiplying the number of repetitions performed in an exercise session by the resistance used (17). Therefore, similar training volumes are achieved when light resistance is used for high repetitions and when heavy resistance is used for low repetitions. In periodized programs, it is appropriate to begin with high training volumes (off-season) and progress to lower volumes at higher intensity (preseason) leading to more sport-specific skills, with concurrent programs aimed at maintaining strength and conditioning while in-season.

■ Intensity is analogous to power and is therefore dependent on the amount of resistance and the speed of the movement (28). High training intensities are appropriate in the preseason and can coincide with sport-specific training.

■ Overtraining can result in decreases in muscle strength and function. It usually occurs when either training volume or intensity is too great and the body cannot appropriately adapt (4).

■ When designing an exercise or weightlifting program, it is important to include activities that are specific to the athlete's goals. For example, if an athlete wants to perform movements that require high muscle strength and power, the athlete should train with weights that are closer to his or her 1-RM and perform fewer repetitions per set (29). Likewise, if an athlete wants to perform movements that require endurance, the athlete should use less weight with higher repetitions.

■ The athletic year is divided into in-season, postseason and off-season, and preseason segments. During the postseason and off-season, training should concentrate on recovery from the competitive season and maintain fitness and strength. Strength training can begin in the off-season and gradually progress to power training and sport-specific training during preseason. Strength, endurance, and power maintenance should be performed in-season.

REST PERIODS

■ Structured rest periods between sets are important to maximize the effectiveness of a resistance training program. Appropriate rest frequency and duration can allow for maximal performance during each set of a specific task and positively affect the metabolic effects of resistance training (18,25).

| Table 110.2 | Summary of Progressive Resistance Training Recommendations from the ACSM Position Stand (25). Each Recommendation is Listed with an A, B, C or D Indicating the Quality or Quantity of Research Supporting that Statement; A is the Best |

Evidence Statement	Grade
Strength training	
CON, ECC, and ISOM actions should be included for novice, intermediate, and advanced training.	A
Training with loads ~60%–70% of 1-RM for 8–12 repetitions for novice to intermediate individuals and cycling loads of 80%–100% of 1-RM for advanced individuals.	A
When training at a specific RM load, it is recommended that a 2%–10% increase in load be applied when the individual can perform the current workload for 1–2 repetitions over the desired number on 2 consecutive training sessions.	B
It is recommended that 1–3 sets per exercise be used by novice individuals.	A
Multiple-set programs (with systematic variation of volume and intensity) are recommended for progression to intermediate and advanced training.	A
Unilateral and bilateral single- and multiple-joint exercises should be included, with emphasis on multiple-joint exercises for maximizing strength in novice, intermediate, and advanced individuals.	A
Free-weight and machine exercises should be included for novice to intermediate training.	A
For advanced strength training, it is recommended that emphasis be placed on free-weight exercises with machine exercises used to compliment program needs.	C
Recommendations for sequencing exercises for novice, intermediate, and advanced strength training include large muscle group exercises before small muscle group exercises, multiple-joint exercises before single-joint exercises, higher intensity exercises before lower intensity exercises, or rotation of upper and lower body or opposing exercises.	C
It is recommended that rest periods of at least 2–3 minutes be used for core exercises using heavier loads for novice, intermediate, and advanced training. For assistance exercises, a shorter rest period length of 1–2 minutes may suffice.	B C
For untrained individuals, it is recommended that slow and moderate CON velocities be used.	A
For intermediate training, it is recommended that moderate CON velocity be used.	A
For advanced training, the inclusion of a continuum of velocities from unintentionally slow to fast CON velocities is recommended and should correspond to the intensity.	C
It is recommended that novice individuals train the entire body 2–3 days a week.	A
It is recommended that for progression to intermediate training, a frequency of 3–4 days a week be used (based on how many muscle groups are trained per workout).	B
It is recommended that advanced lifters train 4–6 days a week.	C
Muscle hypertrophy	
It is recommended that CON, ECC, and ISOM muscle actions be included.	A
For novice and intermediate training, it is recommended that moderate loading be used (70%–85% of 1-RM) for 8–12 repetitions per set for 1–3 sets per exercise.	A
For advanced training, it is recommended that a loading range of 70%–100% of 1-RM be used for 1–12 repetitions per set for 3–6 sets per exercise in a periodized manner such that the majority of training is devoted to 6- to 12-RM and less training devoted to 1- to 6-RM loading.	A
It is recommended that single- and multiple-joint free-weight and machine exercises be included in novice, intermediate, and advanced individuals.	A
For exercise sequencing, an order similar to strength training is recommended.	C
It is recommended that 1- to 3-minute rest periods be used in novice and intermediate training; for advanced training, length of rest period should correspond to the goals of each exercise such that 2- to 3-minute rest periods may be used with heavy loading for core exercises and 1- to 2-minute rest periods may be used for other exercises of moderate to moderately high intensity.	C
It is recommended that slow to moderate velocities be used by novice and intermediate-trained individuals; for advanced training, it is recommended that slow, moderate, and fast repetition velocities be used depending on the load, repetition number, and goals of the particular exercise.	C
It is recommended that a frequency of 2–3 days a week be used for novice training.	A
For intermediate training, the recommendation is similar for total body workouts or 4 days a week when using an upper/lower body split routine.	B
For advanced training, a frequency of 4–6 days a week is recommended.	C

(Continued)

| Table 110.2 | Summary of Progressive Resistance Training Recommendations from the ACSM Position Stand (25). Each Recommendation is Listed with an A, B, C or D Indicating the Quality or Quantity of Research Supporting that Statement; A is the Best (*continued*) |

Evidence Statement	Grade
Muscle power	
The use of predominately multiple-joint exercises performed with sequencing guidelines similar to strength training is recommended for novice, intermediate, and advanced power training.	B
It is recommended that concurrent to a typical strength-training program, a power component is incorporated consisting of 1–3 sets per exercise using light to moderate loading (30%–60% of 1-RM for upper body exercises, 0%–60% of 1-RM for lower body exercises) for 3–6 repetitions not to failure.	A
Various loading strategies are recommended for advanced training. Heavy loading (85%–100% of 1-RM) is necessary for increasing force, and light to moderate loading (30%–60% of 1-RM for upper body exercises, 0%–60% of 1-RM for lower body exercises) performed at an explosive velocity is necessary for increasing fast force production.	B
A multiple-set (3–6 sets) power program integrated into a strength-training program consisting of 1–6 repetitions in a periodized manner is recommended.	A
Rest periods of at least 2–3 minutes between sets for core exercises are recommended when intensity is high. For assistance exercises and those of less intensity, a shorter rest interval (1–2 minutes) is recommended.	D
The recommended frequency for novice power training is similar to strength training (2–3 days a week).	A
For intermediate power training, it is recommended that either a total-body or upper/lower body split workout be used for a frequency of 3–4 days a week.	C
For advanced power training, a frequency of 4–5 days a week is recommended using predominantly total-body or upper/lower body split workouts.	C
Local muscular endurance	
It is recommended that unilateral and bilateral multiple- and single-joint exercises be included using various sequencing combinations for novice, intermediate, and advanced local muscular endurance training.	A
For novice and intermediate training, it is recommended that relatively light loads be used (10–15 repetitions) with moderate to high volume.	A
For advanced training, it is recommended that various loading strategies be used for multiple sets per exercise (10–25 repetitions or more) in a periodized manner, leading to a higher overall volume using lighter intensities.	C
It is recommended that short rest periods be used for muscular endurance training, *e.g.*, 1–2 minutes for high-repetition sets (15–20 repetitions or more) and less than 1 minute for moderate (10–15 repetitions) sets. For circuit weight training, it is recommended that rest periods correspond to the time needed to get from one exercise station to another.	C
Low frequency (2–3 days a week) is effective in novice individuals when training the entire body.	A
For intermediate training, 3 days a week are recommended for total-body workouts, and 4 days a week are recommended for upper/lower body split routine workouts.	C
For advanced training, a higher frequency may be used (4–6 days a week) if muscle group split routines are used.	C
It is recommended that intentionally slow velocities be used when a moderate number of repetitions (10–15) are used.	B
If performing a large number of repetitions (15–25 or more), then moderate to faster velocities are recommended.	B
Motor performance	
It is recommended that multiple-joint exercises be performed using a combination of heavy and light to moderate loading (using fast repetition velocity) with moderate-to-high volume in periodized fashion 4–6 days a week for maximal progression in vertical jumping ability. The inclusion of plyometric training (explosive form of exercise involving various jumps) in combination with resistance training is recommended.	B
It is recommended that the combination of heavy resistance and ballistic resistance exercise (along with sprint and plyometric training) be included for progression in sprinting ability.	B
Older adults	
For further improvements in strength and hypertrophy in older adults, the use of both multiple- and single-joint exercises (free weights and machines), with slow to moderate lifting velocity, for 1–3 sets per exercise with 60%–80% of 1-RM for 8–12 repetitions with 1–3 minutes of rest in between sets for 2–3 days a week, is recommended.	A
Increasing power in healthy older adults includes (a) training to improve muscular strength and (b) the performance of both single- and multiple-joint exercises for 1–3 sets per exercise using light-to-moderate loading (30%–60% of 1-RM) for 6–10 repetitions with high repetition velocity.	B
Similar recommendations may apply to older adults as to young adults, *e.g.*, low to moderate loads performed for moderate-to-high repetitions (10–15 or more), for enhancing muscular endurance.	B

CON, concentric; ECC, eccentric; ISOM, isometric; RM, repetition maximum.

■ Rest time should increase as the intensity of the exercise increases. Currently, there is no gold standard for rest time between sets. It has been suggested that for low resistance (11- to 13-RM), a 1- to 2-minute rest is appropriate; however, for moderate-resistance (8- to 10-RM) and high-resistance exercise ($<$ 5-RM), rest times of 3–5 and $>$ 5 minutes, respectively, may be better (16).

SPECIAL CONSIDERATIONS

■ Strength describes the maximum force that can be generated by a muscle, whereas power is the ability of a muscle to generate large forces quickly. Endurance is the ability of a muscle to contract repeatedly and generate forces for long periods of time.

■ Training for muscle strength should include training with resistance that is closer to maximum ability with lower repetitions. This type of training is most appropriate in the athletic off-season.

■ Training for muscle power involves coordinated movements that encourage speed, accuracy, and fluency. Power training is most appropriate in the athletic preseason and gradually progresses to the competitive season (in-season).

■ Strength training in both the anterior and posterior musculature or training both agonist and antagonist muscle groups is important in an effective strength-training program. It may improve sport- or activity-specific performance and reduce the risk of injury (27).

■ It is important to incorporate gradual warm-up, cool-down, and flexibility exercises into a strength-training regimen to maintain muscle health and fitness, reduce the likelihood of injury or postexercise soreness, and improve athletic and weightlifting performance. Dynamic activity-specific warm-up and cool-down plans are commonly used to prepare the athlete for resistance training while including specific activities from the athlete's sport (23).

■ Supervised and guided strength-training programs yield greater strength gains than those that are unsupervised (21). Recruiting assistance from certified strength and conditioning specialists (CSCSs), exercise physiologists, certified personal trainers (CPTs), or certified athletic trainers (ATCs) may facilitate strength gains and improve overall outcomes and sport-specific preparedness.

■ Finally, athletes are encouraged to participate in weightlifting programs with at least one partner. Weightlifting partners can motivate each other, provide constructive feedback on technique and form, and provide "spotting" for heavy or potentially dangerous lifts. An athlete should never participate in weightlifting alone.

REFERENCES

1. Adams GR, Hather BM, Baldwin KM, Dudley GA. Skeletal muscle myosin heavy chain composition and resistance training. *J Appl Physiol.* 1993;74(2):911–5.

2. Anderson T, Kearney JT. Effects of three resistance training programs on muscular strength and absolute and relative endurance. *Res Q Exerc Sport.* 1982;53(1):1–7.

3. Baker D, Wilson G, Carlyon R. Periodization: the effect on strength of manipulating volume and intensity. *J Strength Cond Res.* 1994:235–42.

4. Brown LE. Nonlinear versus linear periodization models. *J Strength Cond Res.* 2001;23:42–4.

5. Conroy BP, Earle RW. Bone, muscle, and connective tissue adaptations to physical activity. In: Baechle TR, editor. *Essentials of Strength Training and Conditioning.* Champaign (IL): Human Kinetics; 1994. p. 435–46.

6. Deschenes MR, Kraemer WJ. Performance and physiologic adaptations to resistance training. *Am J Phys Med Rehabil.* 2002;81(11 Suppl):S3–16.

7. Ebbeling CB, Clarkson PM. Exercise-induced muscle damage and adaptation. *Sports Med.* 1989;7(4):207–34.

8. Ebben WP, Kindler AG, Chirdon KA, Jenkins NC, Polichnowski AJ, Ng AV. The effect of high-load vs. high-repetition training on endurance performance. *J Strength Cond Res.* 2004;18(3):513–7.

9. Gibala MJ, MacDougall JD, Tarnopolsky MA, Stauber WT, Elorriaga A. Changes in human skeletal muscle ultrastructure and force production after acute resistance exercise. *J Appl Physiol.* 1995;78(2):702–8.

10. Hather BM, Tesch PA, Buchanan P, Dudley GA. Influence of eccentric actions on skeletal muscle adaptations to resistance training. *Acta Physiol Scand.* 1991;143(2):177–85.

11. Higbie EJ, Cureton KJ, Warren GL III, Prior BM. Effects of concentric and eccentric training on muscle strength, cross-sectional area, and neural activation. *J Appl Physiol.* 1996;81(5):2173–81.

12. Ivey FM, Roth SM, Ferrell RE, et al. Effects of age, gender, and myostatin genotype on the hypertrophic response to heavy resistance strength training. *J Gerontol A Biol Sci Med Sci.* 2000;55(11):M641–8.

13. Knight KL. Knee rehabilitation by the daily adjustable progressive resistive exercise technique. *Am J Sports Med.* 1979;7(6):336–7.

14. Knight KL. Quadriceps strengthening with the DAPRE technique: case studies with neurological implications. *Med Sci Sports Exerc.* 1985;17(6):646–50.

15. Kraemer WJ. General adaptations to resistance and endurance training programs. In: Baechle TR, editor. *Essentials of Strength Training and Conditioning.* Champaign (IL): Human Kinetics; 1994. p. 127–50.

16. Kraemer WJ. Strength training basics: designing workouts to meet patients' goals. *Phys Sportsmed.* 2003;31(8):39–45.

17. Kraemer WJ, Adams K, Cafarelli E, et al. American College of Sports Medicine position stand. Progression models in resistance training for healthy adults. *Med Sci Sports Exerc.* 2002;34:364–80.

18. Kraemer WJ, Noble BJ, Clark MJ, Culver BW. Physiologic responses to heavy-resistance exercise with very short rest periods. *Int J Sports Med.* 1987;8(4):247–52.

19. Liu Y, Cseresnyés Z, Randall WR, Schneider MF. Activity-dependent nuclear translocation and intranuclear distribution of NFATc in adult skeletal muscle fibers. *J Cell Biol.* 2001;155(1):27–39.

20. Lorenz T, Campello M. Biomechanics of skeletal muscle. In: Nordin M, Frankel VH, editors. *Basic Biomechanics of the Musculoskeletal System.* Philadelphia (PA): Lippincott Williams & Wilkins; 2001. p. 148–74.

21. Mazzetti SA, Kraemer WJ, Volek JS, et al. The influence of direct supervision of resistance training on strength performance. *Med Sci Sports Exerc.* 2000;32(6):1175–84.

22. McCall GE, Byrnes WC, Dickinson A, Pattany PM, Fleck SJ. Muscle fiber hypertrophy, hyperplasia, and capillary density in college men after resistance training. *J Appl Physiol.* 1996;81(5):2004–12.

23. McHugh MP, Cosgrave CH. To stretch or not to stretch: the role of stretching in injury prevention and performance. *Scand J Med Sci Sports.* 2010;20(2):169–81.

24. Narici MV, Hoppeler H, Kayser B, et al. Human quadriceps cross-sectional area, torque and neural activation during 6 months strength training. *Acta Physiol Scand.* 1996;157(2):175–86.

25. Ratamess NA, Falvo MJ, Mangine GT, Hoffman JR, Faigenbaum AD, Kang J. The effect of rest interval length on metabolic responses to the bench press exercise. *Eur J Appl Physiol.* 2007;100(1): 1–17.

26. Stamford B. Weight training basics part 2: a sample program. *Phys Sportmed.* 1998;26(3):91–2.

27. Wathen D. Exercise selection. In: Baechle TR, editor. *Essentials of Strength Training and Conditioning.* Champaign (IL): Human Kinetics; 1994. p. 416–30.

28. Wathen D. Load assignment. In: Baechle TR, editor. *Essentials of Strength Training and Conditioning.* Champaign (IL): Human Kinetics; 1994. p. 435–46.

29. Wathen D, Roll F. Training methods and modes. In: Baechle TR, editor. *Essentials of Strength Training and Conditioning.* Champaign (IL): Human Kinetics; 1994. p. 403–15.

Wheelchair Sports

Arthur Jason De Luigi, Kevin F. Fitzpatrick, and Paul F. Pasquina

111

INTRODUCTION

- Athletes with disabilities have been participating in organized sports competition since at least 1948.

- A variety of organized athletic events are available for athletes with disabilities. Some involve the use of the wheelchair. Many others are available for patients with disabilities who do not require the use of a wheelchair.

- Events and competitions are structured to ensure optimal competition by creating groups of athletes with similar levels of disability. The classification systems vary depending on the event.

- Disabled athletes present different medical concerns as compared with able-bodied athletes.

- A review of specific medical concerns in various causes of disability is presented in the Chapter 117 (The Disabled Athlete). This chapter will summarize some of the athletic events and competitions available to disabled athletes. In addition, a summary of providing medical care to athletes participating in wheelchair sports will be provided.

HISTORY OF WHEELCHAIR SPORTS

- In 1948, Sir Ludwig Guttmann organized a sports competition involving World War II veterans with a spinal cord injury in Stoke Mandeville, England. This event is considered the first organized athletic competition for athletes with disabilities.

- Four years later, competitors from the Netherlands joined the games, and an international movement was born.

- Olympic-style games for athletes with disabilities were organized for the first time in Rome in 1960, now called Paralympics. In Toronto in 1976, additional disability groups were added. The idea of merging together different disability groups for international sport competitions was born. In the same year, the first Paralympic Winter Games took place in Sweden.

PARALYMPIC GAMES

- The Paralympic Games is currently the world's elite sporting event for athletes with disabilities. Emphasis is placed on the participants' athletic achievements rather than their disabilities.

- The term "Paralympics" derives from the Greek preposition "para" (beside or alongside) and Olympics. The name was originally intended as a pun combining "paraplegic" and "Olympic." However, the term is now used as a combination of "parallel" and "Olympic" to illustrate how the two movements exist side by side.

- Paralympic athletes are divided into six different groups based on the nature of their disabilities: amputee, cerebral palsy, visual impairment, spinal cord injuries, intellectual disability, and a group that includes all athletes who do not fit into the aforementioned groups ("les autres").

- The Paralympics movement has grown dramatically since its first days. The games originated in Rome in 1960 and included 400 athletes from 23 countries. In Beijing in 2008, 3,951 athletes from 146 countries competed. The fact that more countries competed at the Beijing 2008 Paralympics than in the Munich 1972 Olympic Games speaks to the growing popularity and scope of the Paralympic Games.

- Since their founding, the Paralympic Games have been held in the same year as the Olympic Games. Since 1988 (Summer Paralympic Games in Seoul, Korea) and 1992 (Winter Paralympic Games in Albertville, France), the Paralympic Games have used the same venues as the Olympic Games. In 2001, an agreement was reached between the International Olympic Committee (IOC) and the International Paralympic Committee (IPC) securing this practice for the future.

- From 2012 onward, the host city chosen to host the Olympic Games will be obliged to also host the Paralympics.

GROUPS AND CLASSIFICATIONS

- Disabled athletes are grouped in disability categories (http://www.paralympics.org, IPC Classification Code) and compete against athletes with similar disabilities. As previously identified, the groups currently defined by the IPC are amputee, cerebral palsy, visual impairment, spinal injury, intellectual disability, and les autres.

- Les autres (French for "the others") includes all athletes with disabilities who do not fit into any of the other five groups. Examples include dwarfism, multiple sclerosis, congenital limb deformities, and others.

- In 2000, the intellectual disability group was suspended by the IPC after allegations of cheating in the intellectual disability basketball competition. It was revealed that several athletes were not disabled. In November 2009, the IPC voted to reinstate the intellectual disability group.

- To ensure fairness in competition, athletes within a group are classified based on the extent of their disability. Athlete classification is intended to determine an athlete's eligibility to compete and to group athletes for competition.

- To be eligible for competition in the Paralympics, an athlete "must have an impairment that leads to a permanent and verifiable Activity Limitation," and the impairment "should limit the Athlete's ability to compete equitably in elite sport with Athletes without impairment." (IPC Classification Code) (5).

- Athletes are assessed based on their medical records, evaluation of physical capabilities, and observation of the athlete in training and competition.

- Each sport has its own rules and classification systems. An example is wheelchair basketball, which is governed by the International Wheelchair Basketball Federation (IWBF).

- Wheelchair basketball athletes are assigned a point value that is equal to their class (3). An athlete may be assigned a class from 1.0 to 4.5. The rules of wheelchair basketball state that a team must have no more than 14 "points" on the court at any one time.

- To determine the athlete's class, each player is observed during a team's practice and games. A classification panel assigns a class to the athlete based on the following points system:

  - The class 1.0 player: Little or no controlled trunk movement in the forward plane; no active trunk rotation; balance in both forward and sideways directions is significantly impaired; players rely on their arms to return to the upright position when unbalanced.

  - The class 2.0 player: Partially controlled trunk movement in the forward plane; active upper trunk rotation but no lower trunk function; no controlled sideways movement.

  - The class 3.0 player: Good trunk movement in the forward direction; good trunk rotation; no controlled trunk movements sideways.

  - The class 4.0 player: Normal trunk movements, but usually due to limitations in one lower limb, the player has difficulty with controlled movement to one side.

  - The class 4.5 player: Normal trunk movement in all directions; able to reach side to side with no limitations.

MEDICAL CARE OF ATHLETES WITH DISABILITIES

- Athletes with disabilities and athletes in wheelchairs are subject to many of the same injuries and complications from participation in sporting events as able-bodied athletes.

However, many additional considerations make the treatment of disabled athletes unique.

- The Chapter 117 (The Disabled Athlete) contains a complete list of conditions that may affect athletes participating in wheelchair sports, and thus, this will not be discussed here.

- Wheelchair athletes have often experienced previous traumatic injuries that may affect their medical condition during competition. For example, wheelchair athletes may have hardware including screws, plates, or pins that could predispose to further injury; x-rays for new injuries may be complicated by the appearance of previous skeletal injuries; and athletes with a history of traumatic brain injury, splenectomy, or nephrectomy require special attention and safeguards. Awareness of previous traumatic history and injuries is crucial to providing medical care to wheelchair athletes.

- Wheelchair athletes are often insensate below the level of a spinal cord injury or other neurologic insult. This may create difficulty and confusion in identifying or diagnosing neuromusculoskeletal injuries. For example, in a wheelchair athlete with a complete lumbar spinal cord injury who is insensate in the lower limbs, the athlete may not immediately realize the severity of the injury due to lack of sensation and pain in the ankle. This situation requires increased vigilance when screening for and diagnosing neuromusculoskeletal injuries in wheelchair athletes.

- In addition to musculoskeletal injuries, athletes with loss of sensation are at increased risk for other complications including skin breakdown, skin infections, and septic arthritis.

- Because of the high rate of spinal cord injuries among wheelchair athletes, there is a need to increase the awareness and monitoring for conditions associated with spinal cord injuries when caring for wheelchair athletes. Among the conditions that may complicate athletic participation for wheelchair athletes are autonomic dysreflexia, orthostatic hypotension, deep venous thrombosis, skin breakdown, spasticity, thermoregulation abnormalities, and heterotopic ossification.

COMMON INJURIES AND PREVENTION

- Wheelchair athletes and disabled athletes have approximately the same incidence of injuries as able-bodied athletes.

- Due to the adaptive equipment used by disabled athletes, different patterns and types of injuries may be experienced as compared with able-bodied athletes. These patterns and injuries may change with changes in equipment and technology.

- A survey (1) of participants in the 1989 national championships of the National Wheelchair Athletic Association (NWAA), U.S. Association of Blind Athletes (USABA), and U.S. Cerebral Palsy Athletic Association (USCPAA) showed the following incidence of injury during the competitions:

  - NWAA: 26% of athletes reported injuries; 57% of injuries involved the shoulder and arm/elbow.

- USABA: 37% of athletes reported injuries; 53% of injuries involved the lower limb.
- USCPAA: 37% of athletes reported injuries; 21% were knee injuries.

- In disabled skiing, the incidence of injury is similar to the incidence in able-bodied skiers. A survey published in 1992 (4) showed that disabled skiers are injured at a rate of about 3.7 per 1,000 skiing days, whereas able-bodied skiers were injured at a rate of about 3.5 per 1,000 skiing days. However, there were significant differences in the types of injuries sustained. Able-bodied skiers sustained more fractures and lacerations, whereas disabled skiers sustained more bruises and abrasions. Another study (2) of disabled skiers showed that these athletes are 1.4 times more likely to injure their upper extremity as compared to the lower extremity. This may be related to inherent instability in three-track skis, which are often used by disabled skiers, and the inability of many disabled skiers to break a fall with the lower limbs as an able-bodied skier would.

- Elite wheelchair athletes may have different risks for traumatic injuries and overuse injuries due to the demands of training, intensity of competition, and differences in physical conditioning as compared with recreational athletes.

- Several studies of injuries in elite disabled athletes at the Paralympic Games have been published.

- At the 2002 Winter Paralympic Games (6), 9% of athletes experienced injuries. The most common injuries were sprains (32% of injuries), fractures (21%), and lacerations (14%). Following 2002, it was noted that many of the fractures sustained were lower limb fractures in athletes participating in the sledge hockey event. As a result, regulations were modified to require increased protection for the lower limbs and also to change the sledge design to reduce the chance of one sledge overriding another.

- At the 2006 Winter Paralympic Games (7), 8% of athletes were injured, including 8% of males and 8.5% of females. Incidence of injuries was significantly higher in the alpine (12%) and sledge hockey (11%) events as compared with the Nordic/biathlon (4%) and curling (0%) events. Notably, no lower limb injuries were reported in the sledge hockey competition.

- No concussions were reported at the 2002 or 2006 Winter Paralympic Games.

REFERENCES

1. Ferrara MS, Buckley WE, McCann BC, Limbird TJ, Powell JW, Robl R. The injury experience of the competitive athlete with a disability: prevention implications. *Med Sci Sports Exerc.* 1992;24(2):184–8.

2. Ferrara MS, Buckley WE, Messner DG, Benedict J. The injury experience and training history of the competitive skier with a disability. *Am J Sports Med.* 1992;20(1):55–60.

3. International Wheelchair Basketball Federation Official Player Classification Manual. Ver#1 01.09.2010 [Internet]. [cited 2010 Oct]. Available from: http://www.iwbf.org.

4. Laskowski ER, Murtaugh PA. Snow skiing injuries in physically disabled skiers. *Am J Sports Med.* 1992;20(1):55–60.

5. Official Website of Paralympic Movement [Internet]. [cited 2011 Dec 7]. Available from: http://www.paralympic.org/export/sites/default/IPC/IPC_Handbook/Section_2/2008_2_Classification_Code6.pdf.

6. Webborn N, Willick S, Reeser JC. Injuries among disabled athletes during the 2002 Winter Paralympic Games. *Med Sci Sports Exerc.* 2006;38(5):811–5.

7. Webborn N, Willick SE, De Luigi AJ, et al. Incidence of injuries among the participating disabled athletes during the 2006 Winter Paralympic Games. Tromso, Norway: World Congress on Sports Injury Prevention; June 2008, Abstract.

112 Wrestling

Michael G. Bowers and Thomas M. Howard

INTRODUCTION

- Wrestling is a contact sporting event that matches two competitors against each other physically and mentally. The origins of the sport date back to ancient Greek and Roman times near 500 B.C.
- There are approximately 400,000 wrestlers of all ages in the United States. As the sport has grown in popularity and participation has increased, it has been noted that there are injuries and conditions that are unique to the sport.

DEFINITION OF TERMS

- **Takedown:** Points given to a wrestler when advantage is gained from a neutral position on feet. This may be achieved by a trip or throw. Dependent on the style of wrestling, higher point values may be given for the more skillful maneuver to achieve the takedown (3).
- **Fall:** Also known as a *pin*. Determined by the referee when both shoulders are held to the mat for 1 second. The match is over at this time (3).
- **Time advantage:** This is popularly called riding time. Time of control is recorded for both wrestlers and compared. A point is given to the wrestlers if their time is 1 or more minutes greater than their opponent's (6).
- **Sparring:** An activity participated in when both of the competitors are in a neutral position on their feet. Usually comprises grappling and blocking in an attempt to achieve a takedown (3).
- **Leg wrestling:** Term used to describe the use of legs while on the mat to attempt to control an opponent (3).
- **Injury timeout:** Amount of time allowed to a wrestler to attempt to recover from an illness or injury. The time allotted is a maximum of 90 seconds throughout the match. Additionally, a competitor may have two timeouts during the match to tend to injuries as long as 90 seconds of total time is not taken (6).
- **Bleeding timeout:** Time allowed for the evaluation of a bleeding injury. This is different from an injury timeout. The amount of time is at the referee's discretion. Generally, blood timeout has no time limit, but an excessive bleeding injury may be cause for disqualification as determined by the referee and trainer or physician (6).

WRESTLING STYLES

- **Greco-Roman:** A style that was developed and popularized in Europe. Upper body throws are executed with the goal to touch the opponent's shoulders to the mat simultaneously. Points are awarded for skill of throws. At no time are the wrestlers allowed to use their own legs to gain advantage or contact their opponent's legs (3).
- **Freestyle:** Used worldwide and in international wrestling meets. A style of wrestling that combines the use of the upper body and legs to execute maneuvers. Points are awarded for exposure of opponent's back to the mat, takedowns, and reversals. Execution of a more difficult takedown with emphasis on exposure of opponent's back to the mat will increase points awarded. The main objective is to pin the opponent's shoulders to the mat for a 1-second count (3).
- **High school/collegiate:** The style of wrestling that is used in the United States. Considered similar to freestyle because of the use of upper body and legs. A major difference is that points are awarded for time advantage. Also, a wrestler must ensure the safe return of their opponent to the mat after a throw or a takedown. Emphasis is placed on pinning the opponent (3).

INJURY DATA

- Recent National Collegiate Athletic Association (NCAA) Injury Surveillance System (ISS) data conclude that collegiate wrestling has a relatively high rate of injury at 24.3 per 1,000 athlete exposures for competition and 9.7 per 1,000 athlete exposures for practice, second only to football (7,8). The incidence of injury seems to be highest at the beginning of the season, compared with the latter part of the season. Although injuries are common, there seems to be a consensus that most injuries are not serious on the basis of time lost (> 7 days) or injuries that require surgery. Comparison of the different weight classes has yielded no statistical difference in injury percentages (2).

- The knee is the most commonly injured body part in both practice and competition, followed by the shoulder and ankle. The face and neck are the least injured. Sprain is the most common type of injury in practice and competition, with fracture being the least common (2).
- Most injuries occur during takedowns and sparring (2).
- Contact with the opponent, as compared to contact with the mat, was the most common mechanism of injury (2).

MECHANISM OF INJURIES

- A direct blow from the mat or body contact may result in a laceration or contusion during a takedown or sparring. Potential serious injury may occur after a fall, especially if a competitor lands on an opponent after attempting a throw or other types of takedowns (3).
- A friction injury may result in lacerations or abrasions. This can occur with continuous body contact or contact with the mat. This may later result in skin infections or bursitis (3).
- Sprains and strains may occur after a wrestler uses twisting or leverage maneuvers to gain advantage over an opponent (3).
- A competitor may also incur injury to his or her own person while attempting maneuvers (3).
- An often overlooked potential mechanism is overuse injuries (3).

HEAD INJURIES

- Concussions occur with direct contact with a body part or contact with the mat or floor (3). (See Chapter 43.)
- Concussions may occur without loss of consciousness. It is important to evaluate the athlete for any change in behavior or thinking or for physical signs and symptoms (6).
- The competitor should be removed from play, evaluated by a trained medical professional who has experience in concussions, and returned to play dependent on the institution's concussion management protocol (6).
- Lacerations and contusion occur frequently from direct blows from the mat and body parts, such as the head, elbow, and knee. The most common areas are the bony areas around the orbits, zygoma, and scalp. Soft tissues around the mouth and ears are also potential sites. During the match, an injury timeout will be called to evaluate the area. Treatment during the injury timeout may include using Steri-strips to provide temporary closure of the wound. Dressing the wound may also be required at this time. The match can continue as deemed by the referee depending on the severity of the injury. After the match, lacerations should be cleaned and dressed properly. Closure of wounds with heavy nylon suture is recommended if necessary (3).

- Epistaxis may occur with a direct blow from an opponent or the mat. Blood timeout will be taken to determine the extent of the injury. Direct pressure and ice may be applied to the nares to reduce the hemorrhage. A pledget or nose plug may be inserted to enable the wrestler to continue the match. Nosebleed QR is a recently developed product that can be inserted into the nose with a swab (9). Direct pressure to the involved nostril for 15–30 seconds is required for the product to work properly. If the hemorrhage continues even after the above treatments are implemented, then proper medical attention must be sought.
- Nasal fractures with epistaxis are treated as above. A competitor should be evaluated for nasal bone displacement before return to play. Activity may be resumed when indicated. A protective facemask with proper nasal padding may be used to protect the nose from further injury during competition (3).

EAR INJURIES

- Auricular hematomas, also known as *cauliflower ear*, are a common injury for many competitive wrestlers. The advent of wearing properly fitted protective headgear has reduced but not eliminated the incidence of this injury. The pathogenesis of this injury is usually from a direct blow to the soft tissues of the auricle. Fluid collects between the auricular cartilage and the perichondrium, disrupting blood flow to the auricular cartilage (3).
- Treatment of auricular hematomas requires aspiration or incision and drainage. Without early aspiration, new auricular cartilage will form that is tightly encased. This can cause discomfort and eventual disfigurement. Compressive dressings after aspiration are usually applied. These dressings are worn for a period of 3–5 days before reevaluation. Return to play is individualized based on pain and a discussion of risk/benefits of continuing competition with possible fluid reaccumulation (3).
  - One technique described involves suturing the pressure dressing to the auricle with resultant return to play in 24 hours with a low incidence of complications (10). This technique involves suturing dental roll on both sides of the pinna with 1.0 nonabsorbable suture.
  - A second technique involves aspiration followed by a collodion pressure dressing in the antihelix and an Ace wrap to ensure uniform pressure in the area of the hematoma. The athlete is then reevaluated in 3–5 days. Earlier return to play is preceded by a careful discussion of risks and benefits.
  - A dry aspiration represents an organization of the hematoma and the early stages of formation of neocartilage consistent with cauliflower ear. Long-term management (otoplasty) is generally deferred until completion of the wrestling season.

NECK INJURIES

- Neck injuries usually occur during takedowns, especially throws, or when a wrestler is diving for the opponent's legs and the head is the first part of the body that strikes the mat. This may cause injuries such as strains/sprains, stingers, disc injuries, degenerative joint disease, and even fractures or spinal cord injuries (3).
- The etiology of neck injuries is most commonly from hyperextension (3).
- A stinger is a neck injury in which the participant has transient burning or shooting pain or paresthesia in an arm directly related to neck or shoulder trauma. This may be from traction on the brachial plexus or from cervical nerve root impingement. Wrestling is second only to football in regard to stinger injuries (5). (See Chapter 44.)
- If cervical fracture or spinal cord injury is suspected, then prompt medical attention should be sought (3).

BACK INJURIES

- Acute back injuries occur most often during takedowns and throws. Mechanisms that may lead to back injury include torsional movements, exertion against resistance, and hyperextension while in the standing position or hyperflexion while on the mat with an opponent (3).
- Chronic or recurrent back pain is not unusual in wrestlers and may include spondylolysis, spondylolisthesis, or sacroiliac dysfunction (3).

CHEST INJURIES

- Chest wall injuries may occur in a variety of ways. Strains from torsion, direct blows, compression, and exertion against resistance are the most common mechanisms (3).
- These mechanisms may cause rib contusions/fractures, costochondral separations, and abdominal wall strains. Competitors often present with pain on breathing and moving or point tenderness. If a rib fracture is suspected, then careful monitoring of the patient must be initiated because of the possibility of a hemothorax or pneumothorax. Prompt medical attention must be sought if this is suspected. Treatment with rest, anti-inflammatory medications, and local steroid injections may be beneficial. Taping or padding of ribs may be instituted after the initial symptoms have been treated (3).

SHOULDER INJURIES

- Shoulder injuries comprise approximately 14% of all injuries and rank second to knee injuries. Injuries may include acromioclavicular strain, shoulder dislocation, shoulder subluxation, and sternoclavicular strain. Shoulder instability is not uncommon in wrestlers (3).

EXTREMITY INJURIES

- Extremity injuries include injuries to fingers, thumbs, hands, and elbows. Injuries to fingers are relatively common. These include finger proximal interphalangeal dislocations or sprains and subluxation. Sprains may be taped to the adjacent finger to allow use during competition. Dislocations often needed splinted and padded to be functional (3).
- Thumb injuries may be much more disabling. Forceful adduction of the thumb during takedowns may damage the ulnar collateral ligament resulting in a *gamekeeper's thumb*. The competitor may not have the grasp strength to be effective against an opponent. Patient will need to be evaluated for possible thumb spica casting and may even need surgery (3).
- The elbow may be injured when an outstretched arm contacts the mat in an attempt to break a fall. The elbow at this time will be hyperextended, leading to ligamentous injury or even possible dislocation or fracture. Other common injuries include olecranon bursitis from direct trauma (3).

KNEE INJURIES

- The most common body part injured. Knee injuries composed 21% of all injuries in a recent study. The most common of these injuries are strains/sprains, meniscal/cruciate tears, fractures, subluxation, and bursitis. Collateral ligament injury is the most common type of injury, accounting for over 30% of knee injuries. Cruciate ligament injury conversely is much lower (approximately 5%) (2).
- Takedowns and leg wrestling are the most common etiologies of ligament damage (3).
- The lead leg used for defense and initiating takedowns is the most vulnerable (3).
- Wrestlers tend to have a predilection to injure the lateral meniscus or to have isolated lateral/medial collateral sprains as compared to other sports. Etiologies such as overuse, torsion, hyperextension, and shearing all have additive effects toward injury (3).
- Prepatellar bursitis is a common injury because of time spent on the knees while wrestling on the mat or performing takedowns (3).

SKIN INFECTIONS

- A problem that is unique to the sport of competitive wrestling is skin infections from various bacteria, viruses, and fungi.

Modes of transmission include person-to-person contact on exposed skin, especially abraded skin, and contact with poorly disinfected wrestling mats or equipment (3). According to recent NCAA ISS reports, skin infections are associated with at least 17% of the time-loss injuries in wrestling (6).

- All participating competitors are subject to entire body examinations including the hair on the scalp and in the pubic area at weigh-in. If an abraded area or an infectious skin condition cannot be adequately protected, the participant can be medically disqualified. Adequately protected is deemed where skin conditions are diagnosed as noninfectious and treated as per guidelines stipulated by a governing body such as the NCAA and are able to be covered with bandage that will withstand the competition (6).

- Documentation of a competitor's condition will be made available with diagnosis, culture results, and current medical therapy. The decision of the physician or trainer is considered final (6).

- Bacterial infections of the skin include folliculitis, impetigo, furuncle/carbuncle, cellulitis, erysipelas, staphylococcal disease, hidradenitis suppurativa, and community-acquired methicillin-resistant *Staphylococcus aureus* (MRSA). Competitors must not have any new skin lesions for at least 48 hours. No moist or draining lesions at time of match are allowed. Seventy-two hours of antibiotic therapy must be completed in order to compete (6).

- Pediculosis- and scabies-infected participants must have been treated with the proper medication and examined before being allowed to participate in any competition (6).

- Viral infections include herpes gladiatorum, herpes zoster, molluscum contagiosum, and verrucae. Herpes gladiatorum has received much attention because of the high incidence of being contagious and potential for morbidity (4). Wrestlers must be free of systemic illness at the time of competition. Competitors must have been treated for at least 120 hours, with proper antiviral therapy before and at the time of the event. No new active blisters or lesions may be present 72 hours before the medical examination (6).

  - Dry lesions must be covered with an impermeable bandage (6).

  - It is recommended that wrestlers with a history of recurrent herpes gladiatorum or labials be on prophylactic therapy after consultation with a team physician (6).

  - Herpes zoster infections must have crusted over lesions, and the patient cannot be systemically ill before competition (6).

  - Molluscum lesions must be removed by the time of the competition. Localized lesions may be covered with a permeable membrane followed by stretch tape (6).

  - Verrucae-infected wrestlers are allowed to compete under the following conditions. Lesions on the face must be adequately covered by a mask. Solitary lesions on the face must be removed before the match to allow participation. Verrucae on the hands must be covered (6).

- Fungal infections such as tinea have also come under scrutiny because of their high mode of transmission. A minimum of 72 hours of topical bactericidal-type antifungal treatment is required for all tinea corporis. Tinea capitis infections must be treated with a minimum of 2 weeks of systemic antifungal therapy. Treated lesions may be examined with a KOH preparation at the discretion of the examining provider. Lesions should be washed with a fungal shampoo followed by an antifungal cream before being covered with a gas-permeable dressing and stretch tape. A competitor will be disqualified if the lesion cannot be covered adequately (6).

- There is controversy about the spread of infection among teams during outbreaks. Stanforth et al. (11) reported on the prevalence of positive MRSA surface cultures in training rooms and wrestling facilities and suggested that teams with recurrent or widespread infections should thoroughly evaluate procedures for mat maintenance in cleaning and disqualifications of infectious wrestlers. Anderson (1) reported on the Minnesota experience of a herpes gladiatorum outbreak in 2007 favoring more aggressive management of cases and restriction of infected athletes as more important. It is clear that properly cleaned facilities and identification and restriction of infected athletes are important.

WEIGHING IN

- Competitors are placed into separate categories based on their body weight called weight classes. These are predetermined in advance by a governing body such as the NCAA. Currently, there are 10 weight classes ranging from 125 lb to heavyweight (183–235 lb) under the NCAA guidelines. High school participants compete in 14 different weight classes ranging from 103–275 lb (6).

- At the beginning of the season, each wrestler is weighed, and a minimum weight for the competitor is established (6). Nevertheless, one study indicated that many wrestlers compete below the minimum weight established (12). Perceived notions such as being stronger at a lighter weight have a major influence on these decisions.

- The minimum wrestling weight is established by a comparison of several different factors. Hydrated body weight is calculated by checking urine specific gravity. If the urine specific gravity is less than 1.020, then the weight is recorded as the hydrated weight. Skinfold measurements of triceps, subscapular areas, and abdomen are measured to calculate the body fat percentage. Fat-free body weight is calculated and divided by 0.95. This establishes the lowest allowable weight–1 (LAW1), which is a measurement of body weight with allowable 5% body fat. This weight is compared to the lowest allowable weight–2 (LAW2), which is calculated over a set period of time as established by the NCAA with no more than a 1.5% body weight decrease per week. LAW1 is compared to LAW2, with the higher weight being the set minimal weight. This will be the absolute minimum weight set for the wrestler for the season. A competitor must certify by mid-December in a weight class. At no time after this is a competitor allowed to wrestle at a weight class below the certified weight (6). The above guidelines encompass the current recommendation of the American College of Sports Medicine that competitors should not compete at a weight in which body fat levels would be less than 5% of their pre-season weight (12).

- During the season, wrestlers use many methods to lose weight to make their respective weight classes. These include vigorous exercise before weigh-in to lose water weight and self-imposed dehydration and fasting, and some athletes may even use weight-loss pills or diuretics. Acute effects of the above may be loss of strength and stamina, hypovolemia, heat exhaustion or heat stroke, and electrolyte imbalances. Long-term effects of continued rapid weight loss with weight gain may chronically compromise cardiac and renal blood flow. Neuropsychiatric disorders, such as depression, anxiety, bulimia, and anorexia nervosa may become prevalent. Other sequelae may include decreased growth and maturation, especially in younger wrestlers (3).

- It is important for coaches, trainers, and physicians to properly educate the competitors on the dangers of rapid weight loss. Adequate counseling on nutrition and emphasis on conditioning during the season are paramount. The NCAA attempts to dissuade competitors from the practice of rapid weight loss and gain by decreasing the time between weighing in and the actual match (3). By NCAA rules, competitors must weigh in no more than an hour before dual, triangular, and quadrangular matches. In multiteam tournaments, wrestlers must be weighed no more than 2 hours before the first match (6).

REFERENCES

1. Anderson BJ. Managing herpes gladiatorum outbreaks in competitive wrestling: the 2007 Minnesota experience. *Curr Sports Med Rep.* 2008;7(6):323–7.

2. Jarrett GJ, Orwin JF, Dick RW. Injuries in collegiate wrestling. *Am J Sports Med.* 1998;26(5):674–80.

3. Kelly TF, Suby JS. Chapter 58: wrestling. In: Mellion MB, editor. *Team Physician's Handbook.* 3rd ed. Philadelphia (PA): Hanley & Belfus; 2002. p. 614–28.

4. Kohl TD, Giesen DP, Moyer J Jr, Lisney M. Tinea gladiatorum: Pennsylvania's experience. *Clin J Sport Med.* 2002;12(3):165–71.

5. Lillegard WA, Butcher JD, Rucker KS. *Handbook of Sports Medicine: A Symptom-Oriented Approach.* 2nd ed. Boston (MA): Butterworth-Heinemann; 1999. 69 p.

6. National Collegiate Athletic Association. *2010 and 2011 Wrestling Rules and Interpretations.* Indianapolis (IN): National Collegiate Athletic Association; WR 10, WR 68–70, WR 87–88, WA 3–8, WA 28–33, 2009.

7. National Collegiate Athletic Association. Injury surveillance system for wrestling. In: *2002–03 NCAA Sports Medicine Handbook.* Indianapolis (IN): National Collegiate Athletic Association; 2002. p. 1–21.

8. National Collegiate Athletic Association. Injury surveillance system for wrestling. In: *2010–11 NCAA Sports Medicine Handbook.* Indianapolis (IN): National Collegiate Athletic Association; 2010. p. 113–116.

9. Nosebleed QR. Biolife [Internet]. Available from: http://www.biolife.com.

10. Schuller DE, Dankle SD, Strauss RH. A technique to treat wrestler's auricular hematoma without interrupting training or competition. *Arch Otolaryngol Head Neck Surg.* 1989;115(2):202–6.

11. Stanforth B, Krause A, Starkey C, Ryan TJ. Prevalence of community-associated methicillin-resistant *Staphylococcus aureus* in high school wrestling environments. *J Environ Health.* 2010;72(6):12–6.

12. Wroble RR, Moxley DP. Weight loss patterns and success rates in high school wrestlers. *Med Sci Sports Exerc.* 1998;30(4):625–8.

The Pediatric Athlete

Andrew McMarlin, Amanda Weiss Kelly, and Terry Adirim

113

EPIDEMIOLOGY

- Each year, 20–30 million children participate in organized athletic programs (20).
- There were over 7.6 million high school–age adolescents participating in organized competitive sports in 2009–2010 (17).
- About three million pediatric sports injuries occur annually in the United States (13).
- High school athletes account for an estimated 2 million injuries, 500,000 doctor visits, and 30,000 hospitalizations annually (19).
- Twenty-five to thirty percent of these injuries occur during participation in organized sports, and 40% occur in unorganized sports (13).

SPORT-RELATED CONCUSSION IN THE PEDIATRIC ATHLETE

Concussion Incidence

- The Centers for Disease Control and Prevention (CDC) estimate that traumatic brain injuries in children 14 years old and younger result in 435,000 emergency department (ED) visits annually, with approximately half of these injuries being sports related (8). Because many athletic and play activities in this age group are unmonitored and a high proportion of injuries do not result in ED visits, the actual incidence of head injury is likely much higher.
- The pediatric neuropsychology and neurosurgery literature indicates that pediatric athletes are more susceptible to concussion than adults and take longer to recover (4,12,23).

Concussion Management and Return to Play

- Because of the longer recovery time and greater risk for long-term neurologic sequelae in pediatric athletes (4), concussion should be co-managed with the assistance of a sports medicine physician and/or neurologist experienced in the management of pediatric concussion.
- The current international guidelines for this management are reflected in the consensus statement of the Third International Conference on Concussion in Sport, held in Zurich, Switzerland in November 2008 (16).

- At this time, the consensus is that any pediatric athlete suspected of having suffered a concussion should be immediately removed from that game or activity with no return to that activity that day.
- The consensus outlines a return-to-play protocol consisting of six rehabilitation stages: 1) no activity until symptom free (complete physical and cognitive rest); 2) light aerobic exercise; 3) sport-specific exercise; 4) noncontact training drills; 5) full-contact practice; and finally, 6) return to play. There should be 24 hours between each stage, and if any return of concussion symptoms occurs during a rehabilitation stage, the patient returns to the previous stage and level of rehabilitation.
- Many experts recommend neuropsychological testing prior to full return to play, whereas the Zurich consensus emphasizes that this testing should be used as an informational aid to the clinician rather than being the sole basis for return-to-play decisions.
- There is significant variability in concussion management for athletes younger than age 18 years in the number of symptom-free days with no activity between the injury and the beginning of stage 2. This varies among different practices from a minimum of 1 day to 30 days.
- A vital point for clinicians to remember is that children may still demonstrate deficits during neuropsychological testing for a period of time after they are "symptom free." The safest approach in athletes who have had baseline testing and the protocol currently used in many high schools across the United States is to begin stage 2 when their postconcussion neuropsychological testing returns to baseline level (with an age-standardized baseline level for athletes who had no prior testing). An important caveat to this treatment strategy is that current computer-based neuropsychological testing is only valid down to age 10.
- There is no consensus regarding when an athlete with a history of multiple concussions should be restricted from further participation in contact sports. Our understanding of the long-term sequelae of different levels of traumatic brain injury is still evolving. With this lack of complete evidence, a conservative approach to management is appropriate. Evaluation for disqualification from further contact sport activities for a pediatric athlete should be considered on an individual basis. The younger the athlete, the lower the threshold should be for minimizing the risk of further brain injury.

FRACTURES IN THE PEDIATRIC ATHLETE

Physeal Fractures

- The physis is the weakest structure in the growing skeleton, making it more susceptible to injury than the surrounding muscles, tendons, and ligaments.

Salter-Harris Classification

- The Salter-Harris classification is the most widely used method of describing physeal fractures:
  - Type I: Through the physis
  - Type II: Through the physis and metaphysis
  - Type III: Through the physis and epiphysis (therefore involves the articular surface)
  - Type IV: Through the metaphysis, across the physis, through the epiphysis, and involving the articular surface
  - Type V: Crush injury to the physis
  - Type VI: Injury to the perichondrium
- Type I fractures have the best prognosis, with minimal risk for growth arrest in these fractures.
- In type II fractures, growth arrest may occur, especially at specific sites, such as the distal femoral physis.
- In type III injuries, growth arrest is rare, but since the joint surface is involved, anatomic reduction must be maintained to ensure articular cartilage congruity and prevent future joint degeneration.
- In type IV injuries, there is concern for both growth arrest and articular cartilage congruity.
- Type V injuries are usually diagnosed retrospectively after growth arrest or angular deformity has occurred.
- Finally, in type VI injuries, angular deformities may occur if a bony bridge develops in the perichondrium on one side of the physis.
- Salter-Harris fractures can usually be diagnosed with plain films, but magnetic resonance imaging (MRI) and computed tomography (CT) are sometimes used to more accurately delineate physeal injuries.

Apophyseal Avulsion Injuries

- Apophyses are growth plates that add shape and contour, rather than length, to a bone. They are often sites for muscle attachment.
- Apophyseal avulsions typically occur as a result of violent contraction of the attached muscle (23).
- The pelvis is a common site for avulsion fractures. The anterior superior iliac spine (ASIS) can be avulsed by the sartorius muscle with violent flexion of the hip, such as when a sprinter is accelerating in the first few strides from the starting block.
- Violent flexion of the hip or extension of the hip when combined with knee extension can also lead to avulsion of the anterior inferior iliac spine (AIIS) by the rectus femoris.

- Diagnosis of both injuries can be made with plain radiographs. Treatment is conservative including symptom-limited weight bearing until pain free, followed by rehabilitation and gradual return to activities.
- Recovery from an avulsion injury of the AIIS injury is typically more prolonged than that of an ASIS injury.
- Abrupt contraction of the abdominal muscles or tensor fascia lata (muscle of the iliotibial band), as with a rapid direction change, can lead to avulsion of the iliac crest. Direct trauma can also fracture the iliac crest apophysis. This commonly occurs when an athlete is tackled in football. Plain radiographs may not be as useful for diagnosis in this injury, because displacement may be minimal. MRI may be helpful in diagnosing iliac crest avulsion. Treatment is conservative and includes protected weight bearing until the athlete is not in pain followed by rehabilitation and progressive return to activity.
- Other sites of avulsion injury in the hip and pelvis include the greater trochanter (gluteus medius), lesser trochanter (iliopsoas), and ischial tuberosity (adductors, hamstrings). Diagnosis and treatment are similar to that mentioned for ASIS and AIIS injuries.
- Tibial tubercle avulsions typically occur while an athlete is landing or jumping, as a result of a violent contraction of the quadriceps. Excessive bleeding and swelling can cause an anterior compartment syndrome, so a careful neurovascular examination is essential. Diagnosis can be made with plain radiographs. Long leg cast immobilization with the knee in extension for 3–4 weeks is adequate treatment for nondisplaced fractures. Open reduction with internal fixation (ORIF) is required if there is significant displacement of the fracture fragment.
- Avulsions of the medial epicondyle are common in throwing athletes. The athlete typically reports feeling a snap or pop during the throwing motion. Anteroposterior (AP) radiographs will demonstrate the avulsion. Minimally displaced fractures can be treated with immobilization, whereas fractures displaced more than 5 mm should receive surgical referral (12).
- Vertebral end-plate fractures are an avulsion of the ring apophysis of the vertebra. If the avulsion is from the posterior inferior portion of the vertebra, the apophyseal attachment of the associated disc and the apophysis can be displaced into the vertebral canal, causing neurologic symptoms. This injury can be difficult to distinguish from disc herniation. Plain radiographs can show the separated bony fragment, and MRI can demonstrate marrow edema. For symptomatic displacement of the apophysis into the vertebral canal, treatment is operative removal of the disc and bony fragment. Without neurologic symptoms, initial treatment is conservative management.

Torus Fractures

- Torus or buckle fractures are compressive fractures that lead to failure of the bone at the junction of the metaphysis and diaphysis.

- This type of injury only occurs in children and is possible because of the porous nature of their bones.
- Torus fractures are stable and heal well. They can be treated with splinting or casting for comfort.

Greenstick Fractures

- Another fracture that only occurs in children, the greenstick fracture, refers to an incomplete fracture in the shaft of a long bone. There is disruption of one cortex of the bone and bending of the other. The ability of the pediatric bone to plastically deform allows for the occurrence of this type of fracture.
- Greenstick fractures with minimal angulation can be treated with immobilization.
- Surgical intervention may be required for fractures with significant angulation.

Complete Fractures

- Complete fractures are fractures through both cortices that are often displaced and/or angulated, requiring closed reduction or ORIF.

Wrist/Forearm Fractures

- Wrist and forearm fractures are some of the most common fractures in children.
- Most of these fractures can be treated with casting or splinting but may require reduction or ORIF.
- Carpal navicular or scaphoid fractures can occur in children with open growth plates and have a high rate of nonunion.

Supracondylar Fractures

- Supracondylar fractures are very common among 3- to 11-year-old children.
- Supracondylar factures are one of the pediatric fractures with the highest risk of complications, with neurovascular complications being particularly common.
- These fractures are usually sustained from a fall on an outstretched hand, but can also occur as a result of direct trauma. A thorough neurovascular examination is imperative if a supracondylar fracture is suspected.
- The diagnosis can typically be made with plain lateral radiographs of the elbow.
- Any child with a supracondylar fracture should be referred for evaluation by a pediatric orthopedist, because many require surgical fixation.

OVERUSE INJURIES

- Overuse injuries have become more common in children with the growth of competitive youth sports programs (9).

- The risks of overuse are more serious in the pediatric/adolescent athlete because the growing bones of the young athlete cannot handle as much stress as the mature bones of adults (5).
- The American Academy of Pediatrics (AAP) recommends encouraging athletes to incorporate 1–2 days per week of rest from competitive athletics, sports-specific training, and competitive practice to allow for children and adolescents to recover both physically and psychologically. The AAP also emphasizes that the focus of sports participation should be on fun, skill acquisition, safety, and sportsmanship.
- Risk factors for overuse injuries are often divided into **intrinsic** and **extrinsic** factors.

Intrinsic Risks for Overuse Injuries

- Some issues specific to immature skeletons contribute to the risk for overuse injuries in children. For instance, children have growth cartilage in several areas of the skeleton, and it is particularly susceptible to injury from repetitive stress.
- Growth cartilage is found at the physes (epiphysis and apophysis).
- Also, as children experience growth spurts, there are rapid changes in bone length, which can lead to a relative inflexibility of the muscle-tendon units that cross joints. This may predispose the growing athlete to muscular, joint, and physeal injury (9).
- Abnormalities in alignment may also predispose an athlete to overuse injuries. Pes planus or cavus, overpronation, patellofemoral malalignment, tibial torsion, femoral anteversion, and leg length discrepancies may be related to increased risk for overuse injuries in athletes (9).

Extrinsic Risk Factors for Overuse Injury

- Improper training technique can contribute to the risk for overuse injury.
- Increasing intensity, duration, or frequency of training too quickly can lead to overuse injury.
- In runners, injury may also result from persistently running the same direction around the track or on the same side of the street due to angulation of the running surface.
- Also, parental and coaching pressures to increase the intensity of a child's training can contribute to injuries.
- Improperly fitting or worn out equipment may increase the risk of injury. For example, using worn out running shoes or adult-sized weight-training equipment may predispose the pediatric athlete to overuse injury.
- Year-round participation in the same sport may increase the risk of overuse injury.

Common Overuse Injuries

Traction Apophysitis

- A traction apophysitis occurs where a muscle group attaches to a secondary center of ossification.

- It is caused by repetitive stress at these sites that can lead to pain and swelling.

- The diagnosis of an apophysitis can usually be made on physical examination. In nonclassic cases, radiographs may help rule out other conditions.

- Osgood-Schlatter disease is an apophysitis of the tibial tubercle. It is associated with inflexibility of the quadriceps and hamstrings. Jumping and kicking activities exacerbate Osgood-Schlatter disease, so it is commonly diagnosed in basketball and soccer players. Treatment involves relative rest, as well as quadriceps stretching. Strengthening may aggravate the condition.

- Sinding-Larsen-Johansson syndrome is an apophysitis of the inferior pole of the patella and is similar in cause and treatment to Osgood-Schlatter disease.

- Apophysitis of the medial epicondyle of the elbow is common in throwing athletes. It is often termed "little league elbow." Traction on the medial epicondyle occurs as a result of the valgus stress placed on the elbow during the throwing motion.

- Treatment includes relative rest followed by progressive strengthening and gradual return to throwing activities. The athlete's throwing frequency, effort, and technique should be evaluated, and any errors should be corrected. Pitch counts should be monitored closely to ensure that the volume of effort does not exceed an age-appropriate level.

- Sever disease, or calcaneal apophysitis, is a condition resulting in pain at the site of the Achilles tendon insertion on the calcaneus. This is associated with growth spurts and occurs mainly in active 8- to 15-year-olds.

- Treatment includes application of cold packs to the area, bilateral heel lifts in shoes to reduce strain on the Achilles tendon insertion site, and relative rest followed by gradual return to play.

- Iselin disease is an apophysitis of the insertion site of the peroneus brevis tendon on the lateral aspect of the base of the fifth metatarsal (28).

- This condition may appear on x-ray as a widening of the apophysis on the inferior lateral base of metatarsal. This has an orientation parallel to the fifth metatarsal diaphysis. This parallel, rather than more perpendicular, orientation helps differentiate this condition from Jones fractures and completed stress fractures.

Pelvis Apophysitis

- Apophysitis of the pelvis/hip usually affects 14- to 18-year-old runners, sprinters, dancers, soccer players, and ice hockey players. Adolescents with excessively tight hip and thigh muscles are more prone to this overuse condition.

- The apophyses most commonly affected are the ASIS, AIIS, and iliac crest. The muscles that attach to these apophyses flex the hip and rotate and twist the pelvis and trunk.

- Differentiating between this and apophyseal avulsion injury is both clinical (slow onset of dull pain in the groin or side of the hip that worsens with activity rather than an acute or traumatic onset of pain) and radiologic. Both x-ray and ultrasound should show a symmetric width of the affected apophysis relative to the asymptomatic side.

- Differentiating pelvic apophysitis from muscle strain can be challenging but is also managed similarly, with relative rest, ice, gentle stretching, and gradual progression of activity as the symptoms resolve.

Osteochondritis Dissecans

- Osteochondritis dissecans (OCD) is a disorder of growth cartilage where there is a separation of cartilage and subchondral bone from underlying well-vascularized bone. Because this condition may not actually have an inflammatory component, the term osteochondral lesion (OCL) is coming into more common usage.

- Common sites for OCD in children include the knee, ankle, and elbow.

- OCD lesions are usually noted on plain radiographs, although MRI may be needed to identify early or subtle lesions. MRI is also used to assess the stability of the fragment and viability of subchondral bone.

- In general, younger patients and patients with stable lesions have the best prognosis.

- OCD in the knee is most often found on the lateral aspect of the medial femoral condyle but may also be found on the lateral femoral condyle or trochlea. Patients usually complain of vague knee pain and intermittent swelling. If the affected fragment has detached from the underlying bone, creating a loose body, there may be complaints of locking and catching. If the fragment is stable, a period of rest and a gradual return to activity with physical therapy to improve leg strength may be adequate for treatment. If the articular cartilage is disrupted or a loose body is present, a surgical referral is indicated.

- The capitellum of the elbow is a common site for OCD lesions in throwing athletes and gymnasts. In young patients with stable lesions, treatment includes rest, physical therapy, and instruction in proper throwing technique. If the affected fragment is unstable, surgical referral is indicated.

OCD of the Talus

- The talus is the third most common site of OCD/OCL (28). These defects are thought to be primarily due to trauma but can also be idiopathic. Approximately two-thirds of the defects are posteromedial, which tend to be deeper, and one-third are shallower anterolateral lesions (29).

- Both locations of OCLs present with joint line tenderness and an effusion.

- Radiographically, these lesions are best seen on mortise view with plantarflexion or dorsiflexion of ankle. The following classification system by Berndt and Harty is commonly used:

  - Type I: Small area of compression
  - Type II: Partially detached osteochondral lesion

- Type III: Completely detached, nondisplaced fragment
- Type IV: Detached and displaced fragment
- Treatment for type I lesions is typically conservative management with weight bearing as tolerated. For type II and III lesions, casting for 6–10 weeks was slightly more effective than simple non–weight bearing in resolution of the lesions (53% vs. 45% resolution) (29).
- For nonresolution of symptoms with conservative treatment after 8–12 weeks, a negative bone scan rules out OCL, whereas a positive scan should be followed with CT or MRI to more accurately stage the lesion for surgical treatment (28).

Scheuermann Disease

- Scheuermann disease is a common adolescent condition that causes painful thoracic kyphosis, loss of anterior vertebral body height, and wedging of the vertebral bodies (28).
- Most patients have tightness of the hamstrings, gluteals, and lumbodorsal fascia (28).
- The etiology is unclear, but it may be an overuse syndrome.
- Diagnosis can be made with plain radiographs of the thoracic spine, which demonstrate anterior wedging of at least three vertebral bodies, irregular vertebral end-plates (Schmorl nodes), and narrow disc spaces.
- Treatment includes physical therapy for strength and flexibility. Bracing may be used for a period of 9–12 months if kyphosis with Cobb angle > 50 degrees is present and the patient is skeletally immature (3).

Stress Fractures

- Stress fractures occur when there is an accumulation of damage from repetitive stresses that outstrips the bone's ability to repair and remodel.
- Stress fractures are most commonly found in the lower extremities but can also be found in the spine and upper extremity.
- Stress fractures may be diagnosed with plain radiographs but single photon emission CT (SPECT), CT, or MRI may be needed.
- Many stress fractures are similar in the adult and pediatric populations, and only stress fractures specific to the pediatric population are discussed here.

Spondylolysis

- The term spondylolysis refers to a stress fracture of the pars interarticularis of the spine.
- If there is a fracture of both pars, then it may become unstable, and forward displacement of one vertebra on another may result, which is termed *spondylolisthesis*.
- Athletes participating in sports that require repetitive hyperextension, like gymnastics or football, may be at increased risk for spondylolysis.
- Most patients complain of low back pain, which is worse with extension and is relieved by rest.

- Spondylolysis can often be diagnosed with plain radiographs and is best seen on oblique views. It can, however, occur without changes on plain radiographs. In this case, SPECT, MRI, or CT can be used to detect the abnormality (15).
- Treatment includes activity restriction until the patient is asymptomatic followed by a gradual return to activity. A program of core/lumbar strengthening and flexibility should also be instituted. Some practitioners recommend bracing at diagnosis, whereas others recommend bracing only if the patient continues to have pain, despite adequate rest.
- Prognosis is best in cases where only SPECT scan is positive and there is not yet plain radiographic evidence of disease. In cases where radiographic evidence of spondylolysis is present, the likelihood of healing is lower.
- If spondylolisthesis has occurred, there is no chance for healing.
- Conservative therapy, similar to that for spondylolysis, is the most widely recommended treatment for spondylolisthesis.
- The role of surgery is controversial. In cases where neurologic compromise is evident or slipping of the vertebra progresses, surgical stabilization is recommended (22).

Proximal Humeral Physeal Stress Fracture

- The proximal humeral stress fracture is often referred to as "little league shoulder," although it is also seen in other overhead athletes, such as tennis or volleyball players.
- The throwing motion places torsion and distraction forces on the proximal humerus, which when done repetitively, can result in proximal humeral stress fracture. AP internal and external rotation views of the shoulder with comparison views of the opposite shoulder on radiograph can demonstrate widening, sclerosis, or cystic changes of the affected physis.
- Treatment involves cessation of throwing or other overhead activities until the child is asymptomatic, usually about 3 months (25). At that time, progressive return to activity is allowed. Throwing mechanics should be evaluated, and parents and coaches should be warned not to encourage excessive throwing. Age-appropriate pitch counts should be followed.

Distal Radius Physeal Stress Fractures

- Distal radius physeal stress fracture is a Salter-Harris type V stress fracture that typically occurs in gymnasts.
- It is caused by the unusual amount of weight-bearing activities that gymnasts perform with their upper extremities.
- Radial-sided wrist pain is the most common symptom early on.
- The diagnosis may be made with plain radiographs by comparing the affected side to the nonpainful side. Abnormal widening of the physis, "beaking" of the epiphysis, and cystic changes on the metaphyseal side of the bone may be noted on the affected radius; however, MRI may be needed to make the diagnosis if plain radiographs are normal.
- Treatment includes rest until the athlete is asymptomatic, usually 1–3 months. Splinting or casting may be helpful.

- When pain has completely resolved, a gradual return to upper extremity weight bearing is permitted. Attention to technique errors upon return to sport may help prevent reinjury.

Lunatomalacia (Kienböck Disease)

- Kienböck disease is a painful, unilateral condition of the wrist that radiates up the forearm in 15- to 40-year-olds (28). It involves collapse of the lunate from vascular insufficiency and avascular necrosis after single or repetitive microfractures of the bone. These fractures are thought to occur during recurrent compression of the lunate from loads to the wrist while in extremes of flexion and/or extension.
- Negative ulnar variance increases risk for this condition.
- Radiographic findings may be normal initially and progress to demonstrating total lunate collapse and fragmentation.
- If not corrected surgically, this may progress to severe wrist disability and chronic pain.

ANATOMIC VARIANTS

- Several anatomic variants may predispose the pediatric athlete to pain and injury.

Discoid Lateral Meniscus

- Athletes with discoid lateral meniscus often complain of a snapping sensation with extension of the knee.
- Some discoid menisci are not diagnosed until they are torn, in which case the athlete tends to complain of pain, swelling, and mechanical symptoms.
- Diagnosis can often be made on clinical examination.
- MRI can also be used to diagnose meniscal tears and discoid lateral menisci.
- A torn discoid lateral meniscus requires surgery. If a discoid lateral meniscus is found incidentally, surgery is not indicated.

Tarsal Coalition

- Tarsal coalition is a bony or fibrocartilaginous connection of two or more tarsal bones.
- The most common examples are calcaneonavicular and talocalcaneal coalition. They are often bilateral.
- Symptomatic patients typically complain of vague pain that is insidious in onset. The diagnosis of calcaneonavicular coalition can usually be made on the oblique view of the plain radiograph, but CT scan may be necessary to provide a more detailed view of the anatomy or to see talocalcaneal coalition.
- Conservative therapy includes rest, immobilization, rigid shoe inserts, and anti-inflammatory medication.

- In patients who fail conservative therapy, surgical resection of the coalition can be undertaken.

Accessory Ossicles

- Quite common in the foot, the accessory navicular is an accessory ossicle of the proximal medial foot into which a portion of the posterior tibialis tendon inserts.
- Athletes involved in sports that stress the posterior tibialis tendon with running and jumping, like basketball, may develop accessory navicular pain. Flexible flat feet (excessive foot pronation) are often present.
- Diagnosis can be made on the external oblique radiograph of the foot.
- Treatment is typically conservative, with rest, shoe inserts, ice, nonsteroidal anti-inflammatory drugs, and rarely, immobilization. Excision can be performed if conservative therapy fails.
- The os trigonum is another common accessory ossicle that is found posterior to the talus.
- Sports that involve repetitive plantarflexion, such as ballet or soccer, can lead to impingement of the os trigonum between the posterior tibia and calcaneus.
- An os trigonum can usually be seen on lateral radiograph of the ankle.
- Conservative therapy is usually effective. This includes physical therapy for strengthening and flexibility, relative rest, anti-inflammatory medication, and, sometimes, injection. Surgical excision can be performed if conservative therapy fails.

THE OSTEOCHONDROSES

- The osteochondroses are a group of chronic disorders that involve the epiphyses or apophyses.
- They begin as an avascular necrosis of the epiphyseal center followed by eventual repair and replacement of the ossification center.

Panner Disease

- Panner disease is an osteochondrosis of the capitellum associated with repetitive trauma from throwing. It involves variations in the normal ossification of the capitellum of the humerus (26).
- This condition typically affects children between 5 and 11 years of age, a younger age group than that which is typically affected by OCD of the capitellum.
- The athlete complains of pain with activity and may have swelling of the elbow.
- Fragmentation of the capitellum is noted on radiograph of the elbow.
- This is a self-limiting disease and can be treated conservatively with activity modification.

Legg-Calve-Perthes Disease

- Osteochondrosis of the femoral head is referred to as Legg-Calve-Perthes disease.
- Symptoms include knee, groin, or anterior thigh pain and limping after activity.
- AP and frog lateral radiographs of the hip confirm the diagnosis.
- The main goal of treatment is to maintain range of motion and prevent deformity of the femoral head by keeping it contained in the acetabulum.
- Orthopedic referral is indicated.

Freiberg Disease

- Freiberg disease is an osteochondrosis of the metatarsal head.
- It usually affects adolescents.
- Forefoot pain is the typical complaint.
- Flattening of the metatarsal head and fragmentation of the epiphysis can be seen on plain radiographs. However, MRI or bone scan may be necessary for diagnosis early in the disease process.
- With early diagnosis, conservative therapy, including relative rest, padding of the affected metatarsal head, and orthotics, may be successful. With failure of conservative therapy, surgical referral should be made.

Kohler Disease

- Kohler disease is a unilateral avascular necrosis of the navicular bone occurring in 4-year-old boys and 5-year-old girls. This presents as a painful limp with shifting of weight to the lateral aspect of the foot. The navicular is the last bone in the foot to ossify, which may make it more vulnerable to compressive damage during weight bearing.
- Radiographically, the appearance of the navicular bone in Kohler disease may be normal to completely collapsed (the opposite, asymptomatic side may have the same radiologic appearance). The prognosis is typically complete recovery with conservative treatment, including control of pain and swelling, reduced strenuous activity, and longitudinal arch supports and/or medial heel wedges.

SAFETY

Heat and Cold Illness

- Exercising children may not adapt to extremes of temperature as effectively as adults when exposed to a high climatic heat stress. The adaptation of adolescents falls in between.
- According to the CDC-funded National High School Sports-Related Injury Surveillance Study, there were 9,000 cases of heat illness reported in children and adolescents between 2005 and 2009.

- Children have a larger body surface area to body mass ratio than adults, making children more likely to gain heat from the environment in hot conditions and lose it in cold environments (26).
- Heat loss in children is even more apparent in water because of the high thermal conductivity of water.
- Compared to adults exercising at a given level, children have increased heat production per kilogram of body mass. This leads to faster increases in body temperature in warm weather, but can be protective when exercise is performed in cold environments (24).
- Another disadvantage for children exercising in warm environments is that the sweating rate in children is lower than in adults. This is particularly important when the temperature of the environment exceeds the skin temperature. In this type of environment, sweat evaporation from the skin is the only means for cooling the body.
- When dehydrated, a child's temperature rises faster than an adult's, increasing the risk for serious heat injury (26).
- Considerable effort has been made over the past several years to reduce heat injury in sports. The National Athletic Trainers' Association (NATA) has developed heat acclimatization guidelines designed specifically to prevent deaths in high school football players (7).

Hydration

- Children should be well hydrated prior to starting any physical activity (26).
- During activity, children should be encouraged to drink 120 mL (5 oz) of water every 20 minutes. Older, heavier children will require 250 mL (9 oz) every 30 minutes (26).
- For activities lasting longer than 1 hour, a 6% carbohydrate solution with sodium and chloride should be used.
- Beverages should be cold to improve palatability.
- Lightweight clothing should be worn to facilitate sweat evaporation.

Sun Exposure

- Sunscreen with sun protection factor (SPF) of 15 (or higher) should be applied 20 minutes prior to sun exposure to reduce the risk for sunburn and should be reapplied because sweating and activity mechanically reduce the amount of sunscreen coverage.
- Sun exposure during childhood has been linked to the development of skin cancer in adulthood.

Proper Equipment

- Children should be provided with appropriately sized equipment in good condition for sport participation.
- Padding for football, hockey, and soccer is made in children's sizes.

- Weight-training equipment can be found in sizes and with weight increments appropriate for children.
- Mouthguards should be worn for all contact sports to prevent dental injury.

Preseason Medical Evaluation

- The preparticipation physical examination may prevent injury by identifying medical conditions that can be exacerbated by sports participation and musculoskeletal issues that can be addressed and rehabilitated before sports participation.
- Primary objectives for this visit include detection of conditions that may predispose to injury; detection of conditions that may be life threatening or disabling; identification of musculoskeletal problems that need rehabilitation prior to participation; and meeting of legal and insurance requirements.
- Other important objectives include review of general health including psychological health, counseling on health-related issues, and assessment of fitness level for specific sports (2).

Growth and Development

- Some debate exists over whether or not sports participation has an effect on growth.
- Regular physical activity does not appear to have any adverse effects on growth (26).
- There is some evidence that intense, high-volume training may adversely affect growth.
- It appears that young athletes who experience attenuated growth during training will exhibit catch-up growth when training levels decrease. High-intensity exercise, alone, may not account for these effects on growth; inadequate nutritional compensation for a given training volume may also play a role.

Female Athlete Triad

- The female athlete triad (FAT) refers to the interrelationship between energy availability, changes in menstrual function, and bone mineral density,
- A spectrum exists for each component of the triad, and an athlete may sit anywhere along the spectrum for each component. For energy availability, an athlete may have normal energy availability, reduced availability, or low availability, with or without an eating disorder. For menstrual function, an athlete may be eumenorrheic, have subclinical menstrual dysfunction, or functional hypothalamic amenorrhea. And for bone density, an athlete may have optimal bone density, low bone density, or osteoporosis.
- The prevalence of FAT is unknown. One study found eating disorders in 31% of elite female athletes in "thin-build" sports compared to 5.5% of the control population (6). Another found that 25% of female elite athletes in endurance sports, aesthetic sports, and weight-class sports had clinical eating disorders compared to 9% of the general population (27).

- Sustained low energy availability, with or without disordered eating, can impair health.
- Psychological problems associated with eating disorders include low self-esteem, depression, and anxiety disorders.
- Medical complications of eating disorders involve the cardiovascular, endocrine, reproductive, skeletal, gastrointestinal, renal, and central nervous systems.
- Sustained low energy availability can lead to menstrual cycle changes including amenorrhea.
- Bone mineral density (BMD) declines as the number of missed menstrual cycles accumulates, and the loss of BMD may not be fully reversible. Stress fractures occur more commonly in physically active women with menstrual irregularities and/or low BMD, with a relative risk for stress fracture two to four times greater in amenorrheic than eumenorrheic athletes (18).
- Screening for FAT can be challenging because its health consequences are not always readily apparent. Optimal screening times for FAT occur at the preparticipation physical exam and annual health checkups (18).

Strength Training

- Strength training by children and adolescents, when properly supervised, is considered safe and efficacious.
- Strength training is often recommended for improvement in sports performance, injury rehabilitation, injury prevention, and general health benefits (1).
- Studies have shown that when properly structured, strength training can increase strength in preadolescents and adolescents (10,11).
- In preadolescents, strength training increases strength but does not result in muscle hypertrophy (14,21).
- The 2008 position statement from the AAP Committee on Sports Medicine and Fitness concludes that there is not enough evidence to assert that strength-training programs help prevent sports-related musculoskeletal injuries in preadolescents and adolescents except for specific plyometric training programs for adolescent girls for the reduction of anterior cruciate ligament injuries.

REFERENCES

1. AAP Committee on Sports Medicine and Fitness. Strength training by children and adolescents. *Pediatrics.* 2008;121(4):835–40.
2. Adirim TA, Cheng TL. Overview of injuries in the young athlete. *Sports Med.* 2003;33(1):75–81.
3. Ali RM, Green DW, Patel TC. Scheuermann's kyphosis. *Curr Opin Pediatr.* 1999;11(1):70–5.
4. Anderson V, Moore C. Age at injury as a predictor of outcome following pediatric head injury: a longitudinal perspective. *Child Neuropsychol.* 1995;1:187–202.
5. Brenner JS, Council on Sports Medicine and Fitness (American Academy of Pediatrics). Overuse injuries, overtraining, and burnout in child and adolescent athletes. *Pediatrics.* 2007;119(6):1242–5.

6. Byrne S, McLean N. Elite athletes: effects of the pressure to be thin. *J Sci Med Sport.* 2002;5(2):80–94.

7. Casa DJ, Csillan D; Inter-Association Task Force for Preseason Secondary School Athletics Participants, et al. Preseason heat-acclimatization guidelines for secondary school athletics. *J Athl Train.* 2009;44(3): 332–3.

8. Centers for Disease Control and Prevention. What is traumatic brain injury? [Internet]. [cited 2010 Dec]. Available from: http://www.cdc.gov/ncipc/tbi/TBI.htm.

9. DiFiori JP. Stress fracture of the proximal fibula in a young soccer player: a case report and a review of the literature. *Med Sci Sports Exerc.* 1999;31(7):925–8.

10. Faigenbaum AD, Westcott WL, Micheli LJ, et al. The effects of strength training and detraining on children. *J Strength Cond Res.* 1996;10:109–14.

11. Falk B, Tenenbaum G. The effectiveness of resistance training in children. A meta-analysis. *Sports Med.* 1996;22(3):176–86.

12. Field M, Collins MW, Lovell MR, Maroon J. Does age play a role in recovery from sports-related concussion? A comparison of high school and collegiate athletes. *J Pediatr.* 2003;142(5):546–53.

13. Hergenroeder AC. Prevention of sports injuries. *Pediatrics.* 1998;101(6): 1057–63.

14. Kraemer WJ, Fry AC Frykman PN, Conroy B, Hoffman J. Resistance training and youth. *Pediatr Exerc Sci.* 1989;1:336–50.

15. Maxfield BA. Sports-related injury of the pediatric spine. *Radiol Clin North Am.* 2010;48(6):1237–48.

16. McCrory P, Meeuwisse W, Johnston K, et al. Consensus statement on concussion in sport — the 3rd International Conference on Concussion in Sport, held in Zurich, November 2008. *J Clin Neurosci.* 2009;16(6):755–63.

17. National Association of High School Associations. 2009–10 High School Athletics Participation Survey [Internet]. [cited 2011 Jan]. Available from: http://www.nfhs.org.

18. Nattiv A, Louks AB, Manore MM, Sanborn CF, Sundgot-Borgen J, Warren MP. American College of Sports Medicine position stand. The female athlete triad. *Med Sci Sports Exerc.* 2007;39(10):1867–82.

19. Powell JW, Barber-Foss KD. Injury patterns in selected high school sports: a review of the 1995–1997 seasons. *J Athl Train.* 1999;34(3):277–84.

20. Radelet MA, Lephart SM, Rubinstein EN, Myers JB. Survey of the injury rate for children in community sports. *Pediatrics.* 2002;110 (3):e28.

21. Ramsey JA, Blimkie CJ, Smith K, Garner S, MacDougall JD, Sale DG. Strength training effects in prepubescent boys. Issues and controversies. *Med Sci Sports Exerc.* 1990;22(5):605–14.

22. Richardson WJ, Furey CG. Low back and lumbar spine injuries. In: Garrett WE, Speer K, Kirkendall DT, editors. *Principles and Practice of Orthopaedic Sports Medicine.* Philadelphia (PA): Lippincott Williams & Wilkins; 2000.

23. Sim A, Terryberry-Spohr L, Wilson KR. Prolonged recovery of memory functioning after mild traumatic brain injury in adolescent athletes. *Neuro Rehab.* 2007;22:207–16.

24. Smolander J, Bar-Or O, Korhonen O, Ilmarinen J. Thermoregulation during rest and exercise in the cold in pre- and early pubescent boys and in young men. *J Appl Physiol.* 1992;72(4):1589–94.

25. Stanitski CL, DeLee JC, Drez D. *Pediatric and Adolescent Sports Medicine.* Philadelphia (PA): WB Saunders; 1994.

26. Sullivan JA, Anderson SJ, editors. *Care of the Young Athlete.* Rosemont (IL): American Academy of Orthopaedic Surgeons; 2000.

27. Sundgot-Borgen J, Torstveit MK. Prevalence of eating disorders in elite athletes is higher than in the general population. *Clin J Sport Med.* 2004;14(1):25–32.

28. Wheeless CR. *Wheeless Textbook of Orthopedics* [Internet]. 2003. [cited 2011 Nov]. Available from: http://www.ortho-u.net/o2/157.htm.

29. Zengerink M, Struijs PA, Tol JL, van Dijk CN. Treatment of osteochondral lesions of the talus: a systematic review. *Knee Surg Sports Traumatol Arthrosc.* 2010;18(2):238–46.

The Geriatric Athlete

Brian K. Unwin

INTRODUCTION

- Although the challenges of age-related changes may require training modifications and a reassessment of goals, exercise rarely requires complete elimination secondary to a medical disorder.
- This chapter will discuss the following:
  - The demographic shift in aging of the American population
  - Normal age-related physical and physiologic changes related to aging
  - Physiologic and functional benefits of exercise and activity
  - Preparticipation screening
  - General exercise prescription for the older athlete

THE OLDER ATHLETE

- For purposes of discussion, an older athlete will be defined as age 65 years or greater.
- By 2030, about 20% of all Americans (70 million) will be age 65 or older and will outnumber the pediatric population (15).
- The average 75-year-old has three chronic conditions and is on five prescription medications. Exercise has been demonstrated to have positive effects in preventing a number of chronic diseases and is also an important tool to treat the very same conditions (22).
- Sedentary lifestyle is the most prevalent modifiable risk factor for heart disease, a condition present in approximately 50% of individuals age 55–64 and 65% of those age 65–74. One-third of all men age 75 or greater and half of all women of the same age report no or limited physical activity (22).
- Runners age 65 or greater currently make up only 1%–2% of American marathon runners (9,18). Individuals age 50 and older make up 23% of health club members. Adults born from 1946–1964 ("Baby Boomers") attending health clubs are more likely to cross-train and more likely to attend the club regularly—112 days per year (24).
- Although less likely to suffer from acute traumatic injury related to exercise, Baby Boomers are more likely to experience overuse injuries (5).

- The benefits of sports and athletics shift from recreation and cardiovascular fitness in the young to middle-aged individual to preserving physical, cognitive, social, and emotional functioning in the older adult.
- Preserving function in late life helps mitigate the direct and indirect costs related to the chronic care of older adults. Numerous studies support the contention that exercise is the key factor to minimize late-life disability and premature mortality (6,11,13,19,25).

PHYSICAL AND PHYSIOLOGIC CHANGES RELATED TO AGING

- Normal physiologic changes related to aging are discussed elsewhere in detail (15). These changes intertwine with common comorbidities in older adults such as hypertension, diabetes, hyperlipidemia, and arthritis (Table 114.1). The key physiologic change for athletes is the decrease in $\dot{V}O_{2max}$ and maximal heart rate.
- The older adult additionally copes with aging-associated syndromes such as dementia, depression, disability, falls, incontinence, and frailty. See Table 114.1 for a synopsis of these conditions.
- An appreciation of this intersection of normal aging changes, common medical comorbidities, and geriatric syndromes is crucial to assist the aging athlete. Examples of this include:
  - The older golfer with hypertension and aortic valvular sclerosis who develops syncope
  - The older postmenopausal female cyclist who develops incontinence
  - Delirium manifesting in an older athlete who has just completed a marathon
  - A runner with refractory gastroesophageal reflux that results in malnutrition

PHYSIOLOGIC AND FUNCTIONAL BENEFITS OF EXERCISE

- Some of the physiologic effects of exercise are listed in Table 114.1. In addition to the direct effects on the heart and

Table 114.1 | Common Conditions and Exercise Effect in Older Adults

Aging-Related Physiologic Changes	Common Comorbid Conditions	Common Geriatric Syndromes	Exercise Effects
Cardiovascular: Decreased $\dot{V}O_{2max}$ Decreased maximal heart rate Decreased maximal cardiac output Rise in systolic blood pressure Widening pulse pressure Increased large artery stiffness Increased fibrosis Decreased innervation Valve fibrosis Myocyte dropout *Skeletal muscle:* Sarcopenia Loss of Type I and II muscle fibers Decreased basal metabolic rate Decreased fiber volume Muscle denervation Decreased mitochondrial volume; increased collagen Decreased flexibility *Pulmonary:* Lower maximal expiratory flows Stable total lung capacity Lower diffusing capacity Increased ventilation/perfusion mismatch Lower respiratory muscle strength Loss of lung elastic recoil Stiffer chest wall Increased airway reactivity Lower respiratory drive Declining partial pressure of arterial oxygen to age 65 *Bone, ligament, cartilage, meniscus, and tendon* Bone: loss of mineral density; "tubularization" of diaphyseal bone Cartilage: chondromalacia; disuse activity with inactivity Ligaments and tendons: stiffness; increased risk for complete failure; decreased vascularity Meniscus: degeneration; subject to tears; less stress dissipation *Renal:* Decreased renal blood flow and glomerular filtration rate Age-related glomerulosclerosis Impaired concentrating capacity Impaired sodium preservation Impaired response to vasopressin Decreased thirst perception Decreased total-body water Decreased plasma renin and aldosterone production *Gastrointestinal:* Drug interaction Cholelithiasis Decreased anal sphincter pressure Delayed transit Decreased lower esophageal pressure Dysphagia *Hematologic:* Decreased hematopoietic response to stress *Sensory:* Presbyopia Presbycusis Cataracts	Anemia Arthritis Atrial fibrillation Cancer Chronic kidney disease Chronic obstructive pulmonary disease Constipation Diabetes Heart disease Hyperlipidemia Hypertension Osteoporosis Thyroid disorders Vascular disease	Delirium Dementia Depression Dizziness Falls Frailty Health illiteracy Iatrogenic injury Immune deficiency Impairments of instrumental activities of daily living (IADLs) and activities of daily living (ADLs) Incontinence Infection Insomnia Instability (falls) Irritable bowels Polypharmacy Pressure ulcers Social isolation Syncope Temperature dysregulation	*Cardiovascular:* Increased $\dot{V}O_{2max}$ No change in maximal heart rate Increased stroke volume Increase in arterial-venous oxygen difference Reduced mortality from cardiovascular disease and stroke Decreased risk of type 2 diabetes, high blood pressure, dyslipidemia, metabolic syndrome, colon and breast cancers Moderate evidence for decreased risk of lung and endometrial cancers *Metabolic:* Prevention of weight gain Weight loss Weight maintenance after weight loss Reduced abdominal obesity *Neuromuscular:* Increased strength Increased Type I and II fibers No change in number of fibers Increased muscle fiber size and area Increased muscle oxidative capacity Increased motor unit function Fewer falls *Bone and connective tissue:* Increased bone mass Increased bone strength Decreased bone reabsorption Decreased risk of hip fracture *Mood:* Effective in treatment of depression Enhanced self-efficacy *Cognition:* Suggestion of preserved cognition *Function:* Reduced falls Improvements in ADL/IADLs Improved quality of life Improved sleep quality

muscular system, exercise improves an older adult's likelihood of preserved long-term, independent functional status (11,19,25).

■ Exercise increases high-density lipoprotein cholesterol levels, lowers low-density lipoprotein cholesterol levels, lowers blood pressure, improves insulin sensitivity, and decreases blood coagulability (3).

■ Direct effects on the heart muscle include increased myocardial oxygen supply, increased myocardial contraction, and electrical stability (3).

AGE-ASSOCIATED REDUCTIONS IN ENDURANCE EXERCISE PERFORMANCE

■ Masters athletes are older adults (generally defined as age 35 or greater) who have strived to preserve or exceed their prior athletic performance and serve as a model to understand the limits to endurance performance with regard to aging.

■ Peak athletic performance is maintained to approximately age 35, followed by gradual decline to age 60, and accelerated decline thereafter. Examples here are marathon running times and swimming performance (21). See Tables 114.2 and 114.3 for examples of performance levels of older athletes.

■ The primary physiologic determinants to endurance exercise performance are exercise economy, lactate threshold, and maximal aerobic capacity.

  ■ Exercise economy is the steady-state oxygen consumption that occurs during submaximal exercise below the lactate threshold. Multiple cross-sectional and longitudinal studies demonstrate that running economy does not change in masters athletes trained for endurance activities (20).

  ■ Lactate threshold does not appear to change with advancing age in masters athletes (20).

  ■ Maximal aerobic capacity is the primary determinant of decreased endurance exercise performance (10).

PREPARTICIPATION SCREENING OF THE OLDER ATHLETE

■ Responsibility for the preparticipation screening first begins with the athlete contacting a health care provider for assessment. Screening recommendations vary based on the individual's:

  ■ General health
  ■ Medical comorbidities
  ■ Desired level of activity

■ The clinician should have a clear understanding of the patient's exercise plan for development of endurance, strength, speed, flexibility, and balance.

Table 114.2 | Examples of Performance Records by Older Athletes (26)

Women:	Men:
Outdoor 100 m	*Outdoor 100 m*
Age 35: 10.74 (Merlene Ottney)	Age 35: 9.97 (Linford Chritie)
Age 50: 11.67 (Merlene Ottney)	Age 50: 10.88 (Willie Gault)
Age 65: 14.10 (Nadine O'Connor)	Age 65: 12.37 (Stephen Robbins)
Age 80: 18.42 (Hanna Gilbrich)	Age 80: 14.35 (Payton Jordan)
Outdoor 1 Mile	*Outdoor 1 Mile*
Age 35: 4:17.33 (Maricica Puica)	Age 35: 3:51.38 (Bernand Lagat)
Age 50: 5:00.59 (Gitte Karlshoj)	Age 50: 4:27.90 (Nolan Shaheed)
Age 65: 6:16.28 (Marie-Louise Michelson)	Age 65: 4:56.40 (Derek Turnbull)
	Age 80: 7.09.60 (Joseph King)
Outdoor Marathon	*Outdoor Marathon*
Age 35: 2:21.29 (Lyudmila Petrova)	Age 35: 2:03.59 (Haile Gebrselassie)
Age 50: 2:48.47 (Edeltraud Pohl)	Age 50: 2:19.29 (Titus Mamabolo)
Age 65: 3:28.10 (Lieselotte Schultz)	Age 65: 2:41.57 (Derek Turnbull)
Age 80: 4:49.50 (Helen Klein)	Age 80: 3:25.43 (Ed Whitlock)
Outdoor High Jump	*Outdoor High Jump*
Age 35: 2.01 (Inga Babakova)	Age 35: 2.31 (Dragutin Topic)
Age 50: 1.60 (Debbie Brill)	Age 50: 1.98 (Thomas Zacharas)
Age 65: 1.37 (Ursula Stelling)	Age 65: 1.66 (Phil Fehlen)
Age 80: 1.06 (Christel Happ)	Age 80: 1.37 (Richard Lowery)
Outdoor Shot Put	*Outdoor Shot Put*
Age 35: 21.46 (Larisa Peleshenko)	Age 35: 22.19 (Brian Oldfield)
Age 50: 15.15 (Alexandra Marghieva)	Age 50: 18.45 (Klaus Liedtke)
Age 65: 12.21 (Sirgrin Kofink)	Age 65: 15.90 (Kurt Goldschmidt)
Age 80: 8.87 (Rachel Hanssens)	Age 80: 13.98 (Leo Saarinen)
Outdoor Javelin Throw	*Outdoor Javelin Throw*
Age 35: 68.34 (Steffi Nerius)	Age 35: 92.80 (Jan Zelezny)
Age 50: 44.20 (Ingrid Thyssen)	Age 50: 71.01 (Luis Nogueiera)
Age 65: 38.07 (Evaun B. Williams)	Age 65: 57.67 (Gary Stenlund)
Age 80: 21.83 (Rachel Hanssens)	Age 80: 39.06 (William Platts)

■ Summary recommendations for preexercise cardiac evaluation of older adults are presented in Table 114.4. Preparticipation cardiovascular screening includes assessment of:

  ■ Family history (longevity, premature sudden death, heart disease in surviving relatives)

  ■ Personal history (heart murmur, hypertension, congenital and valvular heart disease, myocarditis, Chagas disease, cardioactive medications and over-the-counter

Table 114.3	Older Athletes in Professional Sports by Gender

Men:	Women:
American Football: George Blanda (48) (Last year 1975); http://www.profootballhof.com/history/stats/40_and_over_club.aspx	Basketball: Nancy Lieberman (50) (Last year 2008); http://www.basketball-reference.com/wnba/players/l/liebena01w.html
Baseball: Satchel Paige (59) (Last year 1965); http://www.baseball-reference.com/players/p/paigesa01.shtml	Golf: Sherri Steinhauer (43) (2006 Women's British Open); http://www.lpga.com/content/Chronology2000–2008.pdf
Basketball: Robert Parish (43) (Last year 1997); http://en.wikipedia.org/wiki/List_of_oldest_and_youngest_National_Basketball_Association_players#cite_ref-8	Soccer: Kristine Lilly (39) (Twenty-four year career, 352 international appearances); http://www.womensprosoccer.com/news/press_releases/110105-lilly-retirement
Ice Hockey: Gordie Howe (69) (Last year 1997); http://www.legendsofhockey.net/LegendsOfHockey/jsp/LegendsMember.jsp?mem=p197204&type=Player&page=bio&list=ByName	Tennis: Billie Jean King (At age of 39, won the singles title at the 1983 Birmingham tournament); http://www.itahalloffame.com/

agents, fatigability, syncope, falls, exertional dyspnea, or chest pain)

■ Physical examination (postural vital signs, heart murmur, femoral pulses, findings of Marfan syndrome) (12)

■ The preparticipation assessment then focuses on problems identified in the health history. Identified difficulties are managed on a case-by-case basis. Physical and occupational therapy can confer significant benefits to individuals with functional limitations (limited use of extremities), balance problems, and fall risks.

■ Assessment should consider case-by-case screening for common geriatric syndromes such as dementia, depression, and disablement.

■ Vision and hearing are important to assess due to their roles in injury prevention and personal safety. Older runners who wear glasses or contacts should consider wearing single-vision lenses to reduce their risk of outdoor falls (7).

■ Orthopedic examination should focus on upper and lower extremity joints for pain and limitation in range of motion.

■ The neurologic exam should include assessment of static balance (Romberg testing) and dynamic balance (observation of gait with walking and, ideally, with running).

Table 114.4	Preexercise Evaluation of Older Adults (12)

American Heart Association, World Heart Federation, and International Federation of Sports Medicine (Preparticipation Screening and Assessment of Cardiovascular Disease in Masters Athletes):

■ Masters athletes having moderate-to-high cardiovascular risk profile for coronary artery disease and who desire to enter vigorous competitive situations, should undergo exercise testing.

■ Exercise testing is recommended for masters athletes of any age with symptoms suggestive of coronary artery disease.

■ Exercise testing is advised in masters athletes age 65 and older, even in the absence of risk factors or symptoms.

U.S. Department of Health and Human Services:

■ Asymptomatic adults without diagnosed chronic conditions (diabetes, heart disease, chronic obstructive pulmonary disease, etc.) do not need to consult a physician about engaging in physical activity.

■ Inactive people who gradually progress over time to relatively moderate-intensity activity have no known risk of sudden cardiac events and low risk of bone, muscle, or joint injury.

■ A habitually active, asymptomatic individual engaging in moderate-intensity activity can gradually increase to vigorous intensity without needing to consult with a health care provider.

■ People who develop new symptoms when increasing their levels of activity should consult with the health care provider.

American College of Sports Medicine (2010) and American Heart Association (2000):

Absolute contraindications to aerobic and resistance exercise and training programs include recent myocardial infarction or electrocardiogram changes, unstable angina, uncontrolled hypertension, acute heart failure, severe aortic stenosis and complete heart block. (Other noncardiac contraindications to exercise include acute febrile illness, uncontrolled diabetes, new falls, or musculoskeletal pain)

American College of Cardiology/American Heart Association (2002):

■ Physicians should consider exercise stress testing before initiation of vigorous exercise in healthy men older than 45 years and in healthy women older than 55 years.

■ All sedentary older adults with known coronary artery disease or cardiac symptoms and those individuals with two or more coronary artery disease risk factors should undergo exercise stress testing before initiation of a vigorous exercise program.

GENERAL EXERCISE PRESCRIPTION FOR THE OLDER ATHLETE

- General recommendations for physical activity are presented in Table 114.5. Modifications of these general recommendations are taken on a case-by-case basis for the needs of the individual athlete.

- It is important to emphasize the need for muscle strengthening exercises in the older athlete to preserve bone density and muscle mass. Muscle-strengthening exercises should focus on core muscle groups (shoulders, back, chest, arms, abdomen, hips, and legs) and consist of one set of 8–12 repetitions per activity. More sets may offer additional benefit (22).

- Specific recommendations for balance exercises are presented in the Federal Exercise Guideline.
  - Older adults at risk of falls should do balance training 3 or more days a week. Examples of these exercises include backward walking, sideways walking, heel walking, toe walking, and standing from a sitting position.
  - The exercises can increase in difficulty by progressing from holding onto a stable support (like furniture) while doing the exercises to doing them without support and then with eyes closed (22).

- Promotion of flexibility via stretching exercises is advised for all major muscle groups, as are warm-up and cool-down activities before all exercise events. Stretching should include three to five nonpainful repetitions of a static stretch for each major muscle group, with each stretch lasting 10–30 seconds.
  - A warm-up before moderate- or vigorous-intensity aerobic activity allows a gradual increase in heart rate and breathing at the beginning of the exercise session.
  - A cool-down after activity allows a gradual decrease at the end of the episode.
  - Time spent doing warm-up and cool-down may count toward meeting the aerobic activity guidelines if the activity is at least moderate intensity (22).

- The National Institute of Aging offers a free exercise guide for older adults. This guide includes general education, advice on goal setting, sample exercises, nutritional advice, and tracking tools. It is available online (14).

- *ACSM's Guidelines for Exercise Testing and Prescription* has specific recommendations for advising the older adult in safe exercise (see Table 114.4) (1).

COMMON INJURIES ENCOUNTERED IN OLDER RUNNERS

- Acute traumatic injuries
  - Older adults have a lower incidence of acute traumatic injuries than younger adults due to greater experience and lower intensity of exercise performance (5).
  - The muscle-tendon junction is particularly vulnerable to injury, with the most common injuries involving the Achilles and quadriceps tendons, attributable in part to:
    - ❑ Decreased flexibility and increased muscle fatigue from endurance sports such as running
    - ❑ Extrinsic factors such as training errors, training surface, and incorrect shoe choice

- Chronic and overuse injuries
  - Overuse injuries are common in older adult athletes, accounting for 70% of injuries in older athletes in one study. Common injuries include stress fractures, focal cartilage injuries, plantar fasciitis, and degenerative meniscal tears (5).
  - Despite this increased incidence of injury, running has been clearly demonstrated to:
    - ❑ Protect against disability and increased mortality
    - ❑ Prolong a disability-free life (25)
  - Approaches to treatment in the older adult are similar to those for a younger adult, except that:
    - ❑ Healing and recovery are prolonged.
    - ❑ Training and competition practices are possibly altered to a greater degree.

Table 114.5	General Exercise Prescription for the Older Runner (22)

Minimum activity to achieve health benefits:

- 150 minutes of moderate-intensity aerobic activity (*e.g.*, brisk walking) a week, plus muscle-strengthening activities on at least 2 days a week or

- 75 minutes of vigorous-intensity aerobic activity (*e.g.*, jogging, running) a week, plus muscle-strengthening activities on at least 2 days a week or

- A combination of moderate- and vigorous-intensity aerobic activity equivalent to the above recommendations, plus muscle-strengthening exercises at least 2 days a week

Increased activity for achieving increased health benefits:

- 300 minutes of moderate-intensity aerobic activity a week, plus muscle-strengthening activities on at least 2 days a week or

- 150 minutes of vigorous-intensity aerobic activity a week, plus muscle-strengthening activities on at least 2 days a week or

- A combination of moderate- to vigorous-intensity aerobic activity equivalent to the above recommendations, plus muscle-strengthening activities on at least 2 days a week

- Osteoarthritis (OA)
  - A comprehensive review of the studies evaluating exercise risk factors for the development of OA have shown conflicting results. Potential mediating factors include age, gender, body mass index, body composition, and muscle strength.
  - Development of OA is more closely related to previous joint injury, training intensity, occupational stresses, altered biomechanics, and incomplete rehabilitation (23).
  - The evidence for using exercise as an effective treatment for OA is well established.
    - ❏ The systematic review conducted by the MOVE consensus showed that both strengthening and aerobic exercise can reduce pain and improve function in individuals with hip and knee OA (16).
    - ❏ In general, themes of improved pain and function were noted for aerobic walking programs, and patient preference between home or group exercise programs should be considered.

NUTRITION

- Aging is associated with reductions in all components of energy expenditure (resting metabolic rate, thermic effect of food, and energy expenditure), and masters level athletes have unique nutritional needs. Little data exist on the nutritional needs of older athletes, and nutritional needs are determined by training intensity.
- The Dietary Reference Intakes (DRIs) serve as a guide in establishing energy and micronutrient intake. Estimated energy requirements for active adults by age and gender are presented in Table 114.6 (17).
- Carbohydrate intake can be estimated:
  - As a percentage of total calories (45%–65%)
  - By grams per kilogram of body weight and level of training intensity.
    - ❏ For general training, 5–7 g · kg^{-1} a day of carbohydrate are needed.
    - ❏ Endurance athletes require 7–10 g · kg^{-1} a day.
    - ❏ Ultra-endurance athletes need more than 10 g · kg^{-1} a day.
    - ❏ 30–60 g of carbohydrate should be consumed for every hour of training.
    - ❏ If training occurs daily, recovery from vigorous exercise is enhanced by ingestion of 1.5 g · kg^{-1} of carbohydrate immediately after exercise and an additional carbohydrate feeding 2 hours later (17).
- Protein ingestion for older adults matches that of younger adults (approximately 1.2–1.7 g · kg^{-1} a day).
  - Recovery from endurance and resistance exercise may be enhanced by small amounts of protein (0.1–0.2 g · kg^{-1} an hour).

Table 114.6 | Nutritional Requirements of Older Adults (17)

Estimated energy requirements of older active adults:

Age group in years	Men (kcal · d^{-1})	Women (kcal · d^{-1})
50–59	2,757	2,186
60–69	2,657	2,116
70–79	2,557	2,046
80–89	2,457	1,967

Micronutrient requirements for older active adults:

Vitamin D		
50–70 years	10 μg · d^{-1}	10 μg · d^{-1}
> 70 years	15 μg · d^{-1}	15 μg · d^{-1}
Calcium		
> 50 years	1,200 mg · d^{-1}	1,200 mg · d^{-1}
Vitamin B$_6$		
> 50 years	1.7 mg · d^{-1}	1.5 mg · d^{-1}
Folate		
> 50 years	400 μg · d^{-1}	400 μg · d^{-1}
Vitamin B$_{12}$		
> 50 years	2.4 μg · d^{-1}	2.4 μg · d^{-1}
Iron		
> 50 years	8 mg · d^{-1}	8 mg · d^{-1}
Thiamine	1.2 mg · d^{-1}	1.1 mg · d^{-1}
Riboflavin	1.3 mg · d^{-1}	1.1 mg · d^{-1}
Choline	550 mg · d^{-1}	425 mg · d^{-1}
Zinc	11 mg · d^{-1}	8 mg · d^{-1}
Magnesium	420 mg · d^{-1}	320 mg · d^{-1}
Vitamin C		
> 50 years	90 mg · d^{-1}	75 mg · d^{-1}
Vitamin E		
> 50 years	15 mg · d^{-1}	15 mg · d^{-1}

- Snacks that meet this need include milk, eggs, cheese, yogurt, lean meats, fish, and poultry (17).
- Fat intake should involve 20%–35% of total calories (17).
  - There is no demonstrated benefit to low-fat diets for athletes, and therefore, the American Dietetic Association recommends that athletes do not restrict fat intake.
  - Monounsaturated and long-chain polyunsaturated fats ("heart healthy fats") are recommended (17).
- Micronutrient intake is included in Table 114.6. Little research on micronutrient intake has been performed on masters athletes to determine optimal amounts (17).
  - Nutritional requirements for thiamine, riboflavin, choline, zinc, and magnesium do not appear to be different in older versus younger adults.
  - No evidence suggests there are additional vitamin C requirements in athletes, and the Tolerable Upper Intake Level (UL) is 2,000 mg · d^{-1} for this vitamin.

- Athletes taking supplements should adhere to the ULs of all vitamins and minerals to prevent toxicity.
- Ideally, whole foods are the preferred source of micronutrients, but research has shown that athletes often do not meet Recommended Daily Allowances (RDAs) through their diet.

OSTEOPOROSIS

- Exercise is important in both the treatment and prevention of osteoporosis, which is defined as bone mass loss of 2.5 standard deviations below that of a young adult female.
- Type I osteoporosis is a condition of postmenopausal women affecting trabecular bone. Fractures of the thoracic and upper lumbar vertebrae and wrist are common with this condition.
- Type II osteoporosis affects both genders and is due to age-associated loss of cortical bone, such as the hip and femoral neck.
- Osteoporosis is either:
  - Primary (due to aging).
  - Secondary to an identifiable cause. Identification of secondary causes of osteoporosis is critical to prevent (and reverse) further bone loss. Causes include genetic syndromes, hypogonadal states, endocrinopathies, deficiency states, inflammatory conditions, hematologic and neoplastic conditions, common medical conditions (*e.g.*, renal disease, congestive heart failure, liver disease, alcoholism, diabetes, chronic obstructive lung disease), disuse, and medications (15).
- Prevention and treatment of osteoporosis are multifaceted and include weight-bearing exercises such as walking or running.
- Athletes who have an established diagnosis of osteoporosis or are developing stress fractures should minimize their running activity in favor of cross-training and modified weight-bearing exercises (15).

FLUID REPLACEMENT

- Healthy older adults are generally adequately hydrated but have a blunted thirst response when deprived of water, increasing the risk of becoming dehydrated.
- Older adults:
  - Have age-associated increase in plasma osmolality.
  - Achieve homeostasis more slowly after dehydration.
  - Have slower water and sodium excretion following fluid loads. This results in possible increases in blood pressure or development of hyponatremia.
- Given sufficient time and access to fluids, older adults are able to appropriately rehydrate and should be encouraged to do so during and after exercise.
- Excessive fluid or sodium ingestion is inadvisable.

- Body weight changes can be used to calculate individual fluid replacement needs, with euhydration reflecting a weight within 1% of baseline readings.
- Urine specific gravity measurements of less than 1.020 likely reflect euhydration (4).

TEMPERATURE REGULATION

- Heat stress in older adults results in higher core temperatures, heart rate and fluid losses, and lower sweating rates.
- Cold exposure is associated with blunted vasoconstrictor response and greater loss of heat in older adults.
- These observed physiologic phenomenon are related to age, medical comorbidities, lifestyle choices, medications, acclimatization, and physical conditioning.
- Physicians should identify older athletes with these risk factors in common sense actions to reduce their risk of heat- or cold-related injury (Table 114.7) (2).

JOINT REPLACEMENT

- Joint arthroplasty is expected to dramatically increase in the United States over the next 20 years due to the success of these procedures and the demands of the "Baby Boomer" population.
- Baby Boomers are having these procedures performed at a younger age and at less severe stages of arthritis to preserve lifestyle and to reduce pain.
- In general, individuals decrease the number or intensity of athletic activities after joint replacement.
- There are no controlled studies evaluating appropriate athletic activities after joint replacement. The concern is that high levels

Table 114.7	General Strategies for Prevention of Heat- and Cold-Related Injuries (2)

Appropriate clothing for temperature

Adequate fluid intake and nutrition

Adequate sleep

Not running when acutely ill with viral illness or diarrhea

Avoidance of sunburn

Acclimatization for 10–14 days in the heat

A running partner to monitor each other's well-being

Avoidance of temperature extremes

Recognition of early symptoms of heat/cold injury (clumsiness, stumbling, headache, nausea, dizziness, apathy, confusion, and altered consciousness)

Regular clinician monitoring of overall health and medication regimen of activity may compromise the durability of the joint replacement and result in premature revision of the implant (8).

- Expert opinion from the American Association of Hip and Knee Surgeons, the Knee Society, and the Hip Society has been developed.
  - Low-impact aerobic activities (including stationary cycling, dancing, golf, normal walking, speed walking, and hiking) are "allowed" in the 2005 surveys of Hip Society and Knee Society members.
  - Skating, skiing, horseback riding, and weight-lifting exercises are "allowed" if the patient has prior experience with these activities.
  - Jogging, football, basketball, soccer, and volleyball are specifically not recommended (8).
- The review conducted by Healy et al. (8) comments that many surgeons allow their patients to participate in athletic activities as they wish, as long as:
  - Education on risks is performed.
  - The patient trains for the specific sports activity.
- Stretching and strengthening of core muscles and back, hip, and knee rehabilitation are felt to improve athletic performance after joint replacement (8).

CONCLUSION

- Despite age-related physiologic changes that may adversely affect goals and personal performance, older athletes can enjoy the activity for a lifetime with adaptations.
- Providers should seek to look for ways to keep older athletes moving, rather than preclude their participation.
- The evidence strongly supports the recommendation that choosing to not exercise is more dangerous that staying active.

REFERENCES

1. American College of Sports Medicine. *ACSM's Guidelines for Exercise Testing and Prescription*. 8th ed. Baltimore (MD): Lippincott Williams & Wilkins; 2010. 380 p.
2. American College of Sports Medicine, Armstrong LE, Casa DJ, et al. American College of Sports Medicine position stand. Exertional heat illness during training and competition. *Med Sci Sports Exerc*. 2007;39(3):556–72.
3. American College of Sports Medicine, Chodzko-Zajko WJ, Proctor DN, et al. American College of Sports Medicine position stand. Exercise and physical activity for older adults. *Med Sci Sports Exerc*. 2009;41(7):1510–30.
4. American College of Sports Medicine, Sawka MN, Burke LM, et al. American College of Sports Medicine position stand. Exercise and fluid replacement. *Med Sci Sports Exerc*. 2007;39(2):377–90.
5. Chen AL, Mears SC, Hawkins RJ. Orthopedic care of the aging athlete. *J Am Acad Orthop Surg*. 2005;13(6):407–16.
6. Daly RM, Ahlborg HG, Ringsberg K, Gardsell P, Sernbo I, Karlsson MK. Association between changes in habitual physical activity and changes in bone density, muscle strength, and functional performance in elderly men and women. *J Am Geriatr Soc*. 2008;56(12):2252–60.
7. Haran MJ, Cameron ID, Ivers RQ, et al. Effect on falls of providing single lens distance vision glasses to multifocal glasses wearers: VISABLE randomised controlled trial. *BMJ*. 2010;340:c2265.
8. Healy WL, Sharma S, Schwartz B, Iorio R. Current concepts review. Athletic activity after total joint arthroplasty. *J Bone Joint Surg Am*. 2008;90(10):2245–52.
9. Jokl P, Sethi PM, Cooper AJ. Master's performance in the New York City Marathon 1983–1999. *Br J Sports Med*. 2004;38(4):408–12.
10. Maharam LG, Bauman PA, Kalman D, Skolnik H, Perle SM. Masters athletes: factors affecting performance. *Sports Med*. 1999;28(4):273–85.
11. Manini TM, Pahor M. Physical activity and maintaining physical function in older adults. *Br J Sports Med*. 2009;43(1):28–31.
12. Maron BJ, Araújo CG, Thompson PD, et al. American Heart Association Science Advisory. Recommendations for preparticipation screening and the assessment of cardiovascular disease in masters athletes: an advisory for healthcare professionals from the working groups of the World Heart Federation, the International Federation of Sports Medicine, and the American Heart Association Committee on Exercise, Cardiac Rehabilitation, and Prevention. *Circulation*. 2001;103(2):327–34.
13. Middleton LE, Barnes DE, Lui LY, Yaffe K. Physical activity over the life course and its association with cognitive performance and impairment in old age. *J Am Geriat Soc*. 2010;58(7):1322–6.
14. National Institute on Aging. Exercise and physical activity. National Institutes of Health, 2010 [Internet]. Available from: http://www.nia.nih.gov/NR/rdonlyres/E2A819E3–8BAA–46AA–89E8–321B527D8A2B/0/ExerciseGuide_FINAL_Aug2010.pdf.
15. O'Connor FG, Wilder RP, Nirschl R. Chapter 35: the geriatric runner. In: O'Connor FG, Wilder RP, editors. *Textbook of Running Medicine*. New York (NY): McGraw-Hill Professional Publishing; 2001.
16. Roddy E, Zhang W, Doherty M, et al. Evidence-based recommendations for the role of exercise in the management of osteoarthritis of the hip or knee — the MOVE consensus. *Rheumatology (Oxford)*. 2005;44(1):67–73.
17. Rosenbloom CA, Dunaway A. Nutrition recommendations for masters athletes. *Clin Sports Med*. 2007;26(1):91–100.
18. Running USA. 2010 Marathon, Half-Marathon and State of the Sport Reports. Running USA's Annual Marathon Report [Internet]. Available from: http://www.runningusa.org/node/57770#57771.
19. Stessman J, Hammerman-Rozenberg R, Cohen A, Ein-Mor E, Jacobs JM. Physical activity, function, and longevity among the very old. *Arch Intern Med*. 2009;169(16):1476–83.
20. Tanaka H, Seals DR. Endurance exercise performance in masters athletes: age-associated changes and underlying physiological mechanisms. *J Physiol*. 2008;586(1):55–63.
21. Tanaka H, Seals DR. Invited review: dynamic exercise performance in masters athletes: insight into the effects of primary human aging on physiological functional capacity. *J Appl Physiol*. 2003;95(5):2152–62.
22. United States Department of Health and Human Services. *2008 Physical Activity Guidelines for Older Americans*. Washington (DC): United States Department of Health and Human Services; 2008.
23. Urquhart DM, Soufan C, Teichtahl AJ, Wluka AE, Hanna F, Cicuttini FM. Factors that may mediate the relationship between physical activity and the risk for developing knee osteoarthritis. *Arthritis Res Ther*. 2008;10(1):203.
24. Veciana-Suarez A. A growing number of baby boomers see sports as a way to feel young again [Internet]. [cited 2010 May 28]. Available from: http://www.bellinghamherald.com.
25. Wang BW, Ramey DR, Schettler JD, Hubert HB, Fries JF. Postponed development of disability in elderly runners: a 13-year longitudinal study. *Arch Intern Med*. 2002;162(20):2285–94.
26. World Masters Athletics [Internet]. Available from: http://www.world-masters-athletics.org/records.

115

The Female Athlete

Courtney A. Dawley and Rochelle M. Nolte

INTRODUCTION

- In 1971, there were fewer than 300,000 girls participating in high school athletics, compared to 3.7 million boys. Title IX was passed in 1972, mandating nondiscrimination in all extracurricular activities and varsity athletics that received federal funding. In 2000, there were 2.7 million girls involved in high school sports compared to 3.8 million boys (30).
- Benefits of exercise for girls and women include improved cardiovascular health, less obesity, improved physical and psychological development, improved self-image, decreased school dropout rates, and decreased rates of unwanted or unplanned pregnancy (13,17,29).

ANATOMY AND PHYSIOLOGY

- Menarche occurs approximately 1 year after peak height velocity, which ranges from 10.5–13.0 years for girls, compared to 12.5–15.0 years for boys (28).
- Adult height is reached by age 17–19 years for girls and by age 20–22 for boys.
- Skeletal maturity is completed by age 18–19 for girls and age 21–22 for boys.
- $\dot{V}O_{2max}$ averages around 50 mL $\cdot$ kg $\cdot$ min^{-1} in prepubescent children and changes little in boys throughout puberty, but decreases in girls with puberty secondary to a change in body composition and a decreased percentage of lean body mass.
- After puberty, metabolically active muscle averages 40%–45% of total body weight in boys, but only 35%–38% in girls (16).
- Girls develop smaller heart size, cardiac stroke volume, left ventricular mass, lung volume, aerobic capacity, and hemoglobin levels (13,21).
- Women on average are shorter, weigh less, and have shorter limbs and smaller articular surfaces, narrower shoulders and smaller thoraces, and a wider pelvis in relation to their waist and shoulders than men. Women have less muscle mass per total body weight than equally trained and conditioned men. The average young adult female has approximately 20%–27% body fat, while the average young adult male has 12%–18% body fat (12,28).

THE FEMALE ATHLETE TRIAD AND DISORDERED EATING

- The female athlete triad has three components: (a) low energy availability (with or without an eating disorder), (b) menstrual dysfunction, and (c) decreased bone mineral density (BMD) (23).
- Eating disorders are characterized by disturbances in eating behavior, body image, emotions, and relationships. Tables 115.1 to 115.3 exhibit diagnostic criteria of eating disorders.
  - Anorexia nervosa is an extreme version of restrictive eating behavior in which an individual continues to starve and feel fat, even though she (female athlete) is 15% or more below her ideal body weight.
  - Bulimia nervosa has cycles of recurrent binge eating with a feeling of loss of control followed by inappropriate compensatory behavior.
  - Eating disorder not otherwise specified (ED-NOS) is also included in the *Diagnostic and Statistical Manual of Mental Disorders, 4th Edition* (DSM-IV) and includes patients who have eating disorders but do not meet the exact diagnostic criteria of anorexia nervosa or bulimia nervosa.
  - Disordered eating includes the entire spectrum of abnormal eating behaviors that may not fit any of the DSM-IV criteria for eating disorders.
- Disordered eating can have devastating effects on psychological well-being, skeletal health, and other physiologic problems such as dehydration, electrolyte disturbances, thermoregulatory and cardiac disturbances, loss of muscle mass, and decreased performance in addition to other medical complications.
- Disordered eating can lead to an energy deficit that contributes to menstrual irregularity and an increased risk of stress fractures and decreased BMD.
- Sports or activities that emphasize a lean physique or low body weight, such as gymnastics, swimming, or track and field, have a greater number of athletes who develop the female athlete triad.
- Risk factors for disordered eating and the female athlete triad include the following:
  - Chronic dieting
  - Low self-esteem

Table 115.1 | Diagnostic Criteria for Anorexia Nervosa

A. Refusal to maintain body weight at or above a minimally normal weight for age and height (*e.g.*, weight loss leading to maintenance of body weight < 85% of that expected; or failure to make expected weight gain during period of growth, leading to body weight < 85% of that expected).

B. Intense fear of gaining weight or becoming fat, even though underweight.

C. Disturbance in the way in which one's body weight or shape is experienced, undue influence of body weight or shape on self-evaluation, or denial of the seriousness of the current low body weight.

D. In postmenarchal females, amenorrhea, *i.e.*, the absence of at least three consecutive menstrual cycles. (A woman is considered to have amenorrhea if her periods occur only following hormone, *e.g.*, estrogen, administration.)

Restricting Type: During the current episode of anorexia nervosa, the person has not regularly engaged in binge-eating or purging behavior (*i.e.*, self-induced vomiting or the misuse of laxatives, diuretics, or enemas).

Binge-Eating/Purging Type: During the current episode of anorexia nervosa, the person has regularly engaged in binge-eating or purging behavior (*i.e.*, self-induced vomiting or the misuse of laxatives, diuretics, or enemas)

SOURCE: American Psychiatric Association. *Diagnostic and Statistical Manual of Mental Disorders.* 4th ed. Arlington (VA): American Psychiatric Association; 2000.

Table 115.2 | Diagnostic Criteria for Bulimia Nervosa

A. Recurrent episodes of binge eating. An episode of binge eating is characterized by both of the following:

   a. Eating, in a discrete period of time (*e.g.*, within any 2-hour period), an amount of food that is definitely larger than most people would eat during a similar period of time and under similar circumstances.

   b. A sense of lack of control over eating during the episode (*e.g.*, a feeling that one cannot stop eating or control what or how much one is eating).

B. Recurrent inappropriate compensatory behavior to prevent weight gain, such as self-induced vomiting; misuse of laxative, diuretics, enemas, or other medications; fasting; or excessive exercise.

C. The binge eating and inappropriate compensatory behaviors both occur, on average, at least twice a week for 3 months.

D. Self-evaluation is unduly influenced by body shape and weight.

E. The disturbance does not occur exclusively during episodes of anorexia nervosa.

Purging Type: During the current episode of bulimia nervosa, the person has regularly engaged in self-induced vomiting or the misuse of laxatives, diuretics, or enemas.

Nonpurging Type: During the current episode of bulimia nervosa, the person has used other inappropriate compensatory behaviors, such as fasting or excessive exercise, but has not regularly engaged in self-induced vomiting or the misuse of laxatives, diuretics, or enemas.

SOURCE: American Psychiatric Association. *Diagnostic and Statistical Manual of Mental Disorders.* 4th ed. Arlington (VA): American Psychiatric Association; 2000.

Table 115.3 | Eating Disorder Not Otherwise Specified

The *eating disorder not otherwise specified* category is for disorders of eating that do not meet the criteria for any specific eating disorder. Examples include the following:

1. For females, all the criteria for anorexia nervosa are met except that the individual has regular menses.

2. All the criteria for anorexia nervosa are met except that, despite significant weight loss, the individual's current weight is in the normal range.

3. All the criteria for bulimia nervosa are met except that the binge eating and inappropriate compensatory mechanisms occur at a frequency of less than twice a week or for a duration of less than 3 months.

4. The regular use of inappropriate compensatory behavior by an individual of normal body weight after eating small amounts of food (*e.g.*, self-induced vomiting after the consumption of two cookies).

5. Repeatedly chewing and spitting out, but not swallowing, large amounts of food.

6. Binge-eating disorder: Recurrent episodes of binge eating in the absence of the regular use of inappropriate compensatory behaviors characteristic of bulimia nervosa.

SOURCE: American Psychiatric Association. *Diagnostic and Statistical Manual of Mental Disorders.* 4th ed. Arlington (VA): American Psychiatric Association; 2000.

- Family dysfunction
- Physical abuse
- Biologic factors
- Perfectionism
- Lack of nutrition knowledge
- An emphasis on body weight for performance or appearance
- Pressure to lose weight from parents, coaches, judges, and peers
- A drive to win at any cost
- Self-identity as an athlete only (no identity outside of sports)
- A sudden increase in training
- Exercising through injury
- Overtraining (especially when undernourished)
- A traumatic event such as an injury or loss of a coach
- Vulnerable times such as an adolescent growth spurt, entering college, retiring from athletics, and postpartum depression

- Any athlete with one of the diagnostic criteria of the female athlete triad should be evaluated for the other two by a thorough history and a physical examination.
  - Laboratory tests that may be helpful include the following:
    - Complete blood count
    - Electrolytes, calcium, magnesium, phosphorus, blood urea nitrogen, creatinine, cholesterol, albumin, and total protein
    - Urinalysis
    - Pregnancy test
    - Follicle-stimulating hormone
    - Estradiol
    - Prolactin
    - Thyroid function tests
    - Erythrocyte sedimentation rate
  - An electrocardiogram may also be indicated because some patients may develop cardiac rhythm disturbances, including prolongation of the QTc.

- Treatment for disordered eating requires a multidisciplinary team, including a physician or other health care provider, mental health counselor, and a nutritionist.
  - Treatment includes the following:
    - Recognition of the problem
    - Identification and resolution of psychosocial precipitants
    - Stabilization of medical and nutritional condition
    - Reestablishment of healthy patterns of eating

- Indications for inpatient treatment for a patient with an eating disorder include the following:
  - Very low body weight ($<$ 75% of expected body weight)
  - $>$ 15% loss of initial body weight
  - Rapid ($>$ 10% in 1–2 months) weight loss
  - Cardiac arrhythmias

- Electrolyte imbalances
- Suicidal ideation
- Temperature $<$ 36°C
- Pulse $<$ 45 bpm
- Orthostatic pulse differential $>$ 30 bpm
- Patient not responding to outpatient treatment (2)

AMENORRHEA

- Pregnancy is the most common cause of amenorrhea in sexually active women and must be excluded.

- Primary amenorrhea is diagnosed in females with secondary sexual characteristics without menarche at the age of 16 or in females without secondary sexual characteristics and no menarche at the age of 14 (5,19).

- Athletes who begin intensive training before puberty, especially gymnasts and ballet dancers, are at risk of developing primary amenorrhea. Athletes who associate more stress with their sport and competition are more likely to be amenorrheic (18).

- Evaluation of a patient with amenorrhea should include a thorough medical history, including pubertal milestones in the patient and other female relatives, a thorough menstrual history in patients presenting with secondary amenorrhea, a training and dietary history, medications (including over-the-counter medications such as diuretics, laxatives, ipecac, herbals, or supplements), a thorough family history, and psychological screening for evidence of increased stress, depression, anxiety, obsessive or compulsive personality traits, or symptoms of an eating disorder.
  - A lack of any pubertal development can indicate hypothalamic, pituitary, or gonadal failure.
  - An interruption of normal pubertal development can indicate ovarian failure or pituitary failure, as happens with a pituitary neoplasm.
  - Normal breast and pubic development in the absence of menstrual periods can indicate an abnormality of the reproductive organs.

- A thorough physical should include vital signs, height, weight, body fat, arm span, Tanner stage, any characteristics of chromosomal anomalies, any traits of androgen excess, funduscopic examination and visual field confrontation, evaluation for galactorrhea, palpation of the thyroid, and a pelvic examination. Imaging studies may include a computed tomography or magnetic resonance imaging to rule out a pituitary adenoma if indicated.

- Laboratory testing for amenorrhea is shown in Figure 115.1. During a progestin challenge, the patient is given medroxyprogesterone 10 mg daily for 5–10 days and then assessed for withdrawal bleeding. This testing is appropriate for both primary and secondary amenorrhea.

- If a woman over the age of 30 is presenting with secondary amenorrhea, etiologies to be considered are premature ovarian failure, endometrial hyperplasia, and carcinoma. In all patients,

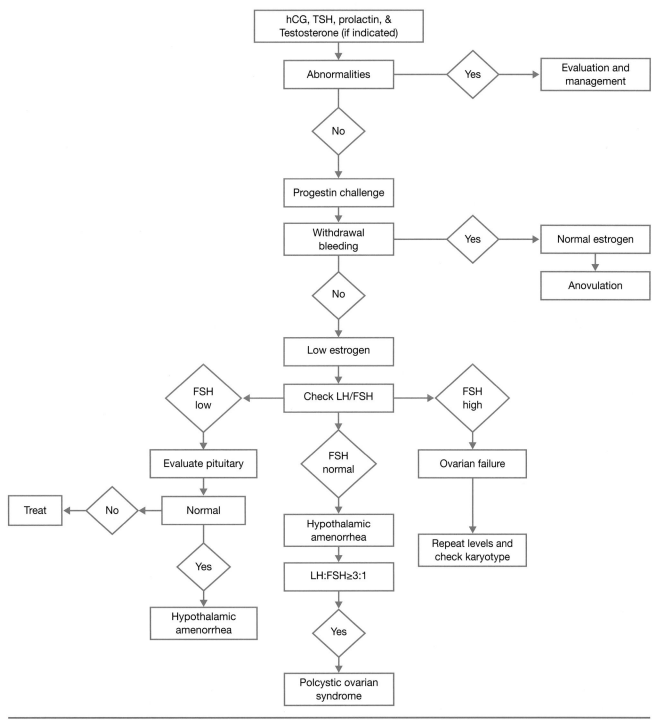

Figure 115.1: Laboratory evaluation of amenorrhea. FSH, follicle-stimulating hormone; hCG, human chorionic gonadotropin; LH, luteinizing hormone; TSH, thyroid-stimulating hormone. Adapted from Fieseler CM. Special considerations for the female runner. *J Back Musculoskel Rehabil.* 1996;6:37–47.

diagnoses to rule out include polycystic ovarian syndrome, Asherman syndrome, and thyroid or pituitary abnormalities.

- In hypothalamic amenorrhea, the pulsatile gonadotropin-releasing hormone (GnRH) is abnormal. Rarely, this can be caused by a tumor, trauma, or a developmental defect. More commonly, it is thought that psychological and/or physical stress affects neurohormones that regulate GnRH, leading to hypothalamic amenorrhea (18).

- Exercise-related amenorrhea can be considered a subset of hypothalamic amenorrhea, which also includes amenorrhea related to anorexia nervosa, weight loss, and psychological stress. It is, however, a diagnosis of exclusion. Exercise-related amenorrhea is thought to be secondary to an energy deficit from an inadequate caloric intake in relationship to energy expenditure. It is thought that girls or women who are having menstrual irregularities secondary to an energy deficit are at risk of decreased

BMD as well. The primary treatment that is recommended at this time is correcting the energy deficit by increasing caloric intake to the point that there is a spontaneous return of menses. This has been associated with an increase in bone mass as well.

LOW BONE MINERAL DENSITY

- Osteoporosis is characterized by microarchitectural deterioration of bone tissue, leading to enhanced skeletal fragility, low bone mass, and an increased risk for fracture.
    - The World Health Organization has established diagnostic criteria for osteoporosis based on bone density measurements.
    - Osteoporosis is defined as a BMD greater than 2.5 standard deviations (SD) below the mean BMD of a young adult woman at her peak bone mass (T-score).
    - Osteopenia is defined as a BMD between 1.0 and 2.5 SD below the mean.
    - A BMD within 1 SD of the mean is considered normal.
    - The U.S. Preventive Services Task Force (January 2011) currently recommends screening for osteoporosis in women age 65 years or older and in younger women whose fracture risk is equal to or greater than that of a 65-year-old white woman who has no additional risk factors.
- There is some controversy about whether the criteria for osteoporosis are appropriate to use when evaluating adolescents and young women with low bone mass, because they were developed to assess postmenopausal women.
- The female athlete triad leads to decreased BMD because bone growth and development are dependent on mechanical, nutritional, and hormonal influences. Women and girls with an energy deficit resulting from decreased caloric intake are at risk of having decreased BMD. Studies have also found a linear relationship between the degree of menstrual dysfunction and vertebral bone density (32).
- The standard method of diagnosing osteoporosis is by dual x-ray absorptiometry (DEXA), which is used to measure bone density at various places, usually the hip, spine, and distal radius. These measurements are used to generate the previously mentioned T-score and an age-matched Z-score.
- The U.S. Preventive Services Task Force recommends BMD screening by DEXA for women over age 65 or women over age 60 who are identified as being at high risk for developing osteoporosis (31).
- Nonmodifiable risk factors for osteoporosis (15) include:
    - Age
    - Sex
    - Race
    - Family history of osteoporosis
    - Past history of low-trauma fracture
- Modifiable risk factors for osteoporosis (15) include:
    - Low body weight
    - Low calcium intake
    - Tobacco use
    - Excessive alcohol use
    - Lack of weight-bearing exercise
    - Low muscle mass
    - Estrogen deficiency (including history of oligomenorrhea, amenorrhea, and delayed menarche)
- Nonpharmacologic measures used in the prevention and treatment of osteoporosis include the following (2,10,15,20):
    - Ensuring adequate caloric intake to meet energy needs and maintaining regular menses if premenopausal
    - Weight-bearing exercise (although it has been shown that weight-bearing exercise cannot overcome the bone loss associated with amenorrhea secondary to inadequate caloric intake) (14,22)
    - Decreasing tobacco and alcohol use
- Nutritional measures used in the prevention and treatment of osteoporosis include the following:
    - Calcium intake of 1,500 mg daily — divided into three doses containing at least 500 mg of elemental calcium to ensure absorption
    - Vitamin D 800 IU daily
- Pharmacologic treatments for pre- and postmenopausal osteoporosis include estrogen, bisphosphonates, selective estrogen receptor modulators, and calcitonin. These antiresorptive agents are indicated for the prevention and treatment of postmenopausal osteoporosis.
- It is thought that the primary problem in the young female athlete is decreased bone formation rather than premature bone loss, so the antiresorptive treatments may not address the problem of adolescent osteopenia/osteoporosis and are not indicated in this population. There is also the concern of possible teratogenic effects if bisphosphonates are used in women of childbearing age.
- Adequate nutrition and weight-bearing exercise during the adolescent years are important for achieving peak bone mass. On average, 92% of the total-body BMD is attained by age 18, and 99% is attained by age 26.
- Different sites appear to mature at different ages. Peak bone mass appears to be complete by age 16 in the femoral neck, whereas the bone mass in the lumbar spine appears to increase into the third decade (33).
- Although amenorrhea is associated with osteopenia, using oral contraceptive pills to induce menses has not been shown to increase bone mass in the absence of improved nutrition and calcium intake. In fact, some studies have shown that oral contraceptives may actually cause a further decrease in BMD in adolescent athletes (33).
- In a study of estrogen administration in young women with anorexia nervosa, overall there was no significant difference in bone mass after 1.5 years between the treatment and control groups, although it appeared that the estrogen did help a subgroup of patients who had body weights less than 70% of ideal body weight; however, a more marked improvement in BMD was obtained with recovery from the eating disorder

and gaining weight to 85% of ideal body weight and having spontaneous return of normal menstrual function without administration of estrogen (14).

■ When assessing overall bone health, vitamin D levels need to be checked, because insufficient and deficient levels have potential negative impact on athletes' health and ability to maximally train (34).

URINARY INCONTINENCE

■ Urinary incontinence is defined as "the complaint of any involuntary leakage of urine" (3). Stress urinary incontinence (SUI) is the most common type of urinary incontinence (3,4,24,25,26).

■ SUI is the involuntary loss of urine related to increased intra-abdominal pressure with such activities as sneezing, coughing, running, jumping, or heavy lifting.

■ Risk factors for SUI include anything that increases intra-abdominal pressure and anything that could weaken the pelvic floor muscles, such as pregnancy and delivery or decreased estrogen.

■ Athletes involved in high-impact activities such as gymnastics (dismount/tumbling), basketball, or volleyball are at risk for SUI during competition or practice (11,27,28).

■ Management of SUI is directed at correcting the underlying pelvic relaxation. Treatment for mild SUI usually includes pelvic floor–strengthening exercises. For women with evidence of vaginal and urethral atrophy secondary to estrogen deficiency, topical or systemic estrogen can be prescribed. For women with severe pelvic relaxation and prolapse, a temporizing measure such as a pessary may be used, but definitive therapy will often require an invasive treatment such as injection therapy or surgical repair.

EXERCISE IN PREGNANCY

■ Physiologic changes of pregnancy can impact the maternal response to exercise as early as the first trimester (7).

■ Increases in pulse, cardiac output, blood pressure, and temperature that are normally seen during exercise are slightly blunted in pregnancy.

■ Blood pressure usually falls slightly, reaching a nadir in the second trimester, and then slowly rises to prepregnancy levels by term.

■ Resting heart rate increases 10–15 bpm during pregnancy, in conjunction with an increase in stroke volume and cardiac output (6).

■ Blood volume increases by almost 50% at term.

■ A dilutional anemia develops in the second trimester that is partially corrected at term due to the increase in plasma volume occurring before the increase in red cell mass.

■ Tidal volume, minute ventilation, and oxygen consumption all increase in pregnancy.

■ Progesterone and relaxin increase pelvic and joint laxity in pregnancy.

■ The increased oxygen consumption of pregnancy will lead to most women experiencing a decline in their exercise tolerance.

■ There is no evidence that exercise has a detrimental effect on pregnancy or labor or fetal well-being (7).

■ Exercise during and after pregnancy has been shown to have a positive psychological effect (6).

■ The babies of regularly exercising women appear to tolerate labor well and have been shown to have a similar head circumference and length but lower body fat than babies born to nonexercising mothers (9).

■ Positive effects of exercise reported during pregnancy include: a tendency to deliver 1 week earlier than nonexercising women; a decreased rate of interventions during labor, including Pitocin use and cesarean section; and decreased pain perception. Mothers who exercise are also more than twice as likely to progress from 4 cm to completely dilated in under 4 hours, and their average second stage of labor is 36 minutes versus 60 minutes in controls (6,7).

■ Long-term benefits of exercising throughout pregnancy include maintenance of long-term fitness and a low cardiovascular risk profile in the perimenopausal period (8).

■ Exertion at altitudes up to 6,000 feet appears to be safe, but engaging in physical activities at higher altitudes carries various risks (1).

■ Scuba diving should be avoided throughout pregnancy as the fetus is at increased risk of decompression sickness secondary to the inability of the fetal pulmonary circulation to filter bubble formation (1).

■ Absolute contraindications to aerobic exercise during pregnancy:
  ■ Hemodynamically significant heart disease
  ■ Restrictive lung disease
  ■ Incompetent cervix/cerclage
  ■ Multiple gestation at risk for premature labor
  ■ Persistent second- or third-trimester bleeding
  ■ Placenta previa after 26 weeks of gestation
  ■ Premature labor during the current pregnancy
  ■ Ruptured membranes
  ■ Preeclampsia/pregnancy-induced hypertension

■ Relative contraindications to aerobic exercise during pregnancy:
  ■ Severe anemia
  ■ Unevaluated maternal cardiac arrhythmia
  ■ Chronic bronchitis
  ■ Poorly controlled type 1 diabetes
  ■ Extreme morbid obesity
  ■ Extreme underweight (body mass index < 12)
  ■ History of extremely sedentary lifestyle
  ■ Intrauterine growth restriction in current pregnancy
  ■ Poorly controlled hypertension
  ■ Orthopedic limitations

- ▪ Poorly controlled seizure disorder
- ▪ Poorly controlled hyperthyroidism
- ▪ Heavy smoker
- Warning signs to terminate exercise while pregnant:
  - ▪ Vaginal bleeding
  - ▪ Dyspnea prior to exertion
  - ▪ Dizziness
  - ▪ Headache
  - ▪ Chest pain
  - ▪ Muscle weakness
  - ▪ Calf pain or swelling (need to rule out thrombophlebitis)
  - ▪ Preterm labor
  - ▪ Decreased fetal movement
  - ▪ Amniotic fluid leakage
- After the first trimester, the uterus can cause obstruction of venous return in the supine position, so athletes will have to adjust weight-training and floor exercises appropriately.
- Motionless standing also causes a significant decrease in cardiac output and should be avoided as much as possible.
- There are currently no definitive guidelines for elite or endurance athletes during pregnancy. All athletes have to deal with the changing physiology of pregnancy, which may necessitate changing their exercise regimen.

REFERENCES

1. ACOG Committee Obstetric Practice. ACOG committee opinion. Number 267, January 2002: exercise during pregnancy and the postpartum period. *Obstet Gynecol.* 2002;99(1):171–3.
2. Becker AE, Grinspoon SK, Klibanski A, Herzog DB. Eating disorders. *N Engl J Med.* 1999;340(14):1092–8.
3. Bø K. Urinary incontinence, pelvic floor dysfunction, exercise and sport. *Sports Med.* 2004;34(7):451–64.
4. Bø K, Borgen JS. Prevalence of stress and urge urinary incontinence in elite athletes and controls. *Med Sci Sports Exerc.* 2001;33(11):1797–802.
5. Bruckner P, Fricker P. Endocrinologic conditions. In: Fields KB, Fricker PA, editors. *Medical Problems in Athletes.* Oxford (UK): Blackwell Science; 1998.
6. Christian JS, Christian SS, Stamm CA, et al. Physiology and exercise. In: Ireland ML, Nattiv A, editors. *The Female Athlete.* New York (NY): Elsevier Science; 2002.
7. Clapp JF 3rd. Exercise during pregnancy. A clinical update. *Clin Sports Med.* 2000;19(2):273–86.
8. Clapp JF 3rd. Long-term outcome after exercising throughout pregnancy: fitness and cardiovascular risk. *Am J Obstet Gynecol.* 2008;199(5):489.e1–6.
9. Clapp JF 3rd, Kim H, Burciu B, Schmidt S, Petry K, Lopez B. Continuing regular exercise during pregnancy: effect of exercise volume on fetoplacental growth. *Am J Obstet Gynecol.* 2002;186(1):142–7.
10. Cundy T, Cornish J, Roberts H, Reid IR. Menopausal bone loss in long-term users of depot medroxyprogesterone acetate contraception. *Am J Obstet Gynecol.* 2002;186(5):978–83.
11. Elia G. Stress urinary incontinence in women removing the barriers to exercise. *Phys Sportsmed.* 1999;27(1):39–52.
12. Fieseler CM. The female runner. In: O'Connor FG, Wilder RP, editors. *Textbook of Running Medicine.* New York (NY): McGraw-Hill; 2001.
13. Greydanus DE, Patel DR. The female athlete. Before and beyond puberty. *Pediatr Clin North Am.* 2002;49(3):553–80, vi.
14. Klibanski A, Biller BM, Schoenfeld DA, Herzog DB, Saxe VC. The effects of estrogen administration on trabecular bone loss in young women with anorexia nervosa. *J Clin Endocrinol Metab.* 1995;80(3):898–904.
15. Lane JM. Osteoporosis. In: Ireland ML, Nattiv A, editors. *The Female Athlete.* New York (NY): Elsevier Science; 2002.
16. Lillegard WA. Special considerations for the pediatric running population. In: O'Connor FG, Wilder RP, editors. *Textbook of Running Medicine.* New York (NY): McGraw-Hill; 2001.
17. Lopiano DA. Modern history of women in sports. Twenty-five years of title IX. *Clin Sports Med.* 2000;19(2):163–73, vii.
18. Marshall LA. Clinical evaluation of amenorrhea in active and athletic women. *Clin Sports Med.* 1994;13(2):371–87.
19. Master-Hunter T, Heiman DL. Amenorrhea: evaluation and treatment. *Am Fam Physician.* 2006;73(8):1374–82.
20. Meier DE. Osteoporosis and other disorders of skeletal aging. In: Cassel CK, Cohen HJ, Larson EB, et al., editors. *Geriatric Medicine.* 3rd ed. New York (NY): Springer-Verlag; 1997.
21. Mittleman KD, Zacher CM. Factors influencing endurance performance, strength, flexibility and coordination. In: Drinkwater BL, editor. *The Encyclopedia of Sports Medicine: Women in Sport: vol. 8, Chap. 2.* London (UK): Blackwell Science; 2000.
22. Nattiv A, Callahan LR, Kelman-Sherstinsky A. The female athlete triad. In: Ireland ML, Nattiv A, editors. *The Female Athlete.* New York (NY): Elsevier Science; 2002.
23. Nattiv A, Loucks AB, Manore MM, et al. American College of Sports Medicine position stand. The female athlete triad. *Med Sci Sports Exerc.* 2007;39(10):1867–82.
24. Nygaard IE. Does prolonged high-impact activity contribute to later urinary incontinence? A retrospective cohort study of female Olympians. *Obstet Gynecol.* 1997;90(5):718–22.
25. Nygaard IE, DeLancey JO, Arnsdorf L, Murphy E. Exercise and incontinence. *Obstet Gynecol.* 1990;75(5):848–51.
26. Nygaard IE, Glowacki C, Saltzman CL. Relationship between foot flexibility and urinary incontinence in nulliparous varsity athletes. *Obstet Gynecol.* 1996;87(6):1049–51.
27. Resnick NM. Urinary incontinence. In: Cassel CK, Cohen HJ, Larson EB, et al., editors. *Geriatric Medicine.* 3rd ed. New York (NY): Springer-Verlag; 1997.
28. Sanborn CF, Jankowski CM. Physiologic considerations for women in sport. *Clin Sports Med.* 1994;13(2):315–27.
29. Slater CA, Stone JA. Participation and historical perspective. In: Ireland ML, Nattiv A, editors. *The Female Athlete.* New York (NY): Elsevier Science; 2002.
30. Strickland SM, Metzl JD. Growth and development. In: Ireland ML, Nattiv A, editors. *The Female Athlete.* New York (NY): Elsevier Science; 2002.
31. U.S. Preventive Services Task Force. Screening for osteoporosis in postmenopausal women: recommendations and rationale. *Ann Intern Med.* 2002;137(10):834–9.
32. Vuori I, Heinonen A. Sport and bone. In: Drinkwater BL, editor. *Women in Sport: Volume VIII of the Encyclopaedia of Sports Medicine.* London (UK): Blackwell Science; 2000.
33. Weaver CM, Teegarden D, Lyle RM, et al. Impact of exercise on bone health and contraindication of oral contraceptive use in young women. *Med Sci Sports Exerc.* 2001;33(6):873–80.
34. Willis KS, Peterson NJ, Larson-Meyer DE. Should we be concerned about the vitamin D status of athletes? *Int J Sport Nutr Exerc Metab.* 2008;18(2):204–24.

The Athlete with Intellectual Disabilities

116

James H. Lynch

TERMINOLOGY

- *Intellectual disability* is a disability characterized by significant limitations both in intellectual functioning (reasoning, learning, problem solving) and in adaptive behavior, which covers a range of everyday social and practical skills (20).

- Intellectual disability is a common developmental disorder that affects approximately 7.5 million Americans.

- An individual is considered to have an intellectual disability if he or she experiences the following three criteria:

  - The individual has a below average intellectual functioning level (2 years or more behind peers).

  - Significant limitations exist in two or more adaptive skill areas.

  - The condition manifests itself before the age of 18.

- Adaptive skill areas are those daily living skills needed to live, work, and play in the community. They include communication, self-care, home living, social skills, leisure, health and safety, self-direction, functional academics, community use, and work.

- Adaptive skills are assessed in the person's typical environment across all aspects of an individual's life. A person with limits in intellectual functioning who does not have limits in adaptive skill areas may not be diagnosed as having intellectual disability (20).

- Definition of *mental retardation*: According to the *Diagnostic and Statistical Manual of Mental Disorders*, mental retardation refers to an intelligence quotient (IQ) of approximately 70 or less on an individually administered standardized test of intelligence concurrent with deficits in adaptive function in two skills areas such as communication, self-care, or home living. Onset of disability occurs before 18 years (2).

- Mental retardation and intellectual disability are two names for the same condition, but intellectual disability is gaining currency as the preferred term.

- In 2007, the American Association on Mental Retardation changed its name to the American Association on Intellectual and Developmental Disabilities.

- The term "mental retardation" is still used in some laws and public policy to determine eligibility for state and federal programs with regard to legal status, education, training, employment, income support, and health care (20).

PHYSIOLOGIC CONSIDERATIONS

- Athletes with intellectual disabilities may have a variety of health-related issues that impact their participation in competitive athletics. With such a diverse population of athletes, there is no unifying list of diagnoses or conditions; however, there are some important points for the sports medicine team to consider.

- Epidemiologic studies of organized athletics for intellectually disabled athletes reveal some patterns and conditions that are more prevalent in this population. Generally speaking, intellectually disabled athletes, as compared to general population athletes, have:

  - A higher prevalence of hearing and visual impairment

  - Decreased measures of strength and endurance

  - Poorer agility, balance, speed, flexibility, and reaction time

  - Higher rates of obesity (half of all with intellectual disability)

  - Lower peak heart rate

  - Lower peak oxygen uptake (7,13,16)

- Using preparticipation screening exam data for Special Olympics athletes, the incidence of sports-significant abnormalities detected is roughly 40%.

  - The most common categories of problems detected among intellectually disabled athletes are neurologic (16%), ophthalmologic (15%), musculoskeletal (6%), and medical (5%).

  - The most common diagnoses are seizure disorder and vision loss (11).

- As a comparison, the incidence of sports-significant abnormalities detected among nondisabled athletes is historically 1%–3%.

PREPARTICIPATION EVALUATION

- The goal in performing a preparticipation physical evaluation (PPE) is to promote the health and safety of the athlete in training and competition.
- The *PPE: Preparticipation Physical Evaluation, Fourth Edition* monograph was updated in 2010 by all major American sports medicine societies. The authors stress that PPE for the athlete with special needs should be similar to any athlete without physical or cognitive disability (1).
  - The PPE should address the particular concerns of the athlete with special needs.
  - The health care provider should:
    - ❏ Be aware of common problems associated with different disabilities
    - ❏ Be able to diagnose abnormalities that may endanger the athlete
    - ❏ Provide support and encourage physical activity
- The preparticipation history has been shown to be helpful in detecting 88% of medical conditions and 67% of musculoskeletal conditions detected during the PPE (1,5).
- Careful attention to the neurologic, musculoskeletal, and cardiopulmonary examination is essential, in particular with the athlete with an intellectual disability.

INJURY AND ILLNESS PATTERNS

- Injury rates for individuals with intellectual disabilities are less than those reported for physically disabled and general population athletes.
- Epidemiologic data have been reported for state, national, and international events (4,12,15,18).
  - Studies have shown that 3%–4% of all athletes are treated at Special Olympics events.
  - Track and field, followed by softball, account for more sports injuries than other events.
  - The most commonly injured site is the knee.
  - Injury rates calculated per 1,000 participant-hours are:
    - ❏ 0.4 for Special Olympics athletes
    - ❏ 2.0 for special education high school students in organized contact sports
    - ❏ These rates can be compared to the following nondisabled adult athletes' injury rates (per 1,000 participant-hours):
      - ▪ 0.03 for swimming
      - ▪ 2.9 for badminton
      - ▪ 3.65 for soccer
      - ▪ 4.1 for football
      - ▪ 4.7 for ice hockey

Table 116.1	Intellectually Disabled Athletics: Sport Injuries and Illnesses (15)		
Summer Sports		**Winter Sports**	
Injuries	Illnesses	Injuries	Illnesses
Abrasion	Heat related	Abrasion	Respiratory
Strain	Gastrointestinal	Strain	Dehydration
Sprain	Seizure	Sprain	Behavioral
Contusion	Headache	Contusion	Gastrointestinal
Epistaxis	Asthma	Laceration	Dermatologic
Laceration	Diabetes control	Blister	Canker sores
Blister	Sunburn	Fracture	Gingivitis
Nail avulsion	Conjunctivitis		
Fracture	Dermatitis Insect bite		

- Frequently encountered injuries and illnesses are listed in Table 116.1.
- In a study of Special Olympics injuries in Texas, athletes with Down syndrome had a relative risk of injury or illness 3.2 times greater than the other athletes (11).

DOWN SYNDROME

- The athlete with Down syndrome (trisomy 21) requires special consideration due to well-described conditions associated with increased risk in athletics.
- Down syndrome is the most common human chromosomal abnormality.
  - Its incidence is estimated at 1 in 600–800 live births.
  - Up to 30% of Special Olympics athletes have Down syndrome.
  - Phenotypically, Down syndrome can vary greatly, but frequent findings include intellectual disability, orthopedic issues, cardiac anomalies, vision problems, epilepsy, and obesity (19).
- National Health Interview Survey data of children with Down syndrome in the United States from 1997–2005 revealed the following general health information:
  - Children with Down syndrome were more than twice as likely as children in the general population to have seizures, recent food allergy, frequent diarrhea, or three or more ear infections.
  - Children with other causes of intellectual disability had higher risks for frequent severe headaches and seizures than did children with Down syndrome (21).

- Cardiac anomalies are prevalent in roughly 50% of persons with Down syndrome as compared to about 1% in the general population.
  - Endocardial cushion defects make up the majority of these, most of which are surgically repaired at a young age.
  - Isolated ventricular septal defects, atrial septal defects, and patent ductus arteriosus compose another 20% of the congenital heart disease associated with Down syndrome.
  - Pulmonary hypertension is also more common in individuals with Down syndrome (14).
  - With or without cardiac malformations, athletes with Down syndrome have been found to have lower cardiovascular fitness levels than their peers due to average lower peak heart rates (19).
- Persons with Down syndrome have a high prevalence of vision and eye health problems. Many eye problems are undetected secondary to infrequent examinations. Down syndrome is associated with an increased frequency of keratoconus, cataract, high refractive error, glaucoma, strabismus, and macular disease.
  - In studies screening Down syndrome athletes, about 20% were observed to have significant uncorrected refractive errors (> 1 diopter).
  - About one-third to one-half of Down syndrome athletes screened prior to participation are observed to have pathology sufficient to affect vision (8,24).
- Due in part to inherent ligamentous laxity, the musculoskeletal system is a frequent cause of disability in Down syndrome athletes. The major areas of concern include the neck, hips, knees, and feet.
  - Cervical spine instability is the most significant musculoskeletal issue for the athlete with Down syndrome.
    - Atlantoaxial instability (AAI), which affects 10%–30% of individuals with Down syndrome, denotes laxity of the articulation between C1 (atlas) and C2 (axis).
    - Although atlantoaxial dislocation can be a significant cause of cord compromise, approximately 98% of AAI cases are asymptomatic (9).
      - Symptoms of AAI include neck pain, cervical deformity, fatigability, abnormal gait, clumsiness, or altered sensation.
      - Neurologic signs include sensory deficits, spasticity, hyperreflexia, clonus, and extensor-plantar reflex.
    - AAI is due to odontoid abnormalities or laxity of the transverse ligament that holds the odontoid process in place against the inner aspect of the arch of the atlas (6).
    - Radiographic evaluation is necessary to detect AAI. Lateral cervical spine radiographs in flexion, extension, and neutral will allow for examination of the atlanto-dens interval (ADI), which is measured from the anterior aspect of odontoid to the posterior surface of anterior arch of atlas.
    - In the early 1980s, the Special Olympics and the American Academy of Pediatrics (AAP) began recommending cervical spine radiographic screening of Special Olympians with Down syndrome before participation in "high-risk" sports (10).
    - These recommendations remain in effect today. The high-risk sports include pentathlon, diving (either as a sport or in swimming starts), butterfly swimming stroke, high jump, gymnastics, soccer, judo, snowboarding, and alpine skiing.
    - Currently, the AAP recommends obtaining screening x-rays between the ages 3 and 5 years for all children with Down syndrome, not just Special Olympians (9).
    - Using Special Olympics' guidelines, AAI is diagnosed when the ADI is more than 4.5 mm.
    - Athletes with asymptomatic AAI should be restricted from high-risk activities that place undue stress on the neck, but no further intervention is warranted.
    - For athletes with symptomatic AAI or an ADI greater than 5 mm, magnetic resonance imaging evaluation is recommended.
    - The guidelines do not recommend continued radiographic screening for children with an ADI less than 4.5 mm.
    - Because some studies have shown AAI progresses over time, especially with young patients, it may be reasonable to obtain repeat evaluations until skeletal maturity is achieved, although there is no consensus on the proper interval (22).
    - Special Olympics does permit athletes with known AAI to play with a signed release only after they are evaluated and counseled in writing by two licensed physicians who determine that the athlete is not medically precluded from participation (10).
  - Acquired hip instability is seen in about 5% of persons with Down syndrome.
    - The natural history of this condition is to progress from acute dislocation to recurrent dislocation, then eventually to fixed dislocation.
    - If treated nonoperatively, caution should be used to modify sports participation to avoid complete hip dislocation (23).
  - Patellofemoral dislocation occurs in 4%–8% of persons with Down syndrome.
    - Progression to fixed dislocations may occur but may do well with nonoperative management.
    - No restriction is necessary for asymptomatic instability.
    - A neoprene knee brace with patellar window and activity restriction may be helpful for an athlete with symptoms (23).

- Foot deformities are very common in athletes with Down syndrome due to generalized ligamentous laxity.
  - ❑ Athletes with Down syndrome are prone to pes planovalgus, metatarsus primus varus, and bunions.
  - ❑ Surgery is rarely necessary because these conditions are well tolerated in athletes with Down syndrome with appropriately fitting shoes (23).
- Life expectancy for individuals with Down syndrome has increased from 12 years of age in 1949, to 35 years of age in 1982, to 55 years of age currently. Hence, there are many older persons with Down syndrome participating in athletics now (3).
- Several health-related changes are associated with aging in athletes with Down syndrome. The following conditions apply to adults with Down syndrome:
  - 40% will develop hypothyroidism.
  - 46%–57% have mitral valve prolapse.
  - 50% have sleep apnea.
  - 70% have conductive hearing loss.
  - 70% over the age of 65 years have visual impairments.
  - Alzheimer disease increases with age from rates of 10% for ages 30–39 years up to 55% for ages 50–59 years (3).

SPECIAL OLYMPICS

- It would be difficult to discuss athletics for those with intellectual disabilities without a general understanding of the Special Olympics.
- Special Olympics International is a nonprofit, international program developed in the 1960s to provide athletic opportunities for people with intellectual disabilities.
  - Mission: "to provide year-round sports training and athletic competition in a variety of Olympic-type sports for children and adults with intellectual disabilities, giving them continuing opportunities to develop physical fitness, demonstrate courage, experience joy and participate in sharing of gifts, skills and friendship with their families, other Special Olympics athletes and the community" (10).
  - Provides opportunities for over 2 million athletes to develop physical fitness and to experience camaraderie in 30 different sports programs in almost 180 countries.
  - Athlete's Oath: "Let me win. But if I cannot win, let me be brave in the attempt" (10).
- To be eligible to participate, an individual must be at least 8 years old, and:
  - Be identified by a professional agency as having an intellectual disability
  - Have a cognitive delay determined by standardized measures
  - Have significant learning or vocational problems due to cognitive delays that require special instruction (17).

- For many athletes, Special Olympics is a path to empowerment, competence, acceptance, joy, and friendship (10).

EVENT COVERAGE

- Coverage of events for intellectually disabled athletes, such as Special Olympics events, frequently relies on volunteers who may or may not have experience with past events.
- As with any other athletic event, systematic planning can help ensure success. Some considerations are outlined below (15).
  - Know the minimal medical facility requirements. Special Olympics requires the following for large competitions (10):
    - ❑ A qualified emergency medical technician (EMT) must be in attendance or readily available at all times.
    - ❑ A licensed medical professional must be on site or on call at all times.
    - ❑ First aid areas must be clearly identified, adequately equipped, and staffed by a qualified EMT for the entire event.
    - ❑ An ambulance with advanced cardiac life support capabilities must be readily available at all times.
  - Estimated crowd attendance must be factored into planning.
  - Seizure precautions should be followed in all activities where there might be a risk of severe injury if a convulsion were to occur, such as in swimming, diving, skiing, or equestrian, for example.
  - Environmental concerns such as adequate shelter, water, and restrooms must be addressed while accounting for the climate and time of day. Fluids must be provided, and drinking breaks encouraged.
  - Preparticipation screening results may assist in planning for unique issues and identifying specific athletes at increased risk.
  - Medical records should be readily available to medical staff. Medical conditions, allergies, medications, and emergency contact information should be located in a central location or on identification badges or race bibs.
  - For monocular athletes, eye protection with polycarbonate lenses should be worn, especially for missile-type sports.
  - Supplies and equipment needed are comparable to other community sporting events. Automated external defibrillators (AEDs) and antiepileptic injectable medications are recommended per Special Olympics guidelines. Some requirements vary by state and may require medical staff to know the location of the closest AED. As with other events, it is important to know local policies.
  - Most care will involve general first aid. Advanced emergency care by trained providers will usually involve initial stabilization and rapid transport of those who require more than basic first aid.

CONCLUSION

- Athletes with intellectual disabilities have a variety of health-related issues that impact their participation in sports.
- Knowledge of illness and injury patterns in athletes with intellectual disabilities allows the sports medicine physician to effectively provide care for these athletes.
- Preparticipation evaluation for the athlete with special needs should be similar to any athlete without intellectual or physical disability but must consider specific conditions that are more prevalent in this population.

REFERENCES

1. American Academy of Family Physicians, American Academy of Pediatrics, American College of Sports Medicine, et al. *PPE: Preparticipation Physical Evaluation*. 4th ed. Washington (DC): American Academy of Pediatrics; 2010. pp. 131–9.
2. American Psychiatric Association Task Force on DSM-IV. *Diagnostic and Statistical Manual of Mental Disorders: DSM-IV-TR*. 4th ed. Washington (DC): American Psychiatric Association; 2000. 943 p.
3. Barnhart RC, Connolly B. Aging and Down syndrome: implications for physical therapy. *Phys Ther*. 2007;87(10):1399–406.
4. Batts KB, Glorioso JE Jr, Williams MS. The medical demands of the special athlete. *Clin J Sport Med*. 1998;8(1):22–5.
5. Birrer RB. The Special Olympics athlete: evaluation and clearance for participation. *Clin Pediatr (Phila)*. 2004;43(9):777–82.
6. Cope R, Olson S. Abnormalities of the cervical spine in Down's syndrome: diagnosis, risks, and review of the literature, with particular reference to the Special Olympics. *South Med J*. 1987;80(1):33–6.
7. Durstine JL, Moore GE, Painter PL, Roberts SO. *ACSM's Exercise Management for Persons with Chronic Diseases and Disabilities*. 3rd ed. Champaign (IL): Human Kinetics; 2009. pp. 359–67.
8. Gutstein W, Sinclair SH, North RV, Bekiroglu N. Screening athletes with Down syndrome for ocular disease. *Optometry*. 2010;81(2):94–9.
9. Hankinson TC, Anderson RC. Craniovertebral junction abnormalities in Down syndrome. *Neurosurgery*. 2010;66(3 Suppl):32–8.
10. International Special Olympics Web site [Internet]. Washington (DC): Special Olympics International; [cited 2010 Dec 19]. Available from: http://www.specialolympics.org/.
11. McCormick DP, Ivey FM Jr, Gold DM, Zimmerman DM, Gemma S, Owen MJ. The preparticipation sports examination in Special Olympics athletes. *Tex Med*. 1988;84(4):39–43.
12. McCormick DP, Niebuhr VN, Risser WL. Injury and illness surveillance at local Special Olympic Games. *Br J Sports Med*. 1990;24(4):221–4.
13. Murphy NA, Carbone PS; American Academy of Pediatrics Council on Children With Disabilities. Promoting the participation of children with disabilities in sports, recreation, and physical activities. *Pediatrics*. 2008;121(5):1057–61.
14. National Association for Child Development Web site [Internet]. Congenital heart disease in children with Down syndrome; [cited 2010 Dec 19]. Available from: http://downsyndrome.nacd.org/heart_disease.php.
15. O'Connor FG. *Sports Medicine: Just the Facts*. New York (NY): McGraw-Hill; 2005. pp. 581–6.
16. Patel DR, Greydanus DE. Sport participation by physically and cognitively challenged young athletes. *Pediatr Clin North Am*. 2010;57(3):795–817.
17. Platt LS. Medical and orthopaedic conditions in special olympics athletes. *J Athl Train*. 2001;36(1):74–80.
18. Ramirez M, Yang J, Bourque L, et al. Sports injuries to high school athletes with disabilities. *Pediatrics*. 2009;123(2):690–6.
19. Sanyer ON. Down syndrome and sport participation. *Curr Sports Med Rep*. 2006;5(6):315–8.
20. Schalock RL. *Intellectual Disability: Definition, Classification, and Systems of Supports*. 11th ed. Washington (DC): American Association on Intellectual and Developmental Disabilities; 2010. 259 p.
21. Schieve LA, Boulet SL, Boyle C, Rasmussen SA, Schendel D. Health of children 3 to 17 years of age with Down syndrome in the 1997–2005 National Health Interview Survey. *Pediatrics*. 2009;123(2):e253–60.
22. Tassone JC, Duey-Holtz A. Spine concerns in the Special Olympian with Down syndrome. *Sports Med Arthrosc*. 2008;16(1):55–60.
23. Winell J, Burke SW. Sports participation of children with Down syndrome. *Orthop Clin North Am*. 2003;34(3):439–43.
24. Woodhouse JM, Adler P, Duignan A. Vision in athletes with intellectual disabilities: the need for improved eyecare. *J Intellect Disabil Res*. 2004;48(Pt 8):736–45.

117 The Disabled Athlete

Kevin F. Fitzpatrick and Paul F. Pasquina

INTRODUCTION

- There are an estimated 54.4 million disabled people in the United States (27).
- There are approximately two million recreational and competitive disabled athletes in the United States (20).
- Among those with disabilities, as many as 60% never participate in any physical activity or sports.
- Although many opportunities exist for individuals with disabilities, the two most limiting factors for participation in athletics are awareness and access (30). Health care practitioners should make every effort to inform these individuals of the multiple opportunities and encourage their safe participation.
- Athletes with disabilities demonstrate increased exercise endurance, muscle strength, cardiovascular efficiency, and flexibility; improved balance; and better motor skills compared with individuals with disabilities who do not participate in athletics.
- In addition to physical benefits, psychological benefits of exercise include self-image, body awareness, motor development, and mood.
- Disabled athletes have fewer cardiac risk factors and higher high-density lipoprotein cholesterol and are less likely to smoke cigarettes than those who are disabled and nonactive (7).
- Individuals with amputations who participate in athletics have improved proprioception and increased proficiency in the use of prosthetic devices (29).
- Athletes with paraplegia are less likely to be hospitalized, have fewer pressure ulcers, and are less susceptible to infections than nonactive individuals with paraplegia (26).
- Injury patterns for disabled athletes are similar to those for athletes without disabilities; however, location of injuries appears to be disability and sport dependent. Lower extremity (LE) injuries are more common in ambulatory athletes (visually impaired, amputee, cerebral palsy), whereas upper extremity (UE) injuries are more frequent in athletes who use a wheelchair (12).
- A 3-year, cross-disability prospective study found the injury rate of disabled athletes to be 9.30/1,000 athlete exposures (10) — an injury rate less than what has been reported in college football (12.0–15.0/1,000) and college soccer (9.8/1,000), but higher than that reported in men's and women's college basketball (7.0/1,000 and 7.3/1,000, respectively) (4,5).

- A 6-year longitudinal study on reported injuries from disabled sports organizations revealed that illnesses (29.8%) were the most common, followed by muscular strains (22.1%), tendonitis (9.5%), sprains (5.8%), contusions (5.6%), and abrasions (5.1%). The body part most commonly injured was the thorax/spine (13.3%), followed by the shoulder (12.8%), the lower leg/ankle and toes (12.0%), and the hip/thigh (7.4%) (11).
- Wheelchair users are at a significant increased risk of UE entrapment neuropathies, like carpal tunnel syndrome (CTS), with a reported prevalence rate of between 50% and 73%; however, it appears that wheelchair athletes have a lower prevalence than nonathletes (2,6).
- With regard to winter sports, studies have shown that disabled athletes have a lower incidence of injuries than able-bodied skiers (19).

PREPARTICIPATION ASSESSMENT

- Preparticipation assessments (PPA) should be performed in a systematic comprehensive fashion similar to that performed for able-bodied athletes.
- Sports medicine practitioners should not be overly focused on the athlete's impairment/disability and miss common medical issues.
- Careful evaluation of the athlete's wheelchair, prosthetics, orthotics, and assistive/adaptive devices should also be performed prior to competition. This is usually facilitated by consultation with the individual's orthotist, prosthetist, or other health care specialists with experience in this area.
- Sports medicine practitioners who are not familiar with certain impairments should solicit assistance from practitioners with more experience. This often requires a team approach. For example, a physician specializing in sports medicine may have little experience in spinal cord injuries (SCIs), whereas an SCI specialist may have even less experience in sports medicine. Together, however, they can jointly assess an individual and clear him or her safely for participation.
- Practitioners should avoid mass screening stations for individuals with disabilities in favor of private office setting visits.
- It is recommended that the PPA be performed by a medical team that is involved in the longitudinal care of the disabled athlete, because knowledge of baseline functioning is essential.

- The specific elements required in the PPA are determined by the sport, the level of participation, the athletic organization, the clinical indications, and the athlete. The PPA should provide information to guide the athlete, trainer, coach, and team physician toward safe participation, activity limitations, and disability-specific training.
- The objectives of the examination include the following:
  - Identify conditions that may require further medical evaluation before the athlete enters into training, require close supervision during training, and may predispose to injury.
  - Determine the athlete's general health to assess fitness level and performance.
  - Counsel on health-related issues and methods for safe participation.
  - Provide referral for identified conditions that require further evaluation and/or monitoring to physicians familiar with the disability and the management of the identified conditions.
- In addition to the standard components of a history, the elements of the history for an athlete with a disability also should include athletic goals, predisability health, present level of training, sports participation, medications and supplements used, presence of impairments, past and family cardiopulmonary history, level of functional independence for mobility and self-care, and needs for adaptive equipment.
- The elements of the disability and sports-specific physical examination are tailored for the individual. Sensory deficits, neurologic deficits, joint stability and range of motion (ROM), muscle strength, flexibility, skin integrity, medications, and adaptive equipment needs must be assessed. During the musculoskeletal examination of an athlete who uses a wheelchair, evaluate the stability, flexibility, and strength of the commonly injured sites (*e.g.*, shoulder, hand and wrist, and LEs) as well as the trunk.
- Special attention should be paid during the PPA to skin breakdown on insensate pressure areas as well as sites that come in contact with orthotics/prosthetics. Also, a careful history of heat/cold injuries and changes in neurologic function should be solicited.
- During the musculoskeletal examination of an individual who has had an LE amputation, assess the stability, flexibility, and strength of the trunk, as well as the hip girdle and the unaffected and affected LE with or without the prosthesis.
- For individuals with UE amputations, the stability, flexibility, and strength of the shoulder girdle must be assessed in the unaffected and affected extremity with and without prosthesis, in addition to a trunk and LE evaluation.
- For the athlete with brain injury, stroke, or multiple sclerosis, it is prudent to assess the limitations of the unaffected and affected areas based on mobility and sports-specific tasks.
- Cardiovascular and pulmonary examinations can identify conditions that can cause cardiopulmonary collapse or disease progression. Suggested guidelines for cardiovascular screening of the athlete are available from the American College of Sports Medicine, American Heart Association, and American College of Cardiology.
- A PPA is performed upon entry into sports and should be repeated at least every 2–3 years. An interim examination prior to each sport season may be necessary if the athlete's health condition changes.

INJURIES AND COMPLICATIONS BY CAUSE OF DISABILITY

- Disabled athletes are subject to many of the same injuries and complications from physical exertion as the able-bodied population.
- In addition, some specific diagnoses that result in disability also lead to increased risk of particular injuries and complications. These will be discussed here.
- There is certainly overlap between the categories of diagnoses resulting in disability. For example, many patients with SCIs are wheelchair users. For the purposes of this discussion, the following conditions will be considered: SCI, major limb loss, and wheelchair use.

WHEELCHAIR USE

- Given the degree to which wheelchair users rely on their upper limbs for mobility and activities of daily living, the importance of recognizing, treating, and preventing upper limb injuries is magnified when compared with the able-bodied population. Because relative rest of the upper limb may be impossible or nearly impossible in this population, other measures should be considered. These may include splinting and orthotic prescriptions, admission to an inpatient setting if rest is required, or home modifications or additional assistance (21).

Shoulder Injuries

- Wheelchair users are at increased risk for shoulder pathology including pain, rotator cuff injuries, subacromial bursitis, acromioclavicular joint abnormalities, coracoacromial ligament thickening, subacromial spurs, distal clavicle osteolysis, and impingement syndrome (1,3).
- Factors contributing to the increased risk in this population include repetitive motion, increased pressure in the shoulder joint during wheelchair propulsion, and muscle imbalances in the shoulder girdle due to weakness (1,9,25,28).
- In wheelchair users, upper limb injuries, including shoulder injuries, are particularly disabling due to the fact that these patients rely on their upper limbs for weight

bearing, transfers, and ambulation in addition to all of the demands placed on the upper limbs in the able-bodied population.

■ Despite increases in repetitive use and high-intensity activity, wheelchair athletes do not have a higher incidence of shoulder pain than nonathletic wheelchair users. In fact, participation in athletic competition appears to be protective from shoulder pain (13). This is likely due to increased strength and endurance in the athletic population.

■ Shoulder complaints among wheelchair users can be reduced by appropriate wheelchair design and the use of ideal propulsion techniques.

Elbow Injuries

■ The elbow is a very common site of ulnar nerve entrapment, representing the second most common upper limb nerve entrapment syndrome.

■ Wheelchair users are an increased risk for ulnar neuropathy at the elbow (14). There is no evidence to suggest that wheelchair athletes are at a greater risk as compared with nonathlete wheelchair users.

■ Symptoms of ulnar neuropathy at the elbow include numbness and tingling in the fifth digit and the ulnar half of the fourth digit, weakness and atrophy in the hand intrinsic muscles, and pain and tenderness in the ulnar groove. Diagnosis of ulnar neuropathy is made based on history, physical examination, and electrodiagnostic testing.

■ Other sources of elbow pain that are reported in wheelchair users are lateral epicondylitis, osteoarthritis, and olecranon bursitis (21).

■ Treatment of elbow pain and injuries in wheelchair users must be tailored to the individual needs of the patient, keeping in mind that many wheelchair users will be non-mobile if they are required to restrict weight bearing or otherwise limit activity involving their upper limb.

Wrist Injuries

■ The carpal tunnel is the most common site of nerve entrapment in able-bodied and disabled persons.

■ Long-term wheelchair users have a prevalence of CTS of 49%–73% (31).

■ Wheelchair users with symptoms and physical examination findings of CTS have lower functional status as compared with wheelchair users without CTS (31).

■ Symptoms of CTS include numbness and tingling in the radial three digits and the radial half of the fourth digit, weakness in thumb abduction, clumsiness, wrist pain, and nocturnal paresthesias. Diagnosis is based on history, physical examination, and electrodiagnostic testing.

■ In addition to CTS, wheelchair users are at increased risk for other wrist overuse injuries and syndromes including ulnar nerve entrapment in Guyon's canal (14), osteoarthritis, tendinitis, and de Quervain tenosynovitis (21).

Upper Limb Fractures

■ The incidence of upper limb fractures in wheelchair athletes or wheelchair users is not known.

■ Wheelchair athletes may be at greater risk for upper limb fractures due to repetitive falls associated with many wheelchair sports, propulsion requiring positioning the hand in a location that is susceptible to injury from nearby wheelchairs or collisions, and relatively high speeds achieved during certain wheelchair sports.

■ Fractures should be treated as in the able-bodied population.

■ Restricted upper limb weight bearing in a wheelchair user may result in immobility.

MAJOR LIMB LOSS

Skin Complications

■ Following amputation and prosthetic fitting, the skin of the distal portion of the residual limb becomes a weight-bearing surface where it had not previously been such. As a result, the distal residual limb is at increased risk for skin breakdown and other skin disorders.

■ Verrucous hyperplasia is a wart-like lesion that may develop at the distal end of the residual limb. It may occur as a result of proximal residual limb constriction from a socket or wrap that causes decreased pressure in the distal residual limb. Prevention consists of equal distribution of pressure through the residual limb, as in a total contact socket (18).

■ Skin breakdown may occur when pressure is applied disproportionately to a pressure-sensitive area of skin on the residual limb, such as the tibial tubercle in a transtibial amputee. The risk may be compounded by the fact that many amputees may have impaired sensation in the residual limb, and sweating with athletic activity can increase moisture at the skin-socket interface and make skin breakdown more likely.

■ Skin breakdown can be particularly disabling in an amputee, who relies on weight bearing through the residual limb for ambulation. If restricted weight bearing is required, ambulation will not be possible. Prevention of skin breakdown involves prosthetic socket design that distributes pressure equally throughout the entire circumferential surface of the residual limb and reduces pressure over pressure-sensitive skin. In addition, silicone liners, padded sleeves, socks, and additional padding can be preventive.

■ In amputee athletes, increased frequency and intensity of weight bearing associated with athletic training and competition likely increase the risk of skin breakdown.

Heterotopic Ossification

■ Heterotopic ossification (HO) is the formation of bone in tissues that are not normally ossified. It has been traditionally reported to occur following traumatic brain injury (TBI), SCI, burns, and total arthroplasty.

- Recently, HO has been reported to occur at high rates in the residual limbs of traumatic amputees (23).

- HO in residual limbs may increase the risk of skin breakdown or cause pain with weight bearing.

- Following TBI, SCI, burns, and arthroplasty, HO typically develops around major joints, thus restricting ROM and limiting mobility. In contrast, following amputation, HO occurs in injured tissues in the residual limb and may not be in the vicinity of a joint.

- Recognition of HO in residual limbs allows for modifications in the design of a prosthetic socket to accommodate for the ectopic bone. Furthermore, monitoring for skin breakdown should be increased in amputees with HO.

- Surgical excision of HO may be required if conservative measures fail to restore adequate levels of function.

Neuroma

- A neuroma occurs at the distal end of a resected nerve in the residual limb of an amputee. When a neuroma is exposed to pressure, it creates paresthesias, dysesthesias, and radiating pain in the phantom distribution of the resected nerve.

- When a neuroma occurs at or near a weight-bearing structure, it can create severe pain with ambulation and weight bearing, limiting an athlete's ability to train and compete.

- Treatment may involve prosthetic modifications to relieve pressure on the neuroma, oral medications including antiepileptic and tricyclic antidepressants, and injection of corticosteroids and local anesthetic into the neuroma. Surgical excision may be necessary if conservative treatments fail.

SPINAL CORD INJURY

Thermoregulation

- Following SCIs, there is disruption of neuroregulatory systems that are involved in control of body temperature. Below the level of the lesion, athletes with SCI have impaired shivering to produce heat and impaired sweating and vasodilation to dissipate heat. Athletes with tetraplegia are at greater risk compared with those with paraplegia (24).

- Paraplegic and tetraplegic athletes are expected to see greater increases in body temperature with exertion and greater decreases in temperature with exposure to cold weather.

- Prevention of temperature-related injuries requires heightened awareness and monitoring, use of appropriate clothing and equipment, availability of rehydration, and avoidance of extremes of temperature when possible.

- Frostbite is of particular concern during cold weather events. Athletes with SCIs have impaired sensation and require frequent visual monitoring to prevent cold injuries.

Autonomic Dysreflexia

- Autonomic dysreflexia (AD) is a condition that occurs when sympathetic outflow in response to a noxious stimulus is unregulated due to interruption of neural pathways after SCI.

- Patients with SCIs at the level of T6 and above are at risk for AD.

- Symptoms include paroxysmal hypertension, bradycardia, facial flushing, and headache. If hypertension continues to increase without treatment, stroke or death may occur (22).

- Common noxious stimuli that lead to AD include tight clothing, urinary or fecal retention, renal or bladder stones, pressure ulcers, infections, or intra-abdominal pathology (e.g., appendicitis).

- Treatment involves sitting the patient upright, loosening clothing, and identifying and eliminating the noxious stimulus. For acute blood pressure control, chewable nifedipine or nitropaste can be used.

- "Boosting" describes the practice of intentionally inducing AD in order to improve athletic performance (15). This dangerous practice should be discouraged and may be life threatening.

Skin Breakdown

- Following SCI, insensate skin leads to a risk of skin breakdown or pressure ulcer.

- Regardless of the level of the injury, the skin over the sacrum, coccyx, and ischial tuberosities is frequently insensate. These areas represent the highest risk for skin breakdown in athletes with SCI.

- Specific athletic events may result in increased risk of skin breakdown in additional areas. For example, wheelchair racers may have increased risk of skin breakdown if the medial surface of the arm and forearm rubs against the wheelchair during propulsion. This may require customized equipment and padding to prevent skin breakdown in activity-specific high-risk skin areas.

- Athletic wheelchairs commonly sacrifice pressure relief for higher performance. This should cause the athlete and caregivers to increase vigilance in monitoring for skin breakdown, changing position frequently, and limiting time in the wheelchair. This is particularly important when an athlete is transitioning to a new piece of equipment (e.g., a new wheelchair). Prevention is of paramount importance in this population.

- At the first sign of skin breakdown or pressure ulcer, weight bearing and athletic activities should be modified or restricted to prevent further injury. Pressure ulcers can be a significant cause of morbidity and mortality in the SCI population.

Heterotopic Ossification

- Following SCI, ectopic bone formation, called HO, may develop in soft tissues surrounding major joints. This can result in pain, edema, fever, restricted ROM, risk of skin breakdown, and activity limitations.

- The most common site of HO after SCI is the hip, but the knee, elbow, and shoulder may also be affected, depending on the level of injury (HO forms below the level of injury).
- The initial presentation may mimic deep venous thrombosis or joint infection. Diagnostic testing is often required to exclude other diagnoses.
- Diagnosis of HO may be made by x-rays, bone scan, or trends in alkaline phosphatase levels.
- Prevention of HO involves frequent ROM exercises. Pharmacologic prophylaxis may be considered in high-risk populations and may consist of nonsteroidal anti-inflammatory drugs or bisphosphonates.
- Extensive HO in athletes may limit participation by limiting ROM, causing pain, or contributing to skin breakdown.
- Surgical excision may be required if conservative and adaptive treatments are not successful.

Spasticity

- Spasticity is a velocity-dependent increase in muscle tone that occurs after injury to the upper motor neuron. It is a common complication of SCI that may limit athletic participation by interfering with voluntary movements and restricting ROM.
- An increase in spasticity may be an indicator of a systemic or otherwise asymptomatic condition. For example, infections, intra-abdominal pathology (*e.g.*, appendicitis), skin breakdown, or bladder distension may have few symptoms that are sensed by a patient with SCI. Therefore, a sudden increase in spasticity should lead to a search for underlying pathology.
- Treatment for spasticity consists of oral medications, including baclofen, dantrolene, tizanidine, and benzodiazepines; injectable medications such as botulinum toxin; and intrathecal medications such as baclofen. If spasticity is resistant to conservative treatment, surgery for tendon lengthening may improve hygiene, activities of daily living, and functional activities including participation in athletics.

Osteoporosis

- Osteoporosis is a nearly universal complication of SCI.
- Decreased weight bearing predisposes to osteoporosis; however, many risk factors are independent of alterations in weight bearing. These risk factors include severity of the injury, spasticity, and time since injury (16).
- Osteoporosis results in increased fracture risk in athletes with SCI.
- Because of impaired sensation below the level of the injury, SCI athletes may not immediately complain of pain after a fracture. Other warning signs may include increases in spasticity or AD.
- Prevention of osteoporosis should include calcium and vitamin D supplementation for all athletes with SCI. Bisphosphonates may also be used for prevention.

Orthostatic Hypotension

- Orthostatic hypotension occurs in most SCI patients.
- Symptoms include light-headedness and dizziness, and syncope may occur if uncorrected.
- Orthostatic hypotension occurs after SCI because of decreased sympathetic efferent activity in vasculature below the level of the injury and also because of decreased reflex vasoconstriction. The result is venous pooling in dependent areas (lower limbs or abdomen) that occurs with changes in position (17).
- Prevention includes the use of lower limb compression stockings and abdominal binders, maintenance of hydration, and salt supplementation. If these measures are insufficient, pharmacologic treatment with midodrine, fludrocortisone, or ephedrine may be helpful (17).
- In SCI athletes, nonpharmacologic prevention should be attempted before the use of pharmacologic agents is considered.

ACUTE MOUNTAIN SICKNESS

- Acute mountain sickness involves a constellation of symptoms (headache, nausea, weakness, shortness of breath) and occurs with exposure to high altitudes. Incidence increases with increasing altitude.
- In many winter sports, competition at high altitudes increases the risk of acute mountain sickness.
- Acute mountain sickness is thought to be caused by alterations in the blood–brain barrier and cerebral vasculature that occur at high altitudes (8).
- Given their altered neurophysiology and anatomy, SCI athletes may be at higher risk of acute mountain sickness (8).
- Acetazolamide may be used as prophylaxis in high-risk scenarios. Treatment may include return to low altitude, acetazolamide, or dexamethasone.

REFERENCES

1. Bayley JC, Cochran TP, Sledge CB. The weight-bearing shoulder. The impingement syndrome in paraplegics. *J Bone Joint Surg Am.* 1987; 69(5):676–8.
2. Boninger ML, Robertson RN, Wolff M, Cooper RA. Upper limb nerve entrapments in elite wheelchair racers. *Am J Phys Med Rehabil.* 1996; 75(3):170–6.
3. Brose SW, Boninger ML, Fullerton B, et al. Shoulder ultrasound abnormalities, physical examination findings, and pain in manual wheelchair users with spinal cord injury. *Arch Phys Med Rehabil.* 2008;89(11):2086–93.
4. Buckley WE. Five year overview of sport injuries: the NAIRS model. *J Phys Educ Rec Dance.* 1982;17:36–40.
5. Buckley WE, Powell JP. NAIRS: an epidemiological overview of the severity of injury in college football. *J Athl Train.* 1982;18:279–82.
6. Burnham RS, Steadward RD. Upper extremity peripheral nerve entrapments among wheelchair athletes: prevalence, location, and risk factors. *Arch Phys Med Rehabil.* 1994;75(5):519–24.

7. Dearwater SR, LaPorte RE, Robertson RJ, Brenes G, Adams LL, Becker D. Activity in the spinal cord-injured patient: an epidemiologic analysis of metabolic parameters. *Med Sci Sports Exerc.* 1986;18(5):541–4.

8. Dicianno BE, Aguila ED, Cooper RA, et al. Acute mountain sickness in disability and adaptive sports: preliminary data. *J Rehabil Res Dev.* 2008;45(4):479–87.

9. Donovan WH, Kraft GH. Rotator cuff tear versus suprascapular nerve injury: a problem in differential diagnosis. *Arch Phys Med Rehabil.* 1974; 55(9):424–8.

10. Ferrara MS, Buckley WE. Athletes with disabilities injury registry. *Adapt Phys Act Q.* 1996;13:50–60.

11. Ferrara MS, Palutsis GR, Snouse S, Davis RW. A longitudinal study of injuries to athletes with disabilities. *Int J Sports Med.* 2000;21(3):221–4.

12. Ferrara MS, Peterson CL. Injuries to athletes with disabilities: identifying injury patterns. *Sports Med.* 2000;30(2):137–43.

13. Fullerton HD, Borckardt JJ, Alfano AP. Shoulder pain: a comparison of wheelchair athletes and nonathletic wheelchair users. *Med Sci Sports Exerc.* 2003;35(12):1958–61.

14. Groah SL, Lanig IS. Neuromusculoskeletal syndromes in wheelchair athletes. *Semin Neurol.* 2000;20(2):201–8.

15. Harris P. Self-induced autonomic dysreflexia ('boosting') practised by some tetraplegic athletes to enhance their athletic performance. *Paraplegia.* 1994;32(5):289–91.

16. Jiang SD, Dai LY, Jiang LS. Osteoporosis after spinal cord injury. *Osteoporos Int.* 2006;17(2):180–92.

17. Krassioukov A, Eng JJ, Warburton DE, Teasell R; Spinal Cord Injury Rehabilitation Evidence Research Team. A systematic review of the management of orthostatic hypotension after spinal cord injury. *Arch Phys Med Rehabil.* 2009;90(5):876–95.

18. Kuiken TA, Miller L, Lipschutz R, Huang ME. Rehabilitation of people with lower limb amputation. In: Braddom RL, editor. *Physical Medicine and Rehabilitation.* Philadelphia (PA): Elsevier; 2007.

19. Laskowski ER, Murtaugh PA. Snow skiing injuries in physically disabled skiers. *Am J Sports Med.* 1992;20(5):553–7.

20. Micheo WF. Concepts in sports medicine. In: Braddom RL, editor. *Physical Medicine and Rehabilitation.* Philadelphia (PA): Elsevier; 2007.

21. Paralyzed Veterans of America Consortium for Spinal Cord Medicine. Preservation of upper limb function following spinal cord injury: a clinical practice guideline for health-care professionals. *J Spinal Cord Med.* 2005;28(5):434–70.

22. Pasquina PF, Houston RM, Belandres PV. Beta blockade in the treatment of autonomic dysreflexia: a case report and review. *Arch Phys Med Rehabil.* 1998;79(5):582–4.

23. Potter BK, Burns TC, Lacap AP, Granville RR, Gajewski D. Heterotopic ossification in the residual limbs of traumatic and combat-related amputees. *J Am Acad Orthop Surg.* 2006;14(10 Spec No.):S191–7.

24. Price MJ, Campbell IG. Effects of spinal cord lesion level upon thermoregulation during exercise in the heat. *Med Sci Sports Exerc.* 2003;35(7): 1100–7.

25. Silfverskiold J, Waters RL. Shoulder pain and functional disability in spinal cord injury patients. *Clin Orthop Relat Res.* 1991;272: 141–5.

26. Stotts KM. Health maintenance: paraplegic athletes and nonathletes. *Arch Phys Med Rehabil.* 1986;67(2):109–14.

27. U.S. Census Bureau. *Americans with Disabilities: 2005, Current Population Reports.* Washington (DC): U.S. Census Bureau; 2008.

28. Waring WP, Maynard FM. Shoulder pain in acute traumatic quadriplegia. *Paraplegia.* 1991;29(1):37–42.

29. Wetterhahn KA, Hanson C, Levy CE. Effect of participation in physical activity on body image of amputees. *Am J Phys Med Rehabil.* 2002;81(3): 194–201.

30. Wu SK, Williams T. Factors influencing sport participation among athletes with spinal cord injury. *Med Sci Sports Exerc.* 2001;33(2): 177–82.

31. Yang J, Boninger ML, Leath JD, Fitzgerald SG, Dyson-Hudson TA, Chang MW. Carpal tunnel syndrome in manual wheelchair users with spinal cord injury: a cross-sectional multicenter study. *Am J Phys Med Rehabil.* 2009;88(12):1007–16.

118 The Athlete with a Total Joint Replacement

Robert W. Engelen and Jennifer L. Reed

PREVALENCE AND OUTCOME

- In 2003, a total of 202,500 primary total hip arthroplasties and 402,100 primary total knee arthroplasties were performed in the United States (10).

- By 2030, the demand for total hip arthroplasty (THA) is estimated to grow by 174% to 572,000, and the demand for total knee arthroplasty (TKA) is estimated to grow by 673% to 3.48 million procedures (10).

- The prevalence of shoulder arthroplasty in 1998 was 15,266, with 8,556 hemiarthroplasties and 6,710 total shoulder arthroplasties (19).

- On average, a modern total joint replacement has a > 90% chance of surviving 10–15 years (1,10).

- Dislocation, periprosthetic fracture, and implant breakage are possible, but uncommon, complications of athletic activity. More salient concerns include implant loosening from periarticular osteolysis and excessive joint-bearing surface component wear.

- Athletic activity increases stress on implant fixation, and several studies have suggested that use and activity levels contribute to loosening rates associated with total joint arthroplasty (21).

- Activity levels can vary tremendously from patient to patient. Implant wear has been shown to be related to use of the joint as opposed to duration of implantation (21).

- Active, high-demand patients place arthroplasty implants at increased risk for loosening and wear.

- Patients under 60 years of age are 30% more active on average than patients 60 years of age or older (24).

- In the Swedish National Hip and Knee Arthroplasty Registers, 10-year revision rates among younger men were three to four times greater when compared to older patients (9,15).

- Published guidelines concerning activity after total joint arthroplasty discourage high levels of activity (2).

- Prospective, randomized studies on athletic activity after joint replacement and its effect on implant survivorship are not available (6).

- Current recommendations are largely based on the opinions of orthopedic surgeons. Tables 118.1 through 118.5 represent revised recommendations from surveys of the Hip, Knee, and American Shoulder and Elbow Societies conducted in 1999 and from repeat survey completed in 2005 (7).

- A recently published review article by Kuster (11) suggests that recommendations be made according to scientific knowledge including a biomechanical analysis of the joint loads during the sport in question.

- The following sections discuss issues that should be taken into account for each patient and sporting activity.

WEAR OF TOTAL JOINT REPLACEMENTS

- Up to 500,000 submicron-sized polyethylene particles are released with each step (20). These small particles can activate macrophages that produce factors such as prostaglandins and interleukins thought to explain the progressive osteolysis and subsequent implant loosening.

- Another major long-term problem is polyethylene wear itself. The total volume of wear particles produced strongly depends on the number of steps, the load applied, and the roughness of the joint surfaces (13). Standard metal on polyethylene has shown elevated levels of wear, greater than 0.2 mm per year (14).

- In a study evaluating the results of 5,700 TKAs recorded in a community joint registry, polyethylene wear accounted for 15% of all revisions and 30% of revisions after the knee survived greater than 5 years (13).

- The most common reason for TKA revision in a community joint registry prospectively following 1,047 patients under the age of 55 was aseptic loosening, but the study showed a 14-year survival rate of 74.5% (3).

- A study by Gschwend et al. (5) followed two cohorts of patients after THA, one cohort active in Nordic and/or Alpine skiing and the other cohort inactive. At 10 years, the wear rate was higher in the active group but loosening remained higher in the inactive group of patients (5).

Table 118.1	Activity After Total Hip Arthroplasty — 1999 Hip Society Survey		
Recommended/Allowed	**Allowed with Experience**	**Not Recommended**	**No Conclusion**
Stationary bicycling	Low-impact aerobics	High-impact aerobics	Jazz dancing
Croquet	Road bicycling	Baseball/softball	Square dancing
Ballroom dancing	Bowling	Basketball	Fencing
Golf	Canoeing	Football	Ice skating
Horseshoes	Hiking	Gymnastics	Roller/inline skating
Shooting	Horseback riding	Handball	Rowing
Shuffleboard	Cross-country skiing	Hockey	Speed walking
Swimming		Jogging	Downhill skiing
Doubles tennis		Lacrosse	Stationary skiing*
Walking		Racquetball	Weightlifting
		Squash	Weight machines
		Rock climbing	
		Soccer	
		Singles tennis	
		Volleyball	

*NordicTrack, Logan, Utah.
SOURCE: Adapted with permission from Healy WL, Iorio R, Lemos MJ. Athletic activity after joint replacement. *Am J Sports Med.* 2001;29(3):377–88.

Table 118.2	Activity After Total Hip Arthroplasty — 2005 Hip Society Survey		
Recommended/Allowed	**Allowed with Experience**	**Not Recommended**	**No Conclusion**
Stationary bicycling	Aerobics	Soccer	Fencing
Ballroom dancing	Rowing	Jogging	Baseball
Golf	Bowling	Basketball	Gymnastics
Shuffleboard	Canoeing	Football	Handball
Swimming	Hiking		Hockey
Doubles tennis	Horseback riding		Rock climbing
Walking	Cross-country skiing		Squash/racquetball
Bowling	Doubles tennis		Singles tennis
Canoeing	Roller skating		Volleyball
Road cycling	Ice skating		
Square dancing	Downhill skiing		
Hiking	Stationary skiing*		
Speed walking	Weightlifting		
	Weight machine		

Note: The 1999 survey asked about croquet, horseshoes, shooting, and lacrosse, which were not included in the 2005 survey.
*NordicTrack, Logan, Utah.
SOURCE: Adapted with permission from Healy WL, Sharma S, Schwartz B, Iorio R. Athletic activity after total joint arthroplasty. *J Bone Joint Surg Am.* 2008;90(10):2245–52.

Table 118.3	Activity After Total Knee Arthroplasty — 1999 Knee Society Survey		
Recommended/Allowed	**Allowed with Experience**	**Not Recommended**	**No Conclusion**
Low-impact aerobics	Road bicycling	Racquetball	Fencing
Stationary bicycling	Canoeing	Squash	Roller blade/inline skating
Bowling	Hiking	Rock climbing	Downhill skiing
Golf	Rowing	Soccer	Weightlifting
Dancing	Cross-country skiing	Singles tennis	
Horseback riding	Stationary skiing*	Volleyball	
Croquet	Speed walking	Football	
Walking	Tennis	Gymnastics	
Swimming	Weight machines	Lacrosse	
Shooting	Ice skating	Hockey	
Shuffleboard		Basketball	
Horseshoes		Jogging	
		Handball	

*NordicTrack, Logan, Utah.
SOURCE: Adapted with permission from Healy WL, Iorio R, Lemos MJ. Athletic activity after joint replacement. *Am J Sports Med.* 2001;29(3):377–88.

INDICATIONS

- Pain remains the primary indication for joint replacement operations; however, disability and reduced function associated with a painful or stiff joint are increasingly seen as appropriate indications for joint replacement.

- Frequently, the desire for functional improvement includes a desire for athletic activity, and many patients choose to have joint replacement to enable them to return to a specific sport (23).

- Mancuso et al. (16) documented that patients who undergo joint replacement have multiple expectations, including relief of symptoms, improvement in physical function, and improvement in psychosocial well-being.

Table 118.4	Activity After Total Knee Arthroplasty — 2005 Knee Society Survey		
Recommended/Allowed	**Allowed with Experience**	**Not Recommended**	**No Conclusion**
Low-impact aerobics	Road bicycling	Racquetball	Fencing
Stationary bicycling	Canoeing	Squash	Roller blade/inline skating
Bowling	Hiking	Rock climbing	Downhill skiing
Golf	Rowing	Soccer	Weightlifting
Dancing	Cross-country skiing	Singles tennis	
Horseback riding	Stationary skiing*	Volleyball	
Croquet	Speed walking	Football	
Walking	Tennis	Gymnastics	
Swimming	Weight machines	Lacrosse	
Shooting	Ice skating	Hockey	
Shuffleboard		Basketball	
Horseshoes		Jogging	
		Handball	

Note: The 1999 survey asked about croquet, horseshoes, shooting, and lacrosse, which were not included in the 2005 survey.
*NordicTrack, Logan, Utah.
SOURCE: Adapted with permission from Healy WL, Sharma S, Schwartz B, Iorio R. Athletic activity after total joint arthroplasty. *J Bone Joint Surg Am.* 2008;90(10):2245–52.

Table 118.5	Activity After Total Shoulder Arthroplasty — 1999 American Shoulder and Elbow Society Survey		
Recommended/Allowed	**Allowed with Experience**	**Not Recommended**	**No Conclusion**
Cross-country skiing	Golf	Football	High-impact aerobics
Stationary skiing*	Ice skating	Gymnastics	Baseball/softball
Speed walking and jogging	Shooting	Hockey	Fencing
Swimming	Downhill skiing	Rock climbing	Handball
Doubles tennis			Horseback riding
Low-impact aerobics			Lacrosse
Bicycling, road and stationary			Racquetball, squash
Bowling			Skating, roller/inline
Canoeing			Rowing
Croquet			Soccer
Shuffleboard			Tennis, singles
Horseshoes			Volleyball
Dancing: ballroom, square, and jazz			Weight training

*NordicTrack, Logan, Utah.
SOURCE: Adapted with permission from Healy WL, Iorio R, Lemos MJ. Athletic activity after joint replacement. *Am J Sports Med.* 2001;29(3):377–88.

JOINT LOAD AND MOMENTS DURING SPORT ACTIVITIES

- Tables 118.6 and 118.7 summarize published data regarding hip and knee joint loads during various daily and athletic activities (11).

- As a general guide, the following hip and knee joint loads can be assumed. During daily activities, loads of up to 3–4 times body weight occur, whereas during sporting activities, loads of 5–10 times body weight might occur.

- Cycling appears to be the most joint friendly, with forces averaging between 1.2 and 1.5 times body weight at the hip and knee (less than the forces experienced while walking).

- A key consideration for both walking and jogging is that the hip and knee joint loads increase as speed increases. During fast running, the knee joint load can reach 10 times body weight or more.

- For activities such as skiing, joint loads can vary significantly depending on style, terrain, and experience. Short turns, large moguls, and inexperience all translate into larger joint loads.

RECREATION OR EXERCISE

- It is important to consider whether an activity will be performed for exercise or for recreation.

- In order to maintain cardiovascular fitness, the American College of Sports Medicine recommends aerobic exercise at least three times a week for 30 minutes or more.

- Joint wear shows a strong correlation to load. Therefore, the most prudent recommendation would be to engage in activities with lower joint loads, such as cycling, swimming, and walking, to maintain cardiovascular fitness.

- Activities with high joint loads, such as running or tennis, should not be performed as regular endurance activities; however, if patients would like to resume certain high-load activities for recreation, such as skiing 1 or 2 weeks a year or hiking on the weekends, this may be acceptable (11).

- Even when engaging in high-load sports recreationally, every effort should be made to reduce the joint forces as much as possible. For example, using ski poles while hiking downhill can reduce the load at the knees by as much as 20% (22).

EXPERIENCE AND PREOPERATIVE ACTIVITY LEVEL OF PATIENT

- The preoperative activity level is a strong predictor of sporting activities postoperatively.

- Patients who have achieved high levels of skill in athletics have the best chance of safely resuming these activities. Patients who have not previously participated in a specific sport or recreational activity may have an increased risk of injury when participating in a new sport after joint replacement (6).

- Preliminary evidence from Switzerland suggests that individuals not regularly active, out of practice, or inexperienced are at higher risk for sporting accidents (17).

- Joint loads can be significantly increased for beginners compared with experienced individuals.

Table 118.6	Hip Joint Loads During Different Activities

Activity	Hip Joint Load (× BW)
Standing on two legs	0.8
Standing on one leg	3.2
Straight leg raise	1.9
Walking at 1 km · h^{-1}	2.9
Walking at 5 km · h^{-1}	4.7
Jogging at 5 km · h^{-1}	5.0
Jogging at 7 km · h^{-1}	5.4
Stumbling	8.7
Cycling low resistance (40 W)	0.5
Cycling high resistance	1.4
Jogging at 12 km · h^{-1}	6
Alpine skiing long turns, flat slope	4.5
Alpine skiing long turns, steep slope	6
Alpine skiing short turns, flat slope	5.5–6.0
Alpine skiing short turns, steep slope	7–8
Alpine skiing small moguls	8–9
Alpine skiing large moguls	10–15
Cross-country skiing classical	4–5
Cross-country skiing skating	4.5
Walking at natural speed	3.2–6.2
Stair ascent	3.4–6.0
Car entry	5–8
Car exit	4.5–8.0
Bath entry	4.6–6.6
Stair ascent	5
Stair descent	5.6
Ramp ascent	6.8
Ramp descent	6.5

BW, body weight.
SOURCE: Adapted with permission from Kuster MS. Exercise recommendations after total joint replacement: a review of the current literature and proposal of scientifically based guidelines. *Sports Med.* 2002;32(7):433–45.

Table 118.7	Knee Joint Forces During Different Activities

Activity	Knee Joint Load (× BW)
Walking at 5.4 km · h^{-1}	3.4–4.0
Walking	3.0
Walking at 5 km · h^{-1}	2.8
Walking at 7 km · h^{-1}	4.3
Walking	3.5
Cycling at 120 W	1.2
Stair ascent	4.3–5.0
Stair descent	3.8–6.0
Ramp ascent	4.5
Ramp descent	4.5
Ramp descent at 5.4 km · h^{-1}	7.0–8.5
Squat descent	5.6
Isokinetic knee extension	Up to 9
Jogging at 9 km · h^{-1}	8–9
Jogging at 12.6 km · h^{-1}	10.3
Running at 16 km · h^{-1}	Up to 14
Bowling on asphalt alleys	Up to 12
Skiing medium steep slope	
Beginner skier	10
Skilled skier	3.5

BW, body weight.
SOURCE: Adapted with permission from Kuster MS. Exercise recommendations after total joint replacement: a review of the current literature and proposal of scientifically based guidelines. *Sports Med.* 2002;32(7):433–45.

DIFFERENCES BETWEEN JOINT TYPES

- When considering appropriate sporting activities for total *knee* joint replacement patients, one must consider not only joint loads, but also the knee flexion angle of the peak load.
- In many total knee designs, the femoral and tibial components are conforming near extension and nonconforming in flexion (12). Hence, delamination and polyethylene destruction can occur during activities like hiking or running where high joint loads occur between 40 and 60 degrees of knee flexion (11).
- It is prudent to be more conservative after TKA than after THA when considering activities with high joint loads in knee flexion. Return to athletic activity 5 years after surgery increased from 36% to 52% after THA but decreased from 42% to 34% after TKA (8).
- In a study by McCarty et al. (18) on return to athletic activity after *shoulder* arthroplasty, there was a high rate of return to swimming (86%), golf (77%), and tennis (75%), but a lower rate of return was seen in sports such as weightlifting (43%), bowling (40%), and softball (20%).
- The rate of sports activity after total ankle replacement (TAR) was 56% and significantly increased the overall sports activity rate by 20%. Hiking was the most reported sports activity after TAR (21).

SURGICAL FACTORS

- A comprehensive discussion of surgical factors is beyond the scope of this chapter; however, some important factors to consider include (a) the importance of an anatomically and biomechanically accurate joint reconstruction with a well-designed implant and a properly balanced soft tissue or muscular envelope; (b) the surgical approach (*e.g.*, lateral vs. posterolateral for THA); (c) fixation (cemented vs. uncemented); and (d) component selection materials (ceramic vs. polyethylene vs. metal).

CONCLUSIONS

- In the absence of prospective randomized controlled trials, physicians have a duty to use the currently available scientific knowledge to educate their patients regarding the risks and benefits of individual athletic activities following joint replacement.

- Patients should not be discouraged from participating in reasonable athletic activity when they prepare and train for the activity and when they understand the risks.

- In general, patients with total joint replacements are encouraged to participate in low-impact, low-demanding sports and to avoid high-impact, high-demanding sports.

- Ultimately, whether to engage in a particular sporting activity after total joint replacement is up to each individual patient. The patient must make the final decision.

REFERENCES

1. Diduch DR, Insall JN, Scott WN, Scuderi GR, Font-Rodriguez D. Total knee replacement in young, active patients. Long-term follow-up and functional outcome. *J Bone Joint Surg Am.* 1997;79(4):575–82.
2. Engh EA, Ing CA. Activity after replacement of the hip, knee or shoulder. *Orthopaedic Special Edition.* 1999;5:61–5.
3. Gioe TJ, Killeen KK, Grimm K, Mehle S, Scheltema K. Why are total knee replacements revised? Analysis of early revision in a community knee implant registry. *Clin Orthop Relat Res.* 2004;428:100–6.
4. Gioe TJ, Novak C, Sinner P, Ma W, Mehle S. Knee arthroplasty in the young patient: survival in a community registry. *Clin Orthop Relat Res.* 2007;464:83–7.
5. Gschwend N, Frei T, Morscher E, Nigg B, Loehr J. Alpine and cross-country skiing after total hip replacement: 2 cohorts of 50 patients each, one active, the other inactive in skiing, followed for 5–10 years. *Acta Orthop Scand.* 2000;71(3):243–9.
6. Healy WL, Iorio R, Lemos MJ. Athletic activity after joint replacement. *Am J Sports Med.* 2001;29(3):377–88.
7. Healy WL, Sharma S, Schwartz B, Iorio R. Athletic activity after total joint arthroplasty. *J Bone Joint Surg Am.* 2008;90(10):2245–52.
8. Huch K, Müller KA, Stürmer T, Brenner H, Puhl W, Günther KP. Sports activities 5 years after total knee or hip arthroplasty: the Ulm Osteoarthritis Study. *Ann Rheum Dis.* 2005;64(12):1715–20.
9. Knutson K, Lewold S, Robertsson O, Lidgren L. The Swedish knee arthroplasty register. A nationwide study of 30,003 knees 1976–1992. *Acta Orthop Scand.* 1994;65(4):375–86.
10. Kurtz S, Ong K, Lau E, Mowat F, Halpern M. Projections of primary and revision hip and knee arthroplasty in the United States from 2005 to 2030. *J Bone Joint Surg Am.* 2007;89(4):780–5.
11. Kuster MS. Exercise recommendations after total joint replacement: a review of the current literature and proposal of scientifically based guidelines. *Sports Med.* 2002;32(7):433–45.
12. Kuster MS, Horz S, Spalinger E, Stachowiak GW, Gächter A. The effects of conformity and load in total knee replacement. *Clin Orthop Relat Res.* 2000;375:302–12.
13. Kuster MS, Stachowiak GW. Factors affecting polyethylene wear in total knee arthroplasty. *Orthopedics.* 2002;25(2 Suppl):S235–42.
14. Long WT, Dorr LD, Gendelman V. An American experience with metal-on-metal total hip arthroplasties: a 7-year follow-up study. *J Arthroplasty.* 2004;19(8 Suppl 3):29–34.
15. Malchau H, Herberts P, Ahnfelt L. Prognosis of total hip replacement in Sweden. Follow-up of 92,675 operations performed 1978–1990. *Acta Orthop Scand.* 1993;64(5):497–506.
16. Mancuso CA, Graziano S, Briskie LM, et al. Randomized trials to modify patients' preoperative expectations of hip and knee arthroplasties. *Clin Orthop Relat Res.* 2008;466(2):424–31.
17. Martin BW, Beelwer I, Szucs T, et al. Economic benefits of the health-enhancing effects of physical activity: first estimates for Switzerland [position statement]. *Schweiz Z Sportmed Sport Traumatol.* 2001;49(3):131–3.
18. McCarty EC, Marx RG, Maerz D, Altchek D, Warren RF. Sports participation after shoulder replacement surgery. *Am J Sports Med.* 2008;36(8):1577–81.
19. Mendenhall S. Editorial. *Orthopedic Network News.* 2000;11:7.
20. Schmalzried TP, Callaghan JJ. Wear in total hip and knee replacements. *J Bone Joint Surg Am.* 1999;81(1):115–36.
21. Schmalzried TP, Shepherd EF, Dorey FJ, et al. The John Charnley Award. Wear is a function of use, not time. *Clin Orthop Relat Res.* 2000;381:36–46.
22. Schwameder H, Roithner R, Müller E, Niessen W, Raschner C. Knee joint forces during downhill walking with hiking poles. *J Sports Sci.* 1999;17(12):969–78.
23. Weiss JM, Noble PC, Conditt MA, et al What functional activities are important to patients with knee replacements? *Clin Orthop Relat Res.* 2002;404:172–88.
24. Zahiri CA, Schmalzried TP, Szuszczewicz ES, Amstutz HC. Assessing activity in joint replacement patients. *J Arthroplasty.* 1998;13(8):890–5.

119 The Athlete with Cancer

Jason M. Matuszak and Tracey O'Connor

INTRODUCTION

- Cancer can strike individuals in the prime of their lives, and athletes are no exception.

- With advances in screening, diagnosis, and management, people increasingly survive cancer and return to activities that are important to them. According to the National Cancer Institute, there are over 11 million cancer survivors in the United States (44).

- Studies indicate that regular exercise can help to prevent certain types of cancer, with the best evidence supporting colon, breast, and endometrial.

- Exercise in a cancer patient or survivor has benefits to both health and general well-being.

- American College of Sports Medicine (ACSM) position stand on exercise in the cancer survivor was published in 2010 (69).

  - This was created to highlight new evidence that shows cancer survivors — including those currently undergoing treatment — can experience a multitude of benefits from exercise. They should avoid inactivity and, as closely as possible, adhere to the 2008 federal Physical Activity Guidelines for Americans.

  - Exercise recommendations should be tailored to the individual cancer survivor to account for exercise tolerance and specific diagnosis. There are certain recommended alterations to the federal physical activity guidelines for specific types of cancer, including breast, prostate, colon, and hematologic (blood or bone marrow).

- Sports medicine physicians are ideally positioned to:

  - Educate athlete about cancer risk

  - Screen for detectable cancers

  - Evaluate musculoskeletal pain for potential malignant causes

  - In conjunction with an athlete and their health care team, develop an exercise program/prescription

  - Educate on the benefits of exercise in the cancer patient and in cancer prevention

ATHLETES POTENTIALLY AT INCREASED RISK OF CANCER

- Environmental exposure

  - Many sports are played outdoors, and as such, there is sun exposure. Multiple studies have shown an increased risk of skin cancer in outdoor sports, including aquatic and traditionally winter sports (3,34,76).

  - Radiation exposure may be higher for athletes that travel frequently by airplane and who have multiple x-rays or, especially, computed tomography scans (1,20,24,47).

  - Skin exposure to trihalomethanes or other carcinogens in swimming pool water has been suggested to be a risk factor for cancer (62).

- Drugs or ergogenic aids that may predispose for cancer

  - Anabolic steroids have traditionally been implicated in hepatoma, and studies show there are sex hormone receptors in liver cancer cells (6,73).

  - Growth hormone

    - Evidence shows individuals with acromegaly have pathologically increased tumor risk.

    - Supplementation for medical or ergogenic reasons may lead to increases in colorectal cancer, second tumors in previous cancer patients taking growth hormone, and in primary tumors as a result of the anabolic effects and resulting abnormal proliferation of malignant cells (6,33,59,60,73).

  - Erythropoietin (EPO) may lead to angiogenesis and inhibit apoptosis of abnormal cells.

  - Oral contraceptive pills may increase risk of breast cancer, especially when started before the age of 20 (41,42). Early menarche has also been implicated, and some have theorized that this is an effect of increased estrogen.

  - Some supplements, including creatine and chromium, are being evaluated for carcinogenicity.

- Other risky behaviors

  - Tobacco use — lung, oropharyngeal cancers (12,55)

  - Sexually transmitted diseases that increase risk of cancer (55)

    - Human papillomavirus — cervical cancer, penile cancer

- Prolonged strenuous exercise
  - Most studies show a reduced risk of cancer with exercise; however, there continue to be concerns that prolonged strenuous exercise, such as that encountered by endurance athletes, may lead to an increased risk in certain individuals.
  - It is theorized that this could be an effect of increased oxidative stress leading to an increased burden of free radicals and significant increases in DNA damage, in conjunction with an observed reversal of the increased activity seen with moderate exercise of macrophages, natural killer cells, and polymorphonuclear neutrophils, which are the first line of defense against cancer.
  - One study of world-class Norwegian athletes showed a three-fold increased risk of thyroid cancer in female athletes (66).
  - In vitro and animal studies do suggest that there is an increased incidence of DNA damage as a result of strenuous exercise; however, strenuous exercise has been demonstrated to shrink tumor size (5,7,65).
  - Human data remain incomplete and inconclusive at this time.

FINDING CANCER IN ATHLETES

Screening (59)

- A history of night sweats, fatigue, unintentional weight loss, decreasing performance, treatment-resistant pain, and recurrent infections suggest the need for further investigation.
- Social history should be reviewed for risk factors for cancer such as tobacco, environmental exposures, or anabolic steroid use.
- A family history of malignancy is important, particularly in cancers that have a strong genetic link.

- The physical examination should include a skin examination to exclude melanoma or other skin cancers. Adenopathy, particularly if a mass is enlarging, nontender, and fixed, suggests lymphoma or metastatic disease. Excessive ecchymoses can represent leukemia. Conjunctival pallor from anemia can be present with neoplasm that infiltrates the bone marrow or from occult blood loss in gastrointestinal malignancies. Testicular cancer frequently presents as testicular mass or swelling. The abdomen should be examined for masses and organomegaly.

Malignancy as Musculoskeletal Pain

- Cancer can present as musculoskeletal pain and should be considered in the differential diagnosis, especially when certain warning signs are seen, including pain unrelieved by rest, unrelenting pain, night pain, or pain that does not improve despite appropriate treatment. It should also be considered when there are constitutional symptoms that suggest malignancy (10).
- Cancers that commonly present as musculoskeletal pain
  - Metastases, most often from breast, lung, thyroid, kidney, and prostate
    - Bone is third most common site of metastases after lung and liver (10).
    - More common than primary tumors of the bone.
    - More likely to cause significant clinical disease due to pain, pathologic fractures, hypercalcemia, and bone marrow replacement (61).
  - Solitary primary musculoskeletal tumors including osteosarcoma, chondrosarcoma, Ewing sarcoma, giant cell tumors, and rhabdomyosarcoma (Table 119.1)
  - Leukemia, lymphoma, and multiple myeloma

Table 119.1	Malignant Solid Tumors of the Musculoskeletal System	
Tumor	**Population Notes**	**Radiographic/Disease Notes**
Primary osteosarcoma	< 30 years of age; male predominance	60% in the knee; also consider in hip, pelvis, shoulder "Moth-eaten" or "sunburst" appearance Codman's triangle
Chondrosarcoma	> 20 years of age	Hip, pelvis, femoral diaphysis, ribs, and proximal humerus Pathologic fracture
Ewing sarcoma	< 30 years of age; male 2:1 predominance	Pelvis, femur, humerus; lucency/lysis; "onion-skin layering"
Giant cell tumors	20–40 years of age; female predominance	Lytic; "soap bubble lesion" Nonsclerotic, sharply defined borders Pathologic fracture; Epiphyseal predilection
Rhabdomyosarcomas	90% < 20 years of age	Enlarging, painful, soft tissue mass Most occur in areas naturally lacking significant skeletal muscle (head, neck, genitourinary tract)
Multiple myeloma	> 50 years of age	Spine or ribs Mechanical back pain Bence-Jones protein Lytic, punched out lesions

PREPARTICIPATION EVALUATION FOR THE ATHLETE PARTICIPATING WITH CANCER

■ There are no specific guidelines for the types of preparticipation evaluation that should be performed on athletes wanting to participate with active cancer; ACSM position stand on exercise guidelines for cancer survivors addressed the preexercise evaluation of survivors.

■ Consider using multidisciplinary approach to evaluate for individual risk, perceived complications, and clinical status.

■ Understand that athletes undergoing active cancer treatment can feel profoundly different over short periods of time. They should remain flexible with their exercise program to their changing condition.

■ Cancer treatments may result in different complications. Chemotherapy, radiation, and hormone therapy can all have side effects that will have a bearing on an individual's ability to participate in activities. The profile of the specific agents should be understood prior to starting an exercise program.

■ If surgery has already been performed, evaluate for possible site-specific or regional complications (*i.e.,* wound integrity, lymphedema of the arm or leg with lymph node dissection).

■ Cardiac complications can be seen with a number of chemotherapy agents, and these may place the athlete at high risk for arrhythmias or cardiomyopathy. There is some evidence to show that stress testing or submaximal stress testing can be used to determine ability to start an exercise program (52).

■ In the cancer survivor without risk of cardiotoxicity or other specific indications, follow ACSM guidelines for exercise testing before moderate to vigorous aerobic exercise training (69).

■ Resistance training can be safely undertaken by athletes with active cancer and cancer survivors. Consideration should be given for fracture risk with osteoporosis related to cancer treatment or bony metastases. Also, care must be taken when performing resistance training with abdominal wounds or an ostomy following cancer surgery to decrease risk of herniation by avoiding excessive intra-abdominal pressure (19,69).

■ Flexibility training may be undertaken safely. Avoid excessive intra-abdominal pressure for athletes with ostomies (69).

THE BENEFITS OF EXERCISE IN THE CANCER PATIENT

■ There is substantial documentation that physical activity has positive effects on physical and psychological health and overall quality of life (72), and that there is an association between physical activity and breast cancer survival (38,74).

■ Physical activity is generally well tolerated during and following cancer treatment. A recent meta-analysis showed that the majority of studies find a positive and significant impact of physical activity intervention during treatment for upper and lower body strength and self-esteem. Following treatment, a positive and significant impact of physical activity interventions was seen for aerobic fitness, upper and lower body strength, lower body flexibility, lean body mass, overall quality of life, and cancer-related fatigue (CRF) (72). Although the power of this study may be limited by the fact that approximately 80% of the patients in these studies had breast cancer, there have been promising results noted for prostate and hematologic cancers as well (69).

■ Despite the documented benefits of exercise, only 25%–30% of cancer survivors are reported to be physically active (defined as meeting the public health exercise guidelines) (30). Young age, higher education, male gender, healthy weight, and absence of comorbidity are positively associated with physical activity among cancer survivors (8,13,40,50).

■ Exercise is safe both during and after most types of cancer treatments, including life-threatening treatments such as bone marrow transplant, with attention to infection risk among those immunocompromised due to treatment (*e.g.,* care to avoid spread of infection through use of equipment at public gyms) (69)

■ Recently reported randomized controlled trials have demonstrated that a slowly progressive weightlifting program in breast cancer patients with lymphedema had no significant effect on limb swelling and resulted in a decreased incidence of lymphedema exacerbations, reduced symptoms, and increased strength (68). In breast cancer patients who are at risk for but have not yet developed lymphedema, a progressive program of resistance training and aerobic activity did not increase the risk for or increase symptoms of lymphedema (2,15). Similar safety data do not yet exist for patients suffering from lymphedema as a consequence of gynecological cancer.

■ Exercise before and after a breast cancer diagnosis has been associated with a decreased risk of recurrence and/or death from breast cancer in observational studies (26,39,43). Two reported observational studies suggest that exercise after a colon cancer diagnosis may reduce the risk of colon cancer–specific and overall mortality (53,54).

EXERCISE FOR THE PREVENTION OF CANCER

■ Physical activity and exercise are important health behaviors in the prevention and management of many acute and chronic diseases (14). Research in cancer over the past 20 years has resulted in physical activity receiving a prominent place in

Table 119.2	Level of Supporting Evidence for Benefit of Physical Activity on Lifetime Risk of Cancer

Cancer Type	Level of Evidence (SORT Criteria)
Colon	1
Breast	2
Endometrial	2
Lung	3
Ovary	3
Prostate	3
All others	Insufficient evidence

SORT, Strength of Recommendation Taxonomy.

many cancer control and exercise science guidelines including the American Cancer Society's guidelines for cancer prevention (48) and survivorship (21).

■ Physical activity is a complex behavior to assess since the type of activity, dose (intensity, duration, frequency), and timing (younger vs. older age) all need to be considered when assessing how this factor influences cancer risk (27).

■ Exercise can be safely advised for most individuals given its large benefit and relatively low risk. Although exercise can be safely recommended, the level of epidemiologic evidence varies by cancer site (Table 119.2) (14).

■ Colon cancer

   ▪ A meta-analysis of case-controlled and cohort studies by Wolin et al. (79) examined the association between physical activity and colon/colorectal cancers. From these data, it is estimated that physical activity reduces colon cancer risk by 20%–25% in both men and women who have the highest levels of physical activity versus the lowest levels of activity (79). Based on the evidence of studies of recreational activity, it is estimated that 30–60 minutes per day of moderate- to vigorous-intensity physical activity may be required to lower colon cancer risk significantly (48).

   ▪ The association between physical activity and a decreased risk of colon cancer is supported by several biologic mechanisms. Physical activity may decrease inflammation, reduce intestinal transit time (and decrease mucosal exposure to carcinogens), decrease insulin-like growth factors, reduce insulin levels, modulate immune function (35,67), and increase vitamin D levels (31). Some of the association may be related to obesity; however, there continues to be statistically significant differences when body composition is controlled for (78).

■ Breast cancer

   ▪ Physical activity as a means of reducing breast cancer risk was first reported in 1985 with an observation that the lifetime incidence of breast and other reproductive cancers was lower in college athletes (29). Since breast cancer is a major cause of mortality and cancer incidence in developed nations and because most risk factors for breast cancer are not able to be modified, there has been considerable research and public interest in reducing breast cancer risk through increased activity (28).

■ Twenty-nine (40%) of 73 studies reviewed found a statistically significant reduction in breast cancer risk when comparing the highest versus the lowest levels of activity. In addition, eight other studies (11%) observed a risk reduction that was of borderline significance, and 14 (19%) had risk reductions that did not achieve statistical significance. No association was found between physical activity and breast cancer in 19 studies (26%), and 3 studies (4%) showed a nonsignificant increased risk. The magnitude of the risk reduction across all studies was 25% (51).

■ Recently, randomized controlled exercise intervention studies have begun to investigate how exercise may influence breast cancer risk by examining the effect on hypothesized biomarkers of breast cancer risk. Evidence is accumulating that physical activity has a beneficial effect on breast cancer risk by decreasing body fat, sex and metabolic hormones, insulin resistance, and inflammation (28).

■ Physical activity reduces breast cancer risk when performed at any age, but activity done after the age of 50 has a stronger effect than activity earlier in life, and sustained lifetime activity is of benefit (25). Current public health recommendations for breast cancer risk reduction are at least 4–7 hours per week of moderate- to vigorous-intensity activity (63).

■ Endometrial cancer

   ▪ Many risk factors are similar for the development of breast and endometrial cancer. Epidemiologic evidence suggests that physical activity is likely to protect against the development of endometrial cancer, and this effect is independent of adiposity and exhibits a dose-response relationship (18).

   ▪ A systematic review of 20 studies found a consistent reduction in endometrial cancer risk with a range of 20%–30% (75). Higher intensity and longer duration activity may be more beneficial than lower intensity, shorter duration activity. Based on the studies conducted to date, about 1 hour of moderate-intensity activity appears to decrease endometrial cancer risk (27).

■ Prostate cancer

   ▪ Prostate cancer is the most frequently diagnosed cancer and the second leading cause of cancer death among men in the United States (44). Risk factors include age, race, and family history; modifiable risk factors are not yet established (32).

   ▪ The evidence for an association between physical activity and prostate cancer is less established than for breast, colon, and endometrial cancer, and the link is classified as possible. In a recent review of 39 epidemiologic studies of physical activity and prostate cancer, an average decrease of 9% in prostate cancer risk was seen when comparing high versus low levels of physical activity (49).

■ Based on a limited number of studies, there was no strong protective effect of earlier life physical activity on risk for prostate cancer. Similarly, the association did not vary substantially between population subgroups. Studies that assessed activity intensity and those that considered fatal prostate cancer as an endpoint reported the strongest inverse association between physical activity and prostate cancer risk (49).

SPECIAL CONSIDERATIONS OF EXERCISE IN THE ATHLETE WITH CANCER

■ The pediatric athlete
  ■ Studies suggest that children and adolescents have different levels of satisfaction with their athletic performance compared with other aspects of their life and in comparison with their peers (46,57). Children with cancer also score their athletic competence lower than their parents do (22).
  ■ Identifiable risk factors for physical performance limitations include (56):
    ❑ Original diagnosis of bone tumor, brain tumor, or Hodgkin disease; female sex; and an income less than $20,000 per year
    ❑ Treatment that included radiation and treatment with a combination of alkylating agents and anthracyclines
    ❑ Musculoskeletal, neurologic, cardiac, pulmonary, sensory, and endocrine organ system dysfunction
■ Exercise programs and CRF
  ■ Fatigue is a common symptom in patients with cancer and is nearly universal in those undergoing cytotoxic chemotherapy, radiation therapy, bone marrow transplantation, or treatment with biologic agents (9). Patients perceive CRF to be the most distressing symptom they suffer, more distressing even than nausea and vomiting or pain, which can often be managed with medications (37,74).
  ■ Current research evidence suggests that both aerobic and resistance exercise programs are beneficial at improving CRF. Recent evidence suggests that greater benefits may be seen when exercise programs are implemented in the survivorship phase rather than the active treatment phase (17,72).
  ■ In a recent randomized controlled trial, a 12-week supervised aerobic exercise program versus usual care in 122 lymphoma patients was shown to offer significant benefit for symptoms of CRF and cardiorespiratory fitness, lean body mass, and depression (16).
  ■ In prostate cancer patients, both resistance and aerobic exercise was found to significantly attenuate CRF over the short term. Only resistance exercise, however, was found to significantly improve CRF in the long term (70).

■ Exercise and immune function
  ■ Macrophages, natural killer (NK) cells, and polymorphonuclear neutrophils are the first line of defense against cancer. It is unclear what effects exercise can have on the function of these cells (77). Schmitz et al. (69) examined two randomized controlled trials that evaluated exercise training on intrinsic factors after breast cancer treatment. They noted one study showed no significant increases in NK cells or their cytotoxic activity after 8 weeks of aerobic exercise training, whereas the other did show significant improvement in NK cell cytotoxic activity after 15 weeks of weekly aerobic exercise three times a week (69).
  ■ Human cross-sectional studies demonstrate an inverse relationship between regular physical activity and inflammatory biomarkers, including C-reactive protein (CRP), tumor necrosis factor-alpha (TNF-α), and interleukin-6 (IL-6). Reductions in CRP levels with exercise training have also been reported (45).
  ■ Animal model data show a positive effect of exercise on macrophage function, with enhanced clearance of lung metastases. Additionally, training results in greater in vitro NK cell cytotoxicity, enhanced in vivo mechanisms of natural immunity, and reduced pulmonary tumor metastases in mice (77).
    ❑ No change in NK cell cytotoxicity was observed after a 12-month walking intervention in healthy postmenopausal women.
  ■ Moderate exercise enhances antigen-specific T-cell–mediated cytokine function, production, and proliferation following vaccination (77).
    ❑ May translate into better protection from infectious agents and greater immunosurveillance
    ❑ Adaptive immune responses in relation to exercise may have a clinically significant impact on virally induced cancers, for example, cervical cancer and human papillomavirus.
  ■ The effect of exercise on lymphomas (Hodgkin lymphoma [HL] and non-Hodgkin lymphoma [NHL]) has been examined in limited studies. It is felt that because of the role of immune mediation, that if there is a significant exercise-induced enhancement of antitumor mechanisms, it would be evident in lymphoma (77).
    ❑ Participation in collegiate sports was associated with a trend of reduced risk of HL, although this did not reach statistical significance.
    ❑ Women who participated in strenuous physical activity at various time points in adult life had a lower risk of HL.
    ❑ A case-control study on NHL and occupational physical activity (measured as energy expenditure or sitting time) found no significant association.

- Studies examining the effect of immune function during cancer treatment have mixed results (58).
  - In a study examining children with acute lymphocytic leukemia, there were nonsignificant decreases in T cells (71).
  - Another study looking at participation in an exercise program after peripheral-blood stem cell transplantation found that exercise did not facilitate or delay immune cell recovery (36).
  - Fairey et al. (23) evaluated studies that looked at immune function status in cancer survivors and reported that several showed significant improvements in immune function as a result of exercise.
- Ergogenic aids in the athlete with cancer
  - It is important to be aware of regular restrictions for use of ergogenic aids for athletes in competition.
  - Androgen receptor agonists, including anabolic androgenic steroids and nonsteroidal agonists (selective androgen receptor modulators), can help with cancer cachexia (11).
  - Growth hormone use may lead to increased risk of second cancer (59,73).
  - EPO is considered for anemia related to cancer treatment.
  - Orchiectomy has been suggested to lead to enhanced athletic performance (4).

REFERENCES

1. Agredano YZ, Chan JL, Kimball RC, Kimball AB. Accessibility to air travel correlates strongly with increasing melanoma incidence. *Melanoma Res.* 2006;16(1):77–81.
2. Ahmed RL, Thomas W, Yee D, Schmitz KH. Randomized controlled trial of weight training and lymphedema in breast cancer survivors. *J Clin Oncol.* 2006;24(18):2765–72.
3. Andersen PA, Buller DB, Walkosz BJ, et al. Environmental cues to UV radiation and personal sun protection in outdoor winter recreation. *Arch Dermatol.* 2010;146(11):1241–7.
4. Atwood CS, Bowen RL. Metabolic clues regarding the enhanced performance of elite endurance athletes from orchiectomy-induced hormonal changes. *Med Hypotheses.* 2007;68(4):735–49.
5. Bacurau AVN, Belmonte MA, Navarro F, et al. Effect of a high-intensity exercise training on the metabolism and function of macrophages and lymphocytes of walker 256 tumor bearing rats. *Exp Biol Med (Maywood).* 2007;232(10):1289–99.
6. Bain J. The many faces of testosterone. *Clin Interv Aging.* 2007;2(4):567–76.
7. Barnard RJ, Ngo TH, Leung PS, Aronson WJ, Golding LA. A low-fat diet and/or strenuous exercise alters the IGF axis in vivo and reduces prostate tumor cell growth in vitro. *Prostate.* 2003;56(3):201–6.
8. Bellizzi KM, Rowland JH, Arora NK, Hamilton AS, Miller MF, Aziz NM. Physical activity and quality of life in adult survivors of non-Hodgkin's lymphoma. *J Clin Oncol.* 2009;27(6):960–6.
9. Berger AM, Abernethy AP, Atkinson A, et al. Cancer-related fatigue. *J Natl Compr Canc Netw.* 2010;8(8):904–31.
10. Bruera ED, Portenoy RK. *Cancer Pain Assessment and Management.* Cambridge (UK): Cambridge University Press; 2003.
11. Burckart K, Beca S, Urban RJ, Sheffield-Moore M. Pathogenesis of muscle wasting in cancer cachexia: targeted anabolic and anticatabolic therapies. *Curr Opin Clin Nutr Metab Care.* 2010;13(4):410–6.
12. Connolly GN, Orleans CT, Blum A. Snuffing tobacco out of sport. *Am J Public Health.* 1992;82(3):351–3.
13. Coups EJ, Park BJ, Feinstein MB, et al. Correlates of physical activity among lung cancer survivors. *Psychooncology.* 2009;18(4):395–404.
14. Courneya KS, Friedenreich CM. Physical activity and cancer: an introduction. *Recent Results Cancer Res.* 2011;186:1–10.
15. Courneya KS, Segal RJ, Mackey JR, et al. Effects of aerobic and resistance exercise in breast cancer patients receiving adjuvant chemotherapy: a multicenter randomized controlled trial. *J Clin Oncol.* 2007;25(28):4396–404.
16. Courneya KS, Sellar CM, Stevinson C, et al. Randomized controlled trial of the effects of aerobic exercise on physical functioning and quality of life in lymphoma patients. *J Clin Oncol.* 2009;27(27):4605–12.
17. Cramp F, Daniel J. Exercise for the management of cancer-related fatigue in adults. *Cochrane Database Syst Rev.* 2008;2:CD006145.
18. Cust AE, Armstrong BK, Friedenreich CM, Slimani N, Bauman A. Physical activity and endometrial cancer risk: a review of the current evidence, biologic mechanisms and the quality of physical activity assessment methods. *Cancer Causes Control.* 2007;18(3):243–58.
19. De Backer IC, Schep G, Backx FJ, Vreugdenhil G, Kuipers H. Resistance training in cancer survivors: a systematic review. *Int J Sports Med.* 2009;30(10):703–12.
20. Downs NJ, Schouten PW, Parisi AV, Turner J. Measurements of the upper body ultraviolet exposure to golfers: non-melanoma skin cancer risk, and the potential benefits of exposure to sunlight. *Photodermatol Photoimmunol Photomed.* 2009;25(6):317–24.
21. Doyle C, Kushi LH, Byers T, et al. Nutrition and physical activity during and after cancer treatment: an American Cancer Society guide for informed choices. *CA Cancer J Clin.* 2006;56(6):323–53.
22. Eapen V, Mabrouk A, Bin-Othman S. Attitudes, perceptions, and family coping in pediatric cancer and childhood diabetes. *Ann N Y Acad Sci.* 2008;1138:47–9.
23. Fairey AS, Courneya KS, Field CJ, Mackey JR. Physical exercise and immune system function in cancer survivors: a comprehensive review and future directions. *Cancer.* 2002;94(2):539–51.
24. Friedberg W, Copeland K, Duke FE, O'Brien K 3rd, Darden EB Jr. Radiation exposure during air travel: guidance provided by the Federal Aviation Administration for air carrier crews. *Health Phys.* 2000;79(5):591–5.
25. Friedenreich CM, Cust AE. Physical activity and breast cancer risk: impact of timing, type and dose of activity and population subgroup effects. *Br J Sports Med.* 2008;42(8):636–47.
26. Friedenreich CM, Gregory J, Kopciuk KA, Mackey JR, Courneya KS. Prospective cohort study of lifetime physical activity and breast cancer survival. *Int J Cancer.* 2009;124(8):1954–62.
27. Friedenreich CM, Neilson HK, Lynch BM. State of the epidemiological evidence on physical activity and cancer prevention. *Eur J Cancer.* 2010;46(14):2593–604.
28. Friedenreich CM, Woolcott CG, McTiernan A, et al. Alberta physical activity and breast cancer prevention trial: sex hormone changes in a year-long exercise intervention among postmenopausal women. *J Clin Oncol.* 2010;28(9):1458–66.
29. Frisch RE, Wyshak G, Albright NL, et al. Lower prevalence of breast cancer and cancers of the reproductive system among former college athletes compared to non-athletes. *Br J Cancer.* 1985;52(6):885–91.
30. Gjerset GM, Fosså SD, Courneya KS, Skovlund E, Thorsen L. Exercise behavior in cancer survivors and associated factors. *J Cancer Surviv.* 2011;5(1):35–43.

31. Gorham ED, Garland CF, Garland FC, et al. Vitamin D and prevention of colorectal cancer. *J Steroid Biochem Mol Biol.* 2005;97(1–2):179–94.

32. Grönberg H. Prostate cancer epidemiology. *Lancet.* 2003;361(9360):859–64.

33. Gullett NP, Hebbar G, Ziegler TR. Update on clinical trials of growth factors and anabolic steroids in cachexia and wasting. *Am J Clin Nutr.* 2010;91(4):1143S–7S.

34. Haley A, Nichols A. A survey of injuries and medical conditions affecting competitive adult outrigger canoe paddlers on O'ahu. *Hawaii Med J.* 2009;68(7):162–5.

35. Harriss DJ, Cable NT, George K, Reilly T, Renehan AG, Haboubi N. Physical activity before and after diagnosis of colorectal cancer: disease risk, clinical outcomes, response pathways and biomarkers. *Sports Med.* 2007;37(11):947–60.

36. Hayes SC, Rowbottom D, Davies PS, Parker TW, Bashford J. Immunological changes after cancer treatment and participation in an exercise program. *Med Sci Sports Exerc.* 2003;35(1):2–9.

37. Hinds PS, Quargnenti A, Bush AJ, et al. An evaluation of the impact of a self-care coping intervention on psychological and clinical outcomes in adolescents with newly diagnosed cancer. *Eur J Oncol Nurs.* 2000;4(1):6–17; discussion 18–9.

38. Holick CN, Newcomb PA, Trentham-Dietz A, et al. Physical activity and survival after diagnosis of invasive breast cancer. *Cancer Epidemiol Biomarkers Prev.* 2008;17(2):379–86.

39. Holmes MD, Chen WY, Feskanich D, Kroenke CH, Colditz GA. Physical activity and survival after breast cancer diagnosis. *JAMA.* 2005;293(20):2479–86.

40. Hong S, Bardwell WA, Natarajan L, et al. Correlates of physical activity level in breast cancer survivors participating in the Women's Healthy Eating and Living (WHEL) Study. *Breast Cancer Res Treat.* 2007;101(2):225–32.

41. Hunter DJ, Colditz GA, Hankinson SE, et al. Oral contraceptive use and breast cancer: a prospective study of young women. *Cancer Epidemiol Biomarkers Prev.* 2010;19(10):2496–502.

42. Iodice S, Barile M, Rotmensz N, et al. Oral contraceptive use and breast or ovarian cancer risk in BRCA1/2 carriers: a meta-analysis. *Eur J Cancer.* 2010;46(12):2275–84.

43. Irwin ML, Smith AW, McTiernan A, et al. Influence of pre- and postdiagnosis physical activity on mortality in breast cancer survivors: the health, eating, activity, and lifestyle study. *J Clin Oncol.* 2008;26(24):3958–64.

44. Jemal A, Siegel R, Ward E, Hao Y, Xu J, Thun MJ. Cancer statistics, 2009. *CA Cancer J Clin.* 2009;59(4):225–49.

45. Kasapis C, Thompson PD. The effects of physical activity on serum C-reactive protein and inflammatory markers: a systematic review. *J Am Coll Cardiol.* 2005;45(10):1563–9.

46. Keats MR, Courneya KS, Danielsen S, Whitsett SF. Leisure-time physical activity and psychosocial well-being in adolescents after cancer diagnosis. *J Pediatr Oncol Nurs.* 1999;16(4):180–8.

47. Kim JN, Lee BM. Risk factors, health risks, and risk management for aircraft personnel and frequent flyers. *J Toxicol Environ Health B Crit Rev.* 2007;10(3):223–34.

48. Kushi LH, Byers T, Doyle C, et al. American Cancer Society Guidelines on Nutrition and Physical Activity for cancer prevention: reducing the risk of cancer with healthy food choices and physical activity. *CA Cancer J Clin.* 2006;56(5):254–81; quiz 313–4.

49. Leitzmann MF. Physical activity and genitourinary cancer prevention. *Recent Results Cancer Res.* 2011;186:43–71.

50. Lynch BM, Cerin E, Newman B, Owen N. Physical activity, activity change, and their correlates in a population-based sample of colorectal cancer survivors. *Ann Behav Med.* 2007;34(2):135–43.

51. Lynch BM, Neilson HK, Friedenreich CM. Physical activity and breast cancer prevention. *Recent Results Cancer Res.* 2011;186:13–42.

52. May AM, van Weert E, Korstjens I, et al. Monitoring training progress during exercise training in cancer survivors: a submaximal exercise test as an alternative for a maximal exercise test? *Arch Phys Med Rehabil.* 2010;91(3):351–7.

53. Meyerhardt JA, Giovannucci EL, Holmes MD, et al. Physical activity and survival after colorectal cancer diagnosis. *J Clin Oncol.* 2006;24(22):3527–34.

54. Meyerhardt JA, Heseltine D, Niedzwiecki D, et al. Impact of physical activity on cancer recurrence and survival in patients with stage III colon cancer: findings from CALGB 89803. *J Clin Oncol.* 2006;24(22):3535–41.

55. Nattiv A, Puffer JC, Green GA. Lifestyles and health risks of collegiate athletes: a multi-center study. *Clin J Sport Med.* 1997;7(4):262–72.

56. Ness KK, Hudson MM, Ginsberg JP, et al. Physical performance limitations in the childhood cancer survivor study cohort. *J Clin Oncol.* 2009;27(14):2382–9.

57. Noll RB, Gartstein MA, Vannatta K, Correll J, Bukowski WM, Davies WH. Social, emotional, and behavioral functioning of children with cancer. *Pediatrics.* 1999;103(1):71–8.

58. O'Connor FG. *Sports Medicine: Just the Facts.* New York (NY): McGraw-Hill Medical Pub. Division; 2005.

59. Ogilvy-Stuart AL, Gleeson H. Cancer risk following growth hormone use in childhood: implications for current practice. *Drug Saf.* 2004;27(6):369–82.

60. Ogilvy-Stuart AL, Shalet SM. Tumour occurrence and recurrence. *Horm Res.* 1992;38(Suppl 1):50–5.

61. Orr FW, Kostenuik P, Sanchez-Sweatman OH, Singh G. Mechanisms involved in the metastasis of cancer to bone. *Breast Cancer Res Treat.* 1993;25(2):151–63.

62. Panyakapo M, Soontornchai S, Paopuree P. Cancer risk assessment from exposure to trihalomethanes in tap water and swimming pool water. *J Environ Sci (China).* 2008;20(3):372–8.

63. Physical Activity Guidelines Advisory Committee Report, 2008. To the Secretary of Health and Human Services. Part A: executive summary. *Nutr Rev.* 2009;67(2):114–20.

64. Pierce JP, Stefanick ML, Flatt SW, et al. Greater survival after breast cancer in physically active women with high vegetable-fruit intake regardless of obesity. *J Clin Oncol.* 2007;25(17):2345–51.

65. Poulsen HE, Weimann A, Loft S. Methods to detect DNA damage by free radicals: relation to exercise. *Proc Nutr Soc.* 1999;58(4):1007–14.

66. Robsahm TE, Hestvik UE, Veierød MB, et al. Cancer risk in Norwegian world class athletes. *Cancer Causes Control.* 2010;21(10):1711–9.

67. Rogers CJ, Colbert LH, Greiner JW, Perkins SN, Hursting SD. Physical activity and cancer prevention: pathways and targets for intervention. *Sports Med.* 2008;38(4):271–96.

68. Schmitz KH, Ahmed RL, Troxel A, et al. Weight lifting in women with breast-cancer-related lymphedema. *N Engl J Med.* 2009;361(7):664–73.

69. Schmitz KH, Courneya KS, Matthews C, et al. American College of Sports Medicine roundtable on exercise guidelines for cancer survivors. *Med Sci Sports Exerc.* 2010;42(7):1409–26.

70. Segal RJ, Reid RD, Courneya KS, et al. Randomized controlled trial of resistance or aerobic exercise in men receiving radiation therapy for prostate cancer. *J Clin Oncol.* 2009;27(3):344–51.

71. Shore S, Shepard RJ. Immune responses to exercise in children treated for cancer. *J Sports Med Phys Fitness.* 1999;39(3):240–3.

72. Speck RM, Courneya KS, Mâsse LC, Duval S, Schmitz KH. An update of controlled physical activity trials in cancer survivors: a systematic review and meta-analysis. *J Cancer Surviv.* 2010;4(2):87–100.

73. Tentori L, Graziani G. Doping with growth hormone/IGF-1, anabolic steroids or erythropoietin: is there a cancer risk? *Pharmacol Res.* 2007;55(5):359–69.

74. Vogelzang NJ, Breitbart W, Cella D, et al. Patient, caregiver, and oncologist perceptions of cancer-related fatigue: results of a tripart assessment survey. The fatigue coalition. *Semin Hematol.* 1997;34(3 Suppl 2):4–12.

75. Voskuil DW, Monninkhof EM, Elias SG, Vlems FA, van Leeuwen FE; Task Force Physical Activity and Cancer. Physical activity and endometrial cancer risk, a systematic review of current evidence. *Cancer Epidemiol Biomarkers Prev.* 2007;16(4):639–48.

76. Walkosz BJ, Buller DB, Andersen PA, et al. Increasing sun protection in winter outdoor recreation a theory-based health communication program. *Am J Prev Med.* 2008;34(6):502–9.

77. Walsh NP, Gleeson M, Shephard RJ, et al. Position statement. Part one: immune function and exercise. *Exerc Immunol Rev.* 2011;17:6–63.

78. Wolin KY, Tuchman H. Physical activity and gastrointestinal cancer prevention. *Recent Results Cancer Res.* 2011;186:73–100.

79. Wolin KY, Yan Y, Colditz GA, Lee IM. Physical activity and colon cancer prevention: a meta-analysis. *Br J Cancer.* 2009;100(4):611–6.

120 Human Immunodeficiency Virus and Sports

Robert J. Dimeff

PATHOPHYSIOLOGY

Definition

- Human immunodeficiency virus (HIV) is a human retrovirus that targets and infects $CD4^+$ T-helper cells. It replicates within the CD4 cells and causes cell death.
- Acquired immunodeficiency syndrome (AIDS) is a chronic illness with an average natural history of > 10 years. It is the result of a progressively immunocompromised state due to quantitative and functional defects in $CD4^+$ T-helper cells. The decline in CD4 cells results in decreased function of the immune system and the development of opportunistic infections and various malignancies (16).

Natural History

- Following a 10- to 28-day incubation period after exposure to HIV, the individual may develop an acute and self-limited viral-like syndrome, followed by seroconversion.
- Seroconversion may occur with the development of the viral syndrome.
- After seroconversion, a clinical latency period occurs that may last over 10 years. During this time, the infected person has normal immune and exercise function.
- As immunocompromise develops, the individual may experience otherwise unexplained fevers, fatigue, weight loss, and lymphadenopathy.
- AIDS occurs as the immune system continues to fail, and opportunistic infections ranging from mild candidiasis to life-threatening *Pneumocystis carinii* pneumonia may occur. Malignancies such as lymphoma and Kaposi sarcoma may develop. Muscle wasting occurs through mechanisms that are still not completely understood (16).

EPIDEMIOLOGY

Worldwide (73)

- 33.3 million people were living with HIV/AIDS as of December 2009, compared with 42 million in 2002.

- In 2010, it was estimated that there were 2.6 million new cases of HIV/AIDS and 1.8 million AIDS deaths.
- Two-thirds of the total cases are in sub-Saharan Africa.
- HIV testing and treatment of pregnant females has decreased the transmission of disease to newborns and infants.

United States (8,73)

- According to the Centers for Disease Control and Prevention (CDC), there were 17,000 deaths from HIV in 2009, and there have been approximately 500,000 HIV-related deaths in the United States since the onset of the disease.
- It is estimated that there have been approximately 48,000 new cases annually since 2006.
- At the end of 2008, it was estimated that there were 1,178,350 persons over the age of 13 in the United States living with HIV infection, and this number continues to increase annually. It is estimated that 20% are unaware of their positive status.
- Men having sex with men (MSM) account for 75% of the HIV cases in the United States. MSM represent 2% of the U.S. population but 50% of all new cases. MSM have a 44 times greater rate of HIV infection than men having sex with women.
- African Americans represent 14% of the U.S. population and 44% of the new cases annually. The rate of infection in African Americans is three times greater than Hispanics and six times greater than Caucasians. African American females have a 15 times higher rate of infection than Caucasian females.

Athletics

- The incidence and prevalence of HIV/AIDS in athletes are unknown, but there are several high-profile elite and professional athletes who have acquired HIV, including Earvin "Magic" Johnson in 1991 (competed in National Basketball Association [NBA] and 1992 Summer Olympics with HIV) and Greg Louganis (competed in 1988 Olympics with HIV), who attribute their infection to personal behaviors unrelated to sports participation.
- Tommy Morrison (professional boxing) was banned from sports after testing positive for HIV in 1996. He was reinstated

in 2006 after apparently becoming HIV negative and has subsequently fought professionally. Controversy regarding his true testing and disease status continues to exist.

- Several professional athletes have died from AIDS contracted from nonsports activities including sexual activity, drug abuse, and blood transfusion. Prominent HIV-positive athletes include Bill Goldsworthy (National Hockey League [NHL]), Jerry Smith (National Football League [NFL]), Alan Wiggins (Major League Baseball [MLB]), Esteban DeJesus (boxing), Tim Richmond (NASCAR driver), Robert McCall and Rudy Galindo (figure skating), and Arthur Ashe (professional tennis).

- HIV-infected athletes have participated in professional American-style football in the United States as well as Canada (26).

- Fears of the widespread dissemination of HIV throughout professional sports have been fueled by reports such as in 1991 when two Canadian physicians announced a woman who had died of AIDS had disclosed that she had sexual intercourse with 30–70 different hockey players in the NHL (33).

- HIV-positive athletes have participated in intercollegiate sports and the 2011 Ironman World Championship (36,43).

TRANSMISSION

- HIV is found in all body fluids of the infected individual including blood, semen, vaginal and cervical secretions, breast milk, and amniotic fluid. The highest concentration of HIV is in the cerebrospinal fluid. The virus is also found in low concentrations in tears, sputum, saliva, and urine, but it is not considered to be infectious in these forms unless they are blood tinged. HIV has not been found in sweat (38).

- The primary routes of transmission are through sexual contact; parenteral exposure to blood, blood products, or blood-containing body fluids; and maternofetal transmission at birth.

- HIV is not transmissible through casual contact, swimming pools, mosquitoes, saliva, sweat, tears, urine, feces, or inanimate object (13).

- With the advances in diagnoses and treatment, the transmission rate has dropped from 92% in the early 1980 to 5% in 2008. This means that at the onset of the epidemic in the 1980s, 92 of 100 HIV-positive patients transmitted the disease to uninfected individuals; the rate is now less than 5 per 100 HIV-positive patients (73).

- There are currently no reports of transmission of HIV from an athlete to a health care provider on the sidelines or in the training room. The theoretical risk to the athletic health care provider is based on data on health care professionals exposed to HIV by needlestick and is estimated at 0.3%. There have been several reports of health care workers who have contracted HIV from infected blood splashed onto their mucous membranes. This is extremely rare and requires prolonged exposure to large amounts of blood; the risk has been estimated at approximately 0.1%. The risk of transmission following exposure to nonintact skin of HIV-infected blood is less than 0.1%, and small amounts of blood on intact skin pose no risk (25,73).

- No transmission of HIV during sports has ever been documented. However, two reports of transmission of HIV during bloody fistfights have been verified by the CDC (19). In determining theoretical risk of on-field HIV transmission, the following are necessary: (a) the presence of an infected athlete; (b) a bleeding wound or exudative skin lesion in the infected athlete; (c) a skin lesion or exposed mucous membrane on a susceptible athlete; and (d) sustained contact between the portal of entry on the susceptible athlete and the infective material (13,43).

- The potential risk of HIV transmission during professional football has been estimated at less than 1 per 85 million game contacts (4).

- Athletes are more at risk of contracting HIV from nonathletic activities. Off-of-the-field situations in which athletes may more commonly put themselves at risk for contracting HIV include: sexual contact, use of injectable steroids or other drugs with shared needles or paraphernalia, tattoos, and body piercings.

- There is a higher proportion of risky lifestyle behaviors among intercollegiate male athletes compared to nonathletes. These include number of sexual partners, sexual activity, intravenous drug use, and episodes of sexually transmitted diseases (51). Although female intercollegiate athletes also show high levels of risky health behaviors, this is less than nonathlete peers (35).

- In the realm of the professional athlete, the rate of risky behavior is unknown, but anecdotal evidence suggests that their celebrity status may lead to higher risks (33).

TESTING

Screening Test

- HIV antibodies are low or absent in the first few weeks of infection but are usually present within 6 weeks. However, antibody production may not be detectable until 6 months after infection. Therefore, antibody testing following possible exposure is recommended at 6 weeks, 3 months, 6 months, and 1 year (16).

- The most common screening test is the enzyme-linked immunosorbent assay (ELISA), which can identify HIV antibodies in the blood with a sensitivity of up to 99.5%. If the ELISA test is positive, it is automatically repeated. If the second screen is positive, infection is confirmed by the Western blot analysis, which identifies antibodies to proteins of a specific molecular weight. It is only after these confirmatory tests are positive that an HIV antibody test should be reported as being positive.

- The U.S. Food and Drug Administration recently approved four rapid HIV antibody tests (28). The OraQuick Advance Rapid test of oral fluid and blood has a sensitivity of 99.6% and specificity of 99.8%–100.0%. The Reveal G-2 Rapid HIV-1 test of serum or plasma has a sensitivity of 99.9% and specificity of 98.6%–99.1%. The Uni-Gold Recombigen test of serum, plasma, and whole blood has a sensitivity of 100.0% and specificity of 99.8%. The Multispot HIV-1/HIV-2 test of serum and plasma has a sensitivity of 100.0% and specificity of 99.93%.

- Detection of p24 core antigen is possible 1–3 weeks after exposure. It is only present for a short interval and thus has been largely replaced by HIV RNA or DNA viral load to determine recent HIV exposure.

Confirmatory Testing

- HIV viral load is performed via polymerase chain reaction or branched DNA testing and is useful at detecting recent exposure as well as monitoring response to treatment.

- It is suggested that a baseline measurement be obtained at the time of diagnosis and then rechecked within 2–8 weeks of initiating or changing treatment. Viral loads are then followed every 3–4 months.

- Viral genotype and phenotypic resistance assays may be used to guide specific antiretroviral therapy.

- T-cell tests can identify the total CD4 count and the CD4:CD8 ratio in the blood, which can assist with HIV diagnosis, management, and treatment and the initiation of prophylaxis therapy for opportunistic infections (24). Normal CD4 cell counts range from 500–1,600 cells $\cdot$ μL^{-1}. CD4 levels ranging from 200–500 cells $\cdot$ μL^{-1} are considered low, and levels below 200 cells $\cdot$ μL^{-1} are considered extremely low and diagnostic of AIDS. Most experts recommend initiation of antiretroviral therapy if the CD4 level is below 350 cells $\cdot$ μL^{-1}. The normal CD4:CD8 ratio is 30%–60%; if the ratio is less than 14%, it is considered diagnostic of AIDS.

Mandatory Testing in Sports

- The American College of Sports Medicine, National Collegiate Athletic Association (NCAA), Canadian Academy of Sport and Exercise Medicine, CDC, International Federation of Sports Medicine, International Olympic Committee, and the World Health Organization do not recommend mandatory screening of athletes for HIV. Any testing that is performed must be accompanied by pre- and posttest counseling, incorporate confidentiality measures, address the frequency of testing, and adhere to local and federal law.

- The 1993 survey of NCAA institutions concerning HIV/AIDS policies found that routine HIV testing for athletes occurred in 4% of institutions and only two were mandatory (44).

- None of the four major professional sports leagues in North America (NFL, NBA, MLB, or NHL) have adopted mandatory HIV testing, but they do recommend routine screening

for athletes engaging in high-risk behaviors. In the NFL, the New York Giants and the Philadelphia Eagles reportedly tested players and personnel in 1991 and 1992 despite some of the players being unaware of the testing (33).

- In 1988, the Nevada Boxing Commission mandated HIV testing for all boxers fighting in Nevada, and a positive result would disqualify a boxer from fighting. Numerous boxing commissions followed the lead, and currently boxers with a positive HIV test are not allowed to box in the United States, although several have fought in other countries (19).

TREATMENT

General Recommendations

- Treatment regimens of HIV-positive patients focus on improving overall general health and slowing the disease progression. Treatment goals should include suppression of viral replication and evolution of resistant strains, increased CD4 cell counts, prevention of disease progression, improved energy levels, maintenance of a healthy weight, improvement in quality of life, and prolongation of overall survival.

- In addition to engaging in a regular exercise program, other general health measures should be reinforced. Eating a healthy, well-balanced diet with high carbohydrates and moderate protein and avoidance of saturated fats and cholesterol is recommended. The HIV-positive patient should be encouraged to obtain adequate sleep, stop smoking, use alcohol in moderation, lose weight if obese, and treat other medical diseases such as hypertension and diabetes.

Highly Active Antiretroviral Therapy

- Highly active antiretroviral therapy (HAART), including nucleoside reverse transcriptase inhibitors, nonnucleoside reverse transcriptase inhibitors, and protease inhibitors, is the cornerstone of treatment of HIV-infected patients. Many drug protocols have been developed, and there are a number of combined medications available to decrease the number of pills that must be consumed. The ultimate goals of HAART are to optimize the immune system and decrease viral load while minimizing the toxicity and development of drug-resistant HIV strains. The main effect of these agents is to suppress viral replication. This allows the immune system to recover and delays and protects the infected individual from developing AIDS (66).

- Treatment regimens are constantly changing to achieve these goals, and thus consultation with HIV experts is necessary.

- Current guidelines now recommend initiation of HAART when CD4 counts drop to 350 cells $\cdot$ μL^{-1} and may be given with counts of 350–500 cells $\cdot$ μL^{-1} (66). Earlier treatment may improve immunologic and virologic outcomes but may also increase drug toxicity and the rate of development of drug resistance. Only 20%, 26%, and 46% of those starting

HAART with CD4 counts of less than 50, 50–200, and 200–350 cells $\cdot$ μL^{-1}, respectively, achieved cell counts over 800 cells $\cdot$ μL^{-1} 7 years after initiation of therapy. If CD4 cell counts were 350–500 or over 500 cells $\cdot$ μL^{-1}, the rates improved to 73% and 87%, respectively (27).

■ Treatment may also be considered in those with high viral loads, rapidly decreasing CD4 cell counts, or low CD4 percentage. Deaths from non-AIDS causes are increased with lower CD4 cell counts. Those on intermittent HAART had higher rates of cardiovascular, renal, hepatic, and pancreatic disease than those on continuous HAART. Patients must adhere to antiretroviral regimens to obtain optimum outcome (1,65,66).

■ Drug toxicities include myopathy, neuropathy, pancreatitis, cardiomyopathy, bone marrow suppression, nephrotoxicity, lactic acidosis with hepatic steatosis, osteonecrosis, osteoporosis, insulin resistance, hyperglycemia, hyperlipidemia, and lipodystrophy. All of these, even in their mildest forms, could have adverse effects on athletic performance (9,61,63,70).

■ The fusion inhibitors enfuvirtide, maraviroc, cenicriviroc, and ibalizumab may prove to be a tremendous advancement in HIV therapy. These attach to cell surface proteins of the CD4 cells or HIV to prevent the virus from entering the immune system. This may be especially beneficial in the treatment of drug-resistant HIV. Current drawbacks include subcutaneous administration, cost, and experimental status (61).

Other Medications and Supplements

■ Testosterone supplementation (transdermal or injection) has been used to improve hypogonadism, loss of lean body mass and muscle wasting, and increased visceral fat in HIV-positive males. Injection of 300 mg of testosterone enanthate for 16 weeks resulted in significant increase in lean body mass, strength, mental health, and quality-of-life scores compared to placebo; however, walking speed, stair climbing ability, fatigue, and mood scores were no different between the groups (34,48).

■ Growth hormone and the growth hormone analog tesamorelin have been shown to decrease visceral fat and increase lean mass in HIV-positive patients suffering from lipodystrophy associated with use of antiviral therapies (2,48). Glutamine and arginine are amino acids essential for immune system function. Both are used during exercise, and deficiencies may have a detrimental effect on tissue recovery and immune function. Supplementation may improve cytokine profile and immunologic function in HIV-positive patients. High-dose arginine supplementation (12 g $\cdot$ d^{-1}) may increase weight gain in HIV-positive patients and may benefit those suffering from chronic or acute infection (20). Preliminary studies have shown that cysteine supplementation in HIV-positive individuals may slow disease progression and prevent muscle wasting, but further research is needed before recommendations can be made (14).

■ Creatine supplementation during a 14-week resistance exercise program in HIV-positive patients resulted in nonsignificant increase in lean body mass but no difference in strength gains compared to placebo. Both groups had improved muscle size, strength, and overall function. Creatine supplementation may be considered in HIV-positive patients engaged in resistance training (67).

■ Oral nutritional supplementation may increase protein synthesis, body weight, and fat mass in HIV-positive individuals (39).

■ Future therapy for HIV treatment and prevention will focus on the development of new antiretroviral agents, genetic engineering, stem cell research, immunotherapy, and vaccine therapy (62).

HIV AND EXERCISE

Effects of Exercise on the Healthy Immune System

■ Physical and psychological stresses are known to alter immune function.

■ Brisk exercise, as short as 30 seconds in duration, causes an increase in leukocyte, monocyte, lymphocyte, and natural killer cell count. This increase is due to increased cardiac output; displacement of leukocytes from reserve pools in the lung, liver, and spleen; and release of epinephrine in response to exercise. Natural killer cell function increases due to the release of cytokines; this response is blunted as a person adapts to the exercise load (16).

■ Lymphocytosis during exercise is brief, and the lymphocyte count will drop within 5 minutes of exercise cessation. The levels fall below baseline over the next hour due to cortisol effects, which after exercise is no longer opposed by epinephrine. The lymphocyte count gradually returns to baseline within 24 hours (16).

■ During exercise, leukocyte count gradually increases as a result of cortisol release; cortisol causes demargination of leukocytes as well as release from bone marrow. These levels return to baseline in about 24 hours. Strenuous exercise also evokes an acute-phase reactant response with activation of complement and release of tumor necrosis factor, interferons, interleukins, and other cytokines (16).

■ Chronic exercise with periods of intense training can have a negative effect on immune function. Natural killer cell count and leukocyte function have been shown to decline in swimmers and runners during periods of intense training. Overtraining is also associated with an increase in upper respiratory tract and gastrointestinal infections (42).

Effects of Exercise on the Immune System of HIV-Positive Patients

■ Moderate exercise improves immune response in HIV-positive subjects. Aerobic exercise increases CD4 levels in asymptomatic HIV-positive patients. Individuals with advanced stages of HIV infection may experience increased CD4 counts and CD4:CD8 ratio in response to aerobic exercise (16).

- At rest, HIV-positive patients have lower antioxidant activity (glutathione *S*-transferase) compared to noninfected controls, but following aerobic and resistance exercise, the levels are the same (11).

- Intense exercise may impair the ability of HIV-positive patients to mobilize neutrophils and natural killer cells. This has been shown in response to 1 hour of exercise at 75% $\dot{V}O_{2max}$ and after 20 minutes of aerobics followed by a set of six resistance exercises (11,72).

Effects of Exercise on HIV-Positive Patients

- There are a number of nonimmunologic effects of HIV that may impair the ability to exercise and must be taken into account when prescribing an exercise program for HIV-positive athletes and patients. These include cardiac effects (decreased $\dot{V}O_{2max}$ due to deconditioning, which may be reversible with aerobic training), pulmonary effects (opportunistic pulmonary infections may have restrictive ventilatory effects), hematologic effects (anemia due directly to HIV disease or as an adverse effect of medications may decrease $\dot{V}O_{2max}$ and lower the lactic acidosis threshold), and muscular effects (some medications may induce mitochondrial myopathies or cause resting lactic acidosis) (69).

- A recent systematic review concluded that although there are limited, high-quality exercise studies in HIV-positive patients, aerobic exercise decreases body fat and improves lipid profiles, whereas resistance training increases body mass and strength (21).

Effects of Aerobic Exercise on HIV-Positive Patients

- Numerous studies and systematic reviews have concluded that 20 minutes of aerobic exercise, three times per week, for as little as 5 weeks improve oxygen consumption, body composition, insulin sensitivity, and depressive and other psychological symptoms (9,11,29,37,40,54). This is especially important in the older HIV-positive patient. In a recent study, 12 HIV-positive males, age 40–49 had near-normal $\dot{V}O_{2max}$, whereas 20 HIV-positive males over age 50 had a 40% decrease in $\dot{V}O_{2max}$ compared to age-matched controls (57).

- Participation in a 6-month cardiorespiratory exercise program was shown to decrease body fat, total cholesterol, triglycerides, and glucose levels and increase $\dot{V}O_{2max}$ in HIV-positive patients in Rwanda, providing an economical treatment to improve overall patient health (59).

- The addition of three times weekly participation in 1-hour gym classes along with monthly counseling sessions for 6 months has been shown to significantly improve quality of life compared with monthly counseling alone in HIV-positive patients (56). Adherence to an aerobic exercise program has been shown to be improved more when HIV-positive patient have better overall general health, whereas perceived self-efficacy and expected outcome are not predictive of continued exercise. Thus, it is important to recommend exercise early in the disease course (58). In addition, simple adherence to a 10-week aerobic exercise

program improves perception of well-being of HIV-positive patients (60).

- HIV-positive patients who self-report being physically active have less central body fat compared to sedentary controls (23).

- Eighteen obese HIV-positive females treated with a 12-week program of aerobic exercise and decreased calorie intake had less visceral and subcutaneous fat and improved overall strength, fitness, and quality of life but no change in levels of blood glucose, insulin, lipids, tissue plasminogen activator, or plasminogen activator inhibitor and no change in insulin sensitivity. Although exercise improves overall health, this study suggests that additional interventions may be necessary to decrease the risk of diabetes and cardiovascular disease in obese HIV-positive females (17).

Effects of Resistance Exercise on HIV-Positive Patients

- Weightlifting exercise training increases muscle mass, strength, function, and insulin sensitivity and decreases body fat in HIV-positive individuals without causing additional adverse effects. It may be useful to combat AIDS-related muscle wasting and should be recommended for athletes with HIV (13,29,40,55).

- The addition of a 16-week resistance training program decreased body mass index and improved lipid profile, had a variable effect on CD4 cell counts, but did not affect viral load in a small series of HIV patients (45).

- A recent study of HIV-positive patients over the age of 60 engaged in 1 year of resistance exercises twice weekly had improvement in strength, glucose control, and lipid profiles compared to nonexercising controls. This effect was most marked if the patients were not on protease inhibitors, and the exercises resulted in no additional adverse effects (68).

Effects of Combined Aerobic and Resistance Exercise on HIV-Positive Patients

- Early studies found that involvement in either an aerobic or resistance weight-training regimen in HIV-positive patients will increase lean mass, upper and lower extremity strength, and $\dot{V}O_{2max}$ (41). The combination of aerobic and resistance exercise should further improve overall health; however, the precise recommendations are difficult based on the available research. It does appear that combined programs are safe for HIV-positive patients of either sex at nearly any age, and there will be significant overall improvement in health.

- Systematic reviews have concluded that combining aerobic exercise with progressive resistance exercise in HIV-positive patients resulted in no additional health benefits beyond those achieved with either program alone (21,29,55,64).

- However, as little as 6 weeks of combined aerobic and resistance exercise significantly improved endurance, exercise time to exhaustion, and $\dot{V}O_{2max}$ of HIV-positive patients compared to nonexercising controls (30). A study of 40 HIV-positive males over age 18 randomized to twice weekly aerobic and resistance exercise or unsupervised walking program found greater decreases in resting heart rate and improved overall health and cognition in those participating in the combined program (22). In addition, a 16-week pilot study of five HIV-positive patients engaged in 20 minutes of aerobics three times weekly and resistance exercise of 8–10 repetitions of seven exercises two times weekly showed increased aerobic capacity, total body weight, and lean body mass; decreased truncal fat and triglycerides; and improved insulin sensitivity (64).

- A recent 12-week study of exercise (three sets of 12 repetition of five resistance exercises, 30 minutes of aerobics, and 10 minutes of general stretching three times weekly) in 27 HIV-positive patients on HAART showed significant improvement in muscle and aerobic fitness and life satisfaction with no alteration of CD4 cell counts compared to nonexercising controls (18).

- Forty HIV-positive females were randomized to either participate in a 16-week combined home-based aerobic and resistance exercise program or maintain current lifestyle. Those in the exercise group had significant improvement in lean mass, strength, and endurance but no change in lipid profile, blood pressure, or visceral fat compared to the control group (12).

- HIV-positive patients participating in 30 minutes each of aerobic and resistance exercise had higher levels of growth hormone and interleukin-6 and lower levels of cortisol and tissue necrosis factor than those completing 60 minutes of aerobics only (15).

- HIV-positive prisoners coinfected with hepatitis C engaged in a 4-month trial of aerobic and strength training had improvement in overall fitness and strength compared to controls (59).

- Twelve HIV-positive children, with an average age of 15 years, completed a 24-session supervised aerobic and resistance exercise program followed by a home-based maintenance program and had improvement in lean body mass, strength, and endurance with no adverse effects (47). Two females, 10 and 17 years of age with lifelong HIV infection, were engaged in a 12-week hospital-based aerobic and strength program and experienced significant increases in muscle mass and strength and a decrease in body fat with no adverse effects (46). These studies suggest that exercise has overall health benefits with minimal risk in young HIV-positive patients.

Effects of Exercise on the Adverse Effects of HIV Therapy

- Aerobic exercise has been shown to improve insulin sensitivity and decrease central adiposity in HIV-positive patients on HAART (50,74). However, HIV-positive patients on HAART have also been shown to have decreased lipolysis and fatty acid oxidation during moderate aerobic exercise compared to those not on medications; this further complicates the treatment of HAART-associated central adiposity (6).

- Thirty HIV-positive patients with HAART-associated lipodystrophy were randomized to a low-fat diet with the addition of either a 12-week moderate aerobic exercise program or a stretching and relaxation program. Those on the aerobic program had improvement in $\dot{V}O_{2max}$ but no change in body weight, body fat, or lipid profile compared to the stretching and relaxation group (71).

- The addition of metformin to an aerobic exercise program may further improve central lipodystrophy (48).

- Aerobic exercise improves quality of life in patients on HAART (50).

Miscellaneous Effects of Exercise on HIV-Positive Patients

- Exercise lowers anxiety and tension levels in HIV-positive individuals (37).

- Yoga and meditation improve overall well-being and have resulted in decreased blood pressure in those with cardiovascular disease (3,7). Exercise has *not* shown benefit in the treatment of peripheral neuropathy in HIV-positive patients (53).

Exercise Recommendations for HIV-Positive Athletes

- Moderate exercise is beneficial to the physical and psychological well-being of the HIV-positive patient, but strenuous exercise may be detrimental (19). Although the exercise demands of high-level and professional athletes may be safe and beneficial, the possible psychological stress must be assessed on an individual basis (16).

- A complete physical exam should be performed to assess the overall health and status of HIV infection before beginning an exercise program. Measurements of lymphocyte levels, CD4 levels, CD4:CD8 ratio, and viral load should be obtained. Cardiopulmonary exercise testing with gas exchange measurements should be considered before determining an exercise prescription, especially in patients with low CD4 counts or high viral loads (16,69). HIV-infected individuals should begin exercising while healthy and attempt to maintain their exercise program. HIV-infected persons can use exercise to help manage their illness and improve their quality of life.

- For healthy, asymptomatic, HIV-positive individuals, unrestricted exercise is acceptable. Avoidance of overtraining should be emphasized. Stress related to competition should be minimized. Moderate exercise (40%–60% $\dot{V}O_{2max}$) or heavy aerobic exercise (60%–80% $\dot{V}O_{2max}$) can be recommended depending on patient preference and motivation. An exercise program prescription should include 30–60 minutes of aerobic exercise most days of the week with resistance training 2–5 days per week depending on the routine.

- For individuals with advanced HIV infection with mild to moderate symptoms or lower CD4 counts (< 200), competition, restrictive training schedules, and exhaustive exercise should be avoided. Physical activity and moderate exercise training should be encouraged under close supervision.

- Athletes with frank AIDS may remain active on a symptom-related basis but should avoid strenuous exercise and reduce or stop training during acute illness.

Recommendations and Restrictions for the HIV-Positive Athlete

- The most widely used recommendations regarding restriction of the HIV-positive athlete from competition come from the American Academy of Pediatrics (AAP) and the NCAA (31,52).

- AAP recommendations: Athletes infected with HIV should be allowed to participate in all competitive sports. Physicians should respect the right to confidentiality including not disclosing infection status to participants or to staff of athletic programs. Physicians should counsel the known HIV-infected athlete of the theoretical risk of contaminating others during sports involving blood exposure, especially wrestling and boxing. Physicians should strongly encourage the HIV-positive athlete to consider another sport (31).

- The NCAA recommendations state that HIV-positive student athletes should be allowed to participate in intercollegiate athletics based on the individual's health status. The athlete should be allowed to play if asymptomatic with no evidence of immunodeficiency. However, the intensity of training and stress of competition should be taken into account to prevent the deterioration of the athlete's health status (52). Despite this recommendation, a number of NCAA institutions may restrict the HIV-positive athlete from participation in selected sports (44).

- HIV-positive boxers are not allowed to box in any U.S. state or territory, are stripped of their title, and must relinquish any championship belt. While not specifically barred from participation in the four major professional sports in North America, given the demands of training and competition on overall health, adverse effects of therapy, and theoretical risk of transmission, most experts recommend against continued participation (16,19).

PREVENTION

- Physicians should educate athletes about risky behaviors and consider HIV testing on a voluntary basis. Education should include discussions on abstinence, safe sex, and use of shared needles or personal items such as razors, clippers, and earrings that may be contaminated with blood. Participation in the Mathare Youth Soccer Association in Kenya, which emphasizes education and sports participation, has been shown to decrease high-risk behavior such as unprotected sexual activity and drug abuse (10).

- Coaches and athletic trainers should receive training in universal precautions and prevention of HIV transmission. The Occupational Safety and Health Administration (OSHA) has standards concerning occupational exposure to bloodborne pathogens, which are applicable to the athletic training room.

- Athletes with skin wounds and potentially infectious skin lesions should be securely covered with bandages and wraps before competition.

- Athletes participating in sports with extensive skin-to-skin contact (*i.e.*, wrestling) should be excluded from matches or practice when skin wounds or lesions are contagious or cannot be securely covered.

- Ambu bags and oral airways should be available for use for cardiopulmonary resuscitation.

- Athletic trainers and health care personnel should use disposable, preferably sterile, examination gloves when treating athletes who are bleeding. Hands should be washed after glove removal.

- Immediate treatment is indicated when an athlete sustains a laceration or wound with substantial bleeding. The blood should be washed off thoroughly with soap and water. Emergency care should not be delayed if gloves are not available. A bulky towel may be used to cover the wound until an off-the-field location is reached and gloves can be used for definitive treatment. The athlete should be allowed to return only after the bleeding is controlled and the wound has been securely covered or wrapped.

- Small amounts of dried blood on uniforms or equipment do not constitute a risk for transmission and do not warrant changing. However, if uniforms or equipment appear wet with blood or if blood has penetrated both sides of the uniform fabric, it should be changed at the next stoppage of play.

- After each practice or game, any uniforms or equipment soiled with blood should be laundered using standard laundry cycles.

- Disposable towels or absorbent cleaning material should be used to clean environmental surfaces. Clean with soap and water, a germicide registered with the Environmental Protection Agency, or a 1/100 dilution of bleach in tap water (1 cup of bleach to 4 gallons of water).

- Receptacles should be available for uniforms soiled with bodily fluids. Sharps containers should be used for needles or scalpel blades.

- Rules forbidding activities such as biting, scratching, fighting, or other unsportsmanlike behaviors that may lead to bloody contact should be strictly enforced (31,43,52).

- Circumcision has also been suggested as a method to decrease the spread of HIV infection (62).

ETHICAL AND LEGAL IMPLICATIONS

Mandatory Testing

- Does the proposed testing policy serve an ethically acceptable purpose? The protection of the HIV-infected athlete and the protection of uninfected athletes from transmission are ethical purposes. Using test results for discrimination against HIV-infected athletes is unethical.

- Is mandatory testing necessary and effective for achieving that purpose? Because HIV transmission on the playing field has never been documented and the risk is theoretically low, mandatory testing is not necessary.

- Does mandatory testing violate the individual rights of the athlete? Mandatory testing does violate the individual athlete's right to privacy, but the question for the professional athlete is if this intrusion is permitted under the collective bargaining agreement of that profession.

- Arguments in favor of permitting violations of the right to privacy cite existing exceptions to HIV testing without consent including criminal justice settings, life insurance underwriting purposes, defense department and military recruits, immigrants to the United States, State Department foreign service personnel, and the Federal Bureau of Prisons for prison inmates.

- A professional team player contract defines the consequences of failure to maintain physical fitness or pass the preseason medical exam, which may include suspension or termination. Proponents of mandatory testing argue that the acceptance of their contract negates any invasion of privacy. It can be argued that the player's privacy is no more violated by HIV testing than by other routine medical tests required by team and league policies. It can also be argued that the team owner should know the overall health status of a player who may be signed to a long-term, multimillion-dollar contract.

- Professional boxers are subjected to mandatory HIV testing to theoretically protect the safety of the infected athlete or other competitors, and the mandatory testing program has yet to be contested in court (19).

- However, most law theorists conclude that mandatory testing is both unethical and illegal (33).

Competition Exclusion

- Courts have ruled that without sufficient medical reason, an HIV-positive athlete cannot be excluded from sports participation (School Board of Nassau County, Florida vs. Arline, 480. U.S. 273 [1987]).

- The Americans with Disabilities Act and the Rehabilitation Act of 1973 do not allow discrimination against people who have contagious diseases who are otherwise qualified to participate. Concern regarding the potentially harmful effects of competition on the immune system of the HIV-positive athlete has not been viewed as legally valid grounds for exclusion from sanctioned athletic events (33).

- Courts have permitted schools to prohibit HIV-positive students from school-sponsored contact sports because of the perceived risk of transmission (Doe vs. Dolton Elementary School District Number 148, 694 F supp. 440 [1988]) and have upheld the decision to exclude an HIV-positive athlete from contact karate (Montalov vs. Radcliffe, 167 F. 3d 873 [4th Cir. 1999], cert. Denied, 120 S Ct. 48 1999).

- Ruben Palacio won the World Boxing Organization Featherweight World Championship in 1993 after 12 years in boxing. On the eve of his first title defense, he was subjected to mandatory HIV testing and tested positive. They stripped him of his title and refused to allow him to compete. Other boxers have suffered a similar fate, being forced to retire from their sport (33).

- In cases in which HIV-positive individuals fail to disclose their status to sexual partners, the courts have ruled in favor of the plaintiff and have fined and sentenced the HIV-positive individual to prison. Canadian Football League Saskatchewan Roughriders player Trevis Smith, who played professional football while he was HIV positive, was convicted of sexual assault and sentenced to 6 years in prison for failure to disclose his HIV status to a sexual partner (5). If an athlete fails to disclose their HIV-positive status and infects another player on the playing field, it is not known how the court may respond (33).

REFERENCES

1. Armstrong W, Calabrese L, Taege A. HIV update 2002: delaying treatment to curb rising resistance. *Cleve Clin J Med.* 2002;69(12):995–9.
2. Benedini S, Terruzzi I, Lazzarin A, Luzi L. Recombinant human growth hormone: rational for use in the treatment of HIV-associated lipodystrophy. *BioDrugs.* 2008;22(2):101–12.
3. Brazier A, Mulkins A, Verhoef M. Evaluating a yogic breathing and meditation intervention for individuals living with HIV/AIDS. *Am J Health Promot.* 2006;20(3):192–5.
4. Brown LS Jr, Drotman DP, Chu A, Brown CL Jr, Knowlan D. Bleeding injuries in professional football: estimating the risk for HIV transmission. *Ann Intern Med.* 1995;122(4):273–4.
5. Brownlee K. Saskatchewan court dismisses former Roughrider Smith's appeal. *Canada Leader Post.* 2008 May 15.
6. Cade WT, Reeds DN, Mittendorfer B, et al. Blunted lipolysis and fatty acid oxidation during moderate exercise in HIV-infected subjects taking HAART. *Am J Physiol Endocrinol Metab.* 2007;292(3):E812–9.
7. Cade WT, Reeds DN, Mondy KE, et al. Yoga lifestyle intervention reduces blood pressure in HIV-infected adults with cardiovascular disease risk factors. *HIV Med.* 2010;11(6):379–88.
8. Centers for Disease Control and Prevention (CDC). HIV Surveillance — United States, 1981–2008. *MMWR Morb Mortal Wkly Rep.* 2011;60(21): 689–93.
9. Das S. Insulin resistance and diabetes in HIV Infection. *Recent Pat Antiinfect Drug Discov.* 2011;6(3):260–8.
10. Delva W, Michielsen K, Meulders B, et al. HIV prevention through sport: the case of the Mathare Youth Sport Association in Kenya. *AIDS Care.* 2010;22(8):1012–20.
11. Deresz LF, Sprinz E, Kramer AS, et al. Regulation of oxidative stress in response to acute aerobic and resistance exercise in HIV-infected subjects: a case–control study. *AIDS Care.* 2010;22(11):1410–7.
12. Dolan SE, Frontera W, Librizzi J, et al. Effects of a supervised home-based aerobic and progressive resistance training regimen in women infected with human immunodeficiency virus: a randomized trial. *Arch Intern Med.* 2006;166(11):1225–31.
13. Dorman JM. Contagious diseases in competitive sport: what are the risks? *J Am Coll Health.* 2000;49(3):105–9.
14. Dröge W, Holm E. Role of cysteine and glutathione in HIV infection and other diseases associated with muscle wasting and immunologic dysfunction. *FASEB J.* 1997;11(13):1077–89.
15. Dudgeon WD, Phillips KD, Durstine JL, et al. Individual exercise session alter circulating hormones and cytokines in HIV-infected men. *Appl Physiol Nutr Metab.* 2010;35(4):560–8.

16. Eichner ER, Calabrese LH. Immunology and exercise. Physiology, pathophysiology, and implications for HIV infection. *Med Clin North Am.* 1994;78(2):377–88.

17. Engelson ES, Agin D, Kenya S, et al. Body composition and metabolic effects of a diet and exercise weight loss regimen on obese, HIV-infected women. *Metabolism.* 2006;55(10):1327–36.

18. Farinatti PT, Borges JP, Gomes RD, Lima D, Fleck SJ. Effects of a supervised exercise program on the physical fitness and immunological function of HIV-infected patients. *J Sports Med Phys Fitness.* 2010;50(4):511–8.

19. Feller A, Flanigan TP. HIV-infected competitive athletes. What are the risks? What precautions should be taken? *J Gen Intern Med.* 1997;12(4):243–6.

20. Field CJ, Johnson I, Pratt VC. Glutamine and arginine: immunonutrients for improved health. *Med Sci Sports Exerc.* 2000;32(7 Suppl):S377–88.

21. Fillipas S, Cherry CL, Cicuttini F, Smirneos L, Holland AE. The effects of exercise training on metabolic and morphological outcomes for people living with HIV: a systemic review of randomized, controlled trials. *HIV Clin Trials.* 2010;11(5):270–82.

22. Fillipas S, Oldmeadow LB, Bailey MJ, Cherry CL. A six-month, supervised, aerobic and resistance exercise program improves self-efficacy in people with human immunodeficiency virus: a randomized controlled trial. *Aust J Physiother.* 2006;52(3):185–90.

23. Florindo AA, De Oliviera Latorre Mdo R, Jaime PC, Segurado AA. Leisure time physical activity prevents accumulation of central fat in HIV/AIDS subjects on highly active antiretroviral therapy. *Int J STD AIDS.* 2007;18(10):692–6.

24. Gallant JE, Hoffmann DJ. CD4 cell count. *Johns Hopkins HIV Guide.* 2007. [Internet] Available from: http://www.hopkinsguides.com/hopkins/ub/view/Johns_Hopkins_HIV_Guide/545031/all/CD4_Cell_Count.

25. Gerberding JL. Management of occupational exposures to blood-borne viruses. *N Engl J Med.* 1995;332(7):444–51.

26. GJ, MD, Confidential Personal Communication, August, 2002.

27. Gras L, Kesselring AM, Griffin JT, et al. CD4 cell counts of 800 cell/mm^3 or greater after 7 years of highly active antiretroviral therapy are feasible in most patients starting with 350 cells/mm^3 or greater. *J Acquir Immune Defic Syndr.* 2007;45(2):183–92.

28. Greenwald JL, Burstein GR, Pincus J, Branson B. A rapid review of rapid HIV antibody tests. *Curr Infect Dis Rep.* 2006;8(2):125–31.

29. Hand GA, Lyerly GW, Jaggers JR, Dudgeon WD. Impact of aerobic and resistance exercise on the health of HIV-infected persons. *Am J Lifestyle Med.* 2009;3(6):489–99.

30. Hand GA, Phillips KD, Dudgeon WD, Lyerly GW, Durstine LJ, Burgess SE. Moderate intensity exercise training reverses functional aerobic impairment in HIV-infected individuals. *AIDS Care.* 2008;20(9):1066–74.

31. Human immunodeficiency virus and other blood-borne viral pathogens in the athletic setting. Committee on Sports Medicine and Fitness. American Academy of Pediatrics. *Pediatrics.* 1999;104(6):1400–3.

32. Johnson RJ. HIV infection in athletes: what are the risks? Who can compete? *Postgrad Med.* 1992;92(7):73–5, 79–80.

33. Johnston JL. Is mandatory HIV testing of professional athletes really the solution? *Health Matrix Clevel.* 1994;4(1):159–203.

34. Knapp PE, Storer TW, Herbst KL, et al. Effects of a supraphysiological dose of testosterone on physical function, muscle performance, mood, and fatigue in men with HIV-associated weight loss. *Am J Physiol Endocrinol Metab.* 2008;294(6):E1135–43.

35. Kokotailo PK, Koscik RE, Henry BC, Fleming MF, Landry GL. Health risk taking and human immunodeficiency virus risk in collegiate female athletes. *J Am Coll Health.* 1998;46(6):263–8.

36. Laird R, MD. Personal communication. October 8, 2011.

37. LaPerriere A, Fletcher MA, Antoni MH, Klimas NG, Ironson G, Schneiderman N. Aerobic exercise training in an AIDS risk group. *Int J Sports Med.* 1991;12(Suppl 1):S53–7.

38. LeBlanc KE. The athlete and HIV. *J La State Med Soc.* 1993;145(11):493–5.

39. Leyes P, Martínez E, Forga Mde T. Use of diet, nutritional supplements and exercise in HIV-infected patients receiving combination antiretroviral therapies: a systematic review. *Antivir Ther.* 2008;13(2):149–59.

40. Lindegaard B, Hansen T, Hvid T, et al. The effect of strength and endurance training on insulin sensitivity and fat distribution in human immunodeficiency virus-infected patients with lipodystrophy. *J Clin Endocrinol Metab.* 2008;93(10):3860–9.

41. Lox CL, McAuley E, Tucker RS. Aerobic and resistance exercise training effects on body composition, muscular strength, and cardiovascular fitness in an HIV-1 population. *Int J Behav Med.* 1996;3(1):55–69.

42. Mackinnon LT. Chronic exercise training effects on immune function. *Med Sci Sports Exerc.* 2000 Jul;32(7 Suppl):S369–76.

43. Mast EE, Goodman RA, Bond WW, Favero MS, Drotman DP. Transmission of blood-borne pathogens during sports: risk and prevention. *Ann Intern Med.* 1995;122(4):283–5.

44. McGrew CA, Dick RW, Schniedwind K, Gikas P. Survey of NCAA institutions concerning HIV/AIDS policies and universal precautions. *Med Sci Sports Exerc.* 1993;25(8):917–21.

45. Mesquita Soares TC, Glavão de Souza HA, De Medeiros Guerra LM, et al. Morphology and biochemical markers of people living with HIV/AIDS undergoing a resistance exercise program: clinical series. *J Sports Med Phys Fitness.* 2011;51(3):462–6.

46. Miller TL. A hospital-based exercise program to improve body composition, strength, and abdominal adiposity in 2 HIV-infected children. *AIDS Read.* 2007;17(9):450–2, 455, 458.

47. Miller TL, Somarriba G, Kinnamon DD, Weiberg GA, Friedman LB, Scott GB. The effect of a structured exercise program on nutrition and fitness outcomes in human immunodeficiency virus-infected children. *AIDS Res Hum Retroviruses.* 2010;26(3):313–9.

48. Moyle G, Moutschen M, Martínez E, et al. Epidemiology, assessment, and management of excess abdominal fat in persons with HIV infection. *AIDS Rev.* 2010;12(1):3–14.

49. Mutimura E, Crowther NJ, Cade TW, Yarasheski KE, Stewart A. Exercise training reduces central adiposity and improves metabolic indices in HAART-treated HIV-positive subjects in Rwanda: a randomized controlled trial. *AIDS Res Hum Retroviruses.* 2008;24(1):15–23.

50. Mutimura E, Stewart A, Crowther NJ, Yarasheski KE, Cade WT. The effects of exercise training on quality of life in HAART-treated HIV-positive Rwandan subjects with body fat redistribution. *Qual Life Res.* 2008;17(3):377–85.

51. Nattiv A, Puffer JC. Lifestyles and health risks of collegiate athletes. *J Fam Pract.* 1991;33(6):585–90.

52. NCAA Guideline 2h: Blood-borne Pathogens and Intercollegiate Athletics. Indianapolis (IN): National Collegiate Athletic Association; August 2000.

53. Nicholas PK, Kemppainen JK, Canaval GE, et al. Symptom management and self-care for peripheral neuropathy in HIV/AIDS. *AIDS Care.* 2007;19(2):179–89.

54. O'Brien K, Nixon S, Tynan AM, Glazier R. Aerobic exercise interventions for adults living with HIV/AIDS. *Cochrane Database Syst Rev.* 2010;8:CD001796.

55. O'Brien K, Tynan AM, Nixon S, Glazier RH. Effects of progressive resistive exercise in adults living with HIV/AIDS: systematic review and meta-analysis of randomized trials. *AIDS Care.* 2008;20(6):631–53.

56. Ogalha C, Luz E, Sampaio E, et al. A randomized, clinical trial to evaluate the impact of regular physical activity on the quality of life, body morphology and metabolic parameters of patients with AIDS in Salvador, Brazil. *J Acquir Immune Defic Syndr.* 2011;57(Suppl 3):S179–85.

57. Oursler KK, Sorkin JD, Smith BA, Katzell LI. Reduced aerobic capacity and physical functioning in older HIV-infected men. *AIDS Res Hum Retroviruses.* 2006;22(11):1113–21.

58. Pavone RM, Burnett KF, LaPerriere A, Perna FM. Social cognitive and physical health determinants of exercise adherence for HIV-1 seropositive, early symptomatic men and women. *Int J Behav Med.* 1998;5(3):245–58.

59. Pérez-Moreno F, Cámara-Sánchez M, Tremblay JF, Riera-Rubio VJ, Gil-Paisán L, Lucia A. Benefits of exercise training in Spanish prison inmates. *Int J Sports Med.* 2007;28(12):1046–52.

60. Petróczi A, Hawkins K, Jones G, Naughton DP. HIV patient characteristics that affect adherence to exercise programmes: an observational study. *Open AIDS J.* 2010;4:148–55.

61. *Prescriber's Letter.* Jellin JM, ed. 2003;10(4):23.

62. Proceeding of the 4th IAS Conference on HIV Pathogenesis, Treatment and Prevention: Male circumcision, new antiretrovirals, genetic engineering most promising HIV prevention, treatment methods conference delegates say; July 2007. [Internet] Available from: http://www.thebody.com/content/art42440.html.

63. Rhoads MP, Lanigan J, Smith CJ, Lyall EG. Effect of specific ART drugs on lipid changes and the need for lipid management in children with HIV. *J Acquir Immune Defic Syndr.* 2011;57(5):404–12.

64. Robinson FP, Quinn LT, Rimmer JH. Effects of high-intensity endurance and resistance exercise on HIV metabolic abnormalities: a pilot study. *Biol Res Nurs.* 2007;8(3):177–85.

65. Rodríguez-Arenas MA, Jarrín I, del Amo J, et al. Delay in initiation of HAART, poorer virologic response, and higher mortality among HIV-infected injecting drug users in Spain. *AIDS Res Hum Retroviruses.* 2006;22(8):715–23.

66. Sabin CA, Philips AN. Should HIV treatment be started at a CD4 cell count above 350 cells/microl in asymptomatic HIV-1 infected patients? *Curr Opin Infect Dis.* 2009;22(2):191–7.

67. Sakkas GK, Mulligan K, Dasilva M, et al. Creatine fails to augment the benefits from resistance training in patients with HIV infection: a randomized, double-blind, placebo controlled-study. *PLoS One.* 2009;4(2):e4605.

68. Souza PM, Jacob-Filho W, Santarém JM, Silva AR, Li HY, Burattini MN. Progressive resistance training in elderly HIV-positive patients: does it work? *Clinics (Sao Paulo).* 2008;63(5):619–24.

69. Stringer WW. Mechanisms of exercise limitation in HIV+ individuals. *Med Sci Sports Exerc.* 2000 Jul; 32(7 Suppl):S412–21.

70. Stringer WW, Sattler FR. Metabolic syndromes associated with HIV: mitigating the side effects of drug therapy. *Phys Sports Med.* 2001;29(12):19–26.

71. Terry L, Sprinz E, Stein R., Medeiros NB, Oliveira J, Ribeiro JP. Exercise training in HIV-1-infected individuals with dyslipidemia and lipodystrophy. *Med Sci Sports Exerc.* 2006;38(3):411–7.

72. Ullum H, Palmø J, Halkjaer-Kristensen J, et al. The effect of acute exercise on lymphocyte subsets, natural killer cells, proliferative responses, and cytokines in HIV-seropositive persons. *J Acquir Immune Defic Syndr.* 1994;7(11):1122–33.

73. Web site of CDC. HIV/AIDS [Internet]. Available from: http://www.cdc.gov/hiv/resources/factsheets/index.htm.

74. Yarasheski KE, Cade WT, Oerton ET, et al. Exercise training augments the peripheral insulin-sensitizing effects of pioglitazone in HIV-infected adults with insulin resistance and central adiposity. *Am J Physiol Endocrinol Metab.* 2011;300(1):E243–51.

Index

Page numbers with "f" and "t" denotes figures and tables, respectively.

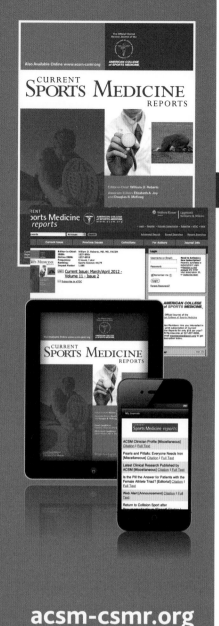